Aravind FAQs in Ophthalmology

Aravind FAQs in Ophthalmology

THIRD EDITION

N Venkatesh Prajna DNB FRCOphth
Director–Academics
Aravind Eye Hospital
Madurai, Tamil Nadu, India

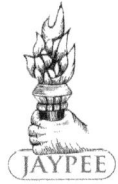

JAYPEE BROTHERS MEDICAL PUBLISHERS
The Health Sciences Publisher
New Delhi | London

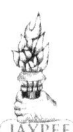

Jaypee Brothers Medical Publishers (P) Ltd

Headquarters

Jaypee Brothers Medical Publishers (P) Ltd
EMCA House, 23/23-B
Ansari Road, Daryaganj
New Delhi 110 002, India
Landline: +91-11-23272143, +91-11-23272703
+91-11-23282021, +91-11-23245672
Email: jaypee@jaypeebrothers.com

Corporate Office

Jaypee Brothers Medical Publishers (P) Ltd
4838/24, Ansari Road, Daryaganj
New Delhi 110 002, India
Phone: +91-11-43574357
Fax: +91-11-43574314
Email: jaypee@jaypeebrothers.com

Overseas Office

JP Medical Ltd
83 Victoria Street, London
SW1H 0HW (UK)
Phone: +44 20 3170 8910
Fax: +44 (0)20 3008 6180
Email: info@jpmedpub.com

Website: www.jaypeebrothers.com
Website: www.jaypeedigital.com

© 2024, Jaypee Brothers Medical Publishers

The views and opinions expressed in this book are solely those of the original contributor(s)/author(s) and do not necessarily represent those of editor(s) or publisher of the book.

All rights reserved. No part of this publication may be reproduced, stored or transmitted in any form or by any means, electronic, mechanical, photocopying, recording or otherwise, without the prior permission in writing of the publishers.

All brand names and product names used in this book are trade names, service marks, trademarks or registered trademarks of their respective owners. The publisher is not associated with any product or vendor mentioned in this book.

Medical knowledge and practice change constantly. This book is designed to provide accurate, authoritative information about the subject matter in question. However, readers are advised to check the most current information available on procedures included and check information from the manufacturer of each product to be administered, to verify the recommended dose, formula, method and duration of administration, adverse effects and contraindications. It is the responsibility of the practitioner to take all appropriate safety precautions. Neither the publisher nor the author(s)/editor(s) assume any liability for any injury and/or damage to persons or property arising from or related to use of material in this book.

This book is sold on the understanding that the publisher is not engaged in providing professional medical services. If such advice or services are required, the services of a competent medical professional should be sought.

Every effort has been made where necessary to contact holders of copyright to obtain permission to reproduce copyright material. If any have been inadvertently overlooked, the publisher will be pleased to make the necessary arrangements at the first opportunity.

Inquiries for bulk sales may be solicited at: jaypee@jaypeebrothers.com

Aravind FAQs in Ophthalmology

First Edition: 2013

Second Edition: 2019

Third Edition: **2024**

ISBN: 978-93-5696-335-1

Dedicated to
*The following trustees of the Aravind Eye Care System (AECS)
who played a stellar role behind the scenes and were
instrumental in the growth of the institution
without expecting anything in return.*

Mrs Lalitha Srinivasan
Mr RS Ramasamy
Mrs Janaki Ramasamy

Preface to the Third Edition

The book *Aravind FAQs in Ophthalmology* continues to be an invaluable asset to the postgraduate students in ophthalmology, as evidenced by the overwhelming response from across India and abroad. The existing topics have been updated to reflect contemporary advancements in this ever-growing field of ophthalmology. Two entirely new sections have been created, one on instrumentation and the second on question bank, which will further help the exam-going students to face the examinations with confidence. The section on the management of ophthalmic conditions can be used as a rehearsal tool for the oral examinations. This book will be a valuable adjunct along with the existing textbooks of ophthalmology and will remove the fear of examinations for the students in ophthalmology.

N Venkatesh Prajna

Preface to the First Edition

The specialty of ophthalmology has developed by leaps and bounds in the recent past. Excellent, comprehensive books are being brought out at regular intervals, which help an ophthalmologist to keep abreast with the times. In my 15 years experience as a residency director, I have often found the need for a concise, examination-oriented ready-reckoner, which would be of use to the postgraduates to answer specifically to the point. This book aims to fill this gap and serves as a compilation of the frequently asked questions (FAQs) and the answers expected in a postgraduate clinical ophthalmology examination. This book should not be misconstrued as a replacement to the existing standard textbooks. These questions have been painstakingly gathered over a 10-year period from the collective experience of several senior teachers at Aravind Eye Hospital, Madurai, Tamil Nadu, India. Apart from the examination-oriented questions, this book also contains examples of case sheet writing and different management scenarios, which will help the students to logically analyze and answer in a coherent manner. I do sincerely hope that this book helps the postgraduate to face his/her examination with confidence.

N Venkatesh Prajna

Acknowledgments

I have received tremendous support from all the faculty and students of the Aravind Eye Care System (AECS) in improving the existing popular edition of the FAQs in Ophthalmology. Without their help and insights, it would not have been possible to bring out a revised edition. I would also like to thank the student community from across the country, who continue to give their feedback and their appreciation through emails and letters, which have encouraged me to think of ways and means to expand the scope of this book. I would also like to sincerely acknowledge and thank the secretarial help rendered to me by Mrs Uma Devi and Kalyani, from the central office of the AECS, who patiently helped in editing the book and making sure that all changes are incorporated. I am very grateful to the management of the AECS for giving me unlimited time and support for making this exercise possible. I would also like to acknowledge the tremendous support of my immediate family for patiently supporting my professional career. My parents, Drs Namperumalsamy and Natchiar, were excellent teachers in their own right and I have learnt a lot from them. My wife, Dr Lalitha, and my children, Dr Meera Lakshmi and Aravind Krishna, have been a source of joy and pride in my professional journey. I do sincerely hope that this book takes the fear factor out of the examinations.

I especially appreciate the constant support and encouragement of Mr Jitendar P Vij (Group Chairman) and Mr Ankit Vij (Managing Director) of M/s Jaypee Brothers Medical Publishers (P) Ltd, New Delhi, India, in publishing the book and also their associates, particularly Ms Chetna Malhotra (Senior Director—Professional Publishing, Marketing, and Business Development) and Ms Pragati Singh (Development Editor) who have been prompt, efficient, and most helpful.

Contents

1. Introduction 1
1.1 Visual Acuity 1
1.2 Color Vision 11
1.3 Anatomical Landmarks in Eye 15
1.4 Embryology 21
1.5 Pharmacology 22
1.6 Microbiology 31
1.7 General Pathology 46
1.8 Slit-lamp Biomicroscope 52
1.9 Direct Ophthalmoscope 60
1.10 Indirect Ophthalmoscope 63
1.11 X-rays in Ophthalmology 67
1.12 Computed Tomography and Magnetic Resonance Imaging 75

2. Cornea 83
2.1 Keratometry 83
2.2 Corneal Vascularization 86
2.3 Corneal Anesthesia 89
2.4 Corneal Deposits 92
2.5 Bacterial and Fungal Corneal Ulcers 95
2.6 Acanthamoeba Keratitis 102
2.7 Viral Keratitis 107
2.8 Interstitial Keratitis 110
2.9 Mooren's Ulcer 113
2.10 Band-shaped Keratopathy 122
2.11 Adherent Leukoma 125
2.12 Bowen's Disease 128
2.13 Keratoconus 132
2.14 Stromal Dystrophies 143
2.15 Fuchs' Endothelial Dystrophy 153
2.16 Endothelial Disorders and Bullous Keratopathy 157
2.17 Keratoplasty 161

3. Uvea 172
3.1 Uveitis—History and Clinical Features 172
3.2 Sympathetic Ophthalmia 195
3.3 Fuchs' Heterochromic Iridocyclitis 197
3.4 Vogt–Koyanagi–Harada Syndrome 199
3.5 Behçet's Disease 201
3.6 Investigations in Uveitis 203
3.7 Treatment of Uveitis 218

4. Glaucoma 224

    4.1 Basic Examination of Glaucoma and Tonometry 224
    4.2 Gonioscopy 237
    4.3 Glaucoma Diagnostic with Variable Corneal Compensation 243
    4.4 Glaucoma Visual Field Defects 245
    4.5 Ultrasound Biomicroscopy and Anterior Segment Optical Coherence Tomography in Glaucoma 256
    4.6 Angle-closure Glaucoma 259
    4.7 Primary Open-angle Glaucoma 270
    4.8 Neovascular Glaucoma 283
    4.9 Pigmentary Glaucoma 292
    4.10 Pseudoexfoliation Glaucoma 297
    4.11 Uveitic Glaucoma 303
    4.12 Steroid-induced Glaucoma 306
    4.13 Lens-induced Glaucoma 309
    4.14 Medical Management of Glaucoma 313
    4.15 Newer Drugs in Glaucoma 326
    4.16 Lasers in Glaucoma 333
    4.17 Trabeculectomy 343
    4.18 Modulation of Wound Healing in Glaucoma Filtering Surgery 359
    4.19 Glaucoma Drainage Devices 364
    4.20 Cyclodestructive Procedures 373
    4.21 Important Glaucoma Studies 379

5. Lens and Cataract 381

6. Retina..403

    6.1 Differential Diagnosis of Retinal Findings 403
    6.2 Fundus Fluorescein Angiography 408
    6.3 Ultrasonography 422
    6.4 Diabetic Retinopathy 427
    6.5 Lasers in Diabetic Retinopathy 443
    6.6 Hypertensive Retinopathy 457
    6.7 Central Retinal Vein Occlusion (CRVO) 462
    6.8 Central Retinal Artery Occlusion 473
    6.9 Retinal Detachment (RD) 479
    6.10 Endophthalmitis 505
    6.11 Retinitis Pigmentosa 514
    6.12 Retinoblastoma 523
    6.13 Age-related Macular Degeneration 530
    6.14 Vitrectomy 539
    6.15 Central Serous Chorioretinopathy 546
    6.16 Angiogenesis 550
    6.17 Intravitreal Injections 552

7. Neuro-ophthalmology 560

    7.1 Normal Pupil 560
    7.2 Abnormal Pupils 564

7.3 Optic Nerve Head 567
7.4 Optic Neuritis 575
7.5 Papilledema 583
7.6 Optic Atrophy 601
7.7 Optic Disk Anomalies 613
7.8 Anterior Ischemic Optic Neuropathy 620
7.9 Oculomotor Nerve 625
7.10 Fourth Nerve Palsy 638
7.11 Abducens Nerve Palsy 643
7.12 Myasthenia Gravis 649
7.13 Nystagmus 658
7.14 Visual Fields in Neuro-ophthalmology 665
7.15 Cavernous Sinus Thrombosis 671
7.16 Caroticocavernous Fistulas 679
7.17 Carotid Artery Occlusion 682
7.18 Ophthalmoplegia 687
7.19 Malingering 694

8. Orbit 700
8.1 Ectropion 700
8.2 Entropion 709
8.3 Ptosis 714
8.4 Eyelid Reconstruction 727
8.5 Blepharophimosis Syndrome 736
8.6 Thyroid-related Orbitopathy and Proptosis 737
8.7 Blowout Fractures of the Orbit 759
8.8 Orbitotomies 765
8.9 Botulinum Toxin 769
8.10 Lacrimal Secretory and Drainage Systems 771
8.11 Contracted Socket 778
8.12 Orbital Implants and Prosthesis 781
8.13 Miscellaneous Ocular Surgeries 784

9. Pediatric Ophthalmology and Strabismus 788
9.1 Pediatric–Ophthalmic Management 788
9.2 Diplopia Charting 804
9.3 Hess Charting 806

10. Optics and Refraction 811

11. Miscellaneous 847
11.1 Vitamin A Deficiency 847
11.2 Localization of Intraocular Foreign Bodies 852
11.3 Genetics 862
11.4 Community Ophthalmology 868
11.5 Traumatic Hyphema and Glaucoma 877
11.6 Sterilization 883
11.7 Landmark Studies in Ophthalmology 885

- 11.8 Diabetic Retinopathy 891
- 11.9 Clinical Trials in Glaucoma 924
- 11.10 Uveitis Studies 931
- 11.11 Pediatric Ophthalmology 937
- 11.12 Studies in Neuro-ophthalmology 942
- 11.13 Cataract Surgery 947

12. Management Summary of Commonly Kept Examination Cases 953

- 12.1 Nonproliferative Diabetic Retinopathy with Clinically Significant Macular Edema 953
- 12.2 Proliferative Diabetic Retinopathy 956
- 12.3 Rhegmatogenous Retinal Detachment 958
- 12.4 Retinitis Pigmentosa 960
- 12.5 Central Retinal Vein Occlusion 963
- 12.6 Optic Atrophy 965
- 12.7 Papilledema 969
- 12.8 Third Nerve Palsy 971
- 12.9 Sixth Nerve Palsy 973
- 12.10 Myasthenia Gravis 974
- 12.11 Thyroid-related Orbitopathy 975
- 12.12 Entropion 978
- 12.13 Ectropion 979
- 12.14 Lagophthalmos 980
- 12.15 Ptosis 981
- 12.16 Blepharophimosis Ptosis Epicanthus Syndrome 986
- 12.17 Medial Canthoplasty 988
- 12.18 Medial Canthal Tendon Shortening with Transnasal Wire 989
- 12.19 Brow Suspension/Frontalis Sling 990
- 12.20 Traumatic Cataract 991
- 12.21 Penetrating Injury with Traumatic Cataract 992
- 12.22 Marfan Syndrome with Subluxation of Lens 993
- 12.23 Active Uveitis in Right Eye and Uveitis with Complicated Cataract in Left Eye 995
- 12.24 Pterygium 997
- 12.25 Keratoconus 999
- 12.26 Macular Corneal Dystrophy 1000
- 12.27 Bacterial Corneal Ulcer 1002
- 12.28 Herpes Simplex Virus Keratitis 1006
- 12.29 Acanthamoeba Keratitis 1008
- 12.30 Primary Open-angle Glaucoma 1009
- 12.31 Postfilter Case: Best Eye, Right Eye (Functioning Filter), and Left Eye (Nonfunctioning Filter) 1010
- 12.32 Pseudoexfoliation Glaucoma Right Eye with IMC 1013
- 12.33 Neovascular Glaucoma 1015
- 12.34 Acute Attack of Angle Closure Glaucoma 1017

13. Case Sheet Writing 1018
- 13.1 Third Nerve Palsy—Model Case Sheet 1029
- 13.2 Glaucoma—Model Case Sheet 1035
- 13.3 A Case of Right Eye—Macular Dystrophy—and Left Eye—Acute Corneal Graft Rejection 1046
- 13.4 Uvea: Model Case Sheet 1055

14. Ophthalmology Question Bank 1060
- 14.1 Ophthalmology Question Bank (MS Exam) 1060
- 14.2 Ophthalmology Question Bank (DNB Exam) 1078

15. Instruments Used in Ophthalmology 1103

Index 1145

CHAPTER 1

Introduction

1.1   VISUAL ACUITY

1. **Define visual acuity (VA).**
   Visual angle is defined as the reciprocal of the minimum resolvable angle measured in minutes of arc for a standard test pattern.

2. **Define visual angle.**
   Visual angle is the angle subtended at the nodal point of the eye by the physical dimensions of an object in the visual field.

3. **What are the components of VA?**
   Visual angle has three components:
   i. *Minimum visible:* Detection of presence or absence of stimulus
   ii. *Minimum separable:* Judgment of location of a visual target relative to another element of the same target
   iii. *Minimum resolvable:* Ability to distinguish between more than one identifying feature in a visible target. Threshold is between 30 seconds and 1 minute of arc

4. **What are the components of measurement of vision?**
   i. VA
   ii. Field of vision
   iii. Color vision
   iv. Binocular single vision

5. **Who developed classic test chart?**
   The classic test chart was developed by Professor Herman Snellen in 1862.

6. **What is the testing distance? Why do we check at that distance?**
   The testing is done 6 m (20 ft) away from the target. At this distance, the divergence of rays that enter the pupil is so small that the rays are considered parallel. Hence, accommodation is eliminated at this distance.

7. Describe Snellen's chart.

Snellen's chart comprises the following:
  i. It consists of a series of black capital letters on a whiteboard arranged in lines, each progressively diminishing in size
  ii. The lines comprising the letters have such a breadth that they will subtend at an angle of 1 minute at the nodal point of the eye at a particular distance
  iii. Each letter is designed such that it fits in a square
  iv. The sides of the letter are five times the breadth of constituent lines
  v. At a given distance, each letter subtends at an angle of 5 minutes at the nodal point of the eye

8. What does normal 6/6 VA represent?

Normal 6/6 VA represents the ability to see 1 minute of arc, which is close to theoretical diffraction limits.

9. Explain LogMAR (logarithm of the minimum angle of resolution) charts.

  i. Used for academic and research purposes
  ii. This is a modification of Snellen's chart, where each subsequent line differs by 0.1 log unit in the minimum angle of resolution (MAR) required for that line
  iii. They have an equal number of letters in each line
  iv. They are used at a distance of 4 m

10. What is the procedure of testing VA using Snellen's chart?

  i. Patient is seated at a distance of 6 m from Snellen's chart because at this distance, the rays of light are practically parallel and the patient exerts minimal accommodation
  ii. The chart should be properly illuminated (not <20 ft candle)
  iii. Patient is asked to read with each eye separately
  iv. VA is recorded as a fraction
      - *Numerator:* Distance of the patient from the chart
      - *Denominator:* Smallest letters read accurately
  v. When the patient is able to read up to the 6 m line, the VA is recorded as 6/6—normal
  vi. Depending on the smallest line the patient can read from a distance of 6 m, the VA is recorded as 6/9, 6/12, 6/18, 6/24, 6/36, and 6/60
  vii. If the patient cannot see the top line from 6 m, he/she is asked to walk toward the chart till one can read the top line
  viii. Depending on the distance at which the patient can read the top line, the VA is recorded as 5/60, 4/60, 3/60, 2/60, and 1/60
  ix. *Finger counting:* If a patient is unable to read the top line even from 1 m, he/she is asked to count fingers (CFs) of the examiner,

the VA is recorded as CF-3', CF-2', CF-1', or CF close to the face, depending on the distance (in meters) at which the patient is able to count fingers
x. *Hand movements (HMs):* When the patient fails to count fingers, the examiner moves his/her hand close to the patient's face. If the patient can appreciate the HMs, the VA is recorded as HM positive
xi. *Perception of light (PL):* When the patient cannot distinguish HM, the examiner notes whether the patient can perceive light or not. If the patient can perceive light, then it is recorded as PL+; if the patient cannot perceive light, then it is recorded as P
xii. *Projection of rays (PR):* If PL is +ve, then PR should be checked by shining light in all four directions, and the patient is asked whether he/she is able to recognize the direction of light rays that are shown The patient's responses are recorded in all four quadrants

11. How is a decimal notation represented?

It converts Snellen fraction to a decimal.
For example: Snellen 20/20—decimal 1.0
Snellen 20/30—decimal 0.7
Snellen 20/40—decimal 0.5

12. How is near vision tested?

i. Near acuity testing demonstrates the ability of a patient to see clearly at a normal reading distance
ii. Test is usually performed at 40 cm (16″) with a printed, handheld chart
iii. The following charts are used:
   - Jaeger's chart
   - Roman test types
   - Snellen's near vision test types

13. Explain Jaeger's chart.

i. Jaeger devised it in 1867
ii. It consisted of ordinary printed fonts of varying sizes used at that time. Various sizes of modern fonts that approximate the original chart are used
iii. In this chart, prints are marked from 1 to 7 and accordingly patient's acuity is labeled as J1 to J7, depending upon the print one can read

14. What is Landolt's testing chart?

i. Landolt's testing chart is similar to Snellen's chart, except that instead of letters, broken circles are used
ii. Each broken ring subtends an angle of 5 minutes at the nodal point
iii. It consists of detection of orientation of the break in the circle

15. What is Vernier acuity?
   i. Vernier acuity is the smallest offset of a line that can be detected
   ii. It is measured using a square wave grating
   iii. An offset of 3–5 seconds of an arc is normally discernible
   iv. It is less than the limit of Snellen VA and is therefore called hyperacuity

16. What is potential acuity testing?
Potential acuity testing refers to tests that are used to assess the VA of eyes in which it is not possible to see the macula because of cataract.
   i. Pinhole test
   ii. *Bluefield entopic phenomena:* Ability to see moving white dots when blue light diffusely illuminates the retina. It represents light transmitted by white blood cells (WBCs) in the perifoveal capillaries
   iii. *Interferometers:* They project laser light from two sources onto the retina. Interference occurs when two sources meet. It is seen as a sine wave grating if the macula is functioning

17. What are Roman test types?
   i. Roman test types are devised by the Faculty of Ophthalmologists of Great Britain in 1952
   ii. They consist of "Times Roman" type fonts with standard spacing
   iii. Near vision is recorded as N5, N6, N8, N10, N12, N18, N36, and N48

18. Explain Snellen's near vision test types.
   i. Snellen's equivalent for near vision was devised on the same principle as distant types
   ii. Graded thickness of letters of different lines is about 1/17th of distant vision chart letters
   iii. Letters equivalent to 6/6 line subtend an angle of 5 minutes at an average reading distance (35 cm/14")

19. What is the procedure of testing near vision?
   i. The patient is seated in a chair and asked to read the near vision chart kept at a distance of 25–35 cm with good illumination thrown over his or her left shoulder
   ii. Each eye should be tested separately
   iii. Near vision is recorded as the smallest type that can be read completely by the patient
   iv. A note of approximate distance at which the near vision chart is held should be made
   v. Thus, near vision is recorded as:
   NV = J1 at 30 cm (in Jaeger's notation)
   NV = N5 at 30 cm (in Faulty's notation)

Feet	Meters	LogMAR
20/20	6/6	0.00
20/30	6/9	0.18
20/40	6/12	0.30
20/60	6/18	0.48
20/80	6/24	0.60
20/120	6/36	0.80
20/200	6/60	1.00

20. **What is the principle of pinhole?**

Pinhole admits only central rays of light, which do not require refraction by the cornea or the lens. The patient can resolve finer detail on the acuity chart in this way, without the use of glasses.

21. **What do we infer from pinhole testing?**
    i. If the pinhole improves VA by two lines or more, then there is more likely a chance of refractive error
    ii. If the pinhole does not improve vision, then other organic causes should be looked for

22. **What is the size of pinhole?**
    1 mm/1.2 mm

23. **What are the types of pinholes?**
    i. Single—no >2.4 mm in diameter is used
    ii. Multiple—central opening surrounded by two rings of small perforation

24. **How is the pinhole testing performed?**
    i. Position the patient and occlude the eye not being tested
    ii. Ask the patient to hold the pinhole occluder in front of the eye that is to be tested. The habitual correction should be worn for the test
    iii. Instruct the patient to look at the distance chart through the single pinhole
    iv. Instruct the patient to use little hand or eye movements to align the pinhole to resolve the sharpest image on the chart
    v. Ask the patient to begin to read the line with the smallest letters that are legible as determined on the previous vision test without the use of pinhole

25. **What are the variables used in VA measurements?**

The conditions that may cause variability in acuity measurements for both near and distance are:

External variables:
  i. If the lighting level is not constant during testing
  ii. Variability in contrast: Charts with higher contrast will be seen more easily than those with lower contrast
  iii. If the chart is not kept clean, smaller letters will become more difficult to identify
  iv. When a projector chart is used, cleanliness of projector bulb and lens and condition of projecting screen will affect the contrast of letters viewed
  v. The distance between the projector and the chart will affect the size of letters
  vi. Sharpness of focus of the projected chart
  vii. Incidental glare on the screen

Optical considerations:
  i. If the patient is wearing eyeglasses, be sure that the lenses are clean. Dirty lenses of any kind, whether trial lenses or contact lenses, will decrease VA
  ii. Effects of tear film abnormalities, such as dry eye syndromes, can be minimized by generous use of artificial tear preparation
  iii. Corneal surface abnormalities produce distortions and must be addressed medically
  iv. Corneal or lenticular astigmatism may necessitate the use of special spectacle or contact lens

Neurologic impairments:
  i. Motility defects such as nystagmus or any other movement disorder that interferes with the ability to align the fovea will lower the acuity measurement
  ii. Visual field defects
  iii. Optic nerve lesions
  iv. Pupil abnormalities
  v. Impairment by drugs, legal or illicit

26. What are the causes of poor near acuity than distance acuity?
  i. Presbyopia/premature presbyopia
  ii. Undercorrected/high hyperopia
  iii. Overcorrected myopia
  iv. Small, centrally located cataracts
  v. Accommodative effort syndrome
  vi. Drugs with anticholinergic effect
  vii. Convergence insufficiency
  viii. Adie's pupil
  ix. Malingering/hysteria

Introduction

27. **How to test vision in infants?**
    i. Blink response—in response to sound, bright light/touching the cornea
    ii. Pupillary reflex—after 29th week of gestation
    iii. Fixation reflex—usually present at birth. It is well developed and well elicited by 2 weeks to 2 months
    iv. Follow movements—following horizontally moving targets. It is seen in full-term newborns and is well developed by the first month. Vertical tracking is elicited by 4-8 weeks
    v. *Catford drum test:*
        - It is based on the observation of pendular eye movement that is elicited as the child follows an oscillating drum with dots
        - Test distance: 60 cm (2 ft)
        - Displayed dot size: 15-0.5 mm
        - Dots represent 20/600 to 20/20 vision
        - Smallest dot that evokes pendular eye movement denotes acuity
        - Disadvantage: Overestimate of vision by two to four times. It is unreliable for amblyopia screening
    vi. *Preferential looking tests (PLT):*
        - The principle is based on the behavioral pattern of an infant to prefer to fixate a pattern stimulus rather than a blank stimulus, both being of the same brightness
    vii. *Teller acuity card test:*
        - It is a modification based on PLT designed for simpler and rapid testing
        - It has 17 cards, each 25.5 × 51 cm. Fifteen of these contain 12.5 × 12.5 cm patches of square wave gratings
        - Cycle consists of one black and one white stripe, and an octave is halving or doubling of spatial frequency
        - Testing distance: Infants up to 6 months of age—38 cm; 7 months to 3 years of age—55 cm; more than 55 years—84 cm
        - Advantage: Very useful quick test for infants and preschool children up to 18 months
        - Disadvantage: It tests near acuity, not distance acuity. It measures resolution acuity, not recognition acuity. It overestimates VA
    viii. *OKNOVIS:*
        - Principle: Based on the principle of arresting an elicited optokinetic nystagmus (OKN) by introducing optotypes of different sizes
        - Portable handheld drums moving at 12 rpm with colored pictures to elicit an OKN
        - Testing distance: 60 cm
        - Optotypes of different sizes are then introduced to arrest OKN

ix. *Cardiff acuity cards:*
   - Principle: Based on the principle of preferential fixation on cards that have picture optotypes and a blank located vertically
   - Child identifies picture by verbalizing, pointing, or fixation preference
x. *Visually evoked response (VEP):*
   - It records the change in the cortical electrical pattern detected by surface electrodes monitoring the occipital cortex following light stimulation of the retina
   - Two types of stimuli:
     1. Pattern—checkerboard or stripes
     2. Flash—unpatterned
   - Preferred is pattern reversal type
   - Can be recorded in two modes: Transient or steady state

28. How do you infer VA from fixation pattern?

Fixation pattern	VA
Gross eccentric fixation	<CF 1 m
Unsteady central fixation	<6/60
Steady central fixation but not maintained	6/60–6/36
Central steady fixation can maintain but prefers the other eye	6/24–6/9
Central steady fixation, free alternation or cross fixation	6/9–6/6

To call it as good fixation, it should be central, steady, and maintained. Preference of fixation in one eye denotes poor vision in nonfixating eye.

29. How is vision tested in infants aged about 1–2 years?
   i. *Boeck candy test (cake decoration test):*
      - Initially, the child's hand is guided to the bead and then to his mouth
      - Each eye is alternatively covered and the difference is noted
   ii. *Worth's ivory ball test:*
      - Ivory balls measuring 0.5–1.5" in diameter are rolled on the floor in front of the child
      - He/she is asked to retrieve each ball
      - Acuity is estimated on the basis of the smallest size for the test distance
   iii. *Sheridan's ball test:*
      - Styrofoam balls of different sizes are rolled in front of the child
      - The quality of fixation for each size is assessed
      - The same can be used as mounted balls used at 10 ft distance against black screen. The fixation behavior for each ball is observed by the examiner hidden behind the screen

30. How is vision tested in children of around 3 years of age?
  i. *Miniature toy test:*
    - A component of STYCAR test
    - Pair of miniature toys are used
    - Test distance is 10 ft
    - Child is asked to name or pick the pair from an assortment
  ii. *Coin test:*
    - Coins of different sizes at different distances are shown
    - Child is asked to distinguish between the two faces of the coin
  iii. *Dot VA test:*
    - In a darkened room, the child is shown an illuminated box with printed black dots of different diameters
    - Then, smaller dots are shown
    - Smallest dot identified correctly twice is taken as acuity threshold

31. How is vision tested in children aged 3–5 years?
  i. Vision test using pictures, symbols, or even letters becomes applicable in this age group
  ii. Training by mother at home is helpful
    - Illiterate E-cutout test
    - Tumbling E test
    - Isolated hand figure test
    - Sheridan–Gardiner test
    - Lippmann's HOTV test
    - Pictorial vision test
    - Broken wheel test
    - Boeck candy bead test
    - Light home picture cards
  iii. *Illiterate E-cutout test:*
    - Child is given a cutout of an E and asked to match this with isolated E's of varying sizes
    - When the child starts understanding orientation of E, the VA chart consisting of E's oriented in various directions is used
  iv. *Tumbling E test:*
    - It is preferred for mass screening in preschool children
    - It consists of different sizes of E, in one of the four positions—right, left, up, or down
    - Distance: 6 m
    - Each eye is tested separately
  v. *Landolt's C:* Similar to the E test
  vi. *Sheridan's letter test:*
    - It uses five letters H, O, T, V, and X in five-letter set
    - A and V are added in seven-letter set

- C and L are also added in nine-letter set
- Testing distance is 10 ft (3 m)
- Child is expected to name the letters/indicate similar letters on the card in hand

vii. *Lippman's HOTV test:*
- It uses only four letters H, O, T, V at a test distance of 3 m
- It is a simpler version of Sheridan test

32. What is hyperacuity?

The human eye is capable of seeing more than the ability of the retinal cones to resolve. This ability is called hyperacuity. It is due to the involvement of higher cortical centers in the parietal cortex, for example:
i. Vernier acuity
ii. Stereo acuity

Vernier acuity:
This is the ability to discern the Vernier separation between two lines not in perfect alignment. It is in the range of 10–20 seconds of an arc.

Stereoacuity:
This is the ability to perceive separation in the three-dimension (3D) depth perception.

33. What is Stiles–Crawford effect?

Stiles and Crawford have shown that pencils of light entering the eye obliquely are less effective as stimuli, compared to those entering the pupil centrally. They pointed out that this effect is not due to aberrations in the optical system but is most likely related to the orientation of the receptors in the retina. This directional sensitivity of the retina is referred to as the Stiles–Crawford effect.

Introduction

1.2 COLOR VISION

1. **How will you test color vision by Ishihara chart?**
    i. Room should be adequately lit by daylight
    ii. Nature of the test should be explained to the patient
    iii. Full refractive correction is worn
    iv. It is preferable to do the test before pupillary dilatation
    v. One eye is first occluded and the other eye is tested
    vi. The plates are kept at a distance of 75 cm from the subject, with the plane of the paper at a right angle to the line of vision
    vii. The standard time taken to answer each plate is 3–5 seconds

2. **Explain Ishihara chart.**
    i. It is designed to provide a test that gives a quick and accurate assessment of color vision deficiency of congenital origin
    ii. It consists of a total of 25 plates

Plate number	Normal	Points with red–green defects	Inference
1	12	12	Both subjects with normal and defective color vision read plate 1 as 12
2	8	3	
3	6	5	
4	29	17	
5	57	35	Subjects with red–green defects read these plates as those in abnormal column. Totally color-blind subjects are unable to read
6	5	2	
7	3	5	
8	15	17	
9	74	21	
10	2	X	Majority of subjects with color vision deficiency read these plates incorrectly
11	6	X	
12	97	X	
13	45	X	
14	5	X	Subjects with normal color vision do not see any number. Those with red–green deficiency read the numbers given in the abnormal column
15	7	X	
16	16	X	
17	73	X	
18	X	5	
19	X	2	

Contd...

Contd...

Plate number	Normal	Points with red–green defects		Inference
20	X	45		Subjects with protanopia read these plates as given in abnormal column (1), those with deuteranomaly read them as given in column (2)
21	X	73		
		Protan	Deutran	
22	26	6	2	
23	42	2	4	
24	35	5	3	
25	96	6	9	

3. **Classify color blindness.**
   i. *Congenital color blindness:*
      X-linked recessive inherited affecting predominantly males
      Types:
      – Dyschromatopsia:
         Anomalous trichromatic color vision:
         a. Protanomalous: Defective red color appreciation
         b. Deuteranomalous: Defective green color appreciation
         c. Tritanomalous: Defective blue color appreciation
      – Dichromatic color vision:
         a. Protanopia: Complete red color defect
         b. Deuteranopia: Complete green color defect
         c. Tritanopia: Complete blue color defect
      – Achromatopsia:
         a. Cone monochromatism—presence of only one primary color
         b. Rod monochromatism
   ii. *Acquired color defects:*
      – Type I red-green defects—similar to protan defects
         Seen in progressive cone dystrophies
         a. Stargardt's disease
         b. Chloroquine toxicity
      – Type II red-green defects—similar to deutran defects
         Seen in optic neuropathies, Leber's optic atrophy, ethambutol toxicity
      – Type III tritan defects
         Seen in progressive rod dystrophies, peripheral retinal lesions, macular edema

4. **What are the differences between congenital and acquired color blindness?**

Congenital	Acquired
Present at birth	Present after birth (3 months)
Type and severity constant	Can change with time
Type of deficiency can be diagnosed precisely	Can show combined color vision deficiency features
Both eyes are equally affected	Very rarely both eyes are equally affected
Visual fields and visual acuity are usually normal	Commonly, there is a reduced visual acuity with field changes
Predominantly are red–green defects	Most commonly are tritan defects
Higher incidence in male population	Equal incidence in both sexes

5. **What are the theories of color vision?**
   i. *Trichromatic theory of Young and Helmholtz:* It postulates the existence of three types of cones, each with a different photopigment maximally sensitive to either red, green, or blue. The sensation of any given color is determined by relative frequency in pulse from each of the cone systems
   ii. *Opponent color theory of Hering:* It states that some colors appear to be mutually exclusive, for example, reddish green

6. **Mention the genes associated with color vision defects.**
   i. Gene for rhodopsin—chromosome 3
   ii. Gene for red and green cones—"q" arm of X chromosome
   iii. Gene for blue cone—chromosome 7

7. **Explain the neurophysiology of color vision.**
   i. *Genesis of visual signals in photoreceptors:* Photochemical changes in cone pigments followed by a cascade of biochemical changes produce visual signal in the form of cone receptor potential
   ii. *Processing and transmission of color vision signals:* The action potential generated in photoreceptors is transmitted by electrical induction to other cells of retina across the synapses of photoreceptors, bipolar cells, and horizontal cells, and then across the synapses of bipolar cells, ganglion cells, and amacrine cells
   iii. *Processing of color signals on lateral geniculate body (LGB):* All LGB neurons carry information from more than one cone cell. Color information carried by ganglion cells is relayed to the parvocellular portion of LGB

   Spectrally nonopponent cells (30%) give the same type of response to any monochromatic light

   Spectrally opponent cells (60%) are excited by some wavelengths and inhibited by others

Four types:
- Cells with red/green antagonism
  a. +R/−G
  b. +G/−R
- Cells with yellow/blue antagonism
  a. +B/−Y
  b. +Y/−B

iv. *Analysis of color signals in visual cortex:* Color information from the parvocellular portion of LGB is relayed to layer IVc of striate cortex in area 17. From here, it passes to blobs in layers II and III. It is relayed to thin strips in usual association area and then to lingual and fusiform gyri of the occipital lobe (specialized area concerned with color)

8. **What are the tests for color vision apart from Ishihara chart?**
   i. *Hardy-Rand-Rittler*
      - It is also a pseudoisochromatic chart test. It is useful to identify protan, deutran, and tritan defects. It consists of 24 plates with vanishing designs containing geometric shapes. Four plates are introductory plates, 6 are for screening (4 for protan and deutran and 2 for tritan), 10 are for grading the severity of protan and deutran defects, and last 4 are for grading tritan defect
   ii. *Lantern test:* The subject has to name the various colors shown to him using a lantern. He is judged based on this
      - There are three types: Edridge Green, Holmes Wright types A and B
   iii. *Farnsworth–Munsell 100 hue test* is a spectrographic test where colored chips are arranged in an ascending order
   iv. *City University color vision test* is also a spectrographic test where the central colored plate is matched to its closest hue from four surrounding color plates
   v. *Nagel's anomaloscope test:* The observer is asked to mix red and green colors in a proportion to match the given yellow color hue. It detects red-green deficiency
   vi. *Holmgren's wool test:* The subject is asked to make a series of color matches from a selection of colored wools

9. **What are the causes of acquired blue-yellow defects?**
   Acquired blue-yellow defects can be caused by glaucoma, retinal detachment, pigmentary degeneration of retina, age-related macular degeneration (ARMD), vascular occlusions, diabetic retinopathy, hypertensive retinopathy, papilledema, central serous retinopathy, and chorioretinitis.

10. **What are the causes of acquired red-green defects?**
    Acquired red-green defects can be caused by optic neuritis, toxic amblyopia, Leber's optic neuropathy, Best's disease, optic nerve lesions, papillitis, and Stargardt's disease.

1.3 ANATOMICAL LANDMARKS IN EYE

CORNEA

1. Dimensions of cornea
   Horizontal diameter—11.75 mm
   Vertical diameter—11 mm
   Posterior diameter—11.5 mm
2. Endothelial cell count
   At birth—6,000 cells/mm^2
   In young adults—2,400–3,000 cells/mm^2
   Corneal decompensation—cell count <500/mm^2
3. Thickness of cornea
   Center—about 0.52 mm
   Periphery—about 0.67 mm
4. Refractive index of cornea—1.37
5. Surgical limbus—2 mm wide
   Anterior limbal border—overlies termination of Bowman's membrane
   Mid-limbal line—overlies termination of Schwalbe's line
   Posterior limbal border—overlies scleral spur
   Preferred site for incision—mid-limbal incision

SCLERA

1. Forms posterior five-sixths of eyeball
2. Thickness
   Posteriorly—thickest 1 mm
   Thinnest at insertion of extraocular muscles—0.3 mm
3. Vortex vein—passes through middle apertures 4-7 mm posterior to equator

UVEA

1. Average diameter of iris—12 mm
2. Average thickness—0.5 mm
3. Thinnest part of iris—at the root
4. Pupil diameter—3-4 mm
5. Pars plicata—2-2.5 mm wide
6. Pars plana—5 mm wide temporally and 3 mm wide nasally
7. Ciliary processes 70-80 in number
8. Short posterior ciliary arteries—from ophthalmic artery, 10-20 branches
9. Long posterior ciliary arteries—two in number
10. Anterior ciliary arteries—seven in number

AQUEOUS HUMOR

1. Ciliary body—site of aqueous production
2. Posterior chamber—0.06 mL of aqueous
3. Anterior chamber—0.25 mL of aqueous
4. Depth of anterior chamber—3 mm in the center

LENS

1. Diameter of lens
    i. 6.5 mm at birth
    ii. 9-10 mm in second decade
2. Thickness of lens
    i. 3.5 mm at birth
    ii. 5 mm at extreme age
3. Weight of lens—135-255 mg
4. Refractive index—1.39
5. Lens capsule thicker anteriorly than posteriorly

VITREOUS HUMOR

1. Weight—4 g
2. Volume—4 cc, 99% water
3. Anterior hyaloid membrane starts from approximately 1.5 mm from ora serrata
4. Vitreous base—4 mm wide, 1.5-2 mm area of pars plana anteriorly and 2 mm of adjoining peripheral retina posterior to ora serrata

RETINA

1. Retinal surface area—266 mm^2
2. Macula lutea—5.5 mm in diameter
3. Fovea centralis
    i. 1.85 mm in diameter
    ii. 5° of visual field
4. Foveola
    i. 0.35 mm in diameter
    ii. Situated 3 mm from temporal edge of optic disk to 1 mm below horizontal meridian
5. Parafoveal area—0.5 mm in diameter
6. Perifoveal area—1.5 mm in diameter
7. Ora serrata—2.1 mm wide temporally and 0.7-0.8 mm wide nasally
8. Number of rods—about 120 million
9. Number of cones—6.5 million
10. Highest density of cones at fovea—199,000 cones/mm^2
11. Each rod—40-60 µm long

12. Each cone—40-80 µm long
13. Foveal avascular zone—500 µm in diameter
14. Optic disk—1.5 mm in diameter
15. Length of optic nerve—47-50 mm
    Intraocular—1 mm
    Intraorbital—30 mm
    Intracanalicular—6-9 mm
    Intracranial—10 mm
16. Difference between retinal artery and vein

Characteristics	Artery	Vein
Color	Bright red	Dark red
Size	Thin	Thick
Central light reflex	Wide	Narrow
Spontaneous pulsation	Always absent in normal individuals	Can be present in 80% of normal cases

MUSCLES OF THE EYE

1. Extraocular and intraocular muscles of the eye

Extraocular	Intraocular
• Superior rectus (SR) • Lateral rectus (LR) • Inferior rectus (IR) • Medial rectus (MR) • Superior oblique (SO) • Inferior oblique (IO) • Levator palpebrae superioris (LPS)	• Ciliary muscles • Sphincter pupillae • Dilator pupillae

2. Six extraocular muscles—four recti and two oblique
3. Origin of recti—common tendinous ring (from the limbus) attached at the apex of orbit
4. Insertion of recti:
   MR—5.5 mm
   IR—6.5 mm
   LR—6.9 mm
   SR—7.7 mm
5. SO muscle—longest and thinnest of all extraocular muscles
   i. 59.5 mm long
   ii. Arises from body of sphenoid
   iii. Inserted onto the upper and outer part of sclera behind the equator
6. IO muscle—shortest of eye muscles
   i. 37 mm long
   ii. Arises from the orbital plate of maxilla
   iii. Inserted in the lower and outer part of sclera behind the equator

LACRIMAL APPARATUS
1. Lacrimal gland is situated in lacrimal fossa formed by the orbital plate of frontal bone
2. Lateral horn of levator muscle aponeurosis divides the gland into two parts
3. Upper and lower lacrimal puncta lie about 6 mm and 6.5 mm lateral from canthus, respectively
4. Canaliculi
   i. 0.5 mm in diameter
   ii. 10 mm in length, vertical 2 mm, and horizontal 8 mm
5. Lacrimal sac lies in lacrimal fossa formed by lacrimal bone and frontal process of maxilla
6. Lacrimal sac is 15 mm in length and 5-6 mm in breadth
7. Volume of sac—20 mm
8. Nasolacrimal duct opens in—inferior meatus of nose
   i. 18 mm in length (12-24 mm)
   ii. Intraosseous part 12.5 mm and intrameatal part 5.5 mm
   iii. 3 mm in diameter

EYELIDS
1. Upper eyelid—covers one-sixth of cornea
2. Lower eyelid—just touches the cornea
3. Palpebral fissure—horizontally 28-30 mm and vertically 9-11 mm
4. LPS:
   i. Origin from the lesser wing of sphenoid above the annulus of Zinn
   ii. Inserts onto septa between orbicularis muscle, pretarsal skin of eyelid, and anterior surface of tarsus
5. Length of LPS:
   i. Fleshy part—40 mm long
   ii. Tendinous aponeurosis—15 mm long
6. Tarsal plates—29 mm long, 1 mm thick

ORBIT
1. Lateral wall of each orbit lies at an angle of 45° to the medial wall
2. Lateral walls of two orbits are 90° to each other
3. Depth of orbit—42 mm along medial wall, 50 mm along lateral wall
4. Base of orbit—40 mm in width, 35 mm in height
5. Volume of orbit—29 mL
6. Ratio of volume of orbit to eyeball is 4.5:1
7. Optic canal—length 6-11 mm, lateral wall shortest and medial wall longest

8. **What is the lymphatic drainage of the ocular structures?**
   The lymphatics of the ocular appendages and conjunctiva follow the given route:

   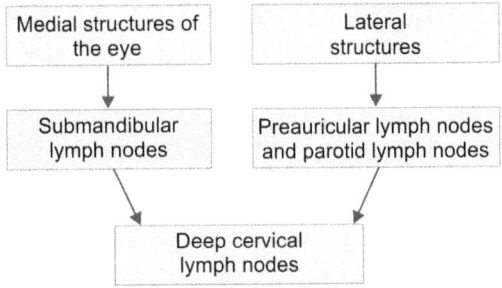

9. *Vascular supply of orbit:*
   Ophthalmic artery: First major branch of internal carotid artery
   Enters the orbit: Within the dural sheath of the optic nerve and passes through the optic canal, below and lateral to the nerve
   In the orbit: Emerges from the meningeal sheath, runs inferolateral to the optic nerve for a short distance, then crosses over it to run along the medial wall
   Termination: Just posterior to the superior orbital margin, gives the terminal branches, the supratrochlear and dorsonasal arteries

10. *Branches of ophthalmic artery:*
    i. Central retinal artery
    ii. Lacrimal artery
    iii. Ciliary arteries
    iv. Ethmoid arteries
    v. Supraorbital artery
    vi. Muscular branches
    vii. Medial palpebral arteries
    viii. Supratrochlear artery
    ix. Dorsonasal artery
    Main supply to the orbit and adnexal structures with few supplementary branches from external carotid artery (ECA).

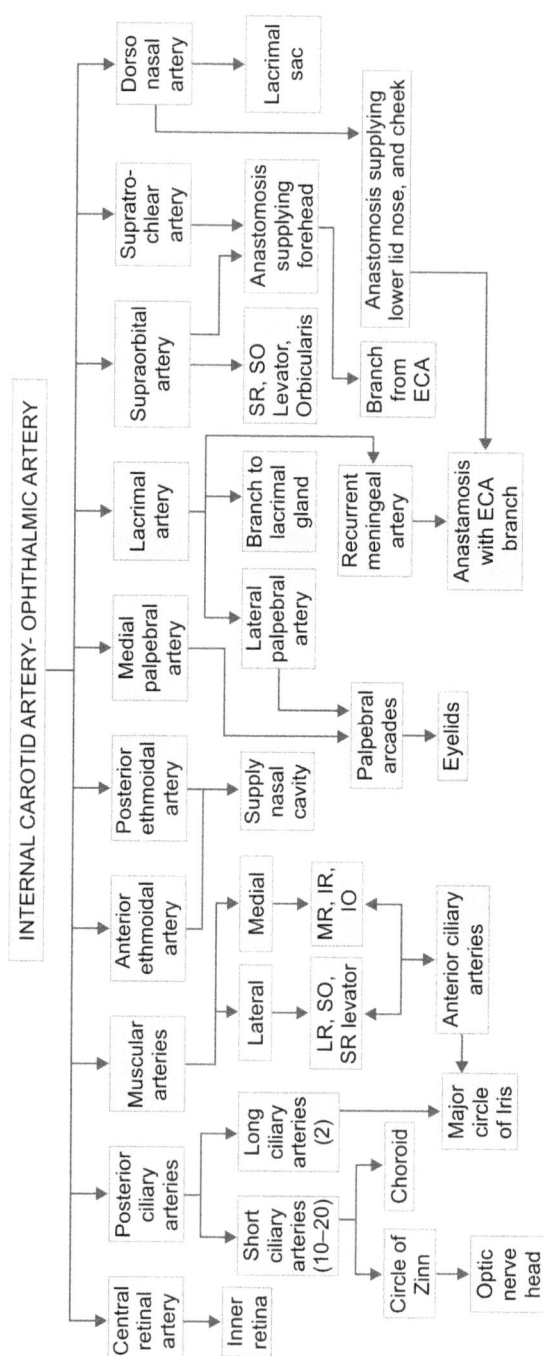

1.4 EMBRYOLOGY

1. **What is the embryologic derivation of ocular structures?**

   Surface ectoderm gives rise to:
   i. Lens
   ii. Corneal epithelium
   iii. Conjunctival epithelium
   iv. Epithelium of eyelids and cilia, meibomian glands, and glands of Zeis and Moll
   v. Epithelium lining nasolacrimal system

   Neural ectoderm gives rise to:
   i. Retinal pigment epithelium
   ii. Neural retina
   iii. Optic nerve fibers (optic nerve, optic chiasm, optic tract)
   iv. Epithelium of ciliary body
   v. Epithelium of iris
   vi. Iris sphincter and dilator muscles

   Mesoderm: Extraocular muscles
   i. A part of choroid
   ii. A part of corneal stroma

   Neural crest gives rise to:
   i. Corneal stroma (which gives rise to Bowman's layer)
   ii. Corneal endothelium (which gives rise to Descemet's membrane)
   iii. Most (or all) of sclera
   iv. Trabecular structures
   v. Uveal pigment cells
   vi. Uveal connective tissue
   vii. Ciliary muscle
   viii. Meninges of optic nerve
   ix. Vascular pericytes.

1.5 PHARMACOLOGY

ANTI-INFECTIVE DOSAGE
Antibiotics

Topical

Cefazolin	5%
Ceftriaxone	10%
Penicillin	100,000 units/mL
Ticarcillin	0.6%
Ciprofloxacin	0.3%
Ofloxacin	0.3%
Moxifloxacin	0.5%
Gatifloxacin	0.3%
Polymyxin B	50,000 units/mL
Vancomycin	2.5–5%
Tobramycin	1–1.4%
Gentamicin	0.3–1.4%
Amikacin	1–2.5%
Chloramphenicol	0.5%

Fortified topical

Cefazolin	50 or 133 mg/mL
Ceftriaxone	50 mg/mL
Cefamandole	50 mg/mL
Penicillin	100,000 units/mL
Methicillin	50 mg/mL
Ampicillin	50 mg/mL
Moxalactam	50 mg/mL
Carbenicillin	4 mg/mL
Ticarcillin	6 mg/mL
Bacitracin	10,000 units/mL
Polymyxin	50,000 units/mL
Vancomycin	50 or 25 mg/mL
Gentamicin	14 or 20 mg/mL
Tobramycin	14 mg/mL
Amikacin	10 mg/mL
Chloramphenicol	5 mg/mL

Subconjunctival

Cefazolin	100 mg
Ceftriaxone	100 mg
Penicillin	0.5 million units
Polymyxin B	10–25 mg
Vancomycin	25 mg
Tobramycin	10–20 mg
Gentamicin	10–20 mg
Amikacin	25–50 mg
Chloramphenicol	100 mg

Contd...

Contd...

Intravitreal	
Cefazolin	2.25 mg/0.1 mL
Ceftriaxone	3 mg
Penicillin	1,000–5,000/unit
Ciprofloxacin	0.1 mg
Ofloxacin	0.1 mg
Vancomycin	1 mg/0.1 mL
Tobramycin	0.2 mg/0.1 mL
Gentamicin	0.1 mg/0.1 mL
Amikacin	0.2–0.4 mg/0.08 mL

Preparations of antifungal topical medications:

Name	Vial size	Strength	Preparation	Refrigeration	Shelf life	Spectrum
Amphotericin B	50 mg	0.15%	Add 10 mL of distilled water to parenteral 50 mg of amphotericin B powder for injection. Draw 3 mL of this and add to 7 mL of artificial tear drops	4°C	1 week at 4°C	Yeasts, filamentous fungi (resistance reported to *Aspergillus*)
Voriconazole	200 mg	1%	Mix 20 mL Ringer lactate (RL) to 200 mg of voriconazole lyophilized powder	4°C	1 week at 4°C	Broad-spectrum activity against molds and yeasts

Preparation of antiprotozoal topical medications:

Name	Strength	Preparation	Storage	Shelf life	Spectrum
Chlorhexidine digluconate	0.02%	Add 5 µL of chlorhexidine digluconate solution (20% in water) in 5 mL of artificial tears using micropipette (1:1,000 dilution)	4°C	1 week at 4°C	*Acanthamoeba*

Contd...

Contd...

Name	Strength	Preparation	Storage	Shelf life	Spectrum
Polyhexam-ethylene biguanide (PHMB)	0.02%	Add 5 µL of PHMB solution (20 %) in 5 mL of artificial tears using micropipette (1:1,000 dilution)	4°C	1 week at 4°C	Acanthamoeba

Intrastromal preparations:

Voriconazole	50 µg/0.1 mL	From 1% topical solution voriconazole, take 1 mL, add 19 mL RL to make 0.05 mg/mL (50 µg/0.1 mL)	To be used immediately	Broad-spectrum activity against molds and yeasts
Amphotericin B	5–10 µg/0.1 mL	Add 10 mL of distilled water to parenteral 50 mg of amphotericin B powder. From 5 mg/mL solution, take 0.2 mL solution and add 0.8 mL balanced salt solution (BSS)/sterile water. Now take 0.1 mL of this solution and add 0.9 mL BSS/sterile water to create 0.1 mg/mL amphotericin B equivalent to 10 µg/0.1 mL	To be used immediately	Yeasts, filamentous fungi (resistance reported to various species of *Aspergillus*)

Intravenous (IV) doses:

Drug	Doses
Vancomycin	2 g daily in 2 doses
Cefazolin	1–6 g daily in 3–4 divided doses
Tobramycin	3–5 mg/kg daily in 2–3 doses
Gentamycin	3–5 mg/kg daily in 2–3 divided doses
Amikacin	15 mg/kg/day in 2–3 divided doses
Ceftazidime	2–6 g daily in 2–3 divided doses
Imipenem	2 g daily in 3–4 divided doses
Voriconazole	• 6 mg/kg IV every 12 hours (24 hours), then 4 mg/kg twice a day • 12 hours or 200 mg/day bd
Amphotericin B	10–20 µg/mL infusion

Intravitreal Injection

Vancomycin (1 mg in 0.1 mL)

- 5– 500 mg powder—add 10 mL of Ringer lactate (RL) → 5,050 mg/mL
- 2 mL of Vancomycin and add 8 mL of RL → 10 mg/mL
- Take 0.1 mL of Vancomycin for injection → 1 mg in 0.1 mL

Cefazolin (2.25 mg in 0.1 mL)

- 5– 500 mg powder—add 10 mL of RL → 5,050 mg/mL
- 1 mL of Cefazolin and add 1.2 mL of RL → 22.7 mg/mL
- Take 0.1 mL of Cefazolin → 2.27 mg

Ceftazidime (2.25 mg in 0.1 mL)

- 500 mg powder—add 10 mL of RL → 50 mg/mL
- 1 mL of Ceftazidime and add 1.2 mL of RL → 22.7 mg/mL
- Take 0.1 mL of Ceftazidime → 22.7 mg

Amikacin (0.4 mg in 0.1 mL)

Use 100 mg vials	Take 0.8 mL of drug (40 mg)
Add 9.2 mL of RL	40 mg in 10 mL
Take 0.1 mL	0.4 mg in 0.1 mL

Amphotericin B (0.005–0.01 mg)

50 mg vial	Add 10 mL of water (5 mg/mL)
Take 1 mL of above	Add 10 mL of water (0.5 mg/mL)
Take 1 mL of above	Add 10 mL of water (0.1 mg/mL)
Inject 0.1 mL of above	(0.01 mg/mL)

Antifungals	
Amphotericin B	1–10 mg/ mL drops, 2.5% ointment
Natamycin	5% suspension
Miconazole	1% drops, 2% ointment
Ketoconazole	1.5%
Fluconazole	0.2–2%
Flucytosine	1%
Antivirals	
5-Iodo-2′-deoxyuridine	0.1% drops, 0.5% ointment
Trifluorothymidine	1% drops
Adenine arabinoside	3% eye ointment
Acyclovir	3% eye ointment

ANTI-INFLAMMATORY DRUGS

I. Nonsteroidal anti-inflammatory drugs
   A. *Topical*

Generic name	Concentration (%)	Normal dosage
Ketorolac tromethamine	0.5%	qid
Flurbiprofen	0.03%	tid to qid
Diclofenac sodium	0.1%	qid
Indomethacin	1%	4–6 times/day
Suprofen	1%	qid

   B. *Systemic*

Generic name	Concentration (%)	Normal dosage
Aspirin	300–600 mg	bd, tds, qid
Acetaminophen	325 mg, 500 mg	bd, tds, qid
Phenylbutazone	100 mg	tds to qid
Oxyphenbutazone	100 mg	tds to qid
Indomethacin	50 mg	tds
Diclofenac sodium	25 mg, 50 mg	bd, tds, qid
Ibuprofen	300–800 mg	tds, qid
Ketoprofen	25 mg, 50 mg, 75 mg	tds, qid
Flurbiprofen	500 mg	bd, tds
Naproxen	250 mg, 500 mg	bd, tds, qid
Etodolac	200 mg, 300 mg	bd, tds, qid
Ketorolac tromethamine	10 mg	qid

II. *Corticosteroids*
   A. *Topical*

Generic name	Concentration (%)
Prednisolone acetate suspension	1%
Prednisolone sodium phosphate solution	1%
Fluorometholone suspension and ointment	0.1%
Dexamethasone phosphate solution	0.1%
Dexamethasone phosphate ointment	0.05%
Hydrocortisone acetate suspension	0.5%
Hydrocortisone acetate solution	0.2%
Hydrocortisone acetate ointment	1.5%
Betamethasone sodium phosphate solution	0.1%
Betamethasone sodium phosphate ointment	0.1%
Loteprednol etabonate	0.5 or 0.2%
Rimexolone	1%
Medrysone	1%

B. *Periocular*

- Methylprednisolone acetate (Depo-Medrol) — Depot preparation
- Triamcinolone acetonide (Kenalog) — Depot preparation
- Triamcinolone diacetate (Aristocort) — Depot preparation
- Hydrocortisone sodium succinate (Solu-Cortef) — Solution
- Betamethasone (Celestone) — Solution

C. *Intraocular*

- Triamcinolone acetonide — 4 mg in 0.1 mL
- Fluocinolone acetonide — Slow-release implants
- Dexamethasone — Slow-release implants

D. *Systemic*
   i. Oral

| Prednisolone (5 or 25 mg tablet) | 1–2 mg/kg/day |

   ii. IV

- Prednisolone — 1–1.5 mg/kg/day
- Triamcinolone
- Dexamethasone — 200 mg/day
- Methylprednisolone — 250–1,000 mg in 100 mL Normal saline for 3 days

III. *Immunomodulators*

A. *Antimetabolites*

- Methotrexate — 7.5–25 mg/week
- Azathioprine — 100–250 mg/day
- Mycophenolate mofetil — 1–3 g/day

B. *Inhibitors of T-cell lymphocytes:*
   i. Oral

- Cyclosporine — 2.5–5 mg/kg/day
- Tacrolimus — 0.1–0.2 mg/kg/day

   ii. IV

- Sirolimus
  - Loading dose 6 mg/day
  - Maintenance dose 4 mg/day

C. *Alkylating agents*

- Cyclophosphamide — 1–2 mg/day
- Chlorambucil — 2–12 mg/day

ANTIGLAUCOMA MEDICATIONS

I. *Cholinergic drugs*
   A. *Parasympathomimetics*

Generic name	Concentration (%)	Normal dosage
Pilocarpine	2%	od to qid
Carbachol	0.75%, 1.5%, 2.25%, 3%	Up to tid

   B. *Anticholinesterases*

Generic name	Concentration (%)	Normal dosage
Echothiophate iodide	0.03%, 0.06%, 0.125%, 0.25%	od to bd
Physostigmine	0.25%	od to tid
Demecarium	0.125%, 0.25%	bd

II. *Adrenergic agents*
   A. *Sympathomimetics*
      i. *Nonselective*

Generic name	Concentration (%)	Normal dosage
Epinephrine	0.25%, 0.5%, 1%, 2%	od to bd
Dipivefrin	0.1%	bd

      ii. *Selective (alpha 2 agonists)*

Generic name	Concentration (%)	Normal dosage
Brimonidine	0.2%	bd
Apraclonidine	1%	od

   B. *Beta-blockers*
      i. *Nonselective*

Generic name	Concentration (%)	Normal dosage
Timolol	0.5%	bd
Carteolol	1%, 2%	bd
Levobunolol	0.5%	od
Metipranolol	0.1%, 0.3%	bd

      ii. *Selective*

Generic name	Concentration (%)	Normal dosage
Betaxolol	0.5%	bd

      iii. *Prostaglandin analogs*

Generic name	Concentration (%)	Normal dosage
Latanoprost	0.005%	od
Travoprost	0.004%	od
Bimatoprost	0.03%	od
Tafluprost	0.0015%	od
Unoprostone	0.12%	od

iv. *Carbonic anhydrase inhibitors*
   a. *Topical*

Generic name	Concentration (%)	Normal dosage
Dorzolamide	2%	bd or tid
Brinzolamide	1%	bd or tid

   b. *Systemic*

Generic name	Concentration (%)	Normal dosage
Acetazolamide	250 mg	bd to qid (available as tablet, sustained-release capsule, and powder for injection)
Dichlorphenamide	50 mg	bd to tid
Methazolamide	50 mg	bd to tid

v. *Hyperosmotic agents*
   a. *Oral:*

Generic name	Concentration (%)	Normal dosage
Glycerol	50%	2 mL/kg body wt
Isosorbide	45%	2 mL/kg body wt

   b. *IV:*

Generic name	Concentration (%)	Normal dosage
Mannitol	20%	5 mL/kg body wt over 30–60 minutes
Urea	45%	

vi. *Neuroprotectors (Experimental)*
   a. NMDA (N-methyl-D-aspartate) receptor antagonists:
      1. Memantine
   b. Nitric oxide synthase inhibitors:
      1. Aminoguanidine
   c. Beta 2 adrenergic agonists:
      1. Brimonidine
   d. Calcium channel blocker:
      1. Nimodipine
   e. Neurotrophic factors:
      1. Neurotrophin-3
   f. Apoptosis inhibitors:
      1. Cytochrome C release inhibitors
      2. Caspase inhibitors
   g. Reactive oxygen species scavenger

NEWER OCULAR HYPOTENSIVE AGENTS (THE DOSAGES OF THESE DRUGS HAVE NOT BEEN GIVEN SINCE THEY ARE CURRENTLY EXPERIMENTAL IN NATURE)

I. *Natural products:*
   A. Cannabinoids
      i. Topical cannabinoid receptor type 1 (CB1) agonists
      ii. WIN 55,212-2
II. *Activators of extracellular matrix hydrolysis:*
   A. Matrix metalloproteinases
   B. Inducers of matrix metalloproteinases
      i. *tert*-butylhydroquinone
   C. Activator of glycosaminoglycan degradation compounds
      i. AL-3037A (sodium ferric ethylenediaminetetraacetate)
III. *Protein kinase inhibitors:*
   A. Broad-spectrum kinase inhibitors
      i. H-7
   B. Inhibitors of protein kinase C
      i. GF109203X
   C. Rho-associated coiled coil-forming kinase (ROCK) inhibitors
      i. Y-27632
      ii. H-1152
IV. *Cytoskeleton modulators:*
   A. Ethacrynic acid
   B. Latrunculin B
   C. Swinholide A
V. *Compounds that increase cyclic guanosine monophosphate (GMP):*
   A. Cyclic GMP analogs
   B. Nitric oxide donors
      i. Nitroglycerin
      ii. Isosorbide dinitrate
      iii. Sodium nitrite
      iv. Hydralazine
      v. Minoxidil
      vi. Sodium nitroprusside
   C. Natriuretic peptides
      i. Atrial natriuretic peptide (ANP)
      ii. Brain-derived natriuretic peptide (BNP)
      iii. C-type natriuretic peptide (CNP)
   D. Compounds that increase natriuretic peptides
      i. Candoxatril.

1.6 MICROBIOLOGY

CULTURE MEDIA

1. **Classify culture media.**
   Based on the nutrient requirements:
   i. Simple media
   ii. Complex media—added ingredients brings out some special features
   iii. Enriched media—egg or blood is added to basal media
   iv. Enrichment media (liquid media)—to selectively enhance the growth of certain bacteria in a mixed culture
   v. Selective media (solid media)—inhibiting substance is added which inhibits other bacteria and enhances growth of particular bacteria
   vi. Indicator media—changes color when there is a particular bacterial growth
   vii. Differential media—brings out differential characters in bacteria

   Based on oxygen requirement:
   i. Aerobic media
   ii. Anaerobic media

   Based on consistency:
   i. Solid media
   ii. Liquid media
   iii. Semi-solid media

2. **How are ocular specimens collected for analysis?**

Site	Method
Conjunctiva	Dry sterile swab is used
Corneal ulcer	Scraping the edge and the base of the ulcer with a Kimura spatula
Lacrimal sac	Specimen is collected in a sterile container and processed within half an hour
Anterior chamber (AC) tap, vitreous	Specimen collected using sterile syringe and immediately sent to laboratory
Orbital tissue	Specimen collected in a sterile container and immediately sent to laboratory

STAPHYLOCOCCUS AUREUS

1. **Describe the morphology of *Staphylococcus aureus*.**
   Staphylococcus aureus is a gram-positive, spherical, aerobic, nonmotile, noncapsulated, and nonsporing organism.

2. **What are the infections caused by *Staphylococci* in the eye?**
   i. Hordeolum internum
   ii. Hordeolum externum

iii. Chalazion
iv. Dacryocystitis
v. Bacterial keratitis
vi. Periorbital cellulitis
vii. Orbital cellulitis
viii. Endogenous endophthalmitis

3. **Why is *Staphylococcus* infection considered a major ocular hazard?**
Resistance to antibiotics [methicillin-resistant *Staphylococcus aureus* (MRSA)] and common disinfectants make them a potential ocular hazard, especially postsurgery.

4. **How will you diagnose *S. aureus* infection in a laboratory?**
   i. *Specimen:* Pus from suppurative lesion
      Swab from conjunctiva/cornea is smeared for the identification of the organism
   ii. *Methods:* Gram staining
      Coagulate test
      Culture and sensitivity

5. **What are the cultural characteristics?**
   i. Growth in a wide temperature range in solid and liquid media
   ii. Commonly used media are blood agar, nutrient agar, and MacConkey agar
   iii. On nutrient agar, colonies are large, circular, convex, smooth, shining, opaque, and easily emulsifiable
   iv. On MacConkey agar, they produce small, pink, lactose fermenting colonies

6. **What antibiotics are used in *S. aureus* infections?**
Antibiotic treatment has to be started according to cultures and sensitivity reports. Empirical treatment includes the use of penicillinase-resistant penicillin (such as methicillin), first-generation cephalosporin, etc.

Drug of choice for MRSA: Vancomycin

Drugs for vancomycin-resistant *Staphylococcus aureus* (VRSA): Daptomycin, linezolid, telavancin, quinupristin, dalfopristin

7. **What are the virulence factors and toxins of *S. aureus*?**
Virulence factors: Coagulase, protein A, lipase, hyaluronidase, nuclease
Toxins: α, β, γ, δ hemolysin, leucocidin, enterotoxin, toxic shock syndrome toxin (TSST), exfoliative toxin

STREPTOCOCCUS PNEUMONIAE (PNEUMOCOCCI)

1. **Describe the morphology and habitat of *Streptococcus pneumoniae*.**
They are gram-positive diplococci, arranged in pairs or short chains, aerobic, facultatively anaerobic, fastidious in growth requirement [growth enhanced by 5–10% (O_2)]. They are nonmotile and capsulated.

2. **What are the cultural characteristics?**
   On blood agar, they form small round colonies, surrounded by a zone of alpha hemolysis. The colony appearance is described as draftsman colonies. Capsulated strains produce mucoid colonies on blood agar.

3. **What are the ocular infections caused by *pneumococci*?**
   i. Dacryocystitis—acute and chronic
   ii. Corneal ulcer
   iii. Conjunctivitis
   iv. Endophthalmitis

4. **What are the laboratory diagnoses of *pneumococci*?**
   i. Gram staining
   ii. Quellung reaction
   iii. Culture on blood agar
   iv. Animal inoculation

5. **What is the treatment modality of pneumococcal infection?**
   Penicillin is the drug of choice. Other drugs include erythromycin, tetracycline, and chloramphenicol.

NEISSERIA SPECIES

1. **What are the *Neisseria* species of ocular importance?**
   i. *Neisseria gonorrhoeae*
   ii. *Neisseria meningitidis*

2. **Describe the morphology and cultural characteristics of *Neisseria*.**
   Gonococci—**kidney-shaped diplococci**
   Meningococci—diplococci with flat surfaces facing each other
   Cultural characteristics: Chocolate agar and 10% CO_2 enhance their growth, whereas toxins in medium inhibit their growth. In chocolate agar/modified Thayer Martin medium, they form 1-5 mm tiny, transparent, convex, glistening, mucoid colonies.

3. **What are the different types of ocular infections caused by *Neisseria* species?**
   Gonococci:
   i. Ophthalmia neonatorum
   ii. Conjunctivitis in adults
   Meningococci:
   i. Conjunctivitis
   ii. Ulcerative keratitis
   iii. Endophthalmitis

4. **How will you differentiate *N. gonorrhoeae* from *N. meningitidis*?**
   N. meningitidis gives positive reaction with maltose, whereas *N. gonorrhoeae* does not.

5. **What are the laboratory diagnoses of *Neisseria* infection?**
   - Gram staining
   - Culture in modified Thayer Martin medium
   - Serology: Enzyme-linked immunosorbent assay (ELISA), fluorescent immunoassay (FIA), immune blotting, latex agglutination

6. **What are the treatment modalities for *Neisseria* infections?**
   Meningococcus:
   - Penicillin
   - Chloramphenicol
   - Cephalosporines

   Gonococcus:
   - Tetracycline
   - Erythromycin
   - Cefoxitin

   Ophthalmic neonatorum:
   - 0.5% erythromycin ointment
   - 1% tetracycline

HAEMOPHILUS INFLUENZAE

1. **Describe the morphology and cultural characteristics of *Haemophilus influenzae*.**
   Morphology: It is a small, gram-negative, nonmotile, nonsporing organism exhibiting pleomorphism.

   Cultural characteristics: Mostly aerobic but can grow anaerobically as well. It requires factors V and X for its growth. When *S. aureus* is stretched across the blood agar plate inoculated with *Haemophilus influenzae*, the growth of *H. influenzae* will be large and well developed near *S. aureus* colonies than those further away from it. This phenomenon is called satellitism, which shows that *H. influenzae* is dependent on factor V for its growth, which is provided by *S. aureus*.

   Other culture media: Fildes agar, Levinthal medium.

2. **What are the diseases caused by *H. influenzae*?**
   Ocular:
   i. Keratitis
   ii. Periorbital cellulitis
   iii. Orbital cellulitis
   iv. Endophthalmitis

Systemic:
  i. Meningitis
  ii. Laryngoepiglottitis
  iii. Conjunctivitis
  iv. Pericarditis
  v. Pneumonia
  vi. Arthritis
  vii. Endocarditis
  viii. Otitis media
  ix. Sinusitis
  x. Bronchitis keratitis, endophthalmitis, orbital and periorbital cellulitis

3. **Is there any other importance regarding *H. influenzae* related to the eye?**
   Yes, it can penetrate the intact cornea.

PSEUDOMONAS AERUGINOSA

1. **Describe the morphology and cultural characteristics of *Pseudomonas aeruginosa*.**
   Gram-negative rod, motile, noncapsulated but many strains have mucoid layer; nonsporing obligate aerobe, can grow anaerobically if nitrate is available. In ordinary media, colonies are large, opaque, and irregular with distinctive, musty odor.

2. **What do you know about the resistance of *P. aeruginosa*?**
   The bacillus is heat resistant and resistant to common antiseptics and disinfectants such as chloroxylenol and hexachlorophene. It is sensitive to acids, glutaraldehyde, silver salts, and strong phenolic disinfectants.

3. **What are the antibiotics effective against *P. aeruginosa*?**
   i. Penicillins—piperacillin, ticarcillin, azlocillin
   ii. Fluoroquinolone—ciprofloxacin, ofloxacin
   iii. Aminoglycosides—gentamicin, amikacin
   iv. Third-, fourth-, fifth-generation cephalosporins
   v. Newer drugs—imipenem and aztreonam

4. **How will you diagnose *P. aeruginosa* in a laboratory?**
   P. aeruginosa grows in most of the media such as MacConkey agar and blood agar. The oxidase reaction is positive in case of mixed infections. Isolation can be done using cetrimide agar on which only *P. aeruginosa* can grow. They produce a characteristic greenish-blue color due to the presence of pyocyanin, pyoverdine, and pyorubin pigments.

NOCARDIA SPECIES

1. **What are the characteristic features of *Nocardia* species?**
   Nocardia are weakly gram-positive, acid-fast, catalase positive, rod-shaped bacteria with beaded branching filaments.

2. **What are the cultural characteristics of *Nocardia*?**
   Colonies have a varied appearance, and most species have aerial hyphae. They are strictly aerobic and can grow slowly on nonselective culture media over a wide temperature range.

3. **Describe the virulence of the organism.**
   They have low virulence but can cause serious opportunistic infections in immunocompromised individuals. The virulence factors are enzymes catalase, superoxide dismutase, and cord factor.

4. **What is its ocular importance?**
   It is the most common acid-fast organism causing bacterial keratitis in India.

5. **Describe the laboratory diagnosis of *Nocardia* keratitis.**
   Specimen: Corneal scraping from the edge and base of the ulcer (without touching the ocular adnexa). Isolation is done using buffered charcoal yeast extract (BCYE) medium. Serological and cutaneous testing is not available.

6. **Discuss drug sensitivity.**
   Amikacin remains the treatment of choice. Other drugs include aminoglycosides, sulfonamide, minocycline, imipenem, linezolid, etc.

7. **What infections can it cause in the eye?**
   i. Keratitis
   ii. Scleritis, sclera abscess
   iii. Dacryocystitis
   iv. Endophthalmitis
   v. Subretinal abscess

CORYNEBACTERIUM DIPHTHERIAE

1. **Describe the morphology and characteristics of *Corynebacterium diphtheriae***
   Morphology and characteristics of *C. diphtheriae* are as follows:
   i. Gram-positive, nonmotile, nonsporing, noncapsulated
   ii. Slender rods with clubbing at one or both ends
   iii. Show pleomorphism
   iv. They contain volutin or Babes–Ernst granules
   v. Cells are arranged as pairs in groups. The arrangement is called Chinese letter pattern on calciferous arrangement

2. What are the cultural characteristics of various media?

Media	Characteristics
Loeffler's serum slope	Small, grayish-white, opaque colonies
Blood agar	Small, grayish-white, opaque, nonhemolytic colonies
Potassium tellurite (selective media)	Black-colored colonies

3. What are the ocular infections caused by *C. diphtheriae*?
   i. Membranous conjunctivitis
   ii. Extraocular muscle palsy
   iii. Ciliary muscle palsy leading to paralysis of accommodation

4. Describe prophylactic measure.
   i. Active, passive, and combined immunization is available
   ii. Active immunization consists of giving diphtheria toxoid along with tetanus toxoid and pertussis vaccine at 6, 10, and 14 weeks of life and booster doses at 1.5 years and 4–6 years

5. How will you treat membranous conjunctivitis?
   i. Any case of membranous conjunctivitis should be treated as diphtheria until proven otherwise
   ii. Treatment includes
      - Antitoxic therapy +
      - Antibiotic therapy
   iii. Antitoxin
      - Moderate cases: 20,000 units diphtheria toxin intramuscular (IM)
      - Severe cases: 50,000–100,000 units—half IM, half intravenous (IV) dose
      - Antiserum instillation into the eye
      Antibiotics include penicillin and erythromycin to be given both topically and systemically

MYCOBACTERIUM TUBERCULOSIS

1. Describe the morphology of *Mycobacterium tuberculosis*.
Mycobacterium tuberculosis is straight or slightly curved rods, occurring singly or in pairs or small clumps. They are acid-fast, nonmotile, nonsporing, noncapsulated, aerobic bacteria.

2. Describe the cultural characteristics of *M. tuberculosis*.
Colonies take 2 weeks to appear. The solid medium most commonly used is Lowenstein-Jensen medium. *M. tuberculosis* forms dry, rough, raised, irregular creamy white colonies with wrinkled surface which are not easily emulsifiable. In liquid media (Middlebrook medium), growth begins at the bottom and creeps to the sides, forming surface pellicle.

3. **What are the ocular manifestations of the infection?**
    i. Tuberculous ulcer of lid margin
    ii. Tuberculous nodule of the lid
    iii. Primary tuberculosis (Tb) of conjunctiva
    iv. Tuberculous dacryocystitis
    v. Phlyctenular keratoconjunctivitis
    vi. Salzmann nodular degeneration
    vii. Interstitial keratitis
    viii. Scleritis
    ix. Granulomatous uveitis
    x. Tuberculous choroiditis
    xi. Eales' disease
    xii. Tb of orbital bone

4. **Describe laboratory diagnosis of Tb.**
    i. Acid-fast staining
    ii. Culture
    iii. Polymerase chain reaction (PCR)-based ELISA
    iv. Western blot
    v. Animal inoculation
    vi. Cell culture
    vii. BACTEC
    viii. Mantoux test

5. **Describe the treatment of Tb.**
    Antituberculosis treatment (ATT) is the treatment of choice consisting of isoniazid, rifampicin, ethambutol, streptomycin, and pyrazinamide. The duration of treatment depends on the primary site of infection as well as the sensitivity of organisms to these first-line drugs.

MYCOBACTERIUM LEPRAE

1. **What are the ocular manifestations of leprosy?**
    i. Thickened eyelids
    ii. Facial nerve palsy
    iii. Conjunctivitis
    iv. Interstitial keratitis
    v. Corneal ulcer/scarring
    vi. Iritis, scleritis, or episcleritis
    vii. Chronic granulomatous uveitis

CHLAMYDIA TRACHOMATIS

1. **What are the characteristic features of *Chlamydia* species?**
    Chlamydia are obligate intracellular gram-negative bacteria. Three species of medical importance are:

i. *Chlamydia trachomatis*
ii. *Chlamydia psittaci*
iii. *Chlamydia pneumoniae*

2. **What are the diagnostic tests for *Chlamydia*?**
   Demonstration of inclusion bodies (Halberstädter-Prowazek bodies) in conjunctival smears using Giemsa stain and direct immunofluorescence.
   i. *Cytology:* Mixed neutrophilic mononuclear infiltrate is characteristic
   ii. *Isolation:* Using conjunctival scrapings, M-coy cells treated with cycloheximide HeLa cell lines
   iii. *Serology:* Complement fixation test, microimmunofluorescent antibody test
   iv. ELISA
   v. Deoxyribonucleic acid (DNA) PCR

3. **How will you treat chlamydial infection?**
   Chlamydial infection can be treated by chemotherapy using tetracycline (in adults) and erythromycin (in children).

ADENOVIRUS

1. **Describe the morphology of adenovirus.**
   Adenovirus has a space vehicle appearance. The capsid consists of capsomeres arranged in an icosahedral pattern.

2. **Discuss adenoviruses of ocular importance.**
   Epidemic pharyngoconjunctival fever—types 3, 4, 7, 14, 21
   Follicular conjunctivitis—types 1, 2, 3, 5, 6, 7
   Epidemic keratoconjunctivitis—types 8, 19, 37

3. **Describe the laboratory diagnosis of adenovirus.**
   i. Electron microscopy
   ii. Viral isolation using primary human embryonic kidney cells, human epithelial cells, and MRC-5 cells
   iii. Serology—complement fixation test—ELISA
   iv. DNA PCR

HERPES SIMPLEX VIRUS

1. **What are the ophthalmic infections caused by herpes simplex virus (HSV)?**
   i. HSV keratitis
   ii. Acute keratoconjunctivitis
   iii. Follicular conjunctivitis
   iv. Chorioretinitis
   v. Acute necrotizing retinitis

2. **Explain the laboratory diagnosis of HSV.**
    i. Microscopy—Tzanck smear
    ii. Antigen detection—fluorescent antibody technique
    iii. DNA PCR
    iv. Viral isolation—human diploid fibroblast
    v. Serology—ELISA, neutralization test, complement fixation tests

3. **What is Tzanck smear?**
   Swab/smears are stained with 1% aqueous toluidine blue "O" for 15 seconds. A positive smear shows multinucleated giant cells with faceted nuclei and homogeneously stained "ground glass" chromatin.

4. **What are the drugs active against HSV keratitis?**
    i. Acyclovir
    ii. Idoxuridine
    iii. Foscarnet

RUBELLA

1. **What are the clinical manifestations of congenital rubella syndrome (CRS)?**
   The triad of CRS consists of:
    i. Congenital heart disease
    ii. Cataract
    iii. Deafness
   Apart from the above, other features may include
   - Ocular:
     - Glaucoma
     - Chorioretinitis
   - Systemic:
     - Hepatosplenomegaly
     - Thrombocytopenia
     - Mental retardation
     - Myocarditis
     - Osteitis

CYTOMEGALOVIRUS

1. **What are the ocular involvement of congenital *Cytomegalovirus* (CMV) infection?**
    i. Cataract
    ii. Glaucoma
    iii. Chorioretinitis
    iv. Microphthalmia

2. How will you differentiate chorioretinitis of CMV from toxoplasmosis?

CMV retinitis	Congenital toxoplasmosis
Multiple foci of involvement	Solitary lesion
Involves periphery mostly	Involves posterior pole
Less destructive chorioretinal lesion	More destructive lesion

3. **What are the features of acquired CMV in the eye?**
    i. Retinal detachment (mostly bilateral)
    ii. Optic atrophy
    iii. Chorioretinitis

HUMAN IMMUNODEFICIENCY VIRUS/ACQUIRED IMMUNODEFICIENCY SYNDROME

1. **What are the ocular manifestations of acquired immunodeficiency syndrome (AIDS)?**

    Anterior segment:
    i. Kaposi sarcoma
    ii. Herpes zoster ophthalmicus
    iii. Herpes simplex keratitis
    iv. Fungal keratitis
    v. Uveitis

    Posterior segment:
    i. Manifestations due to human immunodeficiency virus (HIV) infection itself—HIV retinopathy
    ii. Anterior ischemic optic neuropathy (AION)
    iii. Optic atrophy
    iv. Manifestations due to opportunistic infections such as:
    - CMV retinitis
    - *Toxoplasma* retinochoroiditis
    - *Cryptococcus* chorioretinitis
    - Pneumocystis choroiditis
    - *Candida* endophthalmitis
    - Acute retinal necrosis

2. **What are the features of HIV retinopathy?**
    i. Noninfectious microvascular disorder
    ii. Features include cotton wool spots, microaneurysms, retinal hemorrhages, vascular telangiectasias, and areas of capillary nonperfusion

iii. The most common manifestation is the microvascular changes, whereas the earliest and most consistent finding is the cotton wool spots

iv. Retinal artery and vein occlusion occur rarely. Thus, a case of unexplained retinal artery on vein occlusions should be screened for HIV

CANDIDA ALBICANS

1. **Describe the morphology of *Candida albicans* and its habitat.**
   C. albicans is a yeast, round or ovoid, producing pseudomycelia. It is a normal commensal of oral cavity, lower gastrointestinal tract, and female genital tract. It causes opportunistic infections in human beings.

2. **Describe the diagnosis of candida infection.**
   i. Microscopy: Wet films
   ii. Gram staining
   iii. Culture: Sabouraud dextrose agar (SDA)—colonies are creamy white, smooth, with a yeasty odor
   iv. Corn meal agar forms chlamydospores

3. **What is Reynolds–Braude phenomenon?**
   Reynolds–Braude phenomenon is a rapid method of identifying *C. albicans*. When incubated in human serum at 37°C, *C. albicans* forms germ tubes within 2 hours.

4. **What is the treatment of *Candida* infection?**
   Since *Candida* mostly causes opportunistic infections, eliminating or reducing the predisposing risk factor is important. For local infections, topical nystatin eye drops 5% is used titrating according to response. For systemic infection, amphotericin B and 5 F-U clotrimazole can be used.

5. **What are the ocular manifestations of *Candida*?**
   i. Lid candidiasis
   ii. Pseudomembranous conjunctivitis
   iii. Keratitis
   iv. Endophthalmitis

ASPERGILLUS FUMIGATUS

1. **Discuss the morphology and habitat of *Aspergillus fumigatus*.**
   A. fumigatus is a saprotroph found in soil and decaying organic matter. The fungal colonies produce conidiophore from which minute conidia are disseminated. The spores are found ubiquitously.

2. **Describe the pathogenesis of keratitis by *A. fumigatus*.**

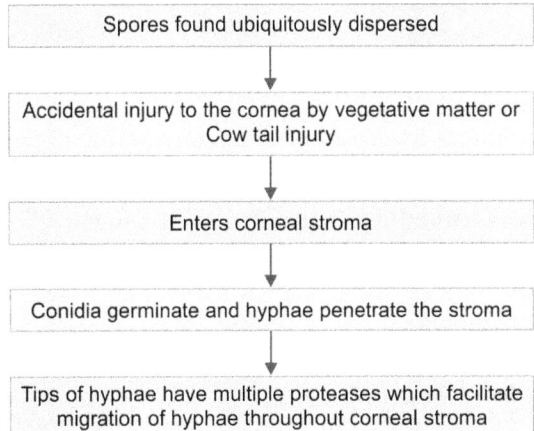

3. **What are the ocular manifestations of *Aspergillus* infection?**
    i. Keratitis
    ii. Endophthalmitis

4. **How will you diagnose *Aspergillus*?**
    i. By the clinical appearance of a fungal corneal ulcer
    ii. Direct examination of fungal hyphae in freshly prepared 10% potassium hydroxide (KOH) mount, periodic acid-Schiff, methenamine silver
    iii. Culturing in Sabouraud's dextrose agar, potato dextrose agar—culture mount with lactophenol cotton blue reveals septate hyphae, conidiophores, and sterigmata bearing conidial chains

FUSARIUM SPECIES

1. **What are the risk factors for *Fusarium* infection?**
    People engaged in agricultural work are more prone to having an infection with *Fusarium* species. Microtrauma to the corneal epithelium leads to the direct implantation of fungal spores into the corneal stroma.

2. **What are the toxins produced by *Fusarium*?**
    i. Moniliformins
    ii. Fusarins
    iii. Fumonisins

TOXOCARA CANIS

1. **What are the definitive and intermediate hosts?**
    i. *Definite host:* Dog
    ii. *Intermediate host:* Man

2. **What are the ocular lesions caused by *Toxocara canis*?**
   i. Diffuse chorioretinitis
   ii. Vitreous abscess
   iii. Peripheral retina and vitreous involvement with vitreous membrane formation
   iv. Posterior pole involvement with preretinal membrane formation
   v. Chronic endophthalmitis

3. **Describe the laboratory diagnosis and treatment.**
   i. Eosinophilia in peripheral smear
   ii. ELISA
   iii. Histopathology
   iv. ELISA
   v. Western blot
   vi. PCR
   vii. Animal inoculation
   Treatment: Thiabendazole and diethylcarbamazine are effective.

TOXOPLASMA GONDII

1. **What are the definitive and intermediate hosts?**
   i. *Definitive host:* Cat (enteric cycle takes place)
   ii. *Intermediate host:* Man (extraintestinal or tissue phase)

2. **What is the mode of transmission of infection?**
   i. Consumption or handling of infected meat
   ii. Contact with carcasses
   iii. Vertical transmission from mother to fetus

3. **What are the ocular lesions of *Toxoplasma gondii*?**
   i. Retinochoroiditis
   ii. Retinal vasculitis
   iii. Retinal iridocyclitis
   iv. Vitritis

4. **Describe the laboratory diagnosis of toxoplasmosis.**
   i. Sabin–Feldman dye test
   ii. Complement fixation test
   iii. Rapid agglutination test
   iv. Indirect hemagglutination test
   v. Indirect immunofluorescence test

5. **What is the basic pathology behind *Toxoplasma* lesions?**
   Hypersensitivity and autoimmune reactions are the basis.

6. **What are the treatment options for toxoplasmosis?**
   i. Sulfamethoxazole + pyrimethamine combination
   ii. Clindamycin

iii. Clarithromycin
iv. Spiramycin (pregnancy)

MICROSPORIDIA

1. **Describe the morphology and habitat of microsporidia.**
   Microsporidia are ubiquitous, intracellular, spore-forming protozoans. The spores are double layered with a thick cell wall. They enclose two nuclei, a polaroplast, a vacuole, and a coiled polar tubule. This coiled polar tubule is the characteristic feature.

2. **What are the ocular diseases caused by microsporidia?**
   i. Stromal keratitis
   ii. Keratoconjunctivitis
   iii. Corneal punctate epithelial keratopathy

3. **What are the methods to diagnose microsporidia in the laboratory?**
   i. Electron microscopy
   ii. Direct microscopy using Gram stain

4. **How will you treat microsporidia keratitis?**
   Antifungals such as fluconazole or voriconazole can be used. Instillation of 0.1% propamidine isethionate has been recommended.

PYTHIUM INSIDIOSUM

1. **Describe the morphology and habitat of *Pythium insidiosum*.**
   Class: Oomycota
   Genus: *Pythium*
   Species: *Pythium insidiosum*
   i. It is mainly found in stagnant freshwater
   ii. It is a pathogen of mammals causing pythiosis

2. **Describe pythiosis in humans.**
   Four forms of the disease are recognized:
   i. Subcutaneous
   ii. Disseminated
   iii. Ocular
   iv. Vascular

3. **What is ocular pythiosis?**
   i. Ocular pythiosis is the only form to infect an otherwise healthy human
   ii. Predisposing factors include contact lens use while swimming in infected fresh water
   iii. It can cause keratitis and periorbital cellulitis
   iv. Prognosis is poor, and the majority of cases may require corneal transplantation or enucleation.

1.7 GENERAL PATHOLOGY

GENERAL DEFINITIONS

Hypertrophy

Hypertrophy is the increase in the size of individual cells, fibers, or tissues without an increase in the number of individual elements.

Hyperplasia

Hyperplasia is the increase in the number of individual cells in tissue. This growth eventually reaches an equilibrium and is never indefinitely progressive.

Aplasia

Aplasia is the lack of development of tissue during embryonic life (e.g., aplasia of optic nerve).

Hypoplasia

Hypoplasia is the arrested development of tissue during embryonic life (e.g., aniridia).

Metaplasia

Metaplasia is the transformation of one type of adult tissue into another type.

Dysplasia

Dysplasia is an abnormal growth of tissue during embryonic life.

Atrophy

Atrophy is the diminution of size, shrinking of cells, fibers, or tissues that previously had reached their full development.

Neoplasia

Neoplasia is a continuous increase in the number of cells in tissue caused by unregulated proliferation and, in some cases, failure of mechanisms that lead to cell death.

1. What are the common fixatives used in ophthalmic pathology?

Fixative	Use
10% neutral buffered formalin (NBF)	Routine fixation of all tissues (e.g., eyelid, conjunctiva, globe, orbit)
Bouin solution	Small biopsies (e.g., conjunctiva)

Contd...

Contd...

Fixative	Use
Absolute ethanol or methanol	Crystals (e.g., corneal urate crystals)
Cytology fixative (ethanol, methanol)	Liquid specimen or smears (e.g., vitreous, aqueous, fine needle aspirates, corneal smears)
Glutaraldehyde	Electron microscopy (corneal microsporidia)
Michael or Zeus transport medium	Immunofluorescence (e.g., conjunctival biopsy for mucous membrane pemphigoid)
Rosewell Park Memorial Institute (RPMI) house culture medium	Tissue culture (e.g., orbital humor for cytogenetics or flow cytometry)

2. **What are the stains commonly used in ophthalmic pathology?**

Stain	Material stained	Example of use
Hematoxylin–eosin	• Nucleus—blue • Cytoplasm—red	General tissue stain
Periodic acid–Schiff (PAS)	Glycogen and proteoglycans	Descemet's membrane, lens capsule, goblet cells
Alcian blue	Acid mucopolysaccharide	Cavernous optic atrophy
Alizarin red	Calcium	Band keratopathy
Colloidal iron	Acid mucopolysaccharide	Macular dystrophy
Congo red	Amyloid	Lattice corneal dystrophy
Masson's trichrome	Collagen/hyaline	Granular corneal dystrophy
Perls' Prussian blue	Iron	Fleisher ring
Oil red O	Fat	
von Kossa	Calcium phosphate salts	Band keratopathy
Giemsa	Some bacteria and parasites	*Chlamydia* and *Acanthamoeba*
Grams stain	Bacteria	Bacterial infection
Gomori or Gorcott Methenamine silver stain	Fungal elements	*Fusarium*
Ziehl–Neelsen	Acid-fast organisms	*Mycobacterium tuberculosis*

■ SQUAMOUS CELL CARCINOMA

1. **What are the sites involved?**
    i. Conjunctiva (most common)
    ii. Eyelids
    iii. Lacrimal sac

2. **What are the predisposing factors?**
    i. Fair-skinned individuals
    ii. Ultraviolet (UV) light exposure
    iii. HPV 16 infection
3. **What are the types of squamous cell carcinoma (SCC)?**
    i. SCC in situ
    ii. Invasive SCC
4. **What are the clinical types of SCC of eyelid?**
    i. Nodular SCC—hyperkeratotic nodule with crusting and erosion
    ii. Ulcerating SCC—ulcer with a red base and sharply defined indurated and everted border
    iii. Cutaneous horn
5. **What is the histopathology of SCC?**
    Histology shows atypical squamous cells (with prominent nuclei and abundant eosinophilic cytoplasm) that form nests and strands that extend beyond the basement membrane into the dermis and incite a fibrotic tissue reaction. Well-differentiated tumors show characteristic keratin pearls and intercellular bridges (desmosomes).
6. **What is the treatment for SCC?**
    i. Treatment of SCC is with surgical excision with adequate tumor clearance
    ii. Frozen section can be done
    iii. Mohs micrographic surgery—involves layered excision of the tumor
7. **What are the variants of SCC?**
    i. Bowen's disease—indolent solitary (or multiple) erythematous sharply demarcated patches
    ii. Adenoacanthoma—a rare pseudoglandular form of SCC

BASAL CELL CARCINOMA

1. **Which is the most common malignant tumor of eyelids?**
    Basal cell carcinoma (BCC)
2. **What are the sites of involvement in order of decreasing frequency?**
    Lower lid > medial canthus > upper lid > lateral canthus
3. **What are the predisposing factors?**
    i. Sunlight
    ii. Genetic factors
    iii. Fair-skinned individuals

4. **What are the clinical types of BCC?**
    i. Nodular BCC—most common
        - Slowly growing, slightly elevated pearly nodule with overlying dilated blood vessels
    ii. Noduloulcerative—centrally ulcerated with pearly raised rolled edges and dilated telangiectatic vessels over lateral margin
    iii. Sclerosing/morpheic—flat or slightly depressed pale yellow indurated plaque
        - This is infiltrative, and the extent is difficult to determine clinically

5. **What is the histopathology of BCC?**
    i. BCC originates from the stratum basale of the epidermis and the outer root sheath of the hair follicle
    ii. Tumor cells have relatively bland monomorphous nuclei and high N:C ratio
    iii. BCC forms cohesive bands with nuclear palisading of peripheral layer.
    iv. In morphea variant, thin cords and strands of tumor cells are seen in fibrotic stroma

6. **What is the treatment of BCC?**
    i. Treatment is complete excision with surgical margin control
    ii. Margin control is achieved with frozen sections or Mohs micrographic surgery

7. **What is Gorlin syndrome/basal cell nevus syndrome?**
    i. Autosomal dominant inheritance
    ii. Defect in tumor suppress gene *PATCHED* in chromosome 9q
    iii. Consists of multiple BCC of skin, odontogenic cyst of jaw, bifid rib, and vertebral anomalies and keratinizing pits on palms and soles

MALIGNANT MELANOMA

1. **What are the common sites of involvement?**
    i. Eyelids
    ii. Conjunctiva
    iii. Uveal tract

2. **What is the common age group affected by choroidal melanoma?**
    i. Median age group is 55 years
    ii. Males > females

3. **What is the most common primary intraocular malignancy in adults?**
Ciliary body and choroidal melanoma

4. **What are the predisposing conditions for uveal melanoma?**
   i. Fair skin
   ii. Lighter iris color
   iii. Numerous atypical cutaneous nevi
   iv. Iris and choroidal nevi
   v. Nevus of Ota
   vi. Uveal melanocytoma

5. **How does choroidal melanoma appear clinically?**
   i. Choroidal melanoma appears as a subretinal gray-brown dome-shaped lesion
   ii. As it grows, it breaks through Bruch's membrane, acquiring a mushroom or collar button shape
   iii. Less commonly, a diffuse pattern is also seen

6. **What are the histologic types of choroidal and ciliary body melanoma?**
   i. Spindle cells—tightly arranged fusiform cells with indistinct cell membranes and slender or plump oval nucleus
      - Consists of a mix of spindle A and spindle B cells arranged in bundles
      - Better prognosis

      Epithelioid melanoma—large pleomorphic cells with distinct cell membranes, large vesicular nuclei with prominent nucleoli and abundant cytoplasm
      - Cells lack cohesiveness and have worst prognosis
         a. Mixed cell type

7. **What is ring melanoma?**
   Ring melanoma is the diffuse variant of melanoma in ciliary body in which the tumor extends for the entire circumference of the ciliary body.

8. **What are the important histologic variables associated with survival?**
   i. Size of tumor in contact with sclera
   ii. Tumor cell type
   iii. Extraocular extension
   iv. Ciliary body involvement

9. **What is the most common site of metastasis?**
   Liver

10. **What are the genetic predispositions for uveal melanoma?**
    i. Mutations in *GNAQ* and *GNA11*
    ii. Monosomy of chromosome 3
    iii. Trisomy of chromosome 8

11. **What are the treatment options available for choroidal melanoma?**
    i. Brachytherapy—for tumors <20 mm in basal diameter and up to 10 mm thick

ii. External beam radiotherapy—for posterior tumors
iii. Transpupillary thermotherapy (TTT)—for treating small tumors when radiotherapy is inappropriate
iv. Enucleation—in case of large tumors, optic disk invasion, extensive involvement of ciliary body or angle, and irreversible loss of useful vision

RHABDOMYOSARCOMA

1. **What is the most common primary malignant orbital tumor in children?**
   Rhabdomyosarcoma

2. **What is the most common age group affected?**
   7–8 years

3. **What are the clinical features?**
   i. Sudden-onset proptosis
   ii. Reddish discoloration of eyelid
   iii. Grape-like submucosal cluster in conjunctiva (Botryoid variant)

4. **What are the histologic types?**
   Rhabdomyosarcomas arise from primitive mesenchymal cells that differentiate toward skeletal muscle.

   Histological types are:
   i. Embryonal (most common)
      - Spindle cells are arranged in loose syncytium with occasional cells bearing cross striation, usually showing frequent mitotic figures
      - Electron microscopy—typical sarcomeric banding pattern is seen
   ii. Differentiated (least common)
      - Best prognosis
      - Feature numerous cells with striking cross striation
   iii. Alveolar
      - Worst prognosis
      - Tumor has a distinct alveolar pattern

4. **What is the role of immunohistochemistry in rhabdomyosarcoma?**
   Immunohistochemistry is positive for desmin, vimentin, muscle-specific actin, and myogenin.

5. **What is the treatment for rhabdomyosarcoma?**
   i. Commonly used guidelines well produced by the Intergroup Rhabdomyosarcoma Study Group
   ii. Treatment comprises a combination of radiotherapy, chemotherapy, and surgical debulking.

1.8 SLIT-LAMP BIOMICROSCOPE

1. **Who discovered the slit lamp?**
   On August 3, 1911, Alvar Gullstrand presented the first rudimentary model of slit lamp and explained its optics and refraction.

2. **Who coined the term slit-lamp biomicroscopy? Why is it called so?**
   The term biomicroscopy was coined by Mawas in 1925. The instrument is called a slit-lamp biomicroscope as it identifies the following basic components:
   Slit lamp—focal narrow beam of light
   Microscope—for stereoscopic magnified observation
   Biomicroscopy—as it is helpful in examination of living eye

3. **List the various steps for carrying out the slit-lamp examination.**
   i. Examination should be carried out in a semi-dark room so that the examiner's eyes are partially dark adapted
   ii. Both the patient and the examiner must be seated in comfortable adjustable chairs
   iii. Slit-lamp table must be stable and flat so that the slit lamp does not slide during the examination and the table should be mounted on a swinging arm or rolling table so that it is adjustable in height
   iv. Adjust the patient's chair high enough so that the patient naturally leans forward with the chin and forehead pressed firmly against the chinrest and headrest without stretching
   v. With the patient's forehead and chin firmly in place, the height of the chinrest can be raised or lowered by means of a nearby knob. In this way, the patient's eye is brought level with the black demarcation line on one of the supporting rods of the patient positioning frame, just below the level of forehead strap
   vi. Adjust the settings on the slit lamp so that the patient is not initially subjected to uncomfortably bright light when the instrument is turned on. This can be accomplished by setting the instrument to provide a very narrow beam of light or by diminishing the light source if it is to provide diffuse illumination
   vii. Oculars of the slit lamp are to be adjusted for the examiner's interpupillary distance

4. **What are the basic principles of slit-lamp illumination?**
   There are three specific principles of slit-lamp illumination:
   i. Focal illumination
   ii. Oblique illumination
   iii. Optical section

5. **Describe the principles.**
    i. Focal illumination—achieved by narrowing the slit beam horizontally or vertically. It permits isolation of specific areas of cornea for observation without extraneous light outside area of examination
    ii. Oblique illumination—light beam is projected from an oblique angle. It is useful for detecting and examining findings in different layers of the cornea
    iii. Optical section—this is the most important and unique feature of slit lamp achieved by making a narrow slit beam. Uses include determining depth or elevation of a defect in cornea, conjunctiva, or locating the depth of opacity within the lens, etc.

6. **What are the types of illumination used for examination?**
    The different illumination in the sequence in which they are used are:
    i. Diffuse illumination
    ii. Sclerotic scatter
    iii. Direct focal illumination
    iv. Broad tangential illumination
    v. Proximal (indirect) illumination
    vi. Retroillumination from the iris
        - Direct
        - Indirect
    vii. Retroillumination from the fundus
    viii. Specular reflection

7. **What is meant by diffuse illumination?**
    Diffuse illumination—also known as wide beam illumination
    i. Principle—a wide unnarrowed beam of light is directed at the cornea from an angle of approximately 15–45°
    ii. Settings—microscope is positioned directly in front of the eye and focused on the anterior surface of the cornea
        - Magnification used is low to medium
        - Illumination is kept at medium to high
    iii. Uses
        - Gross inspection of any corneal scar, irregularities of lid, tear debris, etc.—mainly for obtaining an overview of ocular surface tissues (e.g., bulbar and palpebral conjunctiva)
        - It can be used with cobalt blue or red free filters

        Cobalt blue—introduction of cobalt blue filter without fluorescein will cause corneal iron rings to appear black so it is useful in detecting subtle Fleischer ring in early keratoconus. The cobalt blue filter produces blue light in which the fluorescent dye fluoresces with yellow-green color used for evaluating fluorescein staining of ocular surface tissues or the tear film or during Goldmann applanation tonometry

Red-free filter—produces light-green light for evaluation of rose bengal staining. It is also used to evaluate nerve fiber layer

8. What is sclerotic scatter?
  i. Principle—the optical principle is based on fiber optics—the total internal reflection of light
     - The slit beam is directed at the limbus. The opaque sclera scatters the light and some of the light is directed into the stroma where it travels through the entire cornea by repeatedly reflecting from its anterior and posterior surfaces
     - In normal cornea—it creates a glowing limbal halo but no stromal opacity is visible
     - When opacity is present—the internally reflected light is scattered back to the observer outlining the pattern as in Reis-Bucklers dystrophy
  ii. Settings—slit lamp is about 15° from the microscope. Slit beam is decentered if full view of cornea is desired. Slit height is set at full and slit width at medium broad

9. What is direct focal illumination?
Direct focal illumination is of two types:
  i. *Direct focal illumination with broad beam:*
     - Principle—slit-lamp light is focused directly on an area of interest. The wider the slit beam, the less the information presented to the examiner
     - Settings—slit beam is approximately 30° from microscope
       Slit height is full and slit width is medium broad
     - Uses—crumb-like deposits of granular stromal corneal dystrophy, stand out in direct focal illumination as they are white, reflect light, have sharp margins, and are embedded in clear cornea
  ii. *Direct focal slit illumination with a narrow beam:*
     - Principle—slit lamp is placed obliquely and the slit beam is narrowed. The focused slit creates an optical cross-section of the cornea, allowing the examiner to localize the level of opacities within the cornea and to determine corneal thickness
     - Settings—slit lamp is positioned 30-45° from microscope
       Slit height is full and slit width is narrow
     - Movement—moving the narrow slit systematically across the cornea allows to view serial optical sections and to construct a mental picture of corneal pathology
     - Uses—moderately thin slit is used to identify the pigmentation of Krukenberg's spindle on the posterior surface of cornea

The narrow slit beam localizes
- The net-like opacity in Reis-Buckler's dystrophy to subepithelial area
- Extreme thinning in area of descemetocele in cases of herpes simplex keratitis
- Focal central thinning of cornea in cases of postkeratitis scarring, and keratoconus

10. **What is broad tangential illumination?**
    i. Principle—the examiner focuses the microscope on an area of interest and swings the slit beam far to the side at an extremely oblique angle so that the light sweeps tangentially across the surface of cornea. This enhances surface details by shadowing
    ii. Settings—slit beam is 60-90° from microscope
    Slit height is narrow to one half and slit width is very broad
    iii. Uses:
    - Highlights irregularities on the anterior corneal surface
        a. Corneal intraepithelial neoplasia
        b. Sterile stromal ulcers
        c. Calcific band keratopathy with holes
        d. Diffuse punctate epithelial keratopathy
    - Highlights irregularities on posterior corneal surface, e.g., folds in Descemet's membrane

11. **What is proximal (indirect) illumination?**
    Proximal (indirect) illumination combines features of both sclerotic scatter and retroillumination:
    i. Principle—a moderately wide slit beam is decentered and placed adjacent to an area of interest. Light travels through corneal stroma by internal reflection as it does in sclerotic scatter and accentuates the pattern of opacity
    ii. Settings—slit lamp is about 15° from microscope. Slit height is full and slit width is moderate
    iii. Uses—highlights the internal structures of corneal opacity
    Enables the identification of details within the opacity, e.g., small foreign body within an area of corneal inflammation
    Also useful for observing iris sphincter

12. **What is retroillumination of iris? Give its uses.**
    Retroillumination of the iris can be of two types:
    i. *Direct retroillumination of the iris:*
    - Principle—the slit beam reflects from the surface of the iris and illuminates the cornea from behind and accentuates the refractive properties of corneal pathology

It allows detection of abnormalities not apparent in direct illumination. For example, epithelial basement membrane fingerprint lines
- Settings—slit lamp is separated by 15-30° from microscope
Slit height is reduced and slit width is medium.
ii. *Indirect retroillumination of the iris:*
- Principle—the slit beam is decentered so that it hits the iris near the pupil adjacent to the area of interest in the cornea
Microscope is adjusted so that the area of interest is viewed at the edge of the path of light reflected from iris (marginal retroillumination) or against the adjacent black pupil (indirect retroillumination)
- Settings—the beam can be decentered to allow viewing of object of interest over dark edge of pupil
Slit height is reduced to eliminate background scatter and slit width is narrow to medium.

13. What is retroillumination from fundus?
   i. Principle—slit beam is placed nearly coaxial with microscope and rotated slightly off axis so that it shines in through margin of pupil. This allows the red light reflected from the ocular fundus to pass through cornea to microscope
   ii. Settings—slit lamp is aligned coaxial with microscope and then decentered to edge of pupil
   Slit height is reduced to one-third to avoid striking the iris
   Slit width is medium and curved at one edge to fit in the pupil
   iii. Uses—the following abnormalities are seen:
   - Lattice dystrophy
   - Pseudoexfoliation
   - Keratic precipitates
   - Corneal scars
   - Meesmann's dystrophy
   - Map-dot fingerprint dystrophy
   - Lens vacuoles
   - Cataract
   - Corneal rejection lines

14. What is specular reflection?
   i. Principle—it is based on Snell's law. When the angle of incidence of slit beam equals the angle of observation of microscope, the reflected light from epithelial and endothelial surfaces is viewed
   ii. Settings—beam height is full and beam width is narrow. Microscope and slit beam are 45-60° apart

iii. Movement—place the slit beam adjacent to reflection of slit-lamp filament from the surface of cornea (corneal light reflex)

Slit beam is moved laterally until it overlaps corneal light reflection. Beam is moved further laterally to the edge of corneal light reflection and focuses on the posterior corneal surface to visualize the paving stone-like mosaic of endothelial cells.

15. **What specialized examinations can be carried out with the help of slit lamp?**

    Diagnostic examinations:
    i. Gonioscopy
    ii. Fundus examination with focal illumination
    iii. Pachymetry
    iv. Applanation tonometry
    v. Ophthalmodynamometry
    vi. Slit-lamp photography
    vii. Laser interferometry
    viii. Potential acuity meter test

    Therapeutic uses:
    i. Contact lens fitting
    ii. YAG capsulotomy
    iii. Delivery system for argon, diode, and YAG laser as for retinal lasers, peripheral iridotomy, argon laser trabeculoplasty (ALT), synechiolysis, suturolysis
    iv. Corneal and conjunctival foreign body removal
    v. Corneal scrapings
    vi. Intraoperative slit-lamp illumination:
        There is less risk of phototoxicity because a slit light at 5°, focused on the macula, provides a fixed illumination of 7,000 lm, the same as with an intraocular fiber placed at 17 mm from the macula

16. **Describe optics of slit lamp.**

    Slit lamp is composed of two optical elements:
    i. Objective
    ii. Eyepiece

    Objective lens consists of two planoconvex lenses. With their convexities put together, they provide a composite power of + 22D. Eyepiece has a lens of +10D.

    For good stereopsis, tubes are converged at an angle of 10–15°. The microscope uses a pair of prisms between objective and eyepiece to reinvert the inverted image produced by a compound microscope.

    Most slit lamps provide a range of accommodation from ×6 to ×40.

Modern slit lamps use one of the following three systems to produce a range of magnification:
  i. Czapskiscope with rotating objectives:
     - Oldest and most frequently used
     - Different objectives are placed on a turret type of arrangement that allows them to be fairly rapidly changed during examination
     - Haag-Streit model, Bausch and Lomb, Thorpe model
  ii. Littmann-Galilean telescope principle:
     - Developed by Littmann
     - Sits between objective and eyepiece lenses and does not require either of them to change
     - Provide range of magnification, typically 5
     - It is called Galilean system because it utilizes Galilean telescopes to alter magnification
     - Two optical components are positive and negative lens
     - Zeiss, Rodenstock, American optical slit lamp
  iii. Zoom system:
     - Allows continuously variable degrees of magnification
     - Nikon slit lamp contains zoom system within objective of microscope and offers a range of magnification from ×7 to ×35

17. How to evaluate tear film with the help of slit lamp?

Examination of inferior marginal tear strip can yield information about volume of tears. The tear strip is a line just above the lower lid. It is normally mm in width and has a concave upper aspect. When thin or discontinuous, it is an evidence of deficient aqueous tear volume.

The following are the parameters:

i.	Beam angle	60°
ii.	Beam height	Maximum
iii.	Beam width	Parallel piped
iv.	Filter	None
v.	Illumination	Low or ambient lighting only
vi.	Magnification	10–16×

  vii. Another feature seen in dry eye is increased debris in tear film. Presence of bits of mucus and sloughed epithelial cells is suggestive of delayed tear clearance
  viii. Alteration in morphology of conjunctiva—conjunctivochalasis
  ix. Pathologic signs of meibomian gland disease—ductal orifice pout or metaplasia (white shafts of keratin in orifices), reduced expressibility, increased turbidity, and viscosity of secretions

18. **How to measure lesions with slit lamp?**
    i. Brightness—lowest intensity setting
    ii. Slit-lamp beam—slightly thicker than optical section
    iii. Illuminating arm directly in front of viewing arm
    iv. Focus vertically oriented beam on the lesion to be measured
    v. Vary height of beam till it equals height of lesion. Read the scale
    vi. Rotate the bulb housing 90° to orient the beam horizontally and repeat measurement by varying height of beam to measure horizontal dimensions of lesion
    vii. The bulb housing may be rotated <90° to perform diagonal measurement.

1.9 DIRECT OPHTHALMOSCOPE

1. **Who invented direct ophthalmoscope?**
   Direct ophthalmoscope was invented by Von Helmholtz in 1850.

2. **Explain the procedure for examining with a direct ophthalmoscope.**
   i. It is ideally performed in a dimly lit room
   ii. Patient is asked to look straight ahead at a distant object
   iii. Examiner should be on the side of the eye to be examined
   iv. Patient's right eye to be examined by the examiner's right eye and scope to be held in right hand and vice versa
   v. Examiner should first examine at an arm's distance
   vi. Once the red reflex is appreciated, the examiner should move close to the patient's eye and focus on the structures to be examined

3. **Explain the optics of direct ophthalmoscopy.**
   Principle—in emmetropic patients, the issuing rays will be parallel and will be brought into focus on the retina of the observer.
   Hence, light from the bulb is condensed by a lens and reflected off a two-way mirror into the patient's eye. The observer views the image of the patient's illuminated retina by dialing in the required focusing lens.

4. **At what distance is distant direct ophthalmoscopy performed?**
   Performed at 2 ft (one arm's distance).

5. **What are the applications of distant direct ophthalmoscopy?**
   i. To diagnose the opacities in refractive media
      - Exact location of the opacity can be determined by parallactic displacement
      - Opacities which move in the direction of movement are anterior to pupillary plane and those behind will move in the opposite direction
   ii. To differentiate between a hole and a mole of iris Mole looks black, but a red reflex is seen through hole in iris as in iridodialysis
   iii. To recognize the detached retina or a tumor arising from fundus
   iv. Bruckner's test: In children, refractive error can be assessed by dialing the lens, the power of which will help us focus on the retina clearly

6. **What are the different reflexes seen on distant direct ophthalmoscopy?**
   i. *Red reflex:* Normal
   ii. *Grayish reflex:* Retinal detachment
   iii. *Black reflex:* Vitreous hemorrhage
   iv. *Oil droplet reflex:* Keratoconus
   v. *White reflex (leukokoria):*
      - Retinoblastoma
      - Retinopathy of prematurity

- Congenital cataract
- Toxocariasis
- Persistent primary hyperplastic vitreous
- Retinal dysplasias
- Coats' disease
- Choroidal coloboma

7. **What are the factors determining the field of vision in direct ophthalmoscopy?**
    i. Directly proportional to the size of pupil
    ii. Directly proportional to the axial length of the observed eye/refraction of the patient. A larger area with least magnification is seen in hyperopes and a smaller area with maximum magnification is noted in myopes
    iii. Inversely proportional to distance between observed and observer's eye
    iv. The smaller the sight hole of the ophthalmoscope, the better the field of vision

8. **What are the parts of direct ophthalmoscope?**
    i. On/off rheostat
    ii. View aperture
    iii. Lens power indicator (Rekoss disk)
    iv. Pupil size—large/small
    v. Auxiliary controls—red-free filter, fixation target, slit beam, etc

9. **What is the therapeutic use of direct ophthalmoscope?**
   For xenon laser delivery.

10. **How will you quantify disk edema using direct ophthalmoscope?**
    The direct ophthalmoscope is first focused on the surface of the disk. The dioptric power required for clear disc focussing is noted. Then the ophthalmoscope is used to clearly focus on the adjacent retina. The dioptric power for this maneuver is then noted. The difference between the dioptric powers gives the amount of elevation of the disk, that is, every addition of +3D equals to 1 mm elevation of disk (phakics) 2 mm elevation of disk (aphakics).

    In an emmetropic eye, each diopter of change of focus is equivalent to an axial length of 0.4 mm, or a difference in focusing of 3D indicates a difference in level of 1 mm whereas in aphakics, 3D indicates a difference in level of 2 mm.

11. **What are the characteristics of the image formed?**
    i. V—virtual
    ii. E—erect
    iii. M—magnified

12. **What are the drawbacks of direct ophthalmoscope?**
    i. Lack of stereopsis
    ii. Small field of view
    iii. No view of retinal periphery

13. **What is the magnification of direct ophthalmoscope?**
    15×

14. **What are the advantages of direct ophthalmoscope?**
    i. Safe
    ii. Portable
    iii. Screening tool
    iv. Easy technique

15. **What are the uses of auxiliaries in direct ophthalmoscopy?**
    i. Full spot-viewing through a large pupil
    ii. Small spot-viewing through a small pupil
    iii. Red-free filter change in retinal nerve fiber layer (RNFL) thickness
    iv. Identifying microaneurysms and other vascular abnormalities
    v. Slit-evaluating retinal contour
    vi. Reticule/grid-measuring vessel caliber or small retina lesions
    vii. Fixation target-identifying central/eccentric fixation

16. **How do you find a patient's point of preferred fixation?**
    i. Reduce illumination intensity and dial in fixation target
    ii. Ask the patient to look into the light in center of target
    iii. Determine whether the test mark falls on the central foveal reflex or at an eccentric location
    iv. Ask the patient whether the fixed object is seen as straight ahead off or center

17. **List the differences between direct ophthalmoscope (DO) and indirect ophthalmoscope (IO).**

Points	DO	IO
Stereopsis	Absent	Present
Magnification	15×	3–5×
Static field of view	2 disk diameter	8 disk diameter
Dynamic field of view	Up to equator	Up to ora serrata
Retinal image	Virtual, erect	Real, inverted
Technique	Easy	Difficult
Illumination	Good	Excellent
Uses	Diagnostic mostly	Diagnostic and therapeutic, e.g., PRP, barrage

1.10 INDIRECT OPHTHALMOSCOPE

1. Who invented indirect ophthalmoscope (IO)?
IO was invented by Nagel in 1864.

2. What is the principle behind indirect ophthalmoscopy?
Indirect ophthalmoscopy works on the principle similar to an astronomical telescope.

The principle is to make the eye highly myopic by placing a strong convex lens in front of the patient's eye.

The emergent rays from an area of the fundus are brought to focus in between the lens and observer's eye as a real inverted image.

3. What are the different types of condensing lens used in indirect ophthalmoscopy?
   i. Planoconvex lens
   ii. Biconvex lens
   iii. Aspheric lens

4. What are the advantages and disadvantages of different types of lens?
   i. *Planoconvex lens*
      Advantage: Causes less reflex during examination
      Disadvantage: Plane surface of the lens causes troublesome reflexes when held facing the observer, so the convex side should face toward the observer
   ii. *Biconvex lens*—both surfaces have +10D
      Advantage: Either way, it can be held
      Disadvantage: Reflexes are more as compared to planoconvex lens
   iii. *Aspheric lens*—lenses of greater power (30D/40D)
      Advantage:
      - Helps to obtain less magnification and greater field
      - Minimize aberration
      - Can be used with small pupil and extremely
      - Complicated retinal topography

5. What are the different powers of lenses which could be used as condensing lenses?
The various lenses used are:
   i. 15D (magnifies ×4: Field about 40°)
      It is used for examination of the posterior pole
   ii. 20D (magnifies ×3: Field about 45°)
      It is commonly used for general examination of the fundus
   iii. 25D (magnifies ×2.5: Field is about 50°)

iv. 30D (magnifies ×2: Field is 60°)
It has shorter working distance and is useful when examining patients with a small pupil
v. 40D (magnifies ×2: Field is 60°)
It is used mainly to examine small children

6. **What is the power of accommodation during the examination?**
    i. The working distance is approximately one-third of a meter. This setup enables an emmetropic observer to use only 1D of their accommodation to view the image in the condensing lens
    ii. Myopes can increase or decrease their plus power to suit their refraction
    iii. Presbyopes will need the equivalent of an intermediate range add or their addition for near
    iv. Hypermetropes will need their distance correction

7. **Where is the image formed in IO?**
    The image is formed between the condensing lens and the observer.

8. **Compare different condensing power.**

Features	+14D	+20D	+30D
Distance from eye (inches)	3	2	1.5
Magnification	4–5×	3×	2×
Field	30	50	60
Stereopsis	Normal	¾ normal	½ normal
Illumination	Low	Medium	Bright

9. **What are the advantages of indirect ophthalmoscopy?**
    i. Larger field of retina can be seen
    ii. Lesser distortion of the image of the retina
    iii. Easier to examine if the patient presents with eye movements or with high spherical or refractive power
    iv. Easy visualization of retina anterior to equator
    v. It gives a three-dimensional stereoscopic view of the retina
    vi. It is useful in hazy media because of its bright light and optical property

10. **What are the disadvantages of indirect ophthalmoscopy?**
    i. Magnification in IO is five times using a +20 D lens. This is very less when compared to direct ophthalmoscope (DO), which is 15 times
    ii. Indirect ophthalmoscopy is difficult to perform with small pupil
    iii. It is uncomfortable for the patients due to intense light and scleral indentation

iv. The procedure is more cumbersome and requires extensive practice both in technique and interpretation of the image visualized
v. Reflex sneezing can occur due to exposure to bright light

11. **Discuss the relative position of the image formed in emmetropic, myopic, and hypermetropic eyes.**
    i. Emmetropia—the emergent rays are parallel and thus focused at the principal focus of the lens
    ii. Hypermetropia—the emergent rays are divergent and are therefore focused farther away from the principal focus
    iii. Myopia—the emergent rays are convergent and are therefore focused near the lens

12. **What are the color codings for fundus drawing?**
    For example:

Optic disk	Red
Arteries	Red
Veins	Blue
Attached retina	Red hatching outlined in blue
Detached retina	Blue
Retinal tear	Red with blue outline
Lattice degeneration	Blue hatchings outlined in blue
Retinal pigment	Black
Retinal exudates	Yellow
Choroidal lesions	Brown
Vitreous opacities	Green
Drusen	Black
Nevus	Black
Microaneurysms	Red

13. **How to perform indirect ophthalmoscopy?**
    i. Explain the procedure to the patient
    ii. Reassure him/her of the brightness of the light
    iii. The patient should be lying flat on a stretcher without flexion or extension of the neck in a dark room
    iv. The examiner throws light into the patient's dilated eye from an arm's distance
    v. Binocular ophthalmoscope with a headband or that mounted on a spectacle frame is employed
    vi. Keeping eyes on the reflex, the examiner then interposes the condensing lens in path of the beam of light close to the patient's

eyes and then slowly moves the lens away from the eye until an image of the retina is clearly seen

vii. Use the patient's own hand/finger as target. Patients with sight will then use visual stimuli from his hand for fixation in addition to proprioceptive impulse. This is important in case of blind, monocular, or uncooperative patients

viii. The examiner moves around the head of the patient to examine different quadrants of the fundus

ix. He has to stand opposite to the clock hour position to be examined. For example, to examine inferior quadrant (6 o'clock), the examiner should stand toward the patient's head (12 o'clock)

x. The whole peripheral retina up to the ora serrata can be examined by asking the patient to look in extremes of gaze and using a scleral indentor

14. **How to use scleral indentor?**
    i. It consists of a small curved shaft with a flattened knob-like tip mounted on a thimble
    ii. It can be held between the thumb and the index finger or it can be placed upon the index or middle finger
    iii. The examiner should move the scleral depressor in a direction opposite to that in which he wishes the depression to appear
    iv. It should be rolled gently and longitudinally over the eye surface

15. **What is the role of scleral indentation in examination of fundus?**
    i. Make visible the part of the fundus which lies anterior to the equator
    ii. Making prominent the just or barely perceptible lesions of peripheral retina

16. **What are the factors affecting the field of view?**
    i. Patient's pupil size
    ii. Power of the condensing lens
    iii. Size of the condensing lens
    iv. Refractive error
    v. Distance of the condensing lens held from the patient's eye

17. **How to calculate the magnification of image?**

$$\text{Simple magnification} = \frac{\text{Power of the eye}}{\text{Power of condensing lens}}$$

If power of the eye = 60 D
If condensing lens power = 20 D
Then magnification = 60/20 = 3 times.

1.11 X-RAYS IN OPHTHALMOLOGY

1. **What is the advantage of X-ray skull in ophthalmology?**
   The advantages of plain X-ray skull when compared to other investigations such as a computed tomography (CT) scan are:
   i. Low cost
   ii. Easy availability and usage
   iii. Preliminary test to detect gross abnormality

2. **What are the important structures in X-ray skull to be looked for in ophthalmology?**
   The most important structure to be looked for is the base of the skull. In this, the pituitary fossa is the most important structure. Other landmarks are:
   i. Anterior clinoid process
   ii. Planum sphenoidale
   iii. Chiasmatic sulcus
   iv. Tuberculum sellae
   v. Floor of the pituitary fossa
   vi. Dorsum sellae
   vii. Posterior clinoids

   Occasionally, the pituitary fossa is deep and extends more in the vertical direction than in the anteroposterior direction, and this has been termed the J-shaped sella and has no pathological significance.

3. **When do normal vascular markings of the skull become prominent?**
   Arterial markings in the skull are usually visible as thin wavy lines and may become marked when the external carotid branches supply a vascular lesion like a meningioma or an arteriovenous (AV) malformation.

4. **What are the abnormalities to be looked for in plain X-ray skull?**
   i. Fracture
   ii. Bone erosion: Local, e.g., pituitary fossa; generalized, e.g., Paget's disease
   iii. Abnormal calcification: Tumors, e.g., meningioma, craniopharyngioma, and aneurysm
   iv. Midline shift: If pineal gland is calcified
   v. Signs of raised intracranial pressure: Erosion of posterior clinoids

5. **What are the causes of normal calcification in the X-ray skull?**
   i. Structures in the midline that produce calcification are:
      - Pineal body
      - Falx cerebri
      - Pacchionian granules
      - Habenular commissure

ii. The normal structures away from midline that produce calcification are:
   - Choroid plexus
   - Petroclinoid ligament
   - The lateral edge of diaphragma sellae
   - The carotid artery

6. **What are the abnormal calcifications seen on X-ray skull?**
   Abnormal calcifications seen are:
   i. Tuberculomas may show calcification in 6–7% cases
   ii. The shape and size of the calcification may be diagnostic as in the case of double line wavy (rail road calcification) in Sturge-Weber syndrome
   iii. To position and shape as in the case of suprasellar area or speckled calcification (eggshell) seen in craniopharyngioma
   iv. Meningioma
   v. Retinoblastoma
   vi. Pituitary adenoma
   vii. Mucocele
   viii. Phlebolith
   ix. Other lesions are tuberous sclerosis, toxoplasmosis, oligodendroglioma, aneurysmal sac, subdural hematoma, dermoid, cysticercosis, etc

7. **What are the signs of raised intracranial tension (ICT) in children?**
   i. There is increased separation of the sutures
   ii. Increased convolutional markings
   iii. Thinning of the bone
   iv. Silver beaten appearance—due to pressure of sulci and gyri
       Sutures beyond 2 mm are suspicious of raised ICT, and sometimes this may be seen even in young adults up to 20 years. Conversely, premature fusion of the sutures is seen in craniosynostosis

8. **What are the signs of raised ICT in adults?**
   In adults, there is full ossification of the skull bones, and the sutures are possibly or fully closed, and so sutural separation does not occur. Similarly, abnormal convolution markings are also not seen.
   The changes that occur in the sella turcica constitute the most important signs in raised ICT.
   i. In the earliest phase, there is demineralization of the cortical bone leading to loss of the normal "lamina dura" (white line of the sellar floor)
   ii. This is followed by thinning of the dorsum sellae and the posterior clinoid processes. The dorsum sellae becomes shortened and pointed resulting in a shallow sella turcica

iii. In extreme cases, the sella becomes very shallow, flattened anterior wall gets demineralized, and the floor and dorsum sellae are destroyed

iv. Alternately, the pituitary fossa may enlarge in a balloon-like fashion due to internal hydrocephalus. In such cases, the enlarging III ventricle acts like an expanding intrasellar lesion (empty sella syndrome)

9. **How is X-ray skull lateral view taken and what are the important structures seen in it?**

   With the patient erect or prone, the head is turned with the affected side toward the film. The head is adjusted to true lateral position, with the median plane parallel to the X-ray plate and the interorbital line at right angles to the film.

   The important structures seen are:
   i. Sella turcica
   ii. Pterygopalatine fossa
   iii. Hard palate
   iv. Anterior and posterior walls of frontal sinus

10. **What is Caldwell's view and how is it taken?**

    Caldwell's view is a posteroanterior (PA) (occipitofrontal) view angled 15° caudal to the canthomeatal line, the nose and forehead touching the X-ray film, with the orbitomeatal line perpendicular to the film. It is the best view for frontal sinus.

    It shows:
    i. Shape and size of the orbits
    ii. Superior orbital fissure
    iii. Floor of the sella
    iv. Lamina papyracea

11. **What is Water's view and what structures are seen on it?**

    Water's view is a PA (occipitomental) view inclined with the tragocanthal line forming an angle of 37° with central ray, and the X-ray plate touching the chin.

    It is the best view for maxillary sinus. It shows:
    i. Roof of the orbit
    ii. Superior and inferior orbital rims
    iii. Maxillary antrum
    iv. Ethmoidal air cells

12. **What is base view and what structures are seen on it?**
    i. Submentovertical view
    ii. With the patient erect or supine, the head is hyperextended touching the vertex to the couch and the shoulders raised. The film

is placed lengthwise with its lower border just below the occipital protuberance. The baseline and the film are parallel. The central ray passes submentally and perpendicular to the X-ray plate and the tragocanthal line

iii. Structures seen on it are:
- Anterior wall of middle cranial fossa
- Posterior wall of maxillary antrum
- Basal foramina
- Petrous temporal bones
- Posterior wall of orbit
- Foramen ovale and spinosum

13. What is Rhese's view and what structures are seen on it?
i. In PA position, the chin is raised till the orbitomeatal line is 40° to the film. Then the head is rotated 40° away from the side to be X-rayed
ii. It is also called the optic foramen view as it shows:
- Optic foramen
- Superior orbital fissure
- Lacrimal fossa

14. What is Towne's projection and what structures are seen on it?
i. In supine position, the canthomeatal line and the median sagittal line are perpendicular to the film (fronto-occipital/half axial)
ii. With the patient erect or supine, and the chin well down on the chest, the head is adjusted so that the radiographic baseline is at right angles to the film. The film is placed lengthwise with its upper border 5 cm above the vertex
iii. This view is not used commonly because of increased X-ray radiation to the eyes
iv. Structures seen are:
- Infraorbital fissure
- Superior orbital fissure

15. What is orbitomeatal line?
Orbitomeatal line is the line drawn from the lower margin of the orbit to the superior border of the external auditory canal.

16. What is the significance of optic foramen?
i. Optic foramen is seen in Rhese's view
ii. It lies in the posteroinferior quadrant of the orbit
iii. The average normal diameter of the optic canal is 6–7 mm (<2 mm and >7 mm are pathological)
iv. Both optic canals have to be taken always for comparison. Difference >1.5 mm is significant

17. **What are the causes of small optic canal?**
    i. Congenital
    ii. Inflammatory—osteitis
    iii. Dysostosis like fibrous dysplasia, Paget's disease

18. **What are the causes of optic canal expansion?**
    i. Raised ICT
    ii. Vascular—AV malformation
    iii. Inflammatory—arachnoiditis, sarcoid granuloma, tuberculoma
    iv. Tumors—meningioma, neurofibroma, retinoblastoma

19. **What are the causes of optic canal erosion?**
    Medial wall:
    i. Carcinoma
    ii. Mucocele
    iii. Granuloma of the sphenoid sinus
    Lateral wall:
    i. Pituitary tumors
    ii. Craniopharyngioma
    iii. Roof—tumor of anterior cranial fossa

20. **What are the normal dimensions of the sella turcica?**
    Anteroposterior diameter: 4-16 mm. Average—10.5 mm
    Depth: 4-12 mm. Average—8.1 mm

21. **What is the most common lesion causing enlargement of the sella?**
    Pituitary adenoma

22. **What are the X-ray findings in chromophilic adenoma?**
    i. Enlargement of the sella
    ii. Erosion of the floor of sella
    iii. Erosion of the undermargins of the anterior clinoid process

23. **What is meant by double flooring of the sella?**
    Irregular and asymmetrical enlargement of the fossa mainly in posterior sellar lesions giving the appearance of double flooring on X-ray skull lateral view.

24. **How is calcification in sella best seen?**
    X-ray skull lateral view

25. **What is the most common cause of calcification in midline?**
    Craniopharyngioma

26. **Enumerate causes of calcification in and around sella.**
    i. Atheroma
    ii. Meningioma

iii. Arterial aneurysm
iv. TB meningitis
v. Optic disk glioma

27. **What is empty sella syndrome?**
Empty sella syndrome is an asymmetric enlargement of the sella due to downward herniation of the subarachnoid space into sella due to raised ICT.

28. **Enumerate the causes of enlarged sella.**
    i. Chromophobe adenoma and other pituitary tumors
    ii. Gliomas
    iii. Teratomas
    iv. Craniopharyngiomas
    v. Empty sella syndrome
    vi. Arachnoid cyst
    vii. Ectopic pinealomas

29. **What is the most common cause of suprasellar calcification?**
Craniopharyngioma

30. **Name some common views used in orbital diseases.**
    i. Caldwell's view—supraorbital rim and medial orbital wall
    ii. Water's view—roof and floor of the orbit
    iii. Lateral view—face and orbits
    iv. PA view—paranasal sinuses
    v. Towne's view—supraorbital fissure

31. **What is oblique orbital line?**
Oblique orbital line is a roentgenographic structure formed by the junction of medial and lateral portions of the greater wing of sphenoid.

32. **Enumerate the causes of small orbit.**
    i. Anophthalmos
    ii. Postenucleation
    iii. Microphthalmos
    iv. Mucocele

33. **Enumerate the causes of large orbit.**
    i. Pseudotumor
    ii. Tumors in muscle cone
    iii. Congenital serous cysts
    iv. Dysplasia

34. **Enumerate the causes of bare orbits.**
This is seen in X-ray orbit PA view
    i. Due to hypoplasia of the lesser wing of sphenoid
    ii. Seen in neurofibroma

35. **What is blowout fracture?**
    Fracture of the infraorbital plate without the fracture of the infraorbital rim is blowout fracture.

36. **What is the view used to diagnose blowout fracture?**
    Water's view

37. **What are the X-ray findings on Water's view in blowout fracture?**
    i. Fragmentation of the orbital wall
    ii. Depression of the bone fragments and prolapse of orbital soft tissue into the maxillary sinus—trap door deformity
    iii. Opacification of the maxillary antrum due to hemorrhage and emphysema

38. **What is the most common site of blowout fracture?**
    Posteromedial portion of the orbital floor medial to the inferior orbital fissure.

39. **In what view can superior orbital fissure be best seen?**
    Towne's projection

40. **Name some conditions in which superior orbital fissure is widened?**
    i. Pituitary adenoma
    ii. Intracavernous aneurysm
    iii. Carotid-cavernous fistula
    iv. Mucocele of the sphenoid sinus
    v. Backward extension of intraorbital mass
    vi. Forward extension of intracranial mass

41. **Enumerate some causes of narrowing of superior orbital fissure.**
    Diseases causing increased density and thickness of bone such as:
    i. Fibrous dysplasia
    ii. Paget's disease

42. **Enumerate some causes of hyperostosis of the orbit.**
    i. Acromegaly
    ii. Osteopetrosis
    iii. Anemia in childhood
    iv. Sphenoid ridge meningiomas
    v. Craniostenosis
    vi. Paget's disease

43. **Name some causes of diffuse osteolysis of the orbit.**
    i. Hyperparathyroidism
    ii. Osteomyelitis
    iii. Wegener's granulomatosis
    iv. Malignant neoplasms invading the bone, etc

44. What are the causes of bone destruction with clear-cut margins?
   i. Dermoid cyst—most common
   ii. Histiocytosis
   iii. Meningioma

45. Enumerate some causes of enlargement of the orbit.
   i. *Symmetrical:*
      - Congenital myopia
      - Buphthalmos
      - Mass in muscle cone
      - Optic nerve glioma
      - Optic nerve meningioma
      - Neurofibroma
   ii. *Asymmetrical:*
      - Hemangioma
      - Lacrimal gland tumor
      - Dermoid cyst
      - Schwannoma

46. What are the causes of intraorbital calcification?
   i. *Ocular causes:*
      - Retinoblastoma—most common
      - Meningioma
      - Hemangioma
      - Phlebolith
      - Dermoid cyst
      - Cataract
   ii. *Ocular manifestation of systemic diseases:*
      - Toxoplasmosis
      - Von Hippel–Lindau disease
      - Tuberous sclerosis
      - Sturge–Weber syndrome

1.12 COMPUTED TOMOGRAPHY AND MAGNETIC RESONANCE IMAGING

1. **Who invented computed tomography (CT)?**
   GN Hounsfield invented CT in 1972. It was initially known as electrical and musical industries (EMI) scan.

2. **What is the principle of CT?**

   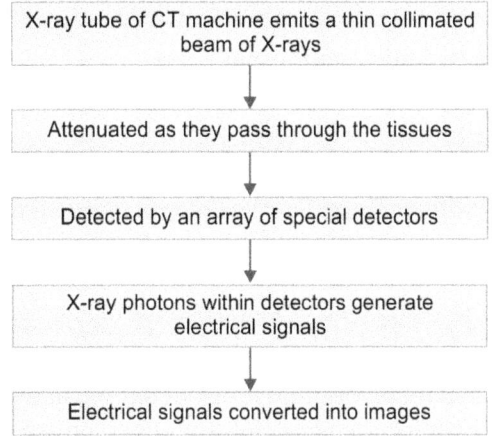

   High-density areas are depicted as white and low-density areas are depicted as black.

3. **What is the radiation dose used in CT?**
   The X-ray dose for a standard CT is 3–5 rads, and for high-resolution CT, it is 10 rads.

4. **What are all the different types of orbital planes employed during CT?**
   i. *Axial plane:* Parallel to the course of the nerve
   ii. *Coronal plane:* Showing the age, optic nerve, and extraocular muscles
   iii. *Sagittal plane:* Parallel to the nasal septum

5. **What influences the resolution of CT?**
   The spatial resolution of a CT scan depends on slice thickness.
   Thinner the slice, higher the resolution, require higher radiation dose.
   2 mm cuts are optimal for the eye and orbit. In evaluation of the orbital apex, 1 mm slice is more informative.

6. **What are the indications of CT?**
   i. Palpable orbital mass
   ii. Unexplained proptosis, ophthalmoplegia, or ptosis
   iii. Preseptal cellulitis with orbital signs

iv. Orbital signs associated with paranasal sinus disease
v. Unexplained afferent dysfunction
vi. Ocular surface or lid tumor with suspected orbital spread
vii. Intraocular tumor with proptosis
viii. Orbital trauma
ix. When magnetic resonance imaging (MRI) is contraindicated

7. **What is Reid's baseline?**
Reid's baseline is a line extending from the inferior orbital rim to the upper margin of the external auditory meatus.

8. **What view best depicts optic canal?**
The plane inclined at 30° to the orbitomeatal line depicts the optic canal and the anterior visual pathway.

9. **What are Hounsfield units?**
Hounsfield units represent a scale of radiation attenuation values of tissues. The number assigned is called Hounsfield number. This number can range from –1,000 to +1,000 HU or above. The higher the number, the greater the attenuation of X-rays and the higher the tissue density.

10. **What is contrast enhancement?**
A contrast-enhancing lesion is one which becomes bright or more intense after contrast medium infusion. An increase in its Hounsfield value is a more reliable indicator of contrast enhancement than an increase in brightness.

11. **What are the views for evaluation of bony orbit?**
    i. *Axial view:* Lateral and medial walls, superior orbital fissure, and optic canal
    ii. *Coronal view:* Orbit floor and roof

12. **What are the causes of enlargement of superior orbital fissure?**
    i. Optic nerve meningioma with intracranial extension
    ii. Carotid-cavernous fistula
    iii. Infraclinoid aneurysm

13. **What are the causes of extraocular muscle enlargement?**

Type of involvement	Common causes
Unilateral, single-muscle involvement	• Thyroid ophthalmopathy • Primary and secondary orbital tumors • Myositis
Unilateral, multiple muscle involvement	*Symmetrical:* • Arteriovenous (AV) shunts • Vascular engorgement • Thyroid ophthalmopathy

Contd...

Contd...

Type of involvement	Common causes
	Asymmetrical: • Myositis • Metastatic tumors • Thyroid ophthalmopathy
Bilateral, single-muscle involvement	• Thyroid ophthalmopathy • Metastatic tumors • Myositis
Bilateral, multiple-muscle involvement	• Thyroid ophthalmopathy • Metastatic tumors • Cavernous sinus thrombosis

14. **Which part of the optic nerve is readily visualized?**
    Optic chiasma is readily visualized because it is surrounded by cerebrospinal fluid in the suprasellar region.

15. **Which part of the optic nerve is poorly visualized?**
    The intracanalicular portion of the optic nerve is poorly imaged on CT due to the absence of intrinsic contract material and partial volume averaging from the adjacent bone.

16. **What is the diameter of the optic foramen?**
    i. The optic foramen is about 3 mm in diameter
    ii. Anterior part of the optic canal—vertically oval in shape
    iii. Middle part of the canal—round
    iv. Posterior part of the canal—horizontally oval

17. **What are the causes of the increase or decrease in the size of optic foramen?**
    Enlargement of the optic canal—tumors of intracanalicular part of the optic nerve—glioma, meningioma
    Decrease in diameter—fibrous dysplasia
    i. Paget's disease
    ii. Hyperostosis secondary to meningioma

18. **Differentiate between optic nerve glioma and meningioma.**

	Glioma	Meningioma
Origin	Neoplasm of astrocytes	Neoplasm of meningothelial cells
Age	Children	Middle age
Sex	No prediction	More in females
Clinical features	Vision loss ↓ Proptosis	Proptosis ↓ Vision loss

Contd...

Contd...

	Glioma	Meningioma
CT scan	Intraconal fusiform enlargement of the optic nerve	• Tubular enlargement of the optic nerve • Tram track appearance
MRI	No calcification	Calcification may be seen
T1	Hypo- to isointense	Hypointense
T2	Variable intensity	Hyperintense

19. **What are the features to be evaluated in case of orbital mass?**
    The following aspects should be evaluated on CT to aid diagnosis:
    i. Assessment of proptosis: Using an amid-orbital scan, a straight line is drawn between the anterior margins of the zygomatic processes. Normally, it intersects the globe at or behind the equator. The distance between the anterior cornea and the interzygomatic line is 21 mm normally. If >21 mm or asymmetry >2 mm—proptosis
    ii. Size, shape, and site of the tumor
    iii. Circumscription of the tumor
    iv. Margin of the tumor—smooth (benign) or irregular (malignant)
    v. Effect on surrounding structures—fossa formation (benign) or hyperostosis
    vi. Internal consistency—homogeneous (benign) or heterogeneous (malignant)

20. **Which is the most common site of bony metastasis?**
    The greater wing of sphenoid is the most common site of bony metastasis in the orbit.

21. **What are the CT findings in Graves' ophthalmopathy?**
    Graves' ophthalmopathy typically shows unilateral or bilateral involvement of single or multiple muscles causing fusiform enlargement with smooth muscle borders, especially posteriorly. Tendons are usually spared.

22. **What are the factors to be assessed in case of an orbital trauma?**
    i. Evaluation of fractures
    ii. Number, location, degree, and direction of fracture fragment displacement
    iii. Evaluation of soft-tissue injury: Muscle entrapment, hematoma, emphysema, etc
    iv. Presence and location of foreign bodies

23. **Where is "empty delta sign" seen?**
    Sigmoid sinus thrombosis.

24. **What are the causes of ring-enhancing lesions?**
    i. Cysticercosis
    ii. Tuberculoma
    iii. Toxoplasmosis
    iv. Metastasis
    v. Abscess

25. **How does blood appear in CT?**
    Acute bleeding (<6 hours)—hyperdense
    Subacute bleeding—isodense with brain (intraparenchymal changes)
    Chronic (>2 weeks)—hypodense

26. **What are the conditions where CT is preferred over MRI?**
    i. Acute trauma
    ii. Bony lesions
    iii. Metallic foreign body

27. **What are all the recent advances in CT scanning?**
    i. Spiral or helical CT scanner
    ii. Three-dimensional CT

28. **What is the principle of MRI?**
    An MRI depends on the rearrangement of hydrogen nuclei when tissue is exposed to a strong electromagnetic pulse. When the pulse subsides, the nuclei return to their normal position, reradiating some of the energy they have absorbed. Sensitive receivers pick up this electromagnetic echo. The signals are analyzed, computed, and displayed as a cross-sectional image.

29. **What are the imaging parameters?**
    T1 → longitudinal or spin–lattice relaxation
    T2 → transverse or spin–spin relaxation

30. **What is the basis of T1 and T2 imaging?**
    When the radiofrequency pulse is switched off, the T1 increases and T2 decreases.
    T1:
    i. Depends on the tissue composition, structure, and surroundings
    ii. It is an expression of the time it takes for the energy imparted by the radiofrequency (RF) pulse to be transferred to the lattice of atoms that surround the nuclei
    iii. T1-weighted images are good for delineating ocular anatomy
    iv. Contrast-weighted images are done with T1
    T2:
    i. Comes about when the protons go out of phase due to inhomogenicity of the external and internal magnetic fields

ii. T2-weighted images are best to discern pathology
iii. The difference in the brightness seen on T2 images can be helpful in differentiating melanotic lesions and hemorrhagic process

31. List some T1 and T2 characteristics of some common tissues.

	T1 signal	T2 signal
Air	Dark (hypointense)	Dark (hypointense)
Bone		
Dense calcification		
Water, edema, cerebrospinal fluid (CSF), vitreous	Dark	Bright
High protein paramagnetic substances (gadolinium, melanin)	Bright	Dark
Fat	Bright	Dark
Gray matter	Dark gray	Light gray
White matter	Light gray	Gray

32. What are the strengths of magnets used in MRI?
0.3, 0.5, 1, 3, and 5 Tesla

33. What is gadolinium?
Gadolinium is a paramagnetic substance (unpaired electrons) that shortens the relaxation time of T1- and T2-weighted sequences. Administered intravenously, it remains intravascular unless there is a breakdown of the blood–brain barrier. It is visualized only in T1-weighted images appearing bright.

34. What are the structures that enhance with gadolinium?
Enhancement of tissues typically occurs with the blood–brain barrier breakdown, which is caused by a neoplasm, infection, or inflammation. The pituitary gland, extraocular muscle, choroid plexus, and nasal mucosa normally lack a blood–brain barrier; hence, they enhance with gadolinium.

35. What are fat-suppression techniques?
Fat-suppression techniques are applied for imaging the orbit. They eliminate the bright signal of orbital fat and delineate normal structures (optic nerve and extraocular muscles), tumors, and inflammatory lesions.

36. What are the types of fat-suppression techniques?
i. T1 fat saturation (used with gadolinium)
ii. Short T1 inversion recovery

37. What is STIR?
STIR is short T1 inversion recovery. It is considered as an optimal sequence for detecting intrinsic lesions of the intraorbital optic nerve

(e.g., optic neuritis). STIR images have very low signal from fat but have high signal from water.

38. **What is FLAIR?**
FLAIR is fluid attenuated inversion recovery. This method teliminates bright signals from fluid, allowing a strong T2-weighted image to remain, which is useful for identifying multiple sclerosis (MS) plaques and ischemia. CSF looks dark (unlike in typical T2), allowing bright MS plaques to be visualized better.

39. **What is diffusion-weighted imaging (DWI) sequence?**
DWI sequence is used to image acute cerebral infarctions within the first hour of a stroke. Ischemia looks bright on DWI. These abnormalities are not detected on other MRI sequences or CT scans.

40. **List few indications of MRI.**
    i. Optic nerve lesions—intraorbital part of optic nerve and intracranial extensions of optic nerve tumors
    ii. Optic nerve sheath lesions (e.g., meningioma)
    iii. Sellar masses
    iv. Cavernous sinus pathology
    v. Intracranial lesions of the visual pathway
    vi. Intracranial aneurysm

41. **What are the contraindications of MRI?**
    i. Presence of metal (aneurysm clips, cochlear implants, pacemakers)
    ii. Cardiac bypass surgery patients (up to 1 month following surgery as there may be local bleeding at the site of metallic materials)
    iii. Claustrophobic patients (difficult to perform)

42. **Differentiate between CT and MRI.**

CT	MRI
• Better for bony lesions	• Better for soft-tissue delineation
• Sensitive to acute hemorrhage	• Insensitive to acute hemorrhage
• Posterior fossa degraded by artifact	• Posterior fossa well visualized
• Poor resolution of demyelinating lesions	• Demyelinating lesions well seen at all stages
• Degraded image of orbital apex because of bony artifact	• Good view of orbital apex
• Metal artifacts	• Ferromagnetic artifacts
• Axial and coronal images	• Axial, coronal, sagittal, and angled images
• Iodinated contrast agent	• Paramagnetic contrast agent
• Risk: Ionizing radiation	• Risk: Magnetic field
• Less claustrophobic	• More claustrophobic
• Less expensive	• More expensive

43. What structures are better delineated on MRI than CT?
  i. Distinction between optic nerve and its surrounding subarachnoid space
  ii. Intracanalicular optic nerve
  iii. Contents of superior orbital fissure
  iv. Intraorbital branches of cranial nerves
  v. Lens, choroids, and ciliary apparatus

44. What is the finding in pituitary macroadenoma?
A classic "snow-man" or "figure of eight" appearance of pituitary macroadenoma is seen in gadolinium-enhanced T1-weighted image as it passes through the diaphragma sellae to extend into suprasellar cistern.

45. How do you differentiate optic neuritis and optic nerve meningioma in MRI?
Optic nerve enhancement (T1 with gadolinium) can differentiate between optic nerve sheath meningioma and optic neuritis. In optic neuritis, gadolinium enhancement is transient, remitting in days, whereas the optic nerve enhancement in optic nerve sheath meningioma persists.

46. What is MR angiography?
MR angiography is a noninvasive method of imaging intra- and extracranial carotids and vertebrobasilar circulation to demonstrate stenosis, dissection, occlusion, AV malformations, and aneurysms.

47. What are the advantages and disadvantages of MR angiography over CT angiography?
Advantage: Does not require contrast
Disadvantage: Small aneurysms and thrombosed aneurysms may be missed.

CHAPTER 2

Cornea

2.1 KERATOMETRY

1. **Define keratometry.**
   Keratometry is the measurement of the curvature of the anterior surface of the cornea across a fixed chord length, usually 2-3 mm, which lies in the optical spherical zone of the cornea.

2. **Who first invented the keratometer?**
   The keratometer was first invented by Helmholtz in 1854. He called it the ophthalmometer. His instrument was made of two glass plates.

3. **Who modified Helmholtz's instrument for clinical use?**
   Javal and Schiotz

4. **Explain the optical principle of the keratometer.**
   The principle of the keratometer is based on the geometry of a spherical reflecting surface. The anterior surface of the cornea acts as a convex mirror, and the size of the image formed (first Purkinje image) varies with its curvature—inversely.

   An object of known size and distance is reflected off the corneal surface, and the size of the reflected image is determined with a measuring telescope. From this, the refracting power of the cornea can be calculated based on an assumed index of refraction.

5. **What is the principle of visible doubling? Why is it necessary to have double images?**
   The image formed on the corneal surface is made to double using prisms. The keratometric reading is calculated by adjusting it such that the lower edge of one image coincides with the upper edge of the other. From the amount of rotation needed to coincide the edges, the image size is measured by the instrument, and thereby the corneal curvature can be calculated.

   It is necessary to have double images to overcome the problem of movement of the eyes during measurements. If the eye moves, both images move together and equally.

6. **How is doubling achieved in the Javal–Schiotz keratometer?**
   In the Javal–Schiotz keratometer, doubling is achieved by a Wollaston prism, which is incorporated in the viewing telescope. A Wollaston prism consists of two rectangular quartz prisms cemented together. Quartz, being a doubly refractive substance, splits a single beam of light to form two polarized light beams.

7. **Name some keratometers.**
   i. Helmholtz keratometer (not used now)
   ii. Reichert (Bausch and Lomb keratometer)—constant object size, variable image size
   iii. Javal–Schiotz keratometer—variable object size, constant image size

8. **What is the relationship between the radius of curvature and dioptric power of the cornea?**
   $$D = (n - 1)/r$$
   where D is the dioptric power of the cornea.
   n is the index of refraction of the cornea.
   r is the radius of the cornea in meters.
   n is usually taken as 1.3375.

9. **What range of corneal curvature can be measured by keratometry?**
   The Bausch and Lomb keratometer measures the radius of curvature from 36.00 to 52.00 D.

10. **What are the keratometric findings in a spherical cornea?**
    There is no difference in power between the two principal meridians. The mires are seen as a perfect sphere.

11. **What are the findings in astigmatism?**
    In astigmatism, there is a difference in power between the two meridians. With-the-rule (WTR) corneal astigmatism—mires will be vertically oval. Against-the-rule (ATR) corneal astigmatism—mires look like a horizontal oval.
    Oblique astigmatism—the principal meridian is between 30–60° and 120–50°. Irregular astigmatism—mires are irregular or doubled.

12. **What are the keratometric findings in keratoconus?**
    Pulsating mires are indicative of keratoconus.
    i. *Early signs:* Inclination and jumping of mires (While attempting to adjust the mires, they jump. If an attempt is made to superimpose the plus mires, they will jump above and below each other.)
    ii. *Other signs:* Minification of mires: In advanced keratoconus ($K > 52$ D), the mires begin to get smaller due to an increased amount of myopia

Oval mires: They occur due to a large amount of astigmatism. The mires are of normal size and have distinct borders. This is also called egg-shaped mires

iii. *Distortion of mires:* The mire image is irregular, wavy, and distorted

13. **Give some clinical uses of keratometry.**
    i. Objective method for determining the curvature of the cornea
    ii. To estimate the amount and direction of corneal astigmatism
    iii. Ocular biometry for intraocular lens (IOL) power calculation
    iv. To monitor pre- and post-surgical astigmatism
    v. Differential diagnosis of axial versus refractive anisometropia
    vi. To diagnose and monitor keratoconus and other corneal diseases
    vii. For contact lens fitting by base curve selection
    viii. To detect rigid gas permeable lens flexure

14. **What are the sources of error in keratometry?**
    i. Improper calibration
    ii. Faulty positioning of the patient
    iii. Improper fixation by the patient
    iv. Accommodative fluctuation by the examiner
    v. Localized corneal distortion, excessive tearing, abnormal lid position
    vi. Improper focusing of the corneal image

15. **What are the new types of keratometers?**
    i. *Automated keratometer:* The reflected image is focused onto a photodetector, which measures the image size, and then the radius of curvature is computed. Infrared light is used to illuminate the mires, as well as in the photodetector
    ii. *Surgical/operating keratometer:* Keratometer attached to the operating microscope

16. **Name other methods of studying corneal curvature.**
    i. Placido disk
    ii. Corneal topography

17. **What are the limitations of keratometry?**
    i. The keratometer assumes that the cornea is a symmetrical spherical or spherocylindrical structure with two principal meridians separated by 90°, whereas in reality, the cornea is an aspheric structure
    ii. The refractive status of only a very small central area of the cornea is measured, neglecting the peripheral zones
    iii. Inaccurate for very flat or very steep corneas, i.e., effective only for a certain range of corneal curvatures
    iv. Ineffective in irregular astigmatism, thus, cannot be used for corneal surface irregularities.

2.2 CORNEAL VASCULARIZATION

1. **What are the factors maintaining transparency of the cornea?**
   A. *Anatomical factors:*
      i. Regular arrangement of the epithelium, which maintains the homogeneity of the refractive index throughout the cornea
      ii. Uniform arrangements of corneal stromal lamellae
      iii. Avascularity
      iv. Barrier function of the endothelium by active (pump) and passive mechanisms (by preventing fluid ingress)
   B. *Physiological factors:*
      i. Relative state of dehydration
      ii. Metabolism of the cornea
      iii. Higher differences between the refractive index of the cornea and air

2. **What are the factors that make a normal avascular cornea vascular?**
   Anything that breaks the normal compactness of the cornea:
   i. Trauma
   ii. Inflammatory
   iii. Toxic
   iv. Nutritional
   v. Presence of vasoformative stimulus

3. **Classify corneal vascularization according to the depth of involvement.**
   i. *Superficial:* Originates from the superficial limbal plexus
   ii. *Interstitial:* It is derived from anterior ciliary arteries
   iii. *Deep or retrocorneal pannus:* It is seen in syphilitic cause of interstitial keratitis

4. **What is pannus?**
   Pannus is the growth of fibrovascular tissue between the epithelium and Bowman's layer. It literally means cloth. It can be degenerative or inflammatory.

   There are four types of pannus:
   i. Pannus trachomatous
   ii. Pannus leprosus
   iii. Pannus phlyctenulosis
   iv. Pannus degenerativas: Associated with blind eyes, such as in bullous keratopathy

5. **What is micropannus and what are its causes?**
   When vascularization extends beyond 1-2 mm from the normal vasculature. The causes are:

i. Inclusion conjunctivitis
ii. Vernal conjunctivitis
iii. Superficial limbic keratoconjunctivitis
iv. Staphylococcal blepharitis
v. Childhood trachoma
vi. Contact lens wear

6. **What is gross pannus and what are its causes?**
   When vascularization extends beyond >2 mm from the normal vasculature. The causes are:
   i. Trachoma
   ii. Staphylococcal blepharitis
   iii. Atopic keratoconjunctivitis
   iv. Rosacea
   v. Herpes simplex keratitis

7. **What is progressive pannus and regressive pannus?**
   i. *Progressive pannus:* Infiltration is ahead of vascularization
   ii. *Regressive pannus:* Vascularization is ahead of infiltration

8. **How do you treat corneal vascularization?**
   i. By treating acute inflammatory cause, if any, vascularization decreases
   ii. *Radiation:* Applicable to the destruction of superficial rather than deep vessels
   It acts by causing the development of endarteritis resulting from trauma to endothelium
   iii. *Surgery:*
   - *Peritomy:* Removal of an annulus of conjunctival and subconjunctival tissue dissected outward from the limbus for 3-4 mm
   - *Superficial keratectomy:* When vascularization is superficial or circumferential
   - *Argon laser photocoagulation*

9. **How do you differentiate between superficial and deep vessels?**
   i. Superficial vessels are usually arranged in an arborizing pattern, present below the epithelial layer, and their continuity can be traced with the conjunctival vessels. They are dark red in color, and they branch dichotomously
   ii. Deep vessels are usually straight, lie in the stroma, not anastomosing, and their continuity cannot be traced beyond the limbus. They are pink in color

10. **How are deep vessels arranged?**

    Deep vessels may be arranged as:
    i. Terminal loops
    ii. Brush
    iii. Parasol
    iv. Umbel
    v. Network
    vi. Interstitial arcade

11. **What is the role of anti-vascular endothelial growth factor (VEGF) in corneal neovascularization?**

    The anti-VEGF will act on newly formed endothelial buds without pericytes. These drugs are tried in diabetic neovascularization. In corneal vascularization, once the vessels become mature with pericytes, these drugs are of limited value. Subconjunctival injections are tried to prevent new vessel formation after keratoplasty in highly vascularized corneas.

2.3 CORNEAL ANESTHESIA

1. **What is the nerve supply of the cornea?**
   Long ciliary nerve, a branch of nasociliary nerve, which is a branch of the ophthalmic division of the trigeminal nerve, supplies the cornea.

2. **What are the branches of the nasociliary nerve?**
   The nasociliary nerve, a branch of the ophthalmic division of the trigeminal nerve, has the following five branches:
   i. Nerve to the ciliary ganglion
   ii. Long ciliary nerves
   iii. Anterior ethmoidal nerve
   iv. Posterior ethmoidal nerve
   v. Infratrochlear nerve

3. **How is the cornea innervated?**

   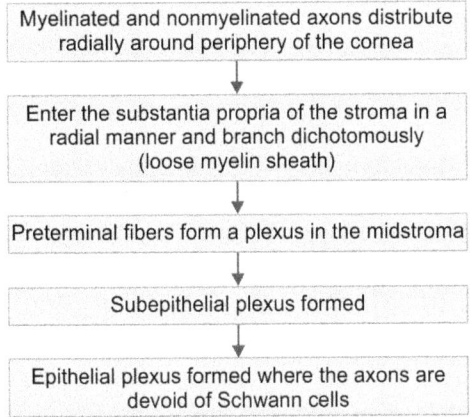

4. **Which part of the cornea is more sensitive?**
   The innervation density is more at the center and decreases fivefold toward the limbus.

5. **How much time does it take for nerves to regenerate?**
   By 4 weeks, a normal innervation pattern is seen, though neural density may be less. The center of the wound is devoid of sensation for >2 weeks.

6. **With which instrument can you measure corneal sensations?**
   Corneal sensations can be tested using a wisp of cotton. In order to quantitate, one can use an instrument called esthesiometer.
   Esthesiometer: Nylon monofilament of 0.08–0.12 mm diameter covers 4–10 corneal epithelial cells. Thus, it stimulates one sensitive nervous unit.

7. **What are the neurotransmitters that play a role in corneal sensations?**
   i. Substance P for pain
   ii. Calcitonin gene-related protein
   iii. Catecholamines—loss of this may lead to epithelial breakdown like that in neurotropic keratitis
   iv. Acetylcholine—levels related to corneal sensations

8. **What are the physiological variations in corneal sensations?**
   i. Most sensitive at apex and least at superior limbus
   ii. Sensitivity lowest in the morning and highest in the evening
   iii. Sensitivity decreases with age

9. **What are the conditions that affect corneal sensitivity?**
   i. *Congenital:*
      - Congenital trigeminal anesthesia
      - Corneal dystrophies—lattice dystrophy, Bassen-Kornzweig syndrome, Pierre-Romberg syndrome, iris nevus syndrome
   ii. *Acquired:*
      - *Diabetes mellitus:* Reduces sensitivity
      - Herpes simplex keratitis
      - Leprosy
      - *Adie's tonic pupil:* Lesion is in ciliary ganglion or short ciliary nerves, where the nerves serving corneal sensations and those supplying the iris sphincter run side by side
      - Myasthenia gravis
      - *Toxic corneal hypoesthesia:* Carbon disulfide, hydrogen sulfide used as pesticides
   iii. *Physiological:*
      - Iris color—lighter the iris color, more the sensitivity
      - Gender—more sensitive in males than females
      - *Eyelid closure:* Decreases sensitivity. This is due to depressed acetylcholine levels with lid close. This is the reason for low corneal sensitivity in the morning after a night's sleep
   iv. *Pharmacological:*
      - Surface anesthetics such as 4% lignocaine and 0.5% proparacaine
      - Beta-blockers—temporary decrease
      - Sodium sulfacetamide—30% solution decreases sensitivity
      - Atropine—decreases sensitivity after 10 minutes of instillation
      This is due to decreased acetylcholine.
   v. *Hormonal:*
      - Preovulatory reduction in corneal sensations due to estrogen rise
      - Decreased corneal sensitivity during pregnancy

vi. *Mechanical:*
   - *Contact lens:* Decreases corneal sensitivity. This may be attributed to the decrease in oxygen pressure at the epithelial level
vii. *Surgical:*
   - *Limbal incisions:* After cataract surgery, the upper half of the cornea may have decreased sensitivity for more than a year
   - *Corneal grafts:* Sensitivity may recover within 2 years
   - *Refractive surgeries:* Laser-assisted in situ keratomileusis (LASIK) decreases sensations
   - *Other procedures:* Photocoagulation and retinal detachment surgeries
   - *Trigeminal denervation:* Decreases sensitivity

10. **When will you suspect corneal anesthesia?**
    i. Persistent nonhealing corneal defect
    ii. Symptoms are very less as compared to the epithelial defect

11. **How will you treat corneal anesthesia?**
    i. A central tarsorrhaphy may be necessary to promote healing
    ii. Corneal grafting will give disastrous results in the presence of corneal anesthesia.

2.4 CORNEAL DEPOSITS

1. **What are the causes of superficial corneal deposits?**
   i. *Pigmented:*
      - Iron lines
      - Spheroidal degeneration
      - Adrenochrome
      - Pigmented (noncalcified) band keratopathy
      - Cornea verticillata
      - Epithelial melanosis
      - Drugs—amiodarone, phenothiazines, epinephrine
      - Metals—iron, gold, copper
      - Blood
      - Bilirubin
      - Corneal tattooing
   ii. *Nonpigmented:*
      - Calcific band keratopathy
      - Subepithelial mucinous dystrophy
      - Coats' white ring
      - Drug deposits—amiodarone
   iii. *Refractile/crystalline:*
      - Meesmann's dystrophy
      - Superficial amyloid
      - Tyrosinemia
      - Intraepithelial ointment
      - Gout

2. **What are the causes of stromal deposits?**
   i. *Pigmented:*
      - Blood staining
      - Siderosis
      - Bilirubin
      - Ochronosis
   ii. *Nonpigmented:*
      - Granular dystrophy
      - Macular dystrophy
      - Fleck dystrophy
      - Lipid deposition
      - Mucopolysaccharidosis
   iii. *Refractile/crystalline:*
      - Lattice dystrophy
      - Schnyder's dystrophy
      - Bietti's crystalline dystrophy

3. **Which are the various iron lines?**
    i. *Stocker's line:* At head of pterygium
    ii. *Hudson-Stahli line:* In palpebral area seen in old age
    iii. *Ferry's line:* At the border of a filtering bleb
    iv. *Fleischer's ring:* Surrounding the cone in keratoconus
    v. Between radial keratotomy incisions
    vi. Adjacent to contour changing pathology, like in Salzmann nodular degeneration

4. **What is the reason for iron staining?**
   Tear pooling at the site of contour change will cause iron deposition.

5. **At what level of the cornea is spheroidal degeneration located?**
   Bowman's layer and anterior stroma

6. **What are the deposits in spheroidal degeneration?**
   Protein-rich matrix containing tryptophan, tyrosine, cystine, cysteine

7. **What kinds of deposits are seen with epinephrine eye drops in glaucoma?**
   Adrenochrome deposits

8. **When does blood staining of the cornea occur?**
   It occurs in the presence of hyphema due to two reasons:
    i. Rise in intraocular pressure
    ii. Compromised endothelium
       The initial appearance of yellow granules within the posterior stroma is a sign of the need of evacuation of hyphema.

9. **How does blood staining in the cornea clear?**
   It clears from the periphery to the center due to the scavenging action of leukocytes, which are present in perilimbal blood vessels.

10. **Where is the Hudson-Stahli line found?**
    Hudson-Stahli line is the most common iron line, located in the lower third of the cornea in the epithelium.
     i. Usually run horizontally, higher nasally, and lower temporally
     ii. Typical bilateral and symmetric
     iii. Altered by various factors such as corneal scar and contact lens wear
     iv. Increases in length and density with time
     v. Seen in as young as 2 years and increases with age up to 70 years

11. **In which condition is the Kayser-Fleischer (KF) ring seen?**
     i. It is seen in Wilson's disease (hepatolenticular degeneration), which is a condition of altered copper metabolism
     ii. It is seen before any nervous symptoms develop

iii. It is a yellow–brown or green ring seen in the peripheral cornea
iv. Deposit is at the level of Descemet's membrane
v. When chelating agents are given, the line disappears

12. How do you differentiate between a picture of arcus senilis and KF ring?

Arcus has a clear intervening space between the limbus and the line called the clear zone of Vogt, whereas the KF ring comes from copper from perilimbal blood vessels. There is no intervening space between the limbus and the line.

13. What are the causes of epithelial melanosis?
   i. *Congenital:* Nevi
   ii. *Sequelae of trachoma and other inflammations* due to migration of conjunctival melanoblasts from the limbus
   iii. *Striate melano keratosis of Cowen:* Normally, it occurs in darkly pigmented individuals. Pigmented lines located in the epithelium extend from the limbus to the central cornea. Probably, they result from migration of pigmented limbal stem cells onto the cornea

14. What are the causes of endothelial melanosis?
   i. *Congenital senile degenerative:* Myopia, diabetes senile cataract, chronic glaucoma
   ii. *Mosaic pigmentation of Vogt:* Outlines the endothelial cells
   iii. *Turk's line:* Due to convection current in the anterior chamber
   iv. *Krukenberg's spindles:* Accentuation of the general atrophic process in which pigment derived from the uveal tract is deposited on the corneal endothelium and aggregated in the shape of a spindle. They are seen in the pupillary axis.

2.5 BACTERIAL AND FUNGAL CORNEAL ULCERS

1. **What are the organisms capable of penetrating intact cornea?**
   i. *Neisseria gonorrhoeae*
   ii. *Haemophilus influenzae*
   iii. *Corynebacterium diphtheriae*
   iv. *Listeria*

2. **What are the common bacteria causing keratitis in India?**
   The most common causes of bacterial keratitis in our country are:
   i. Gram-positive organism:
      – *Streptococcus pneumoniae*
   ii. Gram-negative organism:
      – *Pseudomonas aeruginosa*
   iii. Acid-fast organism:
      – *Nocardia*

3. **What are the common predisposing factors to keratitis?**
   i. Trauma
   ii. Contact lens wear
   iii. Preexisting corneal diseases—trauma, bullous keratopathy, and decreased corneal sensation
   iv. Other factors—chronic blepharoconjunctivitis, dacryocystitis, tear film deficiency, topical steroid therapy, hypovitaminosis A

4. **Which is the most common organism causing keratitis in patients with chronic dacryocystitis?**
   S. pneumoniae

5. **Which is the most common organism among contact lens wearers?**
   P. aeruginosa

6. **What are the typical features of bacterial keratitis?**
   i. Symptoms are more than the signs, and there will be lot of conjunctival congestion, discharge, and chemosis
   ii. Sharp epithelial demarcation with well-defined borders
   iii. Underlying dense, suppurative stromal inflammation

7. **What are the characteristic features of specific bacterial keratitis?**
   i. Gram-positive cocci (such as *S. pneumonia*) cause localized, round, or oval ulcerations with distinct borders
   ii. Ulcus serpens or serpiginous keratitis is also caused by *S. pneumoniae*
   iii. Gram-negative bacilli, such as *Pseudomonas*, cause a rapid, fulminating ulcer with a lot of suppuration and discharge and produce an hourglass appearance in a matter of days

iv. *Moraxella* causes indolent ulcers in debilitated individuals
v. *Nocardia* typically causes a wreath-shaped ulcer that is superficial spreading

8. **How do you do microbiology investigations in a case of corneal ulcer?**
    i. Proparacaine is used as the topical anesthetic of choice since it has the fewest inhibitory effects on the recovery of microorganisms
    ii. Corneal scraping should be performed along the edges and the base of the ulcer. For example, *S. pneumoniae* is recovered from the edges, while *Moraxella* is recovered from the base
    iii. Avoid touching the conjunctiva and eyelashes
    iv. A Kimura spatula can be routinely used. A calcium alginate swab is supposed to give better recovery rates
    v. Smears can be placed on the central part of the slide in an area marked on the reverse
    vi. Culture plates are streaked using a C-shaped design

9. **Name commonly used stains.**
    i. Gram stain
    ii. Acridine orange
    iii. Calcofluor-white
    iv. Giemsa

10. **Which stains require fluorescence microscopy?**
    Acridine orange, calcofluor-white

11. **What are the steps in Gram stain?**
    i. Fix the slide in methyl alcohol
    ii. Flood the slide with crystal gentian violet for 1 minute
    iii. Rinse and flood with Gram's iodine for 1 minute
    iv. Rinse and decolorize with acid alcohol for 20 seconds
    v. Counterstain with dilute carbol fuchsin (safranin) for 1 minute

12. **What is the principle behind Gram stain?**
    Gram-positive organisms have a thicker peptidoglycan layer in their cell wall, which makes them more permeable to the primary stain than gram-negative organisms. Gram-positive bacteria retain the gentian violet–iodine complex and appear purple. Gram-negative bacteria lose the gentian violet–iodine complex with the decolorization step and appear pink when counterstained with safranin.

13. **What is the use of Giemsa's stain?**
    Apart from distinguishing between bacteria and fungi, Giemsa helps to understand the normal and abnormal cellular morphology (such as inflammatory cells).

14. **Name common antibiotics active against gram-positive bacteria.**
    i. Cefazolin (50 mg/mL)
    ii. Chloramphenicol (5-10 mg/mL)
    iii. Moxifloxacin
    iv. Vancomycin (15-50 mg/mL)

15. **Name common antibiotics active against gram-negative bacteria.**
    i. Tobramycin (3-14 mg/mL)
    ii. Gentamicin (3-14 mg/mL)
    iii. Amikacin (20 mg in 0.5 mL)
    iv. Ceftazidime
    v. Ciprofloxacin (3 mg/mL)
    vi. Levofloxacin (3 mg/mL)
    vii. Ofloxacin (3 mg/mL)

16. **How do you make fortified antibiotics?**
    i. *Gentamicin:* Add 2 mL of injectable gentamycin to 5 mL of commercial topical preparation.
    5 mL commercial preparation has—15 mg
    Added drug 2 mL—80 mg
    Total in 7 mL—95 mg
    1 mL contains—13.5 mg
    ii. *Cefazolin:* Add 5 mL or 10 mL of distilled water or sterile saline to a 500 mg vial of cefazolin to obtain a 10% or 5% solution
    iii. *Vancomycin:* Add 10 mL of distilled water or saline to a 500 mg vial of vancomycin and obtain a 5% solution
    iv. *Amikacin:* Add 10 mL of distilled water to 100 mg of amikacin to get 1% solution

17. **What are the advantages of using fortified eye drops?**
    i. For resistant microbial keratitis, to attain an appropriate drug concentration and to stop the fulminant rapid progression of keratitis
    ii. For moderate to severe corneal ulcers
    iii. For pediatric patients as ocular surface bacterial infections affect with a high frequency in newborns and children
    iv. For drugs that are available only in the parenteral form. For example, vancomycin and amphotericin B
    Limitations:
    i. High cost
    ii. Contaminant risk
    iii. Since it is a preservative-free preparation, they have a short shelf-life
    iv. Need for refrigeration

18. **What are the typical features of fungal keratitis?**
    i. Signs more than symptoms
    ii. Feathery margins
    iii. Raised dry surface
    iv. Satellite lesions
    v. Endothelial plaques
    vi. Cheesy hypopyon
    vii. Gritty texture while scraping

19. **Classify fungi.**
    i. *Yeast* (e.g., *Candida, Cryptococcus neoformans, Rhinosporidium*)
    ii. *Filamentous*—septate and nonseptate
    Septate:
    Fusarium, Aspergillus, Curvularia
    Nonseptate:
    Mucor, Rhizopus
    iii. *Dimorphic:*
    Histoplasmosis

20. **What are the most common fungi infecting the cornea?**
    i. *Fusarium*
    ii. *Aspergillus flavus*
    iii. *Aspergillus fumigatus*

21. **How to differentiate *Nocardia* from the fungal filament in KOH mount?**
    Nocardia is slender, branching, and thinner than fungal hyphae.

22. **Name common media used for fungal culture.**
    i. Sabouraud's dextrose agar
    ii. Potato dextrose agar
    iii. Brain-heart infusion
    iv. Blood agar

23. **Classify antifungals.**
    i. *Polyenes*
       - Larger molecular weight:
         Amphotericin, nystatin
       - Smaller molecular weight:
         Natamycin
    ii. *Azoles*
        Clotrimazole, voriconazole, miconazole, ketoconazole, econazole
    iii. *Antimetabolites*
         Flucytosine

24. **What is the drug of choice in filamentous fungal infection?**
    Natamycin 5% suspension (especially for *Fusarium*).

25. **What is the mechanism of action of amphotericin?**
    Amphotericin is effective against *Aspergillus*. It selectively binds to sterol present in the plasma membrane of susceptible fungi and alters membrane permeability.

26. **What is the dose of amphotericin?**
    i. *Topical:* 0.1–0.2% hourly initially
    ii. *Anterior chamber irrigation:* 500 µg in 0.1 mL of normal saline
    iii. *Intravitreal:* 5 µg in 0.1 mL of normal saline

27. **How is amphotericin available?**
    Amphotericin is available as 50 mg dose in a vial. It has to be stored in dark-colored bottles to avoid exposure to light.

28. **What is the mechanism of action of imidazoles?**
    At lower concentration, it inhibits ergosterol synthesis, and at higher concentration, it causes direct damage to the fungal cell membrane.

29. **What are the indications of oral antifungals?**
    i. Deeper ulcers not responding to topical therapy
    ii. Ulcers involving the limbus and extending to the sclera
    In such cases, ketoconazole tablets (200 mg bd) can be used after assessing liver function tests

30. **What are the complications of corneal ulcer?**
    i. Descemetocele
    ii. Perforation
    iii. Anterior synechiae
    iv. Secondary glaucoma
    v. Cataract
    vi. Purulent iridocyclitis
    vii. Endophthalmitis

31. **What is the difference between hypopyon in bacterial and fungal corneal ulcer?**

Hypopyon in bacterial ulcer	Hypopyon in fungal ulcer
Sterile (bacteria cannot invade intact Descemet's membrane)	Infective
Fluid, move according to head posture	Thick and immobile

32. **Write briefly on voriconazole.**
    Voriconazole is a new azole derived from fluconazole. It is active against *Aspergillus*, *Fusarium*, and *Candida*. It inhibits cytochrome

P450-dependent 14-sterol demethylase, an enzyme responsible for the conversion of lanosterol to 14-demethyl-lanosterol.

33. **What are the signs to know whether the ulcer is healing?**
    i. Blunting of the edges of the perimeter of stromal infiltrate
    ii. Decreased density of stromal infiltrate
    iii. Decrease in stromal edema and endothelial plaque
    iv. Decrease in anterior chamber reaction and reduction in the size of hypopyon
    v. Re-epithelization
    vi. Cessation in corneal thinning

34. **What are the causes and signs of nonhealing corneal ulcers?**
    A. *Causes for nonhealing corneal ulcers:*
        i. Inadequate and inappropriate therapy
        ii. Noncompliance to treatment
        iii. Meibomitis
        iv. Trichiasis
        v. Chronic dacryocystitis
        vi. Diabetes mellitus
    B. *Signs of nonhealing ulcer:*
        i. Increase in size of the stromal infiltrate
        ii. Increased density of stromal infiltrate
        iii. Increase in stromal edema and endothelial plaque
        iv. Increase in anterior chamber reaction and increase in size of hypopyon
        v. Absence of re-epithelization
        vi. Progressive corneal thinning

35. **What are the signs of impending corneal perforation and frank perforation?**
    A. *Descemetocele:* Radiating folds in Descemet's membrane are a sign of impending perforation. Descemet folds seen at the base of ulceration. Central clear zone within areas of thinning.
    B. *Signs of perforated ulcer:*
        i. Uveal prolapse
        ii. Positive Seidels test
        iii. Flat or shallow anterior chamber

36. **What are the indications for keratoplasty in infective keratitis?**
    i. Perforated corneal ulcer
    ii. Impending perforation
    iii. Nonhealing corneal ulcer in spite of appropriate and adequate antimicrobial therapy
    iv. Ulcer threatening to involve the limbus

37. **What are the principles in doing therapeutic keratoplasty?**
    i. The aim is to control and eliminate the infection
    ii. The infected tissue along with 1 mm of uninvolved corneal tissue is removed
    iii. A peripheral iridectomy is performed
    iv. Interrupted sutures are used so that selective suture removal can be performed in indicated cases
    v. Postoperatively, antibiotics are used for ulcers caused by bacteria, and antifungals are used for fungal ulcers. Topical steroids are contraindicated in therapeutic keratoplasty done for fungal keratitis

38. **How do you treat nonhealing corneal ulcers?**
    i. First step is to reculture to identify/confirm the initial organism
    ii. Recheck adnexal structures, especially for dacryocystitis
    iii. Intrastromal injection of antimicrobials may be tried
    iv. Tarsorrhaphy

39. **What are the results of the MUTT (Mycotic Ulcer Treatment Trial)?**
    Natamycin is better than voriconazole in treating filamentary fungal keratitis, especially for keratitis caused by *Fusarium*.

2.6 ACANTHAMOEBA KERATITIS

1. **What is *Acanthamoeba*?**
   Acanthamoeba is a freely-living protozoa commonly found in soil, dust, fresh or brackish water, and upper respiratory tract in humans.

2. **What are the different species of *Acanthamoeba*?**
   The different species of *Acanthamoeba* have been classified on the basis of their cyst morphology and isoenzyme into eight species, out of which two of them, namely *Acanthamoeba castellani* and *Acanthamoeba polyphaga*, are implicated in causing corneal infections.

3. **What are the different forms/life cycle of *Acanthamoeba*?**
   i. Cystic (dormant) form
   ii. Trophozoite (active) form

4. **What is the cause of *Acanthamoeba* keratitis (AK)?**
   A. *Western world:* It is commonly associated with contact lens (CL) wear.
      Contact lenses:
      i. CL users (extended wear CL users are at a greater risk)
      ii. Homemade saline as a substitute for CL solution
      iii. CL wears in contaminated waters like swimming with CL
   B. *Indian scenario:* It is commonly associated with contaminated water.
      Trauma:
      Exposure to contaminated water or soil (agricultural population). Tanker-fed water at home, cooling towers, air filters
      Surgery:
      Penetrating keratoplasty
      Radial keratotomy

5. **Why is so much importance given to contact lenses in evaluating a case of AK?**
   This is because AK can spread in numerous ways in relation to contact lenses.
   i. Use of tap water in making CL solutions
   ii. Swimming in a swimming pool/sea (contaminated)
   iii. Shower while wearing lenses
   iv. Minor corneal damage or abrasion, which can happen with CL use itself, can cause AK

6. **What is the pathogenesis of AK?**
   Upon binding to the mannose glycoprotein of the corneal epithelium, *Acanthamoeba* secretes proteins that are cytolytic to the epithelium, as well as proteases, which cause further penetration.

7. **What is the presenting symptom in AK?**
   The common symptom is disproportionate pain compared to the signs, associated with blurred vision.

8. **What is the reason for pain in AK?**
   i. Radial keratoneuritis
   ii. Limbitis
   iii. Scleritis

9. **What are the signs of AK?**
   The signs mimic viral keratitis in many ways; they are classified as early and late.
   Early:
   i. Epithelial irregularity (dirty looking, stippled unhealthy epithelium)
   ii. Pseudodendrites
   iii. Radial keratoneuritis
   iv. Stromal infiltration
   v. Satellite lesions
   vi. Disciform lesion
   Late:
   i. Ring infiltrate (oval-shaped, which is characteristic of this disease)
   ii. Stromal opacification
   iii. Scleritis
   iv. Descemetocele formation

10. **What are the investigations done in AK?**
    Noninvasive:
    i. Confocal microscopy
    Invasive:
    i. Gram and Giemsa stain
    ii. Calcofluor white stain
    iii. 10% KOH mount
    iv. Acridine orange
    v. Immunofluorescent antibody stain
    vi. Periodic acid-Schiff (PAS) and methenamine silver
    vii. Phase contrast microscope
    viii. Polymerase chain reaction (PCR)
    ix. Corneal biopsy

11. **How is *Acanthamoeba* grown in a microbiological environment?**
    The *Acanthamoeba* organism grows well on nonnutrient agar with *Escherichia coli* overlay. The organism creates a track by feeding on *E. coli*.

12. **What are the extracorneal complications of AK?**
    i. Scleritis
    ii. Cataract
    iii. Peripheral ulcerative keratitis
    iv. Glaucoma
    v. Iris atrophy
    vi. Chronic inflammation
    vii. Vascular thrombosis
    viii. Intraocular infection
    ix. The exact etiology of these complications is not known but is likely to be due to drug toxicity (biguanides) or the immune response of the body itself

13. **What are the differential diagnoses of AK?**
    The main differential diagnosis is herpes simplex keratitis (both epithelial and stromal keratitis) and fungal keratitis.

14. **What is the treatment of AK?**
    The treatment of AK can be classified as:
    Medical:
    i. *Biguanides*
        - Polyhexamethylene biguanide (PHMB) (0.02–0.06%)
        - Chlorhexidine 0.02–0.2%
    ii. *Diamidines*
        - Hexamidine 0.1%
        - Propamidine 0.1%
    iii. *Imidazole and triazole antifungals*
    iv. *Aminoglycosides (AMG)*
    v. *Polymyxins*
    Surgical:
    i. Epithelial debridement
    ii. Cryotherapy
    iii. Deep anterior lamellar keratoplasty
    iv. Penetrating keratoplasty

15. **What are the goals of treatment?**
    i. Eradication of trophozoites and cysts
    ii. Rapid resolution of immune response
    iii. Prevent recurrence
    iv. Prevention of complications

16. **What is the mechanism of action of biguanides?**
    Biguanides interact with the cytoplasmic membrane resulting in the loss of cellular components and inhibition of respiratory enzymes.

17. **What is the mechanism of action of diamidines?**
    Diamidines cause structural membrane changes affecting cell permeability. When the molecules enter the amebic cytoplasm, denaturation of cytoplasmic proteins and enzymes occurs. Hexamidine is a faster amebicidal drug than propamidine against trophozoites and cysts.

18. **Which is used as the first line of treatment between the two of the above classes of drugs?**
    Biguanides have shown less toxicity compared to diamidines, so biguanides are used as a first line, but both can be combined in a severe case of AK. It is believed to have an additive or synergistic effect.

19. **How would you prepare a 0.02% solution of PHMB?**
    The 20% parent solution is diluted 1,000 times with saline or sterile water.

20. **What is a major side effect of PHMB?**
    Vascularization of the cornea.

21. **How would you treat a case of limbitis and scleritis in a case of AK?**
    Both can be a cause of significant pain. It is due to severe posterior segment inflammation. Limbitis is an early as well as a late finding. It occurs commonly. It is treated with flurbiprofen 50–100 mg 2–3 times a day.
    Scleritis: It is less common. It responds well to nonsteroidal anti-inflammatory drugs (NSAIDs). If not, then systemic steroids are added.

22. **How would you treat a case of persistent epithelial defect?**
    To exclude superficial bacterial infection, which is very hard to distinguish in the presence of severe AK, topical therapy should be discontinued and nonpreserved prophylactic broad-spectrum antibiotic should be given to prevent bacterial superinfection. After signs of improvement are seen, antiamebic therapy is reintroduced.

23. **How does an epithelial debridement help?**
    Epithelial debridement helps in the following ways:
    i. It serves as a therapeutic and diagnostic tool
    ii. It helps in better drug penetration

24. **How is cryotherapy done?**
    Cryotherapy kills only the trophozoites but not cysts.
    A retinal cryoprobe is taken, and a freeze–thaw method is used until a ball of ice forms near the applicator in the stroma. In this manner, the whole of the cornea is treated. Endothelial failure is a side effect.

25. **When would you perform keratoplasty?**

    Keratoplasty is not required in most cases as medical therapy would suffice, but it is indicated in patients with:
    i. Nonhealing ulcer in spite of appropriate antiamebicidal therapy
    ii. Corneal perforation that does not respond to corneal gluing
    iii. Fulminant corneal abscess
    iv. Intumescent cataract

    Many of these eyes will have associated limbitis and scleritis, so they must be started on prednisolone (1 mg/kg/day) or cyclosporine (3.5–7.5 mg/kg/day), which is tapered in the postgraft period.

26. **What are the newer modes of keratoplasty useful in AK?**

    In the initial stages, the disease is fairly superficial, and hence, a lamellar keratoplasty or deep anterior lamellar keratoplasty can be used to considerably shorten the course of the disease.

2.7 VIRAL KERATITIS

1. **What are the common viruses causing keratitis?**
   i. Adenovirus
   ii. Herpes simplex virus
   iii. Herpes zoster

2. **What are the types of herpes simplex keratitis?**
   Primary infection is extremely rare, and almost all the cases that are seen are due to recurrent infections.
   i. *Epithelial keratitis:*
      - Superficial punctate keratitis
      - Dendritic keratitis
      - Geographic keratitis
   ii. *Subepithelial keratitis:*
      - Neurotrophic keratitis
   iii. *Stromal keratitis:*
      - Necrotizing keratitis
      - Nummular keratitis
      - Disciform keratitis
   iv. *Endothelium:*
      - Endothelitis

3. **What are the differential diagnoses of dendritic keratitis of herpes simplex?**
   i. Herpes zoster
   ii. Healing corneal abrasion
   iii. *Acanthamoeba* keratitis
   iv. Toxic keratitis due to topical drugs
   v. Contact lens-induced abrasions
   vi. Neurotrophic keratopathy

4. **What are the characteristics of a herpes simplex dendrite?**
   Herpes simplex dendrite is usually a central, slender, arborizing lesion with terminal end bulbs. The base of the ulcer stains with fluorescein (due to loss of cellular integrity), while the terminal end bulbs stain with rose bengal (due to lack of mucin binding by the cells).

5. **How will you treat dendritic keratitis?**
   i. *Debridement:* Helps by removing viral-laden cells and can be done for dendritic keratitis. It is not of any value for geographic keratitis
   ii. *Topical acyclovir:* 3% ointment administered five times daily for 2 weeks or topical trifluridine 1% solution eight times daily for 2 weeks

6. **What are the features of neurotrophic keratitis?**
   Neurotrophic keratitis, also called metaherpetic keratitis, is characterized by:
   i. Nonhealing epithelial defect after appropriate and adequate antiviral therapy
   ii. Raised margins
   iii. Underlying gray and opaque stroma
   Treatment is to stop antivirals and to use lubricants. In nonresponsive cases, it may be treated with bandage contact lenses or temporary tarsorrhaphy.

7. **What are the features of disciform keratitis?**
   Disciform keratitis causes defective vision and presents as fusiform stromal edema associated with keratic precipitates underlying the zone of the edema. Few inflammatory cells in the anterior chamber may be seen.

8. **What are the features of necrotizing keratitis?**
   Necrotizing keratitis, a type of viral stromal keratitis, mimics a bacterial or fungal suppurative infection. A previous history of recurrence of infection and the presence of corneal vascularization will help in the diagnosis.

9. **What are the findings of HEDS (Herpetic Eye Disease Study)?**
   i. Topical corticosteroids given together with prophylactic antiviral improve the outcome of stromal keratitis
   ii. There is no benefit of using oral acyclovir in treating stromal keratitis

10. **What are the features of a herpes zoster dendrite?**
    i. Herpes zoster dendrites are pseudodendrites
    ii. They are shorter, stockier, and elevated
    iii. They do not stain with fluorescein but stain with rose bengal

11. **What are the features of herpes-zoster ophthalmicus (HZO)?**
    i. *Lids:*
       - Scarring
       - Trichiasis
       - Marginal notching
       - Cicatricial ectropion or entropion
    ii. *Conjunctiva:*
       - Ischemia with necrosis
       - Circumcorneal congestion
    iii. *Cornea:*
       - Punctate keratitis
       - Dendritic keratitis
       - Stromal keratitis
       - Corneal anesthesia

    iv. *Iris:*
- Sectoral iris atrophy

    v. *Anterior chamber:*
- Hemorrhagic hypopyon

    vi. *Retina:*
- Focal choroiditis
- Occlusive retinal vasculitis
- Retinal detachment

    vii. *Orbit:*
- Ptosis
- Orbital edema
- Proptosis in some cases

    viii. *Central nervous system:*
- Papillitis
- Cranial nerve palsies (commonly third nerve involvement)

12. **What is the treatment for HZO?**
    i. Oral acyclovir 800 mg five times daily for 10–14 days
    ii. There is no use for topical antivirals
    iii. Topical steroids can be used for stromal keratitis
    iv. Oral corticosteroids can be used to reduce zoster pain, especially in older individuals
    v. Lubricants
    vi. Tarsorrhaphy in severe cases of neurotrophic keratitis

13. **How will you treat postherpetic neuralgia?**
    i. Capsaicin cream applied to the skin
    ii. Low doses of amitriptyline or carbamazepine
    iii. Oral gabapentin.

2.8 INTERSTITIAL KERATITIS

1. **What are the types of blepharitis?**
   Blepharitis is a subacute or chronic inflammation of the lid margin. It is clinically classified as:
   i. Bacterial or ulcerative blepharitis
   ii. Seborrheic or squamous blepharitis
   iii. Mixed staphylococcal with seborrheic blepharitis
   iv. Posterior blepharitis or meibomitis
   v. Parasitic blepharitis

2. **What are the corneal lesions caused by blepharitis?**
   i. *Blepharokeratoconjunctivitis:* It is commonly seen in posterior blepharitis, where there is chronic inflammation of the cornea, which may lead to scarring, vascularization, and opacity
   ii. *Marginal keratitis:* It is thought to be caused by a hypersensitivity reaction of staphylococcal toxin in bacterial blepharitis
   iii. *Dry eye:* It is due to tear film instability
   iv. Secondary corneal inflammation

3. **What is interstitial keratitis (IK)?**
   Vascularization and nonsuppurative infiltration affecting the corneal stroma, usually associated with a systemic disease.

4. **What are the causes of IK?**
   i. Congenital syphilis
   ii. Acquired syphilis
   iii. Tuberculosis
   iv. Leprosy
   v. Onchocerciasis
   vi. Infectious mononucleosis
   vii. Lymphogranuloma venereum (LGV)—segmental and highly vascularized
   viii. Cogan's syndrome
   ix. Herpes zoster
   x. Herpes simplex
   xi. Mumps—diffuse rapid involvement of whole cornea, D/D from all others by the rapidity with it clears
   xii. Rubeola
   xiii. Vaccinia
   xiv. Variola
   xv. Leishmaniasis
   xvi. Trypanosomiasis
   xvii. Hodgkin's disease (rare)

xviii. Kaposi's sarcoma (rare)
xix. Mycosis fungoides (rare)
xx. Sarcoid (rare)
xxi. Incontinentia pigmenti
xxii. Toxicity to drugs, such as arsenic
xxiii. Influenza (rare)

5. **What are the nonsystemic conditions that may result in IK?**
   i. Chemical burns
   ii. Chromium deficiency

6. **What is the most common cause of IK?**
   The most important cause is syphilis. Of this, 90% is due to congenital syphilis and the rest is due to acquired syphilis.

7. **When does IK develop in congenital syphilis?**
   IK usually occurs around the age of 5 years to early teens and is bilateral in 80%.

8. **When does IK occur in acquired cases?**
   IK can occur within a few days after the onset of infection, but it generally occurs 10 years later. The majority of the disease is unilateral.

9. **What are the stages?**
   i. *Progressive stage:* With pain, photophobia cloudy cornea, iridocyclitis
   ii. *Florid stage:* Acute inflammation of the eye with deep vascularization of the cornea
   iii. *Regressive stage:* Clearing starts from periphery. Ghost vessels may be present

10. **What are the complications of IK?**
    i. Splits in Descemet's membrane
    ii. Band keratoplasty
    iii. Corneal thinning
    iv. Lipid keratoplasty
    v. Salzmann degeneration
    vi. Glaucoma

11. **What are the systemic features of congenital syphilis?**
    i. History of previous stillbirths
    ii. Frontal bossing
    iii. Overgrowth of maxillary bones
    iv. Hutchinson's teeth—small band-shaped central permanent incisions
    v. Rhagades

vi. Saber shins
vii. Congenital deafness

12. **What is Hutchinson's triad?**
    i. Hutchinson's teeth
    ii. Deafness
    iii. IK

13. **What is Cogan's syndrome?**
    Nonsyphilitic IK, which is bilateral and painful, with vestibuloauditory symptoms.

14. **What are the other causes of IK?**
    i. *Tuberculosis:* Sector-shaped sclerokeratitis
    ii. *Leprosy:* May be associated with pannus.

2.9 MOOREN'S ULCER

1. **Define Mooren's ulcer.**
   Mooren's ulcer is an idiopathic, painful, peripheral ulcerative keratitis (PUK).

2. **What are the other names of Mooren's ulcer?**
   i. Chronic serpiginous ulcer
   ii. Ulcus rodens

3. **What are the symptoms of Mooren's ulcer?**
   i. Severe pain out of proportion to the size of the ulcer
   ii. Decreased visual acuity due to:
      - Central corneal involvement
      - Irregular astigmatism
      - Associated uveitis
      - Perforation

4. **Who described Mooren's ulcer?**
   Mooren's ulcer was first described by Bowman in 1849 and then by McKenzie in 1854 as "chronic serpiginous ulcer of the cornea or *ulcus roden*." Mooren's name, however, became attached to this rare disorder because of his publication of cases in 1863 and 1867. He was the first to clearly describe this insidious corneal problem and define it as a clinical entity.

5. **Describe the clinical presentation of Mooren's ulcer.**
   The initial presentation is a stromal infiltration of the peripheral cornea. The limbus is involved, in contrast to the other PUKs caused by rheumatoid arthritis (RA) and systemic lupus erythematosus (SLE).

   The clinical course of the ulcer is as follows:

   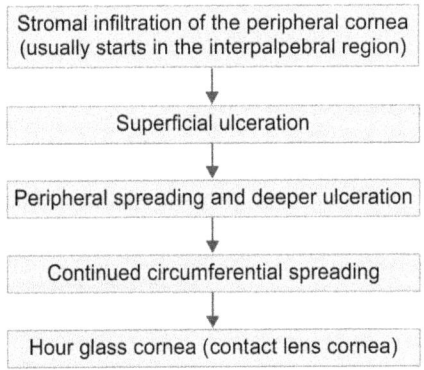

6. **Define PUK.**
   PUK is destruction of juxta-limbal cornea characterized by crescent-shaped destructive inflammation of the corneal stroma associated

with an epithelial defect, presence of stromal inflammatory cells, and progressive stromal degradation and thinning.

7. **Describe the two clinical types of Mooren's ulcer.**
   Type 1:
   i. Occurs in older individuals
   ii. Unilateral
   iii. Mild to moderate symptoms
   Type 2:
   i. Occurs in younger individuals, usually common among the black population
   ii. Bilateral and associated with worm infestation
   iii. Generally responds poorly to therapy

8. **What is Watson classification of Mooren's ulcer?**
   i. Unilateral Mooren's
   ii. Bilateral aggressive Mooren's
   iii. Bilateral indolent Mooren's

9. **What are Watson criteria for Mooren's ulcer?**
   i. Presence of crescent-shaped peripheral corneal ulcer
   ii. Presence of extensive undermining of central edge of ulcer
   iii. Dense corneal infiltrates along the leading edge
   iv. Absence of scleritis
   v. Absence of detectable systemic disease

10. **What are the clinical features of PUK?**
    i. Pain, epiphora, photophobia
    ii. Decreased visual acuity, which can be sudden or gradual
    iii. Crescentic, juxta-limbal epithelial defect
    iv. Stromal yellow–white infiltrates
    v. Stromal thinning
    vi. Circumferential/central spread
    vii. The leading edge of ulcer shows infiltration

11. **What are the anatomic and physiological differences between the center and the periphery of the cornea?**

Central cornea	Peripheral cornea
Avascular	Close to limbal vessels
No inflammatory cells	• Inflammatory cells like • Langerhans cells are present
More prone to infectious disorders	More prone to inflammatory and immune-mediated disorders

12. **Describe the entities associated with Mooren's ulcer.**
    Different entities have been described in association with Mooren's ulcer, but none of the lesions has been proved to have a causal relationship with Mooren's ulcer. Mooren's ulcer is seen associated with:
    i. Helminthiasis
    ii. Hepatitis C infection
    iii. Herpes zoster
    iv. Herpes simplex
    v. Syphilis
    vi. Tuberculosis
    vii. Corneal trauma
    viii. Foreign bodies
    ix. Chemical trauma
    x. Surgical procedures such as cataract extraction and penetrating keratoplasty (PKP)

13. **Name few differential diagnoses for Mooren's ulcer (or PUK).**
    i. *Autoimmune disorders* such as:
       - RA
       - Wegener's granulomatosis
       - Polyarthritis nodosa
       - Inflammatory bowel disease
       - Giant cell arthritis
    ii. *Collagen vascular disorders* such as:
       - SLE
       - Relapsing polychondritis
       - Systemic sclerosis
    iii. *Corneal degenerative conditions* such as:
       - Terrien's marginal keratitis
       - Pellucid marginal degeneration
    iv. *Infectious causes* such as:
       - Herpes simplex keratitis
       - *Acanthamoeba* keratitis
       - Bacterial keratitis

14. **How do we differentiate Mooren's ulcer and PUK caused by RA?**
    RA is a frequent cause of PUK. The clinical picture of PUK in RA is not characteristic to RA, but frequently it is associated with scleritis. Other associated ophthalmic findings include keratoconjunctivitis sicca (the most common ophthalmic finding), episcleritis, and sclerosing keratitis. Advanced systemic involvement is usually apparent at the time of ocular involvement. The patient's clinical profile and positive serologic studies, in particular rheumatoid factor, will help establish the appropriate diagnosis.

15. **What are the ocular conditions associated with PUK?**
    i. Posterior scleritis
    ii. Retinal vasculitis
    iii. Elevation in intraocular pressure
    iv. Keratoconjunctivitis sicca—decreased Schirmer's measurement

16. **Describe the ophthalmic manifestations of Wegener's granulomatosis.**
    Wegener's granulomatosis is a rare multisystem granulomatous necrotizing vasculitis with upper and lower respiratory tract and renal involvement. Ocular involvement may be seen in up to 58% of patients, including proptosis due to orbital involvement, scleritis with or without PUK, PUK alone, uveitis, and vasculitis. Orbital involvement and scleritis are the most common ophthalmic manifestations. Prompt diagnosis is imperative because the initiation of immunosuppressive therapy, such as cyclophosphamide, can be both sight and lifesaving. Serum antinuclear antibody titers are raised in cases of Wegener's granulomatosis.

17. **How are Terrien's marginal degeneration and other corneal degenerations differentiated from Mooren's ulcer?**
    Terrien's marginal degeneration differs from Mooren's ulcer in that it is typically painless, does not ulcerate, and is usually noninflammatory. The disease is usually bilateral but may be asymmetrical. Terrien's degeneration usually begins in the superior cornea, in contrast to Mooren's ulcer, which typically begins in the interpalpebral region as a fine, punctate, stromal opacity. A clear zone exists between the infiltrate and the limbus, which becomes superficially vascularized. Slowly progressive thinning follows. The thin area has a sloping peripheral border and a sharp central edge that is highlighted by a white lipid line. The epithelium remains intact, although bulging of thin stroma causes significant astigmatism.

18. **How is pellucid marginal degeneration differentiated from Mooren's ulcer?**
    Pellucid degeneration causes bilateral, inferior corneal thinning that leads to marked, irregular, against-the-rule astigmatism. Pain and inflammation are lacking, and the epithelium is intact, thus differentiating it from Mooren's ulcer.

19. **Describe the pathophysiology of PUK.**
    i. Any inflammatory stimulus in the peripheral cornea results in a local cellular and humoral response

ii. Which activates complement system, which in turn increase vascular permeability
iii. Increase in neutrophils and release of proteolytic, collagenolytic enzymes (proteases and collagenases) occur, which lyse the stromal collagen and cause corneal thinning

20. **Describe the pathology of Mooren's ulcer.**
    The histopathology of Mooren's ulcer suggests an immune process. The involved limbal cornea consisted of three zones.
    i. The superficial stroma is vascularized and infiltrated with plasma cells and lymphocytes. In this region, there is destruction of the collagen matrix. Epithelium and Bowman's layer are absent
    ii. The midstroma shows hyperactivity of fibroblasts with disorganization of the collagen lamellae
    iii. The deep stroma is essentially intact but contains a heavy macrophage infiltrate. Descemet's membrane and the endothelium are spared
    Heavy neutrophil infiltration, as well as dissolution of the superficial stroma, is present at the leading edge of the ulcer. These neutrophils show evidence of degranulation. The adjacent conjunctiva shows epithelial hyperplasia and a subconjunctival lymphocytic and plasma cell infiltration. Frank vasculitis is not present, and numerous eosinophils may present in the nearby involved conjunctiva during the course of healing.

21. **Describe the pathophysiology of Mooren's ulcer.**
    The precise pathophysiological mechanism of Mooren's ulceration remains unknown, but there is much evidence to suggest that it is an autoimmune process, with both cell-mediated and humoral components.
    On pathological examination, plasma cells, neutrophils, mast cells, and eosinophils have been found in the involved areas. High levels of proteolytic enzymes are found in the affected conjunctiva. Numerous activated neutrophils are found in the involved areas, and these neutrophils are proposed to be the source of the proteases and collagenases that degrade the corneal stroma.

22. **How is cornea immune privileged?**
    A. *Anatomical and molecular barriers*
        i. Blood–retinal barriers and lack of lymphatics
        ii. Paucity of antigen-presenting Langerhans cells
        iii. Dendritic cells and macrophages are absent
        iv. Major histocompatibility complex (MHC) class II proteins are absent, and they express only low levels of MHC class I antigens

B. *Eye-derived immune tolerance (ACAID)*
   i. ACAID is anterior chamber-associated immune deviation
   ii. It acts by identifying any antigens in the anterior chamber with the help of dendritic cells, enters the venous system via trabecular meshwork bypassing lymphatics, and is destroyed in the spleen by regulatory T cells by a complex process
C. *Immune-suppressive intraocular microenvironment*
   i. FAS ligand on endothelial cells causes apoptosis of natural killer cells
   ii. Membrane bound and soluble proteins like transforming growth factor (TGF)-β, thrombospondin, and melanocyte-stimulating hormone (MSH)-α regulate macrophages and dendritic cells

23. **How limbus is different from the rest of the cornea?**
    i. Closer to conjunctiva, sclera, and episclera
    ii. Derives its blood supply and lymphatics from limbal capillary vessels that extend 0.5 mm into the clear cornea
    iii. Source (reservoir) of immunocompetent cells such as macrophages, Langerhans cells, lymphocytes, and plasma cells
    iv. Circulating immune complexes can lodge in the limbal vessels
    v. Contains five times higher levels of C1 than the central cornea, which stimulates chemotaxis of neutrophils
    vi. Large concentration of immunoglobulin M (IgM) directed against immunoglobulin G (IgG) (RA factor) is greater in this site

24. **What are the investigations done to diagnose a case of Mooren's ulcer?**
    Mooren's ulcer is a diagnosis of exclusion.
    Infectious etiologies should be excluded by appropriate smears and cultures.
    This investigation may include a complete blood count with evaluation of the differential count and platelet count—baseline investigations done before starting immunosuppressive therapy.
    i. Erythrocyte sedimentation rate—marker of systemic inflammatory activity
    ii. Rheumatoid factor—to rule out rheumatoid-associated PUK
    iii. Complement fixation, antinuclear antibodies (ANA)—to rule out SLE
    iv. Antineutrophil cytoplasmic antibody (ANCA)—to rule out Wegener's granulomatosis
    v. Circulating immune complexes, liver function tests
    vi. Venereal Disease Research Laboratory (VDRL) and fluorescent treponemal antibody absorption (FTA-ABS) tests—syphilis

vii. Blood urea nitrogen and creatinine
viii. Serum protein electrophoresis
ix. Urinalysis
x. Chest roentgenogram
xi. Additional testing is done as indicated by the review of systems and physical examination

25. **Describe the stepwise management of Mooren's ulcer.**
    The overall goals of therapy are to arrest the destructive process and to promote healing and re-epithelialization of the corneal surface. Most experts agree on a stepwise approach to the management of Mooren's ulcer, which is outlined as follows:
    i. *Topical steroids:* Inflammation can be controlled by topical 1% prednisolone acetate in an hourly basis and tapering it over time, depending on the clinical response. This has to be supplemented with cycloplegic agents and anti-inflammatory drugs to reduce pain and inflammation
    ii. Conjunctival resection
    iii. *Systemic steroids and immunosuppressives:* Prednisolone (1 mg/kg body weight) after assessing systemic factors such as diabetes mellitus, tuberculosis, and other immunosuppressive diseases
    iv. Additional surgical procedure (tectonic grafting)
    v. Rehabilitation

26. **What is the aim of treating PUK?**
    The aim of treatment in cases of PUK is to control the underlying inflammatory process, promote healing of the ulcer, and avoid or prevent progression and complications.

27. **Describe the medical management of PUK?**
    A. *Local treatment:*
        i. *Antibiotics:* To prevent secondary infection
        ii. *Cycloplegics:* To alleviate pain
        iii. Lubricants
        iv. *Collagenase inhibitors:* Tetracycline ointment
        v. Antiglaucoma medications
        vi. Nonsteroidal anti-inflammatory drugs (NSAIDs) are contraindicated as they are
    B. *Systemic treatment:*
        i. Systemic steroids
        ii. Immunosuppressants
        iii. *Systemic collagenase inhibitors:* Tetracycline 250 mg QID or doxycycline 100 mg OD

28. **Describe the surgical management of PUK.**
    i. Glue-assisted bandage contact lens
    ii. Amniotic membrane grafts
    iii. Patch grafts
    iv. Superficial keratectomy
    v. PKP after full immunosuppression
    vi. Conjunctival resection

29. **What parameters should be monitored in patients with chronic systemic steroid therapy?**
    i. Patients should be monitored at 3 monthly intervals
    ii. Monitor weight
    iii. Blood pressure
    iv. Blood glucose
    v. Lipid profile
    vi. Bone scans annually
    vii. *Supplements:* Calcium and vitamin D supplements should be given

30. **When is conjunctival resection advocated?**
    If the ulcer progresses despite the steroid regimen, conjunctival resection should be performed.

31. **What is the rationale for performing conjunctival resection?**
    The rationale of this procedure is that the conjunctiva adjacent to the ulcer contains inflammatory cells that may be producing antibodies against the cornea and cytokines, which amplify the inflammation and recruit additional inflammatory cells.

32. **How is conjunctival resection performed?**
    Under topical and subconjunctival anesthesia, this consists of conjunctival excision to bare sclera extending at least 2 o'clock hours to either side of the peripheral ulcer, and approximately 4 mm posterior to the corneoscleral limbus and parallel to the ulcer. The overhanging lip of ulcerating cornea may also be removed. Postoperatively, a firm pressure dressing should be used.

33. **What are other surgical procedures advocated at the second step?**
    Cryotherapy of limbal conjunctiva, conjunctival excision with thermocoagulation, keratoepithelioplasty, and application of isobutyl cyanoacrylate are the other surgical procedures.

34. **What is keratoepithelioplasty?**
    In this procedure, donor corneal lenticules are sutured onto the scleral bed after conjunctival excision.

35. What is the rationale of keratoepithelioplasty?
It is postulated that the lenticules form a biological barrier between host cornea and the conjunctiva and the immune components it may carry.

36. When is systemic immunosuppression indicated?
The cases of bilateral or progressive Mooren's ulcer that fail the preceding therapeutic attempts will require systemic cytotoxic chemotherapy to bring a halt to the progressive corneal destruction.

37. What are the immunosuppressives and biologicals used in PUK?
   i. The commonly used agents include cyclophosphamide (2 mg/kg/day), azathioprine (2 mg/kg/body weight/day), and methotrexate (7.5–15 mg once weekly)
   ii. *Milder disease:* Antimetabolites (methotrexate, azathioprine, mycophenolate mofetil)
      - Calcineurin inhibitors (cyclosporine A, tacrolimus)
   iii. Wegner's granulomatosis, RA, and sclerokeratitis
      - *First line:* Cyclophosphamide
      - *Second line:* Methotrexate and azathioprine
   iv. Rapidly progressive corneal melting, or one-eyed patient with rapidly deteriorating second eye:
      - Alkylating agents/antimetabolites + biologic response modifiers (infliximab, rituximab)
   v. *Rapidly progressive systemic vasculitis:* Rituximab infusions + antimetabolites/alkylating agents and systemic corticosteroids

38. When is superficial lamellar keratectomy done and how is it useful?
Superficial lamellar keratectomy is done when all the steps of management fail. It arrests the inflammatory process and allows healing of the stroma. After healing, corneal grafting can be done at a later date.

39. When is PKP done in cases of Mooren's ulcer?
An initial tectonic graft is done in the peripheral cornea to strengthen the peripheral cornea. In case the central cornea is involved, a large graft can be performed.

40. How is PKP done in these patients?
In these patients, a 13 mm tectonic corneal graft is first sutured in place of interrupted 10-0 nylon or prolene sutures, with the recipient bite extending into the sclera so that the suture will not pull through the thin host cornea and then a 7.5 or 8.0 mm therapeutic graft is placed.

41. What are the common complications of PKP?
Associated cystoid macular edema and glaucoma may cause defective vision in patients undergoing PKP.

2.10 BAND-SHAPED KERATOPATHY

1. **What are the normal age-related changes of the cornea?**
   i. Flattening in the vertical meridian, leading to increased astigmatism (against the rule)
   ii. Decrease in the thickness of the cornea
   iii. Increase in the thickness of Descemet's membrane
   iv. Arcus senilis
   v. Decrease in the endothelial cell count and luster

2. **What is band-shaped keratopathy?**
   Deposits of calcium and hydroxyapatite in the basement membrane of epithelium, Bowman's, and superficial stroma, usually in the interpalpebral area, are called band-shaped keratopathy (also known as band keratopathy).

3. **What are the causes of band keratopathy?**
   i. *Chronic ocular disease:*
      - Chronic nongranulomatous uveitis—juvenile rheumatoid arthritis
      - Prolonged glaucoma (absolute)
      - Longstanding corneal edema
      - Phthisis bulbi
      - Spheroidal degeneration Norrie's disease—interstitial keratitis
   ii. *Hypercalcemia:*
      - Hyperparathyroidism—primary and tertiary
      - Vitamin D excess
      - Milk alkali syndrome
      - Sarcoidosis
   iii. Normocalcemia—with elevated serum phosphorus
   iv. Hereditary with or without other anomalies
   v. Idiopathic
   vi. *Chronic exposure to mercury:*
      - Vapors
      - Eye drops due to the preservative phenyl-mercuric nitrate/acetate occurs only after months or years of usage. Can be central or peripheral
   vii. Hereditary
   viii. Silicon oil instillation in aphakic eye

4. **What is the pathogenesis of band-shaped keratopathy?**
   Deposits often begin in the periphery and extend to involve the visual axis, thus occupying the interpalpebral area. The deposits are central in cases of chronic ocular inflammation.

The precipitation of calcium salts is due to:
i. Increase in Ca and P levels
ii. Increase in pH due to uveitis, evaporation of tears, and loss of Ca
iii. Concentration by evaporation and thus dry eye is a predisposing factor

The whole process is compounded by the lack of blood vessels, hence preventing the buffering ability of blood serum to inhibit variations in tissue pH.

Small holes are noticed throughout representing the areas in which corneal nerves penetrate Bowman's layer giving a "Swiss cheese appearance".

5. **What are the histopathologic findings in a case of band keratopathy?**
   i. Basophilic staining of the basement membrane of the epithelium
   ii. Calcium deposits in Bowman's membrane and anterior stroma, which coalesce resulting in fragmentation and destruction of Bowman's membrane
   iii. The deposits are initially gray and flat. But with progression, they become white and elevate the epithelium
   iv. The calcium is deposited intracellularly in systemic hypercalcemia
   v. Fibrous pannus separates Bowman's membrane and epithelium

6. **What are the signs and symptoms of band keratopathy?**
   Early stages—asymptomatic
   Late stages:
   i. *Decrease in visual acuity due to:*
      - Decrease in transparency
      - Band across the papillary area
   ii. *Irritation and foreign body sensation* when the deposits either break or elevate the epithelium
      - Tearing and photophobia
      - Calcium may flake off

7. **What are the differential diagnoses of band keratopathy?**
   i. Calcareous degeneration of the cornea is a similar process that involves all layers of the cornea
   ii. Phthisis bulbi
   iii. Intraocular neoplasm
   iv. Extensive trauma

8. **What are the indications of treatment?**
   i. When visual acuity is decreased
   ii. Mechanical irritation of lids
   iii. Epithelial breakdown

9. **What are the methods of treatment?**

Treat the cause of the disease, if known. In addition, the following may be done:

Method I:
   i. 4% cocaine applied over the cornea. Cocaine facilitates the removal of epithelium
   ii. Ethylene diamine tetra-acetic acid (EDTA) is dropped from a 1.5 cm syringe well and allowed to stand for a minute
   iii. Cornea is then scraped with kimura spatula or scalpel blade until the band is removed

Method II:
   i. EDTA is placed on a small strip of cellulose sponge
   ii. Diamond bud is used to polish off the cornea

   If there is no EDTA, just anesthetize the cornea and scrape with a blade until all gritty feeling material is removed.

   Patching in the form of soft contact lenses and collagen shields, along with cycloplegics and mild antibiotic, are used until re-epithelialization.

   Excimer laser phototherapeutic keratectomy can be tried only on smoother lesions.

2.11 ADHERENT LEUKOMA

1. **What are the types of corneal opacities?**
   i. *Nebular (nebula) corneal opacity:* It is a slight opacification of the cornea allowing the details of the iris and pupil to be seen through the corneal opacity
   ii. *Macular (macula) corneal opacity:* It is more dense than nebular corneal opacity; through it, details of the iris and pupil cannot be seen, but the margins can be seen
   iii. *Leukomatous (leukoma) corneal opacity:* It is very dense, white, and totally opaque, obscuring the view of the iris and pupil completely

2. **What is adherent leukoma?**
   Adherent leukoma is a leukomatous opacity in which the iris tissue is incarcerated within the layer of the cornea.

3. **What are the causes of adherent leukoma?**
   i. Perforated corneal ulcer
   ii. Penetrating injury
   iii. Operating wound

4. **What is the mechanism of development of an adherent leukoma?**
   In a cornea that is structurally weak, due to either acute infection or an old scar with thinning, the following events might take place:

   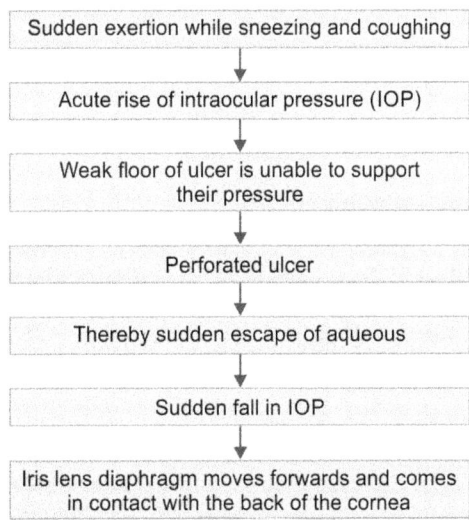

5. **What are the signs and symptoms of adherent leukoma?**
   Symptoms: Visual acuity is decreased if the adherent leukoma affects the central visual axis. In case of peripheral lesions, there may be a chance of *astigmatism*.

Signs:
  i. Corneal surface is flat, leukomatous, and has decreased corneal sensation
  ii. There may be brown pigments dispersed from the iris on the back of the cornea
  iii. The depth of the anterior chamber is irregular
  iv. The pupil is irregular in shape and drawn toward the adhesion
  v. The IOP may be raised

6. **What are the other complications associated with adherent leukoma?**
   i. Perforation
   ii. Pseudocornea formation
   iii. Staphyloma formation
   iv. Ectatic cicatrix
   v. Atheromatous ulcer
   vi. Endophthalmitis
   vii. Panophthalmitis
   viii. Expulsive hemorrhage
   ix. Phthisis bulbi

7. **What are the advantages of perforation in a case of corneal ulcer?**
   i. Pain is reduced due to lowering of IOP and egress of hypopyon
   ii. Rapid healing of the ulcer

8. **What are the reasons of phthisis bulbi?**
   i. Large perforation may cause extrusion of the contents of the eyeball, leading to shrinkage
   ii. Repeated corneal ulcer perforations may be sealed by exudates, which may leak, leading to fistula formation

9. **How do you do tattooing?**
   i. After removing the epithelium, a piece of blotting paper of the same size as the opacity, soaked in fresh 2% platinum chloride solution, is kept over the opacity
   ii. On removing this filter paper, a few drops of fresh 2% hydrazine hydrate solution are applied over the area, which in turn becomes black
   iii. Eye is washed with saline
   iv. A drop of parolene is instilled, and a pad and bandage are applied
   v. The epithelium grows over the black-colored deposit of platinum

10. **What is the treatment of choice for adherent leukoma?**
    i. Optical iridectomy
    ii. Penetrating keratoplasty
    iii. Tattooing and synechotomy

11. **What is the treatment for anterior staphyloma?**
    i. Staphylectomy
    ii. Enucleation and prosthesis fitting

12. **What is the treatment for corneal fistula?**
    i. Cyanoacrylate glue application
    ii. Bandage contact lens
    iii. Penetrating keratoplasty

13. **What is the treatment of choice for panophthalmitis?**
    Evisceration and prosthesis

	Anterior synechia	*Leukoma*	*Adherent leukoma*	*Anterior staphyloma*
i. Definition	Adhesion between iris and cornea	Dense white opacity of the cornea	Adhesion between iris and leukoma	Adhesion between iris and ectatic leukoma
ii. Etiology	• Perforated corneal ulcer • Iridocyclitis • Closed-angle glaucoma	• Healed corneal ulcer • Healed keratitis • Penetrating injury • FB • Corneal dystrophy	• Perforated corneal ulcer • Penetrating injury • Operating wound	• Perforated corneal ulcer • Penetrating injury • Operating wound
iii. Visual acuity	Normal	Impaired	Impaired	Impaired
iv. Corneal surface	Flat	Flat	Flat	Ectatic
v. Pigments	Nil	Fine yellowish-brown lines in the epithelium	Brown pigment from the iris is present	Brown pigment from the iris is present
vi. Anterior chamber	Normal or shallow	Normal	Irregular or shallow	Absent or very shallow
vii. Pupil	Normal	Normal	Drawn toward adhesion	Not seen
viii. Corneal sensation	Normal	Impaired	Impaired	Impaired
ix. Intraocular tension	Normal or raised (closed-angle glaucoma)	Normal	Normal or raised (secondary glaucoma)	Raised

2.12 BOWEN'S DISEASE

1. **What are the old terms used to describe Bowen's disease?**
   i. Intraepithelial epithelioma
   ii. Bowenoid epithelioma

2. **What are the new terms used to describe Bowen's disease?**
   i. Ocular surface squamous neoplasia (OSSN)
   ii. Conjunctival intraepithelial neoplasia (CIN)
   iii. Corneal intraepithelial neoplasia

3. **What is the common site of involvement?**
   Interpalpebral fissure, mostly at limbus

4. **How does Bowen's disease present?**
   Typically, a patient presents with an isolated, slightly elevated, erythematous lesion with well-demarcated borders that fail to heal. The lesion has appearance of a second-degree burn, does not bleed or itch, and is devoid of hairs.

5. **What are the clinical forms of Bowen's disease?**
   i. Gelatinous
   ii. Papilliform
   iii. Leukoplakic
   iv. Nodular
   v. Diffuse

6. **Which form masquerades as chronic conjunctivitis?**
   Diffuse form

7. **What are the risk factors?**
   i. Exposure to sunlight
   ii. Human papilloma virus
   iii. Chronic inflammatory diseases—benign mucous membrane pemphigoid, chronic blepharoconjunctivitis
   iv. Ocular surface injury
   v. Exposure to chemicals—trifluridine, arsenic, petroleum products, cigarette smoking
   vi. Human immunodeficiency virus (HIV)
   vii. Solar keratosis

8. **What is limbal transition zone/stem cell theory?**
   Cells in the limbal area have a highly proliferating and long-living property. Any alteration in this area causes abnormal maturation of conjunctival and corneal epithelial cells, leading to OSSN.

9. **How do you differentiate squamous dysplasia from carcinoma in situ?**
    i. *Squamous dysplasia:* Atypical cells involve only part of epithelium
    ii. *Carcinoma in situ:* Atypia involves throughout epithelium, not involving the basement membrane
10. **What is the histopathological hallmark of Bowen's disease?**
    The histopathological hallmark of Bowen's disease is the lack of penetration of cancerous cells into the dermis.
11. **How does squamous cell carcinoma present?**
    The average age of presentation of squamous cell carcinoma is between 68 and 73 years, but primary squamous cell carcinoma in younger patients may be seen in those who are immunosuppressed.
    They may present as:
    i. Painless plaque/nodules with variable degrees of scale, crust, and ulceration
    ii. Papillomatous growths/cutaneous horns/cysts along the lid margins
12. **What are various histopathological types of OSSN?**
    i. Dysplastic lesions
    ii. Carcinoma in situ
    iii. Squamous cell carcinoma
    iv. Spindle cell variant
    v. Mucoepidermoid carcinoma
    vi. Adenoid squamous carcinoma
13. **Describe spindle cell variant.**
    Spindle cell variant exhibits spindle-shaped cells that may be difficult to distinguish from fibroblasts. Positive immunohistochemical staining for cytokeratin confirms the epithelial nature.
14. **Describe mucoepidermoid carcinoma.**
    Mucoepidermoid carcinoma is a variant of conjunctival squamous cell carcinoma that, in addition to squamous cells, shows mucous secreting cells (stain positively with special stains for mucopolysaccharides such as mucicarmine, Alcian blue, and colloidal iron).
15. **Describe adenoid squamous cell carcinoma.**
    Adenoid squamous cell carcinoma is an aggressive variant with extracellular hyaluronic acid but no intracellular mucin and invades eyeball. Metastasis to distant sites is common.
16. **From where does corneal OSSN arise?**
    The origin of corneal OSSN is controversial. Some investigators suggest that corneal epithelium may undergo dysplastic and cancerous changes, whereas others believe that the origin is in limbus.

17. **When do you suspect intraocular invasion?**
    Intraocular invasion is often heralded by the onset of low-grade inflammation and secondary glaucoma. It is common in older patients.

18. **What are the common sites of metastasis?**
    i. Preauricular, submandibular, cervical lymph nodes
    ii. Parotid
    iii. Lungs
    iv. Bones
    v. Distant organs

19. **What is exfoliative cytology?**
    Using a platinum spatula, brush, and cotton wool tip, cells are obtained from the conjunctival surface, followed by Papanicolaou and Giemsa stains.

20. **What are the advantages and disadvantages of exfoliative cytology?**
    Advantages:
    i. Nature of lesion—benign or malignant
    ii. Sampling from multiple sites
    iii. Deoxyribonucleic acid (DNA) of cells can also be obtained
    Disadvantage:
    Superficial nature of the sample, sometimes containing only keratinized cells

21. **What is impression cytology?**
    Impression cytology is a method of obtaining cells from conjunctival lesions in which filter paper such as cellulose acetate, Millipore filter, or Biopore membrane are placed over the ocular surface to sample superficial cells and then stained by Papanicolaou smear.

22. **What is the treatment?**
    Localized lesion: Excision with autologous conjunctival or limbal transplantation or amniotic membrane graft (Mohs micrographic technique)
    Diffuse:
    i. Topical mitomycin 0.02% twice a day for 15 days followed by a relapsing period
    5-FU:
    ii. Interferon (alternative or adjunct to surgery)
    iii. Very large tumors—enucleation
    iv. Orbital involvement—exenteration

23. **What are the other treatment modalities available?**
    i. Cryotherapy
    ii. Brachytherapy

Cornea

24. **What is the mechanism of cryotherapy?**
    Cryotherapy obliterates microcirculation by lowering temperature within tissues resulting in ischemic necrosis of tumor cells.

25. **What are the side effects of cryotherapy?**
    i. Iritis
    ii. Increase or decrease in intraocular pressure
    iii. Inflammation
    iv. Edema and corneal scarring
    v. Sector iris atrophy
    vi. Ablation of peripheral retina
    vii. Ectropion
    viii. Superficial corneal vascularization

26. **What are the commonly used radioactive materials in brachytherapy?**
    i. Strontium 90
    ii. Ruthenium 106
    iii. Gamma radiation

27. **What are the complications of brachytherapy?**
    i. Conjunctivitis
    ii. Dry eye
    iii. Scleral ulceration
    iv. Corneal perforation
    v. Cataract.

2.13 KERATOCONUS

1. **Name a few corneal ectatic conditions.**

    Keratoconus, keratoglobus, pellucid marginal degeneration, Terrien's marginal degeneration.

2. **What are the signs of keratoconus?**
    i. *External signs:*
        - Munson's sign
        - Rizzuti phenomenon
    ii. *Slit-lamp findings:*
        - Stromal thinning
        - Posterior stress lines (Vogt's striae)
        - Iron ring (Fleischer's ring)
        - Scarring—epithelial or subepithelial
    iii. *Retroillumination signs:*
        - Scissoring on retinoscopy
        - Oil droplet sign ("Charleaux")
    iv. *Photokeratoscopy signs:*
        - Compression of mires inferotemporally ("egg-shaped" mires)
        - Compression of mires inferiorly or centrally
    v. *Videokeratography signs:*
        - *Curvature map:*
            - Localized increased surface power >47 D
            - Inferior superior dioptric asymmetry >1.4 D
            - Relative skewing of the steepest radial axes above and below the horizontal meridian
        - *Elevation map:*
            - Maximum elevation difference in posterior float >50 μ
        - *Pachymetry map:*
            - Thinnest <480 μ

3. **Which gender is commonly affected by keratoconus?**

    Keratoconus has been seen a bit more commonly in males than in females.

4. **What are the biochemical alternations seen in corneas with keratoconus?**

    Various abnormalities suggested include:
    i. Decreased levels of glucose-6-phosphate dehydrogenase (G6PD)
    ii. Relative decrease in hydroxylation of lysine and glycosylation of hydroxylysine
    iii. Decrease in total collagen and a relative increase in structural glycoprotein

iv. In patients with keratoconus, keratan sulfate is decreased and its structure is modified
v. The ratio of dermatan sulfate to keratan sulfate is increased in keratoconus
vi. Decrease in matrix metalloproteinase (MMP) inhibitors leads to increased collagenolytic activity
vii. There is a decreased level of $\alpha 1$ proteinase inhibitor, tissue inhibitor of metalloproteinase (TIMP)-1, and $\alpha 2$-macroglobulin levels in keratoconus cornea
viii. The loss of anterior stromal keratinocytes is due to apoptotic cell death
ix. Keratinocytes have fourfold increased expression of interleukin-1 (IL-1) receptors. IL-1 is released from epithelial and endothelial cells, and IL-1 can cause the loss of keratinocytes through apoptosis and loss of corneal stroma over a period of time

5. **What is Munson's sign?**
Munson's sign is a V-shaped conformation of the lower lid produced by the ectatic cornea in downgaze.

6. **What is Rizzuti's sign?**
Conical reflection on the nasal cornea when a penlight is shown from the temporal side.

7. **What are Vogt's striae?**
Vogt's striae are fine vertical lines in the deep stroma and Descemet's membrane that parallel the axis of the cone and disappear transiently on gentle digital pressure.

8. **What is Fleischer's ring?**
Fleischer's ring is a yellow-brown to olive-green ring of pigment, which may or may not completely surround the base of the cone. The deposition occurs at the level of the basal epithelium. Locating this ring initially may be made easier by using a cobalt filter and carefully focusing on the superior half of the corneal epithelium. Once located, the ring should be viewed in white light to assess its extent.

9. **What is the clinical significance of Fleischer's ring?**
Fleischer's ring delineates the extent of the base of the cone of the keratoconus, which helps to mark the recipient during the penetrating keratoplasty (PKP).

10. **What is acute hydrops?**
Acute hydrops is caused by breaks in Descemet's membrane with stromal imbibition of aqueous through these breaks. The edema may persist for weeks or months, usually diminishing gradually, with relief of

pain and resolution of the redness and corneal edema ultimately being replaced by scarring.

11. **How is acute hydrops treated?**
Acute hydrops is not an ophthalmic emergency and is treated conservatively with topical hypertonic agents, patching or soft contact lens, and mild cycloplegics. The edema usually resolves within a few months.

12. **What is the visual prognosis following healing of acute hydrops?**
Acute hydrops usually heals by scarring. The scarring can flatten the cornea and decrease astigmatism. The flattened cornea can be fitted with a contact lens easier.

13. **Describe scissoring reflex on retinoscopy.**
Scissoring reflex is well appreciated with dilated pupil. The central part of the cone is hypermetropic with regard to its periphery, which is myopic. The scissoring reflex is produced due to the presence of two conjugate foci in the pupillary axis and high astigmatism.

    During retinoscopy, when the neutralization point is approached, the central zone produces a hypermetropic reflex which moves with the streak, and the peripheral zone produces a myopic reflex that moves against the streak, which produces the appearance of scissoring reflex.

14. **Describe oil droplet sign.**
Oil droplet sign is seen with a dilated fundus examination. It is an annular dark shadow separating the bright reflex of the central and peripheral areas. It occurs due to complete internal reflection of the light.

15. **What is swirl staining of the cornea?**
Swirl staining may occur in patients who have never worn contact lenses because basal epithelial cells drop out, and the epithelium slides from the periphery as the cornea regenerates. Thus, a hurricane, vortex, or swirl stain may occur.

16. **What is forme fruste keratoconus?**
Forme fruste keratoconus or subclinical keratoconus is a clinical entity in which there is no frank clinical sign of keratoconus. However, the cornea is at risk of developing keratoconus at a later stage and can be diagnosed only by videokeratography. Cornea is considered suspicious when:
    i. The central keratometry is >47.0 D
    ii. There is presence of an oblique astigmatism of >1.5 D
    iii. Superior-inferior curvature disparity of >1.4 D on videokeratography
    iv. The Massachusetts Eye and Ear Infirmary Keratoconus classification is currently used to detect cases of forme fruste keratoconus and variable grades of clinical keratoconus

17. **What are the systemic disorders associated with keratoconus?**
    i. Crouzon's syndrome
    ii. Down's syndrome
    iii. Laurence-Moon-Bardet-Biedl syndrome
    iv. Marfan's syndrome
    v. Nail-patella syndrome
    vi. Neurofibromatosis
    vii. Osteogenesis imperfecta
    viii. Pseudoxanthoma elasticum
    ix. Turner's syndrome
    x. Xeroderma pigmentosa

18. **What are the ocular associations of keratoconus?**
    The ocular associations of keratoconus can be classified into corneal disorders and noncorneal disorders.

Corneal disorders	Noncorneal disorders
Atopic keratoconjunctivitis	Retinitis pigmentosa
Axenfeld's anomaly	Vernal conjunctivitis
Corneal amyloidosis	Congenital cataracts
Essential iris atrophy	Leber's congenital amaurosis
Fuchs' corneal dystrophy	Gyrate atrophy
Microcornea	Posterior lenticonus
Lattice dystrophy	Aniridia

19. **Why is keratoconus commonly associated with Leber's congenital amaurosis and Down's syndrome?**
    These two disorders are associated with an increased incidence of eye rubbing. This is due to the increased incidence of blepharitis in Down's syndrome and oculodigital sign in Leber's congenital amaurosis. A recent study by Elder suggests that the association might be due to genetic factors rather than eye rubbing.

20. **What is the role of contact lens wear in causing keratoconus?**
    Contact lenses are suggested as a source of mechanical trauma to the cornea. It is extremely difficult to determine which came first, the contact lens wear or the keratoconus. It is possible that mechanical rubbing and hard contact lens wear can act as environmental factors that enhance the progression of the disorder in genetically predisposed individuals.

21. **Describe the three types of cones seen in keratoconus.**
    A. Nipple cone—small in size (<5 mm)
        i. Steep curvature
        ii. Apical center usually lies central or paracentral
        iii. Easiest to fit with contact lens

B. Oval cone—larger (5-6 mm) ellipsoid displaced inferotemporally
C. Globus cone—larger (>6 mm) may involve >75% of the cornea
   i. Most difficult to fit with contact lenses

22. **What is posterior keratoconus?**
Posterior keratoconus is a congenital corneal anomaly unrelated to keratoconus, which is characterized by protrusion of the posterior corneal surface into the stroma and is usually sporadic, unilateral, and nonprogressive.

23. **What are Rabinowitz's criteria for diagnosis of keratoconus?**
    i. Keratometry value >47.2 D
    ii. Steepening of inferior cornea compared with the superior cornea of >1.2 D
    iii. Skewing of the radial axis of astigmatism by >21 D
    iv. Difference in central power of >1 D between the fellow eye

24. **Describe the histopathology of corneas in keratoconus.**
Thinning of corneal stroma, breaks in Bowman's layer, and deposition of iron in the basal layer of the corneal epithelium comprise a triad of the classic histopathologic features found in keratoconus.
    i. *Epithelium*—degeneration of basal cells
       - Breaks accompanied by downgrowth of the epithelium into Bowman's layer
       - Accumulation of ferritin particles within and between basal epithelial cells
    ii. *Bowman's layer*—breaks filled with eruptions of underlying stromal collagen
       - Reticular scarring
    iii. *Stroma*—compactions and loss of arrangement of fibrils in the anterior stroma
       - Decrease in the number of collagen lamellae
    iv. *Descemet's membrane*—rarely affected except in cases with acute hydrops
    v. *Endothelium*—usually normal

25. **Classify keratoconus based on keratometry.**
    i. Mild   <45 D in both meridians
    ii. Moderate   45–52 D in both meridians
    iii. Advanced   >52 D in both meridians
    iv. Severe   >62 D in both meridians

26. **How is a case of keratoconus managed?**
    i. Glasses
    ii. Contact lenses
    iii. Collagen cross-linking

iv. Intracorneal rings
   v. Deep anterior lamellar keratoplasty (DALK)
   vi. PKP

27. **What are the various types of contact lenses used in the management of keratoconus?**
    i. Rigid gas permeable contact lens
    ii. Tricurve flex lens for nipple cone
    iii. Soper lens system
    iv. McGuire lens system
    v. Rose K design
    vi. Nicone design
    vii. Bausch and Lomb C series
    viii. Double posterior curve lenses
        - One central curve to fit the corneal apex
        - Another flatter curve peripheral to the central apical zone to fit the mid-corneal periphery
    ix. Piggy back lenses—gas permeable firm lens is fitted upon a soft lens or flex lens system of a hard lens fitted into the groove of a soft lens. Hard lens with a soft peripheral skirt

28. **What is "three-point touch" technique of contact lens fitting?**
    The lens lightly touches the peak of the cone, then a very low vault over the edges of the cone, and lastly a thin band of touching near the edge of the lens. The name "three-point touch" refers to the edge-peak-edge pattern of the lens touching the cornea. The lens is kept as small as is optically possible. Since the lens will center itself over the peak of the cone, an off-center cone needs a bigger lens than a centered cone.

29. **What is the fluorescein pattern of a well-fit lens in a keratoconus patient?**
    i. Slight central bearing
    ii. Intermediate pooling of tears
    iii. Peripheral bearing or touch over some portion of the lens circumference and perhaps slight peripheral lift at the steepest site of the cone

30. **What are SoftPerm lens?**
    The SoftPerm lens is a hybrid lens with a rigid, gas-permeable center surrounded by a soft, hydrophilic skirt. This lens may be indicated for patients with displaced corneal apexes or for patients who cannot tolerate rigid lenses. However, in advanced keratoconus, in which a lens of larger diameter is useful, the lack of steep base curves in the SoftPerm lens (its steepest base curve is 6.5 mm) limits performance. In addition, the lens material has a low DK value (rigid lens, 14 DK; soft portion, 5.5 DK).

31. What is Soper lens system?

The objective of the Soper lens system is based on sagittal depth. The principle is that a constant base curve with an increased diameter results in increased sagittal depth and a steeper lens. The lenses included in the fitting set are categorized as mild (7.5 mm diameter, 6.0 mm optic zone diameter), moderate (8.5 mm diameter, 7.0 mm optic zone diameter), and advanced (9.5 mm diameter, 8.0 mm optic zone diameter). The initial trial lens is selected on the basis of degree of advancement of the cone. The more advanced the cone, the larger the diameter of the recommended lens; the smaller and more centrally located the apex, the smaller the diameter of the lens.

32. What is thermokeratoplasty?

Thermokeratoplasty is corneal flattening by heat application, which may regularize the corneal surface. It is often used to flatten the cornea at the time of keratoplasty to make trephining easier.

33. What is epikeratoplasty?

A corneal lenticule is sewn over the keratoconus area, flattening the cone, reducing the myopic astigmatism, and improving contact lens fit. It is preferred in conditions such as Down's syndrome because of its noninvasive nature and decreased potential for corneal graft rejection.

34. What is excimer laser phototherapeutic keratectomy?

Excimer laser phototherapeutic keratectomy is useful in the management of patients with keratoconus who have nodular subepithelial corneal scars and who are contact lens intolerant.

35. Why is prognosis of PKP good in cases of keratoconus?

i. Absence of vascularization in the lesion
ii. Keratoconus is a noninflammatory ectatic condition

36. What is collagen cross-linkage?

Corneal collagen cross-linking using riboflavin (C3R) is a noninvasive procedure, which strengthens the weak corneal structure in keratoconus.

This technique works by increasing collagen cross-linking, which are the natural "anchors" within the cornea. Riboflavin eye drops are applied to the cornea, which is then activated by ultraviolet A (UVA) light. This increases the amount of collagen cross-linking in the cornea and strengthens the cornea. The technique uses riboflavin to create new bonds between the adjacent collagen molecules so that the cornea is about one-and-a-half times thicker and less malleable.

37. Explain the mechanism of action of collagen cross-linkage.

Application of riboflavin on the cornea along with penetration for approximately 200 µm and irradiation of the riboflavin molecules through UVA leads to loss of the internal chemical balance of the riboflavin molecules, producing oxygen-free radicals. The riboflavin molecule becomes unstable and only stabilizes when it is linked to two collagen fibrils. A cross bridge is created between the collagen fibrils (i.e., cross-linking) to produce a general strengthening of the cornea.

38. What are the indications for C3R?
   i. *Refractive indications:*
      - Progressive keratoconus:
        - If two topography maps measured at an interval of 6 months or more show the following:
          • Increase in K_{max} by 1 D
          • Increase in astigmatism by 1 D
          • Decrease in pachymetry by 30 μm
          • Marked change in the topographic pattern to crab claw or increase in the hot spot
      - Keratoconus in young patients with borderline pachymetry at the first visit
      - Pellucid marginal degeneration
      - Postrefractive surgery ectasia
   ii. *Nonrefractive indications:*
      - Infective keratitis
      - Pseudophakic bullous keratopathy
      - Scleral C3R in glaucoma

39. What are the contraindications for C3R?
   i. Age <10 years
   ii. Pachymetry <350 μm
   iii. Corneal endothelial count <2,400 cells/mm^2
   iv. Presence of significant corneal opacity
   v. Active vernal keratoconjunctivitis (VKC)
   vi. Corneal epithelial healing disorders
   vii. Any other active disease of the eye
   viii. Pregnancy

40. Which are the modifications of C3R?
   i. *Hypotonic C3R:*
   This uses 0.1% riboflavin (made using water for injection instead of high molecular weight dextran T500 which is used to prepare the isotonic 0.1% riboflavin drops)
   Indication: Thin corneas requiring C3R (350–400 μm)
   Principle: Hypotonic drops when applied to the epithelium debrided cornea lead to transient water retention and hence increase in the corneal thickness to approximately 350 μm. This decreases the endothelial damage from the UV light

ii. *Transepithelial C3R/epi-on technique:*
C3R performed without debriding the epithelium is termed epi-on C3R
Advantages:
- Less painful
- Faster healing
- Reduces chances of corneal infections
- Can be performed in thinner corneas

Disadvantages:
- Less effective than the standard epi-off treatment
- Longer duration

iii. *Accelerated C3R:* The UVA power is increased to 6 mW/cm^2 for 15 minutes or 30 mW/cm^2 and the duration is reduced to 3 minutes, hence keeping the total energy received by the tissue almost the same as in the standard technique
Advantage: Shorter duration and so better patient compliance is achieved
Disadvantage: Still experimental and less effective than the standard technique

41. Compare and contrast the clinical features of keratoconus, keratoglobus, Terrien's, and pellucid marginal degeneration?

	Keratoconus	Keratoglobus	Terrien's	Pellucid
Age group	Progress during adolescence	Presents at birth	Presents at fourth to fifth decade	Presents between second and third decade
Appearance	Progressive thinning of central/ paracentral cornea	Globular deformation of entire cornea	Begins superiorly and spreads circumferentially	Causes inferior thinning of cornea
Vascularization	Absent	Absent	Forms pannus	Absent
Familial inheritance	Most cases are sporadic	Dominant inheritance with incomplete penetrance	Sporadic	Sporadic
Laterality	Bilateral, usually asymmetrical	Bilateral, usually asymmetrical	Unilateral or asymmetrically bilateral	Bilateral
Prognosis after PKP	Very favorable prognosis	Poor prognosis	Good prognosis after lamellar keratoplasty	Moderate

42. **Which are the surgical options for keratoconus treatment?**
    i. DALK—replaces only the stroma up to Descemet's membrane
    Advantage—reduced chances for immune rejection since the endothelial layer is preserved
    Disadvantage—technically difficult procedure
    Visual quality may be inferior to PK because of interface irregularities and astigmatism
    ii. Intracorneal ring segment insertion
    iii. PKP—in the presence of Descemet's scarring, DALK cannot be done. A PKP is the only choice for visual rehabilitation

43. **What are intracorneal rings?**
    Intracorneal ring segments are polymethyl methacrylate (PMMA)/silicon semicircular rings that are inserted in mid-peripheral stroma, which help to reduce high refractive error and provide better fitting of the cornea.

44. **How do intracorneal rings Intacs act?**
    The insertion of a ring of particular thickness in the mid-peripheral stroma will increase the thickness and corneal arc diameter. This will act like a hammock rod to cause central flattening. Two half-ring segments are inserted on either side of the cone. It flattens the cornea, regularizes topography, centralizes the cone, improves uncorrected and best-corrected visual acuity, decreases spherical equivalent and aberrations, and helps redistribute biomechanical stress forces.

45. **What are the types of intrastromal corneal ring segments (ICRSs)?**
    There are four types of ICRS available:
    i. Intacs
    ii. Ferrara rings
    iii. Bisantis segments
    iv. Myoring

46. **What are the indications and contraindications of ICRSs?**
    Indications:
    i. Keratoconus
    ii. Pellucid marginal degeneration
    iii. Postrefractive surgery ectasia
    iv. Myopia (−1 to −3.0 D)
    v. Contact lens intolerance in keratoconus patients
    Contraindications:
    i. Age <21 years
    ii. Corneal scar involving the central optical zone
    iii. Pachymetry <450 μm at the site of insertion
    iv. Associated corneal dystrophy

v. Collagen vascular diseases
vi. Pregnancy and nursing women

46A. What is corneal allogenic intrastromal ring segments (CAIRS)?
CAIRS uses allogenic donor corneal stromal tissue segments, instead of synthetic implants, that are inserted into circular femtosecond dissected channels. Since it is composed of donor cornea, it is biocompatible, can be implanted in thinner corneas, has a lower risk of complications than thinner corneas, and can be implanted more superficially than synthetic implants.

46B. What are the other ways of strengthening the cornea?
Isolated Bowman's membrane transplantation

46C. What are the miscellaneous treatment modalities under research?
i. Small and strong carbon nanoparticles to promote strengthening of the cornea
ii. Tear fluid analysis for detecting biomarkers for keratoconus and targeted treatments such as cyclosporine A to reduce matrix metalloproteinase-9 (MMP-9)

47. What are the causes of prominent corneal nerves?
Ocular causes:
i. Keratoconus
ii. Fuchs' dystrophy
iii. Congenital glaucoma

Systemic causes:
i. Leprosy
ii. Neurofibromatosis
iii. Multiple endocrine neoplasia.

2.14 STROMAL DYSTROPHIES

1. **What is the meaning of the word dystrophy?**
   The word dystrophy is derived from the Greek words, *dys* = wrong, difficult; *trophe* = nourishment.

2. **Define corneal dystrophy.**
   Corneal dystrophies are a group of inherited corneal diseases that are typically bilateral, symmetrical, and slowly progressive without relationship to environmental or systemic factors, causing loss of clarity of one or more layers of the cornea.

3. **Define corneal degenerations.**
   Corneal degenerations may occur from physiological changes occurring from aging or may follow an environmental insult such as exposure to ultraviolet light or secondary to a prior corneal disorder.

4. **What are the differences between corneal dystrophy and degenerations?**

Dystrophy	Degenerations
Bilateral and symmetric	Unilateral or bilateral
Hereditary	Sporadic
Appears early in life	Occur late in life and are considered as aging changes
Noninflammatory	Inflammatory
Avascular and located centrally	Often eccentric and peripheral and are related to vascularity
Usually painless except in recurrent epithelial erosions	Mostly associated with pain
Systemic associations are rare	Local and systemic conditions are common association

5. **Classify corneal dystrophies.**
   Classification according to the layers of the cornea involved (anatomic) is most often used. Other classifications are based on genetic pattern, severity, histopathologic features, or biochemical characteristics.

Layer	Descriptive term
Epithelium	• Epithelial basement membrane dystrophy (EBMD) (map-dot-fingerprint, Cogan's microcystic) • Messman's (juvenile epithelial) dystrophy
Bowman's layer	• Corneal dystrophy of Bowman's layers (CDB) I and II Reis–Bucklers dystrophy (CDB, type I) • Thiel–Behnke dystrophy (CDB, type II)

   Contd...

Contd...

Layer	Descriptive term

Stroma	• Granular dystrophy
	  Type I
	  Type II
	• Lattice dystrophy
	  Type I (Biber-Haab-Dimmer)
	  Type II (Meretoja syndrome)
	  Type III
	• Avellino corneal dystrophy (combined granular-lattice)
	• Macular dystrophy
	  Type I
	  Type II
	• Gelatinous drop-like dystrophy (primary familial amyloidosis)
	• Schnyder crystalline corneal dystrophy
	• Fleck dystrophy
	• Central cloudy dystrophy of Francois
	• Congenital hereditary stromal dystrophy

Endothelium	• Posterior polymorphous dystrophy (PPMD) • Fuchs' hereditary endothelial dystrophy • Congenital hereditary endothelial dystrophy (CHED I and II)

6. What is the age of presentation of the corneal dystrophies?

Most dystrophies become clinically apparent by the second decade of life. There are some that may present in the first few years of life like EBMD and others like Fuchs' dystrophy, which may not become symptomatic until very late in life.

7. What is the mechanism of decreased vision in dystrophies?
  i. Intraocular light scattering in the initial stages
  ii. Disruption of geometric image caused by the corneal deposits and by the anterior corneal surface
  iii. Recurrent corneal erosions and resultant subepithelial scarring
  iv. Opacities causing obstruction to light
  v. By affecting normal endothelial function as in CHED, Fuchs' dystrophy, etc.

8. What are the types of dystrophies affecting vision?
  i. Macular dystrophy
  ii. Lattice dystrophy
  iii. Central crystalline
  iv. CHED
  v. Fuchs' dystrophy

9. What are the types of dystrophies not affecting vision?
  i. Granular
  ii. Fleck dystrophy

10. **What are the modes of inheritance of corneal dystrophies?**
    Most of them are inherited as autosomal dominant, except:
    i. Macular (autosomal recessive)
    ii. CHED (type II)
    iii. Posterior polymorphous (rarely autosomal recessive)
    iv. Type III lattice (recessive)

11. **What is the frequency of recurrence of stromal dystrophy in a graft?**
    Among the stromal dystrophies, the frequency of regraft is highest in lattice dystrophy, followed by granular dystrophy, and then macular dystrophy.
    Of all the dystrophies, the recurrence is very high for gelatinous drop-like dystrophy.

12. **Why is Avellino corneal dystrophy named so?**
    Avellino corneal dystrophy was originally described in a small number of families who traced their roots to a place Avellino in Italy. It is a combination of lattice and granular dystrophies.

13. **How is granular dystrophy inherited?**
    An autosomal dominant transmission with variable expression. It is linked to chromosome 5q31, along with lattice, Avellino, and Reis–Bucklers dystrophy.

14. **What are the features of granular dystrophy?**
    i. Bilaterally symmetric and affects the central cornea
    ii. Glare and photophobia due to light scatter by the opacities
    iii. Vision remains normal till around 40 years. In an affected patient, a diffuse, and irregular, ground-glass haze may appear in the superficial stroma
    iv. It is characterized by discrete, white dense, round-to-oval granular opacities lie in the relatively clear stroma and form a variety of patterns, including arcuate chains and straight lines. *The intervening and peripheral areas of cornea are clear*
    v. They are characterized by focal extracellular aggregates of eosinophilic material occupying all levels of the stroma
    vi. A mutation in the *BIGH3* gene localized to chromosome 5q31 is responsible for granular corneal dystrophy

15. **What are the differential diagnoses of granular dystrophy?**
    Paraproteinemia A, in a patient with leukemia, can produce dense crystalline deposits in the cornea. Serum protein electrophoresis will show an M component spike in the patient with paraproteinemic keratopathy.

16. Classify lattice dystrophies.

Type	Predominant corneal location	Inheritance	Age of onset	Amyloid protein
Type I	Central, full thickness	Autosomal dominant	First–second decade	AA
Type II (coexisting systemic amyloidosis)	Peripheral radial pattern	Autosomal dominant	Third decade	Gelsolin
Type III	Peripheral radial pattern	Autosomal recessive	Sixth decade	AP

17. What are the characteristic features of lattice-I dystrophy?

The characteristic translucent lattice lines vary from a few small comma-shaped flecks to a dense network of large irregular ropy cords that contain white dots. The white dots and lattice lines consist of amyloid. In the corneal stroma, they form fusiform deposits that push aside the collagen lamellae. Lattice dystrophy results from abnormal keratocyte synthesis.

18. What are the slit-lamp findings in lattice-II dystrophy?

Coarse translucent stromal lattice lines radiating centrally from the limbus sparing the central and intervening cornea.

19. What are the systemic features of lattice-II dystrophy?

i. Slowly progressive cranial and peripheral neuropathy
ii. Skin changes such as lichen amyloidosis, cutis laxa, blepharochalasis, protruding lips, mask facies, and variably ventricular hypertrophy and polycythemia vera

20. What are the features of lattice-III dystrophy?

i. Inherited as an autosomal recessive trait and has a late adult onset
ii. The disorder occurs unilaterally or bilaterally
iii. Usually, visual acuity is not greatly affected
iv. The lattice lines are thick and ropy and extend from limbus to limbus
v. Variably sized amyloid deposits accumulate beneath Bowman's layer and in the anterior stroma

21. What are the components of amyloid?

Their chemical composition is unknown, but pre-albumin, transthyretin AP protein, and gelsolin (actin-modulating plasma protein, an amyloidogenic protein) are all associated with the amyloid deposits.

22. Define Avellino dystrophy.

Concurrent granular and lattice dystrophies in the same cornea.

23. **What are the clinical features of combined granular-lattice dystrophy?**

    Combined granular-lattice dystrophy exhibits an autosomal dominant inheritance pattern and appears in the first decade of life.

Granular	Lattice
• The granular lesions resemble the sharply demarcated, round, focal deposits of isolated granular dystrophy, but they occur early in life and may be accompanied by a diffuse haze between the granules • The granular deposits are clustered in the anterior stroma	• The lattice deposits are whiter and more polygonal or speculated, occur later in life, and lack the classic glass-red refractile appearance in retroillumination • The lattice deposits appear in the middle to posterior stroma

24. **What are the characteristic features of gelatinous drop-like dystrophy?**
    i. Gelatinous drop-like dystrophy is a rare, bilaterally symmetric, primary familial corneal amyloidosis
    ii. Inherited as an autosomal recessive mapped to chromosome 1p
    iii. The disorder manifests early in life in the first decade
    iv. Presenting symptoms include photophobia, lacrimation, foreign body sensation, and progressive deteriorating vision
    v. It is characterized by multiple subepithelial gelatinous excrescences that give the corneal surface a mulberry appearance
    vi. The deposits appear opaque on direct illumination and translucent in retroillumination. In advanced case, they are accompanied by neovascularization

25. **What are the characteristics of macular dystrophy?**
    i. Macular dystrophy is an autosomal recessive disease
    ii. It involves both the central and the peripheral cornea and also all the layers of cornea
    iii. It is a heterogeneous disorder, on the basis of the type of an abnormal proteoglycan present
    iv. This condition requires penetrating keratoplasty earlier than other stromal dystrophies
    v. Recurrence after graft is less common when compared to lattice and granular dystrophy. The cornea is thinner than normal

26. **Classify macular dystrophy.**

    Based on the immune histochemical studies, macular dystrophy is classified into two types as:

Type I	Type II
Most common. The antigenic keratin sulfate is absent from both serum and cornea	The antigenic keratin sulfate is present in both serum and cornea
Deficiency of sulfotransferase enzyme (an enzyme that catalyzes the sulfation of kerato amino-glycans) leads to precipitation of less soluble keratin chains in the extracellular matrix, causing loss of transparency	Dermatan sulfate proteoglycan molecule is shorter than that of normal individuals, resulting in abnormal packing of collagen fibers

27. **What is the substance that forms the stromal opacity in macular dystrophy?**

   The stromal opacities correspond to the deposition of abnormal keratin sulfate proteoglycans.

28. **What are the clinical features of central crystalline dystrophy?**
    i. Central crystalline dystrophy is a bilateral disorder with autosomal dominant inheritance
    ii. It is characterized by deposition of subepithelial corneal crystals that appear early in life
    iii. Local disorder of corneal lipid metabolism. Pathologically, the opacities are accumulations of unesterified and esterified cholesterol and phospholipids
    iv. The crystals are generally deposited in an arcuate or circular pattern in the anterior, paracentral stroma. When they are relatively dense, they give the cornea a bull's eye appearance and may reduce vision
    v. Oil Red O stains the globular neutral fats red, whereas the Schultz method stains cholesterol crystals blue–green

29. **What is the Weiss classification of central crystalline dystrophy (Schnyder's crystalline dystrophy)?**
   Weiss has recommended that this dystrophy be reclassified into two major clinical types:
    i. With superficial stromal cholesterol crystals
    ii. With diffuse full-thickness stromal haze alone

30. **What is Schnyder's dystrophy sine (without) crystals?**
   Schnyder's dystrophy is a rare dystrophy with diffuse stromal haze only, called Schnyder's dystrophy sine (without) crystals.

31. **What are associated systemic conditions of central crystalline dystrophy?**
   Central crystalline dystrophy can be associated with hyperlipidemia, thyroid abnormalities, and genu valgum.

32. Describe Bietti's crystalline dystrophy.
i. Bietti's crystalline dystrophy is autosomal recessive disorder
ii. It is characterized by marginal depositions of numerous, small crystals in the anterior peripheral corneal stroma and in the paracentral and peripapillary retina
iii. Visual acuity is retained throughout its course, but pigmentary changes occur at the fovea and in the retinal periphery, which produce poor dark adaption and paracentral scotomata
iv. The demonstration of crystals resembling cholesterol and other lipids suggests a systemic abnormality of lipid metabolism

33. What are the features of fleck dystrophy?
i. Uncommon nonprogressive stromal dystrophy begins very early in life and may be congenital. It shows extreme asymmetry
ii. Affected keratocytes contain two abnormal substances: Excess glycosaminoglycan, which stain with Alcian blue and colloidal iron, and lipids demonstrated by Sudan Black and Oil Red O
iii. Discrete flat gray-white dandruff-like opacities appear throughout the stroma to its periphery. Symptoms are minimal, and vision is usually not reduced

34. What are the features of the central cloudy dystrophy of Francois?
Bilateral, symmetrical, and slowly progressive stromal dystrophy. Autosomal dominant inheritance. Extracellular deposition of mucopolysaccharide and lipid-like material has been described.

Clinically, the opacity is densest centrally and posteriorly and fades both anteriorly and peripherally. Opacities consist of multiple nebulous, polygonal, gray areas separated by crack-like intervening clear zones. Vision is usually not reduced.

35. Write short notes on congenital hereditary stromal dystrophy (CHSD).
i. CHSD is an autosomal dominant disorder and consists of bilaterally symmetric central anterior stromal, flaky feathery opacities that are present at birth
ii. It is nonprogressive but is often accompanied by searching nystagmus and esotropia
iii. Histopathologically, the stroma consists of alternating layers of tightly packed and loosely packed collagen fibrils about 15 nm in diameter
iv. The treatment of choice is penetrating keratoplasty, although amblyopia usually limits visually acuity to 20/200

36. How to differentiate CHSD and CHED?

CHSD	CHED
• Nonprogressive condition • Normal corneal thickness and absence of both epithelial edema and thickening of Descemet's membrane	• Progressive in autosomal recessive condition • Increased corneal thickness to about two to three times and diffuse gray–blue ground-glass appearance, which is the pathological hallmark of the disease

37. What are the various methods of diagnosing corneal dystrophies?
   i. Transmission electron microscopy—accurate method
   ii. Immunohistochemistry—identifies composition of deposits in dystrophic corneas
   iii. Molecular genetics—using common deoxyribonucleic acid (DNA) determinants

38. Name the substances that are found in various stromal dystrophies.
It can be remembered using the acronym.

Marilyn	— Macular
Monroe	— Mucopolysaccharides
Always	— Alcian blue
Gets	— Granular
Her	— Hyaline lipoprotein
Man	— Masson's trichrome stain
L	— Lattice
A	— Amyloid
City	— Congo red

Dystrophy	Material	Stain
Macular	Glycosaminoglycans	Alcian blue
Granular	Hyaline	Mucin
Lattice	Amylin	Congo red

39. What are the stains that are used in stromal dystrophies?
   i. *Stain for amyloid in lattice dystrophy:*
      - Pink to orange by Congo red
      - Alternating red and green color when viewed through a rotating polarizing filter
      - Yellowish green color against black background through two rotating filters
      - Periodic acid Schiff's and Masson's trichrome staining can also be used
   ii. Stain for granular dystrophy (*h*yaline lipoprotein): Masson's trichrome staining gives a bright red color

iii. *Stain for macular dystrophy (glycosaminoglycans or mucopolysaccharides):*
Blue color on staining with Alcian blue, cuprolinic blue, and colloidal iron

40. How to treat a case of stromal dystrophy?
  i. Stromal dystrophy can be treated by observation and best corrected refractive correction by spectacles. Since most of the patients are asymptomatic during their initial stages of presentation, it is better to observe
  ii. *Treatment of symptoms of erosion:* Lubricants
  iii. Excimer laser phototherapeutic keratectomy (PTK):
  Used to treat superficial lesions
  It can also be used to treat recurrence of granular dystrophy in penetrating keratoplasty because the recurrences are almost always superficial
  iv. *Superficial keratectomy:* Dense superficial juvenile variety can be treated by superficial keratectomy or lamellar keratoplasty, an advantage because multiple recurrences can be treated by multiple grafts
  v. *Lamellar keratoplasty:* For diseases involving the superficial stroma
  vi. Deep lamellar keratoplasty
  vii. Penetrating keratoplasty
  Indications: When dense opacities and subepithelial connective tissue reduce visual function to unacceptable levels. But recurrence is common affecting within 5 years.
  Macular dystrophy requires penetrating keratoplasty earlier than other stromal dystrophies.
  Recurrence after graft is less common in macular dystrophy when compared to lattice and granular dystrophy.

41. What is the differential diagnosis of congenital corneal opacity?
Acronym for the differential diagnosis of neonatal cloudy cornea—STUMPED:
S Sclerocornea
T Tears in Descemet's membrane
  Infantile glaucoma—most common cause
  Birth trauma
U Ulcer: Herpes simplex viral keratitis, bacterial, neurotrophic
M *Metabolic disorders:* Rare—mucopolysaccharidosis, mucolipidosis, tyrosinosis
P *Posterior corneal defect:* Posterior keratoconus, Peter's anomaly—most common cause staphyloma

- **E** *Endothelial dystrophy:* CHED, PPMD, congenital hereditary stromal dystrophy
- **D** Dermoid

42. What are the conditions that cause recurrent corneal epithelial erosions?

Primary epithelial dystrophies	Map-dot-fingerprint basement membrane, Franceschetti's recurrent epithelial, epithelial rosette, Meesmann's epithelial
Stromal and endothelial Dystrophies	Reis–Bucklers, gelatinous drop-like, lattice Fuchs' endothelial
Systemic diseases	Epidermolysis bullosa

43. How do you manage recurrent corneal erosions?
  i. Lubricating eye drops and ointments
  ii. Epithelial debridement
  iii. Bandage contact lenses
  iv. Anterior stromal puncture to increase adhesions
  v. Excimer laser PTK.

2.15 FUCHS' ENDOTHELIAL DYSTROPHY

1. **What is Fuchs' dystrophy?**
   Fuchs' dystrophy (combined dystrophy) is defined as a bilateral, noninflammatory, progressive loss of endothelium that results in reduction of vision, the key features being guttae, folds in Descemet's membrane, stromal edema, and microcystic epithelial edema.

2. **Describe the epidemiology of Fuchs' dystrophy.**
   i. Autosomal dominant, occasionally sporadic
   ii. Female preponderance (4:1)
   iii. Elderly; onset of symptoms >50 years
   iv. Increased incidence of primary open-angle glaucoma (POAG) (reason unclear)

3. **Describe the pathogenesis of Fuchs' dystrophy.**
   i. The primary cause of the dysfunctional endothelial cells is unknown
   ii. Corneal swelling is thought to result from the loss of Na–K ATPase pump sites within the endothelium and an increase in permeability
   iii. The deposition of aberrant collagen fibrils and basement membrane with thickening of Descemet's membrane is a result of endothelial cell transformation to fibroblast-like cells

4. **Describe the various hypotheses regarding the pathogenesis of Fuchs' dystrophy.**
   i. Believed to be due to an embryonic defect in the terminal induction or differentiation of neural crest cells resulting in abnormal morphology of Descemet's membrane
   ii. Hormonal influences are suspected as the phenotypic expression is more severe in women
   iii. Endothelial inflammation secondary to trauma, toxins, or infection results in endothelial cell pleomorphism and a thickened abnormal Descemet's membrane

5. **What are the symptoms of Fuchs' dystrophy?**
   i. Initially asymptomatic
   ii. Decrease in vision (related to edema)
   iii. Pain due to ruptured epithelial bullae
   iv. Symptoms are worse upon awakening
   v. Painful episodes subside once subepithelial fibrosis occurs

6. **Why are symptoms worse upon awakening?**
   The decrease in vision and glare in Fuchs' dystrophy is primarily due to varying degrees of epithelial and stromal edema. Decreased evaporation of the tears during sleep decreases their osmolarity, leading to increased edema and decreased visual acuity upon awakening.

7. **Describe the clinical stages of Fuchs' dystrophy.**
   Stage 1:
   i. Asymptomatic
   ii. Central cornel guttae
   iii. Pigments on the posterior corneal surface
   iv. Gray and thickened appearance of Descemet's membrane
   v. In more advanced cases, the endothelium has a "beaten-bronze" appearance due to the associated melanin deposition

   Stage 2:
   i. Painless decrease in vision and glare, severe on awakening
   ii. Stromal edema (ground-glass appearance)
   iii. Microcystic epithelial edema (occurs when stromal thickness has been increased by about 30%)

   Stage 3:
   i. Episodes of pain
   ii. Formation of epithelial and subepithelial bullae, which rupture

   Stage 4:
   i. Visual acuity may be reduced to hand movements
   ii. Free of painful attacks
   iii. Appearance of subepithelial scar tissue

8. **What are the differential diagnoses of Fuchs' dystrophy?**
   i. Posterior polymorphous dystrophy
   ii. Congenital hereditary epithelial dystrophy
   iii. Aphakic/pseudophakic bullous keratopathy
   iv. Chandler's syndrome
   v. Interstitial keratitis
   vi. Trauma
   vii. Intraocular inflammation

9. **How is a diagnosis of Fuchs' dystrophy made?**
   i. Slit-lamp findings of guttae, stromal edema, epithelial bullae
   ii. Increased central corneal thickness on pachymetry
   iii. Specular microscopy

10. **What are the features of Fuchs' dystrophy seen on specular microscopy?**
    i. Pleomorphism (increased variability in cell shape)
    ii. Polymegathism (increased variation in individual cell areas)
    iii. Decreased endothelial cell count
    iv. Guttae are seen as small dark areas with central bright spot in mild disease
    v. Later, severely disorganized endothelial mosaic is seen

11. **What are the histopathological changes in Fuchs' dystrophy?**
    Epithelium:
    i. Initially, intracellular edema in the basal cells
    ii. Later, interepithelial and subepithelial pockets of fluids develop
    iii. Map-dot and fingerprint scarring
    Bowman's membrane:
    i. Usually intact
    ii. Subepithelial fibrosis, thick in advanced disease
    Stroma:
    i. Moderate thickening and edema
    Descemet's membrane:
    i. Diffusely thickened since deposition of collagen basement membrane-like material
    ii. Anterior banded layer—relatively normal
    iii. Posterior nonbanded layer—thinned and irregular
    iv. Followed by a thick banded layer similar to the anterior banded zone and composing the guttae
    Endothelium:
    i. Lower cell density
    ii. Enlarged cells
    iii. Thinning of cells over Descemet's warts
    iv. Fibroblast-like metaplasia in end stage

12. **Why does rupture of bullae cause pain?**
    Rupture of epithelial bullae exposes the underlying nerve ending and hence causes pain.

13. **Describe the medical management of Fuchs' dystrophy.**
    i. Hyperosmotic eyed drops and ointment reduce the epithelial edema and improve both comfort and vision
       - 5% NaCl drops 4–8 times/day
       - 5% NaCl ointment at night
    ii. A hairdryer held at arm's length may help "dry-out" the corneal surface
    iii. Lowering of intraocular pressure (IOP) is useful in some cases
    iv. Bandage contact lens is used to alleviate discomfort from bullae formation and rupture

14. **Describe the surgical management of Fuchs' dystrophy.**
    Indicated when diminished visual acuity impairs normal activities. If there is no corneal opacity due to subepithelial fibrosis, then Descemet's stripping automated endothelial keratoplasty (DSAEK) is done. A recent modification called Descemet's membrane endothelial keratoplasty (DMEK) is also being performed.

15. **What are all the surgical measures for Fuchs' dystrophy done for relief of pain?**
    i. Anterior stromal puncture
    ii. Bowman's membrane cauterization
    iii. Conjunctival hooding
    iv. Amniotic membrane transplantation.

2.16 ENDOTHELIAL DISORDERS AND BULLOUS KERATOPATHY

1. **Classify endothelial diseases.**
   i. *Primary endothelial diseases*
      Endothelial dystrophy:
      - Fuchs' endothelial dystrophy
      - Posterior polymorphous dystrophy (PPMD)
      - Congenial hereditary endothelial dystrophy
      - Iridocorneal endothelial (ICE) syndrome
   ii. *Secondary endothelial diseases*
      - Mechanical trauma to the endothelium
        - Intraocular foreign body
        - Corneal trauma
        - Cataract surgery
          * Preexisting endothelial disease
          * Surgical trauma
          * Intraoperative mechanical trauma
          * Postoperative trauma
          * Vitreous touch
          * Intraocular lens (IOL)
      - Nonmechanical damage to the endothelium
        - Inflammation
        - Increased intraocular pressure (IOP)
        - Contact lens (hypoxia)

2. **What is congenital hereditary endothelial dystrophy (CHED)?**
   CHED is a dystrophy in which there is bilateral corneal edema. The corneal appearance varies from a blue-gray, ground-glass appearance to total opacification.
   Types: CHED 1
   CHED 2

3. **What are the features of CHED 1?**
   Autosomal dominant inheritance with the gene locus on 20p11.2–q11.2. It is less severe developing in the first and second years of life.
   Symptoms: Progressive defective vision is present. Nystagmus is absent.

4. **What are the features of CHED 2?**
   Autosomal recessive inheritance with the gene locus on 20p13. Present at birth. Relatively nonprogressive.
   Symptoms of discomfort are less prominent despite profound epithelial and stromal edema. Nystagmus is common.

5. **What is the pathogenesis of CHED?**
   The association of enlarged stromal collagen fibrils suggests some primary development abnormality of both keratocyte and endothelium quantifying this disorder as an example of mesenchymal dysgenesis.

6. **Is there an association between CHED and glaucoma?**
   A combination of congenital glaucoma and CHED may occur and should be suspected when persistent and total corneal opacification fails to resolve after normalization of IOP.

7. **How do you differentiate between CHED and congenital glaucoma?**

Congenital glaucoma	CHED
Photophobia present	No photophobia
Tearing and redness	Eye white
Megalocornea	Normal-sized cornea
Epithelial edema	More of a thick cornea

8. **What are corneal guttae?**
   Corneal guttae are seen as a primary condition in middle age and old age. They reveal a typical beaten metal appearance of Descemet's membrane (DM). These warts like excrescences are abnormal elaboration of basement membrane and fibrillar collagen by distressed or dystrophied endothelial cells.

9. **What are Hassall–Henle bodies?**
   Guttae located in the periphery of the cornea may be seen in patients as they get older. They are of no clinical significance.

10. **What is PPMD?**
    PPMD is a rare, slowly progressive autosomal dominant or recessive dystrophy that presents early in life. It has been mapped to chromosome 20q11.

    Pathogenesis: The most distinctive microscopic finding is the appearance of abnormal, multilayered endothelial cells that look and behave like epithelial cells or fibroblast.
    These cells:
    i. Show microvilli
    ii. Stain positive for keratin
    iii. Show rapid and easy growth in culture
    iv. Have intercellular desmosomes
    v. Manifest proliferative tendencies
       A diffuse abnormality of the DM is common, including thickening and multilaminated appearance and polymorphous alteration.

11. **What are PPMDs clinical manifestations?**
    The posterior corneal surface shows:
    i. Isolated grouped vesicles
    ii. Geographic-shaped discrete gray lesions
    iii. Broad bands with scalloped edges

12. **What are the associations of PPMD?**
    i. Iris membranes
    ii. Peripheral anterior synechiae
    iii. Ectropion uveae
    iv. Corectopia
    v. Polycoria
    vi. Glaucoma
    vii. Reminiscent of ICE syndrome
    viii. Alport's disease

13. **What are the investigations to detect PPMD?**
    i. Specular microscopy shows typical vesicles and bands
    ii. Confocal microscopy reveals alteration in DM

14. **What is the management of PPMD?**
    i. Most patients are asymptomatic
    ii. Mild corneal edema can be managed as with early Fuchs' dystrophy
    iii. Stromal micropuncture to induce subepithelial pannus can be done to manage localized swelling
    iv. In severe disease, glaucoma must be managed, and the corneal transplant may be required

15. **What is ICE syndrome?**
    ICE syndrome typically unilateral occurring in middle-aged women. It is a spectrum of disorders characterized by varying degrees of corneal edema, glaucoma, and iris abnormalities. It consists of the following three disorders with considerable overlap in presentation.
    i. Progressive iris atrophy
    ii. Iris nevus (Cogan–Reese) syndrome
    iii. Chandler's syndrome

16. **What is the pathogenesis of ICE syndrome?**
    The primary abnormality lies in the endothelial cell, which takes on the ultrastructural characteristics of epithelial cells. The abnormal endothelial cells proliferate and migrate across the angle and onto the surface of the iris, "proliferative endotheliopathy".

    Glaucoma may be due to synechial angle closure secondary to contraction of the abnormal tissue. Herpes simplex virus deoxyribonucleic acid (DNA) has been identified in some ICE syndrome corneal specimens.

17. What are the specific features?

Progressive iris atrophy: Characterized by severe iris changes such as holes and corectopia.

Iris nevus (Cogan-Reese) syndrome: Characterized by either a diffuse nevus which covers the anterior iris or iris nodules. Iris atrophy is absent in 50% of the cases although corectopia may be severe.

Chandler's syndrome:
  i. Characterized by hammered silver corneal endothelial abnormalities
  ii. Presence of corneal edema
  iii. Stromal atrophy is absent in 60% of cases
  iv. Corectopia is mild to moderate
  v. Glaucoma is usually less severe than in the other two syndromes

18. What is the treatment of ICE syndrome?
Management of glaucoma:
  i. Medical treatment is usually ineffective
  ii. Trabeculectomy is frequently unsuccessful
  iii. Artificial filtering shunts are usually required
  iv. Penetrating keratoplasty for the corneal component

19. What are the sequelae of endothelial damage in pseudophakic bullous keratopathy?

Preoperative conditions such as pseudoexfoliation (PXF), angle closure, or surgical insult either due to endothelial injury, anterior chamber intraocular lens (AC IOL), and retained viscoelastics/vitreous can damage the endothelium and cause a deficient working of the Na-K ATPase pump. These leads to:

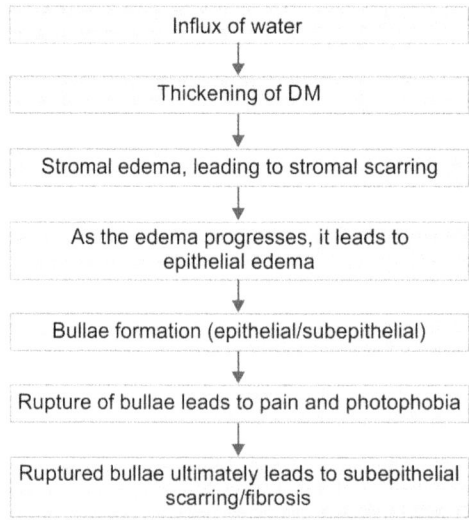

2.17 KERATOPLASTY

1. **What is keratoplasty?**
   Keratoplasty is a surgical procedure wherein the abnormal recipient corneal tissue is replaced by donor corneal tissue, either full thickness or partial thickness.

2. **Why is corneal transplant more successful than the other transplants?**
   The cornea is relatively immune privileged.
   Three factors are:
   i. Absence of blood vessels
   ii. Absence of lymphatics
   iii. Anterior chamber-associated immune deviation (ACAID)

3. **What are the indications for keratoplasty?**
   i. *Optical:*
      - Pseudophakic bullous keratopathy
      - Keratoconus
      - Corneal scars
      - Fuchs' dystrophy
   ii. *Tectonic:*
      - Stromal thinning
      - Descemetocele
      - Ectatic disorders
   iii. *Therapeutic:*
      - Removal of infected corneal tissue refractory to maximal medical therapy

4. **What are the common indications for keratoplasty in our country?**
   i. Corneal scar: Healed infectious keratitis or traumatic scar
   ii. Acute infectious keratitis
   iii. Regrafting
   iv. Aphakic and pseudophakic bullous keratopathy
   v. Corneal dystrophy, especially macular corneal dystrophy
   vi. Keratoconus

5. **What are the common indications for keratoplasty in the West?**
   i. Aphakic or pseudophakic bullous keratopathy
   ii. Fuchs' dystrophy
   iii. Keratoconus
   iv. Corneal scar
   v. Dystrophies

6. **What are the types of keratoplasty?**
   i. Full thickness or penetrating keratoplasty (PKP)
   ii. Partial thickness or lamellar keratoplasty

7. **What are the types of lamellar keratoplasty?**
   i. *Anterior:*
      - Anterior lamellar keratoplasty
      - Deep anterior lamellar keratoplasty (DALK)
   ii. *Posterior:*
      - Posterior lamellar keratoplasty (PLK)
      - Deep lamellar endothelial keratoplasty (DLEK)
      - Descemet's stripping endothelial keratoplasty (DSEK)
      - Descemet's stripping automated endothelial keratoplasty (DSAEK)
      - Descemet's membrane endothelial keratoplasty (DMEK)

8. **What are the conditions having excellent prognosis with keratoplasty?**
   i. Keratoconus
   ii. Central avascular corneal scars
   iii. Granular dystrophy
   iv. Macular dystrophy
   v. Pseudophakic bullous keratopathy

9. **What are the conditions having worst prognosis with keratoplasty?**
   i. Stevens-Johnson syndrome
   ii. Ocular cicatricial pemphigoid
   iii. Severe chemical burns
   iv. Dry eye of any etiology such as collagen vascular disorders

10. **What are the contraindications for donor's selection?**
    i. Death due to an unknown cause
    ii. Rabies
    iii. Certain infectious diseases of central nervous system (CNS) such as Jacob-Creutzfeldt, subacute sclerosing panencephalitis (SSPE), and progressive multifocal leukoencephalopathy
    iv. Human immunodeficiency virus (HIV)
    v. Septicemia
    vi. Systemic infections such as syphilis and viral hepatitis B and C
    vii. Leukemia and disseminated lymphoma
    viii. Intraocular tumors

11. **What is the importance of graft size and how much is it?**
    Usually, the donor cornea should be oversized by 0.5 mm from the recipient cornea. In keratoconus, the same size can be used.
    The graft size is about 7.5–8.5 mm.

12. **What are the disadvantages of larger graft?**
    Larger graft may cause:
    i. Increased intraocular pressure (IOP)
    ii. Rejection
    iii. Anterior synechiae
    iv. Vascularization

13. **What are the disadvantages of smaller graft?**
    Smaller graft would give rise to astigmatism due to subsequent tissue tension.

14. **Why should graft in keratoconus be same size?**
    Using the same diameter trephines for both donor and host tissues helps by decreasing postoperative myopia.

15. **What are the methods of anterior chamber entry in PKP?**
    i. *Trephine:*
       Advantages:
       - Sharp vertical edges
       - Quick
       - Uniform entry in all 360°

       Disadvantage:
       - Not controlled and so chance of damage to intraocular structures
    ii. *Blade:*
       Advantage:
       - Controlled entry

       Disadvantage:
       - May not be uniform

16. **Where are the cardinal sutures placed in PKP?**
    The first suture is placed at 12 o'clock. The second suture is the most important suture and is placed at 6 o'clock position. The third and fourth sutures are put at 3 and 9 o'clock position, respectively. At the end of the four cardinal sutures, a trapezoid should be formed.

17. **What are the indications for interrupted sutures?**
    i. Corneas of uneven thickness
    ii. Corneas with localized areas of inflammation
    iii. Vascularized, inflamed, or thinned corneas where uneven wound healing is expected
    iv. Corneas in which bites on the recipient side are very close to the sclera
    v. Pediatric keratoplasties

18. What are the advantages of interrupted sutures?
i. Technically less difficult
ii. Permit elective removal in case of children and uneven wound healing
iii. Individual suture bites can be adjusted
iv. Selective sutures can be removed in case of infection

19. What are the disadvantages of interrupted sutures?
Stimulate more inflammation and vascularization because of more knots

20. When can continuous sutures be used?
In the absence of inflammation, vascularization, or thinning, continuous sutures can be used.

21. What are the advantages of continuous sutures?
i. Continuous sutures allow more even distribution of tension around the wound
ii. Wound healing is more uniform
iii. They incite less inflammation because of less knots
iv. If double continuous is done, the second running suture can be placed in a manner that counteracts the torque induced by the first

22. What are the disadvantages of continuous sutures?
Sectoral loosening or cheese wiring compromises the entire closure of the cornea.

23. What are torque and antitorque sutures?
When continuous sutures are radially arranged perpendicular to the limbus, they are bound to induce some torque while tightening, and so they are known as torque sutures.

When the sutures are typically placed 30-40° to the donor-recipient interface in the direction of suture advancement, they are known as antitorque sutures.

24. What are combined sutures?
When both types of suturing—continuous and intermittent—are used to secure the graft, it is called combined suture.

25. What is the advantage of combined sutures?
Combined sutures have the advantage of both. Interrupted sutures can be removed as early as 4 weeks later. Continuous suture can remain in situ to protect against wound dehiscence.

26. What are the guidelines for suture removal?
i. Interrupted sutures can be removed before 6-12 months
ii. Combined interrupted sutures in steep meridian at 3 months

iii. Continuous sutures can be removed after 1 year
iv. Always remove suture by pulling on the recipient's side
v. Only loose sutures should be removed. Tight sutures may need to be cut or replaced

27. **What is lamellar keratoplasty?**
Selective replacement of diseased recipient tissue, wherein a partial-thickness donor graft is placed in the recipient corneal bed. This is prepared by lamellar dissection of abnormal corneal tissue, the donor graft being of similar size and thickness as the removed pathological host cornea.

28. **What are the advantages of anterior lamellar over PKP?**
    i. Extraocular procedure and hence devoid of intraocular complications such as hyphema and endophthalmitis
    ii. Large graft can be placed
    iii. Less chances of rejection
    iv. Nonviable tissue (tissue with low endothelial count) can be used
    v. Less stringent donor selection
    vi. Faster recovery
    vii. Better wound strength

29. **What are the disadvantages of lamellar keratoplasty?**
    i. Procedure is technically more demanding
    ii. Visual acuity can be impaired due to uneven dissection of recipient or donor corneal tissue and interface scarring
    iii. Particulate debris trapped in lamellar interface
    iv. Mechanical folds in the posterior layer over the visual axis due to flattening of this layer, especially in keratoconus
    v. Vascularization and opacification at the interface

30. **What are the indications for lamellar keratoplasty?**
    i. *Anterior:*
        - Localized superficial corneal scar
        - Keratoconus
        - Corneal and conjunctival tumors
    ii. *Posterior:*
        - Fuchs' dystrophy without corneal scarring
        - Pseudophakic bullous keratopathy without scarring

31. **When do you prefer anterior lamellar keratoplasty and why?**
Anterior keratoplasties are useful in treating:
    i. Keratoconus
    ii. Scars from refractive surgery or trauma
    iii. Stromal scarring from bacterial or viral infections

Healthy recipient endothelium is preserved, thus decreasing graft rejection and prolonged graft survival.

32. When do you prefer PLK and why?

PLKs are used primarily for endothelial diseases such as:
  i. Fuchs' endothelial dystrophy
  ii. Aphakic or pseudophakic bullous keratopathy

Advantages of PLK are:
  i. Posterior grafts do not require corneal surface incisions and sutures so induced astigmatism is reduced and tectonic stability is greater
  ii. Quicker visual rehabilitation
  iii. Theoretically, lesser chance of stromal rejection
  iv. No suture-related complications as no sutures
  v. Strong wound

33. What are the disadvantages of PLK (DSAEK/DMEK)?
  i. Requires very high-quality donor tissue
  ii. Requires costly instruments such as microkeratome and artificial anterior chamber
  iii. Higher chance of primary graft failure
  iv. Higher chance of resurgeries like rebubbling
  v. Cannot be performed if there is a significant anterior stroma opacity

34. What are inlay and onlay lamellar keratoplasties?

Inlay: Partial thickness of the recipient cornea is removed by lamellar dissection and replaced by partial thickness of the donor cornea

Onlay: Partial-thickness donor cornea is placed over a de-epithelized recipient cornea in which either a small peripheral keratectomy or lamellar dissection has been done (e.g., epikeratoplasty)

35. What are the techniques of DALK?

DALK involves replacing the entire stroma, barring Descemet's membrane (DM). This can be achieved by:
  i. Dissecting with balanced salt solution and ocular viscoelastic device
  ii. Big bubble technique of Anwar, where bubble is used to blow the DM off the rest of the cornea
  iii. Melles' technique, where a series of dissecting blades do a deep dissection to the cornea, almost down to DM

36. What is the difference between DLEK and DSEK?

In DLEK, manual lamellar dissection with corneal depth of 75-85% is done in the recipient. In DSEK, no lamellar dissection is necessary. Instead, the DM is stripped off the central 8 mm of the cornea using a reverse Sinskey's hook, followed by the placement of the folded donor disk via the sclerocorneal tunnel.

37. What is the difference between DSEK and DSAEK?

DSEK: Donor dissection is done using a manual artificial anterior chamber

DSAEK: Donor dissection is done using a microkeratome

38. What is femtosecond DSEK?

In this, the donor tissue is precut with laser. The rest of the steps continue like normal DSEK.

39. How is DSEK superior to DLEK?

DSEK:
  i. Obviates complex recipient trephination and dissection techniques. Better visual outcome
  ii. Less potential for trauma to the anterior chamber and lens
  iii. Ability to perform corneal refractive surgery later on to correct refractive errors

40. What is the advantage of DMEK?

The visual rehabilitation is superior to DSAEK, since only the DM and endothelium are transplanted without any stroma. However, it is technically difficult, and there is a higher chance of graft dislocation.

41. What are the complications of keratoplasty?

Intraoperative complications:
  i. *Improper trephination:* If a smaller-sized trephine is used for donor button instead of the recipient button, complications of smaller graft such as increased IOP may be seen
  ii. Damage to the donor button during trephination
  iii. Incomplete trephination in recipient cornea-retained DM
  iv. Iris or lens damage
  v. Anterior chamber hemorrhage
  vi. Torn posterior capsule during combined keratoplasty with cataract surgery
  vii. Expulsive choroidal hemorrhage

Postoperative complications:
  i. Wound leaks and wound displacement
  ii. Persistent epithelial defects
  iii. Filamentary keratitis
  iv. Suture-related complications:
   - Suture exposure
   - Suture-related infection
   - Suture-related immune infiltrate
  v. Elevated IOP
  vi. Postoperative inflammation
  vii. Anterior synechiae

viii. Pupillary block
ix. Choroidal detachment or hemorrhage
x. Fixed dilated pupil
xi. *Postoperative infection:* Endophthalmitis rates post-PKP: 0.2–0.7%
xii. Primary donor failure

42. **How is the donor tissue evaluated?**
    i. Slit-lamp appearance for luster, presence, or absence of folds
    ii. Specular microscopy data
    iii. Death to preservation time
    iv. Tissue storage time
    v. Serology—hepatitis B and HIV

43. **What is the recommended lower limit for the age of donors?**
    Donor corneas <1 year of age are not used, as these corneas are extremely flaccid and can result in high corneal astigmatism and myopia.

44. **What is the recommended upper limit for the age of donor?**
    The upper limit recommended by the Eye Bank Association of America is 70 years, but as long as the cornea is healthy, donor age does not matter.

45. **What is the difference between graft rejection and failure?**
    Graft rejection is an immunologically mediated, reversible loss of graft transparency in a graft that remained clear for at least 10–14 days following PKP.
    Graft failure is irreversible loss of graft corneal transparency. It can be primary failure or late donor failure or end result of multiple rejection episodes.

46. **Mention the most common types of rejection.**
    i. Endothelial
    ii. Subepithelial
    iii. Epithelial
    iv. Stromal (in decreasing frequency)

47. **What are the risk factors for rejection? Or Who are the high-risk patients?**
    Host factors:
    i. Corneal stromal vascularization
    ii. *Regrafts:* Two or more higher chances
    iii. Coexisting conditions such as uveitis, herpes simplex keratitis, atopic dermatitis, and eczema
    iv. Active ocular inflammation at the time of surgery
    v. *Age:* Young patient

Technical factors:
   i. Larger graft
   ii. Eccentric graft
   iii. Therapeutic keratoplasty
   iv. Suture removal
   v. Loose sutures arching vascularization

48. **What is the Khodadoust line?**
    The linear arrangement of endothelial precipitates, composed of inflammatory cells, originates at the vascularized end of the peripheral donor cornea or at the junction of anterior synechiae with the endothelium and moves toward the center of the cornea. It is seen in the endothelial type of rejection.

49. **What are the conclusions of the Collaborative Corneal Transplant Study (CCTS)?**
       i. Donor–recipient tissue human leukocyte antigen (HLA) typing has no significant long-term effect on the success of transplantation
       ii. ABO compatibility is more useful
       iii. In high-risk patients, high-dose topical long-term steroids, good patient compliance, and close follow-up give successful corneal transplant

50. **What are the symptoms and signs of graft rejection?**
    Symptoms precede the signs.
    Symptoms: Decreased vision
    Photophobia and glare
    Signs: Circumcorneal congestion
    Keratic precipitates
    Localized corneal edema
    Generalized corneal edema

51. **What are the types of graft failure?**
       i. *Primary graft failure:* The graft is irreversibly edematous right from the immediate postoperative period. The causes are:
          – Poor donor tissue
          – Traumatic surgery destroying endothelium
       ii. *Secondary graft failure:* The causes are:
          – Irreversible rejection
          – Infection
          – Trauma

52. **How do you treat endothelial rejection?**
       i. Topical 1% prednisolone acetate eye drops: Titrate according to the response

ii. Subconjunctival injection of 0.5 mg dexamethasone
iii. Oral prednisolone acetate 1 mg/kg body weight
iv. Intravenous methylprednisolone acetate
v. If it is still irreversible, then to plan for a regraft

53. How do you treat graft failure?
Regraft

54. What are the objectives and functions of eye bank?
A. *Objectives:*
   i. Eye banks are maintained and operated for the extraction, removal, care, storage, preservation, and/or use of human eyes or parts thereof for purposes of sight preservation or restoration
   ii. Eye banks are also operated for medical education, instruction pertaining to sight preservation or restoration, or research
   iii. Eye banks must continue to provide a service that ensures the safety and efficacy of donor tissue and ensures fair and equitable distribution of transplantable tissue

B. *Functions:*
   i. Procure, process, and distribute corneal tissue of the highest quality for transplantation
   ii. Provide and process eye tissue for research or teaching as needed
   iii. Provide families of potential donors with the mechanism and operational process to donate a decedent's eyes
   iv. Promote the retrieval of donor tissue from the hospital setting and develop professional in-service programs in order to maximize identification of suitable donors and referral to the eye bank
   v. Provide support and grief counseling to donor families
   vi. Provide for soliciting eye donation from potential donors
   vii. Promote public relation activities

55. Types of corneal preservation in eye bank

Methods	Types	Characteristics	Time limit	Constituents
Short term	Moist chamber	Whole eyes at 4°C	24 hours	–
	McCarey–Kaufman		–	Tc199, dextran,
			2–3 days	$NaHCO_3$, HEPES buffer, gentamycin, phenol red (PH indicator)

Contd...

Contd...

Methods	Types	Characteristics	Time limit	Constituents
Intermediate	K-Sol Dexol Optisol	2–6°C	7–10 days	M-K formulation + 2.5% chondroitin sulfate
	Optisol GS	GS-gentamicin 100 mg/mL and streptomycin 200 mg/mL	14 days	
Long term	Organ culture	31° and 37°C Enables HLA matching	35 days	Minimal essential medium (MEM), supplementing with varying amounts of fetal calf serum (FCS)
Very long term	Cryopreservation	Freezing, vitrification, glycerol	1 year	

Corneal preservatives color change indicators:
  i. Yellow—bacterial contamination
 ii. Red—unacceptable PH
iii. Cloudy—contamination.

CHAPTER 3

Uvea

3.1 UVEITIS—HISTORY AND CLINICAL FEATURES

1. **Why is uvea named so?**
   "Uvea" is derived from the Greek word "*uva*" meaning grape. When the sclera is removed, the center of the eyeball appears like a grape and hence the name.

2. **What does iris mean?**
   Iris is derived from a Greek word meaning rainbow/halo.

3. **What is the normal iris pattern and what are the parts of iris?**
   Iris can be divided into ciliary and pupillary zones by a zigzag line called collarette.
   At the pupillary margin, there is a pigmented frill–fringe of black pigment (due to slight extension of the posterior pigmented epithelium of the iris).
   Pupillary zone is between the pigmented frill and collarette—relatively smooth and flat.
   Ciliary zone consists of radial streaks that are straight when the pupil is small and wavy when the pupil is dilated.

4. **Why do the iris and ciliary body often get involved together?**
   The presence of the major arterial circle causes the involvement of both the iris and ciliary body in pathological conditions. The blood supply to the choroid is essentially segmental, and hence the lesions are also isolated.

5. **What is the importance of age in uveitis?**
   i. *Children:*
      - Juvenile rheumatoid arthritis (JRA)
      - Toxocariasis
   ii. *Young adults:*
      - Behçet's disease
      - Human leukocyte antigen B27 (HLA-B27)-associated uveitis
      - Fuchs' uveitis
      - Sarcoidosis

- Herpes simplex
- Toxoplasmosis

iii. *Middle age:*
- Reiter's disease
- Ankylosing spondylitis (AS)
- Vogt-Koyanagi-Harada (VKH) syndrome
- White dot syndromes
- Toxoplasmosis

iv. *Elderly individuals:*
- VKH syndrome
- Herpes zoster ophthalmicus
- Tuberculosis (TB)
- Leprosy

6. **What is the importance of gender in uveitis?**
   i. *Males:*
   - AS
   - Reiter's disease
   - Behçet's disease
   - Sympathetic ophthalmia (SO)

   ii. *Females:*
   - Rheumatoid arthritis (RA)
   - JRA

7. **What is the importance of race in uveitis?**
   i. *Caucasians:* AS
   ii. *Blacks:* Sarcoidosis
   iii. *Orientals:* VKH syndrome
   iv. *Orientals:* Behçet's disease
   v. *Filipinos:* Coccidioidomycosis

8. **Definitions.**
   i. *Anterior uveitis:*
      It is subdivided into:
      - *Iritis:* Inflammation involving iris only
      - *Iridocyclitis:* Inflammation involving iris and anterior part of ciliary body (the pars plana)
   ii. *Intermediate uveitis:* Predominant involvement of pars plana and extreme periphery of retina
   iii. *Posterior uveitis:* Inflammation beyond the posterior border of vitreous base
   iv. *Panuveitis:* Involvement of the entire uveal tract
   v. *Retinochoroiditis:* Primary involvement of retina with associated involvement of choroid

vi. *Chorioretinitis:* Primary involvement of choroid with associated involvement of retina
vii. *Vitritis:* Presence of cells in the vitreous secondary to inflammation of uvea, retina, optic nerve, and blood vessels
viii. *Diffuse choroiditis:* Generalized inflammation of the choroid
ix. *Disseminated choroiditis:* Two or more scattered foci of inflammation in the choroid, retina, or both
x. *Exogenous infection:* Infection occurring as a result of external injury to uvea, operative trauma, or any other event leading to invasion of microorganisms from outside
xi. *Endogenous infection:* Infection occurring as a result of microorganisms or their products released from a different site within the body
xii. *Secondary infection:* Infection of uveal tract due to spread from other ocular tissue

9. How do you classify uveitis?

International Uveitis Study Group Classification

i. *Anatomical classification*

Term	Primary site of inflammation	Includes
Anterior uveitis	Anterior chamber (AC)	• Iritis • Iridocyclitis • Anterior cyclitis
Intermediate uveitis	Vitreous	• Pars planitis • Posterior cyclitis • Hyalitis
Posterior uveitis	Retina/choroid	• Choroiditis • Chorioretinitis • Retinochoroiditis • Retinitis • Neuroretinitis
Panuveitis	AC/vitreous/retina/choroid	

ii. *Clinical classification*
- *Infectious:*
    - Bacterial
    - Viral
    - Fungal
    - Parasitic
- *Noninfectious:*
    - Known systemic association
    - No known systemic association

- *Masquerade:*
  - Neoplastic
  - Nonneoplastic

Anatomical Classification

Tessler's Classification
  i. Sclerouveitis
  ii. Keratouveitis
  iii. Anterior uveitis
  iv. Iritis
  v. Iridocyclitis
  vi. Intermediate uveitis
  vii. Cyclitis, vitritis
  viii. Pars planitis
  ix. Posterior uveitis
  x. Retinitis
  xi. Choroiditis

Pathological Classification

  i. Granulomatous and nongranulomatous
  ii. Suppurative and exudative

Etiological Classification

Infectious
  i. *Exogenous: Staphylococcus, Pseudomonas, Propionibacterium acnes.* Secondary—iridocyclitis associated with herpetic keratitis, iridocyclitis associated with anterior and posterior scleritis
  ii. *Endogenous:*

Bacterial	- TB - Syphilis - Gonorrhea
Viral	- Herpes simplex - Cytomegalovirus (CMV) - Measles - Influenza
Fungal	- Histoplasmosis - Coccidioidomycosis - Candidiasis
Parasitic	- Toxoplasmosis - Toxocariasis - Onchocerciasis - *Pneumocystis carinii*

Hypersensitivity/autoimmune
  i. Lens-induced—autoimmune reaction to lens protein
  ii. SO—autoimmunity to uveal pigment
  iii. VKH-suspected autoimmune origin
  iv. Behçet's

Toxic
  i. Systemic toxins—onchocercal uveitis
  ii. Endo-ocular uveitis—atrophic uveitis in degenerating eyes
  iii. Iridocyclitis in retinal detachment (RD) due to unusual proteins reaching through retinal tear
  iv. Chemical irritants—miotics and cytotoxic agents

Associated with Systemic Conditions
  i. Associated with arthritis
  ii. AS
  iii. RA
  iv. JRA
  v. Psoriatic arthritis
  vi. *Associated with gastrointestinal tract (GIT) disorders:* Ulcerative colitis
  vii. Associated with anergy: Sarcoidosis, leprosy, TB

Associated with Neoplasms
  i. Retinoblastoma, choroidal melanoma

Idiopathic
  i. Specific—Fuchs'
  ii. Nonspecific—account for 25% of all uveitis

Occurrence of Uveitis
  i. Most common type of uveitis:
     Anterior uveitis is the most common type, followed by intermediate, posterior, and panuveitis
  ii. Most common age group affected, i.e., 20-40 years
  iii. Common causes of uveitis in young adults:
     - Behçet's
     - Sarcoidosis
     - Fuchs' heterochromic iridocyclitis
     - Herpes simplex
     - Toxoplasmosis

iv. Causes of uveitis in middle ages:
   - Reiter's disease
   - AS
   - VKH syndrome
   - White dot syndrome
   - Toxoplasmosis
v. Uveitic entities with sex predilection:

Males	Females
AS	RA
Reiter's syndrome	JRA
Behçet's	

vi. Racial influence on uveitis
   - *Caucasians:* AS, Reiter's syndrome
   - *Black:* Sarcoidosis
   - *Orientals:* VKH, Behçet's
   - *Filipino:* Coccidioidomycosis
vii. Geographic influence on uveitis
   - "Histoplasmosis belt" of Ohio, Missouri, and Mississippi—histoplasmosis
   - Japan and Mediterranean countries—Behçet's disease and VKH
   - San Joaquin Valley of California—coccidioidomycosis
viii. Genetic/familial influence on uveitis
   - RA and collagen disease
   - Syphilis
   - Human immunodeficiency virus (HIV) and CMV
   - TB
   - Pars planitis

Standardization of Uveitis Nomenclature (SUN) Working Group "Activity of Uveitis" terminology:
Inactive: Grade 0 cells in anterior chamber (AC)
Worsening activity: Two-step increase in level of inflammation
Improving activity: Two-step decrease in level of inflammation
Remission: Inactive disease for >3 months after discontinuing all treatment for eye disease

SUN Working Group "Descriptors in Uveitis":
Onset: Sudden/insidious
Duration:
   Limited: <3 months' duration
   Persistent: >3 months' duration

Courses:
   Acute: Sudden onset and limited duration

Recurrent: Repeated episodes separated by periods of inactivity without treatment for a duration of 3 months

Chronic: Persistent uveitis with relapse in <3 months after discontinuing treatment

Remission: Inactive disease for at least 3 months after discontinuing treatment

10. **Name causes of acute and chronic posterior uveitis.**
    i. *Acute posterior uveitis* occurs in toxoplasmosis
    ii. *Chronic posterior uveitis* occurs in pars planitis and toxocariasis

11. **Name causes of acute generalized uveitis.**
    i. Endophthalmitis
    ii. SO

12. **What are the causes of acute suppurative uveitis?**
    i. Panophthalmitis
    ii. Endophthalmitis
    iii. Suppurative iridocyclitis

13. **What are the causes of unilateral nongranulomatous uveitis?**
    i. Fuchs'
    ii. AS

14. **What are the causes of unilateral granulomatous uveitis?**
    i. Viral
    ii. Lens-induced

15. **What are the causes of bilateral granulomatous uveitis?**

Infectious	Noninfectious
TB	Sarcoidosis
Leprosy	Vogt–Koyanagi–Harada (VKH) syndrome
Syphilis	Sympathetic ophthalmia (SO)

16. **What is Fuchs' heterochromic uveitis? What are the gonioscopic findings in Fuchs'? What are its sequelae?**

    Fuchs' uveitis is a unilateral idiopathic nongranulomatous anterior uveitis occurring in young adults. It is associated with heterochromia of the iris.

    Gonioscopic finding in Fuchs'—fine filamentous vessels bridging angle
    Sequelae in Fuchs'—cataract
    　　　　　　　　—glaucoma

17. **What are the causes of uveitis associated with vitritis?**
    i. Pars planitis
    ii. Irvine-Gass syndrome

iii. Active retinitis
iv. Trauma

18. **What is the relevance of eliciting the following history in uveitis?**
    i. Trauma/eye surgery—SO
    ii. Vitiligo, alopecia, poliosis—VKH syndrome
    iii. *Rashes:* Hyper-/hypopigmentation—leprosy
    iv. Low back pain/joint pain—AS, RA, psoriatic arthritis
    v. Painful mouth ulcers—Behçet's syndrome
    vi. Dysentery, altered bowel habits—ulcerative colitis
    vii. Ringing in the ears, hearing loss, headache—VKH
    viii. Respiratory symptoms

19. **Why history of fever is important in uveitis?**
    i. TB
    ii. Syphilis
    iii. Leprosy
    iv. Leptospirosis
    v. Collagen vascular disorders

20. **What are the systemic findings associated with uveitis?**
    Skin:
    i. Rash of secondary syphilis
    ii. Erythema nodosum, sarcoidosis, Behçet's disease
    iii. Psoriasis—plaques, arthritis
    iv. Keratoderma blennorrhagica, Reiter's syndrome
    v. Kaposi sarcoma
    vi. Leprosy
    vii. VKH syndrome
    viii. Sarcoidosis

    Hair:
    i. Alopecia: VKH, secondary syphilis
    ii. Poliosis: VKH

    Nails:
    i. Pitting
    ii. Psoriasis

    Dysentery:
    i. Reiter's syndrome

    Mouth ulcers:
    i. Painful: Behçet's syndrome
    ii. Painless: Reiter's syndrome

Arthritis:
  i. RA
  ii. JRA
  iii. AS

Gut involvement:
  i. Ulcerative colitis
  ii. Crohn's disease

Lungs:
  i. TB
  ii. Sarcoidosis

Urethritis/urethral ulcers:
  i. VKH
  ii. CMV infections
  iii. Congenital toxoplasmosis
  iv. Syphilis

Central nervous system (CNS) involvement:
  i. VKH
  ii. CMV
  iii. Behçet's disease
  iv. Congenital toxoplasmosis

21. **Why do we ask for history of contact with pet animals/livestock?**
    i. Cat—toxocariasis, toxoplasmosis
    ii. Cattle—leptospirosis, cysticercosis, toxoplasmosis
    iii. Pigs—cysticercosis, leptospirosis
    iv. Rat—leptospirosis

22. **What is the mechanism of pain in uveitis?**
    Pain is an acute spasmodic ciliary neuralgia superimposed on a dull ache. Since the iris is richly supplied with sensory nerves from the ophthalmic division of the fifth nerve, pain is very common. It is typically worse at night. It is worse in the acute stage when there is tissue swelling hyperemia and release of high concentration of toxic materials.

23. **What are the symptoms in cyclitis/choroiditis?**
    Cyclitis:
      i. Floaters
      ii. Redness due to ciliary congestion
      iii. Tenderness over pars plana
      iv. Defective vision in chronic cyclitis due to vitreous opacities

    Choroiditis:
      i. Asymptomatic, unless posterior pole is involved
      ii. Photopsia, due to irritation of rods and cones at the periphery of the lesion

iii. Floaters—due to outpouring of exudate
iv. Metamorphopsia due to irregular elevation in the retina. Initially, a positive scotoma develops, following which a negative scotoma develops. Hiatus or negative scotoma is sector-shaped in severe lesions due to destruction of nerve fibers and blockage of retinal vessels causing damage to retinal pigment epithelium (RPE) in the periphery

24. What are the differences between photophobia and blepharospasm?

	Photophobia	*Blepharospasm*
Definition	Increased sensitivity/abnormal intolerance to ambient light	Focal dystonia manifested by forceful, frequent involuntary eyelid closure
Etiology	*Ocular:* Blepharitis, conjunctivitis, keratitis, dry eye, iridocyclitis, vitritis, optic neuritis, papilledema *Nonocular:* Blepharospasm, migraine, traumatic brain injury	• Benign essential • Blepharospasm (BEB)—B/L condition • The exact cause of BEB is unknown and, by definition, it is not associated with another disease entity or syndrome. It is a diagnosis of exclusion
Pathophysiology	*Afferent:* Unmyelinated ciliary branches of ophthalmic nerve (V1)—branch of trigeminal nerve *Center:* Trigeminal nucleus caudalis (TNC) →Thalamus and cortex (nociceptive signals) *Efferent:* Facial nerve → Orbicularis oculi (blinking reflex)	Dysfunction in basal ganglia, overacting facial nerve
Instillation of local anesthetic and exposure to dark	Patient gets relieved of the symptom	Symptom persists
Treatment	Treat the cause	Periodic injection of a botulinum toxin A

25. Differentiate circumcorneal/ciliary and conjunctival congestion.

	Conjunctival	*Circumcorneal*
Site	In fornices	Circumcorneal
Color	Bright red	Pale red/violaceous
Type of discharge	Mucus	Serous

Contd...

Contd...

	Conjunctival	*Circumcorneal*
Branching of vessels	Dichotomous	Radially arranged around the cornea without branching
Origin	Posterior conjunctival vessels	Anterior ciliary vessels
Movement of vessels	Can be moved on moving conjunctiva	Cannot be moved
On pressure	Fill from fornix	Fill from limbus

26. What are the important signs of uveitis?
  i. *Lids and adnexa:*
   - Vesicles—herpes zoster ophthalmicus
   - Poliosis—VKH, SO
   - Nodules—sarcoid, leprosy
   - Madarosis—leprosy
  ii. *Conjunctiva:*
   - Granulomas—foreign body, sarcoidosis, trematode granuloma
  iii. *Cornea:*
   - Keratic precipitates (KP)—granulomatous/nongranulomatous/stellate
   - Dendritic keratitis—viral uveitis
   - Sclerokeratouveitis—syphilis, TB, leprosy
   - Exposure keratopathy—leprosy
   - Band keratopathy—juvenile idiopathic arthritis (JIA), sarcoidosis
  iv. *AC:*
   - Cells, flare
   - Fibrinous membrane—HLA-B27
   - Hypopyon—TB, leptospirosis, endophthalmitis, Behçet's
   - Hyphema—herpetic uveitis, traumatic
  v. *Iris/pupil:*
   - Koeppe, busacca nodules
   - Miotic or irregular/festooned pupils—posterior synechiae
   - Relative afferent pupillary defect—asymmetric disk involvement; disk edema—uveitis or optic atrophy in chronic uveitis
   - Argyll Robertson pupil—neurosyphilis
   - *Iris atrophy:* Sectoral—herpes zoster, patchy—herpes simplex, diffuse—Fuch's heterochromic iridocyclitis, leprosy
  vi. *Lens*—complicated cataract
  vii. *Gonioscopy:*
   - Peripheral anterior synechiae (PAS)—sarcoidosis, TB
   - Iris nodules—sarcoidosis (Berlin's nodule)
   - Neovascularization of angle—Fuch's heterochromic iridocyclitis

viii. *Intraocular pressure (IOP):*
- Secondary glaucoma
- Hypotony

ix. *Vitreous:*
- Inflammatory cells/vitritis
- Traction bands

x. *Pars plana:*
- Snowbanking

xi. *Retina:*
- Snowballs
- Serous detachments
- Cystoid macular edema
- Vasculitis
- RPE clumping
- Choroidal neovascular membrane (CNVM)
- Epiretinal membrane (ERM)

xii. *Optic nerve head:*
- Edema/papillitis
- Neovascularization
- Infiltration
- Optic atrophy

27. **What are the KPs? What is the importance of detecting them? What is their fate?**

    Keratic precipitates comprise lymphocytes, plasma cells, and phagocytes enmeshed in a network of fibrin. Mononuclear phagocytes are common in nongranulomatous KPs. Epithelial and giant cells are common in granulomatous KPs.

    Significance of KPs:
    i. Give clue to diagnosis
    ii. Evidence of inflammatory activity
    iii. Signify involvement of the ciliary body

    Fate of KPs:
    i. Hyalinization
    ii. May disappear after resolution of inflammation
    iii. May reduce in size
    iv. May become pigmented
    v. May get washed away during surgery

    Sometimes, if inflammation becomes chronic, then nongranulomatous KPs may become larger and granulomatous.

28. Describe distribution of KPs.

von Arlt's triangle: A base-down triangle on the inferior aspect of the corneal endothelium, where KPs aggregate due to convection currents of aqueous humor and gravity
Ehrlich Tuck's line: Vertical line along the center of the endothelium
Central: Viral
Diffuse: Fuchs' heterochromic iridocyclitis
In the angle: Sarcoidosis

29. What are the prerequisites for a KP to occur?

i. Defective nutrition of the corneal endothelium so that the cells become sticky and may desquamate in places
ii. The convection currents in the AC (due to the difference of the temperature between the warm iris and the cool cornea)
iii. Gravity

30. Differentiate fresh/old and granulomatous/nongranulomatous KPs.

Fresh		*Old*
White		Pigmented
Round		Flat
Fully hydrated		Dehydrated
Smooth edges		Crenated edges
	Granulomatous	*Nongranulomatous*
Size	Large	Small to medium
Shape	Oval or oblong	Usually circular
Color and appearance	• Yellow and greasy • Mashed potato appearance	White—hydrated
Confluence	Often confluent	Usually nonconfluent
Changes	• Cause alteration of endothelium leading to prelucid halos • May get pigmented	Pigmentation, dehydration, flattening

31. What is flare? What is its significance? How is it examined and graded?

The visualization of the path of the slit lamp when aimed obliquely across the AC is called flare.

Breakdown of blood–ocular barrier and damage to iris blood vessels cause proteins to leak into AC. This causes flare.

Flare in the absence of cells does not indicate active inflammation as damaged blood vessels leak for a long time after inflammation has resolved. Steroids are not indicated in the absence of cells.

Flare is examined at the slit lamp with maximum light intensity and magnification 1 mm long, 1 mm wide beam is directed at 45-60° to ocular surface.

Grading of flare:
Hogan's grading:

Faint—just detectable	= 1+
Moderate—iris details clear	= 2+
Marked—iris details hazy	= 3+
Intense—fibrinous exudates	= 4+

SUN Working Group Grading for AC flare:

Grade	Description
0	None
+1	Faint
+2	Moderate (iris and lens details clear)
+3	Marked (iris and lens details hazy)
+4	Intense (fibrin/plasmoid aqueous)

32. What are the types of AC reaction?

Serous: Flare due to protein exudation
Purulent: Polymorphonuclear neutrophils (PMNs) and necrotic debris causing hypopyon
Fibrinous/plastic: Intense fibrinous exudates, hypopyon
Sanguinoid: Inflammatory cells with red blood cells (RBCs), hypopyon

33. What are the types of cells in AC? How are they graded?

i. Inflammatory cells (lymphocytes and PMN)
ii. RBCs
iii. Iris pigment cells
iv. Malignant cells, e.g., lymphoma

Grading of cells
Hogan's grading:

None	= 0
5–10/field	= 1
10–20/field	= 2
20–50/field	= 3
50/field	= 4

SUN working group grading of AC cells:

Grade	Cells in fields
0	None
+0.5	1–5
+1	6–15
+2	16–25
+3	26–50
+4	>50

34. **How is hypopyon formed in uveitis?**
    Hypopyon is a collection of leukocytes. Sufficient fibrin content in the AC causes cells to clump and settle down as hypopyon.

35. **What are the causes of pseudohypopyon?**
    A collection of cells infiltrating the AC of eye resembles a hypopyon, but caused by tumor or endophthalmitis.

    Causes:
    i. Leukemia
    ii. Masquerade syndrome
    iii. CNS lymphoma
    iv. Melanoma-associated retinopathy
    v. In best macular dystrophy

    Differential diagnosis (D/D):
    i. Emulsified silicon oil in AC D/D
    ii. Phacolytic glaucoma

36. **When is hyphema seen in uveitis?**
    i. Viral uveitis (especially zoster)
    ii. Syphilis
    iii. Ophthalmia nodosum
    iv. Trauma
    v. Masquerade syndrome

37. **What are the iris changes in uveitis?**
    i. Pattern change—iris crypts and furrows are obliterated
    ii. Iris atrophy
    iii. Heterochromia—Fuchs', viral
    iv. Rubeosis
    v. Synechiae
    vi. Seclusio pupillae
    vii. Occlusion pupillae
    viii. Ectropion uveae
    ix. Nodules—Koeppe's and Busaca's
    x. Granulomas and lepra pearls

38. **What are the causes of atrophic patch of iris?**
    i. Sectoral patches—herpes simplex virus, Fuchs' iridocyclitis, chronic uveitis causing posterior synechiae, snakebites, surgical trauma
    ii. Diffuse atrophy—leprosy, herpes zoster, VKH
    iii. Others—pseudoexfoliation syndrome (PXF) and pigment dispersion, iridocorneal endothelial (ICE) syndromes

39. **What are the nodules seen in a case of uveitis? What are leprotic pearls?**
    There are two types of nodules seen in uveitis:

	Koeppe's	*Busacca's*
Location	At pupillary margin	Usually seen along collarette
Pathology	Ectodermal nodules	Mesodermal floccules
Color	Small, usually white, but may be pigmented	Greenish white and larger than Koeppe's nodules
Conditions	Usually seen in granulomatous but may occur in nongranulomatous	Only in granulomatous, never in nongranulomatous uveitis

    Leprotic pearls:
    They are iris nodules, pathognomonic of leprosy, and are situated between collarette and ciliary margin.

40. **What are the types of synechiae?**
    Based on anatomical structures:
    i. Posterior synechiae: Adhesions between the posterior surface of iris and anterior capsule of lens
    ii. PAS: Iris adherent to the cornea adjacent to the angle

41. **What are the types of posterior synechiae?**
    i. Segmental
    ii. Annular posterior synechiae/ring synechiae—360° synechiae which prevents circulation of aqueous from posterior to anterior chamber leading to seclusion pupillae and iris bombe formation
    iii. Total posterior synechiae—plastering of posterior surface of iris to the anterior surface lens; rare occurrence

42. **What are the types of peripheral anterior synechiae (PAS)?**
    Peripheral anterior synechiae in uveitis are typically found inferiorly, while PAS in primary angle closure is more common in superior quadrants initially.
    i. Bridging PAS—discrete high PAS to Schwalbe's line
    ii. Broad-based PAS—seen in TB
    iii. Tent-shaped PAS—sarcoidosis

43. What is seclusio pupillae?
Seclusio pupilla is also called annular or ring synechia. In this condition, the whole circle of the pupillary margin may become tied down to the lens capsule.

44. What is occlusio pupillae?
When the exudate becomes more extensive, it may cover the entire pupillary area, which then becomes filled by a film of opaque, fibrous tissue, and this condition is called occlusio pupillae.

45. What is the differential diagnosis for iris nodules?
   i. Down syndrome (Brushfield spots)
   ii. Epithelial invasion, serous cyst
   iii. Foreign body (retained)
   iv. Fungal endophthalmitis
   v. Iridocyclitis
   vi. Iris freckle
   vii. Iris nevus syndrome (Cogan-Reese)
   viii. Iris pigment epithelial cyst
   ix. Juvenile xanthogranuloma
   x. Leiomyoma
   xi. Malignant melanoma
   xii. Melanocytosis (ocular and oculodermal)
   xiii. Neurofibromatosis
   xiv. Retinoblastoma

46. What are the pupil changes in uveitis?
In the acute stage: Miosis
In the chronic stage: Posterior synechiae

Miosis is due to:
   i. Irritants causing muscle fibers to contract; sphincter effect overcomes dilator leading to constriction
   ii. Vascularity allows unusual amounts of exudation, causing iris to become waterlogged and the pupil to become sluggish
   iii. Radial nature of the vessels

47. What are the causes for synechiae in uveitis?
Inflammation is often accompanied by the release of mediators that promote fibrin deposition, clotting and fibroblast proliferation, which are the probable causes of synechiae.

48. What are the causes for neuro retinitis?
Neuroretinitis is characterized by disk edema, macular star, and retinitis patches. The most common cause is infectious neuroretinitis caused by *Bartonella* (cat scratch disease).

Other infectious diseases include syphilis, Lyme disease, Rocky Mountain Spotted Fever, toxoplasmosis, toxocariasis, histoplasmosis, and leptospirosis.

49. **What are the various causes of complicated cataract?**
    i. Uveitis
    ii. Trauma
    iii. Steroids (systemic steroids)
    iv. Chronic RD
    v. Radiation
    vi. Retinitis pigmentosa (RP)
    vii. High myopia

50. **Why is posterior subcapsular cataract more common in complicated cataract?**
    i. Posterior capsule is thin, and hence toxins can diffuse easily
    ii. Rate of metabolism is low
       Since the metabolism is high in the anterior lens capsule, toxins can be metabolized (easily washed away).

51. **What are the characteristic features of complicated cataract?**
    i. Bread crumb appearance
    ii. Polychromatic luster

52. **What are the vitreous changes in uveitis?**
    Vitreous changes:
    i. Opacities—fine, coarse, stingy snowball
    ii. Posterior vitreous detachment (PVD)
    iii. Cellular precipitation posterior wall of vitreous, flare and cells, fluid in retrovisceral space
    iv. Late shrinkage of vitreous may cause vitreal holes and RD
    v. Vitreous hemorrhage

    SUN Working Group Grading for vitreous cells:

Grade	Number of cells
0	None
+0.5	1–10
+1	10–20
+2	20–30
+3	30–100
+4	>100

53. What are the fundus changes in uveitis?

A. *Optic disk:*
   i. Papillitis (VKH)
   ii. Granuloma (sarcoid)
   iii. Optic atrophy secondary to retinal damage
   iv. Disk hyperemia/edema

B. *Macula:*
   i. Edema (pars planitis, birdshot chorioretinopathy)
   ii. Scar—toxoplasmosis

C. *Peripheral retina:*
   i. Healed retinitis/choroiditis/retinochoroiditis
   ii. RD
      - Serous (VKH)
      - Rhegmatogenous
      - Tractional
   iii. Vascular occlusion
   iv. Perivascular exudates
   v. Candle wax drippings, e.g., sarcoid
   vi. Sheathing, e.g., Eales' disease
   vii. Pars plana exudates—snow banking
   viii. Neovascularization
      - Peripheral—pars planitis
      - Macular—toxoplasmosis
      - Periphery and optic nerve head (ONH) sarcoidosis

54. What are the causes of defective vision in uveitis?

i. *Cornea:*
   - Corneal edema
   - KPs on endothelium

ii. *AC:*
   - Cells and flare

iii. *Pupil:*
   - Miosis

iv. *Lens:*
   - Complicated cataract

v. *Vitreous:*
   - Vitreous cells
   - Vitreous hemorrhage

vi. *Fundus:* Optic disc:
   - Papillitis
   - Papilledema
   - Optic atrophy

vii. *Macula:*
- Edema
- Scar

viii. *Peripheral retina:*
- Retinitis/choroiditis/retinochoroiditis
- RD
- Vascular occlusion

55. **Differentiate choroiditis from retinitis.**

Choroiditis	Retinitis
Yellow patch	White cloudy appearance
Distinct with defined borders	Indistinct borders
Involvement of vessels	Abundant vitreous cells
Vitreous minimal or absent	Sheathing of adjacent vessels
Subretinal hemorrhage	Surrounding retinal edema

56. **What is the difference between active and healed choroiditis?**

Active	Healed
Elevated lesion	Flat
Ill-defined margins	Distinct pigmented margins
Associated with vascular sheathing, hemorrhage, and vitreous inflammation	No associated features

57. **What are the IOP changes that can occur in uveitis?**

Low IOP:
   i. Inflammation of ciliary body and failure to produce sufficient amount of aqueous
   ii. Choroidal detachment
   iii. RD

High IOP:
   i. Trabeculitis
   ii. Neovascular glaucoma (NVG)
   iii. Clogging of trabecular meshwork by inflammatory debris
   iv. Posner-Schlossman syndrome
   v. Sclerosis of trabecular meshwork
   vi. PAS
   vii. Iris bombe
   viii. Steroid-induced glaucoma

58. **What are the uveitic conditions associated with increased IOP?**
   i. Viral
   ii. Toxoplasmosis

iii. Sarcoidosis
iv. Fuchs' heterochromic iridocyclitis
v. Posner–Schlossman syndrome
vi. Steroid-induced uveitis
vii. Lens-induced uveitis

59. What are the characteristic features of Posner–Schlossman syndrome?

Posner–Schlossman syndrome is also known as hypertensive iridocyclitis crisis. The features are:
 i. Quiet eye
 ii. Periodic raised IOP with flare and cells
 iii. Reduced vision during these attacks and mimics angle closure glaucoma
 iv. Treatment is done by using atropine ointment

60. What are the complications of iridocyclitis?

Corneal conditions:
 i. Band keratopathy

AC:
 i. Posterior synechiae
 ii. Iris bombe
 iii. Seclusio pupillae
 iv. Occlusio pupillae

Secondary glaucoma (described above)
Complicated cataract
Cystoid macular edema
Tractional RD
Phthisis bulbi

61. How does phthisis occur in uveitis?

Organization of vitreous forms a cyclitic membrane, contraction of which leads to a RD with base toward lens and apex toward optic disc. As the cyclitic membrane consolidates, the ciliary processes are drawn inward so that the ciliary body detaches, leading to phthisis bulbi.

62. What are the causes of cystoids macular edema in uveitis?

 i. Acute severe iridocyclitis
 ii. Behçet's syndrome
 iii. Pars planitis
 iv. Endophthalmitis
 v. Birdshot chorioretinopathy

63. **Why is the posterior pole of retina involved in uveitis?**
    i. The blood-retinal barrier is composed of tight junctions between the retinal pigment epithelial cells and the endothelium of retinal vessels. Increased permeability at the level of the blood-retinal barrier results in inflammatory cell accumulation and tissue destruction in the retina with or without involvement of the choroid
    ii. Primary retinal vasculitis refers to vasculitis due to direct involvement of vasculature, for example, in diseases characterized by immune complex deposition to the vessel wall
    iii. An occlusive vasculitis is due to egress of inflammatory cells through vessel walls with a resulting periphlebitis
    iv. Neovascularization of the retina can be a manifestation of ischemic uveitis
    v. Accumulation of fluid in the outer plexiform and inner nuclear layers can result in cystoid macular edema with a petaloid pattern on fluorescein angiography

64. **What are the causes of macular chorioretinitis?**
    i. Toxoplasmosis
    ii. TB
    iii. Syphilis
    iv. CMV retinitis
    v. Herpes simplex

65. **What are the causes of retinochoroiditis?**
    i. Toxoplasmosis
    ii. Toxocara granuloma of retina/choroid
    iii. Septic (subacute bacterial endophthalmitis)
    iv. CMV retinitis
    v. Candida retinitis

66. **What are the causes of chorioretinitis?**
    i. TB
    ii. Acute posterior multifocal placoid pigment epitheliopathy (APMPPE)
    iii. Geographical helical polypoidal choroidopathy
    iv. Birdshot choroidopathy
    v. SO
    vi. Presumed ocular histoplasmosis

67. **What is the characteristic description of active toxoplasmic retinochoroiditis?**
    "Headlight in fog" appearances

68. **What are the preoperative concerns while performing cataract surgery in an eye with uveitis?**
    i. The eye should remain quiet for a minimum of 3 months before contemplating surgery under the cover of steroids
    ii. In phacolytic and other lens-induced uveitides, the above does not apply, and cataract surgery could be done immediately

69. **What are the intraoperative steps to be taken while performing cataract surgery in a uveitic eye?**
    i. Inadequate pupillary dilatation (to do sphincterotomy, iris hooks, sector iridectomy)
    ii. Complete cortical removal
    iii. Minimal manipulation of iris
    iv. To perform a prophylactic peripheral iridotomy
    v. Perform capsulorhexis and facilitate in the bag intraocular lens placement
    vi. To preferably use a heparin-coated or an acrylic lens

70. **What are the indications of explanation of intraocular lens (IOLs) in a uveitic eye?**
    i. *Propionibacterium* gene endophthalmitis
    ii. Persistent postoperative uveitis with haptic rubbing of the iris due to "in sulcus" placement

71. **Name a uveitic entity in which intraocular placement of IOL is contraindicated. Why?**
    Juvenile idiopathic arthritis due to persistent severe uveitis causing cyclitic membrane leading to phthisis bulbi.

72. **What are the uses of atropine in a case of uveitis?**
    i. It keeps the iris and ciliary body at rest
    ii. It breaks the preexisting synechia and prevents new synechia from occurring
    iii. It decreases hyperemia

73. **What is mydricaine?**
    Mydricaine is a powerful mydriatic agent and is a combination of procaine, atropine, and adrenaline. 0.3 mL is given through the subconjunctival route.

3.2 SYMPATHETIC OPHTHALMIA

1. **Define sympathetic ophthalmia.**
   Sympathetic ophthalmia is specific bilateral inflammation of the entire uveal tract of unknown etiology, characterized clinically by insidious onset and progressive course with exacerbations and pathologically by a nodular or diffuse infiltration of the uveal tract with lymphocytes and epitheloid cells, almost universally follows a perforating injury involving the uveal tissue.

   Exciting eye—injured eye developing the disease at a variable time after the injury.

   Sympathizing eye—the other eye which develops the disease synchronously or shortly afterward.

2. **What are the predisposing causes for sympathetic ophthalmia?**
   i. *Perforating injuries—65%*
      - Perforating injury involving the uveal tissue and in the vast majority of cases, rapid and reaction-less wound healing is interfered by iris, ciliary body incarceration, or foreign body retention
      - Subacute inflammation in a soft shrunken eye in which delayed or incomplete wound healing is present
      - Wounds in the ciliary region are most dangerous but not very common
   ii. *Operative wounds—25%*
      - Incarceration of iris in the wound
      - Iridectomy, iridencleisis
   iii. *Nonperforating contusions* (subconjunctival scleral rupture)—10%
   iv. *Intraocular malignant melanomata*—rare
      - Complicated by perforation of the globe by invading tumor
      - Necrotic tumors

3. **Discuss the pathology of sympathetic ophthalmia.**
   i. Sympathetic ophthalmia is a clinicopathologic diagnosis and never a histological diagnosis alone
   ii. Focal lymphocytic and plasma cell infiltration around large veins of choroid → coalesce to form multinucleated giant cells → formation of nodules of epitheloid cells with central giant cells surrounded by lymphocytes → infiltration of iris (posterior part) and diffuse infiltration of choroid (especially outer layers)
   iii. Four characteristic histological findings in the sympathizing and exciting eye include:
      - Diffuse granulomatous uveal inflammation composed predominantly of epitheloid cells and lymphocytes; eosinophil and plasma cells may be present—neutrophils are absent

- Sparing of choriocapillaris
- Epitheloid cells containing phagocytosed uveal pigment
- Dalen Fuchs' nodules:
  Collections of epitheloid cells between Bruch's membrane and the retinal pigment epithelium (RPE) with no involvement of the overlying neural retina and sparing of the underlying choriocapillaris
  Some cells may come from transformation of the RPE

4. **What are the clinical features of sympathetic ophthalmia?**

In sympathizing eye:
  i. Mild pain
  ii. Photophobia
  iii. Increased lacrimation
  iv. Blurring of vision
  v. Visual fatigue

In exciting eye:
Decrease in vision and photophobia

Signs in both eyes:
  i. Ciliary injection
  ii. Development of keratic precipitates on corneal endothelium
  iii. Partially dilated and poorly responsive pupil
  iv. Thickened iris
  v. Clouding of vitreous

Posterior segment findings:
  i. Papillitis
  ii. Generalized retinal edema
  iii. Perivasculitis
  iv. Small yellow-white exudate beneath RPE (Dalen–Fuchs' nodule)
  v. Areas of choroiditis
  vi. Exudative retinal detachment.

3.3 FUCHS' HETEROCHROMIC IRIDOCYCLITIS

1. **What are the signs and symptoms of Fuchs' heterochromic iridocyclitis?**

    Symptoms:
    i. Decreased vision—due to cataract formation
    ii. Floaters—due to vitreous opacities
    iii. Discomfort—due to ciliary spasm
    iv. Conjunctival injection
    v. Asymptomatic
    vi. Symptoms due to elevated intraocular pressure (IOP)
    vii. Change in iris color
    viii. Hyphema
    ix. Strabismus from juvenile cataract

    Signs:
    Triad of:
    i. Heterochromia
    ii. Cataract
    iii. Keratic precipitates (KP)

    Heterochromia:
    i. Iris pigments are present in all three layers:
        - Anterior border layer
        - Stroma
        - Posterior pigment epithelium
    ii. There is atrophy of all the three layers
    iii. Atrophy of anterior border layer and stroma—*hypochromia* in many cases and *hyperchromia* in a few due to revealing of the posterior pigment epithelium
    iv. Blue irides—affected eye looks bluer or lighter than the other eye due to loss of orange-brown pigment of the anterior border layer concentrated around the collarette. Rarely show hyperchromia
    v. Brown—usually affected eyes are hypochromic and may appear normal also
    vi. Subtle heterochromia—best observed by naked unaided eye under natural daylight or bright overhead light. Most sensitive method to identify heterochromia is to compare anterior segment photographs taken under standard conditions
    vii. May be congenital/acquired later in life
    viii. Bilateral cases—no heterochromia

    Iris characteristics:
    i. *Anterior border layer:* Depigmentation → lighter, translucent, whitish hazy appearance

ii. Stroma—depigmentation and loss of volume → smooth iris surface → prominent radial vessels → visualization of the sphincter
iii. Pigment epithelium affected: Transillumination defects and abnormalities of the pupillary ruff
iv. Iris nodules: Rare, translucent near the pupillary margin
v. Posterior synechiae are rare
vi. Iris vessels:
   - Due to atrophy—normal iris vessels become conspicuous
   - Radial and orderly dichotomous branching
   - New vessels—fine, filamentous, sinuous, arborizing with anomalous branching pattern
   - Seen on the surface of iris and anterior chamber angle
   - Rarely may form fibrovascular membrane over trabecular meshwork—neovascular glaucoma occasional
   - *Incidence of rubeosis:* 6–22%; more when iris fluorescein angiography is used
   - May cause filiform hemorrhage arising as a fine stream of blood arising in or near the angle usually opposite to the site of puncture during paracentesis—*Amsler sign*
   - Considered to be diagnostic and confirmatory test—but now its clinical utility is questioned
   - Applanation tonometry and cataract surgery may cause bleeding

Iridocyclitis:
Characteristic KPs:
i. Stellate or round, whitish translucent with interspersed wispy filaments precipitated over the entire corneal endothelium diffusely
ii. Minimal anterior chamber cellular activity

Cataract:
i. Posterior subcapsular cataracts
ii. Rapid advance to maturation

Vitreous cells:
Individual cells, aggregates, stingy filaments, and occasional dense vitreous veils.

Glaucoma: 26–59% Mechanism of glaucoma:
i. Rubeosis
ii. Peripheral anterior synechiae
iii. Lens-induced angle closure
iv. Recurrent spontaneous hyphema
v. Steroid response.

3.4 VOGT–KOYANAGI–HARADA SYNDROME

1. **What is Vogt–Koyanagi–Harada (VKH) syndrome?**
   VKH syndrome or uveomeningitic syndrome is a systemic disorder involving many organ systems, including the eye, ear, integumentary, and nervous system.

2. **What are the clinical manifestations of VKH?**
   The American Uveitis Society adopted the criteria for the diagnosis of VKH syndrome in 1978 as follows:
   i. No history of ocular trauma or surgery
   ii. At least three of four of the following signs:
      - Bilateral chronic iridocyclitis
      - Posterior uveitis, including exudative retinal detachment, disk hyperemia or edema, and sunset glow fundus
      - Neurologic signs of tinnitus, neck stiffness, cranial nerve or central nervous system (CNS) problems or cerebrospinal fluid (CSF) pleocytosis
      - Cutaneous findings of alopecia, poliosis, or vitiligo

3. **What are the clinical manifestations of VKH?**
   Typical clinical manifestations of VKH syndrome:
   i. Bilateral panuveitis in association with multifocal serous RD
   ii. CNS manifestations—meningismus, headache, CSF pleocytosis
   iii. Auditory manifestations—hearing loss, tinnitus
   iv. Cutaneous manifestations—vitiligo, alopecia, poliosis

   Most patients present with severe bilateral uveitis associated with exudative retinal detachment and signs of meningismus.

4. **What are the differential diagnoses of VKH?**
   i. Idiopathic central serous choroidopathy
   ii. Nanophthalmos (axial length <19 mm)
   iii. Uveal effusion syndrome
   iv. Bilateral diffuse melanocytic hyperplasia
   v. Toxemia of pregnancy, renal disease
   vi. Posterior scleritis
   vii. Acute retinal necrosis syndrome
   viii. Primary B-cell intraocular lymphoma
   ix. Syphilis, tuberculosis, and sarcoidosis
   x. Sympathetic ophthalmia
   xi. Lupus choroidopathy

5. How will you investigate a case of VKH?

Fluorescein angiography (FA)
  i. Characteristic FA in an acute stage of VKH demonstrates multiple punctate hyperfluorescent dots at the level of retinal pigment epithelium (RPE)
  ii. These hyperfluorescent dots gradually enlarge and stain the subretinal fluid
  iii. 70% of the patients have disk leakage
  iv. In chronic stage, the angiogram shows multiple hyperfluorescent RPE window defects without progressive staining
  v. Alternating hyper- and hypofluorescence from RPE alteration causing "moth eaten" appearance can be found

Ultrasonography:
Echographic manifestations of VKH are described by:
  i. Diffuse thickening of the posterior choroid with low-to-medium reflectivity
  ii. Serous retinal detachment (RD) around posterior pole or inferiorly
  iii. Vitreous opacities without posterior vitreous detachment (PVD)
  iv. Posterior thickening of the sclera or episclera

Lumbar puncture:
Lumbar puncture (LP) has not been used routinely in most recent studies. In a study by Ohno et al., >80% of the patients had CSF pleocytosis consisting mostly of lymphocytes. CSF pleocytosis occurs in 80% of the case within 1 week and resolves within 8 weeks.

MRI discriminates the sclera from the choroid, which is not possible with computerized tomography and allows the detection of subclinical ocular and CNS disease. Choroidal thickening can be demonstrated even when the fundus and fluorescein angiogram appear normal.

3.5 BEHÇET'S DISEASE

1. **Definition of Behçet's disease.**

   Behçet's disease is relapsing and remitting systemic vasculitis of unknown etiology characterized by oral and genital ulcers and ocular inflammation.

   With the triad of:
   i. Recurrent hypopyon—iritis
   ii. Oral ulceration
   iii. Genital ulceration

2. **What is the etiology?**
   i. Viral agent—herpes simplex
   ii. Bacterial—streptococcal species
   iii. Genetic:
      - Human leukocyte antigen (HLA)-B5—ocular type
      - HLA-B12—mucocutaneous
      - HLA-B27—arthritic

3. **What is Behçet's Disease Research Committee Criteria?**

   Major criteria:
   i. Oral aphthous ulceration
   ii. Skin lesions:
      - Erythema nodosum-like skin eruption
      - Subcutaneous thrombophlebitis
      - Cutaneous hypersensitivity
   iii. Ocular lesions
   iv. Recurrent hypopyon iritis or iridocyclitis
   v. Chorioretinitis
   vi. Genital aphthous ulceration

   Minor criteria:
   i. Arthritic symptoms and signs (arthralgia, swelling, redness in large joints)
   ii. Gastrointestinal lesions (appendicitis-like pain, melena, diarrhea, and so on)
   iii. Epididymitis
   iv. Vascular lesions (obliterative vasculitis, occlusions, aneurysms)
   v. Central nervous system (CNS) involvement:
      - Brain stem syndrome
      - Meningoencephalomyelitis syndrome
      - Psychiatric symptoms

4. **What are the anterior segment findings?**
    i. Iridocyclitis with hypopyon—19–31%
    ii. Periorbital pain, redness, photophobia, and blurred vision
    iii. Ciliary injection, fine keratic precipitates (KPs)

    Hypopyon, does not coagulate—changes position with head movement.

    Attack lasts for 2–3 weeks and then subsides; recurrences are the rule with subsequent iris atrophy and posterior synechiae formation.

5. **What are the posterior segment findings?**
    i. Vitritis
    ii. Retinal vasculitis
    iii. Patchy perivascular sheathing and inflammatory exudates surrounding retinal hemorrhages
    iv. Retinal edema
    v. Severe vasculitis—thrombosis—ischemic retinal changes. Branch retinal vein occlusion (BRVO)/central retinal vein occlusion (CRVO)
    vi. Neovascularization—bleeding—fibrosis—retinal detachment (RD) (very rare)
    vii. Optic neuritis in acute phase
    viii. Progressive optic atrophy.

3.6 INVESTIGATIONS IN UVEITIS

1. **What are the indications for investigations in uveitis?**
    i. To arrive at a specific diagnosis
    ii. To choose a correct therapeutic approach
    iii. To rule out infection [steroids are used in majority of uveitic cases; they may exacerbate existing diseases such as tuberculosis (TB) and toxoplasmosis]
    iv. To rule out tumors—because many tumors such as leukemias and retinoblastomas masquerade as uveitis
    v. To rule out presumed autoimmune disease
    vi. To rule out associated systemic conditions, e.g., human leukocyte antigen (HLA)-B27 + juvenile rheumatoid arthritis (JRA) may present as uveitis initially. HLA-B27 positivity forewarns the patient about the systemic nature of the disease and its prognosis
    vii. To evaluate why vision has not improved nonresponders, poor responses, and early recurrences
    viii. To assess the side effects of treatment, e.g., in Behçet's disease, immunosuppressants are used
    ix. For academic and research purposes

2. **Which uveitic entities do not need laboratory investigations for diagnosis?**
    i. Pars planitis
    ii. Fuchs' heterochromic iridocyclitis
    iii. Traumatic uveitis
    iv. Postoperative uveitis

3. **Classify investigations used in uveitis.**

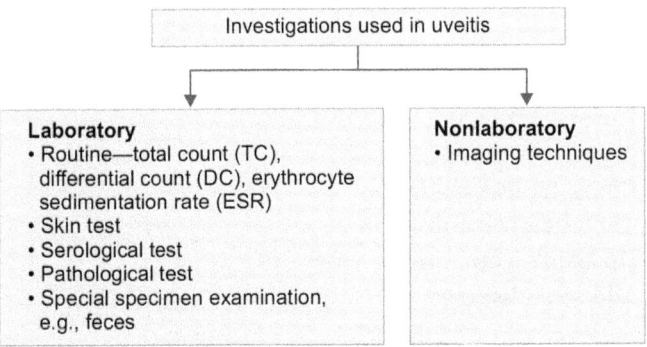

4. **What are the hematological investigations done in uveitis? What is their significance? What is the normal value?**
    White blood cell (WBC) (TC):
    Normal count: 4,500–11,000 cells/μL

Conditions where total count is raised:
  i. Exercise
  ii. Stress
  iii. Infections
  iv. Tissue necrosis (e.g., myocardial infarction, pulmonary infarction)
  v. Chronic inflammatory disorder (e.g., vasculitis)
  vi. Drugs (e.g., glucocorticoids, epinephrine, lithium)

Conditions where TC is decreased
  i. Infections—viral [e.g., influenza, human immunodeficiency virus (HIV), hepatitis]; bacterial (e.g., typhoid, TB)
  ii. Nutritional—B_{12} and folate deficiency
  iii. Autoimmune, e.g., systemic lupus erythematosus (SLE)

5. What are the clinical conditions which can cause raised neutrophils (neutrophilia)?
  i. Inflammatory states
  ii. Nonspecific infections
  iii. Eclampsia
  iv. Hemolytic anemia
  v. Corticosteroids

6. What are the causes of decreased neutrophils (neutropenia)?
  i. Congenital
  ii. Leukemia
  iii. Chemotherapy
  iv. Steroids
  v. Radiation
  vi. Vitamin B_{12}/folate deficiency
  vii. Hemodialysis
  viii. Viral infections

7. What are the causes of raised eosinophils (eosinophilia)?
  i. Parasitic infestation
  ii. Allergic disorders
  iii. Churg–Strauss syndrome
  iv. Cholesterol embolization
  v. Hodgkin's lymphoma
  vi. Addison's disease

8. What are the causes of decreased eosinophils (eosinopenia)?
  i. Congenital
  ii. Leukemia
  iii. Chemotherapy
  iv. Steroids

9. **What are the causes of raised basophils (basophilia)?**
    i. Stress
    ii. Inflammatory states
    iii. Leukemia

10. **What are the causes of decreased basophils (basopenia)?**
    i. Urticaria
    ii. Agranulocytosis
    iii. Ovulation

11. **What are the causes of increased lymphocytes (lymphocytosis)?**
    i. Acute viral infections
    ii. Infectious mononucleosis
    iii. Acute pertussis
    iv. Protozoal—toxoplasmic infections
    v. TB
    vi. Brucellosis
    vii. Chronic lymphocytic leukemia
    viii. Acute lymphocytic leukemia
    ix. Connective tissue disorders
    x. Thyrotoxicosis
    xi. Addison's disease
    xii. Splenomegaly with sequestration of granulocytes

12. **What are the causes of decreased lymphocytes (lymphocytopenia)?**
    i. Common cold
    ii. Corticosteroids
    iii. HIV/viral/bacterial/fungal infections
    iv. Malnutrition
    v. Systemic lupus erythematosus
    vi. Stress
    vii. Prolonged physical exertion
    viii. Rheumatoid arthritis
    ix. Iatrogenic—radiation

13. **What are the causes of increased monocytes (monocytosis)?**
    i. Infections—TB, syphilis, brucellosis, listeria, subacute bacterial endocarditis
    ii. Protozoal infections
    iii. Rickettsial infections
    iv. Myeloproliferative disorders
    v. Autoimmune diseases
    vi. Malignancies: Hodgkin's, leukemia
    vii. Sarcoid
    viii. Lipid storage diseases

14. What are the causes of decreased monocytes (monocytopenia)?
   i. Immunosuppressed states
   ii. Bone marrow suppression
   iii. Radiation states
   iv. Increased destruction: Autoimmune states, carcinoma of hematopoietic system
   v. Hemodialysis

15. What is ESR?
ESR or Biernacki Reaction is defined as the rate at which erythrocytes precipitate in an hour.

16. What are the principles of ESR?
ESR is principally determined by the balance between pro-sedimentary factors and factors that resist sedimentation. The main pro-sedimentary factor is fibrinogen. The negative charge on the surface of red blood cells (RBCs), called potential, is responsible for resisting the sedimentation of erythrocytes.

In inflammatory states, an increase in fibrinogen causes the erythrocytes to stick to each other, thereby causing "rouleaux" formation and raised ESR.

17. What are the causes of raised ESR?
   i. *Physiological:*
      - Pregnancy
      - Exercise
      - Menstruation
   ii. *Pathological:*
      - Anemia
      - Endocarditis
   iii. *Renal disorders*
   iv. *Osteomyelitis*
   v. *Rheumatic fever*
   vi. *Rheumatoid arthritis*
   vii. *Thyroid disorder*
   viii. *Tuberculosis*
   ix. *Syphilis*
   x. *HIV*

Causes of very high-raised ESR:
   i. Giant cell arthritis
   ii. Hyperfibrinogenemia
   iii. Multiple myeloma
   iv. Macroglobulinemia
   v. Necrotizing vasculitis
   vi. Polymyalgia rheumatica

18. **What are the drugs which can cause increased ESR?**
    i. Dextran
    ii. Methyldopa
    iii. Oral contraceptives
    iv. Penicillamines
    v. Theophylline
    vi. Vitamin A

19. **What are the causes of decreased ESR?**
    i. Congestive cardiac failure
    ii. Hyperviscosity syndrome
    iii. Hypofibrinogenemia
    iv. Low plasma protein states
    v. Polycythemia
    vi. Sickle cell anemia
    vii. Very high blood sugar levels
    viii. Severe liver diseases
    ix. Drugs—aspirin, cortisone, quinine

20. **What are the common methods to estimate ESR?**
    i. Westergren's method
    ii. Wintrobe's method

21. **What is tuberculin skin testing (TST)?**
    The Mantoux tuberculin test is the standard method of determining whether a person is infected with *Mycobacterium tuberculosis*. Reliable administration and reading of the TST require standardization of procedures, training, supervision, and practice.

22. **How is the TST administered?**
    The TST is performed by injecting 0.1 mL of tuberculin-purified protein derivative (PPD) into the inner surface of the forearm. The injection should be made with a tuberculin syringe, with the needle bevel facing upward. The TST is an intradermal injection. When placed correctly, the injection should produce a pale elevation of the skin (a wheal) 6-10 mm in diameter.

23. **How is the TST read?**
    The skin test reaction should be read between 48 and 72 hours after administration. A patient who does not return within 72 hours will need to be rescheduled for another skin test.
    The reaction should be measured in millimeters of the induration (palpable, raised, hardened area, or swelling). The reader should not measure erythema (redness). The diameter of the indurated area should be measured across the forearm (perpendicular to the long axis).

24. How are TST reactions interpreted?
Skin test interpretation depends on two factors:
 i. Measurement in millimeters of the induration
 ii. Person's risk of being infected with TB and of progression to disease if infected

25. What are false-positive reactions?
Some persons may react to the TST even though they are not infected with *Mycobacterium tuberculosis*. The causes of these false-positive reactions may include, but are not limited to, the following:
 i. Infection with non-TB mycobacteria
 ii. Previous bacillus Calmette-Guérin (BCG) vaccination
 iii. Incorrect method of TST administration
 iv. Incorrect interpretation of reaction
 v. Incorrect bottle of antigen used

26. What are false-negative reactions?
Some persons may not react to the TST even though they are infected with *Mycobacterium tuberculosis*. The reasons for these false-negative reactions may include, but are not limited to, the following:
 i. Cutaneous anergy (anergy is the inability to react to skin tests because of a weakened immune system)
 ii. Recent TB infection (within 8-10 weeks of exposure)
 iii. Very old TB infection (many years)
 iv. Very young age (<6 months old)
 v. Recent live-virus vaccination (e.g., measles and smallpox)
 vi. Overwhelming TB disease
 vii. Some viral illnesses (e.g., measles and smallpox)
 viii. Incorrect method of TST administration
 ix. Incorrect interpretation of reaction

27. Who can receive a TST?
Most persons can receive a TST. TST is contraindicated only for persons who have had a severe reaction (e.g., necrosis, blistering, anaphylactic shock, or ulcerations) to a previous TST. It is not contraindicated for any other persons, including infants, children, pregnant women, persons who are HIV infected, or persons who have been vaccinated with BCG.

28. How often can TST be repeated?
In general, there is no risk associated with repeated tuberculin skin test placements. If a person does not return within 48-72 hours for a tuberculin skin test reading, a second test can be placed as soon as possible. There is no contraindication to repeating the TST unless a previous TST was associated with a severe reaction.

29. **What is boosted reaction?**

    In some persons who are infected with *Mycobacterium tuberculosis*, the ability to react to tuberculin may wane over time. When given a TST, years after infection, these persons may have a false-negative reaction. However, the TST may stimulate the immune system, causing a positive or boosted reaction to subsequent tests. Giving a second TST after an initial negative TST reaction is called two-step testing.

30. **Why is two-step testing conducted?**

    Two-step testing is useful for the initial skin testing of adults who are going to be retested periodically, such as healthcare workers or nursing home residents. This two-step approach can reduce the likelihood that a boosted reaction to a subsequent TST will be misinterpreted as a recent infection.

31. **Can TST be given to persons receiving vaccinations?**

    Vaccination with live viruses may interfere with TST reactions. For persons scheduled to receive a TST, testing should be done as follows:

    i. Either on the same day as vaccination with live-virus vaccine or 4–6 weeks after the administration of live-virus vaccine
    ii. At least 1 month after smallpox vaccination

32. **Classify the tuberculin skin test reaction.**

    Classification

An induration of *5 or more millimeters* is considered positive in	An induration of *10 or more millimeters* is considered positive in	An induration of *15 or more millimeters* is considered positive in
• HIV-infected persons • A recent contact of a person with TB disease • Persons with fibrotic changes on chest radiograph consistent with prior TB • Patients with organ transplants • Persons who are immunosuppressed for other reasons [e.g., taking the equivalent of >15 mg/day of prednisone for 1 month or longer, taking tumor necrosis factor (TNF) alpha antagonists]	• Recent immigrants (<5 years) from high-prevalence countries • Injection drug users • Residents and employees of high-risk congregate settings • Mycobacteriology laboratory personnel • Persons with clinical conditions that place them at high risk • Children <4 years of age • Infants, children, and adolescents exposed to adults in high-risk categories	any person, including persons with no known risk factors for TB. However, targeted skin testing programs should only be conducted among high-risk groups

33. What is the role of chest X-ray in uveitis cases?
   i. To rule out active pulmonary TB
   ii. To look for sarcoidosis
   iii. To look for secondaries

34. What is the basis of skin tests, and what is the role of skin tests in uveitis?
The basis of all skin tests is delayed hypersensitivity type IV.

Uses of skin tests:
In diagnosis of
   i. Tuberculosis (TB)
   ii. Histoplasmosis
   iii. Coccidomycosis
   iv. To indicate anergy—sarcoidosis
   Pathergy test—Behçet's disease

35. What is Kveim test? How is it done?
   i. Kveim test—a skin test for sarcoidosis
   ii. Suspension of antigenic preparation of human sarcoid tissue prepared from spleen of sarcoidosis patients is injected intradermally
   iii. At the end of 6 weeks—a papule develops
   iv. Papule is biopsied for evidence of granuloma and giant cells
   v. Well-formed epithelial tubercles indicate a positive reaction
   vi. Sensitivity—positive in 80% patients of sarcoidosis

Disadvantages:
   i. Requires standardization by testing in patients with sarcoidosis
   ii. It is usually negative in patients on steroid treatment

36. How is Behçet's skin test done?
   i. The skin test for Behçet's disease is called pathergy test
   ii. Intradermal injection of 0.1 mL of sterile saline solution
   iii. A pustule develops within 18-24 hours
   iv. Patient shows increased sensitivity to needle trauma
   Disadvantage: Only rarely positive in the absence of systemic activity

37. What are the conditions associated with elevated antinuclear antibodies (ANA)?
   i. SLE
   ii. JRA
   iii. Scleroderma
   iv. Hepatitis
   v. Lymphoma
   vi. Polyarteritis nodosa

38. List the conditions in uveitis which are associated with HLA.
   i. HLA-B27—acute anterior uveitis, Reiter's syndrome
   ii. HLA-B51—Japanese with Behçet's disease
   iii. HLA-DR4—VKH
   iv. HLA-B7—macular histoplasmosis
   v. HLA-A29—birdshot chorioretinopathy
   vi. HLA-B8—sarcoidosis

39. What is ELISA?
ELISA is enzyme-linked immunosorbent assay. It is very sensitive and specific.

40. What are uses of ELISA in uveitis?
ELISA is used to detect antibodies of *Toxoplasma, Toxocara,* and *Herpes simplex virus.*

Apart from blood, the test can also be done on aqueous and vitreous sample.

Patients' antibodies are bound to solid-phase antigen and then incubated with enzyme-tagged antibody. Measurement of enzyme activity provides measurement of specific antibody concentration.

41. What are the serological tests for toxoplasmosis?
   i. Toxoplasma dye test/Sabin–Feldman test
   ii. Hemagglutination test
   iii. Indirect fluorescent test
   iv. ELISA
   v. Polymerase chain reaction (PCR)

42. What serological tests for syphilis are commonly done in uveitis?
   i. *Nontreponemal test:* Venereal disease research laboratory (VDRL)
   ii. *Treponemal test:* Fluorescent treponemal antibody absorption (FTA-ABS), treponema pallidum hemagglutination assay (TPHA)

43. What is the role of VDRL and FTA-ABS in case of suspected syphilis?
   i. FTA-ABS is done in syphilis because of its high sensitivity and specificity
   ii. VDRL is done to determine the state of activity of disease and adequacy of treatment

44. What are the two new specific tests for syphilis?
Microhemagglutination assay for treponema pallidum (MHA-TP), i.e., microhemagglutination assay for antibodies to *Treponema pallidum.*
   i. Microhemagglutination assay for treponema pallidum (MHA-TP)
   ii. Hemaggulatination treponemal test (HAATS)

Immunoglobulin G (IgG) titer is more confirmatory than IgM titer.

45. What is the importance of negative ANA?
Negative result is more important as it excludes the diagnosis.

46. When is ANA considered positive?
ANA is considered positive when titers are 1:10 or 1:20.

47. Where is angiotensin-converting enzyme (ACE) produced?
ACE is produced in normal capillary endothelium cells and monocytes

48. What is normal value of ACE?
Normal value
- Males → 12-55 mmol/mL
- Females → 11-29 mmol/mL

49. What conditions are associated with elevated ACE?
i. Increased in active sarcoidosis (falls to normal if there is systemic remission even if ocular inflammation is active; i.e., normal ACE does not rule out sarcoidosis)
ii. Also increased in untreated TB, leprosy, toxoplasmosis (thereby not specific for sarcoidosis)

50. What is HLA?
HLA includes histocompatibility antigens present on the surfaces of most nucleated cells.

51. Where are genes for HLA located?
Human leukocyte antigen genes are located on the short arm of chromosome 6.

Two classes are present:
i. Class I—A, B, C
ii. Class II—D

52. What is the most important HLA in uveitis?
The most important HLA is HLA-B27.
HLA-B27: 58% of normal population
   85% in ankylosing spondylitis (AS)
   70-85% in Reiter's syndrome
In patients with AS, HLA-B27 positivity implies 35% chance of developing acute uveitis, vis-à-vis 7% if negative.

53. What is the importance of serum calcium in uveitis?
Serum calcium—hypercalcemia occurs in 25% of patients with sarcoidosis but is only rarely positive in isolated ocular sarcoidosis with systemic remission.

54. **What is normal A:G ratio? Name conditions where it is reversed.**
    i. Normal A:G ratio is 1.5:1 to 2.5:1.
    ii. Decreased A:G ratio—conditions with elevated antibody concentration, e.g., chronic infections, SLE, rheumatoid arthritis (RA), malignancy, collagen diseases
    iii. Serum globulin is elevated in sarcoidosis

55. **What is the significance of urine culture in CMV infection?**
    It is recovered from urine specimens from 100% patients with acute CMV infection.

56. **What is PCR?**
    PCR works on the principle of amplification of a segment of deoxyribonucleic acid (DNA). It is used to identify infectious agents—bacteria, viruses, and parasites.

57. **What are the uses of PCR in uveitis?**
    PCR is currently used to detect viral DNA in eyes with acute retinal necrosis (ARN) and to diagnose ocular toxoplasmosis and TB.

58. **What is the importance of serum lactate dehydrogenase (LDH) in uveitis?**
    Serum LDH is useful in the diagnosis of retinoblastoma, which can present as uveitis (masquerade syndrome).

59. **What is the importance of serum lysozyme in uveitis?**
    i. Increased in TB, sarcoidosis, leprosy
    ii. Normal level is 1–2 mg/dL

60. **What is rheumatoid factor composed of?**
    i. 7S IgG
    ii. 7S IgM
    iii. 19S IgM

61. **What are the conditions in which rheumatoid factor is positive?**
    i. RA
    ii. JRA
    iii. SLE
    iv. Sjögren's syndrome
    v. Scleroderma
    vi. Infections, e.g., syphilis, infectious mononucleosis, hepatitis

62. **What are the conditions in which rheumatoid factor is negative?**
    i. JRA (pauciarticular variety)
    ii. Seronegative spondyloarthropathies like psoriasis, ulcerative colitis, Crohn's disease, and Reiter's syndrome
    iii. AS

63. What antibody testing methods are used in uveitis?
   i. ELISA
   ii. Indirect fluorescent antibody (IFA)
   iii. Complicated fixation test
   iv. Hemagglutination test

64. How is anterior chamber (AC) paracentesis done?
AC paracentesis is done with a 26-gauge needle attached to a 1 cc tuberculin syringe.

At the limbus, a gutter is made with a blade; care taken to be parallel to plane of iris with bevel up.

It provides a small amount of fluid (200–250 pg).

65. Who proposed AC paracentesis first?
Desmont

66. What are the uses of AC tap?
   i. Detection of organisms by direct exam/culture
   ii. Microscopic study to rule out malignancy
   iii. Assessment of nonspecific biological enzyme, e.g., aqueous ACE
   iv. Immunological test for an infection agent, e.g., ELISA, to show herpes simplex in ARN
   v. Cell cytology

67. How is cell cytology of an aqueous sample done?
A small drop of aqueous is placed on the slide-fixed in absolute methanol for 10 minutes, air dried, stained with Giemsa for 1 hour, rinsed with 95% ethanol, and let to dry.

68. What are the therapeutic investigations done in uveitis?
   i. Vitrectomy
   ii. Trial of antituberculous treatment
   iii. Trial of steroids

69. What are the cells found in AH in different conditions?

Type of cells	Condition
Neutrophils	Bacterial infection
Eosinophils	Parasitic infection
Lymphocytes	Viral, fungal, autoimmune, and hypersensitivity uveitis
Macrophages	Phacoanaphylactic/sympathetic ophthalmia
Tumor cells	Foreign body/masquerade syndrome

70. How is vitreous aspiration done?
   i. Vitreous aspiration is one with a 18–20 gauge needle
   ii. The aspirate is sent for cytology, antibodies, and culture

71. **Why is vitrectomy preferred over vitreous aspiration?**
    i. Collection of more material
    ii. Apart from diagnostic use, it may also prove therapeutic, e.g., in phacoanaphylactic uveitis
    iii. Less complications due to controlled traction on vitreous base
    iv. Avoids long-term hypotony
    v. Chorioretinal biopsy can also be taken with vitrectomy

72. **What are the indications and techniques for chorioretinal biopsy in uveitis?**
    The main indication is bilateral vision-threatening disease not responding to treatment, in which etiology cannot be established.

    It can be done by:
    i. Making scleral flap at the site of lesion by microblade and Vannas scissors
    ii. Can be also done endoretinally while doing vitrectomy with vitrectomy scissors and forceps

73. **What are the contraindications of chorioretinal biopsy?**
    Infections of retina and choroid

74. **What are the complications of chorioretinal biopsy?**
    i. Choroidal hemorrhage
    ii. Retinal detachment
    iii. Infection
    iv. Proliferative vitreoretinopathy

75. **When is lacrimal gland biopsy done in uveitis?**
    Lacrimal gland biopsy is done in suspected sarcoidosis, but only if lacrimal glands are clinically enlarged or show increased uptake on gallium scan.

76. **What are the indications for invasive procedures in uveitis?**
    i. Uncontrolled uveitis
    ii. Endophthalmitis
    iii. Threatened vision
    iv. Doubtful malignancy
    v. Viral retinitis
    vi. Research tool

77. **How is feces examination useful in uveitis?**
    It is useful to diagnose the following organisms:
    i. *E. coli*
    ii. *E. histolytica*
    iii. *Ascariasis*
    iv. *Giardiasis* [can cause cystoid macular edema (CME)]

78. **What X-rays are taken in uveitis?**
    i. *X-ray chest:* TB, sarcoidosis, histoplasmosis
       In TB—X-ray chest may show fibrocavitary lesions or miliary lesions.
       In sarcoidosis—findings can be divided into four stages.
       Stage 1: Bilateral lymphadenopathy and normal parenchyma
       Stage 2: Bilateral lymphadenopathy and reticulonodular parenchymal infiltrates
       Stage 3: Reticulonodular infiltrates alone
       Stage 4: Progressive pulmonary fibrosis
    ii. *X-ray sacroiliac joint:* In all young patients with acute unilateral iritis, irrespective of the presence or absence of low backache. This is because X-ray may be positive before the patient is symptomatic in cases of ankylosing spondylitis
    iii. *X-ray hands and feet:* Sarcoidosis
         Computed tomography/magnetic resonance imaging (CT/MRI) brain is indicated in lymphoma.
    iv. *X-ray skull:* Cerebral calcifications in congenital toxoplasmosis, cytomegalovirus (CMV)

79. **What is the importance of gallium scan?**
    i. Gallium is taken up by mitotically active liposomes of granulocytes
    ii. Scanning is done 48 hours after intravenous injection of labeled gallium citrate

80. **What is the importance of gallium scan in the diagnosis of sarcoidosis?**
    i. In acute systemic sarcoidosis, gallium scan of head, neck, and chest shows increased uptake
    ii. This increased uptake + increased aqueous ACE is highly suggestive of sarcoidosis

81. **In which condition is iris angiography done?**
    Fuchs' heterochromic iridocyclitis—new vessels—in the angle.

82. **What are the indications of FFA in uveitis?**
    i. VKH syndrome
    ii. Acute polypoidal multifocal PPE
    iii. Multiple evanescent white dot syndrome (MEWDS)
    iv. Serpiginous choroiditis

83. **What are the major FFA findings in uveitis?**
    i. Cystoid macular edema
    ii. Subretinal neovascular membrane
    iii. Disk leakage
    iv. Late staining of retinal vessels

v. Neovascularization of retina
vi. Retina vascular capillary dropout and reorganization
vii. RPE perturbation

84. **What are the uses of ultrasonography (USG) in uveitis?**
    i. To diagnose masquerade syndromes like lymphoma, benign lymphoid hyperplasia, and diffuse melanoma
    ii. To plan surgery in hazy media due to complicated cataract
    iii. Vitreal disorders such as hemorrhage, inflammation, pars planitis, retained lens fragments
    iv. Optic disk edema and cupping
    v. Macular edema and exudative detachment
    vi. Choroidal thickening, uveal effusion, scleritis, Harada's disease, sympathetic ophthalmia hypotony
    vii. To rule out Coat's disease and intraocular tumors
    viii. Useful in VKH and toxocariasis

85. **What is the importance of visual fields (VF) in uveitis?**
    i. Association with secondary glaucoma—glaucoma damage can be estimated
    ii. Behçet's syndrome
    iii. Uveitis syndromes are associated with neurologic disorders. VF may be helpful in differentiating papillitis from juxtapapillary uveitis
    iv. Differentiating uveitis from heredodegenerative diseases, e.g., retinitis pigmentosa (RP) from bone spicule pigmentation seen in luetic uveitis
    v. In the early diagnosis and follow-up

86. **What are the indications for lumbar puncture in uveitis?**
    i. VKH
    ii. Reticulum cell sarcoma
    iii. Intraocular lymphoma.

3.7 TREATMENT OF UVEITIS

1. **What are the aims of therapy?**
   i. To prevent vision-threatening complications
   ii. To relieve the patient's discomfort
   iii. To treat the underlying cause, if possible

2. **What are the surgeries done in uveitis?**
   i. Cataract extraction
   ii. Pupillary reconstruction
   iii. Glaucoma surgery
   iv. Peeling of epiretinal membrane (ERM)
   v. Scleral buckling
   vi. Vitrectomy

3. **What is the purpose of using mydriatics/cycloplegics?**
   i. Give comfort by relieving the spasm of ciliary body and sphincter of pupil
   ii. Prevent the formation of posterior synechiae by using a short-acting mydriatic to keep the pupil mobile
   iii. Break down posterior synechiae
   iv. Reduce exudation from the iris:
   One percent atropine—most powerful and longest-acting cycloplegic in severe acute inflammation. It is changed to a short-acting agent once inflammation subsides.

4. **Which short-acting cycloplegics are used, and what is their role?**
   Short-acting cycloplegics are used as they keep the pupil mobile, which is the best mechanism to prevent synechiae formation.

   These agents include:
   i. Tropicamide 0.5%, 1.0%
   ii. Cyclopentolate 0.5%, 1.0%, 2.0%
   (*Note:* Side effect of cyclopentolate—chemoattractant for leukocytes and so it may prove bad for uveitis)

   When long-acting cycloplegics are continued, posterior synechiae occurs in a dilated state, thereby ill serving the very purpose of it.

5. **What are the preparations commonly used topically?**

i. Prednisolone acetate Suspension (Pred Forte)	0.12 and 1%
ii. Prednisolone sodium phosphate solution	0.12 and 1%
iii. Dexamethasone phosphate solution	0.1%
iv. Fluorometholone	0.1 and 1%

Duration and frequency of application depend upon the severity of inflammation.

Initially applied more frequently and tapered slowly over weeks as inflammation subsides.

Steroids should not be used topically more than 2-3 times/day without concomitant antibiotic drops applied once/twice daily. Antibiotic–steroid combinations are usually used.

6. **What are the indications for periocular steroids?**
   i. Severe acute anterior uveitis, especially AS with severe fibrin membrane/hypopyon
   ii. Adjunct to topical/systemic treatment in resistant cases of chronic anterior uveitis
   iii. Intermediate uveitis
   iv. Poor patient compliance

7. **What are the advantages of periocular steroids over drops?**
   i. To achieve therapeutic concentration behind lens
   ii. Drugs not capable of penetrating corneas are able to enter the eye by penetrating sclera
   iii. Long-lasting effect achieved when a depot preparation is used

8. **What are the types of periocular preparations used?**
   i. Anterior sub-Tenon—persistent severe anterior uveitis
   ii. Posterior sub-Tenon—intermediate uveitis, posterior uveitis
   iii. Subconjunctival and retrobulbar injections

9. **What are the types of periocular preparation used?**
   i. Triamcinolone acetonide 40 mg
   ii. Depo-Medrol (methylprednisolone acetate) 40 mg

10. **What are complications of periocular steroids?**
    Topical complication + extraocular muscle fibrosis, scleromalacia, and conjunctival necrosis

11. **Why is posterior sub-Tenon (PST) injection given temporally and in what frequency?**
    PST injection is given temporally because it then reaches the macula. It is given every 4–10 weeks. The injection site is close to the insertion of inferior oblique, which corresponds to anatomical macula.

12. **What are indications for systemic treatment with oral steroids?**
    i. Intractable anterior uveitis (that has not responded to topical medications and anterior sub-Tenon's injections)

ii. Intractable intermediate and posterior uveitis (that has not responded to PST)

13. What are contraindications to steroid treatment?
   i. Inactive disease with chronic flare
   ii. Very mild anterior uveitis
   iii. Intermediate uveitis with normal vision
   iv. Fuchs' uveitis
   v. When antimicrobial treatment is more appropriate, e.g., candidiasis

14. What are indications and dose of intravenous (IV) steroids?
   i. IV pulse methylprednisolone 1 g over 1–2 hours can be employed in cases of a severe inflammatory process that needs to be treated as rapidly as possible
   ii. IV methylprednisolone 1 g/day for 3 days

15. What are the indications for immunosuppressants?
   i. Vision-threatening intraocular inflammation
   ii. Reversibility of the disease process
   iii. No response to steroids
   iv. Intolerable side effects of steroids

16. What are the clinical conditions that need immunosuppressants according to International Uveitis Study Group (IUSG)?

i. Absolute	• Behçet's- Rheumatoid arthritis • Sympathetic ophthalmia • Vogt–Koyanagi–Harada (VKH) • Serpiginous choroidopathy
ii. Relative	• Intermediate uveitis in adults • Preretinal vasculitis • Chronic cystitis

17. What are the classes of immunosuppressives?

i. Antimetabolites	Methotrexate
	Azathioprine
ii. Alkylating agents	Cyclophosphamide
iii. Antibiotics	Cyclosporine
iv. Ergot alkaloid	Bromocriptine
v. Dapsone	
vi. Colchicine	Anti-inflammatory

18. **What are the indications and side effects of different immunosuppressants?**

	Indications	Side effects
Cyclophosphamide	• Behçet's • RA • SO	• Marrow suppression • Hemorrhagic cystitis • Secondary malignancy
Chlorambucil	• Behçet's • SO	• Marrow suppression • Gonadal malignancy • Secondary malignancy • Hepatotoxicity
Methotrexate	• SO • Scleritis	• Marrow suppression • Ulcerative stomatitis • Diarrhea
Azathioprine	• Behçet's SLE • Pemphigoid	• Marrow suppression • Secondary infection
Cyclosporine	• Behçet's • Birdshot chorioretinopathy • Corneal graft rejection	• Hepatotoxicity • Nephrotoxicity • Hyperuricemia
Bromocriptine	Adjunct to cyclosporine in anterior idiopathic uveitis	• Nausea, vomiting • Postural hypotension
Dapsone	Cicatricial pemphigoid	• Hemolytic anemia • Nausea
Colchicine	Behçet's	• Nausea, vomiting • Marrow suspension

19. **What are indications for penetrating keratoplasty (PKP) in uveitis?**
    Corneal scarring caused by herpes simplex keratouveitis

20. **What are indications for vitrectomy?**
    i. Diagnostic—endophthalmitis of suspected infective etiology
    ii. Therapeutic—progressive disease (hypotony) complications needing surgery, e.g., retinal detachment (RD) iris bombe with hypotony

21. **What are the ocular complications of steroids?**
    i. Increased intraocular pressure (IOP)
    ii. Decreased resistance to infection
    iii. Delayed healing of corneal/shear wounds
    iv. Mydriasis—may precipitate angle closure glaucoma
    v. Ptosis
    vi. Complicated cataract
    vii. Blurred vision
    viii. Enhances lytic action of collagenase

ix. Paralysis of accommodation
x. Visual field changes
   - Scotoma
   - Constriction
     - Enlarged blind spot
     - Glaucoma field defect
xi. Problems with color vision
   - Color vision defect
   - Colored halos around lights
xii. Eyelids and conjunctiva
   - Allergic reactions
   - Persisted erythema
   - Telangiectasia
   - Depigmentation
   - Poliosis
   - Scarring
   - Fat atrophy
   - Skin atrophy
xiii. Cornea
   - Superficial punctate keratitis (SPK)
   - Superficial corneal defects
xiv. Irritation
   - Lacrimation
   - Photophobia
   - Ocular pain
   - Burning sensation
   - Anterior uveitis
xv. Corneal/scleral thickness
   - Increased—initial
   - Decreased
xvi. Toxic amblyopia
xvii. Optic atrophy
xviii. May aggravate the following diseases:
   - Scleromalacia perforans
   - Corneal melting disease
   - Behçet's disease
   - Eales disease
   - Presumptive ocular
xix. Retinal embolic phenomena

22. What are the systemic complications of steroids?
i. Endocrine
   - Adrenal insufficiency
   - Cushing's syndrome

- Growth failure
- Menstrual disorders
ii. Neuropsychiatric
    - Pseudotumor cerebri
    - Insomnia
    - Mood swings
    - Psychosis
iii. Gastrointestinal
    - Peptic ulcer
    - Gastric hemorrhage
    - Intestinal perforation
    - Pancreatitis
iv. Musculoskeletal
    - Osteoporosis
    - Vertebral compression fracture
    - Aseptic necrosis of femur
    - Myopathy
v. Cardiovascular
    - Hypertension
    - Sodium and fluid retention
vi. Metabolic
    - Secondary diabetes mellitus
    - Hyperosmotic ketoacidosis
    - Centripetal obesity
    - Hyperlipidemia
vii. Dermatologic
    - Acne
    - Hirsutism
    - Subcutaneous tissue atrophy
viii. Immunologic
    - Impaired inflammatory response
    - Delayed tissue healing.

CHAPTER

Glaucoma

4.1 BASIC EXAMINATION OF GLAUCOMA AND TONOMETRY

1. **What are the methods of measurement of anterior chamber depth (ACD)?**
    i. Clinical method
        - Pen torch or eclipse technique
        - Split limbal technique
    ii. Subjective method
        - *Qualitative:* van Herick's method
        - *Quantitative:* Smith's method
    iii. Objective methods

2. **What is a pen torch shadow or eclipse technique?**
   A pen torch shadow or eclipse technique involves shining a pen torch temporal to the patient's eye and interpreting the light and shadow across the iris front surface.

   This may be done as follows:
    i. In this method, the patient is asked to look straight in primary gaze
    ii. A pen torch is held parallel to the iris plane
    iii. The amount of iris that remains in shadow may then be interpreted as an indication of the depth of the chamber

   With a very narrow angle, the forward bulging iris leaves much of the nasal iris in shadow. A deep chamber with a wide angle allows the reflection of light from most of the iris.

Grade 4	Good spread of light (open angle)	Fully illuminated
Grade 3	Partial shadow of distal iris	>2/3 illuminated
Grade 2	Increasing eclipse	1/3–2/3 illuminated
Grade 1	Large eclipse of distal iris due to forward bulging of iris (narrow angle)	<1/3 illuminated

3. **What is a split limbal technique?**
   van Herick's method can help measure nasal and temporal ACD, but for superior and inferior angles, it gives no clue. Knowing superior angle depth is important as it is the narrowest and most likely to close.

i. In the split limbal technique, the superior anterior chamber angle is illuminated with a slit lamp but assessment is made with the naked eye
ii. With the illumination in the click position, a vertical slit should be placed at 12 o'clock
iii. Observe the arc of light falling on the cornea and iris without the aid of a slit-lamp eyepiece
iv. The angular separation seen at the limbal corneal junction is an estimation of ACD in degrees

Grade	Estimated angle
0	0°
1	10°
2	20°
3	30°
4	≥45°

4. **How do you do van Herick's method of assessment of ACD?**
   van Herick's method is a subjective method of estimation of ACD using a slit lamp by comparing the peripheral ACD with the peripheral corneal thickness.
   Procedure:
   i. The patient is positioned comfortably and looks straight toward the microscope
   ii. The viewing system of the slit lamp is parallel to the visual axis and the illumination system is set at 60° temporal to the viewing system
   iii. The angle is chosen as 60° so that the illuminating beam is approximately perpendicular to the limbus and as the angle is constant whenever the technique is used, this enables consistency of interpretation every time the patient is assessed
   iv. The slit-lamp magnification should be set at 16× and the slit length to maximum to allow an adequate depth of focus
   v. An optical section of the cornea as thin as possible and as close to the temporal limbus as possible is viewed
   vi. A comparison is made between the thickness of the peripheral cornea and the gap between the posterior surface of the cornea and the front of the iris where the beam first touches
   vii. The ratio of these two measurements may be graded and interpreted
   viii. Measurement at the nasal limbus can also be done

van Herick estimate of angle width from ACD at the periphery:

Angle	Depth	Comment
Grade 4 angle	ACD = corneal thickness	Wide open
Grade 3 angle	ACD = 1/4 to 1/2 corneal thickness	Incapable of closure
Grade 2 angle	ACD = 1/4 corneal thickness	Should be gonioscopied
Grade 1 angle	ACD <1/4 corneal thickness	Gonioscopy demonstrates a dangerously narrow angle
Slit angle	ACD = Slit-like (extremely shallow)	
Closed angle	Absent peripheral anterior chamber	

5. What is Smith's method?

Smith's method was described by Smith in 1979. This technique differs from van Herick's in being quantitative.

The procedure is carried out as follows:
  i. The microscope is placed in the straight-ahead position in front of the patient. The illumination is placed at 60° temporally
  ii. To examine the patient's right eye, the practitioner views through the right eyepiece and for the left eye through the left eyepiece
  iii. A beam of 1–2 mm is orientated horizontally and focused on the cornea
  iv. In this position, two horizontal streaks of light are seen: One on the anterior corneal surface and the other on the front surface of the crystalline lens
  v. Altering the slit-height adjustment on the instrument is seen as a lengthening or shortening of the two horizontal reflexes
  vi. Beginning with a short slit, the length is slowly increased to a point at which the ends of the corneal and lenticular reflections appear to meet
  vii. The slit length at this point is then measured (it is assumed that the slit lamp is calibrated for slit length)
  viii. This length may be multiplied by a constant 1.34 to calculate ACD by Smith's method
  ix. Eyes with ACD <2 mm should be dilated with caution

Slit length (mm)	ACD (mm)
1.5	2.01
2.0	2.68
2.5	3.35
3.0	4.02
3.5	4.69

6. **What is adapted Smith's method?**
    i. Adapted Smith's method is used in those situations in which variable slit height is not possible
    ii. In this case, the slit length is noted prior to measurement at a point where it corresponds to 2 mm. The instrument is then set up exactly as in the Smith method but with the initial angle of incidence at 80°
    iii. By gradually closing the angle, the two reflected images on the cornea and lens appear to move closer and the angle at which they first touch is noted
    iv. A corresponding value for the chamber depth for differing angles is then calculated

7. **What are the objective methods?**
    i. Ultrasonography
    ii. Anterior segment optical coherence tomography (AS-OCT), HD-OCT (high-definition optical coherence tomography)
    iii. Oculus Pentacam-Scheimpflug imaging
    iv. Pachometer slit-lamp attachment

8. **What is the normal intraocular pressure (IOP)?**
   The normal IOP is between 10 and 21 mm Hg.

9. **Why is 21 considered as the upper limit?**
   IOP distribution in the general population resembles a Gaussian curve but skewed toward the right. The mean IOP is considered to be 15.5 ± 2.57 mm Hg. 2 standard deviation (SD) above the mean is approximately 20.5 mm Hg as approximately 95% of the area under a Gaussian curve lies between the mean ± 2 SD. The concept of normal IOP limits is viewed as only a rough approximation.

10. **What are the two ways by which aqueous is secreted?**
    i. Active secretion by nonpigmentary ciliary epithelium—80%
    ii. Passive secretion by ultrafiltration and diffusion—20%

11. **What are the factors that determine the level of IOP?**
    i. Rate of aqueous secretion
    ii. Resistance encountered in outflow channels
    iii. Level of episcleral venous pressure

12. **What is normal episcleral venous pressure?**
    The normal range is 8–10 mm Hg.

13. **What are the causes of elevated episcleral venous pressure?**
    i. *Obstruction of venous drainage:*
        - Thyroid eye disease
        - Pseudotumor

- Cavernous sinus thrombosis
- Jugular vein obstruction
- Superior vena cava obstruction
- Pulmonary venous obstruction
- Congestive heart failure
- Radiation

ii. *Arteriovenous anomalies:*
- Carotid-cavernous sinus fistula
- Sturge-Weber syndrome
- Dural fistula
- Venous varix
- Intraocular vascular shunts

iii. *Idiopathic*

14. What are the conditions that influence IOP?
  i. Diurnal variation
  ii. Postural variation
  iii. Exertional influences
  iv. Lid and eye movement
  v. Intraocular conditions
  vi. Systemic conditions
  vii. Environmental conditions
  viii. General anesthesia
  ix. Food and drugs

15. How does IOP vary diurnally?
The most common pattern is that IOP is maximum in midmorning and decreases as the day progresses to become minimum in the late evening or early morning. Some individuals show an elevation at nighttime. This diurnal variation is about 3-6 mm Hg in normal individuals and 10 mm Hg or more in a glaucomatous eye.

16. What is this diurnal variation due to?
The diurnal variation is due to a cyclic fluctuation of blood levels of adrenocortical steroids. Maximum IOP is reached 3-4 hours after the peak of plasma cortisol. The nighttime elevated IOP is due to the supine position along with the fluctuating cortisol levels.

17. What are the types of diurnal variation curves?
There are four types of diurnal variation curves. They are:
  i. *Falling type:* Maximal at 6-8 AM followed by a continuous decline
  ii. *Rising type:* Maximal at 4-6 PM
  iii. *Double variation type:* With two peaks 9-11 AM and 6 PM
  iv. *Flat type* of curve

18. **How does IOP vary with posture?**
    The IOP rises (0.3-6 mm Hg) when the person is lying down. This may be because of an increase in the episcleral venous pressure in the supine posture.

19. **How does IOP vary with exertion?**
    Valsalva maneuvers increase IOP (by increasing episcleral venous pressure), while prolonged exercise decreases IOP (by metabolic acidosis and increased colloid osmotic pressure).

20. **How does IOP vary with lid and eye movement?**
    Forcible eyelid closure raises IOP by 10-90 mm Hg. Repeated eyelid squeezing reduces IOP.
    Widening of the lid fissure increases IOP by approximately 2 mm Hg. Conversely, with Bell's palsy, IOP is slightly reduced.

21. **How does IOP vary with intraocular conditions?**
    Acute anterior uveitis causes a slight reduction in IOP because of decreased aqueous humor production. Rhegmatogenous retinal detachment also causes a reduction because of reduced aqueous humor production as well as shunting of aqueous humor from the posterior chamber through the vitreous and retinal hole into the subretinal space.
    An inflammatory rise in IOP in anterior uveitis.
    Schwartz syndrome—rise in IOP in retinal detachment.

22. **How does IOP vary with systemic conditions?**
    Systemic factors causing increased IOP:
    i. Systemic hypertension
    ii. Systemic hyperthermia
    iii. Adrenocorticotropic hormone and growth hormone stimulation
    iv. Hypothyroidism
    v. Diabetes
    vi. Obesity
    Systemic factors causing decreased IOP:
    i. Pregnancy
    ii. Hyperthyroidism
    iii. Myotonic dystrophy

23. **How does IOP vary with environmental conditions?**
    Exposure to cold decreases IOP (because of lowered episcleral venous pressure), while reduced gravity increases IOP.

24. **How does IOP vary with food and drugs?**
    Agents increasing IOP:
    i. Caffeine
    ii. Corticosteroids

iii. Topical cycloplegics
iv. Water (large volume of water consumption increases IOP: basis of water drinking test)

Agents decreasing IOP:
General anesthesia:
   i. Alcohol
   ii. Heroin and marijuana
   iii. Tobacco smoking

25. **How does IOP vary with anesthetic agents?**
    In general, general anesthetic agents reduce IOP. However, trichloroethylene, ketamine, succinylcholine, and suxamethonium increase IOP.

26. **How does cataract extraction reduce IOP in glaucoma patients?**
    The mechanism of primary angle-closure glaucoma may be principally related to an anteriorly positioned lens and a small anterior segment, which leads to a relative pupillary block and subsequently permanent closure of the anterior chamber angle. Therefore, it seems reasonable that cataract extraction could improve IOP control in eyes with angle-closure glaucoma (ACG). In contrast, although IOP control in primary open-angle glaucoma (POAG) has also been reported to improve after cataract surgery, the mechanisms of the IOP decrease remain unclear. As the trabecular meshwork is compromised in POAG, the IOP reduction after cataract surgery may be transient.

27. **Does heredity influence IOP?**
    IOP tends to be higher in individuals with an enlarged cup-disk ratio and in relatives of patients with open-angle glaucoma.

28. **What is tonography?**
    Tonography is a method used to measure the facility of aqueous outflow. The facility of outflow is called the C value and it ranges from 0.22 to 0.30 μL/min/mm Hg.

29. **How is tonography performed?**
    The clinician first takes the IOP measurement by using a Schiotz tonometer. The tonometer is placed on the cornea, acutely elevating the IOP. The rate at which the pressure declines with time is related to the ease with which the aqueous leaves the eye. The decline in IOP over time can be used to determine the outflow facility.
    Tonography technique:
       i. Patient in a supine position
       ii. Topical anesthetic instilled
       iii. IOP measured with two brief applications of an electronic tonometer

iv. 4-minute tracing of pressure at this position till a smooth tracing is obtained for the full 4 minutes
v. Slope is estimated by placing a free hand line through the middle of oscillations (readings at beginning and end noted)
vi. P_0 and change in readings used to obtain C value from special tonographic tables

$$F = C(P_0 - P_v)$$

F—aqueous outflow rate (microliter/min), P_0—IOP
C—coefficient of outflow facility, P_v—episcleral nervous pressure

30. What is the principle of digital tonometry?
The compressibility of ocular coats is estimated by a sense of fluctuation perceived on palpation.

31. How is IOP measured digitally?
After asking the patient to look down, the sclera is palpated through the upper lid above the tarsal plate using the tip of two fingers. One finger is kept still and the other indents the globe lightly.

32. What are the types of tonometers?
i. *Indentation/impression tonometer:*
   - Schiotz
ii. *Applanation tonometer:*
   - Goldmann, Mackay-Marg, Maklakov, pneumotonometer noncontact
iii. *Newer tonometers:*
   - Dynamic contour tonometer (DCT), ocular response analyzer (ORA)

33. What are the types of weights used in Schiotz tonometry?
A 5.5 g weight is permanently fixed to the plunger, which can be increased to 7.5 or 10 and 15 g by adding additional weights.

34. What are the advantages of Schiotz tonometry?
i. Easy to use
ii. Portable
iii. Useful for screening
iv. Cost-effective

35. What are the disadvantages of Schiotz tonometry?
i. *Ocular rigidity:* The more the scleral rigidity, the higher the reading. Conversely, in conditions like high myopia where the scleral rigidity is low, the IOP is underestimated
ii. *Corneal influences:* A steeper or thicker cornea causes a greater displacement of fluid during indentation tonometry, which leads to a falsely high tonometry reading

iii. *Blood volume alteration:* The variable expulsion of the intraocular blood during indentation tonometry may also influence IOP measurement
iv. *Moses effect:* The hole in the tonometer foot plate can be a source of error

36. **What are all the clinical conditions which cause lower scleral rigidity?**
    i. Myopia
    ii. Application of strong miotics
    iii. Following retinal detachment surgeries and injection of intravitreal gases

    In these conditions of lowered scleral rigidity, a falsely lower IOP estimation is obtained by indentation tonometry.

37. **What are all the clinical conditions which cause higher scleral rigidity?**
    i. Hypermetropia
    ii. Nanophthalmos

    In these conditions of higher scleral rigidity, a falsely higher IOP estimation is obtained by indentation tonometry.

38. **What are the precautions to be taken before using Schiotz tonometry?**
    i. Touch the artificial cornea till the reading is at zero.
    ii. Avoid pressure over the eyelids.
    iii. Sterilize before using.

39. **What are the other types of indentation tonometers?**
    i. Herrington
    ii. Grants
    iii. Maurice

40. **What are the types of applanation tonometers?**
    Applanation tonometers are of two types:

Variable force	Variable area
• Goldmann	• Maklakov–Kalfa
• Perkins	• Applanometer
• Draeger	• Tonomat
• Mackay–Marg	• Halberg

41. **What is the principle of applanation tonometer?**
    The principle of applanation tonometer is based on the Imbert-Fick law, which states that the pressure inside an ideal dry, thin-walled sphere equals the force necessary to flatten its surface divided by the area of the flattening.
    $$P = F/A$$

42. **What is the most common applanation tonometer used?**
    The one designed by Goldmann for use with Haag-Streit slit lamp is the most common applanation tonometer used.

43. **What is the volume of aqueous displaced during application using Goldmann application tonometer?**
    0.5 µL

44. **How much of the anesthetized cornea does the circular plate flatten?**
    3.06 mm of corneal diameter is flattened, which is always constant. Hence, it is called a constant area applanation tonometer.

45. **How is the pressure calculated?**
    When the area is made constant (3.06 mm), then a 0.1 g reading corresponds to a pressure of 1 mm Hg.

46. **What is the rationale behind using a circular plate of a particular (3.06 mm) diameter?**
    At this diameter, the resistance of the cornea to flattening is counterbalanced by the capillary attraction of the tear film meniscus for the tonometer head.

47. **Which dye is used and under what illumination?**
    Fluorescein dye (0.25%) is used and viewed under cobalt blue light.

48. **What should be the angle between the source of illumination and the microscope?**
    The angle should be approximately 60°.

49. **What mark is the knob set before the procedure?**
    The knob is set at 1. If placed at zero, microvibrations are produced which can cause corneal erosions.

50. **What is observed when viewed through the eyepiece?**
    The fluorescence of the stained tear facilitates visualization of the tear meniscus at the margin of the contact between the cornea and biprism. A central blue circle, which is the flattened cornea, surrounded by two yellow semicircles which is the tear meniscus is seen.

51. **What is the desired end point of an applanation tonometer?**
    The biprism which contacts the cornea produces two semicircles that should be equal in size and the inner sides of the two should coincide.

52. **What are the advantages of applanation tonometers over indentation tonometry?**
    i. Reliable and accurate
    ii. Reproducible
    iii. Not influenced by scleral rigidity

53. **What are the disadvantages or source of errors of applanation tonometry?**
    i. *Central corneal thickness:* Thicker corneas produce falsely higher readings, while thinner corneas produce falsely lower readings. However, corneal thickening due to edema causes a falsely lower reading. An average error is 0.7 mm Hg per 10 μm of deviation from the mean of 520 μm
    ii. *Semicircles:* Wider meniscus and improper vertical alignment cause falsely higher readings
    iii. *Corneal astigmatism:* Since astigmatism produces an elliptical area of contact, there is an error in measurement. IOP is underestimated in cases of with-the-rule astigmatism and overestimated in cases of against-the-rule astigmatism with approximately 1 mm Hg for every 4 D of astigmatism
    iv. *Design:* It has a complex design and can be done only in a sitting position
    v. *Corneal irregularity:* It is not useful in case of corneal irregularity
    vi. *Errors following corneal refractive surgery:* It will not be accurate following Lasik surgery

54. **How can errors due to astigmatism be minimized?**
    The tonometer prisms should be rotated so that the axis of the least corneal curvature is opposite the red line on the prism holder.

55. **What are the methods of disinfection of tonometers?**
    The following chemicals can be used to sterilize the tip of applanation tonometers:
    i. 3% hydrogen peroxide
    ii. 70% isopropyl alcohol
    iii. Diluted sodium hypochlorite solution (1:10)
    iv. Heat-sterilized Schiotz tonometer

56. **What are the infections likely to be transmitted?**
    i. Adenovirus of epidemic keratoconjunctivitis (EKC)
    ii. Herpes simplex virus (HSV)—type 1
    iii. Human immunodeficiency virus (HIV)
    iv. Hepatitis B

57. **How is IOP measured in conditions of corneal scarring?**
    The following tonometers can be used:
    i. Noncontact tonometers (NCTs)
    ii. Mackay–Marg
    iii. Tonopen
    iv. Pneumatic tonometers

58. **What are the advantages of tonopen?**
    i. Used in cases of corneal epithelial irregularities
    ii. Measurement of IOP over bandage contact lens
    iii. Useful in edematous and scarred corneas
    iv. Useful in patients with nystagmus and head tremors
    v. Used in operation theater
    vi. Portable

59. **What is the principle of NCTs?**
    A puff of air creates a constant force that deforms the central cornea. The time from an internal reference point to the moment of maximum light detection is measured and converted to IOP.

60. **What are the disadvantages of NCT?**
    i. Tear film damage
    ii. False positives and false negatives

61. **What are the newer modalities of IOP measurement?**
    i. Optical response analyzer
    ii. Dynamic contact tonometer (Pascal)
    iii. Rebound tonometer
    iv. Proview phosphene tonometer

62. **What is the principle behind dynamic contact tonometer (DCT)?**
    Pressure applied to an enclosed fluid is transmitted undiminished to every part of the closed system including the walls of the container. By applying DCT, the cornea is placed in a neutral shape so that pressure on the interior surface equals pressure on the exterior surface.

63. **What are the advantages of DCT over Goldmann applanation tonometer?**
    i. Pressure reading independent of corneal thickness
    ii. No mechanical calibration
    iii. No fluorescein staining
    iv. Direct display of pressure as numerical values

64. **What are the different tonometer measurements independent of corneal variables?**
    i. *PASCAL DCT:* PASCAL has a concave tonometer tip that matches corneal curvature and measures pressure directly by means of a built-in sensor. When it touches the cornea, it allows the cornea to assume its natural shape when pressure on both sides is equal and distortion of the cornea is minimal.

ii. *Reichert ORA:* NCT. The ORA produces a rapid air impulse to apply force to the cornea and uses an electro-optical system to monitor the deformation. The device records two applanation events: The first, while the cornea is moving inward; the other as it returns. The difference between the "in" and "out" pressure values is known as corneal hysteresis, which is a measure of viscoelastic damping, or the ability of the tissue to absorb and dissipate energy.

Glaucoma   237

4.2 GONIOSCOPY

1. **What is gonioscopy?**
   Gonioscopy is a clinical technique that is used to examine structures in the anterior chamber angle and forms an important part of glaucoma evaluation.

2. **What is cycloscopy?**
   Cycloscopy is a technique of direct visualization of ciliary processes under special circumstances such as the presence of an iridectomy, wide iris retraction, aniridia, and some cases of aphakia. The main value is in conjunction with laser therapy to ciliary processes (transpupillary cyclophotocoagulation).

3. **What is the principle of gonioscopy?**
   Under normal conditions, light reflected from the angle structures is incident at the tear-air interface at an oblique angle and is internally reflected. All gonioscopy lenses eliminate the tear-air interface by placing a plastic or glass surface adjacent to the front surface of the eye.

4. **What are the commonly used contact lenses for gonioscopy?**
   i. *Direct gonioscopy (goniolens):*
      - Koeppe
      - Barkan
      - Worst
      - Swan-Jacob
      - Richardson
   ii. *Indirect gonioscopy (gonioprism):*
      - Goldmann
      - Zeiss
      - Posner
      - Sussman

5. **Describe direct gonioscopy.**
   Direct gonioscopy is performed with a hand-held binocular microscope, a fiberoptic illuminator or a pen light, and a direct gonioscopy lens. It is performed with the patient in a supine position (e.g., in an operating room for infants under anesthesia). With direct gonioscopy lenses, an erect view of the angle structures is obtained.

6. **Describe indirect gonioscopy.**
   Instruments:

i. Goldmann single mirror	• Mirror in this lens has a height of 12 mm and a tilt of 62° from the plano front surface • Central well has a diameter of 12 mm, posterior radius of curvature—7.38 mm

Contd...

Contd...

ii.	Goldmann three mirror	Has two mirrors for examination of the fundus and one for the anterior chamber angle • *Equatorial mirror (inclined at 73°):* It is the largest and its oblong shape enables visualization from posterior pole to equator • *Peripheral mirror (67°):* It is intermediate in size and its square shape enables visualization from equator to ora serrata • *Gonioscopy mirror (59°):* It is the smallest and its dome shape is used to visualize extreme periphery and the angle
iii.	Zeiss four mirror (can be used for indentation gonioscopy)	• All four mirrors are tilted at 64° • Original four-mirror lens is mounted on a holding fork called unger or holder • Posner lens has a permanently attached holder rod • Sussman lens is held directly • Patient's own tears are useful as a fluid bridge
iv.	Ritch trabeculoplasty	Two mirrors are titled at 59°. Two are titled at 62°; convex lens is present over one mirror of each set
v.	Trabeculens	It has a 30 D convex lens in a hollow funnel, with four mirrors at 62° angles. It can be used as a diagnostic gonioprism as well as for laser trabeculoplasty and iridotomy

Techniques:
The cornea is anesthetized and with the patient positioned at the slit lamp, topical anesthetic is instilled, and the gonioprism is gently placed against the cornea with or without a fluid bridge (depending on the type). Slit beam is narrowed, carefully avoiding direct illumination of the pupil. A corneal wedge is formed to identify Schwalbe's line.

Visualization into a narrow angle can be enhanced by manipulating the Goldmann gonioprism, by asking the patient to look in the direction of the mirror being used.

7. **Compare direct and indirect gonioscopy.**

Advantages	*Disadvantages*
Indirect	
• Equipment easily available • Quicker procedure • Compression can be done • Slit lamp provides good illumination and magnification	• Orientation is confusing initially • Difficult in narrow angles
Direct	
• Binocular comparison • Simple orientation • Can see over convex iris • Ideal for surgical intervention • Supine position comparable to normal anatomy	• Special equipment • Time-consuming • Expensive

8. **What is compression gonioscopy?**
   Compression gonioscopy is also called indentation gonioscopy. By varying the amount of pressure applied to the cornea by a Zeiss contact lens, the physician can observe the effects since this will cause the aqueous humor to be forced into the angle. This is used to differentiate appositional versus synechial angle closure. Compression gonioscopy can be performed by Zeiss Posner or Sussman lenses.

9. **Describe normal structures of the angle seen in gonioscopy.**
   Starting at the root of the iris and progressing anteriorly toward the cornea, the following structures can be identified by gonioscopy (from behind forward):
   i. *Ciliary body band:* This is a gray or dark brown band and is the portion of ciliary body that is visible in the anterior chamber as a result of the iris insertion into the ciliary body
   ii. *Scleral spur:* This is usually seen as a prominent white line between the ciliary body band and the functional trabecular meshwork. This is the posterior lip of the scleral sulcus
   iii. *Trabecular meshwork:* This is seen as a pigmented band just anterior to the scleral spur. It has an anterior and posterior part. The posterior part is the primary site of aqueous outflow
   iv. *Schwalbe's line:* This is the junction between the angle structures and the cornea. It marks the transition between corneal endothelium and trabecular cells. It also marks the termination of Descemet's membrane

10. **Mention the clinical uses of gonioscopy.**
    i. *Diagnostic:*
       - Differentiate between open-angle and angle-closure glaucoma
       - Early detection of narrow angles
       - Helps in diagnosing secondary glaucomas such as trauma (angle recession), neovascular (new vessels in the angle), pseudoexfoliative [deposition of pseudoexfoliation (PXF) material], and pigmentary glaucoma
       - Helps in identifying tumors, cysts, foreign bodies, or blood in the angle
       - Assess K–F ring (Wilson's disease)
       - Postoperative evaluation:
         - Ostium
         - Cyclodialysis
         - Iridotomy
    ii. *Therapeutic:*
       - Indentation gonioscopy can be used to break an attack of acute angle closure
       - Useful to do goniotomy and goniophotocoagulation

11. **How do you differentiate iris processes and peripheral anterior synechiae (PAS)?**

Iris process	PAS
Lacy, fenestrated	Solid, not fenestrated
Underlying angle structures visible through spaces between strands	Preclude any view of underlying structures

Iris processes are present in one-third of the normal eyes. Generally, they insert at the level of the scleral spur, more in the nasal angle.

12. **How do you differentiate between the normal blood vessel in angle and the pathological angle vessels?**

Normal blood vessel in angle	Pathological angle vessels
Broad	Fine
It will not cross the scleral spur	Crosses the scleral spur
Does not arborize	Branch, arborize in trabecular meshwork

13. **How do you differentiate between Sampaolesi's line and pigmented trabecular meshwork?**

Sampaolesi's line	Pigmented trabecular meshwork
Located anterior to the corneal wedge	Posterior to the corneal wedge
Salt and pepper appearance	Brown sugar
Dark and granular	Fine
Discontinuous	Continuous

14. **Mention the causes of trabecular meshwork pigmentation.**
    i. Pigmentary glaucoma/pigment dispersion syndrome
    ii. PXF
    iii. Pseudophakic pigment dispersion
    iv. Trauma
    v. Following YAG laser iridotomy
    vi. Following acute angle-closure glaucoma
    vii. Anterior uveitis
    viii. Iris melanoma
    ix. Epithelial cysts
    x. Nevus of Ota
    xi. Darkly pigmented iris

15. **What are the causes of blood in the angle?**
    i. Post-traumatic
    ii. Postsurgical
    iii. Postlaser
    iv. Ghost cells recognized as candy stripe pattern

16. **What are the causes of blood in Schlemm's canal?**
    i. *Due to increased episcleral venous pressure*
       - Carotid-cavernous fistula
       - Dural shunt
       - Sturge-Weber syndrome
       - Obstruction of superior vena cava
       - Ocular hypotony
       - Postgonioscopy
    ii. *Due to low intraocular pressure (IOP)*
       - Hypotony following trabeculectomy

17. **What are the causes of PAS?**
    i. Primary angle-closure glaucoma (PACG)
    ii. Anterior uveitis
    iii. Iridocorneal endothelial (ICE) syndrome
    iv. Secondary glaucoma following intraocular surgery (such as wound leak)
    v. Trauma

18. **What are the findings one can expect in gonioscopy following trauma?**
    i. Angle recession
    ii. Trabecular tears
    iii. Iridodialysis and cyclodialysis
    iv. Foreign bodies PAS (late onset)

GONIOSCOPIC GRADING OF ANGLE STRUCTURES
Shaffer's Grading System

Angle grade	Numeric grade	Degrees	Clinical interpretation	Structure visible
Wide open angle	4	35–40°	Closure impossible	Up to the ciliary body
Open	3	25–35°	Closure impossible	Up to the ciliary body
Moderately narrow	2	20°	Eventual closure possible. But unlikely	Trabecular meshwork (pigmented)
Extremely narrow	1	10°	Closure possible	Only Schwalbe's line. May be anterior trabecular meshwork (nonpigmented) seen
Slit angle	S	<10°	Portions appear closed	No angle structures seen. But no obvious iridocorneal contact
Closed angle	0	–	Closure complete	Iridocorneal contact

In grade 0, indentation gonioscopy with Zeiss goniolens is necessary to differentiate appositional from synechial angle closure.

1. **Define occludable angle.**

   This is a condition in which pigmented trabecular meshwork is not visible (Shaffer grade 1 or 0) without indentation or manipulation in at least three quadrants.

2. **What is Scheie's gonioscopic classification?**

Grade	Structure visible
Wide open	All structure visible
Grade 1 narrow	Hard to see the root of the iris
Grade 2 narrow	Ciliary body band obscured
Grade 3 narrow	Posterior trabecular meshwork obscured
Grade 4 narrow	Only Schwalbe's line visible

3. **What is Spaeth classification?**

   Spaeth classification takes four parameters into consideration.
   i. Site of iris root insertion

A	Anterior to trabecular meshwork (i.e., Schwalbe's line)
B	Behind Schwalbe's line (at the level of trabecular meshwork)
C	Centered at the level of the scleral spur
D	Deep to scleral spur (i.e., anterior to ciliary body)
E	Extremely deep inserted into ciliary body

   ii. Width or geometric angle of iris insertion

   The angle between the intersection of imaginary tangents formed by the peripheral third of the iris and the inner wall of the corneoscleral junction is the width or geometric angle of iris insertion. It is graded as 10°, 20°, 30°, and 40°.

   iii. Contour of peripheral iris near the angle

S	Steep or convex configuration
R	Regular or flat
Q	Queer—deeply concave

   iv. Intensity of trabecular meshwork pigmentation—minimal or no pigment (grade 0) to dense pigment deposition (grade 4).

4.3 GLAUCOMA DIAGNOSTIC WITH VARIABLE CORNEAL COMPENSATION

1. **What are the key elements of the printout?**
   i. *Thickness map:*
      - Retinal nerve fiber layer (RNFL) thickness represented on a color-coded map
      - Thick RNFL—yellow, orange, and red
      - Thin RNFL—dark blue, light blue, and green
   ii. *Deviation map:*
      Location and magnitude of RNFL defects over the map
   iii. *TSNIT map:*
      - Displays RNFL thickness over the calculation circle (stands for temporal-superior-nasal-inferior-temporal)
      - Normal TSNIT—map follows a double-hump pattern, i.e., thick RNFL—superior, inferior
      - Thin RNFL—nasal, temporal shows actual values along with a shaded area representing the normal range for that age.
   iv. *Parameters:*
      - TSNIT average
      - Superior average
      - Inferior average
      - TSNIT standard deviation
      - Intereye asymmetry

2. **How is the measurement done? What area is measured and at how many points?**
   It is performed with an undilated pupil of at least 2 mm in diameter. As the scanner has two mirrors that oscillate at 4,000/s, there is a high-pitched noise emitted.

   65,536 points are measured in a full 15 × 150 grid centered at the optic nerve head.

   The central ellipse denotes an area of 1.75 disk diameter in size. The reproducibility of images is 5-8 µm per measured pixel.

   Image quality check: A warning is given if an image fails to meet the criteria. The quality of the image is affected by cataracts and poor media clarity.

3. **What are the abnormal patterns on the thickness map?**
   Abnormal patterns include:
   i. Diffuse loss of NFL, causing areas that should be yellow to fade to red

ii. Focal defects are seen as concentrated dark areas (should be visible on the fundus image as well)
iii. Asymmetry between superior and inferior quadrants
iv. Asymmetry between the two eyes
v. Higher than the normal nasal and temporal thickness (red and yellow where blue should be)

4. **What are the sensitivity and specificity of glaucoma diagnostic with variable corneal compensation (GDx VCC)?**
   i. Sensitivity—96%
   ii. Specificity—93%

5. **What are the advantages of GDx VCC?**
   The advantages of GDx VCC are as follows:
   i. Easy to operate
   ii. Does not require pupillary dilatation
   iii. Good reproducibility
   iv. Does not require a reference plane
   v. Can detect glaucoma on the first examination
   vi. Early detection before standard visual field
   vii. Comparison with age-matched normative database

6. **What are the limitations of GDx VCC?**
   The limitations of GDx VCC are as follows:
   i. It does not provide optic nerve head analysis
   ii. Limited use in moderate/advanced glaucoma
   iii. Does not measure actual RNFL thickness (inferred value)
   iv. No clinical studies on the detection of progression using this technology
   v. No database from the Indian population
   vi. Affected by anterior and posterior segment pathology such as:
      - Ocular surface disorders
      - Macular pathology
      - Cataract and refractive surgery
      - Refractive errors (false positive in myopes)
      - Peripapillary atrophy (PPA; scleral birefringence interferes with RNFL measurement)

7. **What is scanning laser polarimetry?**
   Scanning laser polarimetry is an imaging technology that is utilized to measure peripapillary RNFL thickness. It is based on the principle of birefringence. GDx is the trade name that uses this technology.

8. **What is VCC?**
   VCC stands for variable corneal compensator, which has been created to account for the variable corneal birefringence in patients.

4.4 GLAUCOMA VISUAL FIELD DEFECTS

1. **What is a visual field?**
   Traquair defined a visual field as an island of vision in a sea of darkness. The island of vision is usually described as a three-dimensional graphic representation of differential light sensitivity at different positions of space.

2. **What is the extent of the normal visual field?**

Superior	60°
Inferior	75°
Nasally	60°
Temporally	100–110°

3. **What is a blind spot?**
   A blind spot is a region that corresponds to the optic nerve head, and because there are no photoreceptors in the area, it creates a deep depression within the boundaries of the normal visual field.

4. **What is kinetic perimetry?**
   Kinetic perimetry is one in which a target is moved from an area where it is not seen to an area where it is just seen, keeping the size and intensity of the stimulus constant, e.g., Goldmann perimetry.

5. **What is static perimetry?**
   A stationary stimulus is presented at various locations with variable intensity, e.g., Humphrey's perimetry.

6. **What are the variables that can influence perimetry?**
   i. Alertness of the patient
   ii. Fixation must be constant and centered
   iii. *Background luminance:* Should be maintained between 4 and 31 apostilbs
   iv. Brightness of the stimulus
   v. Patient refraction should be fully corrected
   vi. Pupil size should be constant (2–4 mm)
   vii. Increasing age is associated with a reduction in retinal threshold sensitivity
   viii. High cheekbones and sunken socket
   ix. Media clarity

7. **What are the causes of the generalized decrease in the sensitivity of the visual field?**
   i. Glaucoma
   ii. Cataracts

iii. Use of miotics
   iv. Gross uncorrected refractive errors
   v. Other media opacities

8. **What is an isopter?**

   An isopter is a line on a visual field representation connecting points with the same threshold. It is usually done on a two-dimensional sheet of paper.

9. **What is a scotoma?**

   A scotoma is a localized defect or depression in the visual field. An absolute defect persists even at the maximum stimulus, and a relative scotoma is seen in a weaker stimulus but disappears on increasing the brightness of the stimulus.

10. **What is a depression?**

    A depression is a decrease in expected retinal sensitivity.

11. **What is the sequential progression of visual field defects in glaucoma?**
    i. Generalized depression
    ii. Paracentral scotoma
    iii. Siedel's scotoma
    iv. Arcuate or Bjerrum's scotoma
    v. Double arcuate or ring scotoma
    vi. Nasal step
    vii. Progressive contraction
    viii. Central island and temporal island with or without split fixation

12. **What are angioscotomas?**

    Angioscotomas are long branching scotomas above and below the blind spot, which are presumed to result from shadows created by the large retinal blood vessels.

13. **What is Bjerrum's (arcuate's) area?**

    Bjerrum's (arcuate's) area is an arcuate area extending above and below the blind spot between 10 and 25 of the fixation point.

14. **What is the differential diagnosis for arcuate scotoma?**
    i. *Chorioretinal lesions:*
       - Juxtapapillary choroiditis
       - Myopia with PPA
       - Panretinal photocoagulation
    ii. *Optic nerve head lesions:*
       - Drusen
       - Retinal artery plaques
       - Chronic papilledema

- Colobomas
- Optic pit

iii. *Anterior optic nerve head lesion:*
- Electric shock
- Retrobulbar neuritis
- Cerebral arteritis
- Ischemic optic neuropathy

iv. *Posterior lesions of the visual pathway:*
- Pituitary adenoma
- Optochiasmatic arachnoiditis
- Meningiomas of dorsum sella

15. What is paracentral scotoma?
Paracentral scotoma is the earliest clinically significant field defect. It may appear either below or above the blind spot in Bjerrum's area.

16. What is Seidel's scotoma?
When the disease progresses, paracentral scotoma joins with the blind spot to form a sickle-shaped scotoma known as Seidel's scotoma.

17. What is ring or double arcuate scotoma?
Ring or double arcuate scotoma develops when the two arcuate scotomas join together at the horizontal raphe.

18. What is Roenne's central nasal step?
Roenne's central nasal step is created when the two arcuate scotomas run in different arcs and meet to form a sharp right-angled defect at the horizontal meridian.

19. What are the true baring and false baring of blind spots?
When a small isopter is being studied, a patient with Seidel's scotoma may demonstrate a connection between the blind spot and nonseeing area outside the 25° radius. This is a true baring of the blind spot. A normal patient may exhibit false baring of the blind spot when the isopter is just outside the blind spot.

20. What is scotometry/campimetry?
Estimation of defect of central fields by using a tangent screen is termed campimetry/scotometry.

21. Which part of the visual field is tested using a tangent screen?
Central 300

22. What is the size of the tangent screen board?
1 or 2 m^2

23. At what distance should a patient be seated?
The patient should be seated at a distance of 1 or 2 m according to the tangent screen size.

24. **What is the color and material of the tangent screen?**
    The material of the screen is black felt.
25. **What are the numbers of meridians that should be tested?**
    Eight meridians with one central fixation should be tested.
26. **What is the size of the test object?**
    1–10 mm
27. **How many circles are in a tangent screen?**
    There are six concentric circles from 50 to 300.
28. **What is a wand?**
    A wand is a handle where the object is fixed. Spherical test objects are mounted on the side of the wand near its tip.
29. **What is a meridian?**
    The circles are divided into radial sections by diameter lines called meridians.
30. **What is the color of the test objects used in a tangent screen?**
    White, red, green, and blue
31. **Which is the color maximum used in checking visual fields?**
    White
32. **What is the specific use of colors used in a tangent screen?**
    Red and blue are used for neuro cases and white is used for normal vision and glaucoma.
33. **How to move the target in a tangent screen?**
    i. Normally, it is from nonseeing to seeing area
    ii. When mapping the blind spot, it is from seeing to nonseeing area
34. **What are the types of manual perimeter?**
    i. Goldmann's perimetry
    ii. Bjerrum's perimetry
    iii. Lister's perimetry
35. **What is Bjerrum's perimetry?**
    Bjerrum's perimetry is the quantitative test and subjective method of identifying a central visual field defect.
36. **What is a blind spot?**
    A blind spot is the region of deep depression within the boundaries of the normal visual fields, corresponding to the optic nerve head that lies temporal to the fixation in the visual fields.
37. **What is the location of the blind spot?**
    The center of the blind spot is 120–170 from the point of fixation on the temporal side and is situated 1.50 below the horizontal meridian.

38. What is the size of the blind spot?

The size of the blind spot is 7.5 mm in the vertical direction and 5.5 mm in the horizontal direction.

39. What are the classifications of scotoma?

According to the situation, scotoma is divided into central, peripheral, paracentral, ring, absolute and relative, and positive and negative scotoma.

40. What is central scotoma?

Central scotoma includes the point of fixation. When it has a sufficient density, it interferes with or abolishes central vision altogether. For example, central scotoma caused by macular lesions.

41. What is paracentral scotoma?

Paracentral scotoma is situated to one side of the point of fixation. For example, tobacco amblyopia.

42. What is ring/annular scotoma?

Ring/annular scotoma encircles the point of fixation. For example, retinitis pigmentosa.

43. What is peripheral scotoma?

Peripheral scotoma causes little disturbance of sight and may exist without the patients' knowledge, especially when situated away from the point of fixation.

44. What is a positive scotoma?

A positive scotoma is when the patient sees a black spot in his visual field. For example, changes in eye media or retina.

45. What is negative scotoma?

A negative scotoma is when the scotoma exists as a defect in the visual field but is not perceived by the patient until the visual field of examination.

46. What is mobile scotoma?

If the opacities exist in the vitreous, the scotoma is mobile. For example, muscae volitantes.

47. What is absolute scotoma?

Absolute scotoma refers to the area of the optic nerve head that is devoid of photoreceptors and is seen as vertically oval.

Perception of light is entirely lost over the absolute scotoma.

48. What is relative scotoma?

A scotoma in which there is a visual depression but not complete loss of light perception. For example, toxic amblyopia.

250 Glaucoma

49. What is the importance of the size of the test object?

The size of the scotoma depends on the size of the test object used. By using a large object, it may be impossible to demonstrate a scotoma that is clearly demonstrable when a small test object is used.

50. Describe Bjerrum's screen and its technique.
  i. Bjerrum's screen consists of a black felt screen measuring about 1 or 2 m^2 in size supported on a framework
  ii. The patient should be seated at a distance of 1 or 2 m according to the size of the tangent screen
  iii. The screen has a white object for fixation in its center around which are marked concentric circles from 50 to 300
  iv. The patients fix it on the central dot with one eye occluded
  v. A white target 1-10 mm in diameter is brought from the periphery toward the center in various meridians
  vi. Initially, the blind spot is charged which is normally located about 150° temporal to the fixation point on a 1 m tangent screen

51. How to perform the tangent screen examination?
  i. For a tangent screen examination, it is essential that the patient wears his/her glasses if he/she has a refractive error
  ii. The examiner usually stands toward the side and keeps his/her eye on the patient's eye to ensure that the fixation is absolutely maintained
  iii. The test object, the size of which correlated with the patient's visual acuity, is moved from the periphery toward the center
  iv. The patients indicate when they see the test object, either by making a verbal response such as yes or by tapping the coin
  v. At all times, the fixation of the patient has to be checked
  vi. The easiest way is to map out the patient's blind spot first, which is smaller and closer to the fixation point
  vii. Check the patient's response by rotating the test object, out of view, so that it is not visible to the patient at all
  viii. Transfer the information from the felt screen to the chart carefully
  ix. Make sure to understand the proper degree of eccentricities and the meridian placements in the stitched chart and the recording diagram
  x. Evaluate each scotoma for depth with a small and a larger target

52. How to calibrate Bjerrum's screen?
  i. Bjerrum's screen is calibrated by means of a series of black threads sewn into the black cloth at intervals of 50 along the principal 300 meridians rotating from the fixation point
  ii. These threads cannot be seen by the patients at 2 m, but they are visible to the examiner working at a close range

iii. Alternatively, Sinclair's rule may be used, which translates distance from the fixation point into the appropriate degree and also shows the different meridians

53. What are the differences between neurological and glaucomatous field defects?

Neurological field defects	Glaucomatous field defects
i. It follows the vertical meridian	i. It follows the horizontal meridian
ii. Absolute field defect	ii. Relative field defect, progress to an absolute defect in late stage
iii. Field defects are mostly congruous	iii. Field defects are incongruous

54. What is standard automated perimetry (SAP)?

SAP is also called achromatic automated perimetry. With this procedure, threshold sensitivity measurements are usually performed at a number of test locations using white stimuli on a white background.

55. What is short-wavelength automated perimetry (SWAP)?

SWAP is also known as blue-yellow perimetry. Standard perimeters are available that can project a blue stimulus onto a yellow background. Sensitivity to blue stimuli is believed to be mediated by small bistratified ganglion cells that typically have large receptive fields. This method is more sensitive to detect the early stages of glaucoma.

56. What are the advantages and disadvantages of SWAP?

Advantages:
i. Detects glaucoma early
ii. Can track progression

Disadvantages:
i. Tedious and time-consuming
ii. More affected by refractive error and media opacities

57. What is frequency doubling technology (FDT) perimetry?

The FDT perimeter was developed to measure contrast detection thresholds for frequency-doubled test targets. This test uses a low spatial frequency sinusoidal grating undergoing rapid phase reversal flicker. The instruments employ a 0.25 cycle per degree grating phase reversed at a rapid 25 Hz. It is believed that the stimuli employed in this test preferentially activate the M cells and are most sensitive in the detection of early glaucomatous loss.

58. What are the advantages and disadvantages of FDT perimetry?

Advantages:
i. Portable
ii. Can be used in ambient illumination

iii. Relatively insensitive to refractive error
iv. Shorter learning curve
v. Faster than SAP

Disadvantages:
i. Affected by media opacity
ii. False positives possible
iii. Ability to detect progression is questionable

59. What is false positivity?

When a patient responds at a time when no test stimulus is being presented, a false-positive response is recorded. False positives >33% suggest an unreliable test.

60. What is false negativity?

When a patient fails to respond to a stimulus presented in a location where a dimmer stimulus was previously seen, a false-negative response is recorded. False positive >33% suggest an unreliable test.

61. What is a threshold?

The differential light sensitivity at which a stimulus of a given size and duration of presentation is seen 50% of the time.

62. What is a decibel (dB)?

The measured light sensitivity is expressed in logarithmic units referred to as decibels. It is a 0.1 log unit. It is a relative term used in both static and kinetic perimetry. It refers to log units of attenuation of the maximum light intensity available in the perimeter. The standard staircase strategy used by automated perimeters employs an initial 4 dB step size that decreases to 2 dB on the first reversal and continues until a second reversal occurs.

63. What are the testing strategies in automated perimetry?

Suprathreshold strategy	For screening purposes
Threshold-related strategy	For moderate-to-severe defects
Threshold strategy	Current standard for automated perimetry
Efficient threshold strategies	This is a shorter threshold testing typified by the Swedish interactive thresholding algorithm (SITA) and takes only 50% of the regular threshold strategy. Completes in the shortest time, most practical to use, especially in large clinical settings

64. What are the common programs for glaucoma testing using automated perimetry?

Octopus 32	Central 24° and 30° programs
Humphrey field analyzer (HFA)	24-2 and 30-2 programs

These programs test the central field using a 6° grid. For patients with advanced visual field loss that threatens fixation, serial 10-2 should be used.

65. **What are the test programs of HFA?**

Central field test	Central 30-2 test
	Central 24-2 test
	Central 10-2 test Macula test
Peripheral field test	Peripheral 30/60-1
	Peripheral 30/60-2
	Nasal step
	Temporal crescent
Specialty test	Neurological-20
	Neurological-50
	Central 10-12
	Macular test

66. **What is a central 30-2 test?**
    Central 30-2 test is the most comprehensive form of visual field assessment of the central 30°. It consists of 76 points at 6° apart on either side of the vertical and horizontal axes. The innermost points are 3° from the fixation point.

67. **What is mean deviation?**
    Mean deviation is the mean difference between the normative data for that age and collected data. It is more of an indicator of the general depression.

68. **What is pattern standard deviation?**
    Pattern standard deviation is a measure of variability between two different points within the field, i.e., it measures the difference between a given point and an adjacent point. It determines the localized field effect.

69. **What is glaucoma Hemifield test (GHT)?**
    GHT compares the five clusters of points in the upper field (above the horizontal midline) with the five mirror images in the lower field. These clusters of points are specific to the detection of glaucoma outside normal limits.

70. **What are the indicators in automated perimetry that indicate glaucomatous progression?**
    i. Average fluctuations between two determinations of the visual field will be >3 dB
    ii. Deepening of an existing scotoma is suggested by the reproducible depression of a point in an existing scotoma by >7 dB

iii. Enlargement of an existing scotoma is suggested by the reproducible depression of a point adjacent to an existing scotoma by >9 dB
iv. Development of a new scotoma is suggested by the reproducible depression of a previously normal point in the visual field by >11 dB, or of two adjacent, previously normal points by >5 dB

71. What are the criteria to grade glaucomatous field defects?

Parameters	Early defects	Moderate defects	Severe defects
Mean deviation	<6 dB	−6 to −12 dB	≥12 dB
Corrected pattern standard deviation (CPSD)	Depressed to the $P < 5\%$	Depressed to the $P < 5\%$	Depressed to the $P < 5\%$
Pattern deviation plot			
• Points depressed below $P < 5\%$	<18 (25%)	<37 (50%)	>37 (>50%)
• Points depressed below $P < 1\%$	<10	<20	>20
GHT	Outside normal limits	Outside normal limits	Outside normal limits
Sensitivity in central 5°	No point <15 dB	One hemifield may have a point with sensitivity <15 dB	Both hemifields have points with sensitivity <15 dB

72. What are Anderson's criteria?
i. GHT: Outside normal limits on at least two consecutive occasions
ii. Three or more nonedge points in a location typical of glaucoma, all of which are depressed at $P < 5\%$ and one of which is depressed at $P < 1\%$ level on two consecutive occasions
iii. CPSD (it takes into account the short-term fluctuations, thereby highlighting the localized defects. It accounts for intraobserver variations) at $P < 5\%$ level

73. What are the features of a tangent screen?
i. Tangent screen may be used at 1 or 2 m
ii. It should have a uniform illumination of 7 foot candles
iii. It should be large enough to allow testing of the full 30° of central field

74. What are the features of Goldmann perimetry?
i. Goldmann perimetry is a type of bowl perimetry
ii. The maximum stimulus should be 1,000 apostilbs
iii. The background illumination should be 31.5 apostilbs
iv. A threshold target is initially identified. Careful investigation of the 5°, 10°, and 15° isopters is necessary to detect early glaucoma

75. **What are the other psychophysical tests useful in glaucoma?**
    i. High pass resolution perimetry
    ii. Motion detection perimetry
    iii. Electroretinography (ERG)
    iv. Pattern ERG
    v. Multifocal visual evoked potential

76. **How do glaucomatous visual field defects present with corresponding disk change?**
    i. Localized superior/inferior notching of the optic disk causes localized field defects with an early threat to fixation
    ii. Myopic disk with glaucoma [shallow disk with temporal crescent of PPA along with glaucomatous damage] causes dense superior or inferior scotomas threatening fixation
    iii. Sclerotic disks [shallow saucerized cup and gently sloping neuroretinal rim (NRR)] cause peripheral visual field loss
    iv. Concentrically enlarging disks cause diffuse field loss.

4.5 ULTRASOUND BIOMICROSCOPY AND ANTERIOR SEGMENT OPTICAL COHERENCE TOMOGRAPHY IN GLAUCOMA

1. **What is ultrasound biomicroscope (UBM)?**
   The UBM is a high-frequency ultrasound machine with 50–100 MHz transducers. It is used to image ocular structures anterior to the pars plana region of the eye in living patients.

2. **Give characteristics of the UBM image.**
   The UBM produces cross-sectional images of anterior segment structures providing:
   i. Lateral resolution of 50 µ
   ii. Axial resolution of 25 µ
   iii. Depth of penetration of approximately 4–5 mm
   iv. Field of view of 5 × 5 mm
   v. Vertical image lines of 256
   vi. Scan rate of 8 frames/second

3. **What are the qualitative uses of UBM?**
   i. *Glaucoma:*
      – *Angle-closure glaucoma*
        Angle-closure can occur in four anatomic sites, the iris (pupillary block), the ciliary body (plateau iris), the lens (phakomorphic glaucoma), and behind the iris by a combination of various forces (malignant glaucoma and other posterior pushing glaucoma types). Differentiating these sites is the key to providing effective treatment. UBM is extremely useful in achieving this goal.
         - *Angle occludability*
           Darkroom provocative testing can be done by generating objective results using UBM.
         - *Pupillary block*
           Unbalanced relative pressure gradient between the anterior and posterior chambers results in anterior iris bowing, angle narrowing, and acute or chronic angle closure, seen on UBM.
         - *Plateau iris*
           Indentation UBM shows a double-hump sign (as seen on indentation gonioscopy).
         - *Malignant glaucoma*
           UBM clearly shows that all anterior segment structures are displaced and pressed tightly against the cornea with or without fluid in the supraciliary space.

- *Other causes of angle closure*
  Iridociliary tumor, enlargement of the ciliary body due to inflammation or tumor infiltration, and air or gas bubble after intraocular surgery can be diagnosed on UBM. It can be used in pigment dispersion and pigmentary glaucoma and helps in visualization of the posterior bowing of the iris.
- *Open-angle glaucoma*
  The only type of open-angle glaucoma showing typical finding on UBM is pigment dispersion syndrome. UBM shows a widely open angle, posterior bowing of the peripheral iris, and increased iridolenticular contact.

ii. *Ocular trauma*
  - *Detection of foreign body*
    Wood and concrete: Shadowing artifact
    Metal and glass: Cosmetic artifact
    Detection of the location of intraocular lens for research purposes
  - *Angle recession*
    UBM shows the separation between the longitudinal and circular ciliary muscles.
  - *Cyclodialysis*
    Cyclodialysis cleft confirmed on UBM as an echolucent streak between the sclera and ciliary body, just posterior to the scleral spur.
  - Anterior segment tumors

4. **What are the quantitative uses of UBM in biometry of the anterior chamber?**
   Quantitative uses of UBM in biometry of the anterior chamber are as follows:
   Determination of:
   i. Corneal thickness
   ii. Anterior chamber depth (ACD)
   iii. Posterior chamber depth
   iv. Intraocular lens (IOL) thickness
   v. Scleral thickness

5. **What are the advantages and disadvantages of UBM?**
   Advantages:
   i. Quick
   ii. Convenient
   iii. Minimally invasive investigative tool
   iv. Imaging of the anterior segment structures is possible even in the eyes with corneal edema or corneal opacification that precludes gonioscopic assessment

Disadvantages:
  i. Bulky instrumentation
  ii. Limited penetration into the eye
  iii. Requires immersion technique

6. **How does optical coherence tomography (OCT) work?**
   OCT employs low coherence interferometry to obtain in vivo cross-sectional images of ocular tissues—using light instead of sound (unlike UBM), a beam is shore on structures of the eye and reflections returning from the structures are analyzed to produce real-time images.

7. **What is the wavelength used?**
   i. *For anterior segment*: Longer wavelength (1,310 nm)
   ii. *For posterior segment*: Shorter wavelength (830 nm)

8. **What are the advantages of OCT?**
   i. Noncontact
   ii. Rapid
   iii. Provides a real-time cross-sectional view of the angle structures
   iv. Less observer dependent
   v. Used to diagnose or confirm appositional angle closure
   vi. Used to evaluate the effects of laser peripheral iridotomy (PI)

9. **What are the disadvantages of OCT?**
   i. Poor ability to show details of the ciliary body and posterior surface of the iris
   ii. Cyclodialysis clefts and ciliary body tumors cannot be detected
   iii. Difficult to visualize the superior angle quadrant.

Glaucoma

4.6 ANGLE-CLOSURE GLAUCOMA

1. **Classify angle-closure disease.**
   Many different classifications are cited for angle-closure disease.
   Primary:
   i. *With pupillary block*
      - Primary angle-closure glaucoma (PACG)(acute/subacute/chronic)—(old classification with respect to severity of symptoms)
   ii. *Without pupillary block*
      - Plateau iris syndrome
      - Plateau iris configuration

   Secondary:
   i. *With pupillary block*
      - Miotic induced
      - Swollen lens
      - Mobile lens syndromes (ectopia lentis/microspherophakia)
   ii. *Without pupillary block*
      - Synechiae to lens/vitreous/posterior chamber intraocular lens (PCIOL)
      - Anterior *"pulling"* mechanisms (iris is pulled forward by some membrane)
        - Neovascular glaucoma
        - Iridocorneal endothelial (ICE) syndromes
        - Post-penetrating keratoplasty (PKP)
        - Aniridia
      - Posterior *"pushing"* mechanisms (iris is pushed forward by some posterior segment pathology with anterior rotation of the ciliary body)
        - Ciliary block glaucoma
        - Cysts of the iris/ciliary body
        - Nanophthalmos
        - Intraocular tumors
        - Intravitreal air (pneumoretinopexy)
        - Suprachoroidal hemorrhage
          - Classic (based on clinical symptoms): Acute, subacute, chronic, latent
          - Classification based on the level of obstruction to aqueous flow iris (pupil block/nonpupil block)
          - Ciliary body (plateau iris, cysts)
          - Lens (phakomorphic, phacotopic, anterior subluxation)
          - Posterior segment (malignant, silicone oil induced, vitreous hemorrhage)

2. **What is the classification of primary angle closure (PAC) disease on the basis of natural history?**
    i. *PAC suspect:*
        - >180° of iridotrabecular contact
        - Absence of peripheral anterior synechiae (PAS)
        - Normal intraocular pressure (IOP), disk, and visual fields
    ii. *PAC:*
        - >180° of iridotrabecular contact
        - Either elevated IOP and/or PAS
        - Normal disk and fields
    iii. *Primary angle-closure glaucoma (PACG):*
        - >180° of iridotrabecular contact
        - Elevated IOP plus optic nerve and visual field damage

3. **What are the predisposing factors for angle-closure glaucoma (ACG)?**
    The predisposing factors for ACG include:
    i. *Anatomical factors:*
        - Eyes with small axial length (hypermetropia, nanophthalmos)
        - Smaller corneal diameter
        - Decreased corneal height
        - Shallow anterior chamber
        - Plateau iris configuration
        - Anteriorly placed iris lens diaphragm
        - Thicker and more curved lens (e.g., microspherophakia)
        - More anterior insertion of the iris into the ciliary body
    ii. *Physiological factors:*
        - Mid-dilated pupil (emotional stress)
        - Dim illumination
        - Near work (accommodation)
        - Prone position
    iii. *Demographic factors:*
        - Increasing age
        - Family history
        - *Gender:* More common in females
        - *Race:* Indians, Eskimos, and other Asian groups
    iv. *Psychosomatic factors:*
        - Type-I personality

4. **What are the two forms of iridotrabecular contact?**
    i. Appositional
    ii. Synechial

5. **How does the risk of PACG increase with age?**
    i. Continuing growth of the lens thickness
    ii. More anterior position of the lens
    iii. Pupil becomes increasingly miotic

6. **Why is the mid-dilated pupil a significant cause of increased pupillary block?**
    i. Posterior vector of the force of the iris sphincter muscle reaches its maximum during the mid-dilated time
    ii. Peripheral iris is under less tension and is more easily pushed forward into contact with the trabecular meshwork
    iii. Dilation also causes thickening and bunching of the peripheral iris. With full dilation, there is no contact between the lens and iris and hence there is no pupillary block

7. **What is plateau iris syndrome?**
    The plateau iris syndrome is a form of PACG. It is less common than the pupillary block and is observed most commonly in young adults. Plateau iris syndrome is caused by the anatomically anterior position of the ciliary body with corresponding ciliary processes, which hold the peripheral iris in an anterior position overlying the trabecular meshwork. The iris is commonly located on the same plane as Schwalbe's line and a recess is present in the peripheral angle.

8. **How do you diagnose plateau iris syndrome?**
    Patients with plateau iris syndrome are characteristically asymptomatic but can present with signs and symptoms of acute, intermittent, or chronic angle closure. They demonstrate deep axial anterior chambers but narrow peripheral anterior chambers when examined with a slit lamp.

    On gonioscopic examination, the iris is flat instead of convex with a corresponding narrow anterior chamber angle. If indentation gonioscopy is used, the trabecular meshwork is visible with a sine wave appearance of the rolled-up peripheral iris due to the iris hanging over the anterior ciliary processes.

    To definitively diagnose plateau iris syndrome, a peripheral iridotomy (PI) must be performed; an anterior chamber angle that remains occludable confirms plateau iris syndrome.

    Ultrasound biomicroscope (UBM) definitively reveals the characteristic "plateau" configuration of the peripheral iris, with anterior placement of the ciliary body.

9. **What is plateau iris configuration?**
    Plateau iris configuration occurs when the typical iris configuration is present but without angle closure.

10. **How is plateau iris syndrome treated?**
    Most cases of suspected plateau iris syndrome have at least some component of pupillary block and patients are treated with PI.
    When the diagnosis of plateau iris syndrome is confirmed in a symptomatic patient, argon laser iridoplasty may be used to shrink the peripheral iris and relieve the closed angle.

11. **What are the drugs capable of precipitating angle-closure glaucoma in susceptible eyes?**
    The drugs causing angle-closure glaucoma through the pupillary block mechanism are as follows:
    i. *Adrenergic agonists:*
       - Phenylephrine
       - Ephedrine
    ii. *Noncatecholamine adrenergic agonists:*
       - Naphazoline
       - Salbutamol
    iii. *Anticholinergics:*
       - Tropicamide
       - Ipratropium bromide
       - Promethazine
       - Botulinum toxin
    iv. *Medications with anticholinergic side effects:*
       - Imipramine (tricyclic antidepressants)
       - Fluoxetine [selective serotonin reuptake inhibitor (SSRI)]

    The drugs causing angle-closure glaucoma through the nonpupillary block mechanism are as follows:
    i. *Cholinergics:*
       - Pilocarpine
       - Carbachol
       - Anticholinesterase
    ii. *Sulfonylureas:*
       - Chlorpropamide
       - Gliclazide
       - Glimepiride
       - Tolbutamide
    iii. *Sulfa-based antibiotics:*
       - Trimethoprim-sulfamethoxazole
       - Sulfadiazine
       - Dapsone
    iv. *Other sulfa-based drugs:*
       - Topiramate
       - Sumatriptan
       - Sotalol

v. *Anti-inflammatory:*
   - Mefenamic acid
vi. *Sulfa-based diuretics:*
   - Acetazolamide
   - Furosemide
   - Bumetanide
   - Chlorothiazide
   - Chlorthalidone
   - Metolazone
   - Indapamide
vii. *Rheumatological drugs:*
   - Sulfasalazine
   - Probenecid
   - Celecoxib
viii. *Anticoagulants:*
   - Heparin

12. **What is the mechanism by which drugs can cause angle-closure glaucoma?**

   Drugs can cause either pupillary block or nonpupillary block angle-closure glaucoma.

   Nonpupillary block mechanism:

   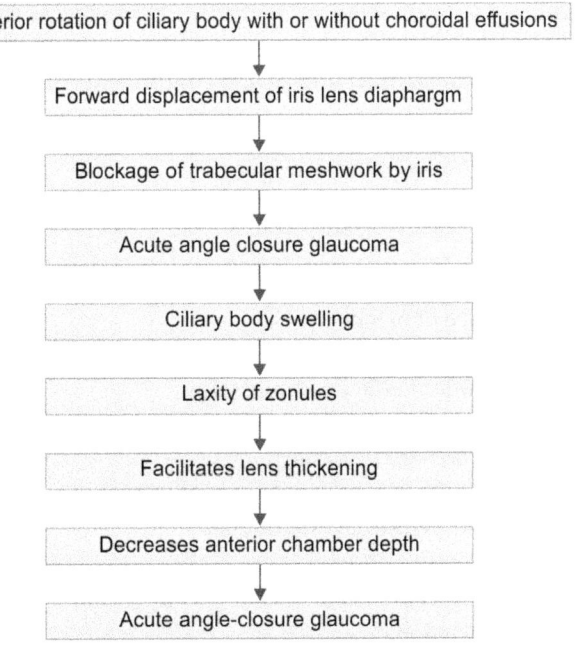

13. **Why is eye pain more in PACG than in primary open-angle glaucoma (POAG), even with the same IOP?**
    The eye pain appears to be related more to the rapid rate of the rise in IOP than the actual pressure.

14. **What is the cause of defective vision in PACG initially?**
    Blurred vision occurs first as a result of distortion of the corneal lamellae and later as a result of corneal epithelial edema.

15. **What are colored haloes due to?**
    Haloes are due to corneal epithelial edema, which acts as a diffraction grating that breaks white light into its component colors.

16. **How do the colored haloes present?**
    Haloes present with blue-green color in the center and yellow-red color in the periphery.

17. **What are the other conditions which can cause colored haloes?**
    i. Mucus on the cornea due to conjunctivitis
    ii. Incipient stage of cataract
    iii. Vitreous opacities
    iv. Snow blindness
    v. Tilt of IOL

18. **What is Fincham test?**
    Fincham or the stenopic test is a test used to distinguish between the haloes seen in incipient cataract and angle-closure glaucoma. A stenopic slit is placed in front of the eye and moved from one end of the pupillary aperture to the other. In glaucoma, the halo remains intact while the halo in incipient cataract breaks into component colors.

19. **What is the incidence of developing angle closure in the fellow eye?**
    About 50% within 5 years.

20. **Describe the clinical features of the various stages of angle-closure glaucoma.**
    i. *Prodromal stage:*
        - Presence of haloes
        - White eye
        - Intermittent attacks of mild pain
        - IOP may rise to 40–60 mm Hg
    ii. *Phase of constant instability:*
        - Intermittency is replaced by regularity
        - Increase in diurnal fluctuations
    iii. *Acute congestive attack:*
        - Circumcorneal congestion
        - Corneal edema

- Pain and vomiting
- Shallow anterior chamber
- Pupil moderately dilated and vertically oval
- Very high IOP

iv. *Chronic closed-angle glaucoma:*
- Presence of PAS
- IOP remains high between attacks
- Decreased vision and fields

v. *Absolute glaucoma:*
- Vision is no perception of light (PL)
- Corneal sensation absent
- Dilated circumcorneal vessels
- Atrophic iris and ectropion uvea
- Optic disk cupped
- Stony hard eye
- Scleral staphyloma

21. **What are the differential diagnoses of acute angle-closure glaucoma?**
    Evidence of compromised angle on gonioscopy or shallow anterior chamber:
    i. Ciliary block glaucoma
    ii. Neovascular glaucoma
    iii. Iridocorneal endothelial (ICE) syndrome
    iv. Plateau iris syndrome with angle closure
    v. Secondary angle closure with pupillary block (phakomorphic glaucoma)

    High-pressure open-angle glaucomas masquerading as acute angle closure:
    i. Glaucomatocyclytic crisis
    ii. Herpes simplex keratouveitis
    iii. Herpes zoster ophthalmicus
    iv. Pigmentary glaucoma
    v. Exfoliative glaucoma
    vi. Phako glaucoma

22. **Why is the pupil in angle-closure glaucoma vertically mid-dilated and nonreacting?**
    The pupil in angle-closure glaucoma is vertically mid-dilated and nonreacting due to iris sphincter ischemia and paresis due to high IOP.

23. **What is inverse glaucoma?**
    In conditions such as spherophakia, miotics increase the iris lens contact area due to slackening of the zonules (due to ciliary muscle contraction)

leading to forward displacement of the lens, thus precipitating or aggravating the pupillary block.

24. **What are the gonioscopic findings in angle-closure glaucoma?**
   In chronic angle closure, PAS is seen late in the course. In the subacute/acute congestive stages, the angle shows an occludable configuration.

25. **How do you do gonioscopy in the presence of corneal edema?**
   Gonioscopy is done after application of one or two drops of anhydrous glycerin. Epithelial bullae are a relative contraindication for gonioscopy.

26. **What are the signs suggestive of previous attacks of angle closure?**
   i. Iris pigments on the back of the cornea and endothelial loss
   ii. PAS
   iii. Sectoral iris atrophy
   iv. Posterior synechiae
   v. Mid-dilated sluggishly reacting pupil
   vi. Glaukomflecken
   vii. Visual field loss
   viii. Diminished outflow facility
   ix. Optic nerve cupping

27. **What are the various provocative tests used to diagnose angle-closure glaucoma?**
   The various provocative tests include:
   i. Mydriatic test
   ii. Darkroom test
   iii. Prone test
   iv. Prone darkroom test
   v. Phenylephrine-pilocarpine test
   vi. Triple test

   Mydriatic test:

   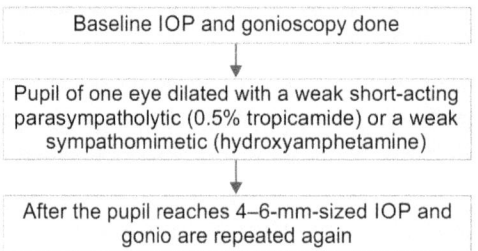

   IOP rise >8 mm Hg or gonio showing angle-closure test is considered positive. Some advocate an additional inclusion of tonography in the test; a decrease of outflow facility by 30% is taken as positive.

Darkroom test:

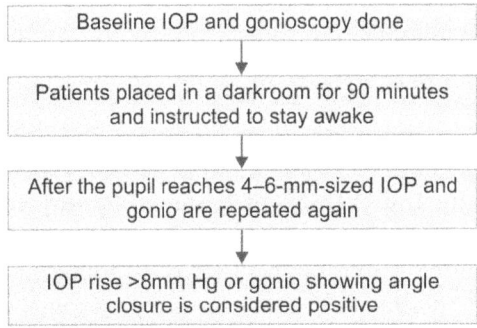

Prone test:

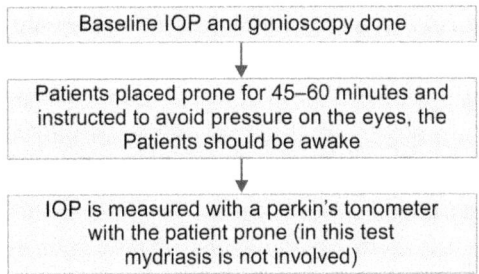

Darkroom prone test:
Darkroom prone test combines the features of darkroom test and prone test.

Phenylephrine-pilocarpine test:
Phenylephrine-pilocarpine test uses 10% phenylephrine and 2% pilocarpine to produce a pupillary block by creating a mid-dilated pupillary state.

Triple test:

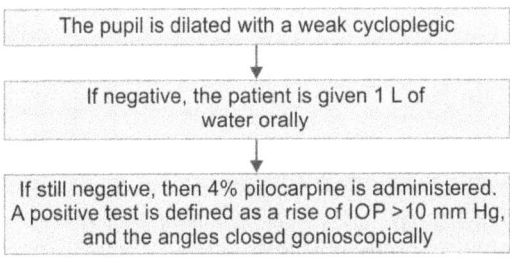

28. **What are the optic nerve head (ONH) changes seen in angle-closure glaucoma?**
    i. In the acute stage, the view is obscured by the corneal edema, but after the corneal edema clears out, the disk is seen to be congested

with or without multiple hemorrhages. In chronic angle closure, the disk changes are similar to the changes seen in POAG

ii. In the chronic congestive stage, the disk will be pale

29. What are the field defects in angle-closure glaucoma during an attack?

There is a generalized constriction of the fields.

30. What are the indications of trabeculectomy in angle-closure glaucoma?

i. Documented progression of ONH cupping inability to achieve target IOP despite laser procedures and maximal tolerable medical therapy

ii. Synechial angle closure (>270°)

31. What is the role of nonpenetrating glaucoma surgeries in angle-closure glaucoma?

Angle-closure glaucoma serves as a relative contraindication to nonpenetrating glaucoma surgeries. Since the trabecular meshwork is very close to the root of the iris, effective filtration may not occur.

32. What is Vogt's triad?

Vogt's triad is a triad of symptoms usually seen in postcongestive glaucoma or any treated case of angle-closure glaucoma. It includes:

i. Glaukomflecken
ii. Patches of iris atrophy
iii. Slightly dilated nonreacting pupil

33. How do we manage the terminal stage of PACG?

The terminal stage of PACG, i.e., absolute glaucoma, is characterized by:

i. Painful blind eye
ii. Ciliary congestion and caput medusa appearance of limbal vessels
iii. Shallow anterior chamber
iv. Atrophic iris
v. Band keratopathy
vi. Very high IOP (stony hard eyeball)
vii. Optic atrophy

Management:

i. Topical antiglaucoma medications
ii. Topical steroids
iii. Cycloplegics (preferably atropine)

If pain still persists:

i. Cryophotocoagulation/cyclophotocoagulation
ii. Retrobulbar alcohol injection
iii. Evisceration/enucleation

34. **How is retrobulbar alcohol given (technique)?**
    Initially, about 2–3 mL of lignocaine is injected in the retrobulbar region. The needle is then held in place, while the syringe is replaced with a 1 mL syringe containing 95–100% alcohol (some prefer to use 50% alcohol). The alcohol is then injected into the retrobulbar space. This is effective for 3–6 months.

35. **What do you anticipate following a retrobulbar alcohol injection?**
    i. Transient ptosis
    ii. Eyelid swelling
    iii. Ocular movement restriction
    iv. Anesthesia (periocular)
    v. Necrosis of ocular tissue

36. **What is combined mechanism glaucoma?**
    An eye with normal IOP and narrow angles, with otherwise normal anatomy, is said to be defined as "anatomically narrow angles." A person like this may present with signs of angle closure such as increased IOP, PAS, iris atrophy, and glaukomflecken. Such symptoms are likely to be diagnosed as PAC/PACG and treated with an iridotomy. Diagnosis of combined mechanism (or POAG with anatomically narrow angles) is typically made in such a patient who experienced an acute attack of angle closure that was treated with a PI. Iridotomy addresses the narrow-angle component, and the ensuing treatment is aimed at the open-angle component of the patient's glaucoma.

37. **What are the newer imaging technologies useful in diagnosis of angle closure?**
    i. UBM
    ii. Anterior segment OCT

38. **What are the causes of increased IOP postlaser iridotomy?**
    i. Inflammation
    ii. Steroid response
    iii. PI not patent
    iv. Plateau iris.

4.7 PRIMARY OPEN-ANGLE GLAUCOMA

1. **Define glaucoma.**

   Glaucoma is a multifactorial chronic progressive optic neuropathy with characteristic optic nerve head (ONH) changes and corresponding visual field defects with an intraocular pressure (IOP) detrimental to that ONH.

2. **What is the electrolyte difference between human plasma and aqueous humor?**

Electrolyte	In aqueous (nM/kgH$_2$O)	In plasma (nM/kgH$_2$O)
Sodium	163	176
Chloride	126	117
Bicarbonate	22	26
pH	7.21	7.40
Ascorbate	0.92	0.06

   i. Aqueous humor is slightly hypertonic and acidic when compared to plasma
   ii. It has marked excess of ascorbate and marked deficit of protein which are considered as its most striking features
   iii. Other reported constituents:
   - Sodium hyaluronate
   - Amino acids
   - Norepinephrine
   - Coagulation components
   - Tissue plasminogen activator
   - Latent collagenase activity

3. **What is the mechanism of aqueous humor outflow?**

   Aqueous humor leaves the eye through conventional and unconventional pathways.

   Conventional pathway or trabecular outflow pathway:
   Contributes to approximately 70–95% of outflow.
   Aqueous humor formed by ciliary processes passes from the posterior chamber to the anterior chamber through the pupil and exits via a trabecular meshwork and Schlemm's canal into the episcleral and conjunctival veins through direct and indirect intrascleral channels.

   Unconventional pathway:
   Contributes to 5–30% of outflow.
   i. *Uveoscleral outflow:*
      Aqueous humor passes through the root of the iris and interstitial spaces of the ciliary muscle to reach the suprachoroidal space.

From there, it passes to episcleral veins via scleral pores surrounding ciliary blood vessels and nerves, vessels of optic nerve membrane, or directly through the collagen substance of sclera.

ii. *Uveovortex outflow:*
Tracer studies in primates have also demonstrated aqueous outflow through vessels of iris, ciliary muscle, and anterior choroid to eventually reach vortex veins. However, the role of net fluid movement is clinically insignificant.

4. **What are the risk factors for primary open-angle glaucoma (POAG)?**
    i. High IOP
    ii. Advanced age
    iii. Family history of glaucoma
    iv. Race (African and Latin ancestry)
    v. Myopia
    vi. Thinner corneas [central corneal thickness (CCT) < 555 μm]
    vii. *Systemic diseases:* Diabetes mellitus and diastolic perfusion pressure < 55 mm Hg

5. **What percentage of risk is associated in family history?**
    i. First-degree relatives are at increased risk
    ii. Siblings are at four times increased risk
    iii. Offsprings are at twice the risk of normal population

6. **What is the prevalence of POAG?**
The prevalence of POAG is 1–2% in persons older than 40 years.

7. **What is ONH?**
    i. ONH extends from the retinal surface to the myelinated portion of the nerve posterior to the lamina
    ii. It extends to 3 mm behind the sclera where the myelination starts

8. **What are the types of axoplasmic flow and which one will be affected in glaucoma?**
    i. Orthograde flow [retina to lateral geniculate body (LGB)]
    ii. Retrograde flow (LGB to retina affected in glaucoma)

9. **What is phasing?**
The measurement of IOP at various times of day and night to record diurnal variation is known as phasing. This is being done since POAG patients manifest greater diurnal variation (≥6 mm Hg).

10. **What is the cause of diurnal variations/fluctuation?**
Fluctuation in aqueous humor production causes mean diurnal IOP measurement variation. The rate of aqueous formation falls to low levels during sleep and increases during the day, most likely in response to circulating catecholamines.

11. **What is the usefulness of diurnal variation measurement?**
    i. For diagnosing glaucoma
    ii. Explaining progressive damage despite apparent good pressure control
    iii. Evaluating the efficacy of therapy
    iv. Distinguishing normal tension glaucoma (NTG) from POAG

12. **What is the pathogenesis of glaucoma damage in POAG patients?**
    The optic nerve damage from glaucoma is multifactorial and may involve genetic susceptibility factors, mechanical forces, ischemia, loss of neurotrophic factors, and neurotoxicity.
    i. Jaeger's schemic theory secondary to raised IOP which causes impaired perfusion of the optic nerve
    ii. Muller's mechanical theory of raised pressure gradient causing direct compression and axonal death
    iii. Susceptibility of ganglion cells
    iv. Loss of architecture of the connective tissue structures within the ONH

13. **What are the genes associated with POAG?**
    MYOC: Myocilin gene (1q21-23)
    WDR36 gene (5q22)
    OPTN optineurin gene (10p)
    NTF4 gene (19q13.3)
    Glaucoma has polygenic or multifactorial transmission.

14. **What is screening in glaucoma?**
    An individual with a first-degree relative with POAG has an approximately eightfold risk of developing glaucoma. Studies have shown that siblings have a higher risk of developing glaucoma than parent/child. Prudence dictates that *anyone* with a first-degree relative with POAG should have regular ocular examinations, including tonometry and ophthalmoscopy, every 1 or 2 years up to age 60 years, with increasing frequency over age 60 years.

15. **What is the normal rate of loss of ganglion cells per year?**
    Five thousand ganglion cells are lost every year in normal individuals by apoptosis.

16. **How do ganglion cells die?**
    Ganglion cells die by a process called apoptosis (preprogrammed genetic mode for individual cellular suicide).

Glaucoma

17. **What are the types of ganglion cells and which cell is susceptible for glaucomatous damage?**

P cells	− M cells
Ratio	− 8:1
P cells	− Motion perception, scotopic information
M cells	− Acuity and color data
"M cells" loss in early glaucoma	

18. **What are the studies done in POAG patients to define systemic risk factors?**
    i. Beaver Dam eye study
    ii. Baltimore eye study
    iii. Blue Mountains eye study

19. **What is the importance of performing gonioscopy every year in open-angle glaucoma patients?**
    With advancing age, the angle-closure component may develop because of increasing thickness of the lens which may warrant peripheral iridotomy to prevent pupillary block.

20. **Define target pressure.**
    Target pressure is defined as the level of IOP below which retinal ganglion cell loss other than due to aging ceases to occur.
    It depends on the IOP at the time of presentation, severity of damage, extent of damage, and rapidity of progression of visual field deterioration.

21. **How is the target IOP set?**
    Other factors that should be considered in establishing the target pressure are as follows:
    i. CCT
    ii. Older age
    iii. Family history of glaucoma (increased risk for presence and progression in POAG)
    iv. African heritage
    v. Myopia
    vi. Asian heritage (increased risk for angle closure)
    vii. Hyperopia
    viii. Ocular ischemia and vasospastic disease (especially in NTG)
    It is individualized for each patient based on IOP at which damage has occurred, rate of progression, and life expectancy/age.

    For minimal damage [early normal neuroretinal rim (NRR) thinning without visual field loss]: Middle to high teens (mm Hg)

    For moderate damage (cupping of the disk with early field loss): Low to middle teens

    For advanced damage: High single digits

22. **How does NTG differ from POAG?**
    i. Mean IOP will always be <21 mm Hg on diurnal testing while ONH damage and glaucomatous field loss are present
    ii. The cup is often shallow with pallor
    iii. Disk hemorrhages are more frequent
    iv. History of migraine, peripheral vasospasm, or chronic blood loss may be reported. Visual field changes are reported to be denser, steeper, and more closer to fixation

23. **What are the sites of maximum resistance to outflow in POAG patients?**
    i. Juxtacanalicular part of trabecular meshwork offers maximum resistance to outflow
    ii. Schlemm's canal

24. **What are the reasons for this maximum resistance?**
    i. Altered corticosteroid metabolism
    ii. Dysfunctional adrenergic control
    iii. Abnormal immunologic process
    iv. Oxidative damage

25. **What is the other reason besides trabecular outflow resistance for elevated IOP in patients with POAG?**
    Obstruction of collector channels by deposition of glycosaminoglycans

26. **What are the histopathological findings in the anterior chamber angles of POAG patients?**
    i. Increase in extracellular matrix (ECM) in the juxtacanalicular region
    ii. Decreased number of pores in Schlemm's canal endothelium
    iii. Increased amount of transforming growth factor (TGF)-β in the aqueous humor
    iv. Alteration in trabecular beams in the form of fragmentation of collagen
    v. Thickened basement membrane
    vi. Fused trabecular beams
    vii. Narrow intertrabecular spaces
    viii. Narrow collector channels
    ix. Decreased number of giant vacuoles

27. **What is unique about the vascular supply of ONH?**
    i. Posterior cerebral artery (PCA) and their branches have a segmented distribution in the choroid ONH (watershed zones)
    ii. Autoregulation
    iii. Blood flow in the ONH is stable until IOP is more than diastolic blood pressure (BP)

28. **What is the size of ONH?**

Vertical	1.88 mm
Horizontal	1.77 mm

29. **What are the ONH changes in glaucoma?**
    i. *Papillary changes (actual changes in the optic disk):*
       - Vertical enlargement of the cup
       - Asymmetric cupping [>0.2 difference in cup-to-disk (CD) ratio]
       - Focal notching/polar notching
       - Concentric enlargement of the cup
       - Deepening of the cup—laminar dot sign
       - Saucerization
       - Disk with sharpened edge/rim
    ii. *Peripapillary changes:*
       - Nerve fiber bundle defects: Types:
         - Localized
         - Wedge-shaped
         - Slit-shaped
         - Diffuse loss
         - Mixed pattern
         - Reversal of pattern
       - Peripapillary choroidal atrophy:
         - Alpha zone
         - Beta zone
       - Disk hemorrhage: Mostly inferotemporal quadrant
    iii. *Vascular changes:*
       - Baring of circumlinear vessels
       - Bayoneting sign
       - Collaterals between two veins at the disk
       - Nasalization of vessels
       - Attenuation of retinal vessels

30. **What are the parapapillary changes in glaucoma?**
    The normal ONH may be surrounded by zones that vary in width, circumference, and pigmentation. There are two zones—alpha and beta. Zone alpha is characterized by irregular hypopigmentation and thinning of the overlying chorioretinal layers. Zone beta is located closer to the optic disk border and is usually more distinctive because of the visible sclera.

31. **What is baring of circumlinear vessels?**
    Vessels that pass circumferentially across the temporal aspect of the cup have been called circumlinear vessels. If they pass the exposed depths of the cup, they are bared. Baring of the circumlinear vessels is seen because, as the cup recedes, it exposes the vessel.

32. **What is nasalization?**
    As the cup enlarges, the retinal vessels are displaced nasally. This can be an indicator of the progression of glaucoma.

33. **What is the significance of disk hemorrhage?**
    Disk hemorrhage is a sign of active disease and it occurs more frequently in NTG and precedes visual field defects by several months. It most commonly occurs inferotemporally and is flame-shaped.

34. **What is saucerization of the optic disk?**
    Occasionally, the glaucomatous damage to the optic disk produces a shallower background bowing of the disk rather than excavation. This is called saucerization.

35. **What is the best method of evaluating the optic disk changes in glaucoma?**
    The best method is slit lamp combined with 60, 78, or 90 D lenses.

36. **What is the best method of documenting the optic disk changes in glaucoma?**
    The best method of documenting the optic disk changes in glaucoma is stereophotographic documentation of ONH.

37. **Why does increased cupping occur?**
    Increased cupping occurs due to:
    i. Backward bowing of the lamina cribrosa
    ii. Elongation of the laminar beams
    iii. Loss of the ganglion cell axons in the rim of neural tissue

38. **Where does the increase in cupping start?**
    Large physiological cups are round in shape, while vertical elongation occurs in glaucoma. The process frequently starts segmentally, often in the lower temporal quadrant. This often causes an early appearance of an upper arcuate scotoma.

39. **What are the types of patterns of glaucomatous cupping?**
    i. Unipolar enlargement of the cup
    ii. Bipolar enlargement of the cup
    iii. Concentric enlargement of the cup
    iv. Nasal cupping—rarely
    v. Cupping in reverse disk

40. **What are the differential diagnoses of glaucomatous cupping?**
    i. *Physiological:*
        - Large physiological cup
        - Optic disk in high myopes

ii. *Pathological:*
   - *Congenital/hereditary:*
     - Coloboma of ONH
     - Morning glory syndrome
     - Congenital pit
     - Tilted disk syndrome
     - Leber hereditary optic neuropathy
   - *Acquired:*
     - Arteritic anterior ischemic optic neuropathy (AAION)
     - Nonarteritic anterior ischemic optic neuropathy (NAION)
     - Compressive optic neuropathy
     - Methanol toxicity—toxic optic neuropathy
     - Shock optic neuropathy
     - Dominant optic atrophy
     - Posterior ischemic optic neuropathy
     - Cupping as sequelae to optic neuritis

41. What is bean pot sign/cupping?
Bean pot cupping is a sign of advanced glaucomatous cupping where there is total cupping clinically seen as a white disk with the loss of all neural rim tissue and bending of all vessels at the margins of the disk.

A cross-section of bean pot cup reveals extreme posterior displacement of the lamina cribrosa and undermining of disk margins.

42. What is the main site of glaucomatous optic nerve damage?
Lamina cribrosa

43. What are the changes in lamina cribrosa in glaucoma?
i. Compression of lamina cribrosa plates
ii. Posterior bowing
iii. Collapse
iv. Increase in lamina pore size occurs due to stretching of collagenous beams or by rupture of smaller beams
v. Decrease in structural support and blockage of axonal transport

44. What is the shape of the NRR?
The NRR is broadest in the inferior disk, then the superior disk, then the nasal disk, and thinnest in the temporal disk [inferior-superior-nasal-temporal (ISNT) rule].

45. What is the shape of the normal cup disk ratio?
Because of the vertically oval optic disk and the horizontally oval optic cup, cup disk ratios are usually larger horizontally than vertically in normal eyes.

46. Why are the superior and inferior poles of the optic disk affected first in glaucoma?

The superior and inferior poles have larger laminar pores, and hence the axon bundles traversing have less support by glial tissue. Thus, they are more prone to damage.

47. Can cupping be reversed?

Reversal of cupping can happen in children and young patients following the lowering of IOP, probably because the sclera is more elastic.

48. What is a laminar dot sign?

Exposure of underlying lamina cribrosa caused by the deepening of the cup and loss of extraneural connective tissue is recognized by the gray fenestra of the lamina which has been referred to as laminar dot sign.

49. How much ganglion cell loss should be there before visual field defects become manifest on white-on-white perimetry?

Forty percent of ganglion cell loss occurs before visual field loss becomes apparent on white-on-white perimetry.

50. Why are temporal and central fields preserved?

i. Lamina septae are closely packed and thick along the horizontal meridian
ii. Resistant to mechanical deformation

51. What are the theories of glaucoma?

i. Multifactorial theory
ii. *Muller's mechanical theory:* Elevated IOP causes direct compression and death of neurons
iii. *Von Jaeger's vascular theory:* Decreased ONH perfusion causes disturbance in autoregulation of ONH, leading to atrophy of neural elements, which pulls the ONH posteriorly (Schnabel's cavernous atrophy)

52. What is the role of glutamate in glaucoma?

i. Glutamate is normally present in the retina and helps in verbal communication between cells
ii. Excessive glutamate is neurotoxic
iii. Elevated IOP renders neurons more permeable to glutamate
    - Activates *N*-methyl-D-aspartate (NMDA) receptors → intracellular calcium influx
    - Activation of nitric oxide pathway → apoptosis

53. What are the modalities to detect preperimetric glaucoma?

i. Optical coherence tomography (OCT)
ii. Glaucoma diagnostic with variable corneal compensation (GDx-VCC) nerve fiber layer (NFL) analyzer

iii. Frequency doubling perimetry (FDP)
iv. Short wavelength automated perimetry (SWAP)
v. Confocal scanning laser ophthalmoscope—Heidelberg retinal tomography (HRT)

54. What is the role of corneal thickness in POAG?

The Goldmann applanation tonometer is accurate only for a CCT measuring 520 µ. Thin corneas have falsely low measured IOP because the force required to applanate is less. Thick corneas have falsely high readings.

55. What is the differential diagnosis of POAG?
i. Pseudoexfoliative glaucoma
ii. Pigmentary glaucoma
iii. Elevated episcleral venous pressure
iv. Postinflammatory glaucoma
v. Steroid-induced glaucoma
vi. AAION and NAAION

56. What is SLT?

SLT is selective laser trabeculoplasty wherein double frequency Nd:YAG 532 nm is used selectively to target melanin cells in the trabecular meshwork.

57. Why are miotics ineffective in angle recession glaucoma?

Due to trabecular scarring, miotics are ineffective while prostaglandin analogs are the drug of choice.

58. What are the types of disk damage in glaucoma?
i. Type I (focal ischemic)
ii. Type II (myopic glaucomatous)
iii. Type III (senile sclerotic)
iv. Type IV (concentrically enlarging)
v. Mixed

59. What is the concept of corneal hysteresis?

Corneal hysteresis measures the elasticity and biomechanical properties of the cornea; hence, IOP is measured more accurately by ocular response analyzer (ORA).

60. When should you suspect an intracranial lesion in a patient with visual field defects?
i. Pallor more than cupping
ii. Asymmetric dyschromatopsia
iii. Fields respecting vertical meridian
iv. Contralateral ONH normal

61. **What are some nonglaucomatous conditions mimicking POAG?**
    i. Chiasmal compression
    ii. AION
    iii. Toxic optic neuropathies
    iv. Hypotension (shock optic neuropathy)

62. **How do you approach the diagnosis and treatment of open-angle glaucoma?**
    i. Identify the risk factors
    ii. Careful optic nerve evaluation and documentation
    iii. Confirm visual field loss with automated perimetry
    iv. Reserve advanced imaging techniques for selected patients
    v. Differentiate ocular hypertension from POAG (may need follow-up for a certain period)
    vi. Educate the patient regarding glaucoma and the side effects of therapy
    vii. Institute therapy—single medication with less side effects and adequate follow-up
    viii. Ensure compliance each time
    ix. Switch over therapy to better drugs before addition
    x. Think of filtering surgery—if maximal tolerable medical therapy fails or in a noncompliant patient

63. **What are the problems associated with myopia and glaucoma?**
    i. Faulty measurement of IOP due to decreased scleral rigidity
    ii. Increased chances of POAG due to:
       - Increasing ovality of the disk due to stretching or tractional vectors not evenly distributed across the myopic optic disk
    iii. Altered scleral rigidity and deformation of the posterior scleral structures can act as contributory factors

64. **What are the most common imaging techniques used for the diagnosis and evaluation of glaucoma?**
    The most common imaging techniques used for the diagnosis and evaluation of glaucoma are as follows:
    i. HRT or confocal scanning laser ophthalmoscope (CSLO)
    ii. OCT
    iii. Scanning laser polarimetry (also called GDx).

65. **What is HRT or CSLO?**
    HRT or CSLO obtains three-dimensional images of the optic disk by acquiring high-resolution images using a 670 μ diode laser.

66. **What are the components of the HRT report?**
    i. Patient demographic data
    ii. Topographic image (on the left upper corner of the printout)

iii. Reflectance image (right upper corner)
  iv. Retinal surface height variation graph
  v. Vertical and horizontal interactive analyses
  vi. Stereometric analysis
  vii. Moorfields regression analysis
  viii. Glaucoma probability score

67. **What are the advantages and disadvantages of HRT?**
    Advantages:
    i. Rapid
    ii. Simple
    iii. No need for pupillary dilatation

    Disadvantages:
    i. Not useful for retinal nerve fiber layer (RNFL) or macula
    ii. Operator-dependent and hence high interobserver variability
    iii. Tends to overestimate rim area in small optic nerves

68. **What are the two types of OCT useful in glaucoma?**
    i. Time domain
    ii. Spectral domain (Fourier domain)

69. **What are the advantages of time domain OCT?**
    i. Possibility of evaluation of ONH topography and RNFL thickness using a single instrument
    ii. Automatic demarcation of the optic nerve borders

70. **Why is spectral domain (SD) OCT superior to time domain OCT?**
    SD-OCT utilizes Fourier transform light to measure the backscattering of light without moving the reference arm which enables the measurements to be more precise.

71. **What are the advantages of SD-OCT?**
    i. Faster
    ii. Higher resolution
    iii. Reduced motion artifacts
    iv. Real-time image quality information which can be compared to a normative database

72. **What are the disadvantages of SD-OCT?**
    i. Expensive
    ii. Quality of images poor in small pupil or media opacities
    iii. Image quality degrades in the deeper regions of the sample

73. **What are the recent developments in OCT technology?**
    i. Adaptive optics
    ii. Swept source OCT

74. **What is the role of OCT in glaucoma?**
    i. *Anterior segment (AS-OCT uses):*
        - Screening for angle closure
        - Plateau iris
        - Malignant glaucoma
        - Efficacy of laser peripheral iridotomy (LPI)
        - Patency of glaucoma drainage device (GDD)
        - Bleb imaging for postoperative bleb management
    ii. *Posterior segment OCT:*
        - To evaluate the RNFL for early (preperimetric) glaucoma detection
        - To evaluate ONH tomography in glaucoma patients
        - To detect, study, and follow the macular changes in hypotony-induced maculopathy after glaucoma surgery
        - To evaluate cystoid macular edema (CME) after combined cataract and glaucoma surgery or following the use of prostaglandin analogs.

4.8 NEOVASCULAR GLAUCOMA

1. **What are the other terminologies for neovascular glaucoma (NVG)?**
   i. Hemorrhagic glaucoma
   ii. Thrombotic glaucoma
   iii. Rubeotic glaucoma
   iv. Congestive glaucoma
   v. 100th day glaucoma

2. **Who coined the term "neovascular glaucoma"?**
   Weiss et al.

3. **Describe the first sign of NVG.**
   i. Clinically new vessel tufts at the pupillary margin
   ii. By using investigative modalities, the first sign is increased permeability of the blood vessels at the pupillary margin as detected by fluorescein angiography on fluorophotometry

4. **Why does ectropion uveae occur?**
   Radial traction due to contraction of the fibrovascular membrane in the angle and the iris pulls the posterior layer of the iris around the pupillary margin onto the anterior iris surface.

5. **What is the etiology of NVG.**
   i. *Ocular vascular diseases:*
      - Diabetic retinopathy
      - Ischemic central retinal vein occlusion (CRVO)
      - Central retinal artery occlusion (CRAO)
      - Branch retinal vein occlusion (BRVO)
      - Branch retinal artery occlusion (BRAO)
      - Leber's miliary aneurysm
      - Sickle cell retinopathy
      - Coats' disease
      - Eales' disease
      - Retinopathy of prematurity (ROP)
      - Persistent fetal vasculature
   ii. *Ocular inflammation:*
      - Chronic uveitis
      - Chronic retinal detachment
      - Sympathetic ophthalmia
      - Endophthalmitis
      - Syphilitic retinitis
      - Vogt-Koyanagi-Harada (VKH)
      - Leber's congenital amaurosis

iii. *Neoplasms:*
   - Malignant melanoma
   - Retinoblastoma
   - Optic nerve glioma with venous stasis retinopathy
   - Metastatic carcinoma
   - Reticulum cell sarcoma
iv. *Systemic diseases:*
   - Diabetes mellitus
   - Sickle cell disease
   - Systemic lupus erythematosus (SLE)
v. *Extraocular vascular disorders:*
   - Carotid artery obstruction
   - Congestive heart failure
   - Giant cell arteritis
   - Carotid cavernous fistula
   - Takayasu (pulseless) disease
vi. *Miscellaneous:*
   - ROP
   - Persistent hyperplastic primary vitreous (PHPV)
   - Eales' disease
   - Coats' disease
   - Rhegmatogenous retinal detachment (RRD) with proliferative vitreoretinopathy (PVR)
   - Retinoschisis
vii. *Precipitating ocular surgical causes:*
   - RD surgery
   - Cataract extraction
   - Vitrectomy
   - Radiation
   - Nd:YAG capsulotomy

6. What is the difference between new vessels and normal iris vessels?

Features	New vessels	Normal vessels
Location	Pupillary margin, angles	Iris stroma
Arrangement	Irregular	Regular
Appearance	Thin	Tortuous
Course	Arborizing	Radial
Character	Fenestrated	Nonfenestrated
Scleral spur	Crosses	Does not cross
Fluorescein	Leakage	No leakage
Histology	Endothelial tube	Has all three coats
Blood–aqueous barrier	Poor	Intact

7. **What are the theories of neovasculogenesis?**
    i. *Retinal hypoxia:* Vascular endothelial cells of blood vessels in the retina release proangiogenic factors such as fibroblast growth factor (FGF), vascular endothelial growth factor (VEGF), transforming growth factor (TGF)-α, tumor necrosis factor (TNF)-α, and angiogenin which incite a cascade leading to activation, proliferation, and migration of endothelial cells—new vessel formation [e.g., proliferative diabetic retinopathy (PDR), ischemic CRVO]
    ii. *Angiogenesis factors:* "Tumor angiogenesis factor" released by tumors into the aqueous and vitreous, increases vasoproliferative activity
    iii. *Chronic dilatation of ocular vessels:* Hypoxia of the iris causes dilatation of its vasculature, which is a stimulus for new vessel formation
    iv. *Vasoinhibitory factors from vitreous and lens:* Loss of these factors, such as in pars plana vitrectomy and pars plana lensectomy, increases rubeosis

8. **What are the most commonly encountered proangiogenesis factors?**
    VEGF, FGF, TNF-α, insulin-like growth factor (IGF), interleukin (IL)-6, platelet-derived growth factor (PDGF), TGF-β, and angiogurin

9. **What are the clinicopathological stages of NVG?**
    i. *Prerubeosis stage:* Patients may have arteriolar/capillary nonperfusion or optic disk neovascularization or retinal neovascularization. Fundus fluorescein angiography (FFA) shows leaking iris vessels and extensive retinal capillary closure. Vitreous fluorophotometry detects increased fluorescein appearance in the vitreous
    ii. *Preglaucoma stage:* It is also called rubeosis stage. Intraocular pressure (IOP) is normal. Slit-lamp examination reveals dilated tufts of preexisting capillaries and new vessels over the iris, especially at the peripupillary area. Neovascularization of the angle (NVA) may also be present
    iii. *Open-angle glaucoma stage:* Rubeosis is more florid with anterior chamber (AC) reaction, high IOP, and open angles on gonioscopy. Angles are covered by a translucent fibrovascular membrane extending to the posterior iris
    iv. *Angle-closure glaucoma stage:* Raised IOP with florid neovascularization of the iris (NVI)/NVA, ectropion uveae, and contracture of the membrane in angles causing peripheral anterior synechiae (PAS) which will lead to eventual total synechial angle closure
    v. *Burnt-out stage*

10. **What is Wand's classification of the stages of NVG?**
    i. *Stage 1:* Vessels at the pupillary margin
    ii. *Stage 2:* Vessels up to collarette
    iii. *Stage 3:* Vessels up to angle
    iv. *Stage 4:* Vessels cross-scleral spur

11. **What are the types of glaucoma occurring in NVG?**
    The types of glaucoma occurring in NVG are open-angle (pretrabecular type) and secondary angle-closure glaucoma.

12. **What is the histopathological feature of open-angle glaucoma stage?**
    The new vessels appear first as endothelial buds from capillaries of the minor arterial circle. The buds then become vascular tufts. The new vessels have thin walls with irregular endothelia and pericytes. A clinically invisible fibrous membrane develops along the vessels, which then covers the angle and iris, obstructing the trabecular meshwork.

13. **What is the cause of angle closure?**
    Contraction of myofibroblasts present in the fibrovascular membrane causes PAS and flattening of the iris surface.

14. **Where do the new vessels arise from?**
    The new vessels arise from the microvasculature (capillaries, venules) of the vascular endothelial cell.

15. **In ischemic CRVO, when does NVG occur?**
    NVG occurs usually between 3 and 5 months (100 days glaucoma) but anywhere from 2 months to 2 years (17–80%).

16. **What are the risk factors in diabetes that cause NVG?**
    In an eye with diabetic retinopathy:
    i. Cataract extraction and vitrectomy
    ii. Cataract extraction with posterior chamber intraocular lens (PCIOL) implantation (increases anterior segment inflammation and disrupts blood–retinal barrier)
    iii. Chronic RD (lens and vitreous provide vasoconstrictive factors and serve as a diffusion barrier for angiogenic factors)
    iv. Longer duration of diabetes, associated hypertension, and hypercholesterolemia
    v. In extracapsular cataract extraction with capsule rupture or loss of zonular support with exposure of vitreous

17. **Name some occlusive vascular diseases causing NVI/NVG.**
    i. Carotid artery ligation
    ii. Internal carotid artery (ICA) obstruction, giant cell arteritis, and Takayasu's disease

18. **What are the differential diagnoses of NVG?**
    i. *Acute congestive stage of PACG* (does not have rubeosis of iris and angles, no fibrovascular membrane over iris and angles, no ectropion uveae)
    ii. *Uveitic glaucoma* [keratic precipitates (KPs) on endothelium, aqueous flare and cells; may have posterior synechiae, complicated cataract, band-shaped keratopathy in chronic cases; acute attack due to pupillary block]
    iii. *Fuchs' heterochromic iridocyclitis* (eye is white and quiet, stellate KPs are present, new vessels are seen at an angle but NVI and NVG are rare, open-angle glaucoma may be present due to trabecular sclerosis)
    iv. *Iridocorneal endothelial (ICE) syndromes* (corneal decompensation, corectopia, pseudopolycoria, iris atrophy)
    v. *Old trauma* (recession of angle, pigment clumps in trabecular meshwork; no NVI)
    vi. *Lens-induced glaucoma*

19. **How is Fuchs' heterochromic iridocyclitis different from NVG?**
    Fuchs' heterochromic iridocyclitis has the following features:
    i. Eye is white and quiet
    ii. New vessels are seen at an angle but new vessels on the iris (NVI) and NVG are rare (filiform vessels)
    iii. Spontaneous hyphemas are common
    iv. Open-angle glaucoma may be present due to trabecular sclerosis
    v. Stellate KPs are present
    vi. Iris heterochromia is present

20. **What are the late complications of NVG?**
    i. Painful bullous keratopathy (due to corneal decompensation or due to high IOP)
    ii. Complete synechial angle closure (due to extensive synechial angle closure or due to the fibrovascular membrane contraction)
    iii. Intractable glaucoma

21. **Name other conditions in which fluorescein leaks from the pupillary margin.**
    i. Exfoliation syndrome (at the site of pupillary ruff defects)
    ii. Fuchs' heterochromic iridocyclitis

22. **Why does fluorescein leak?**
    i. In NVI, gap junctions between the endothelial cells and fenestrations within the basement membrane are present allowing leakage

23. What are the drugs contraindicated in NVG?
   i. Miotics—may increase inflammation and pain
   ii. Epinephrine
   iii. Prostaglandins (relative contraindication as membrane prevents uveoscleral outflow, may cause mild anterior uveitis)

24. What is the role of atropine in the treatment of NVG?
   i. It causes pain relief by relieving ciliary spasm
   ii. It reduces inflammation
   iii. It increases uveoscleral outflow

25. What is the treatment of choice in NVG?
Panretinal photocoagulation (PRP).

26. What is the mechanism of PRP influencing NVG?
Causes destruction of RPE and photoreceptor cells in the posterior segment → reduces oxygen requirement of posterior segment → stimulus for release of angiogenesis factors reduced → decreased proangiogenesis factors → decreased anterior segment neovascularization

27. What are the indications of prophylactic PRP?
   i. In diabetic retinopathy with peripupillary fluorescein leakage undergoing lensectomy or vitrectomy
   ii. Ischemic CRVO with risk factors for developing NVI or NVA (extensive retinal hemorrhage or ischemia) where frequent ophthalmologic follow-up is not possible
   iii. Proliferative diabetic retinopathy

28. What are the LASER treatment options in NVG?
   i. *Anterior segment:*
      - *Gonio-photocoagulation:* It is an inadequate treatment for NVG by itself; it may be a useful adjunct to PRP in certain situations
      Argon laser:
      It eliminates vessels at the angle as they cross scleral spur by direct photocoagulation.
      Exposure time: 0.2 seconds, spot size: 50-100 μm
      Power: 150-500 MW sufficient to blanch and constrict vessels
   ii. *Posterior segment:*
      - *PRP:*
      Parameters: Blue-green-argon laser
      Spot size: 500 μm
      Exposure time: 0.1 seconds
      Power: 300 mW—clear media; 500 mW—lenticular sclerosis
      End point: Moderate intense white burns
      Interburn distance—one half burn width apart

Placement: 2 DD above, temporal and below center of macula 500 mm from the nasal margin of disk extending to or beyond equator

Number: 1,800–2,200 burns in 2–3 divided sittings over 3–6 weeks period.

- *Cyclophotocoagulation:*
  - *Transscleral contact cyclophotocoagulation techniques*

	1,064 nm Nd:YAG	810 nm diode
Power	5–6 J	1.5–2.5 W
Exposure time	0.5–0.7 seconds	1–2 seconds
Applications	30–40	16–18
Distance from limbus	0.5–1 mm	12 mm
Spot size	0.9 mm	100–400 µm

  - *Transscleral noncontact cyclophotocoagulation techniques*

	1,064 nm Nd:YAG	810 nm diode
Power	4–8 J	1,200–1,500 mW
Distance from limbus	1–2 mm	0.5–1 mm
Exposure time	20 ms	1 second
Spot size	0.9 mm	100–400 µm
Depth of focus	3.6 mm beyond surface	3.6 mm beyond surface
Applications	30–40	100–400 µm

  - *Transpupillary:* Argon laser
    - Exposure time: 0.1–0.2 seconds
    - Spot size: 50–100 µm
    - Power: 700–1,500 mW
    - White discoloration and brown concave burn
    - 180° treated
  - *Intraocular:*
    - *Transpupillary visualization:* Argon laser
      » Exposure time: 0.1–0.2 seconds
      » Power: 1,000 mW
      » Three to five per quadrant
      » White reaction with shallow tissue disruption
    - *Endoscopic visualization:* Argon laser
      » Illumination: 20 G probe (670 nm aiming beam)
      » Power of illumination: 1.2 W
      » 3.2 mm at/inside limbus
      » Power: 300 mW
      » 7–8 clock hours treated
      » Whitening and shrinkage of ciliary epithelium

29. **What are the glaucoma surgical procedures in NVG?**
    Filtering surgery: Trab with 5-fluorouracil (5-FU) (50 mg/mL-5 minutes) or mitomycin C (MMC) (0.2–0.4 mg/mL-2 minutes)
    i. *Modified trabeculectomy* with intraocular bipolar cautery of peripheral iris and ciliary processes
    ii. Trabeculectomy after intravitreal/intracameral injection bevacizumab 1.25 mg in 0.05 mL
    iii. *Drainage devices* or valves
    Cyclodestructive procedure (cyclophotocoagulation/cyclocryotherapy)

30. **How will you manage a case of NVG?**
    The main therapeutic goals will be to treat the underlying cause of neovascularization and prevent its further progression, to control the IOP, and to provide symptomatic relief.
    If the IOP is <40 mm Hg, the patient can be started on a combination of aqueous suppressants like topical β-blockers like timolol maleate 0.5% eye drops bid, α-2 adrenergic agonists like 0.2% brimonidine tartrate eye drops TDS, or carbonic anhydrase inhibitors like dorzolamide hydrochloride 2% eye drops TDS.
    i. If the IOP is above 40 mm Hg, for initial control of IOP, start the patient on 100 mL of 20% intravenous mannitol in a dose of 2 g/kg body weight over a period of 20–30 minutes after ruling out systemic hypotension or cardiac disease
    ii. In the absence of history of sulfa allergy, nausea, and vomiting, tab. acetazolamide 250 mg BD or hyperosmotic agents like 50% oral glycerol at 1–1.5 g/kg body weight can be advised after ruling out diabetes mellitus. For symptomatic pain relief, atropine eye ointment 1% and topical prednisolone acetate 1% QID can be instilled
    iii. Once epithelial edema subsides, gonioscopic examination and fundus examination will be performed. If synechial angle closure does not extend for >270° and the patient has definite posterior segment ischemic pathology like PDR or ischemic CRVO, the patient can be advised for PRP in three to four sittings
    iv. Once rubeosis regresses, glaucoma filtering surgery like trabeculectomy using wound modulators like 5-FU (50 mg/mL-5 minutes) or MMC (0.2–0.4 mg/mL-2 minutes) or a glaucoma drainage device like Ahmed valve will be done
    v. If IOP is still not controlled, with hazy media, the patient can undergo panretinal cryotherapy with a cyclodestructive procedure like cyclocryotherapy or transscleral Nd:YAG cyclophotocoagulation

vi. If the IOP is still not controlled and the patient has severe pain in the blind eye, the patient can be advised retrobulbar alcohol injection for pain relief or enucleation after thorough and extensive counseling

31. **What is the indication for transscleral panretinal cryoablation with cryotherapy?**
    Hazy media

32. **What is express shunt?**
    Express shunt is a 3 mm long stainless steel tube with a diameter of 400 μ having a 50 μ diameter lumen, implanted through the limbus.

33. **What is the indication for cyclodestructive procedures in NVG?**
    NVG with pain and poor visual potential with uncontrollable rubeosis and glaucoma.

34. **What are the newer treatments for NVG?**
    i. Anti-VEGF antibodies, e.g., bevacizumab
    ii. α-interferon therapy
    iii. Troxerutin
    iv. Gene transfer of *PEDF* gene

35. **What are probe sizes?**
    i. *Retinal cryotherapy:* 2.5 mm (–70°C)
    ii. *Cyclocryotherapy:* 3.5 mm (–60 to –80°C)

36. **Define rubeosis iridis.**
    Rubeosis iridis refers to new vessels on the surface of the iris regardless of the state of the angle or the presence of glaucoma.

37. **What is the role of bevacizumab (Avastin) in NVG?**
    In NVG, intravitreal bevacizumab (1.25 mg/0.05 mL) (Avastin) can be administered through the pars plana route, 24–78 hours preceding surgery, with near total regression of iris neovascularization within 48 hours and some IOP lowering, an effect lasting for some weeks. Intracameral bevacizumab is also advocated by few experts for decreasing NVI prior to filtering surgery.

    The rapid regression of new vessels allows both panretinal photocoagulation and glaucoma surgery with reduced risk of bleeding.

4.9 PIGMENTARY GLAUCOMA

1. **What is the typical profile of a patient presenting with pigmentary glaucoma (PG)?**
   The typical profile of a patient presenting with PG is young (third decade), myopic, male, and white race.

2. **Mention the chromosomes related to pigment dispersion syndrome (PDS).**
   Chromosome 7q and 18q

3. **How is pigment dispersion glaucoma (PG) caused?**
   PG results from a decreased facility of outflow following pigment deposition in the trabecular meshwork in a subset of patients with PDS.

4. **What is the pathogenesis of PG?**
   i. Pigment release and diminished outflow facility
   ii. *Mechanical theory:* Concave shape of the peripheral iris allows it to rub against the zonules, causing pigment release and dispersion

5. **What are the ocular findings in PG?**
   i. *Cornea:*
      - Krukenberg spindle
      - Increased corneal diameter
      - Corneal endothelial pleomorphism and polymegathism
   ii. *Iris:*
      - *Iris transillumination defects:* Seen in midperiphery [in contrast to pseudoexfoliation (PXF) glaucoma, where it is seen at the pupillary margins]
      - Pigment granules
      - Heterochromia
      - Anisocoria
      - Concave iris configuration
      - Posterior insertion into the sclera
      - Floppier iris stroma
   iii. *Deep anterior chamber*
   iv. *Lens:*
       Pigment deposits on zonules and posterior lens surface (Zentmayer ring or Scheie's line)

6. **What is the characteristic gonioscopic finding in PG?**
   i. The angle is wide open
   ii. Dense, homogeneous dark brown pigment in the full circumference of the trabecular meshwork and pigmented Schwalbe's line is present
   iii. The pigment can cover the entire width of the angle from the ciliary face to the peripheral cornea; a pigment line anterior to Schwalbe's line, often referred to as Sampaolesi line, is seen

7. **What are the differential diagnoses of pigmentation at the angles?**
    i. Aging
    ii. PG
    iii. PXF glaucoma
    iv. Post-trauma
    v. Postintraocular surgery
    vi. Postlaser iridotomy
    vii. Uveitic glaucoma
    viii. Previous attack of angle-closure glaucoma
    ix. Ocular melanosis
    x. Intraocular lens (IOL) placement in sulcus

8. **What are the associated possible fundus findings in PG?**
    i. Retinal detachments (6–7%)
    ii. Lattice degenerations
    iii. Retinal pigment epithelium (RPE) dystrophy

9. **What are the ways by which PG occurs?**
    i. PG is a secondary open-angle glaucoma and is caused by the following mechanisms
    Mechanical theory (Campbell's theory): Rubbing of lens zonules against midperipheral iris due to iris concavity which releases the pigments. These pigments can occlude the angle causing obstruction to the aqueous outflow.
    ii. Anderson et al. postulate that pigment production and mutant melanosomal protein genes may contribute to PG
    iii. Mechanism of glaucoma/IOP elevation in PG

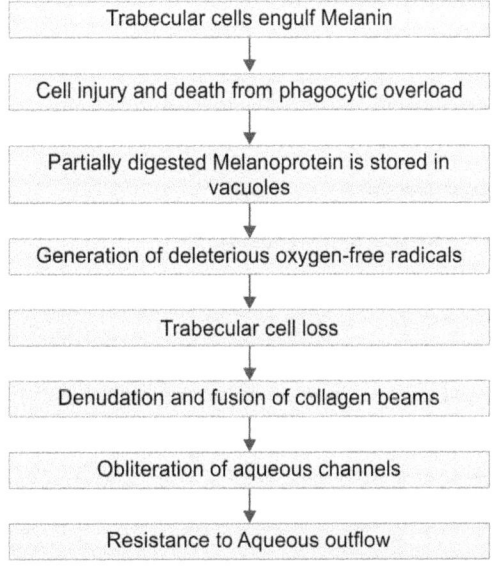

10. **What is a reverse pupillary block?**

   An abnormally great iris–lens contact will prevent equilibration of aqueous between the two chambers, anterior and posterior. Therefore, the iris will assume an even more pronounced concave profile and the rubbing against the zonules will be facilitated. This has been named "reverse pupillary block." Accommodation and exercise will also increase lens concavity and create a reverse block. The reverse block is relieved by a YAG laser iridotomy. The iris profile then loses its concavity to assume a planar configuration.

11. **What is the histopathology of angle structures in PG?**

   Angle structures demonstrate pigment and debris in the trabecular meshwork cells. With advanced disease, the trabecular cell degenerates and wanders from their beams, allowing sclerosis and eventual fusion of the trabecular meshwork.

12. **What are the differential diagnoses of PG?**
   i. PXF glaucoma (PXF material on endothelium, anterior lens capsule angles)
   ii. Chronic uveitis (keratic precipitates on endothelium, aqueous flare, and cells; may have posterior synechiae, complicated cataract, band-shaped keratopathy in chronic cases; acute attack due to pupillary block)
   iii. Angle recession glaucoma
   iv. Ocular melanosis
   v. Trauma
   vi. Herpes zoster
   vii. Siderosis
   viii. Hemosiderosin
   ix. Pigmented intraocular tumors
   x. Previous surgery (including laser surgery)
   xi. Cysts of the iris and ciliary body

13. **What are the differences between PXF and PG?**

Feature	Pseudoexfoliative glaucoma	PG
Profile	Fifth decade and older	Third decade
Severity	Increases with age	Decreases/disappears in later life
Gender	Equal	Males (2:1)
Types of glaucoma	Open-angle and angle-closure	Open-angle glaucoma
Clinical features	Cornea: PXF, pigments on endothelium, guttata	Krukenberg spindle

Contd...

Contd...

Feature	Pseudoexfoliative glaucoma	PG
	Iris: Iris transillumination defects (peripupillary), moth-eaten appearance	Iris transillumination defects (midperiphery), heterochromia, reverse pupillary block
	Pupil: PXF, poor mydriasis	Anisocoria
	Lens: Cataract, phakodonesis, Zonular distribution of PXF	May be normal
Gonioscopy	Sampaolesi line. Uneven distribution of pigments along the meshwork	Increased trabecular pigmentation, dense and homogenously arranged in the full circumference of the trabecular meshwork, more in the inferior angle
Progression	40% with PXF develop glaucoma	35% with PDS develop glaucoma
Management	Surgical in most cases	Medical in most cases
Extraocular involvement	Systemic findings present—amyloid-like material [central nervous system (CNS), cardiovascular system (CVS), kidney, liver]	No systemic association

14. **What are the principles of the medical treatment of PG?**

    The treatment of PG resembles that of primary open-angle glaucoma (POAG) in that the usual progression is from medical therapy to argon laser trabeculoplasty (ALT) to filtering surgery. Adrenergic antagonists, adrenaline (epinephrine), dipivefrin, and carbonic anhydrase inhibitors (CAIs) are useful in the management of PG. Miotic agents reduce IOP in PG and are theoretically appealing because they increase pupillary block and lift the peripheral iris from the zonules.

15. **What is the treatment of PG?**

    Medical:
    i. Pilocarpine 1% eye drops (miosis restricting pupillary movement and pigment release, direct effect on aqueous outflow)
    ii. CAI—dorzolamide 2% eye drops TDS
    iii. β-blockers—timolol maleate 0.5% eye drops BD
    iv. Pilocarpine is poorly tolerated by these young patients and also has chances of higher incidence of retinal detachment

    Laser:
    Nd:YAG laser iridotomy (relieves the posterior bowing of the iris in pigmentary glaucoma) to cure reverse pupillary block

i. Power: 4–8 mJ
ii. One to three pulses per burst

ALT:
i. Power: 200–600 mW increased till blanch/bubble is seen. Low energy settings should be used due to heavy pigmentation
ii. Spot size: 50 µm
iii. Duration: 0.1 seconds
iv. 50 burns over 180°
v. Burn site: Junction of anterior one-third and posterior two-third of trabecular meshwork

Selective laser trabeculoplasty:
i. Frequency-doubled Q switched Nd:YAG laser (532 nm)
ii. Pulse duration: 3 ns
iii. Energy: 0.3–1.7 mJ
iv. Spot size: 400 µm
v. 50 adjacent laser spots over 180°

Surgery:
i. *Filtering surgery*—modified trabeculectomy with 5-fluorouracil (5-FU) (50 mg/mL-5 minutes) or mitomycin C (MMC) (0.2–0.4 mg/mL-2 minutes)
ii. *Drainage devices* or valves.

4.10 PSEUDOEXFOLIATION GLAUCOMA

1. **What is true exfoliation of lens capsule?**
   True exfoliation of lens capsule is a delamination of the anterior capsule. There is a separation of superficial layers of the lens capsule from the deeper layers to form a scroll-like margin, which occasionally floats in the anterior chamber as thin, clear membranes. It was first described in glassblowers; hence, it is called glassblower's cataract.

2. **What is the risk factor associated with capsular delamination?**
   The risk factor associated with capsular delamination is extended exposure to infrared radiation (prophylactic measure—use of protective goggles).

3. **What are the differential diagnoses of capsular delamination?**
   i. Trauma
   ii. Intraocular inflammation
   iii. Idiopathically with advanced age

4. **What is pseudoexfoliation (PXF)?**
   PXF is a gray-white fibrillogranular extracellular matrix (ECM) material composed of a protein core (10–12 fibrils) surrounded by glycosaminoglycans. It is a sticky "Christmas tree" type of protein, aggregating a large number of elastic tissue and basement membrane proteins.

5. **What is glaucoma capsulare?**
   The occurrence of glaucoma in an eye with PXF syndrome is called glaucoma capsulare.

6. **What is the origin of PXF?**
   PXF is thought to be produced by abnormal basement membranes of aging epithelial cells in the trabeculum, equatorial lens capsule, iris, ciliary body, and conjunctiva and then deposited on the anterior lens capsule, zonules, ciliary body, iris, trabeculum, anterior vitreous phase, and conjunctiva.

7. **What are the epidemiological factors of significance?**
   i. ↑ Age → ↑ PXF
   ii. Mostly bilateral but unilateral cases are also present
   iii. More common between 60 and 70 years
   iv. Mostly seen in Scandinavian, Japanese, and Australian populations

8. **What is the incidence of glaucoma in patients with PXF syndrome?**
   Glaucoma is found to occur in 40% of patients with PXF.

9. **List the clinical features of PXF.**
    i. *Corneal changes:*
        - PXF material deposited on the back of the cornea
        - Associated with corneal guttata
        - Associated with spheroidal degeneration
        - Decrease in the endothelial density, polymegathism, and endothelial decompensation
    ii. *Anterior chamber angle:*
        - Increased trabecular meshwork pigmentation (uneven and coarse)
        - *Sampaolesi line:* Deposition of pigment at Schwalbe's line, not pathognomonic of PXF
    iii. *Iris changes:*
        - Material deposited on iris tissue (anterior stroma)
        - Peripupillary iris transillumination defects (moth-eaten appearance)
    iv. *Pupil:*
        - PXF material deposited on the pupillary margin
        - Poor mydriasis (secondary to atrophy of muscle cells)
        - Sphincter atrophy
    v. *Lenticular changes:*
        PXF on the anterior lens capsule has three distinct zones:
        - Translucent, central disk with occasional curled edges (absent in 20% of cases)
        - Central clear zone → corresponds to contact with moving iris
        - Peripheral granular zone → radial striations (most consistent)
    vi. *Zonules and ciliary body changes:*
        - PXF may be detected earliest in the ciliary body or zonules
        - Involvement of zonules

        Subluxation or phakodonesis

10. **What is the mechanism by which PXF causes zonular weakness?**
    i. PXF material erupts through the basement membrane and invades the zonules creating areas of weakness (especially In its origin—nonpigmented ciliary epithelium and insertion—pre-equatorial region of the lens)
    ii. Proteolytic enzymes within the PXF material may facilitate zonular disintegration

11. **What is the target sign in PXF glaucoma?**
    Deposits on the anterior capsule, in a manner resembling a target is the target sign. This is a classic sign. The "target" appearance is caused

by the iris clearing a circular area on the surface of the capsule due to the movement of the iris. These deposits are normally only visible if the pupil is dilated.

12. **What are the findings in iris fluorescein angiography in case of PXF syndrome?**
    i. Hypoperfusion
    ii. Peripupillary leakage

13. **What are the specular microscopy findings in PXF syndrome?**
    i. Decreased cell density of corneal endothelium
    ii. Altered size of endothelial cells
    iii. Altered shape of endothelial cells

14. **Describe the clinical classification of PXF based on morphologic alterations of anterior lens capsule.**
    i. Preclinical stage (clinically invisible)
    ii. Suspected PXF (precapsular layer)
    iii. Mini-PXF (focal defect starts superonasally)
    iv. Classic PXF

15. **What are the differences in gonioscopic findings in PXF and pigmentary glaucoma?**

PXF glaucoma	Pigmentary glaucoma
• Uneven distribution of pigments along the meshwork	• More thicker pigmentation, dense homogenous band of dark pigment in the full circumference of trabecular meshwork more in the inferior angle
• Pigmentation does not extend beyond Schwalbe's line	• Pigmentation extends anterior to Schwalbe's line occluding view of angle structures

16. **What are the intraocular complications of PXF syndrome?**

i. *Trabecular meshwork*	Open-angle glaucoma
	Angle-closure glaucoma
	Acute pressure rise
ii. *Lens or zonules*	Phakodonesis
	Subluxation/dislocation
	Nuclear cataract
	Zonular dialysis
iii. *Iris*	Posterior synechiae
	Uveitis due to impaired blood–aqueous barrier
	Sphincter muscle degeneration

Contd...

Contd...

	Melanin dispersion
	Poor mydriasis
iv. *Cornea*	Early endothelial decompensation
v. *Retina*	Central retinal vein occlusion (CRVO)
	Retinal detachment

17. **How does PXF syndrome cause vein occlusion?**
    There is narrowing of the vessel lumen due to deposition of PXF material produced by the vascular endothelial cells. This in turn leads to occlusion of the veins causing CRVO.

18. **How does open-angle glaucoma in PXF differ from primary open-angle glaucoma (POAG)?**
    i. Greater diurnal fluctuation of intraocular pressure (IOP) in PXF glaucoma
    ii. IOP in PXF glaucoma tends to run higher and more difficult to control
    iii. Glaucomatous neuroretinal rim damage tends to be more diffuse in PXF cases (sectoral preference → primary open-angle glaucoma)
    iv. PXF cases show ↑ tendency for glaucomatous optic atrophy

19. **What are the ways in which PXF causes glaucoma?**
    PXF causes open-angle and angle-closure glaucoma.
    i. *Open-angle glaucoma is caused by the following mechanisms:*
        - Blockage of trabecular meshwork by PXF material by:
            - Active PXF material production within the trabecular meshwork, Schlemm's canal, and collector channels
            - Passive PXF material deposition in intertrabecular spaces Progressive accumulation → Swelling of juxtacanalicular meshwork

            Gradual narrowing of Schlemm's canal
        - Blockage of meshwork by liberated iris pigment
        - Trabecular cell dysfunction
        - Associated open-angle glaucoma
    ii. *PXF causes angle closure by the following mechanisms:*
        - Zonular weakness → anterior movement of lens
        - Lens thickening from cataract formation
        - Increased adhesiveness of the iris to the lens due to PXF material, sphincter muscle degeneration, and uveitis

Glaucoma

20. **Why does a high percentage of PXF cases have occludable angles?**
    Presence of shallower central and peripheral anterior chamber depths (ACDs) due to:
    i. Zonular weakness and forward movement of lens iris diaphragm
    ii. Lens thickening from cataract formation

21. **What is the pathogenesis of PXF?**
    i. *Microfibril theory:* Elastic microfibril hypothesis which states that it is a type of elastosis with elastic microfibrils being secreted abnormally by local ocular cells
    ii. *Basement membrane theory:* PXF may be a basement membrane proteoglycan
    iii. *Glycosaminoglycan theory:* Abnormal metabolism of glycosaminoglycans in the iris

22. **What are the ocular and systemic sites of PXF deposition?**
    Ocular:
    i. Lens capsule epithelium and zonules
    ii. Iris epithelium
    iii. Vascular endothelium
    iv. Corneal endothelium
    v. Schlemm's canal endothelium
    vi. Conjunctiva
    vii. Extraocular muscles
    viii. Orbital septa
    ix. Anterior hyaloid face of the vitreous
    x. Posterior ciliary arteries
    xi. Vortex veins
    xii. Central retinal vessels
    Systemic:
    i. Lungs
    ii. Heart
    iii. Liver
    iv. Kidneys
    v. Skin
    vi. Gallbladder
    vii. Cerebral meninges

23. **What are the differential diagnoses of PXF?**
    i. Uveitis
    ii. Capsular delamination
    iii. Primary amyloidosis
    iv. Pigment dispersion syndrome and pigmentary glaucoma
    v. Melanosis and melanoma

24. What are the important points to be kept in mind while medically managing PXF glaucoma?

i. Tends to respond less well with medical therapy than POAG
ii. Treat aggressively with frequent follow-up
iii. Higher diurnal variation of IOP in PXF to be kept in mind while deciding the target pressure for an individual
iv. Consider argon laser trabeculoplasty/selective laser trabeculoplasty which has a higher success rate in PXF glaucoma than in POAG but shorter duration of effectiveness

25. What is trabecular aspiration?

Surgical modality to remove intertrabecular and pretrabecular debris

26. What are the important findings to be looked for during preoperative evaluation in PXF syndrome patients undergoing cataract surgery?

i. Corneal endothelial compromise
ii. Evidence of zonular dialysis → phakodonesis

Asymmetric ACD
Ultrasound biomicroscope (UBM) to confirm the extent of zonular dialysis
iii. Poor pupillary dilatation
iv. Posterior synechiae
v. Lens subluxation

27. What are the special features to be adopted in PXF cases undergoing cataract surgery to maximize postoperative outcome?

i. Use corneal endothelium-friendly viscoelastics (chondroitin sulfate)
ii. Expand the pupil
   - Kuglen hooks
   - Iris hooks
   - Mini sphincterotomies
   - Sector iridectomy
iii. Use of heparin surface-modified intraocular lens (to minimize postoperative iritis that is common in PXF cases postoperatively)
iv. Capsular tension ring to manage zonular dialysis and stabilize the bag

28. Which gene is associated with exfoliation syndrome?

A polymorphism in exon 1 of the *LOXL1* gene.

4.11 UVEITIC GLAUCOMA

1. **What are the mechanisms of uveitic glaucoma?**
    i. *Open-angle mechanisms:*
        - Clogging of trabecular meshwork and Schlemm's canal by inflammatory cells
        - Trabecular meshwork endothelial cell dysfunction
        - Edema of the trabecular meshwork
        - Prostaglandin-mediated breakdown of the blood–aqueous barrier
        - Steroid-induced glaucoma
    ii. *Closed angle mechanism:*
        Broadly classified as pupillary block and nonpupillary block mechanisms
        - *Pupillary block:*
            - Inflammatory cells, fibrin, and debris collect in the angle
            - The peripheral iris adheres to the trabecular meshwork which leads to the formation of peripheral anterior synechiae
            - Anterior segment inflammation causes posterior synechiae formation
        - *Nonpupillary block:*
            - The ciliary body edema can cause the anterolateral rotation of the ciliary body about its attachment to the scleral spur, which relaxes the lens zonules and causes the forward movement of a rounder lens
            - The anterior face of the ciliary body and peripheral iris is then brought into contact with the trabecular meshwork, causing angle closure
                Chronic inflammation may be associated with angle neovascularization, which causes synechiae to develop.

2. **Describe the development of glaucoma in an acquired immune deficiency syndrome (AIDS) patient.**
    i. Bilateral acute angle-closure glaucoma has been reported in these patients, which is due to choroidal effusion with anterior rotation of the ciliary body
    ii. B-scan echography is helpful in establishing the diagnosis by demonstrating diffuse choroidal thickening with ciliochoroidal effusion
    iii. These cases do not respond to miotics or iridotomy
    iv. Treatment with aqueous suppressants, cycloplegics, and topical steroids is reported to achieve complete resolution of the angle closure

3. **What is Posner–Schlossman syndrome?**
   Posner–Schlossman syndrome is otherwise called glaucomatocyclitic crisis. It is characterized by:
   i. Recurrent attacks of mild anterior uveitis with a marked elevation of IOP
   ii. Virtually always unilateral
   iii. White eye with minimal congestion
   iv. Open angle with occasional debris and the characteristic absence of synechiae
   v. Apraclonidine is especially useful

4. **Describe the management of uveitic glaucoma.**
   There are two components:

   Control of inflammation:
   Topical administration of corticosteroids is preferred for the anterior segment, and commonly used steroids include 1.0% prednisolone acetate or 0.1% dexamethasone. The drops are titrated depending on the response. When the response is insufficient, periocular injections (e.g., dexamethasone phosphate, prednisolone succinate, triamcinolone acetate, or methylprednisolone acetate) or a systemic corticosteroid (e.g., prednisone) may be required.

   Children with uveitis may have unique dosing requirements and drug-associated risks, such as growth retardation with systemic corticosteroids.

   Nonsteroidal anti-inflammatory agents:
   When the use of corticosteroids is contraindicated or inadequate, other anti-inflammatory drugs may be helpful.

   Prostaglandin synthetase inhibitors, such as aspirin, imidazole, indoxyl, indomethacin, and dipyridamole, have been effective.

   In severe cases, *immunosuppressive agents* such as methotrexate, azathioprine, or chlorambucil are used. These patients must be monitored closely for hematologic reactions.

   Newer cyclooxygenase inhibitors such as flurbiprofen, ketorolac, suprofen, and diclofenac may provide useful anti-inflammatory effects without the risk of steroid-induced intraocular pressure (IOP) elevation.

   Mydriatic cycloplegics such as atropine (1%), homatropine (1–5%), or cyclopentolate (0.5–1%) are used to avoid posterior synechiae and to relieve the discomfort of ciliary muscle spasm.

   Control of glaucoma:

   Medical management:
   i. Topical β-blocker, α-2 agonist, and carbonic anhydrase inhibitor are the first-line antiglaucoma drugs in uveitic glaucoma

    ii. An oral carbonic anhydrase inhibitor may be added, and a hyperosmotic agent is used for a short-term emergency measure
    iii. In eyes with acute fibrinous anterior uveitis and impending pupillary block, with or without peripheral anterior synechiae, it may be reasonable to consider the use of intracameral tissue plasminogen activator (6.25–12.5 µg)
    iv. Miotics and prostaglandins are contraindicated in the inflamed eye

Surgical management:
    i. Intraocular surgery should be avoided in active inflammation; the eye should be quiescent for a minimum of 3 months before surgery
    ii. When medical therapy is inadequate, surgery may be required
    iii. Laser iridotomy is safer than an incisional iridectomy but usually fails due to iris inflammation, fibrin exudates, or late neovascularization
    iv. Filtering surgery with heavy steroid therapy is indicated in open-angle cases that are uncontrolled with medical therapy. Additional use of subconjunctival 5-fluorouracil (5-FU) significantly improves the success rate in these cases
    v. Laser trabeculoplasty is not effective in eyes with uveitis and open-angle glaucoma and it may cause an additional, significant rise in IOP and is generally contraindicated in these cases
    vi. Surgical iridectomy during cataract surgery in uveitic cases can be performed to prevent postoperative angle closure due to pupillary block
    vii. Cyclodestructive surgery like transscleral Nd:YAG cyclo-photocoagulation can be done in aphakic and pseudophakic eyes with limited visual potential
    viii. Filtering devices like Ahmed valve may be placed when the inflammation is under control, but steroid cover is important to reduce inflammatory exudates from blocking the lumen during the early postoperative period.

4.12 STEROID-INDUCED GLAUCOMA

1. **Define steroid-induced glaucoma.**
   Corticosteroid-induced glaucoma is a secondary glaucoma of the open-angle type caused by prolonged use of topical, periocular, intravitreal, inhaled, or systemic corticosteroids.
   i. 25% of the general population develops an increase in intraocular pressure (IOP) after 4 weeks of QID topical steroids
   ii. 5% of the population are super-responders—they develop >10–15 mm Hg rise in IOP within 2 weeks
   iii. Approximately 15% of super-responders developing glaucoma require filtering surgery
   iv. There is no racial or sexual predilection for steroid-induced glaucoma

2. **What is steroid responsiveness?**
   The normal population can be divided into three groups on the basis of IOP response to a 6-week course of topical betamethasone:
   i. High—marked elevation of IOP > 30 mm Hg
   ii. Moderate—moderated elevation of IOP 22–30 mm Hg
   iii. Nonresponders—no change in IOP

3. **What is the mechanism of steroid-induced glaucoma?**
   Steroids decrease aqueous outflow by the following mechanisms:
   i. Corticosteroids stabilize the lysosomal membranes, and this inhibits the release of hyaluronidases. Glycosaminoglycans cannot get depolymerized and retain water which leads to narrowing of the trabecular openings
   ii. Endothelial cells lining the trabecular meshwork act as phagocytes of debris; corticosteroids suppress their activity
   iii. In primary open-angle glaucoma (POAG), an abnormal accumulation of dehydrocortisols leads to increased IOP
   iv. Corticosteroids inhibit the synthesis of prostaglandin, whose normal function is to lower IOP
   v. Glucocorticoids alter the trabecular meshwork cell morphology by causing an increase in nuclear size and deoxyribonucleic acid (DNA) content

4. **Who are the people at risk of developing steroid-induced glaucoma?**
   i. Prolonged use of steroid drops for conditions such as vernal conjunctivitis, uveitis, and chronic blepharitis
   ii. Long-term systemic steroid use in conditions such as systemic lupus erythematosus (SLE) and rheumatoid arthritis
   iii. Use of steroid drops in patients with a strong family history of glaucoma

iv. 50% of patients with progressive age-related macular degeneration (AMD) or diffuse macular edema treated with intravitreal injection of 25 mg of triamcinolone acetonide
v. Sub-Tenon depot triamcinolone in the treatment of patients with pars planitis
vi. Diabetic patients
vii. High myopes
viii. Postrefractive surgeries
ix. Asthmatics using inhaled and/or oral steroids

5. **Give an example of a systemic condition causing steroid-induced glaucoma.**
Excessive secretion of endogenous corticosteroids associated with adrenal hyperplasia or adenoma can cause steroid-induced glaucoma.

6. **Discuss the clinical picture of steroid-induced glaucoma in adults.**
   i. Steroid-induced glaucoma in adults resembles chronic open-angle glaucoma with an open, normal-appearing angle and absence of symptoms
   ii. It may have an acute presentation, and IOP rises have been observed within hours after steroid administration
   iii. It may mimic low-tension glaucoma when IOP increase has damaged the optic nerve head

7. **Discuss the clinical picture of steroid-induced glaucoma in children.**
   i. Children, in general, have a lower incidence of positive steroid responses than adults
   ii. Infants treated with steroids develop a condition resembling congenital glaucoma
   iii. Increase in IOP has been reported in infants using steroids for:
       – Nasal and inhalational steroids
       – Eye drops after strabismus surgery

8. **What is the diagnosis of steroid-induced glaucoma?**
Diagnosis requires a high index of suspicion and questioning of patients, specifically about steroid eye drops, ointments, and pills.

9. **Mention a few alternative drugs which have a lesser tendency to cause glaucoma.**
   i. Medrysone
   ii. Loteprednol etabonate
These drugs have a lesser tendency to raise IOP

10. **Are there any genetic influences in the causation of steroid-induced glaucoma?**
The myocilin gene, as well as the optineurin gene, is upregulated in steroid-induced glaucoma.

11. **Mention the prevention of steroid-induced glaucoma.**

    Patient selection:
    i. Good history and systemic conditions
    ii. Avoid steroids when safer drugs are available
    iii. Use the least amount of steroid necessary
    iv. Establish baseline IOP before initiating therapy
    v. Monitor IOP for the duration of steroid therapy

    Drug selection—choose a drug that can achieve the desired response by the safest route, in the lowest concentration, and with the fewest potential side effects.
    i. Topical drops are often associated with raised IOP
    ii. Periocular injection of long-acting steroid—most dangerous
    iii. Systemic steroids—least likely to induce glaucoma

12. **Mention a few words about the relative pressure effects of anti-inflammatory drugs.**
    i. Corticosteroids—pressure-inducing effect is proportional to their anti-inflammatory potency. Hence, betamethasone, dexamethasone, and prednisolone have an increased tendency to induce glaucoma
    ii. Nonadrenal steroids—closely related to progesterone with less pressure-inducing effects. For example, medrysone is used for the treatment of extraocular disorders but has poor corneal penetration. Fluorometholone (0.1%) is more effective than medrysone
    iii. Nonsteroidal anti-inflammatory drugs (NSAIDs):
        - Act as cyclooxygenase (COX) inhibitors
        - May be effective in anterior segment inflammation
        - Act by reducing the breakdown of the blood–aqueous barrier
        - Do not cause an increase in IOP
        - For example, oxyphenbutazone, flurbiprofen, and diclofenac
        - Other drugs in this class are suprofen and ketorolac

13. **Mention the management of steroid-induced glaucoma.**
    i. The first step is to discontinue the drug—IOP returns to normal in a few weeks or replace with a milder anti-inflammatory drug
    ii. Excision of depot steroid if present
    iii. Antiglaucoma drugs can be used to control IOP
    iv. If unsuccessful, filtering surgery should be considered after confirming progression in glaucomatous damages
    v. Patients with steroid-induced glaucoma respond poorly to argon laser trabeculoplasty.

4.13 LENS-INDUCED GLAUCOMA

1. **What is lens-induced glaucoma?**
   A lens-induced glaucoma is a group of secondary glaucoma that shares the lens as a common pathogenic cause.

2. **How will you classify lens-induced glaucoma?**

Open angle	Closed angle
Phakolytic glaucoma	Phakomorphic glaucoma
Lens particle glaucoma	Ectopia lentis
Phakoanaphylaxis glaucoma	

3. **What is the mode of presentation in phakolytic glaucoma?**
   Elderly patients with a history of poor vision and a sudden, rapid onset of pain and redness.

4. **What are the clinical features of phakolytic glaucoma?**
   i. Conjunctiva: Hyperemia
   ii. Cornea: Microcystic corneal edema
   iii. Anterior chamber (AC): Deep prominent cell and flare reaction, no keratic precipitates (KPs), white flocculent material floating in the AC with or without pseudohypopyon
   iv. Iridocorneal angle: Open
   v. Lens: Mature, hypermature/Morgagnian cataract
      1. Wrinkling of the anterior lens capsule
   vi. Intraocular pressure (IOP): High, >35 mm Hg

5. **What is the mechanism of phakolytic glaucoma?**

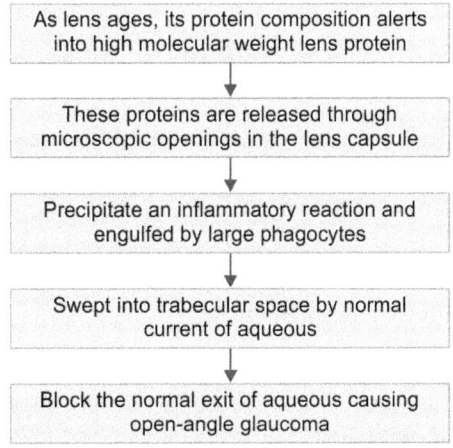

6. **How will you treat phakolytic glaucoma?**
   The ultimate treatment is lens removal after the control of IOP.
   Medical: Reduction of IOP by:
   i. β-blockers
   ii. Apraclonidine
   iii. Carbonic anhydrase inhibitor
   iv. Osmotic agents
   Surgical: Cataract extraction

7. **What are the precipitating events for lens particle glaucoma?**
   i. Remnants of cortical or epinuclear material after cataract surgery
   ii. Nd:YAG laser posterior capsulotomy

8. **Describe the clinical features of lens particle glaucoma.**
   i. *Cornea:* Microcystic corneal edema
      AC: Free cortical material in the AC; dense flare and cells
   ii. *Pupil:* Posterior and peripheral anterior synechiae
   iii. *IOP:* Elevated

9. **What is the treatment for lens particle glaucoma?**
   Medical: Aqueous suppressants (decrease aqueous production), topical steroids (reduce inflammation), and cycloplegics (inhibit posterior synechiae)
   Surgical: Removal of lens debris

10. **Define phakoanaphylactic glaucoma.**
    Phakoanaphylactic glaucoma is a rare entity in which patients become sensitized to their own lens protein following surgery or penetrating trauma resulting in granulomatous inflammation.

11. **Name two criteria to suspect phakoanaphylactic glaucoma.**
    i. Polymorphonuclear leukocytes must be present within the aqueous or vitreous
    ii. Circulating lens protein or particle content of the aqueous must be insufficient to explain glaucoma

12. **What is the clinical feature of phakoanaphylactic glaucoma?**
    i. AC: Moderate reaction
    ii. KPs present on both the corneal endothelium and anterior lens surface
    iii. Low-grade vitritis, synechial formation
    iv. Residual lens material in the AC

13. **What is phakomorphic glaucoma?**
    Secondary angle-closure glaucoma due to lens intumescence is called phakomorphic glaucoma.

14. **What is the differential diagnosis for phakomorphic glaucoma?**
    Primary angle-closure glaucoma (PACG) is the differential diagnosis for phakomorphic glaucoma.

15. **How to differentiate phakomorphic glaucoma from PACG?**

Phakomorphic glaucoma	PACG
Rapid swelling of the lens	Normal lens growth
Occurs in senile cataract and traumatic cataract	Occurs in hypermetropic individual
Asymmetric central shallowing of the AC	Both eyes (BE)—shallow AC
Unilateral mature intumescent cataract	Normal lens

16. **Describe the pathogenesis of phakomorphic glaucoma.**

    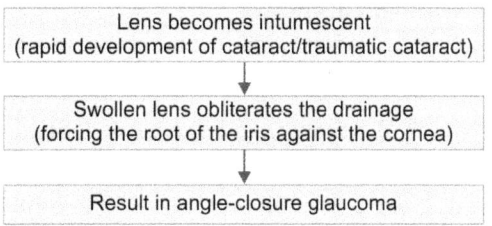

17. **Mention the treatment for phakomorphic glaucoma.**
    i. The definitive treatment is surgery after controlling IOP
    ii. Reduction of IOP by:
       - β-blockers, α-adrenergic agonist, topical or systemic carbonic anhydrase
       - Topical steroids—surgical
         - YAG peripheral iridotomy (PI)
         - Lens extraction

18. **What is ectopia lentis?**
    Ectopia lentis refers to the displacement of the lens from its normal anatomic position.

19. **How does ectopia lentis cause secondary glaucoma?**

    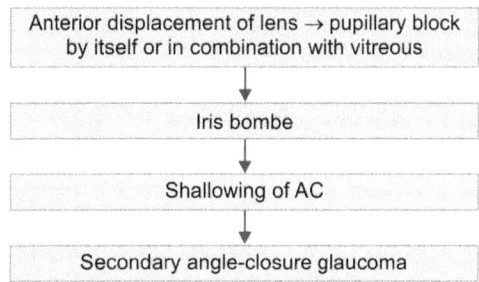

20. What are the causes of ectopia lentis?

Without systemic associations:
   i. Familial ectopia lentis
   ii. Ectopia lentis et pupillae
   iii. Aniridia

With systemic associations:
   i. Marfan syndrome
   ii. Homocystinuria
   iii. Weill–Marchesani syndrome
   iv. Hyperlysinemia
   v. Sulfite oxidase deficiency
   vi. Stickler syndrome
   vii. Ehlers–Danlos syndrome

20. What is the treatment of choice?

The treatment of choice is laser iridotomy since it is PACG with pupillary block.

21. Discuss the medical management of ectopia lentis.

   i. Cycloplegics and mydriatics
   ii. Cycloplegics act by flattening the lens and pulling it posteriorly and breaking the pupillary block
   iii. Miotics should be avoided since they may exaggerate pupillary block and worsen glaucoma

22. Discuss the surgical treatment of ectopia lentis.

   i. Lens removal is not indicated unless the lens is in the AC or there is evidence of lens-induced uveitis
   ii. Pars plana lensectomy is preferable if posterior lens displacement is present.

4.14 MEDICAL MANAGEMENT OF GLAUCOMA

1. **What is the goal of therapy in glaucoma?**
   The goal of therapy in glaucoma is to achieve a target intraocular pressure (IOP) which will arrest or prevent optic nerve head damage and progression of field defects.

2. **What is target pressure?**
   The target pressure is estimated for each patient based on:
   i. Initial IOP
   ii. Degree of existing damage
   iii. Potential side effects, complications, and cost
      Then, it is continually reassessed and reset based on the clinical course. The American Academy of Ophthalmology (AAO) guidelines suggest:
      - For mild damage (optic disk cupping but no visual field loss), the initial target pressure should be 20-30% below baseline
      - For patients with advanced damage, the target pressure range may be a reduction of 40% or more from baseline
      - For patients with normal-tension glaucoma (NTG), a 30% reduction is recommended

3. **What are the advantages of medical therapy for glaucoma?**
   i. Serious side effects are rare
   ii. Most patients are easily controlled

4. **What are the disadvantages of medical therapy?**
   i. Less effective than surgery to lower the IOP
   ii. Prolonged use may interfere with the success of future surgery, if necessary
   iii. Medical therapy tends to escalate with time
   iv. Nuisance factor and side effects may interfere with the quality of life
   v. Costly
   vi. Effects tend to wean away with time
   vii. Difficulty in compliance

5. **Classify drugs used in glaucoma.**
   i. *Cholinergic drugs:*
      - *Parasympathomimetics:* Pilocarpine, carbachol
      - *Anticholinesterases:* Echothiophate iodide, phospholine iodide, physostigmine, demecarium
   ii. *Adrenergic agents:*
      - *Sympathomimetics:*
        Nonselective: Epinephrine, dipivefrine
        Selective (α-agonists): Clonidine, apraclonidine, brimonidine

- *Adrenergic blocking agents:*
  Nonselective: Timolol, levobunolol, metipranolol, carteolol
  Selective (β-1 antagonists): Betaxolol
iii. *Carbonic anhydrase inhibitors (CAIs):*
  Oral: Acetazolamide, methazolamide
  Topical: Dorzolamide, brinzolamide
iv. *Hyperosmotic agents:*
  Oral: Glycerol, isosorbide
  Intravenous (IV): Mannitol, urea
v. *Prostaglandins:*
  Latanoprost, bimatoprost, travoprost, unoprostone
vi. *Neuroprotective agents:*
  - *N*-methyl-D-aspartate (NMDA) receptor antagonists
  - Calcium channel blockers
  - Nitric oxide (NO) synthetase inhibitors
  - Antioxidants
  - Vasodilators

6. **What is the mechanism of action of pilocarpine?**

   Pilocarpine is a directly acting parasympathomimetic.

   In primary angle-closure glaucoma (PACG): Pilocarpine constricts the pupil and pulls the peripheral iris from the trabecular meshwork, thereby relieving the pupillary block and in short-term management, to prepare the eye for iridotomy.

   In primary open-angle glaucoma (POAG): Pilocarpine acts by causing contraction of the longitudinal ciliary muscle, which pulls the scleral spur to tighten the trabecular meshwork, thereby increasing aqueous outflow. It also increases the intertrabecular pore size.

7. **What are the contraindications to the use of pilocarpine?**
   i. Neovascular glaucoma
   ii. Uveitic glaucoma
   iii. Phakolytic glaucoma

8. **What are the adverse effects of pilocarpine?**

   Functional side effects:
   i. Brow ache (due to ciliary body spasm)
   ii. Decreased vision in low illumination due to miosis
   iii. Induced myopia (due to ciliary body contraction)
   iv. Lacrimation due to punctal stenosis

   Anatomical side effects:
   i. Conjunctival congestion
   ii. Corneal epithelial staining
   iii. Increased inflammation

iv. Cataract
   v. Iris pigment cysts
   vi. Retinal holes and detachment
   vii. Increased vascular permeability, formation of posterior synechiae, and postoperative inflammation secondary angle-closure glaucoma on chronic use of pilocarpine

9. **What are the types of adrenergic receptors?**
   The types of adrenergic receptors are α-1, α-2, β-1, and β-2.

10. **Where are they located?**
    α-1: Arterioles, dilator pupillae
    α-2: *Ciliary epithelium*
    β-1: Heart
    β-2: Bronchi, ciliary epithelium

11. **Which is the only cardioselective β-blocker?**
    Betaxolol.

12. **What are the contraindications for β-blockers?**
    i. Congestive cardiac failure
    ii. Second- or third-degree heart block
    iii. Bradycardia
    iv. Asthma
    v. Chronic obstructive pulmonary disease (COPD)

13. **What are the β-blockers used as antiglaucoma medication?**

Timolol	0.5% BD, 0.25%
Betaxolol	0.5% BD
Levobunolol	0.5% BD
Carteolol	1 and 2%
Metipranolol	0.1 and 0.3% BD

14. **What is the mechanism of action of β-blocker?**
    Topical β-blockers inhibit cyclic adenosine monophosphate (cAMP) production in the ciliary epithelium, thereby decreasing aqueous production (20–50%) and hence reducing the IOP (20–30%).

15. **What is the ideal time to use timolol?**
    Timolol reduces aqueous production more when taken in the morning. There is an IOP spike in the early morning due to increasing catecholamines during waking, and hence this can be blunted.

16. **How are β-blockers classified?**

Nonselective	Timolol
	Carteolol
	Levobunolol
	Metipranolol
Selective	Betaxolol

17. **What are the types of decrease in efficacy associated with timolol application?**
    i. Short-term escape—increase in the receptors
    ii. Long-term drift
       This decrease in efficacy may be due to the response of β receptors to constant exposure to an antagonist.

18. **What are the different formulations of timolol?**
    i. Timolol maleate and in gel formulation
    ii. Timolol hemihydrate
    iii. Timolol potassium sorbate

19. **What are the ocular side effects of β-blockers?**
    i. Allergy
    ii. Punctate epithelial erosions
    iii. Decreased tear secretion
    iv. Decreased corneal sensation

20. **What are the systemic side effects?**
    Cardiovascular system (CVS): Bradycardia, hypotension, heart failure

    Respiratory system (RS): Bronchospasm, aggravating asthma, emphysema, bronchitis

    Central nervous system (CNS): Sleep disorders, depression, forgetfulness, rarely hallucinations

21. **What are the ways to decrease systemic absorption of topically administered drugs?**
    i. Lacrimal occlusion following instillation
    ii. Closing the eyes for 3 minutes

22. **Which antiglaucoma drug is contraindicated in children?**
    α-2 agonists are contraindicated in children because they cross the blood–brain barrier (bradycardia, hypotension, apnea, and CNS depression).

23. **What are the advantages of gel-forming solution?**
    i. Stays longer
    ii. Better corneal penetration

iii. Day-long IOP control
iv. Improves compliance
v. Once daily dosing

24. What is 0.5% levobunolol equivalent to?
0.5% timolol (but produces blepharoconjunctivitis more frequently)

25. What is the advantage of betaxolol?
Betaxolol is the only cardioselective β-blocker. It has minimal respiratory side effects. It is also neuroprotective (topical betaxolol seems to increase retinal blood flow).

26. What are the dosages in which brimonidine is available?
i. 0.2% brimonidine tartrate
ii. 0.15% brimonidine purite
iii. 0.1% brimonidine purite

27. What is the action of a highly selective α-2 adrenergic agonist (brimonidine)?
i. Decreases aqueous formation
ii. Increases uveoscleral outflow
iii. Neuroprotection

28. What are the drugs with neuroprotective effects?
Betaxolol and brimonidine

29. What is the mechanism of action of sympathomimetics?
Sympathomimetics decrease aqueous production by the net inhibition of adenylate cyclase and the reduction of intracellular cAMP.

30. What are the side effects of epinephrine and dipivefrine?
Ocular:
i. Black deposits (adrenochrome deposits in conjunctiva and cornea)
ii. Cystoid macular edema (CME)
iii. Pupillary dilatation and hence contraindicated in angle-closure glaucoma

Systemic:
i. Tachycardia
ii. Extrasystoles
iii. Systemic hypertension
iv. Palpitation

31. What is dipivefrine?
Dipivefrine is a derivative prodrug of epinephrine.

32. Why is clonidine not used widely?
i. Narrow therapeutic index
ii. Causes systemic hypotension—worsening blood flow to the optic nerve head

iii. Causes sedation
iv. High incidence of cardiovascular side effects

33. How does apraclonidine work?
Apraclonidine reduces IOP by:
i. Reducing aqueous production
ii. Improving trabecular outflow
iii. Reducing episcleral venous pressure

34. What is the advantage of apraclonidine over clonidine?
Apraclonidine achieves a substantial IOP reduction of clonidine without causing the centrally mediated side effects of systemic hypotension and drowsiness.

35. What are the side effects of α-agonists (brimonidine)?
i. Allergic blepharoconjunctivitis
ii. Dry mouth
iii. Anterior uveitis
iv. Somnolence
v. They should be avoided in children and infants because of the increased risk of somnolence, hypotension, seizures, apnea, and serious derangements of neurotransmitters in the CNS

36. What is apraclonidine?
Apraclonidine is a para-amino derivative of clonidine and is a potent α-2 adrenergic agonist. Clonidine is believed to reduce aqueous humor production, which may be caused by constriction of afferent vessels in the ciliary processes.

37. What is the indication of 1% apraclonidine?
1% apraclonidine has an advantage over clonidine in that it has minimal blood–brain barrier penetration and rapidly brings down the IOP in cases with short-term IOP elevations, such as following laser iridotomies.

38. What are the systemic side effects of α-2 agonists?
CVS: Bradycardia, vasovagal attack, palpitation, postural hypotension
Gastrointestinal tract (GIT): Abdominal pain, nausea, vomiting, diarrhea

39. What is the mechanism of action of CAIs?
CAIs cause a lowering of IOP by decreasing aqueous humor production, by inhibition of carbonic anhydrase II isoenzyme in the ciliary epithelium.

40. What are the forms in which CAIs are available?
Oral: Acetazolamide, methazolamide
Topical: Dorzolamide, brinzolamide

41. **What is the dosage of oral CAI?**
    Acetazolamide, 250 mg tablets, over 6 hours or 500 mg sustained-release capsules twice a day.

42. **What are the side effects of CAI?**
    i. *Ocular:*
       Transient myopic shift
    ii. *Systemic:*
        - *Electrolyte imbalance:*
          - Metabolic acidosis
          - Potassium and chloride depletion
          - Uric acid retention
        - *Gastrointestinal disturbances:*
          - Abdominal discomfort
          - Metallic taste
          - Nausea
          - Diarrhea
          - Anorexia
        - *Genitourinary disturbances:*
          - Nocturia
          - Urolithiasis associated with dysuria
          - Impotence
        - *CNS disturbances:*
          - Drowsiness, headache, fatigue, paresthesias, and tingling sensations
          - Irritability
          - Vertigo
          - Insomnia
        - *Blood dyscrasias:*
          - Agranulocytosis
          - Neutropenia
          - Thrombocytopenia
          - Aplastic anemia
        - *Dermatological side effects:*
          - Exfoliative dermatitis
          - Hair loss
          - Pruritus
          - Stevens-Johnson syndrome

43. **What are the topical CAIs available?**
    2% dorzolamide hydrochloride eye drops used three times a day and 1% brinzolamide used twice a day.

44. **What are the side effects of topical CAI eye drops?**
    i. *Ocular:*
       - Ocular burning
       - Stinging and discomfort
       - Hypersensitivity reactions such as periorbital dermatitis
       - Superficial punctate keratitis
    ii. *Systemic:*
       - Thrombocytopenia

45. **When should CAIs be avoided?**
    CAIs should be avoided in renal transplant patients, renal failure patients, those patients with known allergy to sulfa drugs, and patients with chronic liver disease.

46. **What is the mechanism of action of prostaglandins?**
    Prostaglandins cause increased uveoscleral outflow by three possible mechanisms:
    i. Widen the spaces in the uveoscleral route by degradation of collagen
    ii. Relaxation of the ciliary muscle
    iii. Remodeling the extracellular matrix (ECM) of the ciliary muscle
    iv. In addition, it also has a mild neuroprotective effect

47. **What are the indications for prostaglandins?**
    i. All glaucoma as a first-line medication
    ii. High chance for compliance since once-a-day dose

48. **What are the contraindications for prostaglandins?**
    i. Hypersensitivity
    ii. Contact lens wear
    iii. Relative contraindication in inflammatory glaucoma
    iv. Stopped before cataract surgery

49. **What are the various prostaglandins available?**
    i. Latanoprost (0.005%)
    ii. Travoprost (0.004%)
    iii. Unoprostone (0.12%)
    iv. Bimatoprost (0.03%)

50. **What are the side effects of prostaglandins?**
    i. Increased pigmentation of eyelid skin
    ii. Fat atrophy
    iii. Fornix shortening
    iv. Alterations in eyelid cilia, such as hypertrichosis and increased pigmentation
    v. Conjunctival hyperemia
    vi. Reactivation of dendritic keratitis

vii. Increased iris pigmentation due to upregulation of tyrosinase activity in melanocytes
viii. Uveitis
ix. Cystoid macular edema
x. There are no systemic side effects

51. **What are the effects of prostaglandins on pregnancy?**
    i. First trimester—termination of pregnancy
    ii. Third trimester—premature labor

52. **Why are prostaglandin analogs used at bedtime?**
    Prostaglandin analogs are used at bedtime because they have a peak effect 10-14 hours after administration, bedtime application is recommended:
    i. To maximize efficacy
    ii. To decrease patient symptoms related to vascular dilatation

53. **What are the benefits of prostaglandins?**
    i. Single dosing schedule
    ii. 30-35% reduction in IOP
    iii. Flat IOP curve
    iv. No systemic side effects

54. **What is the specific advantage of travoprost?**
    Travoprost has a good effect over the diurnal variation of IOP. Benzalkonium chloride (BAK)-free formulations are also available.

55. **What is the mechanism of action of hyperosmotic agents?**
    i. Increase the osmolarity of plasma and thereby water from the eye (mainly from the vitreous) moves to the hyperosmotic plasma. This movement of water reduces vitreous volume and causes lowering of IOP
    ii. CNS action decreases the aqueous production

56. **What are the indications for hyperosmotics?**
    i. Any form of acute glaucoma
    ii. To prepare the patient for surgery
    iii. Malignant glaucoma

57. **What is the contraindication for hyperosmotics?**
    i. Anuria
    ii. Severe dehydration
    iii. Severe cardiac decompensation
    iv. Pulmonary edema

58. **What are the side effects of hyperosmotic agents?**
    i. *Ocular:*
        - Rebound of IOP
        - Intraocular hemorrhage
    ii. *Systemic:*
        - GIT:
            - Nausea
            - Vomiting
            - Abdominal cramps
            - Diarrhea
        - CNS:
            - Hyperosmolarity and electrolyte imbalance causes:
                * Thirst
                * Chills
                * Fever
                * Confusion
                * Disorientation
    iii. *Genitourinary system:*
        - Diuresis
        - Electrolyte imbalance
        - Dehydration
        - Hypovolemia
    iv. *CVS:*
        - Angina
        - Pulmonary edema
        - Congestive cardiac failure
    v. *Others:*
        - Hyperglycemia
        - Hypersensitivity

59. **What is the most common instruction given to patients after IV mannitol?**
    Patients are instructed not to get up immediately after the injection, since it may lead to hypo tension and, rarely, even coning of the brain.

60. **What are the dosages of hyperosmotic agents?**

    | Glycerol 50% | Oral route | 1–1.5 g/kg |
    | Isosorbide 45% | Oral route | 1–2 g/kg |
    | Mannitol 20% | IV | 1–2 g/kg |

61. **What is the advantage of isosorbide over glycerol?**
    Isosorbide can be safely given to diabetics unlike glycerol.

62. **Why is mannitol the drug of choice for IV use?**
    i. Less irritating to blood vessels
    ii. Can be used in diabetic patients
    iii. Can be used in renal failure patients

63. **What are the disadvantages of mannitol?**
    i. Large volume
    ii. Dehydration
    iii. Diuresis

64. **What are the advantages of urea?**
    i. Less cellular hydration
    ii. No caloric value
    iii. Penetrates the eye readily

65. **What are the disadvantages of urea?**
    i. Unstable
    ii. Thrombophlebitis and sloughing of skin at the injection site, if extravasation occurs

66. **What are the onset of action and peak action of hyperosmotic agents?**
    i. Mannitol—onset of action: 15-30 minutes, peak action: 30-60 minutes
    ii. Glycerol—onset of action: 10-30 minutes, peak action: 45-120 minutes
    iii. Isosorbide—same as glycerol

67. **What is the percentage reduction of IOP in each class of drugs?**

Prostaglandin analogs	25–32%
β-blockers	20–30%
Adrenergic agonists	15–20%
Parasympathomimetics	15–20%
CAIs	15–20%

68. **What are the disadvantages of using two or more drugs separately?**
    i. Nonadherence to treatment
    ii. Poor compliance
    iii. Difficult scheduling
    iv. Washout effect
    v. Preservative toxicity
    vi. Cost

69. **What are the parameters which need to be addressed when going in for fixed combination (FC)?**
    i. Need
    ii. Is IOP lowering effect superior?

iii. Pharmacologically complementing mechanism of action
iv. Similar dosing schedule

70. What are the advantages of timolol 0.5% + dorzolamide 2% combination?
   i. Reduces IOP more than either drug alone
   ii. Produces maximal or near-maximal efficacy
   iii. Additive in their effect in spite of being aqueous suppressants
   iv. No electrolyte imbalance

71. What is the advantage of timolol and prostaglandin combination?
Prostaglandin increases uveoscleral outflow and timolol decreases aqueous inflow and results in 13–37% IOP reduction.

72. Why should we not combine prostaglandins with pilocarpine?

Pilocarpine	Contracts ciliary muscle
	Decreases uveoscleral outflow
	Increases trabecular outflow
Prostaglandins	Relax ciliary muscle
	Increase uveoscleral outflow

73. What is the FC of prostaglandins?
The FC of prostaglandins is prostaglandins with timolol.

74. What are the advantages of FC?
   i. Simple dosing and easy scheduling
   ii. More patient adherence
   iii. Maintains IOP at a lower level
   iv. Less preservative toxicity
   v. Less systemic toxicity
   vi. Economical

75. What are the disadvantages of FC?
   i. Formulation of both drugs in a single bottle may reduce efficacy due to the time of instillation. For example, for timolol, dosing first thing in the morning is preferred in order to effectively blunt an early morning pressure rise while minimizing the risk of systemic hypotension during sleep, when aqueous production is diminished. Prostaglandin analogs, on the other hand, reach the peak effect 10–14 hours after administration. Hence, bedtime application is recommended to maximize efficacy and decrease patient symptoms related to vascular dilatation. Therefore, when both these drugs are combined, dosage becomes an issue
   ii. Alters the individual potency of the medication
   iii. Without confirming the efficacy of individual components, unnecessary exposure to drugs which will not be beneficial

76. **What are the choices of drugs in uveitic glaucoma?**
    Monotherapy or a combination of any of these drugs: Timolol, brimonidine, or dorzolamide.

77. **What are prostamides?**
    Prostamides are cyclooxygenase-2 (COX-2) derived oxidation products of the endocannabinoids/endovanniloid anandamide.

78. **What is maximal medical therapy?**
    Maximal medical therapy is the use of three drugs over a period of 3 months.

79. **When should one quit and move on to surgery?**
    i. Inability to maintain target IOP
    ii. Progressive glaucomatous damage on maximum medical therapy
    iii. Intolerance
    iv. Poor compliance

80. **What are neuroprotective drugs?**
    Neuroprotective drugs are thought to protect the optic nerve and include:
    i. Memantine
    ii. NO synthetase inhibitors
    iii. Peptides
    iv. Cannabinoids
    v. Calcium channel blockers
    vi. Immunomodulation

81. **Which antiglaucoma medications are contraindicated in uveitis?**
    Miotics and prostaglandin analogs are contraindicated because they increase the blood–aqueous barrier breakdown, thereby increasing inflammation.

82. **What are prostamides closely related to?**
    PGF2α is related to bimatoprost.

4.15 NEWER DRUGS IN GLAUCOMA

1. **Classify new ocular hypotensive agents.**
   i. *Natural products:* Cannabinoids
   ii. *Activators of extracellular matrix (ECM) hydrolysis:* Matrix metalloproteinases (MMPs)
   iii. *Cytoskeleton modulator:* Ethacrynic acid
   iv. Protein kinase inhibitors
   v. Compounds that increase cyclic guanosine monophosphate (cGMP)

2. **What are cannabinoids?**
   Mechanism of action:
   i. Vasodilatation of the efferent vessels in the anterior uvea
   ii. Modification of the surface membrane glycoprotein residues on the ciliary epithelium
   iii. Increased facility of outflow

   Side effects:
   Tachycardia, hypotension, euphoria, and hyperemia of the conjunctiva. Pulmonary fibrosis and impaired neurologic behavior.

   Disadvantages:
   Systemic hypotension, which may be associated with reduced perfusion of the optic nerve head. These side effects of the cannabinoids thus far tested in humans seriously limit their usefulness in the treatment of glaucoma.

3. **What are the activators of the ECM hydrolysis group?**
   Mechanism of action: An excessive accumulation of ECM material in the trabecular meshwork (TM) of glaucomatous eyes likely contributes to decreased aqueous outflow. Therefore, therapeutic manipulations that eliminate the excessive ECM should theoretically improve the outflow facility and consequently lower the intraocular pressure (IOP).

   Current drugs under study from this group:
   i. MMPs:
      Activation of these enzymes reduces the excessive accumulation of ECM molecules, such as proteoglycans, collagens, fibronectins, and laminin, in the glaucomatous eye and in turn decreases hydrodynamic resistance of the outflow pathway.

      Disadvantage:
      MMPs, being proteins of large molecular mass, are not practical as medical treatment.

ii. *Inducers of MMPs:*
   Tert-butylhydroquinone can upregulate MMP-3 expression in the TM cells and increase aqueous outflow facility in glaucoma and nonglaucoma eyes.

iii. *Activator of glycosaminoglycan (GAG) degradation compounds:*
   Products that catalyze the hydrolysis of GAGs stimulate the degradation of ECM in the TM and increase the outflow. GAG-degrading enzymes, hyaluronidase and chondroitinase, consistently increase the outflow facility and decrease the IOP in study models. Similar to MMPs, these GAG-degrading enzymes are not practical for clinical use. AL-3037A (sodium ferri ethylenediamine tetraacetate), a small molecule with a chelated ferric ion, accelerates the ascorbate-mediated hydrolysis of GAGs and enhances outflow facility by 15–20%. Future studies may discover other small molecules that stimulate the production or activation of these enzymes, which are more suitable as clinically useful therapeutic agents.

4. **What are protein kinase inhibitors?**

   Mechanism of action:
   The exact mechanism of action is not fully understood. They likely increase aqueous outflow by affecting the cytoskeleton of the TM or Schlemm's canal endothelial cells.

   Current drugs under study from this group:
   i. Broad-spectrum kinase inhibitors—H-7
   ii. Inhibitors of protein kinase C—GF109203X
   iii. Rho-associated coiled coil-forming kinase (ROCK) inhibitors—Y-27632 and H-1152

   Advantages:
   Topically active and have great IOP-lowering efficacy.

   Disadvantages:
   Since kinases are involved in many cellular functions in most tissues, vigilance is needed for the potential local and systemic side effects of prolonged use of these compounds.

5. **What are cytoskeleton-acting agents?**

   Mechanism of action:
   Compounds that disrupt the cytoskeleton (microfilaments, microtubules, intermediate filaments) can affect the cell shape, contractility, and motility, and these changes may be sufficient to alter the local geometry of the outflow pathway and consequently aqueous outflow.

Current drugs under study from this group:
  i. Ethacrynic acid
  ii. Latrunculin B
  iii. Swinholide A

Disadvantages:
  i. Poor corneal penetration
  ii. Corneal toxicity
  iii. TM toxicity

These side effects have limited its clinical utility as a glaucoma therapeutic agent.

6. What are the compounds that increase cGMP?

Mechanism of action:
cGMP affects both aqueous production and outflow. Activation of cGMP-dependent protein kinases, which by phosphorylation leads to functional changes of various proteins, e.g., inhibition of Na-K ATPase, and leads to a decrease in aqueous production.

Current drugs under study from this group:
  i. *cGMP analogs:*
     Cell permeable analogs of cGMP
  ii. *Nitric oxide (NO) donors:*
     Nitroglycerin, isosorbide dinitrate, sodium nitrite, hydralazine, minoxidil, sodium nitroprusside
  iii. *Natriuretic peptides:*
     Atrial natriuretic peptide (ANP), brain-derived natriuretic peptide (BNP), C-type natriuretic peptide (CNP)

Intracellular cGMP levels can also be increased by the activation of guanylyl cyclases. NO and compounds that release NO by hydrolysis (NO donors) are activators of the soluble guanylyl cyclases. Natriuretic peptides are activators of the membrane-bound guanylyl cyclases. Both NO donors and natriuretic peptides are effective IOP-lowering compounds.

Disadvantages:
Since they are peptides, cornea penetration and degradation by peptidases can be prohibitive hurdles for their clinical usefulness.

Compounds that increase natriuretic peptides:
Candoxatril natriuretic peptides are degraded partly by neutral endopeptidase (NEP) 24.11. Thus, inhibition of this enzyme increases tissue concentration of natriuretic peptides. Oral administration of candoxatril, a prodrug that is metabolized to an NEP 24.11 inhibitor, increases ANP level and significantly lowers IOP by 2–3 mm Hg.

7. **What is neuroprotection?**

    Rationale for using neuroprotection:
    It has been hypothesized that intraretinal or intravitreal glutamate levels that are neurotoxic to ganglion cells play a role in glaucoma, and hence drugs which work against these agents can help in glaucoma management. They are also supposed to enhance the vascular supply and decrease proapoptotic factors.

    Methods for neuroprotection:
    i. *Pharmacologic:*
       - Glutamate receptor antagonists: N-methyl-D-aspartate (NMDA) receptors: Memantine α-amino-3-hydroxy-5-methyl-4-isoxazolepropionic acid (AMPA)/kainate antagonists
       - Calcium channel blocker: Nimodipine
       - β2-adrenergic agonists: Brimonidine
       - Neurotrophic factors: Neurotrophin 3
       - NO synthase inhibitors: Aminoguanidine
       - Reactive oxygen species scavengers
       - Apoptosis inhibitors: Cytochrome C release inhibitors, caspase inhibitors

    ii. *Immune modulation:*
        Focal activation of the immune system in the optic nerve or retina is a way of preserving retinal ganglion cells and their functions. (Activated T lymphocytes primed to optic nerve constituents, e.g., myelin basic protein, would be home to sites of injury and release factors that are neuroprotective.)

    iii. *Preconditioning:*
         Concept: An injury insufficient to cause irreversible damage often may result in increased resistance to future injury. This type of neuroprotection is difficult to translate directly into clinical use, as it requires a series of injuries insufficient to kill retinal ganglion cells and it may not be tolerated by the patient.

    Neurorepair and regeneration:
    Neurorepair is the name given to the production and differentiation of new neurons. Regeneration is the name given to the extension of axons to their appropriate targets. Neurorepair focuses on the use of stem cells (embryonic stem cells, adult stem cells, or more differentiated neural progenitor cells) to repopulate and repair damaged neuronal tissues.

8. **What are neuroprotectors?**
    i. *Memantine*
       Memantine is a NMDA receptor antagonist.

Mechanism of action:
The NMDA receptor is an ion channel that is activated by glutamate, allowing extracellular calcium to enter the cell. In normal physiologic conditions, the NMDA receptor has an important role in neurophysiologic processes, such as memory. However, excessive activation of the NMDA signaling cascade leads to "excitotoxicity," wherein intracellular calcium overloads neurons and causes cell death through apoptosis. Memantine blocks the excessive glutamate stimulation of the NMDA receptor of the regional ganglion cell and protects it from calcium-mediated apoptosis.

Uses: To treat central nervous system (CNS) disorders such as Parkinson's disease and Alzheimer's disease. It is currently being studied as a neuroprotective agent in glaucoma.

ii. *NO synthase inhibitors*
Aminoguanidine:
Mechanism of action:
NO is a gaseous second messenger molecule. It has both physiologic and pathologic functions in blood flow, immune response, and neuronal communication.

The expression of NO is regulated by three different forms of nitric oxide synthase (NOS)—(1) endothelial NOS (eNOS), (2) neuronal NOS (nNOS), and (3) inducible NOS (iNOS).

Role of NO in the eye:
Aqueous humor dynamics, maintaining a clear cornea, ocular blood flow, retinal function, and optic nerve function. Excessive NO generated by iNOS in optic nerve astrocytes and microglia is associated with optic nerve damage. Aminoguanidine by inhibiting iNOS was shown to prevent retinal ganglion cell loss.

iii. *Calcium channel blockers: Nimodipine*
Mechanism of action:
Produces vasodilatation by inhibiting the entrance of calcium ions into vascular smooth muscle cells. Hence, they may protect the optic nerve head by improving vascular perfusion.

They have also been shown to have ocular hypotensive activity.

Current status: The level of evidence at this time, as well as the systemic side effects of calcium channel blockers, does not support the use of this class of drugs for the routine management of glaucoma.

iv. *Neurotrophic factors:*
Neurotrophins are peptides that have an important role in the development and maintenance of various neuronal populations. Brain-derived neurotrophic factor, neurotrophin 3, and nerve growth factor have differential effects on cell survival promotion,

differentiation, or demise. The role of these biologically active peptides and their receptors in relation to the survival and death of ganglion cells is under study.

v. *Apoptosis inhibitors:*
Caspases are a family of proteases that execute the dismantling and demolition of cells undergoing apoptosis. Caspases 8 and 9 have been shown to be activated in experimental glaucoma. Suppression of apoptosis using caspase inhibitors is an approach that has been explored with modest success.

9. **Mention other agents.**
    i. *Tetrahydrocortisol:* A metabolite of cortisol, shown to lower dexamethasone-induced ocular hypertension
    ii. *Mifepristone:* A specific glucocorticoid receptor antagonist, shown to lower IOP, possibly by blocking the glucocorticoid receptor-mediated effects in ocular tissues
    iii. *Spironolactone:* A synthetic steroidal aldosterone antagonist with potassium-sparing diuretic-antihypertensive activity producing significant IOP reduction in glaucoma patients, which persisted 2 weeks after termination of the treatment
    iv. *Antazoline:* An antihistamine of the ethylene diamine class, shown to lower IOP following topical administration apparently by decreasing aqueous production
    v. *Angiotensin-converting enzyme inhibitor:* A topical formulation has been shown to lower IOP in dogs and humans with ocular hypertension or open-angle glaucoma
    vi. *Organic nitrates:* Intravenous nitroglycerin or oral isosorbide dinitrate has been reported to lower IOP in glaucoma and nonglaucoma patients
    vii. *Melatonin:* A hormone produced by the pineal gland, which was shown to lower the IOP in normal subjects
    viii. *Demeclocycline, tetracycline, and other tetracycline derivatives:* Lower IOP in rabbits, which appears to be related to reduced aqueous humor production. Acepromazine, an analog of chlorpromazine that is used as a tranquilizer in veterinary medicine, had no effect on IOP when given topically to normotensive rabbits but reduced the pressure for at least 32 hours in rabbits with chronic IOP elevation produced by argon laser applications to the TM
    ix. *Alternative medicine:* Ginkgo biloba extract (GBE): Leaf extracts of the ginkgo tree have many neuroprotective properties applicable to the treatment of non-IOP-dependent risk factors for glaucomatous damage. GBE exerts significant protective effects against free

radical damage and lipid peroxidation. It preserves mitochondrial metabolism and adenosine triphosphate (ATP) production. It partially prevents morphologic changes and indices of oxidative damage associated with mitochondrial aging. It can scavenge NO and possibly inhibit its production. It can reduce glutamate-induced elevation of calcium concentrations and can reduce oxidative metabolism in resting and calcium-loaded neurons and inhibits apoptosis. GBE has been reported to be neuroprotective for retinal ganglion cells in a rat model of chronic glaucoma.

4.16 LASERS IN GLAUCOMA

1. **What are the applications of lasers in glaucoma?**
   i. *Therapeutic:*
      - To treat internal block:
         - Iridotomy (both argon and Nd:YAG and diode)
      - To treat outflow obstruction:
         - Trabeculoplasty (argon), trabeculopuncture (argon), gonioplasty/iridoplasty (argon)
      - *Miscellaneous uses:*
         - Cyclophotocoagulation (Nd:YAG), cyclodialysis (Nd:YAG), pupilloplasty (argon), sphincterotomy (both)
         - To rupture cysts of the iris and ciliary body (both): Gonio photocoagulation (argon)
         - Laser suturolysis, anterior hyaloidotomy
   ii. *Diagnostic:*
      - Confocal scanning laser ophthalmoscope (optic nerve head evaluation)
      - Laser retinal Doppler flowmetry (optic nerve head perfusions)

2. **Mention the commonly used lasers and their wavelengths.**

Laser	Wavelength (in nm)
Excimer	193
Argon blue-green	488–514
Nd:YAG	1,064
Diode	810
CO_2	10,600

3. **What are the principles used in lasers to treat glaucoma?**
   i. *Photodisruption:*
   When ultrashort pulses of a laser are targeted at the tissue, the latter is reduced to a form of matter called "plasma." This generates fluid forces (both hemodynamic waves and acoustic pulses), which propagate in all directions. This propagating force incises tissue. This forms the basis of Nd:YAG capsulotomies and iridotomies.
   ii. *Photocoagulation:*
   Any chromophore, including iris and trabecular meshwork, absorbs laser light and converts it to heat energy. This causes coagulation of tissue. When collagen is warmed during this process, it contracts and changes the microanatomy of tissues (trabeculoplasty). Likewise, the leaking blood vessels are sealed in neovascular glaucoma (NVG).

4. **What are the indications of laser iridotomy?**
    i. Acute angle-closure glaucoma
    ii. Prodromal stage of angle-closure glaucoma
    iii. Chronic angle-closure glaucoma
    iv. Aphakic or pseudophakic pupillary block
    v. Malignant glaucoma
    vi. Prophylactic laser iridotomy in the fellow eye of angle closure
    vii. Nanophthalmos
    viii. Traumatic secondary angle closure
    ix. Microspherophakia
    x. Pigment dispersion syndrome
    xi. To penetrate nonfunctioning peripheral iridectomy
    xii. Combined mechanism glaucoma
    xiii. Alteration in angle structure due to lens like phakomorphic glaucoma
    xiv. Use of systemic medication like topiramate which may provoke pupillary block
    xv. Family history of primary angle-closure glaucoma (PACG)
    xvi. Patients who cannot come for regular follow-up
    xvii. Need for repeated dilatation due to posterior segment pathology

5. **What are the contraindications of laser peripheral iridotomy (LPI)?**
    i. Corneal edema
    ii. Corneal opacification
    iii. Flat anterior chamber
    iv. A completely sealed angle resulting in angle closure
    v. Primary synechial closure of the angle
    vi. Uveitis
    vii. NVG
    viii. Iridocorneal endothelial (ICE) syndrome

6. **What are the types of peripheral iridectomy?**
    i. *Therapeutic:* Surgical iridectomy or laser PI
    ii. *Optical:*
        - Broad-based or sectoral iridectomy
        - Keyhole iridectomy

7. **What is the mechanism by which argon produces peripheral iridotomy (PI)?**
   Argon laser requires an uptake of light energy by the pigment (thermal effect) and coagulates tissues. However, it requires more energy for iridotomy and is associated with more late closures compared to the Nd:YAG laser.

Glaucoma

8. **What are the conditions where an argon laser is preferred over Nd:YAG in producing PI?**
   i. Brown irises (it is used in sequential contribution with Nd:YAG)
   ii. Patients on chronic anticoagulant therapies (as Nd:YAG works on disruption and not on coagulation)
   iii. Angle-closure stage of NVG
   iv. Patients with blood dyscrasias such as hemophilia

9. **What is the mechanism by which Nd:YAG laser produces PI?**
   Nd:YAG works on the principle of photodisruption and is effective on all iris colors. The laser wavelength is in the near-infrared range (1,064 nm). It is always preferred over the argon laser.

10. **What is the preferred site of PI and why?**
    The preferred site is usually in the *superior quadrant* between 11 and 1 o'clock positions, where it will be covered by the lid. The laser beam should be focused at the base of an iris crypt to facilitate penetration.

    However, *recent studies* comparing superior and temporal LPI concluded the following:
    Temporal placement of LPI is safe and was found to be less likely to result in linear dysphotopsia as compared with superior placement. The temporal iris, therefore, may be considered a preferred location for LPI.

11. **Describe the technique of Nd:YAG PI.**
    i. *Preoperative preparation:*
       Cornea should be clear: Pilocarpine 2%—three times (5 minutes apart), is used to constrict the pupil. (The iris is stretched fully and at its thinnest and easily penetrable.)
       Brimonidine or apraclonidine 0.2%—half hour before the procedure.
    ii. *Role of using a contact lens:* The lens provides firm control over the eyeball and reduces saccades and extraneous eye movements that interfere with the accurate superimposition of burns. The lens assists in:
       - Keeping the lids separated
       - Smoothens out cornea
       - Provides a peripheral magnified view
       - Reduces unnecessary spread of damage by reducing axial expansion of plasma
       - Increases the power density of the spot. The Abraham lens, which is used, consists of a fundus lens with a +55 D planoconvex lens with a D button placed on its anterior surface. The button provides magnification without the loss of depth of focus
    iii. *Gonioscopy solution:* Absorbs excess heat delivered to the cornea, thus decreasing the incidence of corneal burns

iv. *Site:* An iridotomy spot may be placed in the upper nasal iris to avoid diplopia and macular burns. The laser is targeted at the crypts to ensure easy penetration. The red helium-neon laser aiming beam is brought to focus when the multiple beams are brought into a single spot aimed through the center of the contact lens
Energy: 3–10 mJ
1–3 pulses per shot
PI size should be 300–500 µ

v. *Immediate posttreatment:* Prednisolone acetate 1% is used every 2 hours for 1 day and then tapered over a week. The intraocular pressure (IOP) is checked regularly at 1 hour, 1 day, 1 week, and 4 weeks. Gonioscopy is done at 1 week and dilation at 2 weeks. The IOP status of the overlying corneal endothelium, anterior chamber reaction, and iridotomy patency are evaluated. Gonioscopy is always performed to be sure that the pupillary block has been relieved and to determine the extent of posterior anterior synechiae (PAS). The smallest size iris opening that is acceptable following laser iridotomy is 60 µ or greater. More importantly, one must be able to see the lens capsule through the iridotomy to document the relief of pupillary block by gonioscopy. Failing this, repeat treatment is indicated

12. **What are the signs of iridotomy penetration?**
    i. Sudden gush of aqueous
    ii. Retroillumination shows a patent PI
    iii. Deepening of anterior chamber (AC)
    iv. Plomb of iris pigments
    v. Visualization of anterior lens capsule

13. **What are the various techniques used in argon laser PI?**
    i. Hump, drumhead, and chipping are the techniques advocated for producing PI with a continuous wave argon laser
        - *Hump technique:* It involves creating a localized elevation of the iris with large-diameter low-energy burns and then penetrating the hump with a small intense burn.
        - *Drumhead technique:* It involves placing a large-diameter low-energy burn around the intended treatment site to put the iris on stretch, and the area is penetrated with small high-energy burns.
        - *Chipping technique:* It is especially useful in dark brown iris where standard settings may produce black char in iris stroma, making it difficult to penetrate the tissue. This is circumvented by using multiple short-duration burns. This is called the chipping technique.

14. **What are the common complications of LPI?**
    i. Corneal burn
    ii. Uveitis
    iii. Elevated IOP
    iv. Hemorrhage
    v. Pigment dissemination and iris atrophy
    vi. Lens injury
    vii. Posterior synechia
    viii. Retinal damage
    ix. Corectopia
    x. Monocular diplopia
    xi. Malignant glaucoma
    xii. Glare

15. **What is the difference between surgical iridectomy and laser iridotomy?**

	Surgical iridectomy	*Laser iridotomy*
Margins	Clean cut, triangular	Ragged, irregular
Site	Near limbal incision site (mostly 12 o'clock)	Any clock hour on the iris surface
Closure	Not possible	Possible
Surrounding iris tissue	Not altered	May be associated with pigment dispersions

16. **What are the indications for argon laser trabeculoplasty (ALT)?**
    i. Primary open-angle glaucoma (POAG)
    ii. Exfoliative glaucoma
    iii. Pigmentary glaucoma
    iv. Glaucoma in pseudophakia
    v. Combined mechanism glaucoma
    vi. Normal-tension glaucoma (NTG)
    vii. Noncompliance with medications
    viii. Inadequate medical control

17. **What are the contraindications for ALT?**
    i. Inflammatory glaucoma
    ii. ICE syndrome
    iii. NVG
    iv. Synechial angle closure
    v. Developmental glaucoma

18. **Describe the technique of ALT.**
    i. *Preoperatively:* Pilocarpine is used to constrict the pupil. 0.5% apraclonidine and topical xylocaine are instilled

ii. *Contact lens:* Ritch trabeculoplasty/Goldmann 3 mirror can be used
iii. *Site:* Equally spaced burns are applied to the anterior half of the trabecular meshwork at the junction of pigmented functional and nonfunctional trabecular meshwork
iv. *Laser parameters:* 180–360° of angle treated with argon blue-green of 800–1,200 mW; 0.1 seconds exposure, 50 µm spot size, and 24 shots per quadrant
v. *End point:* Blanching of trabecular meshwork or appearance of an air bubble

19. What is the mechanism of action of ALT?
The mechanisms of action of ALT are explained by two theories:
i. *Mechanical theory:* Collagen shrinkage is produced at the site of burns. There is stretching of the trabecular meshwork between the burns which opens the meshwork pores and allows aqueous to flow better. Laser burns attract phagocytes that clean up the debris within the meshwork and allow aqueous to flow better.
ii. *Biological theory:* It causes activation of macrophages to ingest and clear the debris, thereby increasing the outflow facility.

20. What are the complications of ALT?
i. Pressure rise
ii. Visual loss
iii. Peripheral anterior synechiae
iv. Uveitis
v. Hyphema
vi. Increased incidence of Tenon's cyst following trabeculectomy

21. What is the percentage decrease in IOP following argon laser trabeculoplasty in POAG?
The average reduction is about 30%. About 50% of eyes remain well controlled after 5 years of treatment.

22. What is the effect on the success of trabeculectomy following ALT versus eyes in which no laser was done previously?
The risk of encapsulated blebs following filtration surgery is up to three times more in eyes previously treated by ALT.

23. What are the indications for selective laser trabeculoplasty?
i. Open-angle glaucoma
ii. Failed ALT
iii. Pseudoexfoliation (PXF) glaucoma
iv. Pigmentary glaucoma
v. Juvenile glaucoma

vi. Inflammatory glaucoma
vii. Poorly compliant patient
viii. End-stage treatment

24. **What are the contraindications for selective laser trabeculoplasty?**
    i. Angle-closure glaucoma
    ii. Uveitic glaucoma
    iii. Angle recession glaucoma
    iv. Developmental glaucoma
    v. NVG

25. **What is the mechanism of action of selective laser trabeculoplasty?**
    Selective laser trabeculoplasty therapy targets the pigmented melanin-containing cells (yellow) in the trabecular meshwork, preventing thermal transfer to the surrounding tissue.
    A cellular and biochemical model has been proposed.
    Macrophages are recruited to the laser treatment zones which stimulate the release of cytokines. These cytokines upregulate synthetic matrix metalloproteinase (MMP), which increases the porosity of the endothelial layers of the trabecular meshwork and Schlemm's canal and increases aqueous outflow.

26. **What are the laser parameters used in selective laser trabeculoplasty?**
    Frequency-doubled Q-switched Nd:YAG laser is used. 532 nm, pulse duration 3 ms
    Spot size: 400 μ
    Energy: 0.2–1.7 mW, 50–100 adjacent laser spots are applied.

27. **What are the future trends in laser trabeculoplasty?**
    Micropulse laser trabeculoplasty (MLT) using an 810 nm diode laser
    Titanium Sapphire LTP (SOLX 790) using 790 nm; 5–10 μs.

28. **What is laser iridoplasty?**
    Laser iridoplasty is also called gonioplasty and is a technique to deepen the angle. It is an iris flattening procedure done in:
    i. Plateau iris
    ii. Nanophthalmos
    iii. POAG in anatomically narrow angle
    iv. Adjunct to laser trabeculoplasty
    v. After Nd:YAG iridotomy where IOP is still not controlled

29. **What are the settings used for laser iridoplasty?**
    Settings: 500 μm
    200–400 mW power
    0.2–0.5 seconds
    20–24 spots over 360°
    1 mm away from iris root

30. What is the role of lasers in cyclodestructive procedures?

Involves cyclophotocoagulation: A thermal method of destroying part of the ciliary body.

Approaches can be:

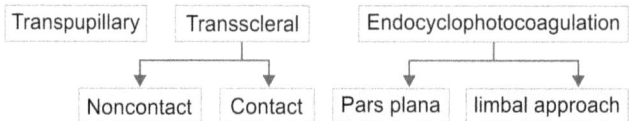

Transpupillary procedures are unpredictable and give disappointing results.

Transscleral route is the preferred modality.

In noncontact: There is slit-lamp delivery of laser energy through air.

Contact method: It involves fiberoptic probe delivery directly to the ocular surface.

Endocyclophotocoagulation: It involves the use of an intraocular laser probe to treat ciliary processes. Two options are available:

Pars plana route: It is particularly useful in NVG in diabetic patients in whom vitrectomy is also needed.

Limbal route: The procedure is carried out through limbal incision. It isseful in phakic, pseudophakic, and aphakic patients. It can be combined with cataract extraction.

30. How is a laser useful in malignant glaucoma?

Laser hyaloidectomy/hyaloidotomy or vitreolysis is done. In malignant glaucoma, the anterior hyaloid acts as a barrier to fluid movement into the anterior chamber. A laser (by Nd:YAG) is used to photodisrupt the anterior hyaloid face and relieve ciliovitreal compression.

Laser parameters: 100–200 µm

Spot size: 1–11 mm

31. What is laser suturolysis?

Laser suturolysis is a technique by which scleral flap sutures applied for closing flap in trabeculectomy can be lysed or cut using lasers.

32. Describe the technique of laser suturolysis.

Lasers used	Solid Nd:YAG laser or argon green
Timing	Within 3–15 days to 2 months or more after use of mitomycin C after trabeculectomy
Indications	When the target IOP is not reached
Lenses used	Zeiss gonioprism or Hoskins laser suturolysis lens
Duration	0.02–0.15 seconds
Spot size	50–100 nm
Power	200–1,000 mW

Gentle pressure over the conjunctiva makes sutures more visible.

33. What are the complications of laser suturolysis?
   i. Conjunctival burns
   ii. Flat anterior chamber
   iii. Conjunctival flap leak
   iv. Hypotonous maculopathy
   v. Iris incarceration, hyphema
   vi. Blebitis, endophthalmitis

34. Describe the technique of digital pressure.
A constant and firm digital compression is applied over the inferior aspect of the globe through the patient's lower lid while the eye is upturned. The duration of each compression should not last for >10 seconds.

35. What is goniophotocoagulation?
Goniophotocoagulation is used to ablate vessels which cross the scleral spur.
Argon laser of 150–500 mW
100 µ spot size is used for 0.2 seconds for this procedure.

36. What are the indications for transscleral cyclophotocoagulation?
   i. In refractory glaucoma when IOP is uncontrolled despite maximum tolerated medical treatment and failed filtration or high risk of failure of the same like in aphakic, pseudophakic, or NVGs
   ii. Glaucoma associated with inflammation
   iii. Eyes with a previous failed filtering procedure or following penetrating keratoplasty

37. Describe diode laser transscleral cyclophotocoagulation.
Anesthesia: Administer local anesthetic. Supplement with retro- or peribulbar injections. It can be done in a supine position or sitting at the slit lamp.
Energy levels of 0.5–2.75 J for 32 applications distributed over 360° of the ciliary body

Treatment quadrants: Over a 270° area involving the inferior, nasal, and superior quadrants (16–18 applications reduce complications). The temporal quadrant is spared to allow for some ciliary production of aqueous humor. The 3 and 9 o'clock meridians are avoided to prevent damage to the long posterior ciliary arteries.

Treatment parameters:

Pigmentation	Starting power (mW)	Starting duration (ms)
Dark	1,500	2,000
Light	1,750	2,000

Pops may be heard during treatment, indicating tissue disruption, but they are not a prerequisite for effective treatment.

The G probe tip (Gaasterland made) and eye surface are kept moist by methylcellulose or artificial tears.

Postoperative care: The eye is patched for 4-6 hours. Topical cycloplegics BD or more and topical steroids QID are given and tapered as inflammation subsides. All preoperative glaucoma medications except miotics are to be continued. Monitor patients at 1, 3, and 6 weeks after treatment.

38. What are the complications of diode cyclophotocoagulation?

Common complications:
 i. Pain
 ii. Inflammation
 iii. Reduced visual acuity due to cystoid macular edema
 iv. Hypotony

Uncommon complications:
 i. Hypopyon
 ii. Corneal epithelial defect
 iii. Scleral thinning
 iv. Graft failure
 v. Malignant glaucoma
 vi. Suprachoroidal hemorrhage
 vii. Hyphema
 viii. Sympathetic ophthalmitis
 ix. Phthisis bulbi.

4.17 TRABECULECTOMY

1. **What are the definitions of anatomical limbus?**
   The anterior limit of the limbus is formed by a line joining the end of Bowman's membrane and the end of Descemet's membrane (Schwalbe's line). The posterior limit is a curved line marking the transition between regularly arranged corneal collagen fibers and haphazardly arranged scleral collagen fibers.

2. **What are the definitions of the surgical limbus?**
   Surgical limbus is an annular band, 2 mm wide with the posterior limit overlying the scleral spur. It is divided into:
   i. Anterior blue zone (between Bowman's membrane and Schwalbe's line)
   ii. Posterior white zone (between Schwalbe's line and scleral spur)

3. **What are the types of filtering surgeries?**
   Filtering surgeries are of three types:
   i. Full thickness
   ii. Partial thickness
   iii. Nonpenetrating

   Full thickness (example):
   i. Sclerectomy
   ii. Trephination
   iii. Thermal sclerostomy (Scheie's procedure)
   iv. Laser sclerostomy (ab externo/interno)
   v. Iridencleisis
   vi. Goniopuncture

   Partial thickness:
   i. Trabeculectomy

   Nonpenetrating:
   i. Viscocanalostomy
   ii. Canaloplasty
   iii. Deep sclerectomy

4. **What are "full-thickness" operations?**
   "Full-thickness" operations are filtering operations without a sclera flap. The entire thickness of the wall from the corneoscleral surface to the anterior chamber (AC) is removed.

5. **What is a "partial thickness" operation?**
   An operation with a partial thickness flap of sclera overlying the opening between the AC and the subconjunctival space, e.g., trabeculectomy.

6. **What is the advantage of a partial thickness flap over a full thickness?**
    i. Uniform control of intraocular pressure (IOP)
    ii. Decreased risk of postoperative hypotony, thus decreased risk of hypotonous maculopathy
    iii. Decreased risk of postoperative complications such as hyphema, iris prolapse, and shallow AC
    iv. Decreased risk of postoperative infection and endophthalmitis

7. **Is the term trabeculectomy a misnomer?**
    Yes, the term trabeculectomy is a misnomer because the block of tissue removed does not need to include trabecular meshwork to be successful. The procedure involves a peripheral posterior keratectomy more than the removal of the trabecular meshwork.

8. **What is the principle?**
    Trabeculectomy works mainly because of filtration. The basic mechanism is by creating a fistula at the limbus, which allows aqueous humor to drain from the AC, around the edges of the sclera flap, and into the subconjunctival space from where it leaves by transconjunctival filtration or by absorption into the lymphatics and vessels of subconjunctival tissue.

9. **What are the indications for trabeculectomy in primary open-angle glaucoma?**
    Failed maximal tolerated medical therapy and failed laser surgery or poor candidates of laser with any of the following:
    i. Progressive glaucomatous optic nerve head (ONH) damage
    ii. Progressive glaucomatous field loss
    iii. Anticipated ONH damage or as a result of excessive IOP
    iv. Anticipated visual field damage
    v. Lack of compliance with anticipated progressive glaucomatous damage

10. **What are the features of a good filtering bleb?**
    The blebs which are associated with good IOP control are:
    i. Avascular and transparent
    ii. Numerous microcysts in the epithelium
    iii. Either low and diffuse or more circumscribed and elevated

11. **What are the signs of a failing bleb?**
    The signs of a failing bleb are:
    i. Reduced bleb height
    ii. Increased bleb wall thickness
    iii. Vascularization of the bleb
    iv. Loss of transparency
    iv. Loss of conjunctival microcysts
    v. Raised IOP

12. What are the types of blebs following trabeculectomy?

There are four types of blebs following trabeculectomy:
  i. *Type 1 bleb:* Thin and polycystic appearance due to transconjunctival flow of aqueous. It is associated with good filtration
  ii. *Type 2 bleb:* Flat, thin, and diffuse with a relatively avascular appearance, associated with good filtration. Conjunctival microcysts are usually visible with high magnification
  iii. *Type 3 bleb:* Flat, not associated with microcystic spaces, contains engorged blood vessels on its surface. This bleb does not filter and hence the IOP is elevated
  iv. *Type 4 bleb/encapsulated bleb/Tenon's cyst:* Localized, highly elevated, dome-shaped, cyst-like cavity of hypertrophied Tenon's capsule with engorged surface blood vessels. This bleb does not filter and hence the IOP is elevated
  v. *Risk factors for Tenon's cyst:*
     - Young individuals
     - Previous conjunctival surgery
     - Secondary glaucoma
     - Laser trabeculoplasty
     - Topical sympathomimetic therapy
     - Tenon cyst in the fellow eye

13. What is preoperative care?

  i. If the IOP is very high, then it is reduced to a safe level
  ii. Treat any ocular inflammation (reduced chances of establishing a lasting bleb)
  iii. Discontinue epinephrine/anticholinesterase to reduce vascular congestion and reduce intraoperative bleeding
  iv. Discontinue aqueous suppressant timolol (2 weeks prior) and carbonic anhydrase inhibitors (1–2 days prior) to prevent ocular hypotony and establish a filtering bleb
  v. Avoid gentamicin, which can irritate conjunctiva and produce congestion of the eyes
  vi. Constrict pupil with pilocarpine 1% 3 times, 1 hour before the operation. It prevents iris prolapse
  vii. If aspirin had been used, it is discontinued for 5 days before surgery
  viii. If eyes have new vessels, preoperative panretinal laser photocoagulation should be done first to induce regression of vessels and improve prognosis

14. What are the steps of trabeculectomy?

  i. *Anesthesia:* Under retrobulbar/peribulbar/sub-Tenon's/general anesthesia (avoid massage in case of advanced glaucoma, can lead to snuff out phenomenon)

ii. A bridle suture is inserted 2 mm anterior to the limbus
iii. A conjunctival flap is fashioned superonasally. The flap may be based either at the limbus or at the fornix
iv. A triangle or rectangle based at the limbus is outlined on the sclera measuring 3 mm radially and 4 mm circumferentially by a wet field cautery. One may make a square/triangular flap. With a sharp pointed knife, incisions are made along the cautery marks through two-third of the sclera thickness starting as anteriorly as possible behind the reflected flap
v. One of the corners of the flap is held up with toolkit Colibri forceps and dissection is started. A natural tissue plane will become apparent at about one-third of the scleral thickness. The dissection is done in an antidirection in the same plane keeping the blade flat until the color turns from white to gray
vi. The dissection is continued until a clear cornea has been reached
vii. Paracentesis is done at this stage
viii. The fistula is begun by entering the AC with a knife just behind the hinge of the scleral flap
ix. This deep block is excised using Kelly Descemet's membrane punch
x. Internal ostium should be 1.5 × 2 mm
xi. A peripheral iridectomy is performed to prevent blockage of the internal ostium by the peripheral iris
xii. The superficial sclera flap is sutured with interrupted 10-0 nylon so that it is apposed lightly to the underlying bed
xiii. If necessary, AC can be reformed by injecting balanced salt solution (BSS) through the paracentesis with a Rycroft cannula
xiv. The conjunctival flap is sutured with 8-0 Vicryl
xv. At the completion of the surgery, one drop of 1% atropine eye drop is instilled and a mixture of betamethasone and gentamicin (0.8 mL gentamycin, 0.3 mL betamethasone) is injected inferiorly under the conjunctiva

15. **What are the structures removed in trabeculectomy?**
From outside to inside:
i. Block of scleral tissue
ii. Schlemm's canal
iii. Trabecular meshwork
iv. Schwalbe's line
v. Block of the peripheral cornea
vi. Iris
(Tenon's removal is optional. Some surgeons prefer to remove it, as it is a source for fibroblasts.)

16. **What are the advantages of a fornix-based flap?**
    i. Easier to create
    ii. Good surgical exposure
    iii. Easier to identify surgical landmarks
    iv. Avoids postconjunctival scarring

17. **What are the disadvantages of a fornix-based flap?**
    i. Harder to excise Tenon's tissue
    ii. Spontaneous aqueous leak at the limbus in the early postoperative period
    iii. Caution when doing argon laser lysis of sclera flap sutures subconjunctival 5-fluorouracil (5-FU) injections and digital pressure in the early postoperative period
    iv. Late postoperative IOP not as low as a limbus-based flap

18. **What are the advantages of a limbus-based flap?**
    i. Easier to excise Tenon's tissue
    ii. Argon laser lysis of sclera flap sutures, subconjunctival 5-FU injections, and digital pressure can be done with more safety in the early postoperative period
    iii. Late postoperative IOP is lower

19. **What are the disadvantages of a limbus-based flap?**
    i. Anterior dissection of the conjunctival flap is difficult as an incision in the conjunctiva is made posterior to the fornix
    ii. Poor surgical exposure
    iii. More conjunctival manipulation

20. **Which are the more preferred limbus/fornix-based flaps?**
    Studies comparing fornix-based or limbus-based trabeculectomies have demonstrated equivalent success in IOP control both with and without antimetabolites.

21. **What is the problem with sclerostomy at 12 o'clock?**
    Bleeding from a perforating branch of an anterior ciliary vessel that passes through the sclera to enter the ciliary body 2–4 mm from the limbus.

22. **What are the preferred sites of sclerostomy for limbus- and fornix-based flaps?**
    i. Limbus-based—superotemporal quadrant as conjunctival incision can be made farther back in the fornix
    ii. Fornix-based—superonasal quadrant is adequate

23. **What is the purpose of a corneal incision?**
    A corneal incision provides an entry for the fluid into the AC at any stage of the operation.

24. What needles can one use for the corneal incision?
A dull needle can be used for corneal incision because the top of a sharp needle will get caught in the corneal stroma.

25. What is the disadvantage of bridle suture under the superior rectus tendon?
Subconjunctival hemorrhage may occur.

26. What are the reasons for doing an iridectomy with trabeculectomy?
i. To prevent iris incarceration in the sclerostomy with blockage of aqueous outflow if it shallows postoperatively
ii. To prevent pupillary block if posterior synechiae or a pupillary membrane develops secondary to postoperative intraocular inflammation

27. What should be the size of an iridectomy?
An iridectomy should be basal and wider than the opening in the AC so that the iris tissue does not block the opening.

28. When should the sclera flap be sutured more tightly?
i. Eyes with primary angle-closure glaucoma (PACG) and those with a history of malignant glaucoma
ii. Aphakic/highly myopic eyes prone to choroidal hemorrhage
iii. Nanophthalmic eye and eyes with elevated episcleral venous pressure prone to suprachoroidal infusion and flat AC

29. Why should a tenonectomy be done?
i. Improves visibility of the nylon sutures in the postoperative period
ii. Partially determines the effectiveness of suture lysis, which determines the final postoperative pressure

30. What should be used to reform the AC?
Usually done with BSS

Healon (sodium hyaluronate), it can maintain anterior chamber depth (ACD), prevent choroidal effusion or suprachoroidal hemorrhage, decrease the rate of postoperative hyphema, and delay scarring of the bleb. However, IOP may be higher in the early postoperative period.

31. Why is hemostasis essential in trabeculectomy surgery?
Hemostasis is essential in trabeculectomy surgery because blood in the AC under the conjunctival flap can produce scarring of the bleb and cause failure of filtration.

32. How can it be prevented?
i. The internal sclerostomy is made as far anteriorly as possible
ii. Ensure effective hemostasis by proper cautery during the operation; overcautery should not be done as the scleral flap will be thin

33. **What should be the postoperative evaluation of the eye?**
    i. Extent of the height of the bleb
    ii. Presence/absence of microcysts
    iii. Presence/absence of aqueous leak
    iv. Visibility of sclera flap sutures through the overlaying conjunctival flap
    v. IOP
    vi. Clarity of cornea
    vii. AC depth
    viii. AC inflammation
    ix. Hyphema
    x. Choroidal detachment/suprachoroidal hemorrhage
    xi. Optic disk and macular appearance

34. **What is the role of atropine 1% and scopolamine 0.25% postoperative?**
    By paralyzing the ciliary muscles, atropine 1% and scopolamine 0.25%:
    i. Tighten the zonular lens-iris diaphragm—maximally deepening the AC
    ii. Maintain blood-aqueous barrier
    iii. Give relief from ciliary spasm
    iv. Dilate the pupil
    v. Prevent the formation of posterior synechiae

35. **What are the factors contributing to poor prognosis in filtering surgery?**
    i. Age < 40 years
    ii. Previous failed filter
    iii. Aphakia/pseudophakia
    iv. Neovascular glaucoma
    v. Active uveitis
    vi. Congenital glaucoma
    vii. Congenital disease, e.g., Stevens-Johnson syndrome, ocular pemphigoid
    viii. Previous penetrating keratoplasty
    ix. Previous scleral buckle for retinal reattachment
    x. Previous topical medications
    xi. Chronic conjunctival inflammation
    xii. Previous conjunctival surgery

36. **What is the most common problem after trabeculectomy?**
    The most common problem after trabeculectomy is shallowing of the AC postoperatively.

37. **What are the main causes of a shallow AC for trabeculectomy?**
    Shallow AC can be associated with:
    i. *Hypotony:*
       - Wound leak
       - Excessive filtration
       - Serous choroidal detachment
    ii. *Raised IOP:*
       - Malignant glaucoma
       - Incomplete peripheral iridectomy with pupillary block
       - Delayed suprachoroidal hemorrhage

38. **What are the characteristics and treatment of wound leak?**
    Characteristics:
    i. Soft eye
    ii. Poor bleb
    iii. Positive Seidel's test

    Treatment:
    i. Immediate pressure dressing
    ii. Simmons scleral shell tamponade
    iii. Therapeutic soft contact lenses
    iv. Cyanoacrylate tissue adhesive covered with collagen shield
        If the defect is large, suturing of the defect, construction of a new conjunctival flap created posterior to the original flap, or a conjunctival autograft can be considered.

39. **What are the characteristics and treatment of excessive filtration?**
    Characteristics:
    i. Very low IOP
    ii. A good bleb
    iii. A negative Seidel's test
    iv. Choroidal detachment may be present

    Treatment:
    i. First step is firm patching
    ii. Simmons scleral shell
    iii. Therapeutic soft contact lenses
    iv. Aqueous suppressants (to promote spontaneous healing by temporarily reducing aqueous flow through the fistula)
    v. Atropine (to prevent pupillary block)
    vi. Steroids
        Surgical: Reformation of the AC with air, sodium hyaluronate or SF6, and drainage of choroidal detachment if they are very deep. Scleral flap and conjunctiva are resutured.

40. **What are the characteristic features, cause, and treatment of ciliary block glaucoma?**

    Features:
    i. Hard eye
    ii. No bleb
    iii. Negative Seidel's test

    Cause:
    - Blockage of aqueous flow at the secreting portion of the ciliary body so that it is forced backward into the vitreous

    Treatment:
    i. Strong topical mydriatics
    ii. If this fails, osmotic agents—intravenous (IV) mannitol
    iii. If the osmotic agent fails, the anterior hyaloid phase is disrupted through a patent iridectomy with an Nd:YAG laser
    iv. Needling of aqueous pockets in vitreous
    v. Removal of aqueous pockets from vitreous through sclerostomy and formation of AC by air through paracentesis
    vi. If laser therapy fails, an anterior vitrectomy via the pars plana should be performed with a vitreous cutter and the entrapped fluid removed

41. **What are the complications of postoperative shallowing of the AC?**
    i. Peripheral anterior synechiae
    ii. Corneal endothelial damage
    iii. Cataract

42. **What are the causes of failure of filtration?**
    i. *Intraocular factors:*
       - Obstruction of fistula by clot, iris, ciliary body, lens, vitreous
       - Bleb failure
       - Poor surgical techniques which prevent the exit of aqueous from the AC
    ii. *Extraocular factors:*
       - Subconjunctival fibrosis
       - Individual racial and genetic factors

43. **What is the most common cause for bleb failure?**
    The most common cause for bleb failure is subconjunctival fibrosis.

44. **What is the management of failure of filtration?**
    Two causes for failure of filtration:
    i. Obstruction of fistula by iris/ciliary body/lens or vitreous
    ii. Failing filtering bleb

If there is obstruction:
  i. Low-energy argon laser therapy can be done surrounding the obstruction.
  ii. Internal bleb revision

If failing bleb:
  i. Increase the steroids to hourly dosing
  ii. Digital pressure
  iii. Argon laser suturolysis: 50 µ spot size, 0.02–0.1 seconds, 250–1,000 mW power
  iv. If fibrin or clot is obstructing, intracameral tissue plasminogen activator (6–12.5 µg)
  v. Restart antiglaucoma medications
  vi. Repeat the filtering procedure with antimetabolites or drainage implants

45. How can the success rate of trabeculectomy be improved?

Preoperative techniques:
  i. Treat surface infections
  ii. Discontinue use of pilocarpine, aqueous suppressants, carbonic anhydrase inhibitor, and aspirin
  iii. Decrease the use of preservatives such as benzalkonium chloride (BAK)

Intraoperative techniques:
  i. Constriction of pupil
  ii. Prevent conjunctival buttonhole or scleral flap disinsertion
  iii. Internal ostium should be 1.5 × 2 mm. Iridectomy should be larger than this ostium to prevent blockage
  iv. Tight wound closure

Postoperative techniques:
By the use of antimetabolites which inhibit the wound healing. Antimetabolites used are as follows:
  i. Corticosteroids
  ii. 5-FU
  iii. Mitomycin C (MMC)
  iv. Suramin
  v. Beta radiation (strontium)
  vi. Tissue plasminogen activator
  vii. Gamma interferon
  viii. Calcium ionophores

46. What are the complications of antimetabolites?

The complications are more with MMC than 5-FU.

Most important complications are as follows:
  i. Early or late hypotony
  ii. Bleb leak
  iii. Bleb-related infection

Others are as follows:
Lids:
  i. Punctal occlusion (more with 5-FU)
  ii. Cicatricial ectropion

Conjunctiva:
  i. Wound and suture track leaks
  ii. Disintegration of Vicryl sutures

Cornea:
  i. Erosion
  ii. Ulcer
  Endothelial toxicity is common with mitomycin and epithelial toxicity is common with 5-FU
  i. Pupillary block
  ii. Cataracts
  iii. Hypotonous maculopathy
  iv. Choroidal hemorrhage
  v. Malignant glaucoma

47. What are the advantages of argon laser suture lysis?
  i. Scleral flap can be closed tightly intraoperatively
  ii. Decreases hypotony
  iii. Decreases choroidal separation
  iv. Decreases suprachoroidal hemorrhage
  v. Decreases the hospital stay

48. What are the instruments used for laser suture lysis?
  i. Hoskins suture lysis lens
  ii. Edge of four mirror gonio prism
  iii. High magnification Mandelkorn lens or Blumenthal lens

49. What is the role of aqueous humor in wound modulation?
Aqueous humor decreases the stimulation of fibroblasts as aqueous humor contains lots of factors to inhibit active inflammation. The bleb is formed permanently without fibrosis.

50. What is the role of postoperative digital pressure?
  i. Encourages flow of fluid through sclerostomy
  ii. Expands the filtering bleb
  iii. Prevents anatomic obstructions to filtration from becoming unalterable

51. When should digital pressure be applied?
Rather than waiting for a bleb to fail, if the IOP rises above 12 mm Hg or if the target pressure is not achieved, digital pressure should be applied.

52. What are the problems due to digital pressure?
　i. Small subconjunctival hemorrhages
　ii. Hyphema
　iii. Rupture of a filtering wound
　iv. Dehiscence of an incisional wound

53. What are the complications of trabeculectomy?
　i. Intraoperative
　ii. Early postoperative
　iii. Late postoperative

Intraoperative:
　i. Conjunctival buttonhole/perforation
　ii. Amputation of sclera flap
　iii. Flap related—thick, thin, irregular, and buttonholing
　iv. Hemorrhage
　v. Damage of lens
　vi. Vitreous loss
　vii. Choroidal effusion
　viii. Cyclodialysis cleft
　ix. Malignant glaucoma

Early postoperative:
　i. *Hypotony and flat AC:*
　　- Conjunctival defect
　　- Excessive filtration
　　- Serous choroidal detachment
　ii. *Hypotony and formed AC:*
　　- Hypotony maculopathy
　iii. *Raised IOP and flat AC:*
　　- Delayed suprachoroidal hemorrhage
　　- Malignant glaucoma
　　- Incomplete peripheral iridotomy (PI) with pupillary block
　iv. *Raised IOP with deep AC:*
　　- Obstruction of fistula
　　- Failing bleb
　v. Uveitis
　vi. Hyphema
　vii. Dellen
　viii. Loss of central vision
　ix. Ocular decompression retinopathy

Late postoperative:
  i. Bleb infection/endophthalmitis
  ii. Cataract
  iii. Dissection of filtering bleb into cornea
  iv. Leaking filtering bleb
  v. Cyst of Tenon's capsule
  vi. Hyphema
  vii. Pupillary membrane
  viii. Corneal edema
  ix. Failure of filtration
  x. Malignant glaucoma
  xi. Upper eyelid retraction
  xii. Scleral staphyloma
  xiii. Sympathetic ophthalmia

54. **What are the methods for repairing a conjunctival buttonhole?**
    i. Small pinpoint leaks can be sealed with cyanoacrylate glues or fibrin glues
    ii. Direct microsurgical repair
    iii. Wing suture technique
    iv. Glaucoma (Simmons) shell technique
    v. Purse string suture

55. **What care should be taken during trabeculectomy surgery in aphakic/highly myopic eyes?**
    Aphakic/highly myopic eyes are hypotonous and can develop intra-/suprachoroidal hemorrhage.

56. **How can a leaking filtering bleb be detected?**
    Many can be detected with 0.25% fluorescein; subtle leaks are seen with 2% fluorescein.

57. **How is a leaking bleb managed?**
    i. If the leak is minimal, chamber is of good depth, and bleb is pale and elevated, then conservative treatment is done.
    ii. Aqueous flow with blockers and carbonic anhydrase inhibitors
    iii. Topical antibiotic—gentamicin which irritates the conjunctiva and facilitates healing of the conjunctival defect
    iv. Patching of the eye to lid movement
    v. If associated with flat AC, glaucoma shells
    vi. If not effective, then surgical repair is done.

58. **What is the earliest evidence of a bleb infection?**
    Mild conjunctival hyperemia around the filtering bleb is the first sign. If treatment is delayed, there is a risk of endophthalmitis.

59. What is the treatment of bleb infection?
   i. Initial treatment is empirical
   ii. Topical antibiotics frequently
   iii. Topical steroids 12–24 hours after starting antibiotics

60. What are the common organisms involved in bleb-related endophthalmitis?
   i. *Haemophilus influenzae*
   ii. *Staphylococcus*
   iii. *Streptococcus*

61. What is the treatment of Tenon's cyst?
   i. Usually resolves spontaneously within 2–4 months
   ii. However, medical therapy may be needed to control IOP during this time

62. How is a corneal dellen formed and what is the treatment?
Localized disruption of the precorneal tear film → corneal dehydration causes stromal thinning and dellen formation
   i. Usually occurs in the horizontal plane within the lid fissure
   ii. Treatment—artificial tears and patching
       If ineffective, steroid drops are decreased

63. Why is trabeculectomy more successful in older patients?
   i. Atrophic Tenon's capsule
   ii. Decreased capacity for fibroblastic proliferation

64. What are the indicators for combined glaucoma and cataract surgery?
May be considered in patients with visually significant cataracts and:
   i. Inadequate control of IOP
   ii. Medication intolerance/poor compliance
   iii. Advanced glaucoma
   iv. Eyes requiring epinephrine compound
   v. Marginally functioning filter

65. What are the advantages of combined cataract surgery?
   i. Earlier visual rehabilitation owing to cataract extraction
   ii. Reduces the risk of early postoperative IOP spikes which is detrimental in the eyes with severely excavated ONH
   iii. A one-time single intervention eliminates the need for further surgery
   iv. Patient compliance is better

66. What are the disadvantages of combined approach?
   i. Long-term IOP control seems questionable owing to loss of bleb function from enhanced episcleral scarring

ii. Increased incidence of postoperative complications—hyphema, uveitis, shallow chambers, and hypotony

67. What are the advantages of two-stage procedure over combined procedure?

There is more decrease in IOP as plain trabeculectomy decreases IOP by 41%. There is a lesser risk of postoperative complications such as hyphema, inflammation, hypotony, and shallow AC.

68. What are the antimetabolites used routinely?

MMC and 5-FU.
Dosage: MMC: 0.2–0.5 mg/mL for 1–5 minutes
5-FU: 30 mg/mL for 5 minutes; subconjunctival dose is 5 mg.

69. What are the indications for adjuvant antimetabolite therapy?

High-risk factors:
  i. Neovascular glaucoma
  ii. Previous failed trabeculectomy or artificial filtering devices
  iii. Certain secondary glaucomas [e.g., inflammatory, post-traumatic angle recession, iridocorneal endothelial syndrome (ICE) syndrome]

Intermediate-risk factors:
  i. Patients on topical antiglaucoma medications (sympathomimetics) for 3 years
  ii. Previous conjunctival surgery
  iii. Previous cataract surgery

Low-risk factors:
  i. Black patients
  ii. Patients under the age of 40 years

70. What is the mechanism of action of 5-FU?

5-FU inhibits deoxyribonucleic acid (DNA) synthesis and is active in the "S" phase of the cell cycle. Fibroblastic proliferation is inhibited, but fibroblastic attachment and migration are unaffected.

71. What is the mechanism of action of MMC?

MMC is an alkylating agent which selectively inhibits DNA replication, mitosis, and protein synthesis. The drug inhibits proliferation of fibroblasts, suppresses vascular ingrowth, and is much more potent than 5-FU.

72. Where are the antimetabolites placed?

The antimetabolites are placed in the sub-Tenon's space as the most common cause for failure is subconjunctival fibrosis.

73. **Why is previous long-term use of medications associated with failure of trabeculectomy?**
    i. Increased fibroblastic proliferation in conjunctiva
    ii. Reduced goblet cells
    iii. Infiltration of conjunctiva with inflammatory cells

74. **What are the advantages of releasable sutures and laser suturolysis?**
    i. Can leave the eye with a firm pressure
    ii. Can protect the eye against low pressure and complications associated with low pressure
    iii. Can titrate the eye pressure postoperatively

75. **Name full-thickness surgeries.**
    i. Thermal sclerotomy (Scheie's procedure)
    ii. Sclerectomy—anterior lip sclerectomy and posterior lip sclerectomy
    iii. Trephination
    iv. Iridencleisis.

4.18 MODULATION OF WOUND HEALING IN GLAUCOMA FILTERING SURGERY

1. **What are the pharmacological techniques that interfere with wound healing to maintain the success of trabeculectomy?**
    i. The preoperative and postoperative administration of glucocorticosteroids to control inflammation and thereby scarring
    ii. The local intraoperative and postoperative administration of antineoplastic agents such as mitomycin C (MMC) and 5-fluorouracil (5-FU) to reduce fibroblast proliferation
    iii. The use of agents to interfere with the synthesis of normal collagen such as β-aminopropionitrile and penicillamine

2. **What is the role of corticosteroids in glaucoma filtering surgeries?**
    i. Corticosteroids control inflammation and immune response at multiple points
    ii. Anti-inflammatory mechanisms of corticosteroids include constriction of blood vessels, stabilization of lysosomes, inhibition of degranulation, impairment of leukocyte chemotaxis, reduction of lymphocyte proliferation, suppression of fibroplasia, inhibition of phospholipase A2 production, which subsequently prevents cyclooxygenase and lipoxygenase from producing prostaglandins, prostacyclins, thromboxanes, and leukotrienes

3. **What is the role of nonsteroidal anti-inflammatory drugs (NSAIDs) in glaucoma filtering surgeries?**
    i. NSAIDs are a heterogeneous group of agents that inhibit the enzyme cyclooxygenase from converting arachidonic acid into prostaglandins and thromboxanes
    ii. They have been demonstrated to inhibit the proliferation of human Tenon fibroblasts in culture

4. **What is the role of MMC in glaucoma filtering surgeries?**
    i. Mitomycin C is an alkylating agent isolated from the fermentation filtrate of *Streptomyces caespitosus*
    ii. It inhibits deoxyribonucleic acid (DNA)-dependent ribonucleic acid (RNA) synthesis and binds to cellular DNA sites on cell membranes, forming free radicals and chelating metal ions
    iii. Like 5-FU, mitomycin inhibits fibroblast proliferation, but unlike 5-FU, it affects cells in all phases

5. **Describe the methods of administration of MMC.**
    i. After outlining and partially dissecting the scleral flap to ensure the integrity of the scleral tissues, the conjunctiva is inspected to rule out the presence of any tears or buttonholes

ii. *MMC dilution:* The drug is available in a vial as purple-colored powder at a concentration of 2 mg/mL. It is further reconstituted with 5 mL of distilled water or normal saline to make 0.4 mg/mL or in 10 mL to make 0.2 mg/mL. When reconstituted to a concentration of 0.2 mg/mL, it is stable for 1 hour at room temperature
iii. An amputated tip of a 4.5 × 4.5 mm sized methylcellulose sponge soaked in a 0.2–0.5 mg/mL solution of MMC is then placed between the conjunctiva/Tenon's capsule and episclera for 1–5 minutes
iv. During this time, the edges of the conjunctival flap are pulled over the sponge so that the tissue edges are not exposed to the drug
v. The area is then rinsed with copious amounts of balanced salt solution
vi. A relatively tight scleral flap is prudent to reduce the likelihood of prolonged postoperative hypotony

6. **What are the side effects of MMC?**

Irritation:
   i. Lacrimation
   ii. Hyperemia
   iii. Photophobia
   iv. Ocular pain

Eyelids and conjunctiva:
   i. Allergic or irritative reactions
   ii. Erythema
   iii. Conjunctivitis
   iv. Avascularity
   v. Hyperemia
   vi. Blepharitis
   vii. Granuloma
   viii. Symblepharon

Cornea:
   i. Corneal melting
   ii. Edema
   iii. Erosion
   iv. Crystalline epithelial deposits
   v. Endothelial decompensation
   vi. Punctate keratitis
   vii. Delayed wound healing
   viii. Perforation
   ix. Recurrence of herpes simplex

Sclera:
   i. Scleral melting (necrotizing scleritis)
   ii. Delayed wound healing

iii. Avascularity
iv. Erosion
v. Perforation
vi. Calcium deposits

Uvea:
i. Iridocyclitis
ii. Hyperemia
iii. Hypopigmentation of the iris

Glaucoma

Punctal occlusion

Hypotony

7. **What is the role of 5-FU in glaucoma filtering surgeries?**
   i. 5-FU is a pyrimidine analog
   ii. It is a folic acid antagonist
   iii. It is active in the "S" phase (synthesis phase) of the cell cycle
   iv. The mechanism of action is to prevent the reduction of folic acid to tetrahydrofolic acid by noncompetitive enzyme inhibition. This results in the inhibition of DNA and RNA synthesis and eventual cell death
   v. Inhibition of fibroblast proliferation has been regarded as the primary mechanism by which 5-FU enhances and maintains bleb function

8. **Describe the methods of administration of 5-FU.**
   5-FU can be given as subconjunctival injections or as an intraoperative application.
   i. *Subconjunctival injection of 5-FU:*
      - Subconjunctival injection of 5-FU may be administered in an undiluted concentration (50 mg/mL), although many prefer to dilute it to 10 mg/mL
   ii. *Dilution:*
      - Five milligrams of the agent is drawn into a tuberculin syringe, after which the tuberculin needle is replaced with a 0.5-inch 30-gauge needle
      - After administration of a topical anesthetic, at least two cotton-tipped applicators soaked in 4% topical lidocaine are used to swab and further anesthetize the tissues at the proposed injection site
      - The injection is then given 90–180° from the trabeculectomy site
   iii. *Dosage:*
      - Twice daily for 1 week and once daily for the second week for a total of 21 injections (105 mg)

9. **What are the side effects of subconjunctival or intradermal 5-FU?**

   Irritation:
   i. Lacrimation
   ii. Ocular pain
   iii. Edema
   iv. Burning sensation

   Eyelids or conjunctiva:
   i. Cicatricial ectropion
   ii. Allergic reactions
   iii. Erythema
   iv. Hyperpigmentation
   v. Keratinization
   vi. Urticaria
   vii. Subconjunctival hemorrhages
   viii. Periorbital edema

   Cornea:
   i. Superficial punctate keratitis
   ii. Ulceration
   iii. Scarring stromal
   iv. Keratinized plaques
   v. Delayed wound healing
   vi. Endothelial damage

10. **How to choose an agent: 5-FU versus MMC?**
    i. Currently, intraoperative 5-FU with supplementary postoperative 5% FU injections are used in most primary filtering surgeries
    ii. 5% FU is also used in selected higher-risk cases, particularly those with MMC complications in a previous surgery or those at risk for hypotonous maculopathy
    iii. MMC is used in most high-risk cases, including aphakic or pseudophakic eyes, eyes with previous filtration failure surgery, eyes with a history of anterior segment neovascularization, and eyes with uveitis
    iv. MMC is also used in selected cases of primary filtering surgery (e.g., when trabeculectomy with 5-FU has failed in the fellow eye)

11. **What is the latest advancement in glaucoma filtering surgery?**
    Photodynamic therapy with diffuse blue light, coupled with a photosensitizing agent to kill fibroblasts, may be another way to control the surface area of treatment and modulate healing. It will be important to determine the effect of these agents on the overlying epithelium, because differentiated stable epithelium may have a suppressive effect on fibroblasts in the wound.

12. **What are the indications for antimetabolites in glaucoma filtering surgery?**
    i. *Patient factors:*
       - Young patients
       - Previous failed trabeculectomy
       - Previous conjunctival surgery (e.g., pterygium surgery)
    ii. *Ocular factors:*
       - Secondary glaucomas (neovascular, uveitic, traumatic, and pseudophakic glaucoma)
       - Congenital/pediatric glaucoma

13. **What are the measures to be taken to prevent antimetabolite toxicity?**
    i. Thorough irrigation after the prescribed time of application
    ii. Water-tight wound closure
    iii. Careful dissection to prevent buttonhole formation

14. **What is the role of Ologen in glaucoma filtering surgeries?**
    i. Composed of three-dimensional (3D) collagen-glycosaminoglycan copolymers (Ologen)
    ii. *Source:* Porcine collagen
    iii. *Mechanism of action:*
       - Provides a scaffold for fibroblasts to grow randomly
       - Absorbs the aqueous and functions like a reservoir
       - Provides pressure on the scleral flap to create controlled drainage of aqueous
       - Gets biodegraded by 90–180 days
    iv. *Advantages:*
       - Limits postoperative hypotony by the tamponading effect
       - Does not produce thin avascular blebs which are at risk for bleb infection and endophthalmitis
       - No special handling and disposal precautions
       - Not teratogenic like MMC
    v. *Disadvantage:* LASER suture lysis is difficult when sutures are covered by the implant and not clearly visible.

4.19 GLAUCOMA DRAINAGE DEVICES

1. **Define glaucoma drainage devices (GDDs) (aqueous shunt devices).**

   GDDs consist of an alloplastic tube leading to a large equatorial reservoir that drains aqueous humor from the anterior chamber (AC).

2. **Define setons.**

   Setons are solid stents or wicks, using the principle of surface-tension flow for fluid to exit the AC, while structurally intended to maintain a patent drainage fistula.

3. **Define shunts.**

   Shunts are hollow tubular structures that allow bidirectional flow. [Open-tubed devices have been synthesized to serve as *shunts*, secured translimbally to allow flow subconjunctivally (e.g., Molteno or Baerveldt implants)].

4. **Define valves.**

   Valves allow unidirectional flow which need an activating pressure to open it. For example, Krupin or Ahmed valves.

5. **What are the common features of all GDDs?**
   i. Manufacturing drainage tubes and explant portions of the devices from materials to which fibroblasts cannot firmly adhere
   ii. Equatorial placement of the explant portion of the device
   iii. Similar diameter of all drainage tubes
   iv. Ridge along the edge of the explant plate where drainge tube inserts ensures optimal functioning of the GDD

6. **What is the principle of GDD?**

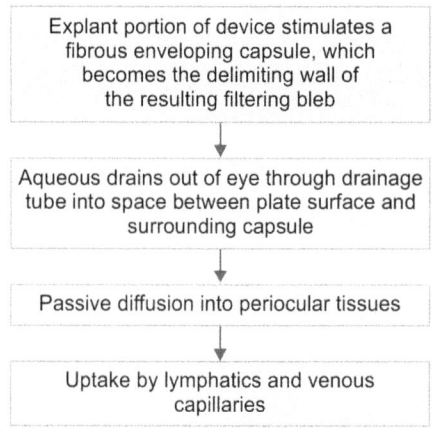

7. What are the factors that decide the hydraulic conductivity of GDD?

The drainage capacity of the bleb is directly proportional to the surface area of the capsule around the explants. The resistance of the capsule to flow is directly proportional to its thickness.

8. What are the indications of GDD?

All refractory glaucomas such as:
  i. Uveitic glaucoma
  ii. Neovascular glaucoma
  iii. Congenital glaucoma
  iv. Refractory juvenile glaucoma
  v. Multiple failed trabeculectomy
  vi. Extensive conjunctival scarring
  vii. Post-penetrating keratoplasty (PKP)
  viii. Aniridia
  ix. Post-traumatic glaucoma

Failed primary glaucomas

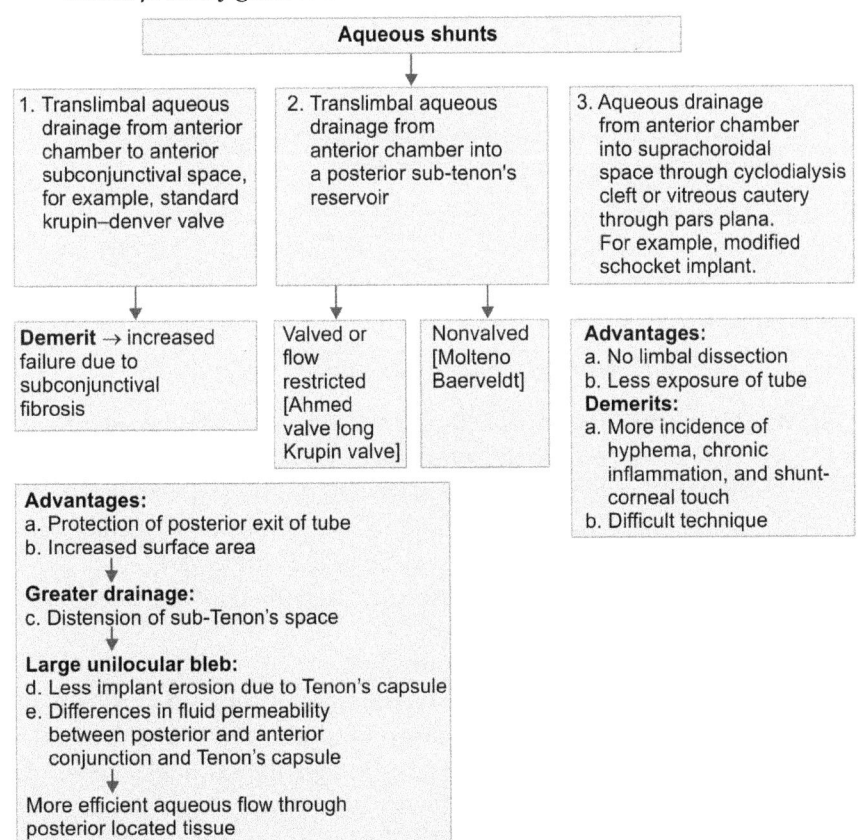

9. **Describe the Molteno implant.**
   i. The first implant with a nonvalved device
   ii. Material—polypropylene
   iii. Consists of a circular plate with a drainage tube
   iv. Outer diameter of drainage tube—0.63 mm
   v. Inner diameter of drainage tube—0.3 mm
   vi. Types—single plate, double plate, and triple plate

10. **Describe the Baerveldt implant.**
    i. Nonvalved
    ii. Material—silicone

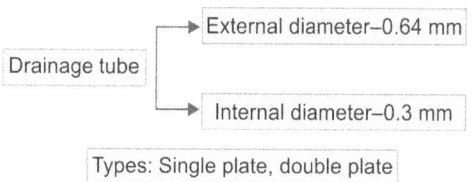

Types: Single plate, double plate

11. **What are the advantages of Baerveldt GDD?**

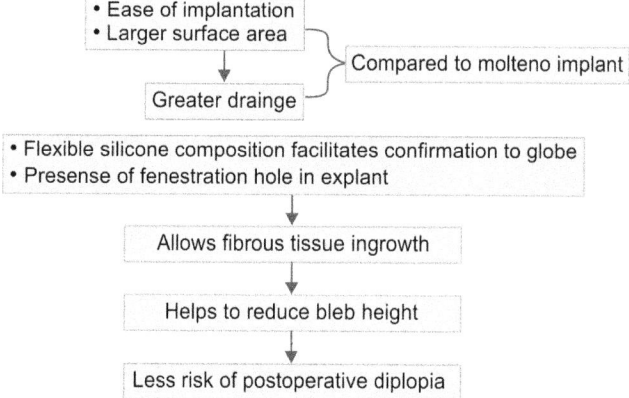

12. **What is the mechanism of action of the Ahmed glaucoma valve?**
    i. An oval-shaped polypropylene plate with 184 mm^2 (double plate—364 mm^2) surface area is connected to a silicone drainage tube via two layers of the silicone elastomer membrane that functions as a one-way valve by Venturi effect (Bernoulli's principle)
    ii. The goal is to keep the intraocular pressure (IOP) between 8 and 10 mm Hg
    iii. Venturi design (Bernoulli's principle)
    The tension on the silicone membranes is designed to only allow outflow when the IOP is above 8–10 mm Hg. When the initial pressure in the anterior chamber is high, the valve fully opens. As the pressure is reduced, the membrane opening automatically reduces in size, diminishing the flow.

13. **Describe the OptiMed glaucoma pressure regulator.**
    OptiMed glaucoma pressure regulator consists of a silicone tube attached to a polymethyl methacrylate matrix of conductive resistors that regulate the flow of aqueous through capillary action.

14. **What is the preoperative evaluation in a case of GDDs.**
    i. Potential for useful vision is a must
    ii. Preoperative IOP
    iii. Upper lid position
    iv. Scleral exposure
    v. Tear film stability
    vi. Blepharitis (risk of late postoperative infection)
    vii. Corneal clarity, especially peripheral cornea, for intraoperative confirmation of tube location
    viii. Eyes with posterior chamber intraocular lens (PCIOL)
        - Shallow AC
        - Post-PKP eyes
        - Endothelial cell function
          (All the abovementioned risk factors are indications for GDD with pars plana tube insertion into the vitreous cavity.)
    ix. Presence of vitreous strands in AC → may occlude the tube tip
    x. Cataract—for concurrent cataract surgery and GDD
    xi. Gonioscopy
        - Assesses peripheral anterior synechiae (PAS) → areas to be avoided for tube insertion (PAS)
        - Neovascularization of the angle
        - Preoperative treatment to halt the

    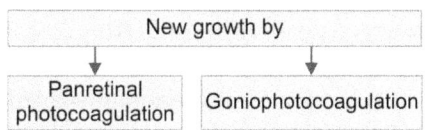

15. **What are the drugs to be stopped preoperatively?**
    i. Pilocarpine or echothiophate
       (to reduce postoperative inflammation)
       Continue all other glaucoma drugs till surgery
    ii. Warfarin

16. **What are the types of surgical techniques for GDD implantation?**

Limbal-based conjunctival flap	Fornix-based conjunctival flap
• Two-layer closure securing	• If tissue coverage over the device is adequate
• Tenon's capsule and conjunctiva with separate running layers of absorbable sutures	↓
	• Suturing only at lateral corners of flap

i. *One-stage installation:*
   - One-stage complete surgical installation with immediate function, done with devices that have flow restrictors or valves
ii. *Two-stage installation:*
   - Temporary ligature of tube on a nonvalved device for 2–3 weeks
   - Time for the development of the capsule and acceptable resistance to outflow

17. **What are the types of temporary ligature sutures?**
    i. Rip cord—intraluminal occluding sutures left beneath the conjunctiva for pulling (4-0 chromic catgut)
    ii. Absorbable 8-0 polyglactin or 10-0 prolene tied around the tube (released by argon laser suturolysis)
    iii. 5-0 nylon tied to the side of the tube and to an adjacent occluding structure, like a spacer, which is removed after 2–3 weeks

18. **What is the cause of hypotony in both single- and double-stage techniques?**
    Hypotony can occur due to leakage around the surface of the tube, where it penetrates the eye wall.

19. **What is the difference between GDD bleb and trabeculectomy bleb?**
    Features of GDD bleb:
    i. More posterior filtering bleb
    ii. More consistently organized surrounding capsule which is distinct and separable from overlying Tenon's capsule
    iii. Absence of conjunctival microcysts as seen in trabeculectomy

20. **What is the preferred positioning of GDD?**
    i. Superotemporal quadrant
    ii. Centered at the equator and equally spaced between adjacent rectus muscles
    iii. Anterior edge of the explant
       ↓
       8–10 mm posterior to the corneoscleral junction
    iv. Explant plates are sutured to the episclera
       ↓
       Complication encountered
       ↓
       Perforation of sclera

21. **How do you manage/identify perforation of the sclera?**
    i. Identification → gush of vitreous gel is seen
    ii. Management → apply cryotherapy to the area
        Under direct observation by an indirect ophthalmoscope

22. **When do you suture the explant to the avascular insertion of the superior rectus (instead of the episclera)?**
    i. Staphyloma
    ii. Quiescent scleritis

23. **What are the complications of the superonasal placement of GDD?**
    i. Vertical strabismus—pseudo-Brown's syndrome
    ii. Impact on the optic nerve

24. **What are the instances where the GDD can migrate?**
    i. Inadequate suturing
       ↓
       Posterior migration of explant
       ↓
       Extrusion of the tube from the AC
    ii. Postoperative hypotony
       ↓
       Drainage tube migrates anteriorly and impacts the cornea, lens, or iris.

25. **Where do you place the second plate in an explant with two plates?**
    The second plate and its interconnecting tube are placed either above or below the superior rectus muscle and attached by suturing in a similar manner to the first plate.

26. **How do you install the drainage tube?**

AC installation	Pars plana installation

• Tube shortened to the appropriate length with a sharp level to facilitate passage through a 23-gauge needle tract
  Tip → Beveled up surface
• Site of insertion
  ↓
  Posterior edge of blue limbus
• Preparation of the site of insertion
  ↓
  Use wet field cautery
• 1.5–2 mm of the tube should extend through the endothelium parallel to the plane of the iris (prevents migration)
	• Indications
	  – Aphakia and PCIOL eyes
	  – Post-PKP eyes
	  – Eyes with shallow AC
	  – Decreased endothelial cell function
	• Tip → Beveled down
	• Needle tract oriented perpendicularly to the scleral surface, 3–4 mm posterior to the limbus
	• Verify tube tip by direct visualization that it is free of vitreous
	• Precautions:
	  – Complete pars plana vitrectomy
	    ↓
	  – Clearance of vitreous base in the quadrant of tube insertion

27. **What are the advantages of the installation of a drainage tube through 21- or 23-gauge needle tract compared to the traditional sclerectomy?**
    i. Ensures a tight fit
    ii. Prevents aqueous leak around the tube

28. **What are the advantages of a scleral patch graft?**
    - Covering the portion of the tube exposed to lid contact (usually 3–5 mm of the tube)

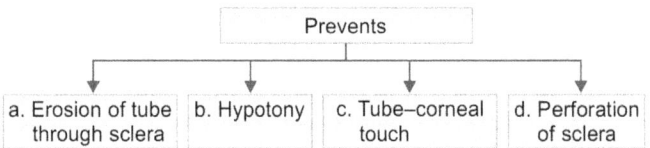

29. **How is the technique of a scleral patch graft performed?**
    A full-thickness scleral patch graft is taken according to the required size.
    ↓
    A nonoccluding mattress suture is usually placed over the tube near its insertion.

30. **What are the complications of a scleral patch graft?**
    i. Abrupt elevation of limbal conjunctiva
        ↓
        Corneal dellen formation
    ii. Scleral melt

31. **What is the role of intracameral hyaluronic acid (Healon)?**
    Reforming the AC with intracameral hyaluronic acid at the end of the procedure through a paracentesis entry helps in:
    i. Decreasing postoperative hypotony and flat AC
    ii. Intraoperative evaluation of tube position
    iii. Slows the process of aqueous drainage in the immediate postoperative period

32. **Compare valved and nonvalved GDD.**
    i. Advantage of valved → simple one-step procedure
    ii. Advantages regarding clinical safety and efficacy not clear over a short-term/long-term follow-up, appear to be equal

33. **What is the principle behind the sizing of nonvalved devices?**
    i. Larger devices → younger, healthier eyes
    ii. Smaller devices → older, sicker eyes

34. How do you implant a modified Schocket device?

A bent 18-gauge needle is inserted into a sharp buckle capsule incision
↓
A segment of side-perforated tubing is fed into the needle bore of the 18-gauge needle and pulled into the buckle capsule. (Segmented side perforated tubing later becomes the intracapsular portion.)
↓
The tube segment is placed between the buckle capsule and the AC.
↓
Tight closure of buckle capsule incision
↓
An anchoring suture of 10° prolene is placed to prevent the tube from slipping.

35. What is the level of IOP reduction as compared to trabeculectomy?

The percentage of IOP reduction achieved in GDD is less compared to trabeculectomy.

36. What are the contraindicated postoperative medications?

Increases vascularization of bleb capsule
  i. Miotics
  ii. α agonists

37. What are the complications of aqueous shunt surgery?

Intraoperative:
  i. *Hyphema:* Injury to the iris root with tube insertion
  ii. *Lens damage:* Improper tube length or direction
  iii. *Lens or corneal endothelial damage:* Needle tip trauma
  iv. Scleral perforation and retinal tear; needle injury while suturing the plate to the globe
  v. *Hypotony:* Sclerotomy site too wide for the tube, incomplete tube occlusion

Early postoperative
  i. *IOP elevation before occluding suture absorbs:* Risk for nerves with advanced damage
  ii. *Dellen:* Elevated conjunctiva over the patch graft causing poor tear lubrication
  iii. *Hypotony:* Excessive aqueous run-off with flat AC and choroidal effusion
  iv. *Intraocular inflammation:* Marked in eyes with chronic uveitis
  v. *Suprachoroidal hemorrhage:* Postoperative hypotony and high preoperative IOP
  vi. *Transient diplopia:* Edema within the orbit and rectus muscles
  vii. *Endophthalmitis:* Direct intraoperative contamination

viii. *Aqueous misdirection:* Initial postoperative hypotony and choroidal swelling

Late postoperative:
  i. *Cataract progression:* With or without direct mechanical injury, prolonged hypotony
  ii. *Chorioretinal folds:* Prolonged hypotony
  iii. *Chronic iritis:* History of uveitis or neovascularization
  iv. Corneal edema and graft failure; with or without cornea touch
  v. Persistent elevated IOP after tube open; thick fibrous capsule
  vi. *Hypotony maculopathy:* Excessive aqueous fluid runoff
  vii. Inadequate IOP control with properly functioning Baerveldt glaucoma drainage device: Hypertensive phase
  viii. *Motility disturbance, strabismus, diplopia:* Bleb displacement of the globe, muscle fibrosis
  ix. *Patch graft melting:* Tube or plate erosion associated with poor lid closure, dry eye
  x. *Retinal detachment:* Scleral perforation, underlying disease such as diabetic retinopathy
  xi. Tube occlusion; blood, fibrin, iris, or vitreous
  xii. *Tube migration:* Poor fixation of the plate to the sclera
  xiii. *Endophthalmitis:* Associated with tube exposure

38. How do you manage erosion of the tube?

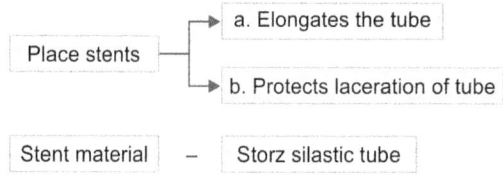

39. What are the phases of GDD surgery postoperatively?
Hypertensive phase
Hypotensive phase
Transient ↑ IOP
in immediate postoperative.

40. What are the recent advances in GDD?
  i. iStent
  ii. Hydrus Schlemm's canal scaffold ivantis insertion
  iii. Cypass (suprachoroidal microstents)
  iv. Trabectome (internal trabeculotomy)

41. What is an Ex-PRESS shunt?
The Ex-PRESS shunt consists of a small stainless steel tube (equivalent to a 26-gauge needle) with a barbed end to anchor it in the trabecular tissue, through which it is placed on a stent and secured without suture.

4.20 CYCLODESTRUCTIVE PROCEDURES

1. **Classify cyclodestructive procedures.**
   Based on the destructive energy source:
   i. Diathermy
   ii. β-irradiation
   iii. Electrolysis
   iv. Cryotherapy
   v. Laser photocoagulation
   vi. Therapeutic ultrasound
   vii. Microwave cyclodestruction

   Based on the route by which the energy reaches the ciliary process:
   i. Transscleral
   ii. Transpupillary
   iii. Intraocular

2. **Describe the technique of penetrating cyclodiathermy.**
   Penetration of the sclera (with or without preparation of a conjunctival flap):
   Site: 2.5–5 mm from the corneolimbal junction
      A 1–1.5 mm electrode is used.
   Current: 40–45 mA
   Duration: 10–20 seconds
   One or two rows of lesions placed several millimeters apart for approximately 180°

3. **What is the mechanism of action in cyclodiathermy?**
   i. Cell death within the ciliary body
   ii. More posteriorly placed lesions create a draining fistula in the area of pars plana

4. **What are the demerits of diathermy?**
   i. Low success rate
   ii. Hypotony
   iii. Phthisical eye

5. **What is the newer diathermy?**
   One pole diathermy unit

6. **Describe the mechanism of action of cyclocryotherapy.**
   The ability of the ciliary process to produce aqueous humor is destroyed by two mechanisms:
   i. Intracellular ice crystal formation
   ii. Ischemic necrosis

7. What is the additional effect of cyclocryotherapy other than intraocular pressure (IOP)?

Cyclocryotherapy also causes destruction of corneal nerves and thus causes relief from pain.

8. Describe the technique of cyclocryotherapy.

Instruments:
 i. Nitrous oxide or carbon dioxide gas cryosurgical units
 ii. Cryoprobe tips ranging from 1.5 to 4 mm. Commonly, 2.5 mm is suggested for cyclocryotherapy

Cryoprobe placement:
 i. Placement of the anterior edge of the probe, firmly on the sclera, 1 mm from the corneolimbal junction temporally, inferiorly, and nasally, and 1 mm superiorly

Number of cryoapplications:
 i. Two to three quadrants → three to four applications per quadrant
 ii. Rule of thumb → treat <180° or 6 applications in each treatment session

Freezing technique:
 i. Temperature: 60–80°C
 ii. Duration: 60 seconds

Postoperative management:
 i. Systemic analgesics
 ii. Topical corticosteroids—frequently
 iii. Cycloplegics
 iv. Preoperative glaucoma medications except miotics

9. What is the minimum time interval between repeated cyclotherapy?

The minimum time interval between repeated cyclotherapy is 1 month.

10. What is the additional measure taken for proper cryoprobe placement over the ciliary process in cases of distorted anatomic landmarks, e.g., buphthalmos?

The additional measure taken is transillumination (for delineating the pars plicata).

11. List the complications of cyclocryotherapy.

 i. Transient rise of IOP
 ii. Uveitis
 iii. Pain
 iv. Hyphema
 v. Hypotony and sometimes phthisis—best avoided by treating a limited area each time

vi. Choroidal detachment
vii. Intravitreal neovascularization causing vitreous hemorrhage
viii. Anterior segment ischemia
ix. Lens subluxation
x. Sympathetic ophthalmia

12. **List the indications for cyclocryotherapy/transscleral photocoagulation.**
    i. Relief for refractory ocular pain secondary to increased IOP in blind eyes
    ii. Repeated failure of other glaucoma surgeries
    iii. Glaucoma following penetrating keratoplasty (PKP)
    iv. Chronic open-angle glaucoma in aphakia
    v. Congenital glaucoma
    vi. High-risk cases in which medical and other glaucoma surgical procedures have failed or not felt to be feasible
    vii. Patient who requires urgent IOP reduction but who is too sick to undergo incisional surgery

13. **Describe the mechanism of action of transscleral cyclophotocoagulation.**
    i. *Reduced aqueous production:* Due to damage of pars plicata due to direct destruction of ciliary epithelium and reduced vascular perfusion
    ii. *Increased aqueous outflow:* Due to increased pars plana or transscleral outflow

14. **What are the types of lasers used in transscleral cyclophotocoagulation?**
    i. Nd:YAG lasers (yttrium–aluminum-garnet): 1,064 nm
    ii. Semiconductor diode lasers: 750–810 nm
    iii. Krypton lasers

15. **What is the advantage of diode laser over Nd:YAG laser in cyclophotocoagulation?**
    i. The energy needed to produce comparable lesions is less with the diode laser than that required with the Nd:YAG laser
    ii. Primarily because of the smaller size and greater durability of diode lasers, transscleral diode cyclophotocoagulation is currently the most commonly performed cyclodestructive procedure
    iii. Transscleral diode cyclophotocoagulation has the advantage of being quick and easy to perform

16. **What are the advantages of semiconductor diode lasers?**
    i. Greater absorption by uveal melanin
    ii. Solid-state construction with compact size (portable)
    iii. Low maintenance requirements

17. **What are the types of cryoprobes?**

Diameter	Indications
1 mm	Intracapsular cataract extraction (ICCE)
2 mm	Retinal cryotherapy
2.5–4 mm	Cyclocryotherapy
>4 mm	Hammerhead probe —Treatment of malignant melanoma

18. **Describe the preoperative preparation of the patient in laser cycloablation.**
    i. Retrobulbar anesthesia is usually preferred over peribulbar
    ii. Contralateral eye is patched to prevent the entry of stray laser light

19. **What is the role of contact lens in the Nd:YAG noncontact thermal mode?**
    i. Maintains lid separation
    ii. Compresses and blanches the conjunctiva. Allows more energy to reach the ciliary body
    iii. Provides measurement from the limbus (applying laser 0.5–1.5 mm behind the limbus is optimum)
    iv. Reduces laser backscatter at the air-tissue interface
    v. A higher incidence of phthisis is observed when the laser is applied with contact lens

20. **What is the protocol commonly followed for noncontact transscleral cyclophotocoagulation (Nd:YAG)?**
    i. 30-40 evenly spaced lesions for 360°
    ii. Approximately eight applications per quadrant
    iii. Spare the 3 and 9 o'clock positions from laser applications due to long posterior ciliary vessels underneath

21. **What is the minimum time interval before retreatment in transscleral laser cyclophotocoagulation?**
    i. 1 month
    ii. Two-third of cases do not require retreatments

22. **In which condition is contact Nd:YAG transscleral cyclophotocoagulation indicated over a noncontact laser?**
    i. Pediatric patients with refractory glaucoma

23. **Describe the complications of transscleral cyclophotocoagulation.**
    i. Conjunctival hyperemia
    ii. Uveitis
    iii. Malignant glaucoma
    iv. Sympathetic ophthalmia
    v. Ocular hypotony

24. **What are the measures taken to prevent full-thickness sclerostomies?**
    i. Use of well-rounded, polished tips
    ii. Prior to treatment, inspect the probes to make sure that they are free of mucus and other debris
    iii. Constantly keep the eyeball moist

25. **What are the factors that influence the variability of tissue response in contact delivery systems?**
    i. Probe pressure
    ii. Probe diameter
    iii. Time of probe contact

26. **What is the prerequisite for transpupillary cyclophotocoagulation?**
    i. A sufficient number of ciliary processes (at least a quarter) must be visualized gonioscopically

27. **Describe the technique of transpupillary cyclophotocoagulation.**
    i. Argon laser
    ii. *Spot size:* 100–200 µ
    iii. *Duration:* 0.1–0.2 seconds
    iv. *Energy level:* 700–1,000 mW
    v. *Desired effect:* Produces a white discoloration as well as a brown concave burn with pigment dispersion or gas bubbles
    vi. All the visible portions of ciliary processes are treated
    vii. Three to five applications for each process
    viii. All visible processes treated up to a total of 180°

28. **What are the factors that decide the outcome of transpupillary cyclophotocoagulation?**
    i. Number of ciliary processes that can be visualized and treated
    ii. Intensity of laser burns to each process
    iii. Angle at which ciliary processes are visualized gonioscopically

29. **What are different types of intraocular photocoagulation?**
    i. With transpupillary visualization
    ii. With endoscopic visualization (argon or diode laser)

30. **Describe the technique of therapeutic ultrasound.**
    i. Immersion applicator or contact ultrasound (contains a distensible rubber membrane that can be inflated)
    ii. Six to seven exposures of ultrasound delivered at an intensity level of 10 kW/cm^2 for 5 seconds each to scleral sites near the limbus

31. **What is transscleral microwave cyclodestruction?**
    Direct application of high-frequency electromagnetic radiation over conjunctiva causes heat-induced damage to the ciliary body and causes a decreased production of aqueous humor.

32. **Describe the mechanism of action by which ultrasound works to decrease IOP.**

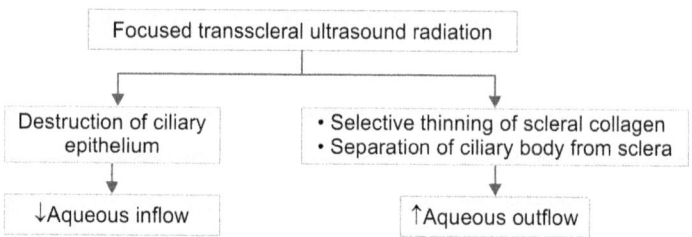

4.21 IMPORTANT GLAUCOMA STUDIES

1. **What are the important landmark studies in glaucoma?**
    i. Ocular Hypertension Treatment Study (OHTS)
    ii. Collaborative Initial Glaucoma Treatment Study (CIGTS)
    iii. Early Manifest Glaucoma Trial (EMGT)
    iv. Advanced Glaucoma Intervention Study (AGIS)
    v. Tube versus Trabeculectomy (TvT) study

2. **What are the findings of the Ocular Hypertension Treatment Study (OHTS)?**
    Treating abnormally elevated intraocular pressure (IOP), especially in high-risk individuals, with topical medications delays or prevents the onset of glaucomatous damage.

3. **What are the findings of the Collaborative Initial Glaucoma Treatment Study (CIGTS)? (Drugs vs surgery)**
    i. Consider surgery first in patients with moderate or advanced disease
    ii. African-American patients and diabetics, however, do not do well with initial surgery
    iii. Filtering surgery is easier before eye drops are used
    iv. Surgery reduces IOP spikes
    v. Major surgical complications were few

4. **What are the findings of the Early Manifest Glaucoma Trial (EMGT)?**
    i. Pressure lowering is beneficial in glaucoma treatment in all clinical situations
    ii. Every 1 mm Hg of IOP reduction was associated with a risk reduction of 10–13%
    iii. Disease progression in patients can be variable
    iv. Mean IOP, not fluctuation, is what matters (in contrast to CIGTS)

5. **What are the results of the Collaborative Normal-Tension Glaucoma Study (CNTG)?**
    i. Glaucoma progression was slower in the treated group
    ii. Patients who had filtering surgery were more likely than the other patient groups to develop cataracts

6. **What are the results of the Advanced Glaucoma Intervention Study (AGIS)?**
    i. Lower mean IOP results in a reduced risk of visual field progression

ii. Patients were randomized to receive argon laser trabeculoplasty (ALT)–trabeculectomy–trabeculectomy (ATT) or trabeculectomy–ALT–trabeculectomy (TAT)
iii. African-American patients were better off with ALT first (ATT)

7. **What are the results of Tube versus Trabeculectomy (TvT) study?**
    i. Tubes were as useful as trabeculectomy even in early cases
    ii. Shunts (tubes) had a higher long-term success rate and lower complications
    iii. Trabeculectomy had quicker pressure control.

CHAPTER 5

Lens and Cataract

1. **What is the size of the adult human lens?**
   The adult human lens measures 9 mm equatorially and 5 mm anteroposteriorly. It weighs approximately 255 mg.

2. **What are the changes in the eye during accommodation?**
   i. Contraction of the ciliary muscle
   ii. Decrease in ciliary ring diameter
   iii. Decrease in zonular tension
   iv. More spherical shape of the lens
   v. Decrease in lens equatorial diameter
   vi. Increased axial lens thickness
   vii. Steepening of the central anterior lens curvature
   viii. Increased lens dioptric power

3. **What is the level of amplitude of accommodation?**
   i. Adolescents have 12–16 D of accommodation
   ii. Adults at 40 years have 4–8 D
   iii. After 50 years, accommodation reduces to 2 D

4. **What is lenticonus?**
   i. Lenticonus is a congenital, localized cone-shaped deformation of the anterior or posterior lens surface
   ii. Anterior lenticonus is uncommon, bilateral, and associated with Alport's syndrome
   iii. Posterior lenticonus is more common, unilateral, and axial

5. **What are the associated ocular anomalies of anterior and posterior lenticonus?**
   i. *Anterior lenticonus-associated ocular anomalies:*
      - Dot-and-fleck retinopathy
      - Posterior polymorphous corneal dystrophy
      - Temporal macular thinning
      - Subcapsular and cortical cataract
   ii. *Posterior lenticonus-associated ocular anomalies:*
      - Amblyopia
      - Subcapsular and cortical cataract
      - Strabismus
      - Glaucoma (in Lowe syndrome)

6. **What are the types of lens coloboma?**
   i. *Primary coloboma:* Isolated wedge-shaped defect or indentation
   ii. *Secondary coloboma:* Defect or indentation of the lens periphery caused by the lack of ciliary body or zonular development

7. **How do you treat presbyopia during cataract surgery?**
   i. Monovision
   ii. Multifocal intraocular lens (IOL)
   iii. Accommodating IOL

8. **What is Mittendorf dot?**
   Mittendorf dot is a remnant of the posterior pupillary membrane of the tunica vasculosa lentis and is located inferonasal to the posterior pole of the lens.

9. **What are the common causes of microspherophakia?**
   i. Weill–Marchesani syndrome
   ii. Marfan's syndrome
   iii. Peter's anomaly
   iv. Alport's syndrome
   v. Lowe syndrome

10. **What is the type of glaucoma seen in microspherophakia?**
    Inverse glaucoma, which is pupillary block glaucoma, is associated with microspherophakia.

    Here, miotics aggravate the condition by stimulating the ciliary muscle contraction, thereby loosening zonules and further increasing anterior displacement.

    Mydriatics tighten the zonules and are the preferred treatment.

11. **What are the common causes of cataracts in children?**
    i. *Bilateral cataracts:*
       - Idiopathic
       - Hereditary cataracts
       - Maternal infections such as rubella, cytomegalovirus (CMV), varicella, and syphilis
       - Ocular anomalies such as aniridia and anterior segment dysgenesis syndrome
    ii. *Unilateral cataracts:*
       - Idiopathic
       - Trauma
       - Persistent fetal vasculature
       - Posterior pole tumors

12. **What are the indications for cataract surgery in children?**
    i. Dense cataract obstructing view of fundus
    ii. Cataract >3 mm in diameter

iii. Associated with strabismus/nystagmus
   iv. Visual acuity <6/24

13. **What is the timing of surgical intervention in pediatric cataracts?**
    i. Bilateral dense cataracts require early surgery within 6-8 weeks
    ii. Unilateral dense cataracts should be operated as soon as possible

14. **What are the surgical challenges faced in pediatric cataract?**
    i. Difficulty in capsulorrhexis formation due to very elastic anterior capsule
    ii. Soft lens
    iii. Positive intravitreal pressure due to well-formed vitreous
    iv. Wound leak due to low scleral and corneal rigidity

15. **What are the conditions which can cause poorer visual results following cataract surgery in children?**
    i. Unilateral cataracts carry a poorer prognosis than bilateral cataracts
    ii. Patients with nystagmus
    iii. If adequate visual rehabilitation or treatment of amblyopia is not carried out

16. **What are the causes of ectopia lentis?**
    i. Marfan's syndrome
    ii. Homocystinuria
    iii. Aniridia
    iv. Congenital glaucoma
    v. Trauma
    vi. Ehlers-Danlos syndrome
    vii. Sulfite oxidase deficiency
    viii. Hyperlysinemia
    ix. Ectopia lentis at papillae

17. **What are the features of Marfan's syndrome?**
    i. *Systemic:*
       - Arachnodactyly
       - Long arm span
       - Chest deformities
       - Mitral valve prolapse
       - Dilated aortic root
       - High arched palate
    ii. *Ocular:*
       - Axial myopia
       - Hypoplasia of dilator pupillae (difficulty in dilatation)
       - Superotemporal subluxation of lens
       - Pupillary block glaucoma
       - Retinal detachment (RD)

18. **What is the lens status in various syndromes?**
    i. *Marfan's syndrome:* Superotemporal subluxation with the presence of zonules
    ii. *Homocystinuria:* Lens subluxation inferiorly with absent zonules
    iii. *Weill–Marchesani:* Lens subluxation inferiorly along with microspherophakia

19. **What are the drugs which can cause cataracts?**
    i. Corticosteroids
    ii. Phenothiazines and other antipsychotics
    iii. Topical miotics
    iv. Amiodarone
    v. Statins.

20. **What is Vossius ring?**
    The imprinting of the pupillary ruff onto the anterior surface of the lens due to blunt trauma is termed Vossius ring.

21. **What are the characteristic types of cataract in specific situations?**
    i. *Trauma:* Rosette cataract
    ii. *Infrared rays (Glassblowers cataract):* Exfoliative cataract
    iii. *Chalcosis:* Sunflower cataract
    iv. *Diabetes:* Snow-flake cataract
    v. *Myotonic dystrophy:* Polychromatic crystals in a Christmas tree pattern.

22. **What are the experimental medical agents tried for reversal of cataracts?**
    i. Aldose reductase inhibitors
    ii. Aspirin
    iii. Glutathione-raising agents

23. **What are the indications for cataract surgery?**
    i. Reduced visual function due to cataract
    ii. Lens-induced disease such as phacolysis, phacoanaphylaxis, and phacomorphic angle closure
    iii. Second eye cataract surgery to improve stereopsis and reduce anisometropia
    iv. Cataract-limiting assessment or treatment of posterior segment disease
    v. Refractive lens extraction (clear lens), particularly in high ametropia

24. **What are the common types of cataract?**
    i. *Cortical cataracts:* Characterized by spokes, water clefts, and vacuoles due to osmotic imbalances in lens epithelial cells

ii. *Nuclear cataract:* Result from accumulation of protein aggregates becoming more harder with time
　　　iii. *Posterior subcapsular cataract:* Associated with diabetes, steroid use, and ocular inflammation

25. **What is posterior polar cataract (PPC)?**
　　PPC forms early in life and may become more clinically significant over time. It is bilateral in 65–80% of cases. PPC often arises at the end of the hyaloid artery remnant, which results in range of pathology from benign Mittendorf dot to more clinically relevant cataract.

26. **Name the classifications of PPC.**
　　Duke Elder classification:
　　　i. Stationary—central opacity with bull's eye ring appearance
　　　ii. Progressive—central opacity with enlarging radiations over time

　　Daljit Singh classification:
　　Type 1: PPC with posterior subcapsular cataract
　　Type 2: Round/oval opacity with ringed appearance-like onion with/without grayish spots at the edge
　　Type 3: Sharply defined round/oval white opacity with dense white spot at the edge associated with a weak, thin/absent posterior capsule. These dense white spots are a diagnostic sign (Daljit Singh sign) of posterior capsule rupture.

　　Schroeder classification:
　　Based on the effect of opacity on pupillary obstruction in the red reflex testing:
　　Grade 1: Small opacity without any effect on the optical quality of the clear part of the lens
　　Grade 2: Two-thirds obstruction without other effects
　　Grade 3: Disk-like opacity in the posterior capsule is surrounded by an area of further optical distortion. Only the dilated pupil shows a clear red reflex surrounding this zone.
　　Grade 4: Opacity is totally occlusive; no sufficient red reflex is obtained by dilation of the pupil.

27. **What is complicated cataract?**
　　Complicated cataract is also known as secondary cataract. It develops as a result of other primary ocular diseases.
　　The cataract mainly begins as a posterior subcapsular cataract.
　　　i. *Inflammatory conditions:* Inflammations of the uveal tract (iridocyclitis, pars planitis, posterior uveitis), corneal ulcer, endophthalmitis
　　　ii. *Degenerative conditions:* Essential iris atrophy, retinitis pigmentosa, myopic chorioretinal degenerations, and other pigmentary retinal dystrophies

iii. *RD:* Long-standing cases of RD can lead to complicated cataracts
iv. *Glaucoma:* Primary or secondary glaucoma
v. *Intraocular tumors:* Retinoblastoma, melanoma, metastatic tumors involving the choroid or the anterior segment

28. **What are the surgical challenges in case of complicated cataracts?**
The various challenges faced intraoperatively include inadequate visualization due to a small pupil, synechiae, pupillary membranes, and corneal opacification. There is a high risk of intraoperative complications such as posterior capsular rent, zonular dehiscence, anterior chamber (AC) hemorrhage, and pigment dispersion.

29. **What are the anterior segment findings to observe in traumatic cataracts?**
    i. *Eyeball:* Ocular deviation and ocular movements
    ii. *Eyelid:* Laceration or scarring may be seen
    iii. *Conjunctiva:* Subconjunctival hemorrhage, chemosis, or scar may be present
    iv. *Cornea:* Corneal clouding/edema, corneal perforation, scar, sutures, intrastromal foreign body
    v. *Sclera:* Repaired scleral perforation or scar
    vi. *Anterior chamber:* AC cells, flare, hyphema, vitreous or lens matter
    vii. *Iris:* Iridodonesis/iridodialysis/posterior synechiae/iris atrophy
    viii. *Pupil:* Sphincter tear, eccentric pupil/traumatic mydriasis, oval/peaking pupil/irregular/vitreous entangling pupillary area
    ix. Direct and consensual light reactions of both eyes should be recorded. Presence of relative afferent pathway defect (RAPD) suggests posterior segment complications such as RD or traumatic optic neuropathy
    x. *Lens:* Anterior lens capsule (ALC) breach, phacodonesis, cataractous lens, posterior capsule breach, status of zonules

30. **What is second sight of the aged?**
Nuclear sclerosis induces progressive index myopia, which results in improvement of near vision. Patients with this form of cataract are able to read without their presbyopic correction, which has been termed "second sight of the aged".

31. **What are the tests by which postoperative acuity can be estimated in the presence of a dense cataract?**
    i. Laser interferometry
    ii. Potential acuity meter

32. **What are the tests to assess macular function in the presence of cataract?**
    i. Maddox rod test
    ii. Photostress recovery time: Normal is <50 seconds

iii. Blue-light endoscopy
iv. Purkinje's entoptic phenomenon
v. Electroretinography (ERG)
vi. Visual evoked potential (VEP)

33. What are cohesive viscoelastics?
Cohesive viscoelastics are high-molecular-weight agents with high surface tensions and high pseudoplasticity. They tend to be easily aspirated from the eye. Examples include Healon, Amvisc, and Healon GV.

34. What are dispersive viscoelastics?
Dispersive viscoelastics are substances with low molecular weight and good coating abilities. They tend to be removed less rapidly. Examples include Viscoat and Vitrax.

35. What are the advantages of peribulbar anesthesia as compared to retrobulbar anesthesia?
i. Lower risk of optic nerve damage
ii. Lower risk of systemic neurological effects

36. What are the disadvantages of peribulbar anesthesia?
i. Needs more anesthetic
ii. More chemosis and congestion
iii. May need more number of injections

37. What are the complications of retrobulbar and peribulbar anesthesia?
i. Retrobulbar hemorrhage
ii. Globe penetration
iii. Optic nerve damage
iv. Extraocular muscle damage
v. Neurological damage due to intrathecal penetration of drugs
vi. Death

38. What is the technique of giving a sub-Tenon's anesthesia?
i. Visualization of sclera—whiter, more fibrous appearance compared to Tenon's capsule, which indicates adequate dissection
ii. Little resistance is felt when the needle is inserted in the sub-Tenon's space. Attempts at injecting into the subconjunctival space offer greater resistance and are accompanied by ballooning of the conjunctiva
iii. Slight proptosis of the eyeball will be noted after completion of sub-Tenon's block
iv. Theoretically, B scan can be used to confirm the position of needle in sub-Tenon's space. T sign indicating the presence of sub-Tenon's fluid will be present after successful administration of sub-Tenon's block

39. **What are the different pump designs in phacoemulsification machines?**
    i. Peristaltic
    ii. Diaphragm
    iii. Venturi

40. **Describe terms in phacodyamics.**
    i. *Phacodynamics:* The various functions of the phaco machine and their interrelationship is called phacodynamics. The basic functions of the machine are two which include ultrasonic power for emulsification and irrigation aspiration for safe suction of the emulsified material. Irrigation aspiration system and the parameters on which it depends together are called fluidics
    ii. *Power:* Phaco power is produced by the ultrasonic vibrations of the quartz crystal in the handpiece. It is created by an interaction between frequency and stroke length
    iii. *Flow rate (FR):* It determines how fast things will happen in the eye. The higher the FR, the lesser the rise time and sooner the debris in the AC is cleared. Most peristaltic machines work best at an optimum FR of 20–36 cc/min
    iv. *Vacuum:* It is generated by the machine and is a measure of the strength of the "hold" that the handpiece has on the nucleus. The level of vacuum and port size will determine how strong the grip is. The holding power is inversely proportional to the port size
    v. *Rise time:* This is the time taken by a machine to reach maximum preset vacuum after occlusion has been achieved. The higher the frame rate (FR), the lesser the response time (RT) though the relationship is not absolutely linear
    vi. *Power delivery:* Pulse mode and burst mode
        - *Pulse mode:* In pulse mode, each pulse of energy is followed by a gap of equal duration. For effective power delivery, the nuclear fragment has to be held, so the interval between the pulses of phaco allows the vacuum to build up, and thus a good hold is developed
        - *Burst mode:* This is useful in hard cataracts where maximum power is delivered at intervals which vary with the amount of depression of foot pedal. Burst mode is a variant of panel mode where the energy is fixed, and the frequency of phaco bursts will increase with increasing depression of the foot pedal in phaco mode
    vii. *Surge:* Sudden withdrawal of fluid from AC after occlusion breaks is called surge. Beyond a certain limit, it may cause collapse of chamber

41. **What are the various techniques of nucleus fragmentation in phacoemulsification?**
    i. Divide and conquer
    ii. Stop and chop
    iii. Direct chop

42. **What are the steps which can be taken to modify astigmatism following phacoemulsification?**
    i. Toric IOLs
    ii. Limbal relaxing incisions (LRIs)
    iii. Astigmatic keratotomy

43. **How do you treat astigmatism in cataract surgery?**
    i. Astigmatism <1 D—LRIs
    ii. Astigmatism 1-3 D—toric IOL or LRIs, although toric IOLs are regarded to give more reliable results
    iii. Astigmatism >3 D—a combination of toric IOL, LRIs (or corneal-relaxing incisions), and/or strategic cataract incision placement

44. **What is toric IOL?**
    Toric IOLs refer to astigmatism-correcting IOLs used at the time of cataract surgery to decrease postoperative astigmatism. Standard toric IOLs are available in cylinder powers of 1.5-6.0 D. They are usually intended for regular corneal astigmatism in a range from 0.75 to 4.75 D, and extended series or customized IOLs are available to achieve higher cylindrical power. Toric IOLs are available as monofocal and multifocal lenses.

45. **How to mark toric IOL before surgery?**
    Prior to beginning the surgical procedure, the precise reference marking of the cornea is done with the patient upright and looking forward. It is important that the patient is sitting for this procedure as cyclotorsion may occur when the patient lies down. The cornea is marked at the 3, 6, and 9 o'clock positions after instillation of a topical anesthetic. This can be done in the preoperative area or in the operating room. Corneal marking instruments are available which ease this step. This can also be marked with a skin-marking pen.

    After the patient is draped, the steep axis should be marked with a degree gauge so as to provide a guide for the orienting marks on the toric IOL later in the procedure. It is wise to double-check the axis with preoperative notes. Then, the surgeon proceeds with the surgery as per routine.

46. **What is Sanders-Retzlaff-Kraff (SRK) formula?**
    SRK formula was developed by Sanders, Retzlaff, and Kraff and is useful for calculating the required IOL power. IOL power $P = A - (2.5 L) - 0.9 K$,

where "A" is the constant specific to the lens implant, "L" is the axial length, and "K" is the average keratometry reading.

47. What are the various formulae used in IOL power calculation?
  i. 1st generation:
     - SRK
     - Binkhorst
  ii. 2nd generation:
     - SRK II
     - Hoffer
  iii. 3rd generation:
     - SRK-T
     - Hoffer Q
     - Holladay 1
  iv. 4th generation:
     - Holladay 2
     - Haigis
     - Olsen

48. What are the types of IOL?
  i. *Based on method of fixation:*
     - Anterior chamber IOL (ACIOL)
     - Iris-supported lens
     - Posterior chamber IOL (PCIOL)
  ii. *Based on material used:*
     - Rigid polymethyl methacrylate (PMMA) IOL
     - Foldable IOL
     - Ultrathin IOL
  iii. *Based on focality:*
     - Monofocal IOL
     - Multifocal IOL
     - Pseudoaccomodative IOL
     - Accommodative IOL
     - Extended depth focus IOL
  iv. *Based on toricity and sphericity:*
     - Toric IOL
     - Aspheric IOL
  v. *Based on edge finish:*
     - Rigid IOL
     - Square-edged IOL
     - Sharp-edged IOL

49. What is biometry?
Biometry facilitates the calculation of lens power to result in desired postoperative refractive outcome. It includes:

i. Keratometry (K reading), which involves determination of curvature of the anterior corneal surface expressed in diopters
   ii. Measurement of axial length

50. **What are the commonly used IOL power calculation formulae?**
    i. Hoffer Q
    ii. SRK/T
    iii. Holladay 1, Holladay 2
    iv. Haigis (especially for post-Lasik patients)

51. **What are the ways to calculate IOL power in a patient who has undergone corneal refractive surgery?**
    i. Refractive surgery technique
       K = Prerefractive surgery average K value + (change in refraction at the corneal plane)
    ii. Contact lens technique (when no pretreatment data exists)
    iii. Special formulae such as Haigis formula

52. **What are the IOL power calculations in children?**
    According to Dahan et al.:
    i. In older children >8 years—emmetropia is the target; hence, the same correction from calculated biometric power is recommended
    ii. Between 2 and 8 years—10% undercorrection from calculated biometric power is recommended to counter myopic shift
    iii. Below 2 years—20% undercorrection from calculated biometric power is recommended

53. **What is surgically induced astigmatism?**
    Surgically induced astigmatism is the range of achieved astigmatism cylinder and axis treatment and is used to compare the achieved astigmatism treatment to the intended treatment. It causes flattening in the meridian of incision and steepening 90° away. It is one of the factors that influence the desirable refractive outcome.

54. **How do you correct astigmatism during cataract surgery?**
    i. Incision placement: At the steepest meridian
    ii. LRIs
    iii. Toric IOLs
    iv. Bio-optics [cataract followed by photorefractive keratectomy (PRK)]

55. **What are the types of cataract incision?**
    A. *Small incision cataract surgery (SICS) (external incision);*
       i. Smiling/antifrown/curved parallel to limbus
       ii. Straight incision
       iii. Frown/curved opposite to limbus/antismile
       iv. Inverted V-shaped
       v. Scleral flap incision

B. *Phaco:*
   i. Clear corneal incision (triplanar, biplanar, uniplanar, hinged)
   ii. Posterior limbal
   iii. Modified temporal (corneolimbal/limboscleral)
   While presenting a pseudophakic case, we have to mention about the SICS/phaco scar in anterior segment examination, with scar description such as size, shape, distance from limbus, and any sutures.

56. **What are the signs of posterior capsular rent?**
    i. Deepening of AC
    ii. Difficulty in rotating the nuclear material that could previously rotate
    iii. Distorting pupil
    iv. Sudden appearance of red reflex
    v. Loss of followability of lens material and phaco efficacy during phaco or I/A
    vi. Visible vitreous strands to the instrument's tip
    vii. Posterior or lateral movement of nucleus
    viii. Unusual movement or stress lines in capsular bag (capsular starring)
    ix. Frank descent of nuclear material into the vitreous
    x. If the lens does not center in the usual manner
    xi. If folded, IOL becomes entangled with the capsular bag
    xii. Difficulty in aspiration of residual cortex

57. **What are the steps during which posterior capsular rent can happen?**
    i. Anterior capsulorhexis
    ii. Hydrodissection
    iii. Cortex aspiration
    iv. Nucleotomy
    v. IOL implantation

58. **What are the steps to be taken in a case of intraoperative posterior capsular tear?**
    i. Stop infusion of irrigating fluid
    ii. Avoid AC collapse by refilling viscoelastics
    iii. Mechanical anterior vitrectomy to take care of vitreous in the AC or in the wound
    iv. Attempt retrieval of fragments only if they are accessible
    v. If a significant amount of cortex or nucleus falls into the vitreous, then pars plana vitrectomy is performed
    vi. The IOL is placed in the bag in the event of a small, well-defined tear. In case of a big tear but with an associated intact peripheral capsular rim, the lens can be placed in the ciliary sulcus

vii. Plan a peripheral iridectomy after IOL implantation
viii. The incision is closed in a watertight manner
ix. In the postoperative period, frequent use of topical steroidal drops and topical nonsteroidal anti-inflammatory drugs (NSAIDs) may be used

59. What are the conditions which can cause shallow AC following cataract surgery?
  i. *Conditions associated with increased intraocular pressure (IOP):*
     - Pupillary block glaucoma
     - Suprachoroidal hemorrhage
     - Malignant glaucoma (ciliary block glaucoma)
  ii. *Conditions associated with decreased IOP:*
     - Leaking incision
     - Choroidal detachment

60. How do you manage a case of aphakia?
  i. *Optical:*
     - Spectacles
     - Contact lens
  ii. *Surgical:*
     - Eyes with poor capsular support
        - Epikeratophakia
        - Iris-supported IOL—iris claw lens, iris-sutured PCIOL
        - Angle-supported IOL
        - Scleral-supported IOL
        - Capsule-supported IOL
     - Eyes with good capsular support
        - In-the-bag placement
        - Simple sulcus placement
        - Membrane optic capture placement
        - Capsule membrane suture fixation of IOL

61. What are the causes of glaucoma after cataract surgery?
The causes can be classified into:
  i. *Secondary open-angle glaucoma:*
     - Early causes (first postoperative week)
        - Retained viscoelastic
        - Big air bubble in AC
        - Aphakia with vitreous block
        - Damage to the angle structures intraoperatively
        - Distortion of angle due to improper suturing technique in extracapsular cataract extraction (ECCE)
        - Preexisting chronic open-angle glaucoma
        - Idiopathic

- *Intermediate causes (1 week to 2 months postoperation):*
  - Preexisting chronic open-angle glaucoma
  - Hyphema
  - Retained lens fragments or cortical matter in AC clogging the trabecular meshwork (TM)
  - Vitreous in AC
  - Postoperative inflammation
  - Steroid-induced glaucoma
  - Ghost cell glaucoma
- *Late (>2 months post-operation):*
  - Preexisting chronic open-angle glaucoma
  - Ghost cell glaucoma
  - Pressure on the angle structures by ACIOL
  - Pigment dispersion syndrome
  - Chronic inflammation
  - Uveitis glaucoma hyphema syndrome [uveitis-glaucoma-hyphema (UGH) syndrome]
  - Pseudophakic neovascular glaucoma (NVG)
  - Late occurring hemorrhages
  - Post-neodymium (Nd):YAG capsulotomy
  - Proliferation of iris melanocytes across TM

ii. *Secondary angle-closure glaucoma:*
- With pupillary block
  - Anterior hyaloid causing pupillary block
  - Optic capture
  - Hyphema blocking the pupil
  - Posterior synechiae following inflammation
  - Fibrinous aqueous
  - Silicon oil
- Without pupillary block
  - Preexisting angle closure glaucoma
  - Inflammation/hyphema
  - Prolonged AC shallowing
  - Iris incarceration in incision
  - IOL haptics
  - NVG
  - Epithelial/fibrous ingrowth
    Aqueous misdirection (malignant glaucoma)

62. What are the types of multifocal IOLs?
   i. *Diffractive:* Incoming light is diffracted by an interference grid producing separate focal points simultaneously
   ii. *Refractive:* Optic composed of concentric rings of different power

iii. Combined refractive and aphorized diffractive
iv. Sector-shaped refractive

63. **What are the disadvantages of multifocal IOLs?**
    i. Full correction may not be obtained
    ii. Night glare and haloes
    iii. Dysphotopsia
    iv. Decreased contrast sensitivity

64. **What is extended depth of focus (EDF) IOL?**
    These is a newer category of IOLs that aims to give an elongated focus of vision without compromising distance visual acuity. It extends the depth of focus through a combination of effects from its echelette design, reduced chromatic aberration, and negative spherical aberration. Intermediate vision is improved compared to standard bifocal multifocal IOLs, but near vision may only be modestly improved. Additionally, while patients may have better levels of contrast sensitivity and less ocular aberrations, they may experience a unique visual phenomenon typically described as "starbursts".

65. **What are the accommodating IOLs?**
    Accommodating IOLs lenses have single optic and utilize a forward-backward axial movement of IOL in response to ciliary muscle contraction (e.g., Crystalens).

66. **What is tackiness of IOLs?**
    Acrylic polymer material of IOL is reported to have a tacky surface which means that the posterior as well as the anterior capsule remains adherent to the lens surface after implantation in the bag and prevents posterior capsule opacification (PCO), capsular fibrosis, and lens decentration.

67. **What are the special steps taken for small pupil in cataract surgery?**
    i. *Optimize mydriasis:*
       - Stop miotics in advance
       - Use topical NSAID along with mydriatics
    ii. Highly cohesive viscoelastics: Used to dilate the pupil
    iii. Posterior synechiolysis
    iv. Iris hooks and pupil expanders

68. **What are the special steps taken for zonule weakness/dehiscence?**
    i. Make the main incision opposite to the area of zonular weakness
    ii. Initiate the capsulorhexis toward the weak zonules using the intact zonules for counter traction
    iii. Use iris hooks
    iv. Careful hydrodissection and hydrodelineation
    v. Sufficient phaco power to avoid pushing the nucleus

vi. Use capsular tension ring to stabilize the bag. If zonular loss is marked, use Cionni ring and fix to sclera
vii. Insert the leading haptic into the bag toward the area of zonular weakness and gently direct the trailing haptic into the bag with McPherson forceps

69. **What are the special steps taken for brunescent cataract?**
    i. Larger capsulorhexis
    ii. Bottle height low to reduce irrigation volume
    iii. Move phaco tip slowly when sculpting
    iv. Use enough power to avoid pushing the lens
    v. Use burst mode of pulse mode to avoid chatter
    vi. Adequate viscoelastics, preferably a soft shell technique

70. **What is capsular tension ring?**
    Capsular tension ring is a supportive device used in eyes with zonulopathy. It is a compressible and flexible circular ring made of PMMA which is 270° with smooth-edged terminals, eyelets at free ends.
    It is used in zonular dialysis <4 clock hours.
    Uses:
    i. Provides support during cataract removal
    ii. IOL stabilization and centration
    iii. Prevents wrinkling of posterior capsule

71. **What are the special steps taken for white cataract?**
    i. Use of Trypan blue 0.06%
    ii. Use smaller capsulorhexis since it may extend to periphery
    iii. Use higher density viscoelastic

72. **What is soft shell technique?**
    i. Inject dispersive viscoelastic adjacent to the endothelium (Viscoat)
    ii. Then expand the AC below using cohesive viscoelastic, thus spreading the dispersive agent against the endothelium

73. **What are the potential risk factors for the development of PCO?**
    i. Younger age at surgery
    ii. Intraocular inflammation
    iii. Round-edged IOLs are more prone to developing PCO than square-edged IOLs
    iv. Smaller capsulorhexis
    v. Residual cortical material and anterior capsular opacity
    vi. Presence of intraocular silicon oil
    vii. PMMA IOLs are more likely to develop PCO than acrylic IOLs

74. **What are the types of PCO?**
    i. *Regeneratory PCO:* It is due to the migration of lens epithelial cells along the posterior capsule behind the IOL

Elschnig pearls—these cells proliferate to form layers of lens material, leading to opacification

Soemmerring's ring—when arranged in a form of ring between anterior capsular rim and posterior capsule

ii. *Fibrotic PCO:* Here, the lens epithelial cells of the anterior capsule undergo transformation to myofibroblasts, causing fibrosis and contraction of the capsule bag. This can lead to decentration of the IOL and hinder visualization of the peripheral retina

75. **What is capsular bag distension syndrome?**
Capsular bag distension syndrome is a rare complication of cataract surgery with IOL placement in the bag where fluid builds up behind the IOL and posterior capsule, leading to distension of the posterior capsule with anterior displacement of the PCIOL. The trapped fluid develops a turbid consistency which leads to decreased visual acuity for the patient and can be associated with either a myopic (more common) or a hyperopic shift.

Symptomatic patients will have decreased visual acuity. If significant anterior displacement of the lens-diaphragm exists, IOP may also be elevated. On slit lamp, when the smoky, turbid fluid is visible between the IOL and clear posterior capsule, a layering effect produces a phenomenon known as a retrolenticular pseudohypopyon. There is shallowing of the AC, tight apposition of the iris to lens implant, anterior bowing of the iris, or late capsular fibrosis.

Anterior segment optical coherence tomography (ASOCT) and anterior segment UBM are useful for early diagnosis. Treatment includes Nd:YAG laser posterior and/or anterior capsulotomy. YAG allows for quick release of the trapped fluid and returns the IOL to its previous position, resolving the patient's myopic shift and visual blurring.

76. **What are the signs of expulsive suprachoroidal hemorrhage?**
    i. Sudden increase of IOP
    ii. Darkening of the red reflex
    iii. Wound gape
    iv. Expulsion of the lens, vitreous, and bright red blood
    v. Severe pain

77. **What are the risk factors for expulsive hemorrhage?**
    i. Uncontrolled glaucoma
    ii. Arterial hypertension
    iii. Patients on anticoagulant therapy
    iv. Bleeding diathesis
    v. Prolonged hypotony

78. How will you manage expulsive hemorrhage?
i. Attempt to close the wound as quickly as possible
ii. Posterior sclerotomies (5–7 mm posterior to the limbus)

79. What is the nature of the fluid used for irrigation in cataract surgery?
Balanced salt solution (isotonic solution)—NaCl 0.64%, KCl 0.075%, CaCl

80. Why is normal saline not used as irrigation solution?
Normal saline, because of its corrosive action, can cause deterioration of metallic components. Hence, it is not used.

81. Why are the IOLs washed before implantation?
This is done to reduce toxic anterior segment syndrome (TASS). TASS is an acute postoperative sterile inflammatory reaction of the anterior segment tissues to a toxic substance. It can occur after any anterior segment surgery.

The most commonly observed risk factors for TASS were:
i. Inadequate flushing of cannulated instruments
ii. Use of enzymatic detergents
iii. Use of reusable cannulas
iv. Poor instrument maintenance
v. Contact of the IOL or instrument tips with gloved hands

The surgical gloves retain a residue of the releasing agent that is used to extract them from the molds during manufacturing. Touching the IOL or other surfaces may transfer this releasing agent from the gloves to the interior of the eye, where inflammation can occur. For this reason, IOLs should be loaded into the cassette using forceps without contact from a gloved finger or hand. Similarly, the injector tip should not be touched with a gloved finger, and it is safer to wash the IOL with BSS before implantation to reduce the incidence of TASS.

82. A. Iris coloboma
The embryonic fissure normally closes around the fifth week of intrauterine life. Improper closure of choroidal fissure or optic fissure anteriorly results in iris coloboma.

B. Treatment of iris coloboma

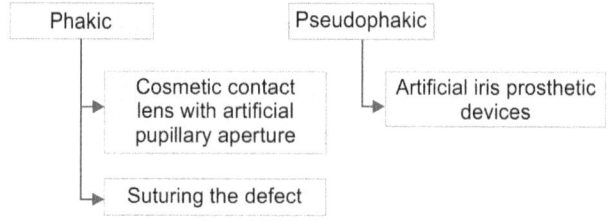

C. **Types of iris coloboma:**
Based on site:
   i. Inferonasal quadrant
   ii. Found elsewhere
Based on involvement:
   i. Complete—involves iris pigment epithelium and stroma—keyhole pupil
   ii. Incomplete—involves pupillary margin

83. **What are the types of IOL used in an iris coloboma/aniridia patient?**
Iris-reconstruction lenses are a combination of artificial iris devices and lenses by Morcher. The optics may vary in their diameters.
   i. 67B model—12.5-mm aniridia implant with a 3-mm optic meant for sulcus placement or scleral suturing
   ii. 50F—10-mm aniridia ring with occluder panels all the way around, meant to be dialed into the capsular bag against another one
   iii. 96F—11-mm partial aniridia ring with an occluder paddle that covers up to 3 clock hours

84. **What are the intraoperative precautions to be taken when cataract surgery is performed on specific situations?**
   A. *Diabetics:*
      i. Phacoemulsification with IOL implantation yields better visual results and less inflammation as compared to extracapsular cataract surgery
      ii. Anterior capsular phimosis is more common in diabetic eyes. The capsulorhexis size should, therefore, be larger than normal but smaller than IOL optic diameter to prevent anterior IOL displacement and PCO
      iii. A large diameter optic (i.e., 6.0 mm or larger) also facilitates diagnosis and treatment of peripheral retinal pathology postoperatively
      iv. Longer duration and complicated cataract surgery are associated with a greater risk of progression of retinopathy and subsequent visual compromise
      v. In diabetic patients, there is a high likelihood of poor pupillary dilatation due to damage to pupillary parasympathetic supply. Thus, iris hooks, Malyugin ring, or other iris expanders should be considered for intraoperative use in these patients
      vi. In addition, complications such as intraoperative hyphema due to the presence of rubeosis iridis need to be kept in mind. Some studies have shown that preoperative intravitreal anti-vascular endothelial growth factor (anti-VEGF) agents may decrease the chances of bleeding from iris neovascularization

vii. The diabetic eye is more prone to keratoepitheliopathy, including corneal epithelial defects/abrasions, which may heal slowly. The impaired corneal wound healing has multiple etiologies including neurogenic (sub-basal nerve abnormalities) and impaired corneal stem cell and epithelial cell division
viii. Studies have also shown greater predisposition to corneal endothelial cell loss in people with diabetes compared to nondiabetics. Hence, routine specular microscopy is recommended for all people with diabetes, and greater care should be taken with regard to endothelial protection when operating on diabetic patients

B. *In human immunodeficiency virus (HIV) patients:*
   i. Phaco in a HIV-positive patient should be done with a phaco machine of newer generation which does not need any internal tubing system and preferably to be done as the last case in an operation theater (OT)
   ii. If the phaco machine has an internal tubing system, it should be properly sterilized after doing a phaco procedure and to be done as the last case in OT for that machine
   iii. It is better to do surgery under topical anesthesia with clear corneal section
   iv. Protective barriers while operating an HIV patient consist mainly of eye wear, gloves, cap and mask, footwear, and impervious gown
      - *Gloves:* Use of double gloves-five-fold reduction of risk of skin contamination or special prick-proof gloves
         Tight gloves tend to get punctured easily.
      - *Footwear:* Wellington boot and calf length plastic over boots are worn rather than shoes or clog
      - *Impervious gown:* Several waterproof fabrics with the ability to breathe available for use and are comfortable to wear

C. *In glaucoma:*
   i. Good control of IOP preoperatively. Avoid preoperative pilocarpine and prostaglandin analogs
   ii. The *bleb* position will determine the approach for the cataract surgery incision, which should avoid the bleb area. Note whether the bleb is functioning and whether it is cystic or flat and/or fibrosed or vascularized. This will determine whether intraoperative bleb revision is required
   iii. The position of the *peripheral iridectomy* and the pupil's ability to dilate. Iris manipulation during cataract surgery with floppy

iris or poor dilation due to posterior synechiae may increase the risk of postoperative inflammation, which may compromise bleb function

iv. *Pseudoexfoliation*, as this may be associated with weak zonules, which is a reason for caution in cataract surgery

v. *Care of the existing bleb*, especially if thin and cystic, during placement of the lid speculum and any physical manipulation or instrumentation of the eye during wound incision and paracentesis

vi. *Bleb revision*, if needed. This can be done using needling and/or additional application of antimetabolites

vii. *Maintaining the AC depth*, especially in patients with a high-functioning bleb. Take extra caution to prevent posterior capsular rent and vitreous loss. Ensure that any tube that is in place is not blocked, obstructed, or displaced

viii. *Review a functioning tube*, if present. It can be repositioned or flushed to improve the chances of it functioning after surgery. It may also be trimmed if too long

ix. *IOL placement.* The aim is to place the IOL in the bag; otherwise, be prepared for a sulcus placement if the capsule or zonules are compromised. Position the lens so that the haptic is away from the primary incision (to avoid it migrating into the AC). Avoid AC IOLs because they can directly affect the bleb and may produce undue postoperative inflammation

x. *AC washout.* Thoroughly remove viscoelastic as well as nuclear and cortical lens material. This will prevent blockage of drainage channels and/or tubes and reduce postoperative inflammation and IOP spikes. However, take care to prevent excessive flushing against the corneal endothelium as this can cause damage

xi. *Wound closure.* Use sutures to produce a watertight wound. A wound leak will increase the risk of bleb failure

85. What is PHAKONIT?

The term PHAKONIT was given as phaco (PHAKO) was done with a needle (N) opening via an incision (I) and with the phaco tip (T).

The titanium tip of the phaco handpiece has a diameter of 0.9 mm. The surrounding infusion sleeve, which occupies most space, is taken out. Thus, the cataract is removed through a 0.9 mm opening.

PHACONIT is further advanced into Microphaconit with 0.7 mm phaco tip.

86. What is femtosecond laser-assisted cataract surgery (FLACS)?

FLACS is a recent development in cataract surgery. It can offer a greater level of precision and repeatability for creation of tissue planes than manual technique. It offers more precise incisional astigmatism management (wounds and arcuate keratotomies), lens centration (capsulotomy), and reduced effective phaco energy (nuclear fragmentation).

The femtosecond laser can be used to create cleavage planes via photodisruption in transparent/translucent tissues, focused with the aid of real-time intraoperative imaging [*optical coherence tomography (OCT)* or Scheimpflug].

It uses neodymium: glass 1,053 nm (near-infrared) wavelength light. It emits ultrashort pulses (10–15 seconds), eliminate the collateral damage of the surrounding tissues, and the heat generation associated with slower excimer and Nd:YAG lasers.

Femtosecond laser energy is absorbed by the tissue, resulting in plasma formation. This plasma of free electrons and ionized molecules rapidly expands, creating cavitation bubbles. The force of the cavitation bubble creation separates the tissue. The process of converting laser energy into mechanical energy is known as photodisruption.

The Food and Drug Administration (FDA) approved three steps in cataract surgery:

i. Corneal incisions
ii. Anterior capsulotomy
iii. Lens fragmentation.

CHAPTER 6

Retina

6.1 DIFFERENTIAL DIAGNOSIS OF RETINAL FINDINGS

1. **Retinal neovascularization**
    i. Diabetes
    ii. Retinal vein occlusion
    iii. Hypertension
    iv. Sickle cell retinopathy
    v. Ocular ischemic syndrome
    vi. Retinopathy of prematurity (ROP)
    vii. Familial exudative vitreoretinopathy
    viii. Norrie's disease
    ix. Eales' disease
    x. *Inflammation:* Vasculitis, posterior uveitis
    xi. Hyperviscosity syndrome
    xii. Radiation retinopathy
    xiii. Talc emboli

2. **Intraretinal hemorrhage**
    i. Diabetes
    ii. Retinal vein occlusion
    iii. Hypertension
    iv. Hyperviscosity syndrome
    v. Anemia
    vi. Ocular ischemic syndrome
    vii. Subretinal neovascularization (SRNV)
    viii. Associated with infections, e.g., human immunodeficiency virus (HIV) microangiopathy, Roth's spots
    ix. Valsalva retinopathy
    x. Eales' disease
    xi. Sickle cell retinopathy

3. **Subretinal choroidal neovascularization**
    i. Age-related macular degeneration (ARMD)
    ii. Postinflammatory
    iii. Presumed ocular histoplasmosis syndrome (POHS)

iv. Myopic degeneration
v. Trauma
vi. Dystrophies (Sorsby's, Best's, etc.)
vii. Optic nerve drusen
viii. Angioid streaks

4. **Retinal telangiectasia**
    i. Diabetes
    ii. Hypertension
    iii. Previous retinal vein occlusion
    iv. Sickle cell retinopathy
    v. Idiopathic juxtafoveal telangiectasia
    vi. Radiation retinopathy
    vii. Coats' disease
    viii. Incontinentia pigmenti

5. **Retinal vascular tortuosity**
    i. Polycythemia
    ii. Leukemia
    iii. Retinal vein occlusion
    iv. Dysproteinemia
    v. Sickle cell disease
    vi. Familial dysproteinemia
    vii. Mucopolysaccharidosis
    viii. Fabry's disease
    ix. Hyperviscosity syndrome
    x. Eales' disease
    xi. Racemose angioma
    xii. Epiretinal membrane

6. **Retinal deposits**
    i. Exudates
        - Diabetes
        - Hypertension
        - Retinal vein occlusion
        - Vascular tumors
        - Coats' disease
    ii. Drusen
        - ARMD
        - Basal laminar drusen
        - Sorsby fundus dystrophy
    iii. Crystals
        - Juxtafoveal telangiectasia
        - Tamoxifen
        - Bietti's crystalline retinopathy
        - Canthaxanthin toxicity

iv.	White dots	- Multiple evanescent white dot syndrome (MEWDS) - Birdshot chorioretinopathy - Hereditary fundus albipunctatus
v.	Flecks	- Stargardt - Fundus flavimaculatus - Hereditary fundus albipunctatus
vi.	Yellow lesions	- Best macular dystrophy - Pattern dystrophy - ARMD - Harada's disease - Metastasis

7. **Cherry-red spots in the macula**
    i. Central retinal artery occlusion (CRAO)
    ii. Sphingolipidoses (Tay-Sachs, Gaucher, and Niemann-Pick)
    iii. Quinine toxicity
    iv. Traumatic retinal edema
    v. Ocular ischemic syndrome
    vi. Macular hole with surrounding retinal detachment

8. **Macular edema**
    i. Diabetes mellitus
    ii. Retinal vein occlusion
    iii. Pseudophakic (Irvine-Gass)
    iv. SRNV
    v. Uveitis/scleritis
    vi. Hypertension
    vii. Choroidal ischemia
    viii. Retinitis pigmentosa
    ix. Vascular tumor
    x. Nicotinic acid toxicity

9. **Macular star**
    i. Hypertension
    ii. Retinal vein occlusion
    iii. Papilledema
    iv. *Inflammation:* Choroiditis, posterior scleritis, vasculitis, neuroretinitis, toxoplasmosis, chronic infection, e.g., syphilis

10. **Macular atrophy**
    i. ARMD
    ii. Pathological myopia
    iii. Stargardt's disease
    iv. Cone dystrophy

    v. Dominant retinal dystrophies
    vi. Best's vitelliform dystrophy
    vii. X-linked retinoschisis
    viii. Chloroquine toxicity
    ix. After pigment epithelial detachment
    x. Solar retinopathy
11. **Bull's eye maculopathy**
    i. Macular, cone, or cone/rod dystrophies
    ii. Drug toxicity—chloroquine
    iii. Batten's disease
    iv. Benign concentric annular macular dystrophy
    v. Bardet-Biedl syndrome
12. **Angioid streaks**
    i. Pseudoxanthoma elasticum
    ii. Paget's disease
    iii. Hemoglobinopathies
    iv. Ehlers-Danlos syndrome
13. **Choroidal folds**
    i. Hypermetropia
    ii. Hypotony
    iii. Papilledema
    iv. Retrobulbar mass lesions
    v. Thyroid eye disease
    vi. Posterior scleritis
    vii. Scleral buckle
    viii. Choroidal tumors
    ix. Choroidal neovascularization
14. **Roth spots (hemorrhage with white center)**
    i. Bacterial endocarditis
    ii. Leukemia
    iii. Severe anemia
    iv. Sickle cell disease
    v. Collagen vascular disease
    vi. Diabetes mellitus
    vii. Multiple myeloma
    viii. HIV retinopathy
15. **Drugs causing toxic maculopathies**
    i. Aminoglycosides
    ii. Canthaxanthin
    iii. Chloroquine and hydroxychloroquine

     iv. Chlorpromazine
     v. Quinine
     vi. Niacin
     vii. Interferon alpha
     viii. Tamoxifen
     ix. Sildenafil (Viagra)

16. **Vascular changes of retina in aging**
    i. Loss of cellularity in peripheral capillaries with attachment of internal limiting membrane (ILM) to the peripheral vascular arcades
    ii. Decrease of capillaries around fovea
    iii. Atherosclerotic changes of vessels (hyalinization, hyperplasia of muscular layer, fibrinoid necrosis of wall)
    iv. Decreased venular blood flow velocity

17. **What is the importance of red infarct and white infarct?**
    Red infarcts are hemorrhagic infarcts caused by artery and vein occlusion and in reperfusion areas in tissues with a dual blood supply.

    White infarct or anemic infarct is caused by arterial occlusion in organ with end arterial circulation replaced by a collagenous scarring, e.g., retina.

6.2 FUNDUS FLUORESCEIN ANGIOGRAPHY

1. **What is luminescence, fluorescence, and phosphorescence?**
    i. Luminescence is the emission of light from any source other than high temperature. This occurs when there is absorption of electromagnetic radiation, and the electrons are elevated to higher energy states. The energy is then reemitted by spontaneous decay of the electrons to lower energy levels. When this decay occurs in the visible spectrum, it is called luminescence
    ii. Fluorescence is luminescence that is maintained only by continuous excitation; thus, emission stops when excitation stops
    iii. Phosphorescence is luminescence where the emission continues long after the excitation has stopped

2. **What are the dyes used in ocular angiography?**
    i. Fluorescein sodium
    ii. Indocyanine green

3. **Describe the chemical properties of fluorescein.**
    i. Orange-red crystalline hydrocarbon, related to phenolphthalein, resulting from the interaction of phthalic acid anhydride and resorcinol
    ii. The chemical name is resorcin phthalein sodium, $C_{20}H_{10}Na_2O_5$
    iii. It has low molecular weight (376 Da), and high solubility in water allows rapid diffusion

4. **Describe the biophysical properties of fluorescein.**
    i. Maximum fluorescence at pH 7.4
    ii. Up to 80% protein bound (mainly albumin)
    iii. Only the remaining 20% is available for fluorescence
    iv. Rapid diffusion through intra- and extracellular spaces
    v. Elimination rapidly through the liver and kidney in 24–36 hours

5. **Describe the absorption and emission peaks of fluorescein.**
    Sodium fluorescein gets excited by light energy between 465 and 490 nm which is a blue spectrum and will fluoresce at a wavelength of 520 and 530 nm which is green–yellow.

6. **What are the other uses of fluorescein in ophthalmology?**
    i. Applanation tonometry
    ii. To identify corneal epithelial defects
    iii. Contact lens fitting
    iv. Seidel's test
    v. Fluorescein dye disappearance test
    vi. Tear film breakup time testing

vii. For nasolacrimal duct obstruction evaluation
viii. Fluorophotometry

7. **What is the common bacterial contaminant of fluorescein solution?**
   Pseudomonas aeruginosa

8. **What is fluorescein angiography?**
   Fluorescein angiography is fundal photography performed in rapid sequence following intravenous injection of fluorescein dye.

   It provides three main information:
   i. The flow characteristics in the blood vessels as the dye reaches and circulates through the retina
   ii. It records fine details of the pigment epithelium and retinal circulation that may not otherwise be visible
   iii. It gives a clear picture of the retinal vessels and assessment of their functional integrity

9. **Describe the history of fundus fluorescein angiography (FFA).**
   i. Ehrlich introduced fluorescein into investigative ophthalmology in 1882
   ii. Chao and Flocks gave the earliest description of FFA in 1958
   iii. Novotny and Alvis introduced this into clinical use in 1961

10. **Describe the principle of FFA.**
    Inner and outer blood–retinal barriers are the key to understanding FFA. Both barriers control movement of fluid, ions, and electrolytes from intravascular to extravascular space in retina.
    i. *Inner blood–retinal barrier:*
       - At the level of retinal capillary endothelium and basement membrane
       - Prevents all leaks of fluorescein and albumin-bound fluorescein
       - Thus, a clear picture of retinal blood vessels is seen in a normal angiogram
    ii. *Outer blood–retinal barrier:*
       - Composed of intact retinal pigment epithelium (RPE) which is impermeable to fluorescein
       - RPE acts as an optical barrier to fluorescein and masks choroidal circulation

11. **What are the requirements to perform FFA?**
    i. Fundus camera with two camera backs, timer, filters, and barrier
    ii. 35 mm black and white film
    iii. 35 mm color film
    iv. 23 gauge scalp vein needle
    v. 5 mL syringe with 1.5-inch needle

vi. 5 mL of 10% fluorescein solution
vii. Tourniquet
viii. Emergency tray with medicines to counter anaphylaxis

12. **Describe the filters used in FFA.**
    i. A *blue excitation filter* through which white light passes from the camera. The emerging blue light excites the fluorescein molecules in the retinal and choroidal circulations, which then emit light of a longer wavelength (yellow–green)
    ii. A *yellow–green barrier filter* then blocks any reflected blue light from the eye allowing only yellow–green light to pass through unimpaired to be recorded

13. **What is the dosage of fluorescein used for FFA?**
    Solutions containing 500–1,000 mg of fluorescein are available in vials of:
    i. 5 mL of 10% fluorescein (most commonly used)
    ii. 10 mL of 5% fluorescein
    iii. 3 mL of 25% fluorescein (preferred in opaque media)

14. **Describe the technique employed in FFA.**
    A good-quality angiogram requires adequate pupillary dilation and clear media.
    i. The patient is seated in front of the fundus camera
    ii. Fluorescein, usually 5 mL of a 10% solution, is drawn up into a syringe
    iii. A red-free image is captured
    iv. Fluorescein is injected intravenously over a few seconds
    v. Images are taken at approximately 1-second intervals, 5–25 seconds after injection
    vi. After the transit phase has been photographed in one eye, control pictures are taken of the opposite eye
    vii. If appropriate, late photographs may also be taken after 10 minutes and, occasionally, 20 minutes if leakage is anticipated

15. **List some of the *main indications* for fluorescein angiography.**
    Fluorescein angiography is used mainly for the study of abnormal ocular vasculature. The following are the main indications for fluorescein angiography:
    i. *Diabetic retinopathy (DR):*
        - Detecting any significant macular edema which is not clinically obvious
        - Locating the area of edema for laser treatment

- Differentiating ischemic from exudative diabetic maculopathy
- Differentiating between intraretinal microvascular abnormality (IRMA) and new blood vessels if clinical differentiation is difficult
- In the presence of dense asteroid hyalosis to detect occult neovascularization elsewhere (NVE) and neovascularization of disk (NVD)

ii. *Retinal vein occlusion:*
- Determining the integrity of the foveal capillary bed and the extent of macular edema following branch retinal vein occlusion
- Differentiating collaterals from neovascularization
- To determine capillary nonperfusion (CNP) areas

iii. *Age-related macular degeneration (ARMD):*
- Locate the subretinal neovascularization and determine its suitability for laser treatment

iv. *Other indications:*
- Locating subretinal neovascular membrane in various conditions (*high myopia, angioid streaks, choroidal rupture, and chorioretinitis*)
- Locating abnormal blood vessels (*e.g., idiopathic retinal telangiectasia*)
- Looking for breakdown of RPE tight junctions (*central serous retinal retinopathy*) or the blood–retinal barrier (*cystoid macular edema*)
- Help with diagnosis of retinal conditions (*e.g., Stargardt's disease gives a characteristic dark choroid*)

16. **What are the contraindications of FFA?**
    i. Renal failure
    ii. Juvenile asthmatics
    iii. Recent cardiac illness
    iv. Previous adverse reactions
    v. Pregnancy (not proven; better to avoid)

    Caution required in:
    i. Elderly patients
    ii. Blood dyscrasia
    iii. Impaired lymphatic system

17. **Which new investigation can be done for chronic renal failure (CRF) patients in which FFA is absolutely contraindicated?**
    Optical coherence tomography angiography (OCTA) is recommended. It enables to study the retinal vasculature without the need for dye injection.

18. **What are the phases described in an angiogram?**
    i. Choroidal (prearterial)
    ii. Arterial
    iii. Arteriovenous (capillary)
    iv. Venous
    v. Late (elimination)

19. **Describe the phases of normal fluorescein angiography.**
    Normally, 10–15 seconds elapse between dye injection and arrival of dye in the short ciliary arteries (arm-to-retina time). Choroidal circulation precedes retinal circulation by 1 second. Transit of dye through the retinal circulation takes approximately 15–20 seconds.
    i. *Choroidal phase:* Choroidal filling via the short ciliary arteries results in initial patchy filling of lobules, very quickly followed by a diffuse (blush) as dye leaks out of the choriocapillaris. Cilioretinal vessels and prelaminar optic disk capillaries fill during this phase
    ii. *Arterial phase:* The central retinal artery fills about 1 second later than choroidal filling
    iii. *Capillary phase:* The capillaries quickly fill following the arterial phase. The perifoveal capillary network is particularly prominent as the underlying choroidal circulation is masked by luteal pigment in the retina and melanin pigment in the RPE. [At the center of this capillary ring is the foveal avascular zone (FAZ) (500 mm in diameter)]
    iv. *Venous phase:* Early filling of the veins is from tributaries joining their margins, resulting in a tramline effect (laminar flow). Later, the whole diameter of the veins is filled
    v. *Late phase:* After 10-15 minutes, little dye remains within the blood circulation. Dye that has left the blood to ocular structures is particularly visible during this phase

20. **What do you mean by laminar flow?**
    Laminar flow happens in the venous phase of FFA. It is due to the following reasons:
    i. Fluorescein from venules enters the veins along their walls
    ii. Vascular flow is faster in the center of the lumen than on the sides, and fluorescein seems to stick to the sides, creating the laminar pattern
    iii. The dark central lamina is nonfluorescent blood that comes from the periphery, which takes longer time to fluoresce because of its more distant location
    iv. As the fluorescent filling increases in veins, laminae eventually enlarge and meet, resulting in complete fluorescence of retinal veins

21. **Under which conditions does the arm-to-retina time increase in FFA?**
    i. Carotid artery occlusion
    ii. Takayasu arteritis
    iii. Ocular ischemic syndrome
    iv. Conditions associated with reduced cardiac output

22. **What is A–V transit time?**
    i. A–V transit time is the time from the appearance of dye in the retinal arteries to complete filling of the retinal veins
    ii. Normal—10–12 seconds

23. **Why does the fovea appear dark on FFA?**
    i. Absence of blood vessels in the FAZ
    ii. Blockage of background choroidal fluorescence due to increased density of xanthophyll at the fovea
    iii. Blockage of background choroidal fluorescence by the RPE cells at the fovea, which is larger and contains more melanin than elsewhere

24. **What is the normal size of FAZ?**
    Average size is 650 μm.
    A size >1,000 μm suggests ischemia.

25. **What are the side effects of FFA?**
    FFAs are transient and do not require treatment.
    i. Staining of skin, sclera, tears, saliva, and urine (lasting 24–36 hours)
    ii. Flushy sensation, tingling of lips, and metallic taste

26. **What are the adverse reactions of FFA?**
    FFAs require medical intervention.
    Mild:
    i. Nausea and vomiting
    ii. Vasovagal responses—dizziness, light-headedness
    Moderate:
    i. Urticaria
    ii. Syncope
    iii. Phlebitis
    iv. Local tissue necrosis and nerve palsies (due to extravasation)
    Severe:
    i. Respiratory—laryngeal edema, bronchospasm, anaphylaxis
    ii. Neurologic—tonic-clonic seizures
    iii. Cardiac—arrest, death

27. **What are the methods to reduce the side effects of FFA?**
    i. Nil per oral
    ii. Slow injection of the drug
    iii. Reduced dosage of the drug
    iv. Antiemetics

28. **What are the abnormal fluorescein patterns?**
    i. *Hypofluorescence:* Reduction or absence of normal fluorescence is hypofluoresence. It is any normally dark area on the positive print of any angiogram

    It is seen in two major patterns:
    - Blocked fluorescence
    - Vascular filling defects

    ii. *Hyperfluorescence:* Appearance of areas that are more fluorescent, which may be due to enhanced visualization of a normal density of fluorescein in the fundus or an absolute increase in the fluorescein content of the tissues

    It is seen in several major patterns:
    - Window defect
    - Pooling of dye
    - Leakage
    - Staining of tissue

    iii. *Pseudofluorescence in FFA:*
    - Normal occurrence in every angiogram
    - Occurs late in angiogram
    - Fluorescein material is activated within aqueous/vitreous, and fluorescence is reflected from fundus structures such as optic disk

    Pseudofluorescence is an artifact of reflected fluorescein activated elsewhere in eye other than apparent fluorescence of structures due to inadequate barrier filters.

29. **What are true and false fluorescence?**
    i. Late fluorescence of optic disk: Combination of true and pseudofluorescence
    ii. Dye bound to plasma protein penetrates vessel wall poorly; hence, only free dye enters aqueous
    iii. Dye in anterior segment is low; hence, pseudofluorescence is also low
    iv. Fluorescence of myelinated nerve fiber in late films is due to activated dye in aqueous/vitreous emitting fluorescence lately. This is called false fluorescence due to overlap of exciter and barrier filter

30. Describe the causes of hypofluorescence.

Hypofluorescence can be because of blocked fluorescence or vascular filling defects.

i. *Blocked fluorescence:*
   - *Pigments*
     RPE hypertrophy
     Melanin, xanthophyll at macula
     Hemoglobin
   - *Exudates*
   - *Edema and transudates*
     Diskiform degeneration
     Central serous retinopathy (CSR)
     Detachment
   - *Hemorrhage*, e.g., choroidal, retinal, subhyaloid

ii. *Vascular filling defects:*
   - Vascular occlusions of retinal, artery, vein, and capillary bed
   - Choriocapillaris—nonperfusion, choroidal sclerosis

31. How to differentiate blocked fluorescence and vascular filling defects?

Blocked fluorescence is most easily differentiated from hypofluorescence due to hypoperfusion by evaluating the ophthalmoscopic view where a lesion is usually visible that corresponds to the area of blocked fluorescence. If no corresponding area is visible clinically, then it is likely an area of vascular filling defect and not blocked fluorescence.

32. Describe the causes of hyperfluorescence.

i. *Preinjection phase:*
   - Autofluorescence
   - Pseudofluorescence

ii. *Increased transmission (window defect):*
   - Atrophic pigment—drusen, RPE atrophy, albino epithelial window defect
   - Leak
   - Pooling (in space)
     New vessels
     Retinal
     Subretinal—choroidal neovascular membrane (CNVM), CSR
   - Staining (in tissue)
     Retinal, e.g., soft exudate
     Subretinal, e.g., drusen, scar tissue

iii. *Abnormal vessels:*
   - Neovascularization
   - Occlusions
   - Micro- and macroaneurysms

- Telangiectasia, e.g., Coats' angiomatosis
- Shunts and collaterals subretinal
- Neovascular membrane tumors
- Retinal—retinoblastoma
- Subretinal—malignant melanoma, choroidal hemangioma

33. **What is autofluorescence and pseudofluorescence?**
    i. *Autofluorescence* occurs when certain structures in the eye naturally fluoresce.
       - Optic nerve head drusen
       - Scar tissue
       - Astrocytic hamartoma
       - Cataractous lens
    ii. *Pseudofluorescence* is a false fluorescence indicating an inefficient filter system.
       - Old filters
       - Brand new filters
       - High humidity
       - Exposure to light

34. **What is the importance of fundus autofluorescence (FAF) imaging?**
    FAF is used to evaluate the diseases such as ARMD, macular dystrophies, and retinitis pigmentosa (RP). It gives a good indication of outer retinal health. Each RPE cell has hundreds of autofluorescent granules, and they show a very characteristic retinal distribution in normal aging. A loss of autofluorescence usually signals significant damage to RPE cells. A recent advancement is quantitative, which helps to see the RPE damage over time.

35. **What is leakage?**
    Leakage refers to the gradual, marked increase in fluorescence throughout the angiogram when:
    i. Fluorescein molecules seep through the pigment epithelium into the subretinal space or neurosensory retina
    ii. Out of retinal blood vessels into the retinal interstitium or
    iii. From retinal neovascularization into the vitreous

    The borders of hyperfluorescence become increasingly blurred, and the greatest intensity of hyperfluorescence is appreciated in the late phases of the study, when the only significant fluorescein dye remaining in the eye is extravascular.

    Examples include:
    i. Choroidal neovascularization
    ii. Microaneurysms

iii. Telangiectatic capillaries in diabetic macular edema or
iv. Neovascularization of the disk

36. **Describe staining.**
    Staining refers to a pattern of hyperfluorescence where the fluorescence gradually increases in intensity through transit views and persists in late views, but its borders remain fixed throughout the angiogram process. Staining results from fluorescein entry into solid tissue or similar material that retains the fluorescein such as:
    i. Scar
    ii. Drusen
    iii. Optic nerve tissue or sclera

37. **Describe pooling.**
    Pooling refers to accumulation of fluorescein in a fluid-filled space in the retina or choroid. The margins of the space trapping the fluorescein are usually distinct, as seen in an RPE detachment in central serous chorioretinopathy.

38. **Explain transmission defect or window defect.**
    Transmission defect or window defect refers to a view of the normal choroidal fluorescence through a defect in the pigment or loss of pigment in the RPE. In this pattern, hyperfluorescence occurs early, corresponding to filling of the choroidal circulation, and reaches its greatest intensity with the peak of choroidal filling. The fluorescence does not increase in size or shape and usually fades in the late phases of the angiogram.

39. **What are the angiographic findings in DR?**
    i. *Indications of FFA in DR:*
       - Clinically significant macular edema
       - Macular ischemia
       - Fellow eye of high risk/severe proliferative diabetic retinopathy (PDR) (asymmetric DR)
       - Suspected severe nonproliferative diabetic retinopathy (NPDR)/PDR—to differentiate IRMA and NVE
       - Asteroid hyalosis
       - Featureless retina
       - To differentiate diabetic papillopathy from anterior ischemic optic neuropathy (AION) and NVD
    ii. *Salient findings:*
        The two most important phases of FFA in a diabetic eye are the mid-arteriovenous phase and the late venous phase.

- AV phase
  - The most important observations are CNP areas outside the arcades and FAZ
  - FAZ changes in DR Irregularity of FAZ margins Capillary budding into FAZ
    * Pruning of the vessels
    * Widening of intercapillary spaces in perifoveal capillary bed
    * Enlargement of FAZ (normal diameter is 500 μm)
  - Leaking microaneurysms—many more than clinically evident are seen and can be differentiated from dot hemorrhages
  - IRMA and new vessels are seen at the borders of CNP areas. The former leak minimally and the latter profusely
- *Late phase:* Emphasizes leakage
  - *Mild NPDR* Microaneurysms—hyperfluorescent dots that may
    * leak in later phases
    * Superficial and deep retinal hemorrhages causing blocked choroidal fluorescence
- *Severe NPDR:*
  - All features as in mild NPDR
  - CNP areas—seen as areas of hypofluorescence and usually outlined by dilated capillaries unlike hypofluorescence caused by hemorrhages
  - IRMAs are segmental and irregular dilatation of capillary channels lying within CNP areas
  - Venous abnormalities—such as dilatation, beading, looping, and reduplication
  - Soft exudates cause blockage of choroidal fluorescence like retinal hemorrhages
- *PDR:*
  - NVD or NVE on retinal surface or elevated into vitreous—these leak the dye profusely which increases in later phase
  - Preretinal (subhyaloid) hemorrhages are well outlined and these block both retinal and choroidal fluorescence
- *Focal diabetic maculopathy:*
  - Focal leaks from microaneurysms in macular area
  - Hard exudates cause blocked choroidal fluorescence
- *Diffuse diabetic maculopathy (cystoid):*
  - Dilated retinal capillaries are seen leaking diffusely in the macular area
  - Typical petaloid or honeycomb pattern of cystoid macular edema (CME) may be seen in late phases
  - Hard exudates typically are not seen

40. **Describe the characteristic features of FFA in other common retinal pathologies.**
    i. *Cystoid macular edema:*
        - Petaloid pattern of staining of cysts in macula
        - Disk may leak or stain
        - Leak into vitreous in late phases
    ii. *CSR:*
        - 95% have one or more typical leakage points
        - Arteriovenous phase shows the leakage point
        - In late phases
            - It spreads in all directions, i.e., ink-blot type of leakage.
            - It first ascends forming smokestack and then spreads like a mushroom or umbrella (7–20%)
        - Scar will show hyperfluorescence with hypofluorescent patches
        - Optic pit shows hyperfluorescence
    iii. *Macular hole:*
        - Pseudohole shows no abnormal fluorescence except for traction-induced retinal vascular leakage
        - Outer lamellar hole—variable degrees of window defect
        - Inner lamellar hole—no transmitted fluorescence or minimal window defect
        - Full-thickness hole—granular hyperfluorescent window defects in the arteriovenous phase. Surrounding elevation produces blockage of choroidal fluorescence, which increases the contrast
    iv. *Branch retinal vein occlusion (BRVO):*
        - Early arteriovenous phase shows delayed filling of involved vein
        - Hemorrhages and cotton wool spots produce blocked fluorescence
        - NVD, NVE, and CNP areas are seen
        - Macular edema (perifoveal capillary leakage) and macular ischemia (broken FAZ)
    v. *Central retinal vein occlusion (CRVO):*
        - Delayed central venous filling and emptying
        - Engorged and tortuous retinal veins
        - NVD, NVE, and CNP areas are seen
        - Blocked fluorescence
        - New vessels (early leakage) and collaterals (no leakage)
    vi. *Anterior ischemic optic neuropathy (AION):*
        - Early arteriovenous phase—hypofluorescence of the disk
        - Mid-arteriovenous phase—patient capillaries leak and show edema
        - Hypofluorescent areas remain as such due to CNP

vii. *Subretinal neovascular membrane (SRNVM)*
   - Early arteriovenous phase shows lacy irregular nodular hyperfluorescence
   - Late phase shows leakage and pooling
   - A lacy network of new vessels suggests a "classic" lesion, whereas diffuse leakage suggests an "occult lesion"

41. **Describe indocyanine green (ICG) angiography.**

    Indocyanine green angiography is of particular value in delineating the choroidal circulation and can be a useful adjunct to FA in the investigation of macular disease in certain circumstances. About 98% of the ICG molecules bind to serum protein, reducing the passage of ICG through the fenestrations of the choriocapillaris, which are impermeable to the larger protein molecules.

    Indications:
    i. Exudative ARMD
       - Occult CNV
       - CNV associated with PED
       - Recurrent CNV adjacent to laser scars
       - Identification of feeder vessels
    ii. Polypoidal choroidal vasculopathy
    iii. Chronic CSR
    iv. Lacquer cracks and angioid streaks
    v. VKH
    vi. White dot syndromes
    vii. Choroidal melanoma

42. **Describe anterior segment angiography.**

    Abnormal blood vessels in the conjunctiva, cornea, and iris may be identified with fluorescein angiography.

    Mainly iris angiography is done to diagnose:
    i. Iris neovascularization
    ii. Iris tumors

    Findings:
    i. Normal iris vessels follow a fairly straight pattern from the iris root to the pupillary border with anastomotic connections between the vessels near the iris root and those of the collarette
    ii. Rubeosis leak of fluorescein dye is extensive and occurs early in the angiography

43. **What is the principle of ICG angiography?**

    ICG is a water-soluble, tricarbocyanine anion dye with a molecular weight of 774.96 Da.

It absorbs near-infrared region of light with maximum absorption at 790 nm with a maximum emission at 835 nm.

Above 98% is bound to globulin such as A1-lipoprotein with negligible extrahepatic removal. High molecular weight in combination with high percentage bound to plasma protein reduces the amount of dye that exits through fenestration in choroidal vessels. Hence, it is suitable for studying the choroidal vascular network. Since it has a longer wavelength, it penetrates more and hence is useful to study choroidal vessels.

44. **Why is CME stellate in the macular area as opposed to the honeycomb appearance of cystoid edema outside the macula?**
    i. The fovea contains only the following four layers of the retina—the internal limiting membrane (ILM), the outer plexiform layer, the outer nuclear layer, and the rods and cones. No intermediate layers exist between the ILM and the outer plexiform layer in the fovea
    ii. The outer plexiform layer is oblique in the foveal region, but outside the macular region, it is perpendicular

45. **What are the other peculiarities in the macular region?**
    i. It is thinner
    ii. The pigment epithelial cells are more columnar and have a greater concentration of melanin and lipofuscin granules than in the remainder of the fundus
    iii. Xanthophyll is present
    iv. Absence of retinal vessels for 400–500 mm in diameter

46. **Why is the macular region black in FFA?**
    i. Absence of vessels
    ii. Differences in pigmentation.

6.3 ULTRASONOGRAPHY

1. **What is an ultrasound?**
   Ultrasound is an acoustic wave that consists of oscillation of particles with a frequency >20,000 Hz and hence is inaudible.

2. **What is the audible range?**
   20–20,000 Hz

3. **What is the frequency of diagnostic ophthalmic ultrasonography (USG)?**
   8–20 MHz

4. **What is an A-scan?**
   A—amplitude
   A-scan is one-dimensional acoustic display in which echoes are represented as vertical spikes. The spacing of spikes depends on the time it takes for the sound to reach an interface, and the height indicates the strength of the returning echoes (i.e., amplitude).

5. **What is B-scan?**
   B—brightness
   B-scan produces two-dimensional acoustic sections. This requires focused beam with a frequency of 10 MHz. The echo is represented by a dot, and the strength of the echo is depicted by the brightness of the dot.

6. **What is standardized echography?**
   The combined use of standardized A-scan and contact B-scan is called standardized echography.

7. **What is M-mode?**
   M-mode [also called time motion (TM)] systems will examine temporal variations in tissue dimension, thus providing data concerning accommodation and vascular pulsations in tumors.

8. **What are the basic probe orientations?**
   i. Transverse
   ii. Longitudinal
   iii. Axial

9. **What are the indications for echography?**
   i. Ocular media

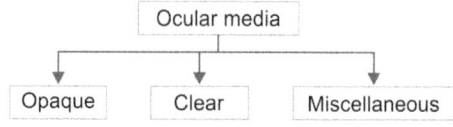

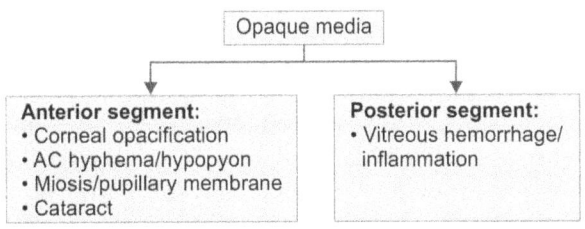

ii. Clear media

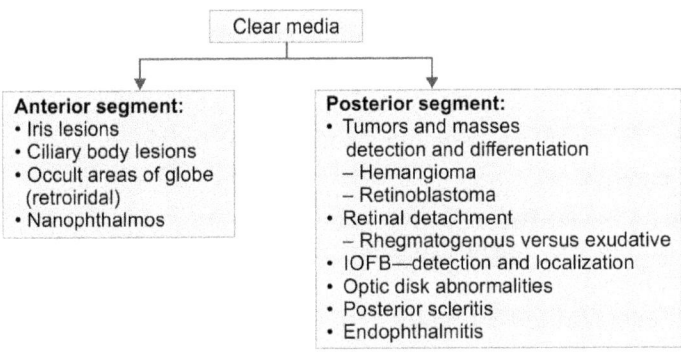

iii. Miscellaneous
- *Biometry:*
    - Axial eye length
    - Anterior chamber (AC) depth
    - Lens thickness
    - Tumor measurement
- *Orbital indications:*
    - Pseudotumor
    - Thyroid myopathy
    - Orbital tumors

10. **How does asteroid hyalosis show up in USG?**
    i. *B-scan:*
        - Bright point-like echo that is either diffuse or focal
        - Clear area of vitreous between the posterior boundary of the opacities and the posterior hyaloid
    ii. *A-scan:*
        - Medium-to-high reflective spikes

11. **How does vitreous hemorrhage (VH) show up in USG?**
    Aim:
    To establish the density and location of the hemorrhage and the cause of an unexplained hemorrhage.

    Mild VH:
    B-scan: Dots and short lines
    A-scan: Chain of low amplitude spikes

More dense hemorrhage:
More opacities on B-scan and higher reflectivity on A-scan

If blood organizes, larger interfaces are formed, resulting in membranous surfaces on B-scan and higher reflectivity on A-scan.

Because of gravity, blood may layer inferiorly, resulting in highly reflective pseudomembrane that may be confused with retinal detachment (RD).

12. **How is USG useful in intraocular foreign body (IOFB)?**
    i. For more precise localization and to determine the extent of intraocular damage
    ii. For determining if a foreign body (FB) which is located next to the scleral wall lies just within or just outside the globe

    Metallic FB
    A-scan → Very high reflective spikes
    B-scan → Very bright signal that persists at low sensitivity and marked shadowing (gain lowest)
    i. Standardized echography can monitor the response of FB to pulsed magnet, to determine if it can be removed magnetically
    ii. Spherical FB (gun pellets/bullets)
       Reduplication/multiple signals due to reverberation of sound
       A-scan: Series of spikes of decreasing amplitude
       B-scan: Multiple short bright echoes in decreasing brightness
    iii. *Glass FB:* Produces extremely high reflection signal, only if the sound wave is perpendicular to the surface. If nonperpendicular, sound is reflected away from probe; hence, it can be missed

13. **How is USG useful in endophthalmitis?**
    i. *A-scan:* Chain of low-amplitude spikes from vitreous cavity
    ii. *B-scan:*
        - Diffuse low-intensity vitreous echoes
        - Diffuse thickening of retina–choroid–sclera (RCS) complex
        - Serous/tractional RD may be seen

14. **What is the normal RCS complex thickness?**
    1–1.5 mm

15. **What are the conditions with increased RCS thickness?**
    May be diffuse or focal
    i. Choroidal edema (high reflective)
       - Uveitis
       - Endophthalmitis
       - Macular edema
       - Vascular congestion
       - Hypotony

ii. Inflammatory infiltration (low reflective)
      - VKH syndrome
      - Sympathetic ophthalmia
      - Lymphoid hyperplasia of uvea
  iii. Choroidal tumors
      - Primary
      - Metastatic
  iv. Nanophthalmos

16. **How does posterior vitreous detachment (PVD) look in USG?**
    i. It can be focal or extensive and may be completely separated or remain attached to disk or at other sites [such as neovascularization elsewhere (NVE)/tears/impact sites in trauma/arcades]
    ii. B-scan—smooth, thick membranous with fluid undulating after movements
    iii. Scan—low (normal eye) to high (as in dense hemorrhage) reflectivity with marked horizontal and vertical spike after movements

17. **How does RD look in USG?**
    i. B-scan—bright, continuous folded membrane with more tethered restricted aftermovement—total RD is attached usually at disk and ora
    ii. A-scan—100% tall single spike at tissue sensitivity
    iii. Less than 100% spike is seen if retina is atrophic, severely folded, or disrupted
    iv. Very mobile RD is seen if it is bullous
    v. Hemorrhagic RD produces echoes in the subretinal space
    vi. Configuration of RD should be determined which varies from very shallow, flat, and smooth membrane to a bullous folded and funnel-shaped membrane. The funnel shape may be open/closed and may be concave, triangular, or T-shaped
    vii. Long-standing RD may develop cyst with cholesterol crystals that produce bright echoes and RD may be echolucent
    viii. Tractional RD
      - Tent like if there is point adherence
      - Tabletop RD

18. **What are the USG findings in nanophthalmos?**
    i. Short axial length (14–20.5 mm)
    ii. Shallow AC
    iii. Diffuse RCS thickening (>2 mm)
    iv. Normal-sized lens

19. **What are the USG findings in choroidal melanoma?**
    i. Collar button or mushroom-shaped appearance
    ii. Regular structure with low-to-medium reflectivity

iii. Marked sound attenuation on A-scan
iv. High vascularity indicated by marked spontaneous motion
v. Choroidal excavation is seen in the base of the mass where the low reflective tumor replaces the normally high reflective choroidal layer
vi. Hemorrhage into globe and serous RD also seen
vii. Extrascleral extension detected by a well-circumscribed area of homogeneity that is situated mostly adjacent to lesion
viii. Treated tumors—more irregular in structure, more highly reflective, and decreases in elevation

20. **What are the USG findings in retinoblastoma?**
A-scan—extremely high reflectivity
B-scan:
    i. Large bright mass at high sensitivity
    ii. At low sensitivity shows multiple bright echoes corresponding to calcium deposits
    iii. Shadowing of sclera and orbit
    iv. Diffuse tumor may not have calcification.

21. **What are the USG findings in choroidal hemangioma?**
    i. Solid, regularly structured, highly reflective
    ii. Internal vascularity—less pronounced than in melanoma
    iii. Lesions—mildly to moderately elevated with a dome-shaped configuration and are normally located posteriorly

22. **How will you differentiate between thyroid myopathy and pseudotumor?**
In thyroid myopathy, tendons are spared, with enlargement of muscle belly, whereas in pseudotumor, there will be diffuse enlargement of muscles (involving tendons) seen. Typical beer belly pattern is seen in thyroid-related myopathy.

23. **What are the limitations of orbital USG?**
    i. Tumors located at the orbital apex are difficult to recognize because of the attenuation of sound and confluence of optic nerve and muscles that are inseparable ultrasonically
    ii. Tumors <2 mm are not seen
    iii. Tumors originating/extending along the bony wall of the orbit do not present a reflecting surface perpendicular to the ultrasonic beam and consequently do not produce distinct echoes (e.g., meningioma, osteoma, pseudotumor)
    iv. Floor fractures, surgical defects of the orbital wall, and hyperostosis of bone are not reliably detectable.

6.4 DIABETIC RETINOPATHY

1. **What are the characteristic features of retinal arteries?**
   Retinal arteries are end arteries.

2. **What are the various anatomical layers of retinal artery?**
   i. *Intima:* The innermost layer is composed of a single layer of endothelium
   ii. *Internal elastic lamina:* It separates the intima from the media
   iii. *Media:* It consists mainly of smooth muscle
   iv. *Adventitia:* It is the outermost layer and is composed of loose connective tissue

3. **What are the outer and inner blood-retinal barriers?**
   i. *Outer blood-retinal barrier:* It consists of basal lamina of the Bruch and zonal occludens between the retinal pigment epithelium (RPE)
   ii. *Inner blood-retinal barrier:* The endothelial cells of the capillaries linked by the tight junctions form the inner blood-retinal barrier

4. **How do the RPE and the photoreceptors derive their nutrition?**
   RPE and layer of rods and cones are avascular and derive their nourishment from the choroidal circulation.

5. **What are the characteristics of retinal capillaries?**
   i. They supply the inner two-thirds of the retina while the outer third is supplied by choriocapillaris
   ii. There are two capillary networks—the inner (located in the ganglion cell layer) and the outer (in the inner nuclear layer)

6. **Why is proliferative diabetic retinopathy (PDR) more prevalent in insulin-dependent diabetes mellitus (IDDM) than in noninsulin-dependent diabetes mellitus (NIDDM)?**
   PDR is the result of prolonged, very high average blood glucose levels, and such levels are seen more in patients with IDDM.

7. **What are the risk factors for developing diabetic retinopathy (DR) in patients with diabetes mellitus (DM)?**
   i. Longer duration of the disease
   ii. Metabolic control—worsening of retinopathy occurs with poor control of hyperglycemia

8. **What are the systemic factors that have an adverse effect on DR?**
   i. Duration of diabetes
   ii. Poor metabolic control of diabetes
   iii. Pregnancy
   iv. Hypertension

v. Nephropathy
vi. Anemia
vii. Hyperlipidemia

9. **What are the ocular conditions which decrease the progression of DR?**
    i. Chorioretinal scarring
    ii. Retinitis pigmentosa
    iii. High myopia
    iv. Optic atrophy
    (It is due to decreased retinal metabolic demand.)

10. **What are the causes of vision loss in diabetes?**
    i. *Anterior segment pathology:*
        - Cornea—superficial punctate keratitis, neurotrophic keratitis
        - Fluctuating refractive error
        - Cataract (snowflakes cataract, rapidly progressing)
    ii. *Posterior segment pathology:*
        - Diabetic macular edema (DME)
        - Vitreous hemorrhage (VH)
        - Tractional and combined mechanism retinal detachment (RD)
        - Ischemic maculopathy
        - Vitreomacular traction
        - Laser or surgery-induced complications
        - Intravitreal injection-related complication
        - Neovascular glaucoma (NVG)
        - Diabetic papillopathy
        - Nonarteritic anterior ischemic optic neuropathy
        - Wolfram's syndrome (type 1 diabetes, optic atrophy, hearing defect)

11. **What are the ocular manifestations of diabetes?**
    i. *Orbit:*
        - Orbital cellulitis
        - Orbital mucormycosis
    ii. *Lid and adnexa:*
        More susceptible for
        - Wart
        - Recurrent hordeolum
        - Blepharitis
        - Xanthelasma
    iii. *Conjunctiva:*
        - Microaneurysm of bulbar conjunctiva
        - Dilatation
        - Tortuosity of vessels

iv. *Cornea:*
   - Reduced corneal sensitivity
   - Superficial punctate keratitis
   - Recurrent erosions
   - Neurotrophic keratitis
   - Tear film abnormality, reduced tear break-up time (TBUT) causing dry eye diseases
   - Endothelial cell changes
v. *Iris:*
   - Rubeosis iridis
   - Iris depigmentation
   - Iris atrophy
vi. *Pupil:*
   - Miotic pupil
   - Rigid pupil responding poorly to mydriatics
vii. *Lens:* Cataract—snowflakes and posterior subcapsular
viii. *Change in refractive error:* Hyperglycemia causes increased refractive index of lens and thus myopic shift, whereas hypoglycemia causes decreased refractive index of lens and thus induces hyperopic shift.
ix. *Transient paralysis of accommodation*
x. *Extraocular movement:* Third, fourth, and sixth nerve palsy
xi. *Retina:*
   DR and its sequelae such as:
   - VH
   - Macular edema
   - Ischemic maculopathy
   - Tractional RD
   - Combined mechanism RD
xii. *Optic disk:*
   - Diabetic papillopathy
   - Nonarteritic ischemic optic neuropathy
   - *Wolfram syndrome:* Optic atrophy, DM type 1, and hearing defect
xiii. *Glaucoma:*
   - More susceptible for development of POAG and its progression
   - NVG secondary to PDR

12. **Explain the pathogenesis of diabetic microangiopathy.**
   Diabetic microangiopathy occurs at the level of capillaries and comprises:
   i. *Capillaropathy:*
      - Degeneration and loss of pericytes

- Proliferation of endothelial cells
- Thickening of basement membrane and occlusion

ii. *Hematological changes:*
- Deformation of erythrocytes and rouleaux formation
- Changes in red blood cell (RBC) leading to defective oxygen transport
- Increased plasma viscosity
- Increased stickiness and aggregation of platelets

These changes result in microvascular occlusion and leakage.

13. **Mention the retinal vascular changes in DR.**
    i. *Capillaries:*
    - Occlusion
    - Dilatation
    - Microaneurysms
    - Abnormal permeability
    ii. *Arterioles:*
    - Narrowing of terminal arterioles
    - Occlusion
    - Sheathing
    iii. *Veins:*
    - Tortuosity
    - Looping
    - Beading
    - Sausage-like segmentation

14. **What are the functions of basement membrane?**
    i. Structural integrity to blood vessels
    ii. Filtration barrier for molecules of various sizes and charges
    iii. Regulate cell proliferation and differentiation

15. **What is the ratio of endothelium cells to pericytes?**
    Normal endothelial cells to pericyte ratio is 1:1, and there is loss of intramural pericytes in DM.

16. **What are the causes of breakdown of blood-retinal barrier?**
    i. Opening of tight junction between adjacent endothelial cell processes
    ii. Fenestration of the endothelial cell cytoplasm (normally absent)
    iii. Increased infoldings of plasma membrane at the basal surface of RPE cells
    iv. Increased transport by endocytic vessels

17. **How does microvascular leakage occur?**
    Loss of pericyte results in distention of capillary walls, which leads to breakdown in blood-retinal barrier and leakage of plasma.

18. **What is the cause of endothelial cell damage in DR?**
    It is due to increased sorbitol level in endothelial cells.

19. **What are the causes of RBC changes in DR?**
    It is due to increased growth hormone.

20. **What is the cause of increased platelet stickiness in DR?**
    It is due to increased factor VIII.

21. **What are the features of nonproliferative diabetic retinopathy (NPDR)?**
    i. Retinal microvascular changes are limited to the confines of the retina and do not extend beyond the internal limiting membrane
    ii. Findings include microaneurysms, areas of capillary nonperfusion, dot and blot retinal hemorrhages, and vascular abnormalities

22. **What are the causes of defective vision in DR?**
    i. *Retinal causes:*
        - Macular edema
        - Macular ischemia
        - Tractional RD involving macula
        - Rhegmatogenous RD involving macula [secondary to contraction of fibrovascular proliferation (FVP) causing retinal break]
        - Combined rhegmatogenous and tractional RD involving macula
        - Macular distortion secondary to contraction of FVP
        - RPE atrophy and subretinal fibrosis (in long-standing DME)
        - Epiretinal membrane
        - Circinate retinopathy
        - Massive lipid exudation in lipemia retinalis
    ii. *Nonretinal causes:*
        - NVG
        - Erythroclastic (RBC-induced) glaucoma
        - Ghost cell glaucoma
        - Snowflake cataract
        - VH
        - Dense premacular subhyaloid hemorrhage
        - Diabetic papillopathy

23. **Of these, what is the most important cause of defective vision?**
    Macular edema

24. **What are the characteristic features of macula?**
    Macula is an area bounded by temporal arcades, 4 mm temporal, and 0.8 mm inferior to the optic disk.

    It is 5 mm in diameter/3.5 disk diameter (DD)/18° of visual angle. Histologically, it has more than one layer of ganglion cells and has xanthophyll pigments. It has high density of cones, more than one layer.

25. **What are the characteristic features of fovea?**

    Fovea is an area of depression inside macula.

    It is 1.5 mm in diameter/1 DD /5° of visual angle. Histologically, it has six to eight layers of ganglion cells, tall RPE cells, and a thick internal limiting membrane. The central 0.5 mm area of fovea is devoid of blood vessels and is called foveal avascular zone (FAZ). It has the special functions of form sense and color vision due to the high density of cones.

26. **What are the characteristic features of foveola?**

    Foveola is the central floor of fovea.

    It is 0.35 mm in diameter/0.2 DD/0.54 minutes of visual angle. It is the thinnest part of retina. There are only three layers of the retina, namely RPE, layer of cones, and nerve fiber layer. It has no ganglion cells or rods. It has only cones ($150,000/mm^2$), which are most densely packed and elongated, which causes a slight bowing internally called the umbo.

27. **Which are the thinnest and thickest parts of the retina?**
    i. *Thinnest part:* Foveola (three layers)
    ii. *Thickest part:* Margin of the fovea, where the inner nuclear layer, outer plexiform layer, and ganglion cell layers are the thickest

28. **How will you classify DR?**
    i. *Mild NPDR:* At least one microaneurysm
    ii. *Moderate NPDR:*
       - Intraretinal hemorrhage or microaneurysm <ETDRS (Early Treatment Diabetic Retinopathy Study) standard photograph 2A
       - Cotton wool spots, venous beading, and intraretinal microvascular abnormality (IRMA)
    iii. *Severe NPDR:* 4:2:1 rule
    iv. *Very severe NPDR:* At least two of the criteria for severe NPDR
    v. *High-risk PDR:*
       - Neovascularization of disk (NVD) >1/2 disk area
       - NVD plus vitreous or preretinal hemorrhage
       - Neovascularization elsewhere (NVE) >1/2 disk area plus preretinal or VH
    vi. *Advanced PDR:* Tractional RD

29. **Where will you find microaneurysms?**

    Microaneurysms are found between superior and temporal vascular arcades and within center of the circinate (wreath)

30. **What is the size of the microaneurysm?**

    The minimum size of the microaneurysm should be 20 µm to be seen by DO.

31. What are microaneurysms?

Microaneurysms are localized saccular outpouchings of the capillary wall, often caused by pericyte loss. They are continuous with the blood vessels. They appear as red, round intraretinal lesions of 30–120 μm in size and are located in the inner nuclear layer of the retina. However, clinically they are indistinguishable from dot hemorrhages. Fluorescein angiogram reveals hyperfluorescence. They are saccular outpouchings of the capillary wall probably arising at the weak points due to loss of pericytes.

32. What are hard exudates and where are they located?

Hard exudates are caused by chronic localized retinal edema and appear at the junction of the normal and edematous retina. They are composed of lipoproteins and lipid-filled macrophages and are located mainly in the outer plexiform layer of the retina. Fundus fluorescein angiography (FFA) shows hypofluorescence.

33. How do you differentiate drusen and hard exudates?

Drusen:
  i. Oval or round in shape
  ii. Whitish or yellowish in color
  iii. Punched-out areas of choroid or pigment epithelial atrophy

Hard exudates:
  i. Waxy yellow lesions with distinct margin
  ii. Other features of DR such as microaneurysms and hemorrhages will be present

34. Why are the retinal superficial hemorrhages flame shaped?

Retinal superficial hemorrhages occur at the nerve fiber layer and are flame shaped since they follow the architecture of the nerve fiber layer. They arise from superficial precapillary arterioles.

35. Why are the inner retinal hemorrhages dot shaped?

Inner retinal hemorrhages are dot shaped is because the inner retinal structures are perpendicular to the retinal surface.

36. What are cotton wool spots?

Cotton wool spots are due to the ischemic infarction of the nerve fiber layer. Because of the ischemia, interruption of axoplasmic flow happens and buildup of transported material within axons occurs.

37. What are the causes of cotton wool spots?

Causes are:
  i. *Systemic diseases:*
     - Diabetes
     - Hypertension
     - Collagen vascular diseases

ii. *Vascular:*
      - Central retinal vein occlusion (CRVO)
      - Branch retinal vein occlusion (BRVO)
   iii. *Infections:*
      - Human immunodeficiency virus (HIV) retinopathy
      - Toxoplasmosis
   iv. *Hematological:*
      - Leukemias
      - Anemia
      - Hypercoagulable states
   v. *Others:*
      - Radiation retinopathy
      - Purtscher's retinopathy
      - Interferon therapy

38. **Describe IRMA.**
    IRMA is frequently seen adjacent to capillary closure, and it resembles focal areas of flat retinal neovascularization clinically. These are arteriovenous shunts that run from arterioles to venules. IRMA indicates severe NPDR and may herald the onset of the preproliferative stage of diabetic retinopathy (PPDR).

39. **What is the difference between retinal collaterals, shunts, and neovascularization?**
    Retinal collaterals: These are vessels that develop within the framework of the existing retinal vascular network. Collaterals originate from the retinal capillary bed, joining obstructed to nonobstructed adjacent vessels, or bypassing obstructions in a single vessel; i.e., veins are linked to veins, arteries are linked to arteries, and, less frequently, arteries are joined to veins. Flow in these channels is generally slow. For example, branched retinal artery occlusion, retinal vein occlusion, sickle cell hemoglobinopathies, and Leber's multiple miliary aneurysms.

    Shunts: These are arteriovenous communications, congenital or developmental, in which blood passes directly from artery to vein without going through the normal capillary bed. Flow in these vessels is usually rapid. These vessels do not leak on FFA except large vascular malformations. For example, retinal angioma, Takayasu disease, and Coats' disease.

    Neovascularization: These are new vessels originating and contiguous with the preexisting retinal vascular bed. They are located either within or adjacent to ischemic areas. These vessels usually leak on FFA. For example, PDR, CRVO, Coats' disease, and Eales' disease.

Retina **435**

40. **Why retinal edema commonly occurs at macula?**
    i. High metabolic activity
    ii. Extremely high concentration of cells
    iii. Central avascular zone creates a watershed arrangement between the retinal and choroidal circulation, thus reducing the absorption of fluid
    iv. Thickness and loose binding of inner connection fibers in Henle's layer
    v. Radial arrangement of Henle's layer
    vi. Lack of inner layers at the fovea

41. **Explain the pathological changes of diabetic maculopathy.**
    Pathological changes are classified into:
    i. *Intraretinal:*
       - Macular edema
       - Macular ischemia
    ii. *Preretinal:*
       - Thickened posterior hyaloid
       - Thickened preretinal membrane
       - Macular traction
       - Macular ectopia

42. **What is normal foveal thickness?**
    According to ETDRS definition
    i. Foveal thickness (212 ± 20 μm)—mean thickness in the central 1,000-μm diameter area
    ii. Central foveal thickness (182 ± 23 μm)—mean thickness at the point of intersection of six radial scans

43. **What are the reasons for focal and diffuse macular edema?**
    The most common causes of visual impairment in diabetic patients are given below:
    i. *Focal edema:* Due to localized leakage from microaneurysm leading to hard exudates ring formation and retinal thickening
    ii. *Diffuse edema (>2 DD size):* Due to generalized leakage from decompensated capillaries throughout the posterior pole

44. **What is clinically significant macular edema (CSME)?**
    i. Retinal thickening at or within 500 μm of the center of macula
    ii. Hard exudates at or within 500 μm of the center of macula with adjacent retinal thickening
    iii. Retinal thickening of 1 DD or larger, any part of which is within 1 DD of the center of the fovea

45. How does macular ischemia look clinically?
i. Signs are variable: Multiple cotton wool spots and attenuated arterioles may be seen
ii. Macula may look relatively normal despite reduced visual acuity

46. What are the FFA characteristics of macular ischemia?
i. Focal capillary dropout
ii. Enlargement of FAZ
iii. Occlusion of arterioles of the macula

47. How do you manage clinically significant DME?
i. Maximize medical control of blood glucose and blood pressure
ii. If it is a noncentric DME, but meeting the criteria of CSME (modified ETDRS classification), then laser can be performed
Spot size: 100 μm
Time: 0.1 second
Space: One spot size apart
iii. Center involving DME > 400 μm is treated with intravitreal injections of ranibizumab (supported by NICE trial). It is given monthly till vision is stable for 3 months. If the patient is pregnant or does not want the injection, then laser can be given
iv. To consider intravitreal fluocinolone acetonide for long-standing nonresponsive DME
v. *Surgery:*
In cases with posterior hyaloid traction, pars plana vitrectomy and detachment of posterior hyaloid may be useful for treating DME

48. What are the protocols for DME management?

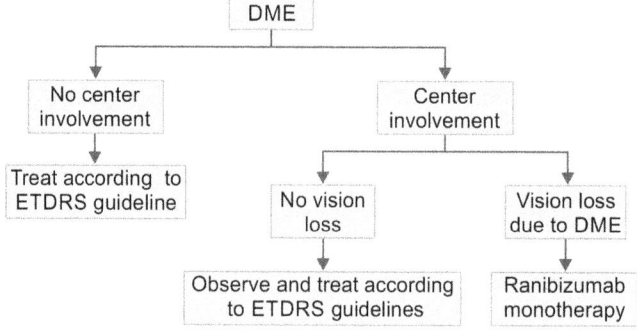

49. What are the treatment considerations for first-line treatment for eyes with PDR in the following situations, based on Diabetic Retinopathy Clinical Research (DRCR) studies?
a. *PDR with central involved DME:* Initiate treatment with anti-VEGF (vascular endothelial growth factor) monotherapy and reevaluate

the need for panretinal photocoagulation (PRP), once the eye does not require anti-VEGF agents

b. *PDR with noncentral involved DME:* Consider using anti-VEGF monotherapy

c. *PDR with no DME:* Anti-VEGF and PRP are equally good alternatives

50. **How do you manage eyes being treated with anti-VEGF for PDR that develops VH?**

    Patients should continue getting anti-VEGF on a monthly basis till the hemorrhage clears. After that, the neovascularization status is reassessed. Regular fundus evaluation and USG should be done to see whether tractional RD is happening or worsening.

51. **What are the characteristic features of PPDR?**
    i. *Clinical features:*
       - Presence of cotton wool spots
       - Presence of IRMA
       - Venous beading
       - Narrowing of vessels
       - Dark blot hemorrhages
    ii. *Fluorescein angiogram features:*
       - Extension of papillary nonperfusion areas

52. **What is the 4:2:1 rule?**

    ETDRS investigators developed the 4:2:1 rule to help clinicians identify patients at greater risk of progression.
    i. Diffuse intraretinal hemorrhages and microaneurysms in *four* quadrants
    ii. Venous beading in *two* quadrants
    iii. IRMAs in *one* quadrant

53. **What is the incidence of PDR in diabetic population?**

    The incidence is 5–10%. Type I patients are typically at risk.

54. **What is the cause of neovascularization?**
    i. Liberation of vasoformative angiogenic growth factors (VEGF, placental growth factor, pigment epithelial factor) elaborated by the hypoxic retina in an attempt to revascularize hypoxic areas is thought to produce neovascularization
    ii. Inhibition of endogenous inhibitors such as endostatin and angiostatin

55. **What is the common site for neovascularization?**

    The common site for neovascularization is mainly along major temporal arcade at the posterior pole and over the disk, arising most frequently from veins. Predilection of neovascularization over the disk to bleed is due to absence of internal limiting membrane; hence, NVD is more dangerous than NVE.

56. What is high-risk PDR?
High-risk PDR was defined in the diabetic retinopathy study (DRS) as any one of the following:
  i. Mild NVD with VH
  ii. Moderate-to-severe NVD with or without VH (≥DRS standard 10A, showing one-fourth to one-third disk area of NVD)
  iii. Moderate NVE (one-half disk area) with VH

57. What is the appearance of VH on ophthalmoscopic examination?
It is black in color

58. What are the various stages in the development of PDR?
  i. Fine new vessels with minimal fibrous tissue cross and extend beyond the internal limiting membrane (ILM)
  ii. New vessels increase in size and extend with an increased fibrous component
  iii. New vessels regress, leaving residual FVP along the posterior hyaloid

59. What are the constituents of FVP?
FVP is the presence of newly formed blood vessels often accompanied by fibrous tissue spreading along the inner surface of retina and optic disk or extending into the vitreous cavity.
Risk factors:
  i. Elevated glycated hemoglobin (HbA1c)
  ii. Elevated serum lipids (triglycerides)
  iii. Diabetic neuropathy
  iv. Decreased hematocrit
  v. Decreased plasma albumin
  vi. Anemia

60. What are the signs of regression of FVP?
  i. Regression of new vessels
  ii. Fibrous tissue becomes thinner and transparent

61. What are the signs of involutional or quiescent DR?
  i. Reduction in caliber of retinal vessels
    – Previously dilated or beaded vessels return to their normal size
    – Small arterioles appear to be white threads without visible blood columns
  ii. Detachment of vitreous from all areas except vitreoretinal adhesion areas
  iii. Clearing VH
  iv. Fibrous tissue becomes more thinner and transparent

62. **What is the most common type of RD that occurs in diabetes?**
    i. Tractional RD
    ii. Combined RD and rhegmatogenous RD also occur

63. **What are the current indications for pars plana vitrectomy in PDR?**
    i. Dense, nonclearing VH
    ii. Tractional RD involving or threatening macula
    iii. Combined tractional and rhegmatogenous RD
    iv. Diffuse DME associated with posterior hyaloid traction
    v. Significant recurrent VH despite maximal PRP

64. **What are the complications of PDR?**
    i. Persistent VH
    ii. Tractional RD
    iii. Development of opaque membranes on the posterior surface of detached hyaloid
    iv. Rubeosis iridis and NVG

65. **What are the landmark studies in DR?**
    i. *Epidemiological studies:*
       - Wisconsin Epidemiology Study of DR (WESDR)
         In type I diabetics, retinopathy was seen in 13% of those with less than 5-year duration of DM and in 90% of those with a duration of 10-15 years
         In type II diabetics, in people not taking insulin, the corresponding rates are 24% and 53%
    ii. *Studies that measured the efficacy of photocoagulation:*
       - DRS—proved the use of photocoagulation in the treatment
       - ETDRS—gave data regarding when to do photocoagulation
    iii. *Study that measured the efficacy of vitrectomy:*
       - Diabetic Retinopathy Vitrectomy Study (DRVS)—proved the advantage of early vitrectomy in VH complicating PDR
    iv. *Studies that measured the efficacy of metabolic control:*
       - Diabetes Control and Complication Trial (DCCT)—intensive glycemic control reduces DR and other microvascular complications of diabetes
       - UKPDS—United Kingdom Prospective Diabetes Study
       - Action to control cardiovascular risk in diabetes (ACCORD): Very intensive control of diabetes (HbA1c <6%) caused an increased rate of death
    v. *Studies measuring the efficacy of intravitreal injections:*
       - DRCR network: It showed that ranibizumab was superior to laser or triamcinolone in DME

- *READ 2 and RESTORE:* They found that ranibizumab was visually superior to laser alone in DME
- *RISE and RIDE, and RESOLVE:* They showed that ranibizumab was superior to sham for the treatment of DME

66. **What are the differential diagnoses for NPDR?**
    i. CRVO
    ii. BRVO
    iii. Ocular ischemic syndrome
    iv. Hypertensive retinopathy
    v. Leukemia
    vi. Anemia
    vii. HIV microangiopathy

67. **What are the differential diagnoses for PDR?**
    i. Vascular obstruction
    ii. Sickle cell retinopathy
    iii. Ocular ischemic syndrome
    iv. Sarcoidosis
    v. Eales' disease
    vi. Tuberculosis
    vii. Embolization from intravenous drug use

68. **What are the differential diagnoses for DME?**
    i. CRVO or BRVO
    ii. Postoperative CME
    iii. Neovascular ARMD
    iv. Uveitic cystoid macular edema
    v. Epiretinal membrane
    vi. Vitreomacular traction
    vii. Hypotony maculopathy

69. **What was the main study objective of DRS?**
    The main study objective was to determine if photocoagulation reduced the risk of severe visual loss in PDR.

70. **What were the major methodology aspects of DRS?**
    i. Randomization
    ii. One eye of each patient was assigned randomly to photocoagulation (argon or xenon) and the other eye for follow-up. Eye on treatment was randomly assigned to argon or xenon arc

71. **What was the inference of DRS?**
    i. Photocoagulation reduced the risk of severe visual loss by 50% or more

ii. Modest risks of decrease in visual acuity and constriction of visual fields (more for xenon)
iii. Treatment benefit outweighs risks for eyes with high-risk PDR

72. **What were the main study questions of ETDRS?**
    i. Is photocoagulation effective in treating DME?
    ii. Is photocoagulation effective for treating DR?
    iii. Is aspirin effective for preventing progression of DR?

73. **What were the results of ETDRS?**
    i. *Aspirin use results:*
       - Aspirin use did not alter progression of DR but reduced the risk of cardiovascular morbidity and mortality
    ii. *Early scatter photocoagulation results:*
       - Early scatter photocoagulation resulted in a small reduction in the risk of severe visual loss
       - It is not indicated for eyes with mild-to-moderate DR
       - It may be most effective in patients with type 2 diabetes
    iii. *Macular edema results:*
       - Focal photocoagulation for DME decreased the risk of moderate visual loss, reduced retinal thickening, and increased the chance of moderate visual gain

74. **What was the main study question of DRVS?**
    The main study question was to evaluate the natural course and effect of surgical intervention on severe PDR and its complications.

75. **What were the clinical recommendations?**
    i. Early vitrectomy is advantageous for severe VH causing a significant decrease in vision, especially in type I diabetics
    ii. Greater urgency for early surgery in uncontrolled FVP or when proliferation has been treated partially by scatter photocoagulation
    iii. Eyes with traction detachment not involving the fovea and producing visual loss do not need surgery until there is detachment of fovea, provided the proliferation process is not severe

76. **What were the main study questions of DCCT?**
    i. *Primary prevention study:* Will intensive control of blood glucose slow development and subsequent progression of DR?
    ii. *Secondary prevention study:* Will intensive control of blood glucose slow progression of DR?

77. **What were the main study outcomes of DCCT?**
    i. Intensive control reduced the risk of developing retinopathy and also slowed the progression of retinopathy
    ii. Intensive control also reduced the risk of clinical neuropathy and albuminuria

78. **What were the study questions of UKPDS?**
    Will intensive control of blood glucose and intensive control of blood pressure reduce the risk of microvascular complications of DR?

79. **What were the main study outcomes of UKPDS?**
    Intensive control of diabetes and blood pressure slowed the progression of DR and reduced the risk of other microvascular complications of DR.

80. **What are the recent newer protocols in DRCR.net?**
    i. *Protocol T*
    To determine relative efficacy and safety of intravitreous aflibercept, bevacizumab, and ranibizumab in the treatment of DME.
    Conclusion:
    When the initial visual acuity loss was mild and there were no apparent differences, at worse levels of initial visual acuity, aflibercept was more effective at improving vision.
    ii. *Protocol S*
    PRP versus intravitreous ranibizumab for PDR.
    Conclusion:
    Among eyes with PDR, treatment with ranibizumab resulted in visual acuity that was not inferior to PRP at 2 years. The ranibizumab group showed better visual acuity, decreased peripheral visual field loss, fewer vitrectomies, and were less likely to develop central-involved DME.
    Although longer-term follow-up is needed, ranibizumab may be a reasonable treatment alternative for patients with PDR.
    iii. *Protocol I*
    Intravitreal ranibizumab for DME with prompt versus deferred laser treatment.
    Conclusion:
    5-year results suggest that focal or grid laser treatment at initiation of intravitreal ranibizumab is no better than deferring laser treatment for >24 weeks in eye with center involving DME with visual impairment.
    More than half of eyes in which laser treatment is deferred may avoid laser for at least 5 years. Such eyes may require more injections to achieve these results.

6.5 LASERS IN DIABETIC RETINOPATHY

1. **What does the word LASER stand for and what is its basic principle?**
   LASER stands for *L*ight *A*mplification by *S*timulated *E*mission of *R*adiation.
   Principle: Electrons in lasing medium are excited to a higher energy level, which then decay to a lower energy state with the release of a photon, which may be spontaneous or stimulated emission. This photon then targets the tissue of interest.

2. **What are the types of laser tissue interaction?**
   i. *Photocoagulation*—absorption of light by pigments causes 10–20°C rise in temperature leading to protein denaturation/coagulation. For example, panretinal photocoagulation (PRP) for high-risk proliferative diabetic retinopathy (PDR)
   ii. *Photoablation*—high-energy ultraviolet (UV) rays are used to break covalent bonds. For example, excimer laser for refractive surgery
   iii. *Photodisruption*—high-energy pulsed laser strip electrons from molecules, which form plasma. This expands causing a mechanical shock wave displacing tissue. For example, Nd-YAG laser capsulotomy
   iv. *Photoactivation*—conversion of a chemical from one form to another using light. For example, photodynamic therapy (PDT) using verteporfin

3. **What are the types of laser tissue interaction in the eye?**
   i. *Photochemical effects:*
      - Photoradiation (dye laser)
      - Photoablation (excimer lasers)
   ii. *Thermal effects:* Photocoagulation (argon, krypton laser)
   iii. *Ionizing effect:* Photodisruption (Nd:YAG laser)

4. **How does laser work?**
   The lasing material is placed in a resonant cavity, which has a mirror at each end. When a photon encounters an excited electron and stimulated emission occurs, the light emitted travels to and fro in the cavity and reinforces itself, producing coherent, monochromatic, and collimated light.

5. **What are the different types of lasers used?**
   i. *Based on types of laser media, lasers are classified as:*
      - *Solid-state lasers:*
        - Ruby laser
        - Nd:YAG laser

- *Gas lasers:*
  - Argon laser
  - Krypton laser
  - CO_2 laser
- *Liquid lasers:*
  Dye laser (not much popular)
- *Semiconductor lasers:*
  - Diode lasers

ii. *Based on types of output modes:*
- *Continuous wave:* Coherent, monochromatic, and collimated light are produced continuously, e.g., argon lasers
- *Pulsed mode*
  - *Mode locked:* Pulses in Q-switched mode are separated from each other by a specific time interval and all the wavelengths are in phase
  - *Q-switched mode:* Single, brief, and very high power pulsed, e.g., Nd:YAG, CO_2
  - *Rerunning mode:* The pulses are not separated by a specific time interval, and the wavelengths are not in place

6. What does solid-state laser use?

Solid-state lasers are ruby laser and Nd:YAG laser. The active element in ruby laser is chromium ion incorporated in sapphire crystal. In the Nd:YAG, the yttrium–aluminum–garnet is doped with neodymium ions.

7. What does gas laser use?

Gas lasers have an ionized rare gas as their active medium. For example, argon and krypton lasers are ion lasers.

8. What does tunable dye laser mean?

A tunable dye laser is a fluorescent organic compound dissolved in liquid solvent which, when optically pumped by a laser/flash lamp laser, can emit laser radiation over a wide range of wavelength. The output wavelength can be changed over the possible lasing band by varying the tuning element.

9. What is phototherapy?

Necrosis of tumor/neovascularization using locally/systematically administered photosensitizer.

10. What is the mechanism by which phototherapy works?

Photochemically sensitized target tissue, when exposed to laser of proper wavelength, releases singlet oxygen. This damages the lesion by lipid peroxidation. For example, photodynamic therapy—verteporfin.

11. Discuss few important lasers and their properties.

Laser type	Wavelength (nm)	Active medium	Primary damage mechanism	Applications
Argon	488–514	Gas	• Photothermal • Photochemical	• Trabeculoplasty • Iridotomy • Iridoplasty • PRP/PDT • Laser • Suturolysis • Sclerotomy
CO_2	10,600 [Far infrared radiation (IR)]	Gas	Photothermal	• Oculoplastic surgery • Laser phacolysis • Sclerostomy
Excimer	193 (UV)	Gas (Ar/F)	Photochemical	• Laser-assisted in situ keratomileusis (LASIK) • Laser epithelial keratomileusis (LASEK) • Photorefractive keratectomy (PRK)/phototherapeutic keratectomy (PTK) • Trabeculoplasty • Sclerostomy
Nd:YAG	532 (green) 1,064 (near IR)	Solid neodymium ion in yttrium–aluminum–*garnet* matrix	• Photodisruption • Photothermal	• Capsulotomy • Iridotomy • Trabeculoplasty • Phakolysis • Sclerostomy • PRP • Cyclophotocoagulation • Oculoplastic • Surgery
Diode	(620–895) Red and IR	Solid *gallium* aluminum	Photothermal	• PRP • Iridotomy • Iridoplasty • Sclerostomy • Suturolysis • Trabeculoplasty • Cyclophotocoagulation
Dye	310–1,200 (UV-visible IR)	Fluorescent dye	• Photothermal • Photochemical	• Penetrating keratoplasty (PKP) • PDT • Iridotomy • Sclerostomy • Suturolysis

12. What are the lenses used in laser photocoagulation?

Negative power plano-concave lens	High plus power lens
Upright image	Real and inverted image
Superior image of small retinal area (focal laser)	Loss of fine resolution with wide field of view (PRP)
Same spot size as that selected	Magnifies the spot size selected
Hruby lens	• Goldmann lens • Rodenstock panfundoscope • Mainster lenses PRP 165, focal/grid • Volk lenses—superquad 160, area centralis

Lenses used for PRP:

Lens	Image magnification	Laser spot magnification	Field of view
Goldmann 3 mirror	0.93×	1.08×	140°
Mainster PRP 165	0.68×	1.96×	165–180°
Volk superquad	0.50×	2.00×	160–165°
Volk quadraspheric	0.51×	1.97×	120–144°

Lenses used in focal/grid laser photocoagulation:

Lens	Image magnification	Laser spot magnification	Field of view
Mainster focal/grid	0.96×	1.05×	90–121°
Mainster high mag	1.25×	0.8×	75–88°
Volk area centralis	1.06×	0.94×	70–84°

13. How can you increase the burn intensity?

$$\text{Burn intensity} = \frac{(\text{Burn duration}) \times (\text{Power setting})}{\text{Spot size}}$$

So, intensity can be increased by:
↑duration
↑power
↑spot size

14. How does Nd:YAG laser work?

Nd:YAG laser uses a trivalent neodymium ion, which is excited in YAG matrix by an external exciting source (flash lamp/other laser diode).

15. What is the special property of Nd:YAG?

Nd ion laser works at 1,064 nm (near infrared) and can be used as a continuous wave laser. Because of longer wavelength, it would penetrate tissue that would otherwise scatter a shorter wavelength.

16. **How can it be frequency doubled?**
    Bypassing through KTP (potassium titanium phosphate) crystal. The emitted wavelength is 532 nm.

17. **What is the use of frequency doubling?**
    At this wavelength, it is well absorbed by hemoglobin and retinal pigment epithelium (RPE) and hardly any by xanthophyll. This property makes it excellent for use in retina and vitreous disorders.

18. **What is Q-switching?**
    Q-switching causes giant pulse formation.
    In this technique, a laser can be made to produce a pulsed output beam. Because the pulse duration is so short, the total power delivered per pulse is not very high, but the peak power per pulse is very high.

19. **What are the uses of Q-switched Nd:YAG laser?**
    i. Capsulotomy
    ii. Iridotomy
    Hyaloidotomy—release of loculated preretinal blood into vitreous cavity

20. **What are the properties of laser light?**
    i. *Coherence:* The photons are in phase with each other in time and space
    ii. *Collimation:* Light amplification of photons produced in parallel beam
    iii. *Monochromatic:* Photons are emitted in a single wavelength
    iv. *High intensity*

21. **What is the difference between photocoagulation and photoablation?**
    Photocoagulation: Process, by which light energy is converted into heat energy, resulting in coagulation of tissue proteins and producing a burn.
    Photoablation: High-energy photons are able to break the intramolecular bonds of the corneal surface tissue enabling a fine layer to be removed with each pulse without thermal damage to remaining cornea.

22. **What are the fundus pigments?**
    i. *Melanin*—in RPE and choroids
    ii. *Xanthophyll*—in macula (ganglion cells)
    iii. *Hemoglobin*—in blood vessels

23. **What is the absorption spectrum of pigments in the retina?**

Pigments in the retina	Absorbs	Reflects
Melanin	All wavelength	
Xanthophyll	Blue	Yellow and red
Hemoglobin	Blue, green, and yellow	Red

24. **What are the various parameters used in laser photocoagulation?**
    i. *Spot size*—ranges 501,000 μm
    ii. *Exposure time*—0.01–5 seconds
    iii. *Power*—0–3,000 mW

25. **What is the relationship between spot size and energy requirements in laser?**
    To decrease energy, spot size is increased except in xenon arc where a decrease of energy is caused by decreasing spot size.

26. **When do we use different time duration laser burns?**
    Shorter duration burns (0.05 seconds) are more comfortable.
    Longer burns (0.1–0.2 seconds) are more effective and less likely to rupture Bruch's membrane.

27. **What are the factors that determine the effectiveness of any photocoagulation?**
    i. Penetration of light through ocular media
    ii. Amount of light absorbed by the pigment and converted to heat

28. **What are the indications of photocoagulation in eye?**
    i. Diabetic retinopathy
    ii. Retinal vascular abnormalities
       - Branch retinal vein occlusion (BRVO) (grid, sector)
       - Ischemic central retinal vein occlusion (ICRVO) with neovascular glaucoma (NVG)
    iii. Subretinal neovascularization
    iv. Retinal break
    v. Vascular tumors
    vi. Iridectomy
    vii. Trabeculoplasty
    viii. Vasculitis
    ix. Coloboma
    x. Optic nerve pit

29. **What are the indications of laser photocoagulation in diabetic retinopathy?**
    i. Clinically significant macular edema (CSME)
    ii. Paramacular edema
    iii. PDR:
       - High-risk PDR
       - Early PDR
          - Patients with poor compliance
          - During pregnancy
          - Patients with systemic diseases

- Pending cataract surgery
- Rubeosis
- Severe/very severe nonproliferative diabetic retinopathy NPDR (irregular follow-up)

30. **What are the laser types used in the treatment of macular edema?**
    i. Direct/focal
    ii. Grid for diffuse leakage
    iii. For circinate leakage, treat within the circinate

31. **Discuss diabetic retinopathy clinical research network (DRCR.net) focal/grid photocoagulation [modified-ETDRS (Early Treatment Diabetic Retinopathy Study] technique.**

Features	Focal	Grid
Wavelength	Green–Yellow	Green–Yellow
Area	Direct treatment of all leaking microaneurysms in areas of retinal thickening 500–3,000 μm from center of macula	Areas of edema not associated with microaneurysms. • 500–3,000 μm superior, and inferior to macula and 500–3,500 μm temporally • No burns within 500 μm from disk or over the maculopapillary bundle
Spot size	50 μm	50 μm
Burn duration	0.05–0.1 seconds	0.05–0.1 seconds
Power	100–400 MW	100–400 MW
Intensity	Grade 3 burn evident beneath all microaneurysms	Bare visible (light gray) 2 visible burn width apart

32. **What is the intensity of photocoagulation burns?**

i. Grade I (light)	Faint retinal blanching
ii. Grade II (mild)	Hazy translucent retinal burn
iii. Grade III (moderate)	Opaque gray/dirty white
iv. Grade IV (heavy)	Dense chalky white

33. **What are the disadvantages of green laser?**
    i. Attenuated by nuclear sclerosis
    ii. Cannot do immediately after fluorescein fundus angiography (FFA), since residual vitreous fluorescein provides troublesome fluorescence with green illumination
    iii. Absorbed by luteal pigments in the foveal region and hence yellow laser is preferable

34. How does laser work in CSME?
   i. Direct closure of leaking vascular microaneurysms due to laser-induced endovascular thrombosis and heat-induced contraction at the vessel wall. It acts by increasing filtration by RPE
   ii. Thermally damaged RPE alters outer retinal–blood barrier, thereby favoring fluid movement from retina to choroid
   iii. Photoreceptor destruction increases inner retinal oxygenation, which results in vasoconstriction decreased blood flow and therefore decreased vascular leakage
   iv. RPE damage causes retinal capillary and venule endothelial proliferation, which restores inner blood–retinal barrier
   v. Decreases the amount of retinal leakage by decreasing the total surface area of leaking retinal vessels

35. What are the side effects of focal photocoagulation?
   i. Paracentral scotoma
   ii. Transient increased edema/decreased vision
   iii. Choroidal neovascularization
   iv. Subretinal fibrosis
   v. Photocoagulation scar expansion
   vi. Inadvertent foveal burn

36. How long should we wait for macular edema to resolve following laser before deciding on retreatment?
Up to 4 months

37. What is the minimal level of visual acuity to give focal treatment in macular edema?
Focal treatment has to be given even if vision is 6/6 or better if the edema is clinically significant.

38. What are the indicators of poor prognosis in CSME for laser photocoagulation?
   i. Extensive macular capillary nonperfusion (ischemic maculopathy)
   ii. Diffuse disease
   iii. Cystoid macular edema (long)
   iv. Lamellar macular hole
   v. Foveal hard exudates plaque

39. What are the indications for PRP?
   i. High-risk PDR
   ii. *Others:*
      - Rubeosis with/without NVG
      - PDR developing in pregnancy
      - Early PDR or severe NPDR with an increased risk for progression (poor compliance, fulminant course in fellow eye, uncontrolled

systemic diseases such as hypertension, nephropathy, and anemia)
- Widespread retinal ischemia/capillary dropouts on FFA of >10 disk diameter (DD) area

40. What is the mechanism of action of PRP?
   i. Conversion of hypoxic areas to anoxic areas
   ii. Greater perfusion from the choroidal circulation by achieving a closer approximation of the inner layer of the retina with choriocapillaris
   iii. Destruction of badly perfused capillaries and grossly hypoxic retina, thus diverting available blood to a healthier retina
   iv. Destruction of leaking blood vessels which create an abnormal hemodynamic situation in the diabetic retina, thereby normalizing the vascular supply of the macular region

41. What are the parameters of PRP?
Blue-green argon/Fd Nd:YAG lasers

Spot size:	200–500 μm
Exposure time:	0.1–0.2 seconds
Power:	200–500 mW
End point:	Moderately intense white burns
Inter burn distance:	One burn width apart
Placement:	2 DD above, temporal, and below center of macula 500 μm from nasal margin of the optic disk and extends to or beyond the equator.

To avoid direct treatment of:
   i. Major retinal vessels
   ii. Macula
   iii. Papillomacular area
   iv. Area of gliosis
   v. Retinal hemorrhage
   vi. Chorioretinal scars

42. What are the approximate number of burns required for completing PRP?
1,800–2,200 burns in two to three divided sittings over 3–6 weeks' period.
Multiple sessions decrease the risk of:
   i. Macular edema
   ii. Exudative retinal detachment (RD)
   iii. Choroidal detachment
   iv. Angle closure glaucoma

43. **What are the indications of additional laser treatment after initial PRP?**
    For recurrent or persisting neovascularization

44. **What is the placement or number for additional burns in PRP?**
    i. In between prior treatment scars
    ii. Anterior to previous scars
    iii. Posterior pole—2 DD away from the macula
    Number at least 500–700

45. **What are the complications of PRP?**
    Functional complications:
    i. Decreased night vision
    ii. Decreased color vision
    iii. Decreased peripheral vision
    iv. Loss of one or two lines of visual acuity
    v. Glare, photopsia

    Anatomical complications:
    i. *Anterior segment:*
        – Cornea burns
            - Erosion
            - Superficial punctate keratitis (SPK)
        – Shallowing of anterior chamber (AC)
        – Iris
            - Iritis
            - Atrophy
            - Damage to sphincter
            - Posterior synechiae
        – Lens
            - Lens opacities
    ii. *Posterior segment:*
        – Foveal burn
        – Occlusion of vein/artery
        – Retinal hemorrhage
        – Choroidal hemorrhage—due to rupture of Bruch's membrane/choroidal detachment
        – Macular edema following extensive PRP
        – Macular pucker
        – Contraction of fibrous tissue leading to tractional RD
        – Choroidal neovascular membrane (CNVM)
        – Subretinal fibrosis
        – Scar expansion

46. **What are the causes of pain during PRP?**
    i. Inadequate anesthesia
    ii. High power or long duration burns
    iii. Large number burns
    iv. Focused on the choroid rather than the retina
    v. Treatment over the long posterior ciliary nerves on the horizontal meridian
    vi. Peripheral treatment

47. **What are the differences between choroiditis pigmentation marks and old laser marks?**

Choroiditis pigmentation	Old laser marks
Irregular	Regular with equal spacing
Pigmentation is peripheral	Pigmentation is in the center
Anywhere	Spare the macular regions and immediately surrounding the disk

48. **What is the goal of PRP?**
    i. To cause regression of existing neovascular tissue
    ii. To prevent new vessel formation

49. **Why is PRP done inferiorly first?**
    PRP is done inferiorly first so that if a hemorrhage occurs, only the superior retina is left to be lasered, which is easier.

50. **What is the wavelength of argon laser?**
    Argon blue-green emits both blue (488 nm) and green (514 nm).

51. **What are the advantages of argon laser?**
    i. Coherent radiation—more efficient delivery
    ii. High monochromaticity
    iii. Very small spot size

52. **What are the disadvantages of argon laser?**
    i. Absorption by cataract lens
    ii. Poor penetration through vitreous hemorrhage (VH)
    iii. Uptake by macular xanthophyll (blue-green)—cannot be used for treatment around macula
    iv. High intraocular scattering leads to less precise retinal focusing

53. **What is the wavelength of krypton red?**
    647 nm

54. **What are the advantages of krypton?**
    i. Useful in treatment of lesions within foveal avascular zone and papillomacular bundle (as not absorbed by xanthophylls)

ii. Better penetration through nuclear sclerotic cataracts (decreased absorption by lens) and through moderate VH (decreased absorption by hemoglobin) because of decreased intraocular scattering

55. **What are the disadvantages of krypton laser?**
    Red light must have melanin for its absorption.
    i. Less effective for treating vascular abnormalities because of poor absorption by hemoglobin
    ii. Less effective for pale fundus
    iii. Increased pain and hemorrhage due to deeper choroid penetration

56. **What are the modes of delivery of lasers?**
    i. Slit lamp
    ii. Indirect ophthalmoscopy
    iii. Endolaser

57. **What are the various lenses used?**
    i. All-purpose fundus contact lens
       - Goldmann contact lens
       - Karickhoff lens
    ii. Contact lens for macular photocoagulation
       - Volk super macula
       - Mainster high magnification
       - Volk area centralis
       - Mainster standard lens
       } Real inverted
    iii. For peripheral photocoagulation
       - Rodenstock panfundoscopic
       - Volk trans equator
       - Mainster widefield
       - Mainster ultrafield
       } Inverted real magnified
    iv. Noncontact lenses
       - 60 D
       - 78 D
       - 90 D

58. **What are the indications of laser photocoagulation through indirect ophthalmoscopy delivery?**
    i. PRP in patients with hazy media, patients unable to sit, early anterior segment postoperative period
    ii. Retinopathy of prematurity
    iii. Peripheral proliferative lesions as in pars planitis, Eales' disease, sickle cell retinopathy, Coats' disease
    iv. Peripheral retinal breaks
    v. Retinal photocoagulation following pneumatic retinopexy
    vi. *Retinal and choroidal tumors:* Choroidal malignant melanoma, retinoblastoma

59. **What are the advantages of laser photocoagulation through indirect ophthalmoscope delivery?**
    Treatment of patients with:
    i. Hazy media
    ii. Poorly dilated pupils
    iii. In presence of intraocular gas bubbles
    iv. For patients unable to sit at a slit lamp
    v. For peripheral lesions

60. **Which is more responsive to treatment, flat or elevated new vessels?**
    i. Flat vessels
    ii. Because absorption of laser energy by elevated lesions is less

61. **Which is more likely to bleed, neovascularization of disk (NVD) or neovascularization elsewhere (NVE)? Why?**
    NVD. Because of the absence of internal limiting membrane over the disk.

62. **What is to be done when bleeding occurs during photocoagulation?**
    i. Bleeding can be stopped by increasing the pressure of the contact lens on the globe
    ii. By increasing the laser energy and hitting the bleeding point repeatedly

63. **What are the relative indications for retrobulbar anesthesia in photocoagulation procedures?**
    i. Significant ocular pain
    ii. Significant eye movement
    iii. Treatment near the foveal center to avoid incidental foveal burns

64. **What are the indications of anterior retinal cryotherapy?**
    i. Progressive proliferative diseases [NVD, NVE, or neovascularization of iris (NVI)] despite full PRP
    ii. When media opacities (cataract, VH) preclude PRP

65. **What are the diameters of various cryoprobes used in ophthalmology?**
    Endocryopexy—1 mm
    ICCE—1.5 mm
    Retina—2-2.5 mm

66. **What are the recent advances in laser photocoagulation?**
    i. Pattern scanning laser—PASCAL® (Topcon Inc.)
        - Laser—double frequency Nd-YAG 532 nm laser and 577 nm yellow laser
        - Uses a microprocessor-driven scanner that produces a variety of scalable patterns, viewable on a computer screen and selected by the physician. Allows the operator to apply multiple spots almost

simultaneously, with a single foot pedal depression, multiple laser burns in a rapid predetermined sequence in the form of a pattern array produced by a scanner
- *Advantages:*
  - Faster 56 spots in 0.6 seconds—reduces treatment duration
  - Lesser pain and better patient comfort
  - Perfect spacing of spots—no accidental confluence/overlapping
  - End point management system—reduction of fluence decreases collateral damage to the surrounding tissue compared with conventional laser
- *Disadvantages:*
  - The efficacy of PASCAL laser, however, appears to be diminished compared to conventional laser therapy when the same number of laser spots was delivered

ii. Micropulse laser—IRIDEX 577 nm
  - Using a micropulse mode, laser energy is delivered with a train of repetitive short pulses (typically 100–300 μs "on" and 1,700–1,900 μs "off") within an "envelope" whose width is typically 200–300 ms.
  - Mechanism of action—stimulates the RPE and has a beneficial effect on its activation
  - Advantages—the length of pulses shorter than the thermal relaxation time of the target tissue and allows tissues to cool before the next pulse to limit damage to adjacent areas, thereby minimizing scarring
  - Uses—macular edema, central serous chorioretinopathy (CSCR), CNVM

iii. Navigated Lase—NAVILAS
  - Combines color fundus photography, fluorescein angiography (FA), and IR imaging with a target locked frequency-doubled solid-state laser (wavelength 532 nm)
  - *Features:*
    - Computer-based treatment planning—superimposed FFA and live retinal images for targeting
    - Safety/eye-tracking feature—minimize inadvertent laser treatment
    - Accuracy
    - Multimodal integration—FA, optical coherence tomography (OCT), indocyanine green (ICG)
    - Patient comfort
    - Treatment ease
    - Documentation.

6.6 HYPERTENSIVE RETINOPATHY

1. **What are the different classifications of hypertensive (HTN) retinopathy?**
   There are two main classifications:
   i. Keith–Wagener–Barker classification
   ii. Scheie's classification

2. **What is the Keith–Wagener–Barker classification?**
   It is divided into four groups:
   Group 1—minimal constriction of the arterioles with some tortuosity
   Group 2—abnormalities in group 1 with definite focal narrowing and arteriovenous (AV) nicking
   Group 3—group 1 and 2 abnormalities and hemorrhages, exudates, cotton wool spots
   Group 4—above findings along with optic disk edema

3. **What is Scheie's classification?**
   Scheie classified changes of hypertension and arteriosclerosis separately. *Scheie's classification of HTN retinopathy:*
   Stage 0—no visible retinal vascular abnormalities
   Stage 1—diffuse arteriolar narrowing
   Stage 2—arteriolar narrowing with areas of focal arteriolar constriction
   Stage 3—diffuse and focal arteriolar narrowing with retinal hemorrhages
   Stage 4—all above findings with retinal edema, hard exudates, and optic disk edema

   Scheie's classification of arteriolosclerosis:
   Stage 0—normal
   Stage 1—broadening of arteriolar light reflex
   Stage 2—light reflex changes and AV crossing changes
   Stage 3—copper wiring of arterioles
   Stage 4—silver wiring of arterioles

4. **What is Salus's sign?**
   Deflection of vein as it crosses the arteriole

5. **What is Gunn's sign?**
   Tapering of veins on either side of AV crossing

6. **What is Bonnet's sign?**
   Banking of veins distal to AV crossings

7. **What is the cause of arteriolar light reflex?**
   It is the light reflected from the convex surface of normal arteriolar wall.

8. **What is copper wiring?**
   When the light reflex from the vessel wall takes on a reddish-brown hue due to an increase in arteriolosclerosis, it is called copper wiring.

9. **What is silver wiring?**
   When there is severe arteriolosclerosis and no blood is seen inside the vessel wall, it is called silver wiring.

10. **What is the reason for arteriolar narrowing?**
    When there is a rise in blood pressure, it excites the pliable and nonsclerotic retinal vessels to increase their vascular tone by autoregulation.

11. **What is a cotton wool spot?**
    Cotton wool spot is an area of focal ischemic infarct of the nerve fiber layer as a result of axon disruption.

12. **What are flame-shaped hemorrhages?**
    Flame-shaped hemorrhages are the hemorrhages present in the nerve fiber layer from superficial precapillary arterioles and hence assuming the architecture of the nerve fiber layer.

13. **What are the differential diagnoses of flame-shaped hemorrhages?**
    They are:
    i. HTN retinopathy
    ii. Diabetic retinopathy
    iii. Central retinal vein occlusion (CRVO)
    iv. Branch retinal vein occlusion (BRVO)
    v. Papilledema
    vi. Glaucoma [especially normal tension glaucoma (NTG)]
    vii. Anterior ischemic optic neuropathy (AION)
    viii. Ocular ischemic syndrome
    ix. Eales' disease
    x. Hemoglobinopathies

14. **What are hard exudates?**
    Hard exudates are caused by chronic retinal edema. They develop at the junction of the normal and edematous retina and are composed of lipoprotein and lipid-rich macrophages located within the outer plexiform layer.

15. **What are the differential diagnoses of hard exudates?**
    They are:
    i. Diabetic retinopathy
    ii. HTN retinopathy
    iii. BRVO
    iv. CRVO
    v. Coats' disease

vi. Retinal artery macroaneurysm
vii. Radiation retinopathy
viii. Eales' disease

16. **What is macular star?**
Macular star is the deposition of hard exudates in a star-shaped pattern around the fovea. This is due to chronic macular edema in HTN retinopathy.

17. **What are the differential diagnoses of macular star?**
They are:
i. HTN retinopathy
ii. Neuroretinitis
iii. Papilledema
iv. CRVO
v. BRVO

18. **What is the hallmark of accelerated hypertension?**
Optic disk swelling

19. **How is hypertensive eye disease divided on the basis of ocular tissue involved?**
Hypertensive eye disease is divided into:
i. HTN retinopathy
ii. HTN choroidopathy
iii. HTN optic neuropathy

20. **What are different phases of HTN retinopathy?**
HTN retinopathy is divided into:
i. Vasoconstrictive phase
ii. Exudative phase
iii. Sclerotic phase

21. **What are the changes in vasoconstrictive phase?**
Fundus changes:
i. Diffuse arteriolar narrowing
ii. Focal arteriolar narrowing
iii. Reduction of arteriole to venule ratio (normal—2:3)

22. **What are the changes in exudative phase?**
Fundus changes:
i. Flame-shaped hemorrhages
ii. Cotton wool spots
iii. Hard exudates

23. **What is the finding in sclerotic phase?**
Fundus changes:
i. Sclerosis of vessel wall (copper wiring and silver wiring)
ii. AV crossing changes (Salus's sign, Bonnet's sign, and Gunn's sign)

24. What are the complications of HTN retinopathy?
Complications are:
   i. Macroaneurysms
   ii. Central retinal artery or vein occlusion
   iii. Branch retinal artery or vein occlusion
   iv. Epiretinal membrane formation
   v. Macular edema
   vi. Retinal neovascularization
   vii. Vitreous hemorrhage

25. What is HTN arteriolosclerosis?
HTN arteriolosclerosis is a progressive increase in the elastic and muscular component in the walls of the arterioles.

26. What is onion skin appearance of the vessel wall?
In long-standing hypertension, elastic tissue forms multiple concentric layers. The muscular layer is replaced by collagen fibers and the intima is replaced by hyaline thickening. These give the appearance of onion skin.

27. What are the risk factors for HTN choroidopathy?
It is commonly seen in acute HTN and young patients. Risk factors are:
   i. Toxemia of pregnancy
   ii. Malignant HTN
   iii. Renal disease
   iv. Pheochromocytoma
   v. Acquired diseases of connective tissue

28. What are the fundus changes in HTN choroidopathy?
Fundus changes are:
   i. Elschnig's spots and Siegrist's streaks
   ii. Serous retinal detachments
   iii. Macular star
   iv. Retinal pigment epithelium (RPE) depigmentation
   v. Subretinal exudates
   vi. Choroidal sclerosis

29. What are Elschnig's spots?
Elschnig's spots are small black spots surrounded by yellow halos representing RPE infarct due to focal occlusion of choriocapillaris.

30. What are Siegrist's streaks?
Siegrist's streaks are flecks arranged linearly along the choroidal vessels, indicative of fibrinoid necrosis.

31. How is choroidal circulation different from retinal circulation?
Choroidal circulation has the following peculiarities:
   i. Profuse sympathetic nerve supply

ii. No autoregulation of blood flow
iii. No blood-ocular barrier

Hence, increased blood pressure is directly transferred to choroidal choriocapillaris, which initially constrict, but further increase in blood pressure overcomes the compensatory tone, resulting in damage to the muscle layer and endothelium.

32. What is HTN optic neuropathy?

HTN optic neuropathy is characterized by:
  i. Swelling of the optic nerve head (ONH)
  ii. Blurring of the disk margins
  iii. Hemorrhages over the ONH
  iv. Ischemia and pallor of the disk

33. What are the differential diagnoses of HTN optic neuropathy?

Differential diagnoses are:
  i. CRVO
  ii. AION
  iii. Radiation retinopathy
  iv. Diabetic papillopathy
  v. Neuroretinitis

34. What is malignant hypertension?

Diastolic blood pressure of >120 mm Hg

It is characterized by fibrinoid necrosis of the arterioles. Choroidopathy and optic neuropathy are more common but retinopathy also occurs in malignant hypertension.

35. What are ocular manifestations in pregnancy-induced HTN (PIH)?

They are divided as:
  i. Conjunctiva—
    - Capillary tortuosity
    - Conjunctival hemorrhages
    - Ischemic necrosis of conjunctiva
  ii. Hypertensive retinopathy changes
  iii. Choroid—serous detachments
  iv. Optic nerve—disk edema and rarely optic atrophy

36. How do you manage PIH?

The fundus findings that occur generally return to normal in response to appropriate medical management or upon spontaneous or elective delivery. The role of an ophthalmologist is limited.

37. What is the management of HTN retinopathy?

Control of hypertension is the key step. An ophthalmologist mainly plays a supportive role to a primary care physician in the diagnosis and management of systemic hypertension with prompt referral.

6.7 CENTRAL RETINAL VEIN OCCLUSION (CRVO)

1. **What are the main types of central retinal vein occlusion (CRVO)?**
   i. *Ischemic CRVO* [nonperfused/hemorrhagic/complete (ICRVO)]
   ii. *Nonischemic CRVO* [perfused/partial/incomplete (NICRVO)]

2. **What is indeterminate CRVO?**
   A CRVO is categorized as indeterminate when there is sufficient intraretinal hemorrhage to prevent angiographic determination of perfusion status.

3. **Which type of CRVO is more prevalent in younger age group?**
   NICRVO

4. **Which type of CRVO is more prevalent in older age group?**
   ICRVO

5. **Which type of CRVO is known to recur in the same eye?**
   NICRVO

6. **What is the crucial period for the development of neovascularization after the ischemic insult?**
   First 7 months (The risk period may span up to 2 years.)

7. **What percentage of patients with neovascularization develops neovascular glaucoma (NVG)?**
   33% of patients with iris neovascularization develop NVG.

8. **What is the need for distinction between the two types of CRVO?**
   i. Prediction of the risk of subsequent ocular neovascularization
   ii. Identification of patients who will have poor visual prognosis
   iii. Determination of the likelihood of spontaneous visual improvement
   iv. Decision as to appropriate follow-up interval

9. **Mention the causes of CRVO.**
   i. *Systemic vascular disease:*
      - Hypertension (HTN) (artery compresses the vein)
      - Thrombosis of the central retinal vein (CRV)
      - Diabetes
      - Hyperlipidemia
      - Hematological alterations such as hyperviscosity syndrome, blood dyscrasias
      - Leukemia
   ii. *Ocular disease:*
      - Primary open angle glaucoma (POAG)
      - Ischemic optic neuropathy

- Events compressing the proximal part of the optic nerve such as retrobulbar hemorrhage, orbital pseudotumor, optic nerve tumors
iii. *Inflammatory/autoimmune vasculitis:*
- Systemic lupus erythematosus
- Behcet's disease
- Sarcoidosis
iv. *Infectious vasculitis:*
- Human immunodeficiency virus (HIV)
- Syphilis
- Herpes zoster
v. *Medications:*
- Oral contraceptives
- Diuretics
- Hepatitis B vaccine
vi. *Others:*
- After retrobulbar block, dehydration, pregnancy

10. **Where is the common site of occlusion in NICRVO?**
    6 mm behind lamina cribrosa

11. **What is the common site of occlusion in ICRVO?**
    At the region of lamina cribrosa or immediately posterior it

12. **How do we check for raised CRV pressure?**
    Digital ophthalmodynamometry

13. **How is this done?**
    In normal eyes, the CRV spontaneously pulses or can be made to wink or collapse with minimal ocular pressure through the eyelids. In CRVO, the vein and artery link together, or in extreme cases, the artery is more easily compressed than the vein.

14. **Why does ICRVO present with a more malignant picture?**
    In ICRVO, the site of occlusion is closer to the disk, i.e., it is at lamina cribrosa or immediately posterior to it, where only a few collaterals are present to drain the blood. So, there is a marked increase in venous pressure with a more malignant picture at presentation. NICRVO has occlusion more proximally with plenty of collaterals to drain the blood.

15. **How does glaucoma cause CRVO?**
    i. The pressure in CRV at optic disk depends upon the intraocular pressure (IOP), the former being always higher than the latter to maintain blood flow. A rise of IOP would produce retinal venous stasis and sluggish venous outflow—one of the factors in Virchow's triad for thrombus formation.

ii. The central retinal artery and veins are subjected to compression from mechanical stretching of lamina cribrosa, while passing through rigid sieve-like openings, especially in POAG.
iii. Nasalization and compression of vessels

16. **How does CRVO cause glaucoma?**
    i. NVG (open-angle and closed-angle types)
    ii. In the management of macular edema in CRVO, intravitreal steroid may cause steroid-induced glaucoma

17. **What are the risk factors for the conversion of NICRVO to ICRVO?**
    i. *Ocular risk factors:*
       - NICRVO with visual acuity at presentation of <6/60
       - Presence of five to nine disk areas of nonperfusion on angiography
    ii. *Systemic risk factors:*
       - Elderly individuals (>60 years)
       - Associated cardiovascular disease
       - Blood dyscrasias
       - Nocturnal hypotension

18. **What are the pathological changes in CRVO?**
    i. Hemorrhagic infarction of the inner layer of retina
    ii. Neovascularization of disk (NVD), retina, iris, angle
    iii. Thickening of retina, reactive gliosis
    iv. Intraretinal edema

19. **What is the most common cause of visual loss in CRVO?**
    Macular edema

20. **Why do patients of CRVO complain of defective vision in the early morning?**
    The fall in the blood pressure (BP) during sleep (nocturnal hypotension) alters the perfusion pressure, and so the venous circulation is further slowed down, converting partial thrombosis to complete thrombosis.

21. **Why do patients with CRVO have amaurosis fugax?**
    The thrombus formation in CRV completely cuts off the retinal vascular blood flow, resulting in transient obscuration of vision with field defects. However, due to the sudden rise in the blood pressure at the arterial end of the retinal vascular blood flow, the freshly formed thrombus is pushed out of the site of block and relieves the ischemia, resulting in the return of vision and field normality.

22. **Which type of CRVO is usually asymptomatic?**
    NICRVO

23. **Which type of CRVO presents with amaurosis fugax?**
    NICRVO

24. **Which type of CRVO presents with sudden loss of vision?**
    ICRVO

25. **What is the most common field defect in CRVO?**
    Central scotoma

26. **What are the clinical tests used in the evaluation of CRVO?**
    Clinical tests can be classified into two categories:
    (COMP: Please set the below list as per the original author input)

    Morphological
    i. Ophthalmoscopy
    ii. Fundus fluorescein angiography (FFA)

    Functional
    i. Visual acuity
    ii. Relative afferent pupillary defect (RAPD)
    iii. Visual fields
    iv. Electroretinogram (ERG)

27. **Differentiate between NICRVO and ICRVO.**

Features	NICRVO	ICRVO
V/A	Better than 6/60	Worse than 6/60 (3/60-HM)
Anterior segment	Normal RAPD++	RAPD+/− neovascularization of iris (NVI), neovascularization of angle (NVA) +/− NVG features
Fundus	Less retinal hemorrhage at posterior pole Cotton wool spot +	Abundant and extensive retinal superficial hemorrhage Cotton wool spot + + +
Field defects	50–75%	100%
ERG changes	+/−	++ (decreased "b" wave amplitude)
FFA changes	Few nonperfusion areas	Nonperfusion areas >10 disk diameter (DD)
Course	Majority resolve completely (48%)	Majority do not resolve, leading to ocular morbidity

28. **What is the importance of RAPD in the setting of CRVO?**
    Uses:
    i. Higher sensitivity at earliest stages
    ii. It gives reliable information in spite of hazy media
    iii. It can detect conversion of nonischemic to ICRVO
    iv. It is a noninvasive and inexpensive diagnostic tool

    Limitations:
    i. To test for RAPD, it is essential to have a normal fellow eye and normal optic disk and pupil in both eyes. For example, it is not useful in pharmacologically miotic or mydriatic pupil, glaucomatous disk damage, or optic neuropathy

ii. The amount of RAPD is influenced by the size of the central scotoma because it is modified more by the number of retinal ganglion cells involved than by the area of the retina. For example, NICRVO with central large, dense, macular edema may show an RAPD.

29. **What will be the fundus picture in ICRVO?**
    i. Widespread retinal hemorrhages (tomato ketchup fundus)
    ii. Retinal venous engorgement and tortuosity
    iii. Cotton wool spots
    iv. Macular edema
    v. Optic disk edema

30. **What is the footprint of asymptomatic NICRVO?**
    Retinocapillary venous collaterals on optic disk

31. **What is the importance of ocular neovascularization in CRVO?**
    i. Ocular neovascularization is seen in 2/3 of ICRVO.
    ii. Ocular neovascularization, if seen in NICRVO, should raise the suspicion of other associated conditions such as:
    - DM and other proliferative retinopathy
    - Carotid artery disease

32. **Which is the most common site of neovascularization in ICRVO?**
    Iris

33. **What is the importance of ischemic index in CRVO?**

    $$\text{Ischemic index} = \frac{\text{Nonperfusion area}}{\text{Total area of retina}}$$

    The risk of developing neovascularization is directly proportional to the degree of ischemic index.
    Ischemic index:
    0–10%   — <1% develop NVG
    10–50%   — 7% develop NVG
    >50%   — 45% develop NVG

34. **What are the indications of FFA in CRVO?**
    FFA should be performed after the acute phase is over since the hemorrhages during the acute phase will not provide accurate information.
    i. To look for any macular ischemia before treatment
    ii. To evaluate the extent of capillary nonperfusion (CNP)
    iii. In cases of NICRVO, follow-up changes can be identified such as conversion to ischemic type.

35. **Discuss FFA findings in ICRVO and NICRVO.**
    ICRVO:
    i. Hypofluorescence due to retinal CNP, blockage from retinal hemorrhages

ii. Increased arteriovenous (AV) transit time
iii. Macular area shows pooling due to edema and nonperfusion areas suggestive of macular ischemia
iv. NVD and neovascularization elsewhere (NVE) show leakage
v. Vessel wall staining

NICRVO:
i. Delayed AV transit time
ii. Blockage by hemorrhages
iii. Nonperfusion areas are minimal
iv. Late leakage
v. FFA may become normal after NICRVO resolves

36. How do you differentiate between ICRVO and NICRVO by FFA?
i. *ICRVO:* >10 DD of CNP area
ii. *NICRVO:* <10 DD of CNP area

37. Is ERG useful in differentiating ICRVO from NICRVO?
Amplitude reduction of "b" wave has 80% sensitivity and specificity in differentiating ICRVO from NICRVO. It does not require normal fellow eye and can be done in patients with optic nerve and pupil abnormalities also. In ICRVO:
i. "b" wave amplitude decreased to <60% of normal
ii. "b" wave amplitude reduced by 1 standard deviation or more, below the normal mean value

38. What are the investigations to be done in patients with CRVO?

History:	Age
	Sex
	Occupation/lifestyle
	Diabetes mellitus (DM)/HTN
Ocular:	Slit-lamp examination
	Direct/indirect ophthalmoscopy
	Field charting
	FFA
	ERG
General:	BP, pulse rate
	Systemic examination
Specific investigations:	BP
	Electrocardiogram (ECG)
	Full blood count and erythrocyte sedimentation rate (ESR)
	Fetal bovine serum (FBS) and lipids
	Urine albumin and serum creatinine
	Plasma protein electrophoresis

Young patients have to be specifically screened for:
Thrombophilia screening
Autoantibodies [anticardiolipin, lupus anticoagulant, antinuclear antibody (ANA), deoxyribonucleic acid (DNA), angiotensin-converting enzyme (ACE)]
Homocysteine

39. **What is the differential diagnosis (D/D) for CRVO?**
    i. D/D of papilledema
    ii. D/D of cotton wool spots

40. **How will you manage CRVO?**
    i. Treat the associated cause such as HTN, diabetes, and elevated cholesterol
    ii. Intravitreal triamcinolone acetonide for treating macular edema
    iii. Intravitreal anti-VEGF agents to reduce macular edema
    iv. Surgical decompression of CRVO via radial optic neurotomy, which involves sectioning the posterior scleral ring and retinal vein cannulation with an infusion of tissue plasminogen activators, has been reported

41. **What are the findings of central vein occlusion study (CVOS) group?**
    The CVOS findings are as follows:
    i. Even though grid laser treatment in the macula reduced angiographic evidence of macular edema, it yielded no benefit in improved visual acuity (VA).
    ii. The most important risk factor predictive of iris neovascularization in CRVO is poor VA. Scatter panretinal photocoagulation (PRP) failed to decrease the incidence of iris neovascularization. CVOS recommended waiting for at least 2 o'clock hours of iris neovascularization to show on undilated gonioscopy before performing photocoagulation.

42. **What is significant anterior segment neovascularization?**
    More than 2 o'clock hours NVI and/or NVA

43. **When is PRP indicated in CRVO?**
    i. Patient presenting with NVI or NVA
    ii. Patient presenting with NVD or NVE, even without NVA or NVI

44. **When is prophylactic PRP indicated in CRVO?**
    Patient with *ICRVO* where regular follow-up is not possible.

45. **Is grid photocoagulation useful in macular edema due to CRVO?**
    No

46. **Why is there no improvement of VA after grid in CRVO as against that seen in branch retinal vein occlusion (BRVO) or early stages of diabetic macular edema (DME)? (CVOS)**
    i. Difference in the pathophysiology of the diseases
    ii. CRVO usually results in the diffuse capillary leakage involving all the macular area, unlikely in BRVO or background diabetic retinopathy (DR)
    iii. In BRVO, macular edema may have more angiographically normal parafoveal capillaries
    iv. Also in BRVO, collateral channels typically develop temporal to the macula crossing the horizontal raphe. This may permit a greater normalization of venous circulation in the recovery phase [as opposed to central vein occlusion (CVO), where collateral channels develop at the optic nerve]
    v. In CRVO—macular edema involves the center of the fovea and additionally includes all four quadrants in the parafoveal region. May adversely affect the recuperative process in the macula

47. **What is the role of steroids in the management of CRVO?**
    Steroids decrease macular edema in NICRVO.
    Treatment of CRVO in young is especially secondary to phlebitis. Dexamethasone implants (*Ozurdex*) have been used and have shown to be of benefit in the GENEVA studies.

48. **What are the other intravitreal injections which can be given?**
    i. *Cruise trial:* Found monthly intravitreal 0.5 mg ranibizumab for 6 months is useful, especially when macular edema is present.
    ii. *COPERNICUS and GALILEO trials:* Found monthly intravitreal 2 mg aflibercept (VEGF trap-eye) to be useful.

49. **What is the role of cyclocryotherapy?**
    Procedure:
    i. 180° of the ciliary body is treated at one time, employing six spots of freezing, 2.5 mm posterior to the limbus.
    ii. The 3.5 mm probe is allowed to reach –60 to –80°C and is left in place for 1 minute each.

50. **What is anterior retinal cryotherapy (ARC)?**
    Indication in NVG: In cases in which the cornea, lens, and vitreous are hazy to allow adequate PRP.
    Procedure:
    i. A 2.5 mm retinal cryoprobe is used. The first row of application is performed 8 mm posterior to limbus, three spots between each rectus muscle

ii. Second row of application is performed 11 mm behind the limbus, four spots between each rectus muscle
iii. Probe is applied for approximately 10 seconds

51. What are the complications of ARC?
i. Tractional and exudative retinal detachment (RD)
ii. Vitreous hemorrhage

52. What is the visual outcome in patients with CRVO?
Depends on the vision on presentation:
NICRVO—final V/A is better than 6/60 in 50% patients
ICRVO—final V/A is worse than 6/60 in 93%, worse than 3/60 in 10%

53. Why is visual prognosis in young patients good?
i. Due to absence of significant retinal ischemia
ii. Young patients with healthy blood vessels may be able to tolerate brief periods of CRVO better than older individuals

54. What is the differential diagnosis of CRVO?
i. Ocular ischemic syndrome
ii. Hyperviscosity retinopathy
iii. Diabetic retinopathy
iv. Papilledema

55. What are the sequela of BRVO/CRVO?
i. *BRVO:*
Most common complication:
Macular edema
Macular ischemia
Neovascularization
ii. *CRVO:*
Most common complication:
Vitreous hemorrhage
Anterior segment neovascularization
NVG

56. What are the evidence of old BRVO and old CRVO?
i. *Old BRVO:*
- Once intraretinal hemorrhage is absorbed, it leads to segmental distribution of retinal vascular abnormalities such as:
  - Capillary nonperfusion
  - Dilation of capillaries
  - Microaneurysms
  - Sclerosed vessels
  - Telangiectatic vessels
  - Collateral vessel formation

- *On FFA:* When hemorrhages have resolved, microvascular changes are seen, giving a clue to old BRVO.
- *On OCT:* Photoreceptor ellipsoid zone and external limiting membrane abnormalities, having long-standing macular ischemia and macular edema

ii. *Old CRVO:*
With time, the extent of intraretinal hemorrhage may decrease/resolve completely with:
- Variable degrees of secondary retinal pigment epithelium alteration
- Macular edema often chronically persists despite resolution of intraretinal hemorrhage
- Epiretinal membrane and foveal pigmentary alterations are seen.
- "Optociliary shunt" vessels form on optic nerve head (ONH) as a sign of newly formed collateral channels and choroidal circulation
- Response to secondary retinal ischemia—NVD, NVE may develop
- NVI, NVA—ICRVO on long-standing—secondary angle closure from peripheral anterior synechiae. Increase in IOP with NVI/NVA

57. Which is the most common site of BRVO and why?
Superotemporal quadrant is the most common site of BRVO due to a large number of AV crossing, which supports the hypothesis of AV nicking as a cause.

58. What are the conditions which can act as precursors of BRVO?
i. HTN
ii. Diabetes
iii. Hyperlipidemia
iv. Hyperhomocysteinemia
v. Ocular HTN/glaucoma
vi. Shorter axial length
vii. *Blood coagulation disorders:* High plasma viscosity due to leukemia, myeloma, changes in protein C pathway, myelofibrosis
viii. Systemic inflammatory disorders such as Behcet's, PAN, Wegener's, and Goodpasture syndrome
ix. Retrobulbar external compression

59. What is the prethrombotic sign of BRVO?
Bonnet sign—deflection of retinal vein at the AV crossing is a prethrombotic sign it may progress to an acute BRVO

60. Can FFA be done in acute BRVO?
Acute BRVOs with the dense intraretinal hemorrhages may make FFA interpretation challenging due to blockage of fluorescence by the hemorrhage. Hence, FFA is not done at the acute stage of BRVO.

61. **Discuss treatment guidelines of BRVO.**
    i. Treatment of risk factors by physician
    ii. Ophthalmic management of BRVO
    i. *Nonischemic BRVO:*
    Baseline:
    If VA is better than 6/12, observe the progress for 3 months
    if VA is worse than 6/12 with macular edema and hemorrhage not masking fovea:
    - FFA is done to assess macular integrity—no macular ischemia—observe for 3 months
    - Mild-to-moderate macular ischemia—consider ranibizumab or Ozurdex
    - Severe macular ischemia—no treatment is recommended, observe for neovascular (NV) formation

    If VA is 6/12 or worse with macular edema and hemorrhage masking macula:
    - Monthly ranibizumab or Ozurdex for 3 months
    - Perform FFA at 3 months to assess foveal integrity
    - If severe macular ischemia is present at 3 months—no treatment will be beneficial and further therapy should be carefully considered.

    At 3 months follow-up:
    - Consider modified grid laser photocoagulation if persistent macular edema, no or minimal macular ischemia, and other treatments unsuccessful or unavailable
    - If VA is ≥6/9 or no macular edema, continue to observe. If the patient is on intravitreal injection, continue monthly intravitreal injections until maximum VA is achieved.

    Further follow-up:
    - If under observation, follow-up in 3 monthly intervals until 18 months.
    - In case of recurrence or new edema, consider reinitiating intravitreal injections.

    ii. *Ischemic BRVO:*
    - Watch carefully for neovascularization
    - If NVE, consider sector laser photocoagulation applied to all ischemic areas. Intravitreal bevacizumab can also be given with laser. Follow up at 3 monthly intervals for 24 months.

6.8 CENTRAL RETINAL ARTERY OCCLUSION

1. **What does central retinal artery supply?**
   Central retinal artery is a branch of ophthalmic artery that enters the eye within the optic nerve and supplies blood to the inner layers of the retina, extending from the inner aspect of the inner nuclear layer to the nerve fiber layer. Therefore, central retinal artery occlusion (CRAO) leads to damage predominantly in the inner layers of the retina.

2. **What are the causes of CRAO?**
   i. Atherosclerosis-related thrombosis
   ii. Carotid embolism
   iii. Giant cell arteritis
   iv. Cardiac embolism, which may be calcific emboli or vegetations or thrombus or myxomatous material
   v. Periarteritis
   vi. Thrombophilic disorders
   vii. Sickling hemoglobinopathies
   viii. Retinal migraine

3. **Where is the occlusion present in CRAO?**
   Occlusion is most commonly present at the level of lamina cribrosa (80%).

4. **What are the features of atherosclerosis?**
   Atherosclerosis is characterized by focal intimal thickening comprising cells of smooth muscle origin, connective tissue, and lipid-containing foam cells.

5. **What are the risk factors of atherosclerosis-related thrombosis?**
   Risk factors are:
   i. Aging
   ii. Hypertension
   iii. Diabetes
   iv. Hyperhomocysteinemia
   v. Increased low-density lipoproteins (LDL) cholesterol
   vi. Obesity
   vii. Smoking
   viii. Sedentary lifestyle

6. **Where does carotid embolism originate from and what are the types of emboli?**
   Carotid embolism mostly originates from an atheromatous plaque at the carotid bifurcation and less commonly from the aortic arch. The emboli may be of:

      i. Cholesterol *(Hollenhorst plaques):* Appear as intermittent showers of minute, bright, refractile, golden to yellow-orange crystals. They rarely cause significant obstruction to the retinal arterioles and are frequently asymptomatic
     ii. *Calcific emboli:* Single, white nonscintillating and are often on or close to the disk. Calcific emboli are more dangerous than the others as they cause permanent occlusion of the central retinal artery or its branches
    iii. *Fibrin-platelet emboli:* Dull, gray, multiple elongated particles that occasionally fill the entire lumen. They may cause retinal transient-ischemic attacks with resultant amaurosis fugax and occasionally complete obstruction

7. **What is the incidence of CRAO?**
   i. 1 per 10,000 outpatients
   ii. Above the age of 60 years
   iii. Bilateral in 2-3% of cases—to rule out cardiac valvular diseases, giant cell arteries, and vascular inflammations

8. **Describe the clinical features of CRAO.**
   Symptoms:
   i. Sudden painless loss of vision
   ii. In a few cases, visual loss is preceded by amaurosis fugax
   iii. Visual acuity—counting fingers to perception of light (PL)+ve in 90% of cases
      – In case of PL-ve—suspect associated ophthalmic artery occlusion or optic nerve damage

   Signs:
   i. Relative afferent pupillary defect (RAPD)—within seconds after CRAO
      – Will be present even when fundus appears normal during the early phases of CRAO
   ii. Anterior segment is usually normal initially
   iii. Rubeosis iridis at the time of obstruction is rare
      – If present, suspect concomitant carotid artery obstruction
      – Rubeosis iridis in CRAO develops at a mean of 4-5 weeks after obstruction, with a range of 1-15 weeks, and is seen in 18% of eyes
   iv. Yellowish-white opacification of superficial retina in the posterior pole except fovea. This loss of retinal transparency is due to ischemia of the inner half of retina. This usually resolves in 4-6 weeks
   v. Cherry-red spot in the foveal area due to extremely thin retina, allowing view of underlying retinal pigment epithelium and choroids

vi. In early stages, the retinal arteries are attenuated. The retinal veins are thin, dilated, or normal
In severe cases, segmentation or "box caring" of blood vessels in arteries and veins are seen
vii. In 20% of CRAO, Hollenhorst plaque (glistening, yellow cholesterol embolus) that arises from atherosclerotic deposits in the carotid artery
viii. Neovascularization of disk (NVD) in 2–3%
ix. Late fundus picture:
- Consecutive optic atrophy
- Attenuated blood vessels to a relatively normal fundus picture
- When present, pigmentary changes may indicate carotid or ophthalmic artery occlusion

9. **Mention the differential diagnosis of CRAO.**
    i. Acute ophthalmic artery occlusion (usually no cherry-red spot)
    ii. Other causes of cherry-red spot such as Tay–Sachs disease, Neimann–Pick disease, and some cone dystrophies
    iii. Berlin's edema
    iv. Anterior ischemic optic neuropathy
    v. Inadvertent intraretinal injection of gentamicin

10. **What is cherry-red spot?**
    Cherry-red spot at the macula is a clinical sign seen in the context of thickening and loss of transparency of the retina at the posterior pole. The fovea being the thinnest part of the retina and devoid of ganglion cells retains relative transparency, due to which the color of the choroids shines through.
    In case of lipid storage diseases, the lipids are stored in the ganglion cell layer of the retina, giving the retina a white appearance. As ganglion cells are absent at the foveola, this area retains relative transparency and contrasts with the surrounding retina.

11. **What are the causes of cherry-red spot?**
    i. CRAO
    ii. Sphingolipidoses such as Gaucher's disease, Neimann–Pick disease, Tay-Sachs disease, Goldberg syndrome, Faber syndrome, gangliosidosis GM1-type 2, and Sandhoff's disease
    iii. Berlin edema/commotio retinae
    iv. Macular retinal hole with surrounding retinal detachment
    v. Quinine toxicity
    vi. Hollenhorst syndrome (chorioretinal artery infarction syndrome)
    vii. Cardiac myxomas
    viii. Severe hypertension

ix. Temporal arteritis
x. Myotonic dystrophy syndrome

12. **What are the systemic diseases associated with CRAO?**
    i. Atheromatous vascular diseases
    ii. Diabetes mellitus
    iii. Hypertension
    iv. Cardiac valvular/occlusive disease
    v. Carotid occlusive disease
    vi. Compressive vascular disease
    vii. Blood dyscrasias
    viii. Embolic disease
    ix. Vasculitis
    x. Spasm following retrobulbar injection

13. **What are the ocular diseases associated with CRAO?**
    i. Precapillary arterial loops
    ii. Optic disk drusen
    iii. Increased intraocular pressure (IOP)
    iv. Toxoplasmosis
    v. Optic neuritis

14. **How do you treat a case of CRAO?**
    CRAO is an ophthalmic emergency. Treatment has to be instituted as soon as the diagnosis of CRAO is made even before workup of the case.
    i. *Bringing down the IOP:*
        - Dislodges the embolus
        - Produces retinal arterial dilation and increases retinal perfusion
            - Ocular massage with gonioscope preferred
            - Paracentesis of anterior chamber
            - IOP-lowering drugs
    ii. *Vasodilation:*
        - Carbogen inhalation
        - Retrobulbar or systemic administration of vasodilators
        - Sublingual nitroglycerin
    iii. *Fibrinolysis:*
        Mode and effects of treatment
        - *Ocular massage:*
            - Done digitally or by direct visualization of the artery by using a contact lens (Goldmann lens)
            - Compression of globe for approximately 10 seconds to obtain retinal arterial pulsation or flow cessation, followed by 5 seconds of sudden release, which is continued for approximately 20 minutes

- Improvement of retinal blood flow is seen as reestablishment of continuous laminar flow and increase in width of blood column and disappearance of fragmented flow
- *Anterior chamber paracentesis:*
  - Causes sudden decrease in IOP. As a result, the perfusion pressure behind the obstruction will push on an obstructing embolus. Technique: Performed at the slit lamp using topical anesthesia with a 25-gauge needle

  Generally, 0.1–0.2 mL of aqueous is removed.
- *IOP-lowering agents:*

  Act in the same mechanism as AC paracentesis
  - 500 mg of intravenous (IV) acetazolamide
  - 20% IV mannitol
  - Oral 50% glycerol
- *Vasodilators:*
  - Carbogen (95% of O_2 + 5% CO_2 mixture)
  - Inhalation of 100% O_2 in the presence of CRAO produces a normal pO_2 at the surface of the retina via diffusion from the choroids
  - CO_2 is a vasodilator and can produce increased retinal blood flow
    - In the absence of CO_2-O_2 mixture, rebreathing into a paper bag can be considered
  - Retrobulbar or systemic papaverine or tolazoline
  - Sublingual nitroglycerin
- *Fibrinolytic agents:*
  - Administered through the supraorbital artery. This produces 100 times higher doses of fibrinolytic agent at the central retinal artery than IV administration due to retrograde flow into ophthalmic artery
  - Injection of urokinase into the internal carotid artery through femoral artery catheterization has been tried
  - Systemic thrombolysis using plasminogen has also shown improvement in CRAO patients

Workup/investigations
  i. A detailed history regarding hypertension, diabetes, cardiac diseases, and other systemic vascular diseases, e.g., giant cell arteritis
  ii. Check pulse (to rule out atrial fibrillation) and blood pressure (BP)
  iii. Erythrocyte sedimentation rate (ESR), fasting blood sugar (FBS) < glycosylated hemoglobin (Hb) < total count (TC), differential count (DC), prothrombin time (PT), and activated partial thromboplastin time (aPTT)

- In young patients (<50 years), consider lipid profile, antinuclear antibody (ANA), rheumatoid factor (RF), fluorescent treponemal antibody absorption (FTA-ABS), serum electrophoresis, Hb electrophoresis, and antiphospholipid antibodies
  iv. Carotid artery evaluation: Digital palpation/duplex ultrasonography (USG)
  v. Electrocardiogram (ECG), echo
  vi. Fundus fluorescein angiography (FFA) and electroretinogram (ERG)

15. What is the FFA picture in CRAO?
  i. Delay in arterial filling
  ii. Prolonged A-V transit time
  iii. Complete lack of filling of arteries is unusual
  iv. Choroidal vascular filling is usually normal in eyes with CRAO
  v. If there is marked delay in choroidal filling in the presence of cherry-red spot, suspect ophthalmic artery occlusion or carotid artery occlusion
  vi. Though the arterial narrowing and visual loss persist, the fluorescein angiogram can become normal after varying time following CRAO

16. What is the ERG picture in CRAO?
  i. "b" wave diminution—due to inner retinal ischemia
  ii. "a" wave is generally normal

17. What are the causes of sudden visual loss?
  i. *Painless loss of vision:*
   - CRAO
   - Retinal detachment
   - Retrobulbar neuritis
   - Methyl alcohol poisoning
   - Vitreous hemorrhage
  ii. *Painful loss of vision:*
   - Acute congestive glaucoma
   - Optic neuritis
   - Traumatic avulsion of optic nerve
   - Meningeal carcinomatosis.

6.9 RETINAL DETACHMENT (RD)

1. **What are the layers of retina?**
   From outer to inner:
   i. Retinal pigment epithelium (RPE)
   ii. Layers of rods and cones
   iii. External limiting membrane
   iv. Outer nuclear
   v. Outer plexiform
   vi. Inner nuclear
   vii. Inner plexiform
   viii. Ganglion cell layer
   ix. Nerve fiber layer
   x. Internal limiting membrane (ILM)

2. **Define macula.**
   Macula is an oval shaped pigmented area, of around 5.5 mm diameter, with its centre shifted slightly laterally from the visual axis by 5 degrees.

3. **Define fovea and foveola.**
   Fovea: It is a depression in the inner retinal surface at the center of the macula with a diameter of 1.5 mm. Ophthalmoscopically, it gives rise to an oval light reflex because of the increased thickness of the retina and ILM at its border.

   Foveola: It forms the central floor of the fovea and has a diameter of 0.35 mm. It is the thinnest part of the retina, is devoid of ganglion cells, and consists only of cones and their nuclei.

4. **What are the layers of Bruch's membrane?**
   i. Basement membrane of RPE
   ii. Inner loose collagenous zone
   iii. Middle layer of elastic fibers
   iv. Outer loose collagenous zone
   v. Basement membrane of the endothelium of the choriocapillaris

5. **What are the layers of choroid?**
   Four layers from without inward:
   i. Suprachoroidal lamina (lamina fusca)
   ii. Stroma of choroids:
      - Outer layer of choroidal vessels—Haller's layer
      - Inner layer of choroidal vessels—Sattler's layer
   iii. Choriocapillaris
   iv. Bruch's membrane or lamina vitrea

6. **What is the blood supply of choroid?**
   Posterior choroid up to the equator: Short posterior ciliary arteries. These arise as two trunks from the ophthalmic artery. Each trunk divides into 10–20 branches that pierce the sclera around the optic nerve and supply the choroid in a segmental manner.

   Anterior choroid: Recurrent ciliary arteries, long posterior ciliary artery, and anterior ciliary artery.

7. **What is the blood supply of retina?**
   Outer four layers (pigment epithelium, layer of rods and cones, external limiting membrane, and outer nuclear layer) get their nutrition from choriocapillaris.

   Inner six layers (outer plexiform layer, inner nuclear layer, inner plexiform layer, layer of ganglion cells, nerve fiber layer, and ILM) get their blood supply from the central retinal artery.

8. **What is vitreous base?**
   Vitreous base straddles ora serrata, extending 1.5–2 mm anteriorly and 1–3 mm posteriorly. Here, it has its strongest attachment at the posterior part of the pars plana and immediate portion of the ora serrata.

9. **What are the normal attachments of vitreous to retina?**
   i. Around vitreous base
   ii. Around the optic disk
   iii. Around the fovea
   iv. Around the peripheral blood vessels

10. **What is the composition of vitreous?**
    Vitreous is composed of 99% water with a volume of 4 cm^3. The liquid phase contains hyaluronic acid. The maximum concentration of hyaluronic acid is seen in the periphery of the vitreous, particularly in the posterior cortical layer.

    Collagen helps in forming a meshwork that intertwines hyaluronic acid, providing rigidity and viscosity to the vitreous. The collagen types are II, IX, and XI.

11. **What are the different portions of the vitreous?**
    i. *Vitreous cortex:* This constitutes the peripheral 0.2–0.3 mm broad dense vitreous zone and covers the entire vitreous body. The fibrous condensations of the vitreous cortex are called anterior hyaloid membrane (extending from the vitreous base to the posterior surface of the lens) and posterior hyaloid membrane (nearer the retina, firmly joining to margins of the optic disk, fovea, and retinal blood vessels).
    ii. *Central or core vitreous:* In this structure, cells are few and fibers are thin and do not attach to the peripheral structures. Wider separation

of collagen fibers provides more transparency to the central vitreous (less dense optically).

12. **Why is the vitreous transparent?**
    i. High water content and low solid content
    ii. Light absorption is negligible since the gel is colorless
    iii. Blood–ocular barrier prevents the entry of formed elements of the blood

13. **What are the two potential spaces in front of the anterior surface of vitreous that may get opened in pathological conditions?**
    i. *Petit's canal:* This is a potential space between the zonules and posterior lens capsule in front and the anterior vitreous face behind
    ii. *Berger's space:* It is an expansion of the anterior end of Cloquet's canal

14. **What is Cloquet's canal?**
    Cloquet's canal is a tubular structure in adult vitreous body representing the fetal hyaloid artery and contains the vestiges of the primary vitreous, which gets localized within the canal due to growth of secondary vitreous around it.

15. **What are the landmarks of vortex vein?**
    Vortex ampullae are located just posterior to the equator in the 1, 5, 7, and 11 o'clock meridian. The average point of emergence of vortex veins varies from 14 to 24 mm (about 20 mm from the limbus). Superior temporal vortex vein leaves the sclera about 8 mm behind the equator. Superior nasal and inferior nasal vortex veins exit 6 mm behind the equator. Inferior temporal vortex vein is placed 5.5 mm behind the equator.

16. **What are the landmarks of posterior ciliary arteries?**
    The posterior ciliary arteries arise below the optic nerve from the ophthalmic artery as two trunks and divide into the following:
    i. *Long posterior ciliary arteries:* Two in number—one on the nasal and the other on the temporal side of the globe in the horizontal meridian. They pierce the sclera about 3-4 mm anterior to the optic nerve, traverse the sclera very obliquely forward for 3-5 mm to suprachoroidal space, and supply ciliary body anastomosing with anterior ciliary arteries to form the major arterial circle of iris
    ii. *Short posterior ciliary arteries:* About 20 in number, pierce the sclera around the optic nerve and supply posterior sclera and choroid

17. **What are the weak areas of sclera?**
    i. Just behind the muscle insertion
    ii. Equator
    iii. Limbus

18. **How does a normal retina remain attached?**
    i. An interphotoreceptor matrix between the cells forms a "glue" that helps to maintain cellular apposition
    ii. RPE functions as a cellular pump to remove ions and water from the interphotoreceptor matrix providing a "suction force" that keeps the retina attached
    iii. Vitreous acts as a tamponade

19. **What is syneresis?**
    Syneresis is contraction of gel, which separates its liquid from solid component

20. **What is synchysis?**
    Synchysis is liquefaction of gel

21. **What is a retinal break?**
    A retinal break is a full-thickness defect in the sensory retina connecting the vitreous cavity and the potential or actual subretinal space.

    They can be tears or holes.
    i. *Tears:* They are caused by dynamic vitreoretinal traction.
    ii. *Holes:* They are caused by chronic atrophy of sensory retina and are less dangerous than tears.
    Operculated holes: When a piece of retina has been pulled away from the rest of the retina and when this piece of retina attached to the detached vitreous face floats internal and anterior to the hole, the piece of retina is called operculum and the hole an operculated hole.

22. **What are the factors responsible for break?**
    i. Dynamic vitreoretinal traction
    ii. Underlying weakness in peripheral retina due to predisposing degeneration

23. **Name the most common site of breaks.**
    Upper temporal quadrant (60%)

24. **What is primary and secondary break?**
    Primary—break responsible for RD
    Secondary—break not responsible for RD

25. **What is retinal dialysis?**
    Retinal dialysis is the disinsertion of neurosensory retina (NSR) from the neuropigment epithelium of pars plana.

26. **What is the most common and pathognomonic site for dialysis in blunt trauma?**
    Upper nasal quadrant

27. What is the most common site for nontrauma dialysis?
Inferior temporal quadrant

28. What are giant tear and horseshoe tear (HST)?
Giant tear: A tear involving 90° or more of the circumference of the globe. It has vitreous gel attached to the anterior margin of the break. Common site is immediate postoral retina.

HST: A retinal tear that takes the shape of a horseshoe with the ends pointing toward the ora. The tongue of retina inside the horseshoe is called a flap. HST is always a sequelae of lattice degeneration. It is formed when an attempt to posterior vitreous detachment (PVD) at lattice edges tears off the retina, creating a horseshoe-shaped tear.

29. What are the peripheral retinal degenerations not associated with RD?
Benign peripheral retinal degenerations are:
 i. Peripheral cystoid degenerations
 ii. Snowflakes
 iii. Paving-stone degenerations
 iv. Honeycomb degenerations
 v. Drusen

30. Which peripheral retinal degenerations predispose to RD?
 i. Lattice degeneration
 ii. Snail track degeneration
 iii. Retinoschisis
 iv. White without pressure
 v. Diffuse chorioretinal atrophy

31. What is lattice degeneration?
Lattice degeneration is sharply demarcated, circumferentially oriented, spindle-shaped areas of retinal thinning. There is discontinuity of ILM with variable atrophy of the underlying sensory retina. It is present in 8% of normal population and 40% of patients with RD and commonly associated with myopia.

Most common location: The most common location is between equator and the posterior border of vitreous base, more in the superotemporal quadrant. Lattice may be complicated by retinal tears or atrophic holes. It should be treated prophylactically in those with a past history of detachment in the fellow eye, family history of detachment, recently acquired HSTs, and aphakic patients.

32. What is snail track degeneration?
Snail track degeneration is sharply demarcated bands of tightly packed snowflakes which gives the peripheral retina a white frost-like

appearance. Round holes may be seen in the snail track and overlying vitreous liquefaction may be present. Snail track degeneration is a predisposing condition for RD.

33. **What are the manifestations of pathological myopia?**
    A. *Anatomical manifestations:*
        i. Corneal astigmatism
        ii. Deep anterior chamber
        iii. Angle iris processes
        iv. Zonular dehiscence
        v. Vitreous syneresis
        vi. Lattice degeneration
        vii. Scleral expansion and thinning
        viii. Decreased ocular rigidity
        ix. Increased axial length
        x. Tilted disk
        xi. Peripapillary detachment
        xii. Temporal crescent
        xiii. Macular lacquer cracks
        xiv. Pigment epithelial thinning
        xv. Choroidal attenuation
        xvi. Foveal retinoschisis
        xvii. Posterior staphyloma
    B. *Ocular manifestations:*
        i. Strabismus—exophoria/exotropia
        ii. Cataract—posterior subcapsular cataract (PSCC), complicated cataract
        iii. Glaucoma—pigmentary/normal tensive glaucoma
        iv. Choroidal retinal atrophy
        v. PVD
        vi. Retinal detachment (RD)
        vii. Fuchs spot
        viii. Macular hole
        ix. Choroidal neovascular membrane

34. **What is retinoschisis?**
    Retinoschisis is the horizontal splitting of the peripheral sensory retina into two layers:
    i. Outer (choroidal layer)
    ii. Inner (vitreous layer)
    There are two main types:
    - *Typical:*
        - Split is at the outer plexiform layer
        - Does not extend posterior to the equator

- Outer layer is uniform
- Less transparent inner layer
- *Reticular:*
  - Split is at the nerve fiber layer
  - Extends posterior to the equator more often, may involve the fovea
  - Outer layer is not homogenous and may have dark areas
  - Greater transparency of the inner layer

Seen in 5% normal population above 20 years and common among hypermetropes. This is a predisposing condition for RD.

35. What is white with pressure (WWP)?
Translucent gray appearance of retina induced by indenting it

36. What is white without pressure?
It is a gray appearance of retina even without indenting it.

37. What is PVD?
It is a separation of cortical vitreous from the ILM. It may be complete or incomplete. Acute PVD may cause retinal tears, rhegmatogenous retinal detachment (RRD), avulsion of blood vessel in the periphery, and vitreous hemorrhage.

38. Why is there tessellation in the fundus?
i. Decreased pigmentation in the RPE
ii. Increased pigmentation in the choroid

39. What is Weiss ring?
Weiss ring is a solitary floater consisting of the detached annular attachment of vitreous to the margin of the optic disk.

40. What are the standard color codes used in fundus drawings?
i. Detached retina—*blue*
ii. Attached retina—*red*
iii. Retinal veins—*blue*
iv. Retinal breaks—*red with blue outlines*
v. Flap of retinal tear—*blue*
vi. Thinned retina—*red hatches outlined in blue*
vii. Lattice degeneration—*blue hatches outlined in blue*
viii. Retinal pigment—*black*
ix. Exudates—*yellow*
x. Vitreous opacities—*green*

41. What is retinal detachment (RD)?
RD is defined as the separation of NSR from the RPE with accumulation of fluid in the potential space between NSR and RPE.

42. **What are the types of RD?**
    i. Rhegmatogenous
    ii. Tractional
    iii. Exudative
    iv. Combined tractional and rhegmatogenous

43. **What is RRD?**
    Rhegma—break
    RRD occurs secondary to a full-thickness defect in the sensory retina, which permits the fluid from synchytic (liquefied) vitreous to enter the subretinal space. There are two types of RRD—primary and secondary.
    i. *Primary:* Retinal break has not been preceded by an antecedent condition (e.g., degenerations) and is usually preceded by PVD.
    ii. *Secondary:* Retinal break has been preceded by an antecedent condition such as lattice.

44. **What are the prerequisites for RRD?**
    i. Presence of retinal break
    ii. Liquefied vitreous gel
    iii. Traction over/at break keeping it open to allow fluid to pass in subretinal space

45. **What are the important causes of liquefaction of vitreous in early childhood that can predispose to RRD?**
    i. Trauma
    ii. High myopia
    iii. Inflammation (vitritis)
    iv. Retinochoroidal coloboma
    v. Genetic predisposition such as Stickler's syndrome, Marfan's syndrome, and Ehlers–Danlos syndrome

46. **What are the symptoms of RRD?**
    i. *Flashes or photopsia:* Due to vitreoretinal traction
    ii. *Floaters:* Due to microbleeding from retinal tear
    iii. *Field defects:* Due to spread of subretinal fluid (SRF) posterior to equator

47. **What are flashes due to?**
    The perception of flashes or photopsia is due to the production of phosphenes by pathophysiological stimulation of retina. During PVD, as the vitreous separates from the retinal surface, the retina is disturbed mechanically, stimulating a sensation of light. Ocular migraine is a differential diagnosis.

48. **What is the significance of floaters?**
    i. Sudden appearance of one large floater near the visual axis is mostly due to PVD (Weiss ring)

ii. Appearance of numerous curvilinear opacities within the visual field indicates vitreous degeneration
   iii. Floaters due to vitreous hemorrhage are characterized by numerous tiny black dots, followed by cobwebs as the blood forms clots

49. **What is the significance of visual field?**
    The quadrant of visual field in which field defect first appears is useful in predicting the location of primary retinal break (which will be in opposite quadrant). Patients tend to be less aware of superior field defects; hence, patients with inferior RD may not be symptomatically aware. High bullous detachments cause dense field defects, while flat detachments produce relative field defects.

50. **What are the symptoms perceived by a patient with acute vitreous hemorrhage?**
    Shower of floaters/reddish smoke

51. **What are the signs of fresh signs of RRD?**
    i. Marcus Gunn pupil
    ii. Intraocular pressure (IOP) lowers by about 5 mm Hg than the other eye
    iii. Mild anterior uveitis
    iv. Tobacco dusting in the vitreous
    v. Retinal breaks
    vi. Detached retina has a convex configuration and a slightly opaque and corrugated appearance with loss of an underlying choroidal pattern

52. **Why is IOP decreased in certain RDs?**
    An eye with RRD typically has decreased IOP and is due to the following factors:
    i. *Early transient pressure drop* may result from inflammation and reduced aqueous production
    ii. *Prolonged hypotony* may be caused by posterior flow, presumably through a break in the RPE

53. **What is Schwartz syndrome?**
    RRD is typically associated with decreased IOP. Schwartz described a condition in which the patient presents with unilateral IOP elevation, RD, and open anterior chamber angle.

54. **Why is IOP raised in certain RDs?**
    Chronic low-grade uveitis in RDs damages the trabecular meshwork in long-standing RDs
    ↓
    Rubeosis iridis [neovascularization of the iris (NVI)]
    ↓
    Increased IOP

55. **What is "tobacco dusting"?**
    i. Pathognomonic of RRD
    ii. Present in the anterior vitreous phase
    iii. The cells represent macrophages containing shed RPE

56. **What is the incidence of RD in myopes?**
    40% of all RDs occur in myopes.

57. **What are the reasons for high myopes to have RRD?**
    i. Increased stretch of the retina over the bigger eyeball
    ii. Incidence of lattice generation is higher
    iii. Incidence of PVD is higher
    iv. Macular hole
    v. Vitreous loss during cataract surgery
    vi. Diffuse chorioretinal atrophy

58. **Which are the systemic conditions associated with RRD?**
    i. Marfan's syndrome
    ii. Ehlers-Danlos syndrome
    iii. Stickler syndrome
    iv. Goldmann-Favre syndrome
    v. Homocystinuria

59. **Why is detached retina gray?**
    Retina is transparent normally, and the normal color of retina is due to the underlying choriocapillaris showing through the transparent retina. However, in detachment, the following factors make the retina look gray:
    i. Detached retina is away from capillaries
    ii. Presence of SRF
    iii. Retinal edema

60. **Why is configuration of SRF important?**
    The configuration of SRF is important because SRF spreads in gravitational fashion and its shape is governed by anatomic limits (ora and optic nerve). It can be used to locate primary break.

61. **What are the factors promoting SRF into the break?**
    i. Ocular movements
    ii. Gravity
    iii. Vitreous traction, at the edge of the break
    iv. PVD

62. **What is Lincoff's rule?**
    Lincoff's rules are a set of guidelines on finding the retinal break based on the configuration of the RD. SRF usually spreads in a gravitational fashion and its shape is governed by anatomical limits and location of

the primary retinal break. If the primary break is located superiorly, SRF first spreads inferiorly on the same side of the break and then spreads superiorly on the opposite side of the fundus.
   i. A shallow inferior RD in which SRF is slightly higher on the temporal side points to a primary break on that side
   ii. A primary break at 6 o'clock will cause inferior RD with equal fluid levels
   iii. In a bullous inferior RD, the primary break usually lies above the horizontal meridian
   iv. If a primary break is in the upper nasal quadrant, the SRF will revolve around the optic disk and then rise on the temporal side until it is level with the primary break
   v. A subtotal RD with a superior wedge of attached retina points to a 1° break located in the periphery nearest its highest borders
   vi. When the SRF crosses the vertical midline above, the primary break is near to 12 o'clock, and the lower edge of the RD corresponds to the side of the break

63. How does a RD progress?
RD can go through any of the following patterns:
   i. Usually, most detachments progress to total detachments
   ii. "Stable detachment" forms demarcation lines and does not settle (commonly in inferior breaks)
   iii. Settling of retinal break spontaneously (only superior retinal breaks) as RD settles inferiorly the site of original break flattens
   iv. Rarely by scarring, spontaneous closure of retinal hole may occur resulting in reattachment

64. What are late secondary changes in RD?
   i. Retinal thinning
   ii. Proliferative vitreoretinopathy (PVR) changes
   iii. Subretinal demarcation line (3 months)
   iv. Intraretinal cyst formation (1 year)
   v. Pigmentation

65. What are demarcation lines?
Demarcation line is formed due to pigment epithelial proliferation and migration at the boundary of the detached and attached retina and is a sign of the chronicity of the condition. It takes about 3 months for the demarcation lines to develop.

66. What is vitreoretinal traction?
Vitreoretinal traction is the force exerted on the retina by structures originating in the vitreous.

Types:
  i. Dynamic—it is induced by rapid eye movement, where there is a centripetal force toward the vitreous cavity. It is responsible for retinal tears and RRD.
  ii. Static—independent of ocular movements and plays an important role in the pathogenesis of tractional retinal detachment (TRD) and PVR.

It may be:
  i. Tangential→ epiretinal fibrovascular membranes
  ii. Anteroposterior (AP) traction → contraction of fibrovascular membranes
  iii. Bridging (trampoline) traction → contraction of fibrovascular membranes which stretch from one part of the posterior retina to another or between vascular arcades which tend to pull the two involved points together.

67. **What is tractional retinal detachment (TRD)?**
    TRD occurs when the NSR is pulled away from the RPE by contracting vitreoretinal membranes in the absence of a retinal break.

68. **What are the conditions causing TRD?**
    i. Diabetes
    ii. Trauma
    iii. Vascular occlusions
    iv. Cataract extraction with vitreous incarceration
    v. Perforating or penetrating injury to the globe
    vi. Sickle cell hemoglobinopathies
    vii. Retrolental fibroplasia
    viii. Persistent hyperplastic primary vitreous (PHPV)
    ix. Pars planitis
    x. Eales' disease
    xi. *Toxoplasma* and *Toxocara* infections

69. **What is the pathogenesis of exudative RD?**

    Diseases of choroids and retina
    ↓
    Damages RPE
    ↓
    Allows passage of fluid (transudate) from choroids into subretinal space

70. **What are the causes of exudative RD?**
    i. *Inflammatory:* Vogt-Koyanagi-Harada (VKH) syndrome
    Peripheral uveitis
    Excessive cryopexy
    Extensive photocoagulation
    Choroidal effusion

ii. *Systemic:* Renal failure
Hypertension
Dysproteinemia and macroglobulinemia
iii. *RPE defect:* RPE detachment
Central serous retinopathy (CSR)
iv. *SRNV:* Age-related macular degeneration (ARMD)
Presumed histoplasmosis
Angioid streaks
Choroidal rupture
v. *Tumors:* Malignant melanoma
Metastasis
Retinoblastoma

71. How do you differentiate between the three types of RD?

Rhegmatogenous, tractional, and exudative

Features	Rhegmatogenous	Exudative	Tractional
History	Photopsia, visual field defects	Systemic factors such as malignant hypertension, eclampsia, and renal failure	Diabetes, penetrating trauma, sickle cell disease
Retinal break	Present	No break or coincidental	No primary break, may develop secondary break
Extent of detachment	Extends to ora early	Gravity dependent, extension to ora is variable	Frequently does not extend to ora
Retinal motility	Undulating bulla or folds	Smoothly elevated bullae, usually without folds	Taut retina, concave surface. Peaks to traction points
Retinal elevation and shape	Low to moderate; convex sometimes	Varies—may be extremely high convex concave	Elevated to level of focal traction
Evidence of chronicity	Demarcation lines, intraretinal macrocysts, atrophic retina	Usually none	Demarcation lines
Pigment in vitreous	Present in 70% of cases	Not present	Present in trauma cases
Vitreous changes	Frequently syneretic, PVD, traction on flap of tear	Usually clear, except uveitis	Vitreoretinal traction

Contd...

Contd...

Features	Rhegmatogenous	Exudative	Tractional
SRF	Clear	May be turbid and shift rapidly to dependent location with changes in head position	Clear, no shift
Choroidal mass	None	May be present	None
IOP	Frequently low	Varies	Usually normal
Transillumination	Normal	Blocked transillumination if pigmented choroidal mass is present	Normal
Examples of conditions causing detachment	Peripheral retinal degeneration, PVD, cytomegalovirus (CMV) retinitis, Stickler syndrome, Marfan's syndrome, Ehlers–Danlos syndrome	Uveitis, metastatic tumor, malignant melanoma, Coats' disease, VKH syndrome, retinoblastoma	Proliferative diabetic retinopathy, retinopathy of prematurity, *Toxocara* sickle cell retinopathy, post-traumatic vitreous traction

IOP: Intraocular pressure; PVD: posterior vitreous detachment; SRF: subretinal fluid; VKH: Vogt–Koyanagi–Harada

72. **What is the differential diagnosis of leukokoria?**
    i. *Congenital:*
        - Norrie's disease
        - Incontinentia pigmenti
        - Autosomal dominant exudative vitreoretinopathy
    ii. *Developmental:*
        - Retinopathy of prematurity
        - Myelinated nerve fiber layer
        - Coloboma
        - PHPV
        - Congenital cataract
    iii. *Inflammatory:*
        - CMV retinitis
        - Toxoplasma
        - *Toxocara*
    iv. *Tumor:*
        - Retinoblastoma

v. *Vasculitis:*
   - Coats' disease
vi. *Others:*
   - RD
   - Vitreous hemorrhage

73. **What are the conditions exhibiting abnormal retinal embryogenesis?**
    i. Retinal dysplasia
    ii. Norrie's disease
    iii. Fundus coloboma
    iv. Optic nerve pits
    v. Persistent fetal vasculature

74. **What are the diseases which simulate RD?**
    i. Retinoschisis
    ii. Choroidal detachment
    iii. Vitreous hemorrhage
    iv. Endophthalmitis
    v. Melanoma of choroid with exudative detachment
    vi. Intraocular cysticercosis
    vii. Uveal effusion syndrome
    viii. Severe vitritis

75. **What are the complications of long-standing RD?**
    i. Uveitis
    ii. Complicated cataract
    iii. Rubeosis iridis
    iv. Glaucoma
    v. Band keratopathy
    vi. Phthisis

76. **What are the types of traumatic RD?**
    i. Tractional
    ii. Rhegmatogenous
    iii. Combined

77. **What is the pathogenesis of traumatic RD?**
    Penetrating trauma → Vitreous incarceration at the site of penetration injuries
    ↓
    Vitreoretinal traction

    The weakest area is in the temporal periphery.

    Blunt trauma → Compression of AP diameter of globe and simultaneous expansion at the equatorial plane. It can cause retinal dialysis (frequent in the upper nasal quadrant) or can cause macular or equatorial holes.
    ↓

Causes
↓
Dialysis, tears (equatorial), macular holes

78. How to differentiate between RRD and retinoschisis?

Features	RRD	Retinoschisis
Symptoms	Photopsia and floaters are present	Photopsia and floaters are absent as no vitreoretinal traction
Visual field defect	Relative scotoma	Absolute scotoma
Detachment	Convex with undulated appearance with mobility	Convex, smooth, thin and immobile, localized
	Presence of tobacco dusting, demarcation, and intraretinal cysts	Absence of such findings
Laser photocoagulation	Does not create burn due to underlying SRF	Will create a burn
Associated refractive error	Myopia	Hypermetropia
Location	Superiotemporal	Inferotemporal

RRD: rhegmatogenous retinal detachment

79. Differentiate between RD and choroidal detachment (CD) clinically.

Features	RD	CD
Symptoms	Photopsia and floaters are present	Absent (no vitreoretinal traction)
Appearance	Convex, undulated, mobile on eye movements. Lighter in color	Brown, convex, smooth, bullous detachment which is relatively immobile. Darker in color
Macula	May be involved	Elevations do not extend to the posterior pole because they are limited by the firm adhesion between the suprachoroidal lamellae and sclera where the vortex veins enter the scleral canals
IOP	Normal/low	Very low
Periphery examinations	Scleral indentation required for periphery examination	Peripheral retina and ora serrata may be seen without scleral indentation
Anterior chamber	Normal depth	Shallow

CD: choroidal detachment; IOP: Intraocular pressure; RD: retinal detachment

80. **How do you classify PVR changes associated with RD?**

Modified Retina Society Classification/Silicone Study Classification		
Grade	Name	Clinical sign
A	Minimal	Vitreous haze, vitreous pigment clumps
B	Moderate	Wrinkling of inner retinal surface, rolled edge of retinal break, retinal stiffness, tortuosity, ↓ motility of vitreous
CP 1–12 (clock hours)	Marked	Posterior to equator focal, diffuse or circumferential full-thickness folds, subretinal strands
CA 1–12 (clock hours)	Marked	Anterior to equator focal, diffuse, circumferential full-thickness folds, subretinal strands, anterior displacement, anterior condensed vitreous strands
D	Massive	Fixed retinal folds in four quadrants; D-1 wide funnel shape; D-2 narrow funnel shape; D-3 closed funnel (optic nerve head, not visible)

81. **What are the factors governing visual function following surgical reattachment?**
    If the macula has been involved, the prognosis is poorer. It is especially poorer if:
    i. The time of involvement is >2 months
    ii. Height of macular detachment and age >60 years negatively affect visual restoration

82. **What is the principle of RD surgery?**
    i. Identify all the breaks (see the break)
    ii. Create a controlled injury to the RPE and retina to produce a chorioretinal adhesion at the site of all retinal breaks (seal the break)
    iii. Employing an appropriate technique such as scleral buckling and/or intravitreal gas to approximate the retinal breaks to the underlying treated RPE

83. **What is an explant?**
    Buckling element (silicon) sutured directly onto the sclera to create a buckle height

84. **What is an implant?**
    Buckling element placed within the sclera to create a buckle height

85. **What are the types of buckles used?**
    i. *Radial explant:* Placed at right angles to limbus
    ii. *Sequential circumferential explants:* Placed circumferentially to limbus to create a sequential buckle

iii. *Encircling circumferential explants:* 360° buckle
iv. Soft silicone sponges for radial or circumferential buckling
v. *Hard silicone straps:* Used for 360° buckling
vi. Hard silicone tires

86. What are the indications for radial buckling?
i. Large U-shaped tears, particularly when "fish mouthing" is anticipated (especially if it is a single break)
ii. Posterior retinal breaks

87. What are the indications for segmental circumferential buckling?
i. Multiple breaks located in one or two quadrants and varying distance from ora serrata
ii. Anterior breaks
iii. Wide breaks, dialysis, and giant tears

88. What are the indications for encircling buckle (360°)?
i. Break involving three or more quadrants
ii. Extensive RD without detectable breaks, particularly in eyes with hazy media
iii. Lattice degeneration, snail track degeneration involving three or more quadrants
iv. Along with vitrectomy

89. What are the preliminary examinations to be done before surgery?
i. Check all clinically important lesions to see if they are correctly indicated in drawing
ii. Assess retinal mobility by moving eye with squint hook. Good retinal motility indicates absence of significant PVR and hence carries a good prognosis
iii. Try to appose the retinal break to the RPE by indenting the sclera with squint hook; if this can be done with ease, drainage of SRF may not be necessary
iv. Assess the dimensions of retinal breaks, by comparing them with the diameter of the optic nerve head (1.5 mm)
v. Assess whether the break is anterior or posterior to the equator

90. What are the steps in scleral buckling surgery?
i. Preliminary examination
ii. 360° peritomy
iii. Traction (bridle) sutures around the recti
iv. Inspection of sclera
v. Localization of the break
vi. Cryotherapy
vii. Scleral buckling

viii. Drainage of SRF
ix. Intravitreal air or balanced salt solution (BSS) injection
x. Closure of the peritomy

91. What precautions should be taken during peritomy?
Care should be taken not to damage the plica semilunaris, tears in conjunctiva and muscle.

92. What is the purpose of bridle sutures?
i. To stabilize the globe
ii. To manipulate it into optimal position during surgery

93. How do you take bridle sutures?
i. Insert a squint hook under rectus muscle
ii. Pass a reverse mounted needle with a 4-0 black silk suture under the muscle tendon
iii. Secure the suture by twisting it around the forceps and cut externally

94. What are the complications associated with taking bridle suture?
i. Damage to vortex veins
 The inferior vortex veins are more anteriorly placed and can be damaged by a posterior insertion of squint hook under inferior rectus. If the vein is damaged, do not cauterize; instead, wait for the bleeding to stop
ii. Rupture of muscle belly due to excessive traction on the sutures
iii. Muscle disinsertion

95. What is the purpose of examining sclera?
i. *To detect scleral thinning:*
 It is characterized by gray color due to underlying choroids. Complications due to it are:
 - Penetration of the needle into choroid and retina while the scleral bite is taken
 - Sutures may cut through the thin sclera after the sutures are tied
ii. *To detect anomalous vortex veins:*
 - As they can be damaged during cryotherapy, scleral buckling, and SRF drainage

96. What are the three modalities used for prophylaxis of RD?
i. Cryotherapy
ii. Laser photocoagulation
iii. Scleral buckling for large tears

97. What are the principles in the prophylactic management of retinal breaks?
i. *Breaks needing treatment:* High myopia, aphakic eyes, symptomatic tear, any break with SRF more than one disk diameter (DD), any

break >1 o'clock hour, family history of RD, systemic conditions such as Marfan's syndrome, Ehlers–Danlos syndrome

ii. *Breaks needing only observation:* Asymptomatic holes, asymptomatic tears

98. What is the principle of cryotherapy?

Cryotherapy is based on the Joule–Thomson effect, which states that when gas is allowed to pass through a narrow passage and under high pressure, it cools to a determined (–70°C) temperature. Cryotherapy causes freezing of the intracellular and extracellular water to ice. This leads to tissue death and sterile with aseptic necrosis and an inflammatory reaction. Scarring will result in stronger than normal bond between the sensory retina, RPE, and choroids. This permanently seals the break.

99. What are the indications for cryotherapy of retinal breaks? What is the temperature generated by cryoprobe and what is the probe size?

Indications:

i. Hazy ocular media

ii. Peripherally located tears near the ora

iii. Tears at the region of vortex veins and at the large ciliary vessels

iv. Small pupils

Temperature of probe: –80°C

Probe size: Standard size of 2.5 mm

100. What is the technique of cryotherapy?

i. By using an indirect ophthalmoscope, locate the break

ii. Indent the sclera gently with cryoprobe and bring the RPE as close as possible to the break

iii. Start freezing until sensory retina has turned "white"

iv. Repeat cryotherapy until the entire break has been surrounded. Cryoprobe position is changed only after complete thawing

101. How is laser retinopexy done?

i. *Laser source:* Double frequency Nd:YAG, diode

ii. *Instruments:* Slit lamp or indirect ophthalmoscope, Goldmann three-mirror lens or wide-angle fundoscopic lens

iii. *Spot size:* 200–500 μm

iv. *Duration:* 0.1–0.2 seconds

v. *Power:* 150–400 mW

vi. *Burn placement:* ½ burn width apart for at least three rows. Lesion should be surrounded 360° or, if closer to the ora, should be treated in a U-shaped pattern around the posterior edge of the lesion

102. What are the indications for SRF drainage?
  i. Difficulty in localization of retinal breaks in bullous detachments
  ii. Long-standing RD as SRF is viscous
  iii. Bullous RD
  iv. Ganglion RD
  v. Glaucomatous cyclitis
  vi. Resurgeries

103. What are the methods of SRF drainage?
  i. *Prang:* Here, digital pressure is applied till the central retinal artery is occluded and choroidal vasculature is blanched. Then, a full-thickness perforation is made with a 27-gauge hypodermic needle to drain SRF. Air is injected to form the globe
  ii. *Cut down:* Radial sclerotomy is made beneath the area of deepest SRF. Mattress suture may be placed across the lips of the sclerotomy. Prolapsed choroidal knuckle is examined with +20 D lens for large choroidal vessels. After ruling this out, light cautery is applied to knuckle to avoid bleeding, and knuckle is perforated with a 25-gauge hypodermic needle

104. What are the advantages of SRF drainage?
SRF drainage provides immediate contact between sensory retina and RPE with flattening of the fovea. If this contact is delayed, the stickiness of RPE wears off and adequate adhesion may not occur, resulting in nonattachment of retina.

105. What are the precautions taken before drainage of SRF?
  i. Examine the fundus to make sure that SRF has not shifted
  ii. Avoid vortex vein
  iii. IOP should not be elevated (it may cause retinal incarceration)

106. How do you know that SRF drainage is completed?
By the presence of pigments

107. What are the complications of SRF drainage?
  i. Choroidal hemorrhage
  ii. Ocular hypotony
  iii. Iatrogenic break
  iv. Retinal incarceration
  v. Vitreous prolapse
  vi. Damage to long posterior ciliary arteries and nerves
  vii. Endophthalmitis

108. What are the indications for internal tamponade in scleral buckling?
  i. Superior break
  ii. Hypotony
  iii. Retinal folds

iv. Fish mouthing
v. Posterior breaks

109. What are the causes of failed scleral buckling surgery?
i. Improper positioning of buckle
ii. Missed holes and iatrogenic inadvertent retinal perforations
iii. Residual vitreous traction
iv. PVR
v. Infection and extrusion of buckle

110. What are the complications of scleral buckling and RD surgery?
Immediate:
i. Failure to reattach retina
ii. Iatrogenic break
iii. Central retinal artery occlusion (CRAO)
iv. Anterior segment ischemia
v. Excessive cryotherapy resulting in exudative RD

Early:
i. Choroidal detachment
ii. Vitritis
iii. Bacterial endophthalmitis
iv. Acute orbital cellulitis

Late:
i. Extraocular muscle (EOM) imbalance
ii. Exposure of implant
iii. Infection
iv. Ptosis
v. Maculopathy
vi. Cataract
vii. PVR
viii. Macular pucker

111. Who are the best candidates for pneumatic retinopexy?
i. A detachment caused by a single break, in superior 8 o'clock hours
ii. The break should not be >1 o'clock hour
iii. Multiple breaks but in 1-2 o'clock hours of each other
iv. Free of systemic disease (rheumatoid arthritis) (who can maintain position)
v. Phakic patients
vi. Total PVD

112. Which are the cases not suitable for pneumoretinopexy?
i. Breaks larger than 1 o'clock hour or multiple breaks extending over >1 o'clock hour of retina
ii. Breaks in the inferior part of the retina

iii. Presence of PVR, grades C and D, since this surgery does not relieve vitreoretinal traction
iv. Physical disability
v. Severe uncontrolled glaucoma cloudy media

113. How is this procedure done?
The eye to be treated is massaged well to reduce the IOP. Selected gas is drawn through a 0.22 μm Millipore filter. Injection is given, 4 mm posterior to the limbus in the region of pars plana temporally. The 30-gauge needle is directed toward the center of the vitreous to ensure penetration of the pars plana epithelium and the anterior hyaloid face. With the injection side uppermost and the needle being vertical, the gas is injected moderately. To prevent leakage, from the injection site, the head is turned to the opposite side.

114. What are the principles of pneumoretinopexy?
Intraocular gases keep the retinal break closed by the following properties:
i. Mechanical closure and thus RPE pump removes excessive SRF
ii. Surface tension
iii. Buoyancy

115. What are the complications of pneumoretinopexy?
i. Subretinal migration of gas
ii. Gas entrapment at the injection site
iii. Iatrogenic macular detachment
iv. New retinal breaks
v. Vitreous incarceration in the paracentesis site
vi. Subconjunctival gas
vii. Cataract and glaucoma
viii. Fish-eggs formation

116. What are the advantages and disadvantages of pneumatic retinopexy with that of scleral buckling?
Advantages:
i. Postoperative vision is better
ii. Morbidity is less
iii. Attachment results are similar
iv. Incidence of cataract is less
v. Economical

Disadvantages:
i. Need for postoperative positioning
ii. Needs closer monitoring

117. What are the indications for vitrectomy in RD?
  i. PVR grade C2 or more
  ii. Giant retinal tear and dialysis
  iii. Posterior break
  iv. Associated with vitreous hemorrhage
  v. Combined RRD with TRD
  vi. Colobomatous detachment
  vii. Inadequate pupillary size
  viii. Associated cataract surgery
  ix. Associated intraocular foreign bodies

118. What are the substances used as vitreous substitutes in RD surgery?
  i. Intraocular gases:

Nonexpansile	Expansile
– Air	– SF6
– SF6: Air mixture	– C3F8
– C3F8: Air mixture	

  ii. Silicone oil
  iii. Perfluorocarbon liquids (PFCL)

119. What are the characteristics of intraocular gases?
  i. *Air:*
    – Average duration of action: 3 days
    – Maximum size: Immediate
    – Average expansion: No expansion
    – Advantages: Low cost and universal availability
    – Disadvantage: Shorter time of action
  ii. *SF6*
    – Average duration of action: 2 days
    – Maximum size: 36 hours
    – Average expansion: Doubles
    – Advantages:
      - Smaller amount of gas required
      - No need for reinjecting the gas in case a new break develops
    – Disadvantage: Air travel contraindicated for a prolonged time
  iii. *C3F8*
    – Average duration of action: 38 days
    – Maximum size: 3 days
    – Average expansion: Quadruples
    – Advantages and disadvantages: Similar to SF6

120. What are the common silicone oils used?
  i. Polydimethylsiloxane (PDMS)
  ii. Trifluoromethyl siloxane

121. What is the mechanism of action of silicone oils?

Silicone oils provide retinal tamponade for a longer period, more than the intraocular gases. Since they are heavier than water, they allow SRF to drain through peripheral retinal break. They can act as a mechanical instrument to cleave planes and also act as an internal tamponade.

122. What are the indications for the use of silicone oil?
   i. RD complicated by PVR changes
   ii. Traumatic RD
   iii. Giant retinal tears
   iv. Tractional and combined RDs
   v. RD associated with choroidal colobomas
   vi. RD associated with infectious retinitis

123. What are the complications of silicone oil?
   i. Silicone oil migration under the retina
   ii. Suprachoroidal silicone oil
   iii. Silicone oil keratopathy
   iv. Inverse hypopyon
   v. Glaucoma
   vi. Vitreous floaters

124. What are the advantages of silicone oil over intraocular gases?
   i. *Intraoperative advantages:*
      - Better intraoperative visualization
      - Easier retinopexy
      - Control of hemorrhage and effusion
   ii. *Postoperative advantages:*
      - Longer lasting tamponade
      - Posturing less critical
      - Better immediate visual acuity
      - Air travel not contraindicated

125. What are PFCLs?

PFCLs are fully fluorinated synthetic analogs of hydrocarbons containing carbon–fluoride bonds.

126. What are the characteristics of PFCL that enable them to be used as a vitreous substitute?
   i. Optical clarity
   ii. Similar refractive index to that of water
   iii. High density
   iv. Biologically inert
   v. High cohesive force

127. What are the commonly used PFCL materials?
   i. Perfluoro-*n*-octane
   ii. Perfluorotributylamine
   iii. Perfluorodecalin

128. What are the indications of PFCL?
   i. RD with PVR
   ii. RD with giant retinal tear
   iii. Traumatic RD
   iv. Lens/intraocular lens (IOL) dislocation into vitreous
   v. Management of suprachoroidal hemorrhage

129. Who is the father of RD surgery?
Jules Gonin (1923) treated retinal break by ignipuncture.

130. Who invented scleral buckling?
Custodis

131. Who invented vitrectomy?
Machemer in 1971.

6.10 ENDOPHTHALMITIS

1. **Define endophthalmitis.**
   Endophthalmitis is an inflammation of the internal layers of the eye resulting from intraocular colonization of infectious agents and manifesting with an exudation into the vitreous cavity.

2. **Classify endophthalmitis.**
   i. *Based on route of entry:*
      - *Exogenous:* Pathogen is introduced from outside
        - Postoperative
        - Post-traumatic
      - *Endogenous:* Pathogen is introduced from ocular circulation
   ii. *Based on microorganisms:*
      - Bacterial
        - *Gram-positive*
          Staphylococcus epidermidis
          Staphylococcus aureus
          Streptococcus pneumoniae
          Streptococcus viridans
          Peptostreptococci
          Corynebacterium
          Propionibacterium acnes
          Actinomyces
        - *Gram-negative*
          Pseudomonas aeruginosa
          Proteus mirabilis
          Klebsiella
          Haemophilus influenzae
          Escherichia coli
      - Fungal
        - *Aspergillus*
        - *Candida*
        - *Cephalosporium*
        - *Penicillium*
        - *Paecilomyces*
   iii. *Based on duration:*

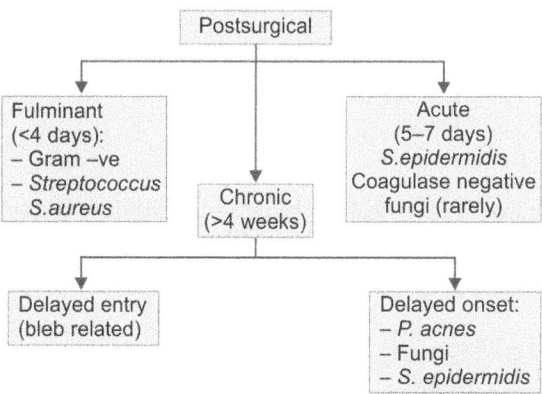

3. **What are the symptoms of endophthalmitis?**
    i. Decrease in vision [94% in Endophthalmitis Vitrectomy Study (EVS) study]
    ii. Pain
    iii. Tearing
    iv. Photophobia
    v. Redness
    vi. Blepharospasm

4. **What are the signs of endophthalmitis?**
    i. Lids
        - Edema
    ii. Conjunctiva
        - Chemosis, circumcorneal congestion
    iii. Cornea
        - May be clear or gross edema
        - Limbal ring abscess
        - Wound dehiscence
        - Suture abscess
    iv. Anterior chamber
        - Flare and cells
        - Hypopyon
        - Exudate
    v. Iris
        - Posterior synechiae
    vi. Pupil
        - Sluggish or absent pupillary reflexes
    vii. Vitreous
        - Cells and exudates

    Fundal glow
    Grading of media clarity (based on EVS):
    i. >20/40 (6/12) view of retina
    ii. 2° order retinal vessel visible
    iii. Some vessels visible but not second order
    iv. No vessels visible
    v. No red reflex

5. **What are the differential diagnoses of endophthalmitis?**

    Surgical
    i. Fibrinous reactions
    ii. Dislocated lens
    iii. Chemical response

    Nonsurgical
    i. Retained intraocular foreign body (IOFB)
    ii. Pars planitis
    iii. Old vitreous hemorrhage

iv. Complicated surgery (manipulation)
v. Microscopic hyphema
vi. Phacoanaphylaxis

iv. Toxoplasmosis/*Toxocara*
v. Necrotic retinoblastoma

6. **What is the role of ultrasonography (USG) in endophthalmitis?**
   To diagnose:
   i. Vitritis
   ii. Choroidal detachment
   iii. Retinal detachment (RD)
   iv. Dislocated lens/nucleus
   v. Radiolucent IOFB
   vi. Parasitic infestation

7. **What are the common organisms implicated in traumatic endophthalmitis?**
   i. *Bacillus* species
   ii. Gram-negative species (*Pseudomonas*)
   iii. Fungi

8. **What are the common organisms implicated in endogenous endophthalmitis?**
   i. *Candida*
   ii. *Neisseria*
   iii. *Bacillus*

9. **What are the common organisms implicated in postoperative endophthalmitis?**
   i. *Pseudomonas*
   ii. *Nocardia*
   iii. *S. epidermidis*
   iv. *H. influenzae* (associated with bleb-related endophthalmitis)

10. **Define "laboratory confirmed growth."**
    i. At least semiconfluent growth on solid media
    ii. Any growth on more than or equal to two media
    iii. Growth on one media supported by gram-positive stain

11. **What are the objectives in endophthalmitis treatment?**
    Primary:
    i. Control/eradicate infection
    ii. Manage complication
    iii. Restoration of vision

    Secondary:
    i. Symptomatic relief
    ii. Prevent panophthalmitis
    iii. Maintain globe integrity

12. **What are the important determinants in outcome?**
    i. Time duration between onset of infection and presentation
    ii. Virulence and load of organism
    iii. Pharmacokinetics and spectrum of drug activity

13. **What are the modalities of treatment?**

    Medical
    i. Antimicrobial
    ii. Anti-inflammatory
    iii. Supportive

    Surgical
    Vitrectomy

14. **What are the steps taken before intravitreal injection?**
    i. Informed consent
    ii. Check if vision is at least perception of light (PL)
    iii. Echography
    iv. To check for wound integrity
    v. Suture abscess
    vi. Lens status
    vii. Intraocular pressure (IOP)

15. **What are the materials for intravitreal injection?**
    i. Clean glass slides
    ii. Culture plates
    iii. Tuberculin syringe
    iv. 26-gauge half-inch, 23-gauge 1-inch needle
    v. Antimicrobial vials
    vi. Lid speculum, sterile cotton-tipped applicator
    vii. Topical xylocaine hydrochloride 4%

16. **What are the steps in intravitreal injection?**
    i. Informed consent is taken
    ii. Paint periocular region with povidone iodine and wash cul-de-sac with the same solution
    iii. Apply topical xylocaine hydrochloride 4% adequately
    iv. Visualize the injection site from limbus (3.0 mm if aphakic, 3.5 mm if pseudophakic, 4 mm if phakic)
    v. Stabilize globe and insert a 26–30 gauge needle with bevel up toward anterior or midvitreous
    vi. Inject drug drop by drop
    vii. If multiple drugs are to be given, replace syringe but not needle
    viii. Check IOP at the end
    ix. Subcutaneous antibiotic is given and eye is patched

17. **What are the advantages of vitrectomy?**
    i. Decrease infection and inflammatory load
    ii. Provides undiluted specimen for culture

iii. Increases antimicrobial drug concentration within the eye
iv. Enables rapid visual recovery by removing media opacities

18. **What are the cardinal principles in vitrectomy?**
    i. Maximum cutting rate
    ii. Minimum suction
    iii. Do not attempt to induce PVD
    iv. Do not attempt to go close to retina

19. **What are the indications for vitrectomy in infectious endophthalmitis?**
    i. Severe cases at manifestation defined as loss of red reflex, loss of light reflex, afferent pupillary defect, and corneal ring infiltrate, etc.
    ii. All cases demonstrating gram-negative bacteria in microbiology
    iii. Cases where vitreous infection precludes retinal examination
    iv. Vitreous abscess
    v. Cases not responding to initial medical therapy

20. **What are the causes of treatment failure?**
    i. Late presentation/delayed diagnosis
    ii. Highly virulent organism
    iii. Drug resistance
    iv. Inadequate drug concentration
    v. Complications (RD)
    vi. Poor visibility for pars plana vitrectomy (PPV)
    vii. Faulty diagnosis
    viii. Failure to recognize a nidus of infection, e.g., dacryocystitis

Endophthalmitis Vitrectomy Study (EVS)

21. **What were the main objectives of the EVS?**
    The main objectives of the EVS were to determine the role of early PPV in comparison to intravitreal injection in patients with postoperative endophthalmitis and also to identify the role of systemic antibiotic treatment in these cases.

22. **What were the outcome measures of this study?**
    Visual acuity and media clarity at the end of 3–9-month follow-up were the outcome measures.

23. **Mention the inclusion and exclusion criteria for this study.**
    Inclusion criteria:
    i. Bacterial endophthalmitis within 6 weeks of cataract surgery or secondary intraocular lens (IOL) implantation.
    ii. Visual acuity of PL or better, but worse than 20/50 with relatively clear cornea and anterior chamber view

Exclusion criteria:
  i. History of other intraocular surgeries
  ii. Presentation after 6 weeks
  iii. Fungal infection
  iv. Previous intraocular antibiotic
  v. Retinal and choroidal detachments
  vi. Drug sensitivity to lactams

24. **What were the drugs used in the study?**
   i. *Intravitreal*:
      - Vancomycin (1,000 µg in 0.1 mL)
      - Amikacin (400 µg in 0.1 mL)
      (No intravitreal corticosteroids were used.)
   ii. *Systemic*:
      - Ceftazidime (2 g, 8 hourly)
      - Amikacin (7-5 mg/kg BD)
      If allergic to lactams, oral ciprofloxacin 750 mg BD was used.
   iii. *Subconjunctival*:
      - Vancomycin   (25 mg/0.5 mL)
      - Ceftazidime   (100 mg/0.5 mL)
      - Dexamethasone   (6 mg/0.25 mL)
   iv. *Topical*:
      - Vancomycin (50 mg/mL)   every 4 hours
      - Amikacin (20 mg/mL)   every 4 hours

25. **What were the major conclusions of the study?**
   i. There was no difference in final visual acuity or media clarity with or without the use of systemic antibiotics.
   ii. In patients whose initial visual acuity was hand motions or better, there was no difference in visual outcome whether or not an immediate vitrectomy was performed.
   iii. In patients with only light perception vision, vitrectomy was much better than intravitreal injections alone.

26. **What is sterile postoperative endophthalmitis?**
   Sterile postoperative endophthalmitis is caused by the following:
   i. Postoperative inflammation to retained lens matter
   ii. Residual chemicals
   iii. Toxicity of residual monomers on polymethyl methacrylate (PMMA)
   iv. Mechanical irritation of iris and ciliary body

27. **Name the most common organisms in bleb-related endophthalmitis?**
   i. *Streptococcus*
   ii. *H. influenzae*

28. **What is the mode of treatment in severe *P. acnes* infection?**
    i. Vitrectomy
    ii. Total capsulectomy
    iii. IOL explantation combined with intraocular and systemic antibiotics

29. **What are the organisms common in endogenous endophthalmitis?**

Fungal	Bacteria
Candida	B. cereus
	Aspergillus

30. **What are the organisms common in post-traumatic endophthalmitis?**

Bacterial	Fungal
S. epidermidis	Fusarium
Bacillus cereus	
In children	
Streptococcal species	

31. **How does treatment of endogenous endophthalmitis differ from other types?**
    i. Both bacterial and fungal infections in the initial phase are treated with intensive intravenous therapy
    ii. Only if infection is not responding to medical intravenous therapy can intravitreal be considered

32. **What drug is contraindicated in endogenous endophthalmitis?**
    Corticosteroids

33. **How to prepare the commonly recommended intravitreal drugs in postoperative endophthalmitis?**
    Antibacterial:
    i. Vancomycin hydrochloride (1,000 μg in 0.1 mL)
       - The drug is available as a powder in strength of 500 μg
       - Reconstitute it with 10 mL of sterile solution for injection or saline
       - This gives a strength of 50 mg in 1 mL and hence 10 mg in 0.2 mL
       - 0.2 mL of this drug is drawn into a tuberculin syringe, and this is further diluted with 0.8 mL of sterile saline to give a strength of 10 mg in 1 mL and hence 1,000 μg (1 mg) in 0.1 mL
    ii. Ceftazidime hydrochloride (2.25 mg in 0.1 mL)
       - The drug is available as a powder in a strength of 500 mg powder
       - Reconstitute it with 2 mL of sterile saline solution for injection to give a strength of 250 mg in 1 mL (225 mg of active ingredient) and 25 mg (22.5 mg) in 0.1 mL
       - 0.1 mL of the drug is drawn into a tuberculin syringe and diluted further with 0.9 mL of sterile solution to give a strength of 25 mg (22.5 mg) in 1 mL and hence 2.25 mg in 0.1 mL

iii. Cefazolin hydrochloride (2.25 mg in 0.1 mL)
    Same as for ceftazidime
iv. Amikacin sulfate (400 µg in 0.1 mL)
    - The drug is available as a solution in a strength of 100 mg in a 2 mL vial (50 mg in 1 mL) and 10 mg in a 0.2 mL vial
    - 0.2 mL of the drug is drawn into a tuberculin syringe and diluted further with 2.3 mL of sterile solution to give a strength of 10 mg in 2.5 mL and hence 4,000 µg in 0.1 mL
v. Gentamicin sulfate (200 µg in 0.1 mL)
    - The drug is available as a solution of 80 mg in a 2 mL vial (40 mg in 1 mL) and 4 mg in a 0.1 mL vial
    - 0.1 mL of the drug is drawn into a tuberculin syringe and diluted further with 1.9 mL of solution to give a strength of 4 mg in 2 mL (2 mg in 1 mL) and hence 200 µg in 0.1 mL

Antifungal:
i. Amphotericin B (5 µg in 0.1 mL)
    - The drug is available as a 50 mg powder vial
    - Reconstitute this with 10 mL of dextrose 5% to give a concentration of 5 mg per mL and 500 µg in 0.1 mL
    - Take 0.1 mL into a tuberculin syringe and dilute further with 9.9 mL of dextrose 5% to give a concentration of 500 µg in 10 mL and 50 µg per mL and 5 µg in 0.1 mL
ii. Voriconazole
    - One vial of voriconazole contains 1 mg of the drug in a powder form
    - It is reconstituted with 1 cm^3 normal saline
    - 0.1 mL of the drug solution now contains 0.1 mg or 100 µg of voriconazole, which is the recommended dose for intravitreal injection
    - 0.1 mL of the drug is withdrawn and injected into the vitreous cavity

Corticosteroids:
Intravitreal dexamethasone (400 µg in 0.1 mL)
i. The drug is available as a solution in strength of 8 mg in 2 mL vial (4 mg in 1 mL) and hence 0.4 mg (400 µg) in 0.1 mL
ii. 0.1 mL of the drug may be withdrawn directly into a tuberculin syringe without any further dilution

34. What are the recommended doses of systemic antibiotics in endogenous endophthalmitis?

Chloramphenicol—1-1.5 mg IV 6 hourly
Cefuroxime—3 g IV 8 hourly
Cefotaxime—2 g IV 4 hourly
Moxalactam—2-4 g IV 6-8 hourly

Ampicillin—2-4 g IV 4 hourly
Vancomycin—500 mg IV 6 hourly
Ceftizoxime—2 g IV 6 hourly
Penicillin G—2 mU IV 2 hourly

Gentamicin—8 mg/kg/day IV

Intravenous (IV) treatment should continue at least for a period of 10-14 days.

35. **What are the differences between panophthalmitis and endophthalmitis?**

Panophthalmitis	Endophthalmitis
Intense purulent inflammation of the whole eyeball. Involves all coats of the eye	Inflammation of inner coats of eyeball, aqueous and vitreous humor
Ocular movements restricted	Ocular movements not restricted
Systemic symptoms more—fever, orbital cellulitis, cavernous, sinus thrombosis, meningitis	Systemic symptoms less. Ocular—corneal clouding, hypopyon (intense)
Management: Evisceration	*Management:* Core vitrectomy

6.11 RETINITIS PIGMENTOSA

1. **Define retinitis pigmentosa (RP).**
   Retinitis pigmentosa is a clinically and genetically heterogenous group of progressive hereditary disorders that diffusely and primarily affects photoreceptor and pigment epithelial function, and that is associated with progressive cell loss and eventually atrophy of several retinal layers.

2. **What are synonyms of RP?**
   i. Tapetoretinal degeneration
   ii. Primary pigmentary retinal degeneration
   iii. Pigmentary retinopathy
   iv. Rod-cone dystrophy
   v. Retinal dystrophy

3. **What is the prevalence rate of RP?**
   Between 1/3,000 and 1/5,000

4. **What is the earliest presentation of RP?**
   Nyctalopia (night blindness) and progressive visual field disturbances are the earliest presentations of RP. By the age of 30 years, more than 75% of the patients become symptomatic.

5. **What are the causes of nyctalopia (night blindness)?**
   i. *Congenital stationary night blindness:*
      - Presenting with normal fundus—autosomal dominant (AD), autosomal recessive (AR), and X-linked forms
      - Presenting with abnormal fundus—fundus albipunctatus and Oguchi's disease
   ii. *Progressive night blindness:*
      - Retinitis pigmentosa
      - Choroidal diseases such as choroideremia, gyrate dystrophy, and diffuse choroidal atrophy
      - High myopia
      - Progressive glaucoma
      - Retinitis punctata albescens
      - Vitamin A deficiency
      - Liver cirrhosis (alcoholic)
      - Tapetoretinal degenerations
   iii. *Spurious night blindness:*
      - Nuclear cataract
      - Postrefractive surgery

6. **What is day blindness (hemeralopia)?**
    i. Posterior subcapsular cataract
    ii. Hereditary retinoschisis
    iii. Intraocular iron

7. **What are the causes of central vision loss in RP?**
    i. Posterior subcapsular cataract
    ii. Cystoid macular edema (CME)
    iii. Cellophane maculopathy
    iv. Diffuse vascular leakage
    v. Macular preretinal fibrosis
    vi. Retinal pigment epithelium (RPE) defects

8. **What are the visual field defects in RP?**
    i. *Paracentral scotoma:* Starts 20° from fixation
    ii. *Ring scotoma:* Outer edge of the ring expands rapidly to the periphery, while the inner ring contracts toward fixation
    iii. *Constricted tunnel field of vision (tubular vision)*

9. **What is the cause of ring-like scotomas in the visual field?**
    The pigmentary changes extend both posteriorly and anteriorly, giving rise to ring-like scotoma in the visual field.

10. **What are the conditions that can cause tubular vision?**
    i. Retinitis pigmentosa
    ii. Glaucoma
    iii. High myopia
    iv. Aphakic glasses
    v. Extensive choroiditis
    vi. Extensive panretinal photocoagulation
    vii. Chronic atrophic papilledema
    viii. Hysteria and malingering
    ix. Alcohol poisoning

11. **What are the diagnostic criteria for RP?**
    i. Bilateral involvement
    ii. Loss of peripheral vision and night vision
    iii. Rod dysfunction
        - Dark adaptation
        - Electroretinogram (ERG)
    iv. Progressive loss in photoreceptor function

12. **Which photoreceptors are involved?**
    Both cones and rods are involved, but the rod is predominantly involved.

13. **What is the mode of inheritance?**
    i. *AR*: 60%
    ii. *AD*: 10–25%
    iii. *X-linked*: 5–18%

14. **Discuss the prognosis of inheritance pattern of RP.**
    i. Best prognosis—AD
    ii. Worst prognosis—X-linked

15. **What is the triad of RP?**
    i. Arteriolar attenuation
    ii. Retinal bone spicule pigmentation
    iii. Waxy disk pallor

16. **What are the causes of retinal vessel attenuation?**
    The exact cause is unknown, but it is thought to be a secondary change. It is thought to be the result of:
    i. Increased intravascular oxygen tension due to decreased oxygen consumption by degenerating outer retinal layers
    ii. Closer proximity of retinal vascular network to the choroidal circulations as a result of retinal thinning

17. **What are the differential diagnoses of retinal vessel narrowing?**
    i. Arteriosclerosis
    ii. Hypertensive retinopathy
    iii. Coarctation of aorta
    iv. Hyperbaric oxygen therapy
    v. Apparent narrowing (hypermetropia, aphakia)
    vi. Inflammatory disorders such as temporal arteritis and polyarteritis nodosa

18. **What is the cause of "bone spicule pigment deposits"?**
    Pigments getting released from the degenerating RPE migrate into the inner retina and accumulates in the inner retina around the blood vessels, especially at the vessel branchings, producing a perivascular cuffing and bone spicule pigment formation.

19. **What are the conditions causing pigmentation in retina?**
    i. Retinitis pigmentosa
    ii. Senile changes (degenerative pigmentation)
    iii. Inflammatory conditions such as rubella, congenital syphilis (salt and pepper fundus), and toxoplasmosis
    iv. Cytomegalovirus (CMV) retinitis
    v. Toxic: Chloroquine, phenothiazines, clofazimine
    vi. Iatrogenic: Photocoagulation, cryotherapy
    vii. Trauma

viii. Spontaneously settled retinal detachment (RD)
ix. Hereditary chorioretinal dystrophies such as fundus flavimaculatus and pigmented paravenous chorioretinal atrophy
x. Choroideremia
xi. Peripheral retinal pigment degeneration

20. **What is the site of pigmentary deposition in the initial stages of RP?**
Pigmentary deposition is found at the midperipheral, equatorial region of the fundus. This part of the retina is the one to develop first and according to the principle of abiotrophy undergoes degeneration first as well.

21. **What are the conditions that cause consecutive optic atrophy (waxy disk pallor)?**
    i. Retinitis pigmentosa
    ii. High myopia
    iii. Extensive photocoagulation
    iv. Diffuse chorioretinitis
    v. Central retinal artery occlusion (CRAO)

22. **What is the cause of waxy disk pallor in RP?**
The waxy disk pallor is due to a thick preretinal membrane centered on the disk that extends over the retina in all quadrants. The preretinal membrane appears to originate from fibrous astroglial cells in the optic nerve. The reorganization of fibrous astrocytes into the thickened retinal membrane over the optic nerve could contribute to the appearance of waxy pallor of the optic disk.

23. **What are the classic fundus appearances in a case of RP?**
    i. *Optic nerve changes:*
        - Variable waxy pallor disk
        - Consecutive optic atrophy
    ii. *Vessel changes:* Arteriolar narrowing
    iii. *General retinal changes:*
        - Pigment within the retina—generalized granularity or discrete
        - Pigment clumps or bone spicule appearing pigment deposits
        - A generalized mottling or moth-eaten pattern of the RPE
        - A refractile appearance to the retina
    iv. *Macular changes:* Loss of foveal reflex
        Maculopathy (three types):
        - Atropic
        - Cellophane
        - CME

v. *Vitreous changes:*
- *Stage 1:* Fine colorless dust particles
- *Stage 2:* Posterior vitreous detachment
- *Stage 3:* Vitreous condensation
- *Stage 4:* Collapse

24. **What are the changes in macula?**
Three types of macular lesions are as follows:
   i. Atrophy of the macular area with thinning of RPE and mottled transmission defects of fluorescein angiography
   ii. Cystic lesion or partial-thickness holes within the macula with radial, inner retinal traction lines and/or various degrees of preretinal membranes causing a "surface wrinkling phenomenon" (cellophane maculopathy)
   iii. CME and increased capillary permeability

25. **What are the vitreous particles seen in RP?**
Fine melanin pigment granules, pigment granules, uveal melanocytes, retinal astrocytes, and macrophage-like cells

26. **What are the associated ocular features?**
   i. Myopia
   ii. Keratoconus
   iii. Open-angle glaucoma
   iv. Posterior subcapsular cataract
   v. Optic disk drusen
   vi. Microphthalmus

27. **What are the causes of cataract formation in RP?**
Cataract formation in RP is possibly caused by pseudoinflammatory pigmental cells in the vitreous and is of the central posterior subcapsular variety. Ultrastructurally, the cataracts of RP are not unique except for focal epithelial degeneration, which may cause osmotic instability.

28. **What is to be kept in mind when performing cataract surgery in retinitis pigmentosa?**
   i. Patients with retinitis pigmentosa and complicated cataract who undergo cataract surgery may suffer from capsular phimosis as a postoperative complication.
   ii. Performing a larger rhexis and use of capsular tension ring (CTR) may be useful approaches to minimizing the complication.

29. **Discuss the theories of RP.**
   i. Vascular theory
      - Sclerosis of choroid and choriocapillaris
      - Sclerosis of retinal vessels

ii. Pigmentary theory
   - Changes in neuroepithelium and pigmentary epithelium
iii. Abiotrophy
iv. Premature senility and death of cells of specified tissues—equatorial parts are affected first because it is the first to attain full development.

30. What are the variants of RP?

i. *Inverse RP or central RP:*
   Pigments are more seen centrally and the equatorial and peripheral retina may be spared
ii. *Sectoral RP:*
   Pigmentary changes are confined to one quadrant. Visual function remains good for many years
iii. *RP with exudative vasculopathy:*
   It is bilateral and consists of vascular anomalies, serous RD, and lipid deposits in retinal periphery
iv. *Unilateral RP:*
   These are patients with unilateral pigmentary degeneration.
v. *RP sine pigmento*
   Typical symptoms and the presence of signs except pigmentary deposition
vi. *Retinitis punctata albescens:*
   Fine white punctate lesions in the midperiphery at the level of pigment epithelium with symptoms of RP

31. What are the tests of visual function done in patients with RP?

i. *Electroretinogram (ERG):*
   - Very useful to determine early loss of photoreceptor function
   - Prognostic information in some cases of RP
   - Useful in evaluating therapeutic modalities of retinal dystrophies
ii. *Dark adaptations and visual sensitivity:*
   To measure visual sensitivity, a test light positioned on a given area of the retina is dimmed to a subthreshold level and is then made gradually brighter. The intensity at which it is perceived is defined as visual threshold and may be expressed in log units.

   Dark adaptation involves the measurement of the absolute thresholds at given time intervals as the retina adapts to the dark. The Goldmann–Weekers adaptometer is the most commonly used.
iii. *Visual fields*
iv. *Fundus reflectometry:*
   Useful technique for quantitative assessment of photopigment regeneration
v. *Contrast sensitivity:*
   It is a more sensitive test of macular function.

vi. *Electrooculogram (EOG):*
   The EOG is thought to measure the functions of both the photoreceptors and RPE. Although EOG is abnormal in RP even in early stages, ERG is more preferred.
vii. *Visually evoked response*
viii. *Fluorescein angiography:*
   It is useful in patients with exudative vasculopathy and cystoid macular edema.
ix. *Vitreous fluorophotometry:*
   It is a method of evaluating the blood–retinal barrier by quantifying the leakage of fluorescein from retinal vessels into the posterior vitreous. It is useful to detect abnormality of the blood–retinal barrier. Patients with RP have a marked elevation of the dye concentration in the vitreous.

32. **What is the significance of the various waves in ERG?**
    i. The a-wave is the initial cornea-negative deflection; it is hypothesized to arise from the photoreceptors.
    ii. The b-wave is the largest wave of the ERG and is a cornea-positive wave. There is general consensus that the b-wave reflects primarily the activity of depolarizing (on) bipolar cells and also from the Muller cells.
    iii. The c-wave is a cornea-positive wave on the ERG. It is generated from the RPE mainly in response to rod photoreceptors.

33. **How is ERG useful in RP?**
    i. Patients with advanced RP have nondetectable rod and cone responses
    ii. In patients with early disease, a and b waves generated by the photoreceptors in response to white light under dark-adapted conditions are reduced in amplitude
    iii. In all genetic subtypes of RP, the pure rod responses have "b" wave amplitudes that are nondetectable or reduced with either prolonged or normal implicit times

34. **What is non-detectable ERG?**
    Nondetectable ERG is defined as <10 µV

35. **What are the conditions that can cause nonrecordable ERG?**
    i. Leber's congenital amaurosis
    ii. Retinal aplasia
    iii. Retinitis pigmentosa
    iv. Total RD

36. **What are histopathological changes of RP?**
    i. Rod and cone outer segments—shortened and disorganized (but inner segment remains normal)

ii. In the area of visual loss from RP, there is total loss and decrease in photoreceptor number
iii. Pigmented cells invade the retina
   - Typical RPE cells away from the RPE layer and macrophage-like cells that contain melanin are also found in retina

37. **What are the systemic associations with RP?**
    i. *Usher's syndrome:*
       Congenital sensory neural deafness with RP
    ii. *Laurence-Moon-Bardet-Biedl syndrome:* Components are
       - Retinal dystrophy
       - Mental retardation
       - Truncal obesity
       - Hypogonadism
       - Polydactyly
    iii. *Cockayne syndrome:*
       RP with infantile onset of growth failure, cutaneous photosensitivity to ultraviolet (UV) light, cachexia, dementia, cerebellar dysfunction, and joint contractures
    iv. *Alstrom syndrome:*
       Cone-rod dystrophy, interstitial nephropathy, and progressive sensory neural deafness
    v. *RP with neurological disorders:*
       These are lysosomal storage diseases with accumulation of insoluble autofluorescent lipopigments in a variety of tissues. They are characterized by symptoms of RP along with cerebellar degeneration and extrapyramidal signs. They are of the following types:
       - *Infantile form:* Haltia-Santavuori syndrome
       - *Late infantile form:* Jansky-Bielschowsky syndrome
       - *Juvenile form:* Batten-Spielmeyer-Vogt syndrome
       - Hallervorden-Spatz syndrome
    vi. *Spinocerebellar degenerations (Pierre-Marie's hereditary cerebellar ataxia)*
    vii. *Kearns-Sayre syndrome (mitochondrial myopathy)*
       Pigmentary degeneration of the retina, external ophthalmoplegia, and complete heart block
    viii. *Refsum's syndrome (phytanic acid storage disease)*
       RP with peripheral neuropathy, cranial neuropathy, cerebellar involvement, cardiomyopathy, and sudden death.
    ix. *Mucopolysaccharidosis: Sanfilippo's and Schie's syndrome*
    x. *Abetalipoproteinemia Bassen-Kornzweig syndrome*
       RP with infantile steatorrhea and failure to thrive

38. What are the types of Usher's syndrome?

Type I: Congenital, bilateral sensorineural deafness, and no intelligible speech

Type II: Nonprogressive moderate to profound congenital sensory neural hearing impairment and late manifestation of RP

Type III: Type I patients with ataxia

39. Why is deafness associated with RP?
   i. Common origin of RPE and the epithelium of organ of Corti
   ii. The cilium of inner air and the cilium of the photoreceptors may fail to develop due to a defective gene in Usher syndrome

40. How do you manage a case of RP?
   i. Clinical evaluation and investigation
   ii. Treatment of allied conditions
   iii. Low vision aids
   iv. Genetic counseling
   v. Psychological and vocational counseling

41. Discuss the treatment of RP.
   i. *Medical*
   Vitamin A 15,000 IU/day, delays the rod photoreceptor degeneration, stalls the progression of RP.
   ii. *Light deprivation*
   Dark glasses during outdoor activities—CPF (corning photochromatic filter)
   iii. *Optical aids*
   - Mirrors and prisms mounted on spectacles for peripheral field *expansion*
   - Field expanders
     - Drawbacks such as distortion of depth perception
   - Reverse Galilean telescopes
     - Diminish central visual acuity to an unacceptably low level
       + Low vision aid
       + Magnifiers and closed-circuit television
       + Image intensifiers
       + High-intensity lantern

42. What are the recent treatment modalities in RP?
   i. Argus II epiretinal prosthesis (bionic eye)
   ii. Retinal chip research
   iii. Stem cell
   iv. Gene therapy
   v. CNTF (ciliary neurotrophic factor)
   vi. Hormone estrogen injection.

6.12 RETINOBLASTOMA

1. **What is the most common intraocular malignancy of childhood?**
   Retinoblastoma (RB)

2. **What are the other common childhood malignancies?**
   i. Rhabdomyosarcoma
   ii. Neuroblastoma
   iii. Ewing's sarcoma
   iv. Wilms' tumor

3. **What is the incidence of RB?**
   1 in 17,000 live births in Western countries

4. **What are the modes of presentations?**
   i. Heritable—40%
   ii. Nonheritable—60%

5. **What is the pathogenesis?**
   RB1 tumor suppressor gene is located on the long arm of chromosome 13 at region 14. It codes for RB nucleoprotein, which normally suppresses cell division. Any mutation in the *RB* gene will cause RB.

6. **What are the nonocular cancers common in heritable RB?**
   i. Pinealoma
   ii. Osteosarcoma
   iii. Melanoma
   iv. Malignancies of brain and lungs

7. **From where does it arise?**
   It arises from primitive retinal cells before differentiation.

8. **What is the common age of presentation?**
   i. The first year of life in bilateral cases
   ii. The second year of life in unilateral cases

9. **Why is RB seldom seen after 3 years of age?**
   Primitive retinal cells disappear within the first few years of life.

10. **What are the patterns of tumor spread?**
    i. Endophytic (vitreous): Retina is not detached
    ii. Exophytic (subretinal space): Retina is detached
    iii. Optic nerve invasion
    iv. Diffuse infiltration of the retina
    v. Metastasis

11. **What is the histopathological hallmark of differentiated RB?**
    Rosette formation

12. **Describe Flexner-Wintersteiner rosette.**
    Flexner-Wintersteiner rosette is an expression of retinal differentiation. Cells surround a central lumen lined by a refractile structure. Refractile lining corresponds to the external limiting membrane of the retina. It is characterized by a single row of columnar cells with eosinophilic cytoplasm and peripherally situated nuclei.

13. **Describe Homer-Wright rosette.**
    Homer-Wright rosette consists of cells which form around a mass of neural fibers. No lumen is present.

14. **What are the differences between Flexner-Wintersteiner and Homer-Wright rosettes?**

Flexner–Wintersteiner rosette	Homer–Wright rosette
It consists of columnar cells around the central lumen	It consists of cells around a mass of neural fibers. No lumen is present
Hyaluronidase is present	Hyaluronidase is absent
It is also seen in medulloepithelioma	It is also seen in neuroblastoma, medulloblastoma, and medulloepithelioma

15. **What are fleurettes?**
    Fleurettes are a cluster of tumor cells with long cytoplasmic processes that project through a fenestrated membrane and resemble a bouquet of flowers. They represent photoreceptor differentiation.

16. **What are the presenting features of RB?**
    i. Leukocoria—56% (white reflex in the pupillary area)
    ii. Strabismus—20%
    iii. Vitreous opacity
    iv. Pseudohypopyon
    v. Iris heterochromia
    vi. Spontaneous hyphema
    vii. Inflammation mimicking orbital cellulitis
    viii. Vitreous hemorrhage (VH)
    ix. Glaucoma
    x. Corneal edema
    xi. Proptosis

17. **What is the differential diagnosis of leukocoria?**
    i. Persistent hyperplastic primary vitreous (PHPV)
    ii. Coats' disease
    iii. Toxocariasis
    iv. Retinopathy of prematurity (ROP)
    v. Coloboma of choroid

vi. Cataract
vii. VH
viii. Retinal detachment (RD)
ix. Retinal dysplasia

18. **What are the signs of regression in case of endophytic RB?**
    i. Pigmented atrophic ring at the circumference of the tumor
    ii. Translucency of tumor

19. **What are the predictive factors of metastasis?**
    i. Orbital invasion
    ii. Optic nerve invasion
    iii. Massive choroidal invasion
    iv. Tumor volume >1 cm^3

20. **What are the investigations useful in the diagnosis of RB?**
    i. X-ray skull
    ii. Ultrasonography (USG)
    iii. Magnetic resonance imaging (MRI)
    iv. Specular microscopy (seeding of tumor cells in the endothelium)

21. **What are the features of RB in X-ray?**
    i. Expansion of optic canal
    ii. Diffuse or finely stippled calcification

22. **How does USG help in cases of RB?**
    i. Tumor dimension
    ii. Orbital shadowing
    iii. Calcification
    iv. Helpful in hazy media

23. **How does computed tomography (CT) help?**
    i. To determine the size and extraocular extent of the tumor
    ii. Calcification
    iii. Optic nerve evaluation

24. **How does RB present in MRI?**
    i. Hyperintense in T1-weighted images
    ii. Hypointense in T2-weighted images

25. **What are the investigations contraindicated in RB?**
    i. Fine needle aspiration cytology (FNAC) and incisional biopsy are contraindicated. It may lead to tumor seeding into the orbit
    ii. CT scan carries a risk of secondary tumor formation

26. **Describe the types of RB based on USG.**
    i. Solid—early lesion
    ii. Cystic—advanced tumor cells floating in the vitreous

27. What are the inflammatory conditions that mimic RB?
  i. Toxocariasis
  ii. Posterior uveitis
  iii. Orbital cellulitis
  iv. Congenital toxoplasmosis

28. What are the neoplastic conditions that mimic RB?
  i. Retinal astrocytic hamartoma
  ii. Medulloepithelioma
  iii. Leukemia
  iv. Rhabdomyosarcoma

29. Name a few diseases having intraocular calcification.
  i. RB
  ii. Toxoplasmosis
  iii. Tuberculosis
  iv. Cysticercosis
  v. Syphilis
  vi. *Toxocara* endophthalmitis
  vii. Coats' disease

30. What are the classification systems used in RB?
  i. Reese–Ellsworth classification
  ii. International classification system

31. What is international classification?

Group A (very-low risk)	Small tumor <3 mm confined to the retina; 3 mm from fovea, 1.5 mm from optic disk
Group B (low risk)	Tumor >3 mm confined to the retina in any location with clear subretinal fluid (SRF) <6 mm from the tumor margin
Group C (moderate risk)	Localized vitreous subretinal seeding (>6 mm in total from tumor margin). If there is more than one site of subretinal/vitreous seeding, then the total of these sites must be <6 mm
Group D (high risk)	Diffuse vitreous and/or subretinal seeding (>6 mm in total from tumor margin). If there is more than one site of subretinal/vitreous seeding, then the total of these sites must be >6 mm; SRF >6 mm from the tumor margin
Group E (very-high risk)	No visual potential or any one of the following: • Tumor in the anterior segment • Tumor in the ciliary body • Neovascular glaucoma (NVG) • VH obscuring tumor of significant hyphema • Phthisical or prephthisical • Orbital cellulitis-like presentation

32. **What are the various treatment modalities available for RB?**
    i. Enucleation
    ii. Chemotherapy
    iii. Radiotherapy
    iv. Cryotherapy
    v. Transpupillary thermotherapy
    vi. Photocoagulation

33. **How do you plan to treat RB?**
    i. *Unilateral nonheritable RB:*
       - Group A: Photocoagulation and cryotherapy
       - Group B: Three to four cycles of chemotherapy. Solitary lesion can be treated using a radioactive plaque.
       - Group C: Six cycles of chemotherapy
       - Group D: Enucleation
    ii. *Bilateral RB:* Symmetrical disease
       - Group A: Photocoagulation and cryotherapy
       - Groups B to C: Same treatment as unilateral disease
       - Group D: Six cycles of three-drug chemotherapy
    iii. *Bilateral RB:* Asymmetrical disease
       If the worst eye is in group E, then primary enucleation is recommended.

34. **What are the precautions to be taken while enucleating retinoblasmic eye?**
    Special considerations for enucleation in RB are as follows:
    i. Minimal manipulation
    ii. Avoid use of clamps, snares, or cautery
    iii. Avoid perforation of the eye
    iv. Harvest long (>15 mm) optic nerve stump
    v. Inspect the enucleated eye for macroscopic extraocular extension and optic nerve involvement
    vi. Harvest fresh tissue for genetic studies
    vii. Place a primary implant
    viii. Avoid biointegrated implant if postoperative radiotherapy is necessary.

35. **What is the role of chemotherapy in the management of RB?**
    i. Chemo reduction of tumor in association with local therapy
    ii. To reduce the possibility of orbital recurrence
    iii. Suspected/documented metastasis

36. **What are the common chemotherapeutic agents used in the management of RB?**
    i. Day 1—vincristine + etoposide + carboplatin

ii. Day 2—etoposide
Standard dose (thrice weekly, six cycles):
- Vincristine—1.5 mg/m^2 (0.05 mg/kg for children <36 months and maximum dose <2 mg)
- Etoposide—150 mg/m^2 (5 mg/kg for children <36 months)
- Carboplatin—560 mg/m^2 (18.6 mg/kg for children <36 months)

High dose (thrice weekly, 6-12 cycles):
- Vincristine—0.025 mg/kg
- Etoposide—12 mg/kg
- Carboplatin—28 mg/kg

37. **What is periocular chemotherapy?**
    Subtenon carboplatin had been tried. 2 mL of 10 mg/mL solution is injected.

38. **What are the side effects of periocular chemotherapy?**
    Orbital myositis and optic atrophy

39. **What are the indications of focal therapy?**
    i. Small tumor <3 mm in diameter and height located in visually noncrucial areas
    ii. As an adjuvant in large tumors/vitreous/subretinal seeding

40. **What are the lasers used in the management of RB?**
    The lasers used in the management of RB are xenon arc and argon laser. Focal consolidation is most often accomplished with transpupillary therapy.

41. **Where do you prefer cryoablation and laser photoablation?**
    Laser photoablation is preferred for posteriorly located tumors and cryoablation for anteriorly located tumors because of the risk of optic nerve and macular damage. RD can occur in cryo scar.

42. **What is the indicator of satisfactory freezing during cryotherapy in RB?**
    The vitreous overlying the tumor must be frozen.

43. **What is the aim of modern treatment?**
    To save life as well as salvage vision

44. **What are the absolute indications for enucleation?**
    i. Tumor >50% of the globe
    ii. Orbital or optic nerve involvement
    iii. Anterior segment involvement with or without NVG

45. **What are the types of radiation therapy?**
    i. External beam therapy
    ii. Intensity-modulated radiation therapy
    iii. Brachytherapy

46. **What are the limitations of external beam radiotherapy?**
    i. Increased risk of second independent primary malignancy, e.g., osteosarcoma
    ii. Radiation-related sequelae such as midface hypoplasia, cataract, optic neuropathy, and vasculopathy

47. **What are the factors that influence the prognosis of RB?**
    i. Tumor size
    ii. Amount of vitreous/anterior chamber seeding
    iii. Presence/absence of choroidal invasion
    iv. Degree of tumor invasion of the optic nerve or subarachnoid space

48. **Name the cryotherapy technique followed in the treatment of RB.**
    Triple freeze-thaw technique

49. **What is the new gene therapy used in the treatment of RB?**
    Targeted therapy uses adenoviral-mediated transfection of tumor cells with thymidine kinase and renders tumor cells susceptible to systemically administered ganciclovir.

50. **What is trilateral RB?**
    Trilateral RB is bilateral RB with pinealoblastoma.

51. **What is the importance of genetic counseling in the management of RB?**
    In patients with a positive family history, 40% of the siblings would be at risk of developing RB and 40% of the offspring of the affected patient may develop RB.

    In patients with no family history of RB, if the affected child has unilateral RB, 1% of the siblings are at risk and 8% of the offspring may develop RB.

    In cases of bilateral RB with no positive family history, 6% of the siblings and 40% of the offspring have a chance of developing RB.

6.13 AGE-RELATED MACULAR DEGENERATION

1. **Define age-related macular degeneration (ARMD).**
   i. ARMD is a spectrum of disease
   ii. Associated with visual loss, retinal pigment epithelium (RPE) changes, drusen, geographical atrophy of the retina, and subretinal neovascular membrane (SRNVM)
   iii. It usually occurs in person aged above 50 years
   iv. Drusen alone without visual loss is not considered as ARMD

2. **Define early ARMD (according to the International Epidemiological Age-related Maculopathy Study Group).**
   Degenerative disorder in persons >50 years characterized by presence of any of the following:
   i. Soft drusen >63 µm
   ii. Area of hyperpigmentation and/or hypopigmentation associated with drusen but excluding pigment surrounding small, hard drusen
   iii. Visual acuity (VA) is not a criterion for diagnosis

3. **What are the risk factors for ARMD?**
   i. Age—incidence, prevalence, and progression all increase with age
   ii. Gender—female > male: 2:1 (Blue Mountains Eye Study)
   iii. Race—more in Whites
   iv. Ocular risk factor—hyperopia
   v. Family history—four times higher risk
   vi. Oxidative stress—accumulation of prooxidant melanin oligomers in RPE is responsible
   vii. Systemic hypertension
   viii. Smoking—increases the risk
   ix. Light exposure—photooxidative damage mediated by reactive O_2 intermediates. Dietary and medication factor—very high doses of zinc, vitamin C, vitamin E, and β-carotene provide a modest protective effect on progression to advanced neovascular ARMD
   x. Genetic factors—1q 25-31 and 10q26 increases risk
   xi. Cataract surgery

4. **What are the clinical features of ARMD?**
   i. Blurred vision—dry ARMD: Asymptomatic or gradual loss of central vision; wet ARMD: Rapid onset of vision loss
   ii. Difficulty in night vision
   iii. Decreased contrast sensitivity
   iv. Decrease saturation of colors
   v. Distorted vision (metamorphopsia)
   vi. Central scotomas
   vii. Slow recovery of visual function after exposure to bright light

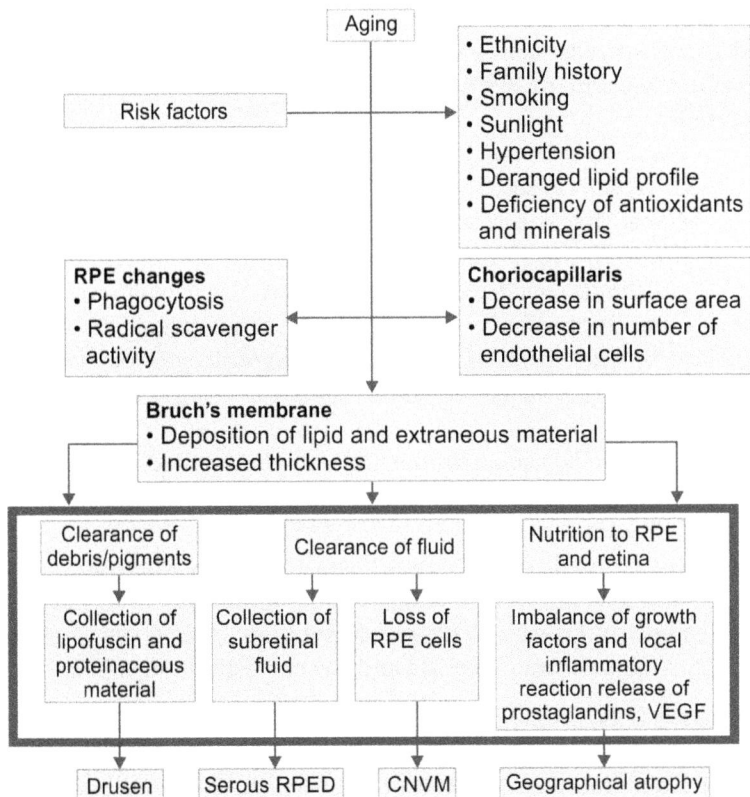

(CNVM: choroidal neovascular membrane; RPE: retinal pigment epithelium; RPED: retinal pigment epithelial detachment; VEGF: vascular endothelial growth factor)

5. **What is the classification of ARMD?**

    AREDS (Age-Related Eye Disease Study) classification:
    i. No ARMD—category 1—control group—no or few small drusen <63 μm
    ii. Early ARMD—category 2—combination of multiple small drusen, few intermediate drusen (63–124 μm), or RPE abnormalities
    iii. Intermediate ARMD—category 3—extensive intermediate drusen, at least one large drusen (125 μm) or geographic atrophy not involving the center of the fovea
    iv. Advanced ARMD—category 4—characterized by one or more of the following in one eye:
        - Geographic atrophy of the RPE and choriocapillaris involving the center of fovea
        - Choroidal neovascularization (CNV)
        - Serous and/or hemorrhagic detachment of sensory retina or RPE
        - Retinal hard exudates
        - Subretinal and sub-RPE fibrovascular proliferation
        - Diskiform scar

6. **What are drusen?**
   Drusen are aggregation of hyaline material located between Bruch's membrane and the RPE.
   Types:
   i. *Small, hard drusen:* Referred simply as drusen <63 μm
   ii. *Large, soft drusen:* >63 μm, ill-defined borders and vary in size and shape. They have a tendency toward confluence
   Three types (on basis of pathogenesis):
   - *Granular soft drusen:* About 250 μm (2× vein width) with a yellow solid appearance, their confluence results in sinuous shapes
   - *Soft serous drusen and drusenoid pigment epithelial detachments (PEDs):* >500 μm, may have pooled serous fluid, appearing blister like
   - *Soft membranous drusen:* Clinically between 63 and 175 μm (0.5-1.5 vein width), appear paler and shallower than the granular drusen
   iii. *Regressing drusen:* Drusen begin to regress when the overlying RPE fails. They become whiter and harder due to inspissation of contents. Hypo- and hyperpigmentation develop over the surface, margins become irregular, and foci of calcification appear

7. **Classify CNV/SRNVM.**
   Histologically, CNV is growth of abnormal, fragile new vessels between Bruch's membrane and RPE or between the RPE and neurosensory retina. These vessels sprout from the choriocapillaris and proceed inward through the defects in Bruch's membrane.
   i. *Topographic classification:*
      - Extrafoveal (>200 μm from foveal center)
      - Juxtafoveal (1–199 μm from foveal center)
      - Subfoveal—under the fovea
   ii. *Angiographic classification:*
      - *Classic CNV*—reveals fairly discrete hyperfluorescence in the early phase of angiogram that progressively intensifies throughout the transit phase, with intense late leakage of dye into the overlying neurosensory retinal detachment
      - *Occult CNV* has two forms:
        - FVPED (Fibrovascular PED)—appears 1–2 minutes after dye injection. It appears as an irregular elevation of RPE with stippled leakage into overlying neurosensory detachment in early and late phases
        - Late leakage of undetermined source: Regions of stippled or ill-defined leakage into overlying neurosensory detachment without a distinct source focus that can be identified in the early frames of angiogram

8. **What is pigment epithelium detachment (PED) and how to identify it in fluorescein angiography?**

   PED appears as sharply demarcated, dome-shaped elevations of RPE. If filled with serous fluid, they transilluminate. Four types of PED (on basis of angiographic pattern) are as follows:
   i. *FVPED*—appears 1-2 minutes after dye injection. It appears as an irregular elevation of RPE with stippled leakage into overlying neurosensory detachment in early and late phases
   ii. *Serous PED*—uniform bright smooth and sharp hyperfluorescence with rapid homogenous filling that starts in the early phase without leakage in the late phase of angiogram. It may or may not overlie CNVM
   iii. *Drusenoid PED*—reveals hyperfluorescence in midphase which increases in the late phase with faint hyperfluorescence of drusen and late staining. It does not have CNVM
   iv. *Hemorrhagic PED*—dark sub-RPE blood, which blocks choroidal fluorescence on angiography

9. **What is RPE rip/tear?**

   RPE rip/tear occurs as a complication in serous or FVPED at the border of attached and detached RPE due to stretching forces of the underlying fluid or from the contractile forces of the fibrovascular tissue. Clinically, it is seen as an area of hypopigmentation with a hyperpigmented wavy border on one side due to rolling in of the free edge of torn RPE.

10. **What is diskiform scar?**

    Diskiform scar is the last stage in the evolution of neovascular ARMD, just as geographic atrophy as in dry ARMD. Clinically apparent white to yellow subretinal scar with intervening areas of hyperpigmentation composed of fibrovascular complex is called diskiform scar.

11. **How do you differentiate dry ARMD and wet ARMD?**

Dry or nonexudative ARMD	Wet or exudative ARMD
More common	Less common
Atrophic and hypertrophic changes in the RPE underlying the central retina (macula) as well as deposits (drusen) on the RPE	Abnormal blood vessels called CNVMs develop under the retina
May progress to the exudative form of ARMD	Leak fluid and blood, and ultimately cause a blinding diskiform scar in and under the retina
Visual loss can occur particularly when geographic atrophy of the RPE develops in the fovea and causes a central scotoma	Causes severe visual loss as a result of leaky CNVMs
(ARMD: age-related macular degeneration; CNVMs: choroidal neovascular membranes; RPE: retinal pigment epithelium)	

12. **What are the investigations for ARMD?**
    i. Fundus fluorescein angiography (FFA)
    ii. Indocyanine green (ICG) angiography
    iii. Optical coherence tomography (OCT)
    iv. Multifocal electroretinography (MERG)
    i. *FFA*
        - *Classic CNV*—reveals fairly discrete hyperfluorescence in the early phase of angiogram that progressively intensifies throughout the transit phase, with intense late leakage of dye into the overlying neurosensory retinal detachment
        - *Occult CNV* has two forms:
            - FVPED—appears 1-2 minutes after dye injection. It appears as an irregular elevation of RPE with stippled leakage into overlying neurosensory detachment in early and late phases
            - Late leakage of undetermined source—regions of stippled or ill-defined leakage into overlying neurosensory detachment without a distinct source focus that can be identified in the early frames of angiogram
    ii. *ICG angiography*—can facilitate visualization of choroidal vasculature and CNVM through hemorrhage. ICG angiography can show CNVM as localized hot spots or as diffuse hyperfluorescent plaques
    iii. *OCT*—high reflective thickened Bruch's/RPE complex that is characteristic of CNV in ARMD. For monitoring the therapeutic response to photodynamic therapy (PDT) and anti-VEGF therapy

13. **What are the differential diagnoses for CNVM?**
    i. Idiopathic polypoidal choroidal vasculopathy (IPCV)
    ii. Myopia
    iii. Angioid streaks
    iv. Presumed ocular histoplasmosis syndrome

14. **What are the treatment options available for ARMD?**
    i. *Early ARMD*—no proven treatment
    ii. *Intermediate ARMD*—the combination treatment of antioxidants, vitamins and minerals causes significant reduction in both the development of advanced ARMD and vision loss

    AREDS 1 supplement:
    - 500 mg of vitamin C
    - 400 international units of vitamin E
    - 15 mg of beta-carotene (equivalent of 25,000 international units of vitamin A)
    - 80 mg of zinc as zinc oxide
    - 2 mg of copper as cupric oxide

AREDS 2 supplement:
- 500 mg of vitamin C
- 400 international units of vitamin E
- 80 mg of zinc as zinc oxide
- 2 mg of copper as cupric oxide
- 10 mg lutein and 2 mg zeaxanthin
- No beta-carotene

Subjects who took AREDS containing lutein/zeaxanthin and no beta-carotene had a slight reduction in the risk of advanced ARMD, compared to those who took AREDS with beta-carotene and no lutein/zeaxanthin. Beta-carotene was excluded in the AREDS 2 supplement as it had a higher risk of bronchogenic carcinoma in smokers/former smokers.

iii. *Neovascular ARMD:*
- VEGF inhibitors have become the first-line therapy for treating neovascular ARMD
- *Pegaptanib (Macugen)*—first drug approved by United States Food and Drug Administration (USFDA) for the treatment of wet ARMD; it is an aptamer, a selective antagonist for a specific VEGF A isoform (VEGF-165); had only limited efficacy; dose: 0.3 mg/90 µL injected every 6 weeks intravitreally
- *Ranibizumab (Lucentis)*—recombinant humanized monoclonal antibody fragment; inhibits all isoforms of VEGF A; dose: 0.5 mg in 0.05 mL every month intravitreally or as needed
- *Bevacizumab (Avastin)*—recombinant humanized monoclonal whole antibody; inhibits all isoforms of VEGF A; used as an off-label drug in the treatment of wet ARMD; dose: 1.25 mg in 0.05 mL monthly or as needed
- *Aflibercept (Eylea)*—recombinant fusion protein; consists of two human VEGF receptors fused with the Fc region of human immunoglobulin; inhibits VEGF A, VEGF B, and PIGF; dose: 2 mg in 0.05 mL injected every 4–8 weeks

Treatment according to the location of CNVM:
  i. *Subfoveal CNV*—anti-VEGFs are the primary therapy; verteporfin PDT only in subjects not responding to anti-VEGFs
  ii. *Juxtafoveal CNV*—anti-VEGFs are the primary therapy; verteporfin PDT only in subjects not responding to anti-VEGFs
  iii. *Extrafoveal CNV*—anti-VEGFs, verteporfin PDT/TTT/thermal laser treatment

PDT:
Mechanism of action: Initially, a drug (verteporfin) is administered. The drug gets concentrated in the immature endothelium of CNVM,

and light activation induces a photochemical reaction in the target area that causes immunologic and cellular damage, including endothelial damage of new vessels causing subsequent thrombosis and occlusion of the vasculature.

Procedure:
  i. Intravenous infusion of verteporfin (a benzoporphyrin derivative monoacid)—light-activated drug
  ii. After 15 minutes, the laser light (689 nm) is applied for 90 seconds

Avoid direct sunlight for about 2–5 days after treatment.

Follow-up every 3 monthly

Contraindicated in porphyria

Transpupillary thermotherapy (TTT):
- Modified infrared diode laser (810 nm) attached to the slit lamp is used
- It is used in treatment of extrafoveal CNVM

15. **What is the composition and mechanism of action of the major anti-VEGF agent?**
     i. Ranibizumab (Lucentis) is a 48 kDa recombinant humanized immunoglobulin G1 kappa isotype antibody fragment that binds all isoforms of VEGF-A
     ii. Bevacizumab (Avastin) is a 149 kDa full length humanized monoclonal immunoglobulin G1 antibody that binds all isoforms of VEGF-A
     iii. Aflibercept (Eylea), previously known as VEGF trap-eye, is a 115 kDa recombinant fusion protein consisting of VEGF extracellular binding domains of the human VEGF receptors 1 and 2 fused to the Fc domain of human immunoglobulin G1
     iv. Pegaptanib sodium (Macugen) is an RNA oligonucleotide ligand that binds to the 165 isoform of VEGF

16. **What are the newer modalities of treatments for ARMD?**
     i. *Ziv-Aflibercept (Zaltrap)*—VEGF trap, recombinant soluble VEGF receptor protein
     ii. *Brolucizumab (Beovu)*—humanized single-chain antibody fragment
     iii. *Faricimab*—simultaneously binds to and neutralizes Angiopoietin-2 (Ang2) and VEGF-A
     iv. *Conbercept*—recombinant fusion protein
     v. *Small interfering RNA (siRNA):*
        Bevasiranib—it silences the gene that promotes the overgrowth of blood vessels that lead to vision loss by shutting down the production of VEGF.

Sirna-027 therapy—modified siRNA that specifically targets VEGF receptor 1, a component of the angiogenic pathway found on endothelial cells.

17. **What surgical treatment options are available for ARMD?**
    i. *Macular translocation*—the aim of the surgery is to relocate the central neurosensory retina (fovea) away from the CNV, to an area of healthier RPE, Bruch's membrane, and choroid
    ii. *Iris/RPE transplantation*—fetal or mature RPE transplanted
    iii. *Surgical removal*—failed to show a beneficial effect on vision in elderly patients with ARMD
    iv. *Retinal rotation*—extrafoveal RPE can maintain foveal function. Surgery has not been widely adopted
    v. *Transplantation*—transplantation of the autologous RPE. It is performed in two different ways—the transplantation of a freshly harvested RPE suspension immediately after membrane removal and transplantation of a full-thickness RPE-choroidal patch excised from the midperiphery of the retina and translocated subfoveally

18. **What are the rehabilitation measures for ARMD patients?**
    i. Provision of low-vision aids
    ii. Visual handicap registration
    iii. Training and coping strategies
    iv. Statutory and voluntary support services in the community

19. **Name the studies for ARMD.**
    i. *MARINA* (Minimally Classic/Occult Trial of the Anti-VEGF Antibody Ranibizumab in the treatment of Neovascular ARMD)
    ii. *ANCHOR* (Anti-VEGF Antibody for the treatment of Predominantly Classic CNV in AMD)
    iii. *VISION* (VEGF Inhibition Study in Ocular Neovascularization)
    iv. *VIP* (Verteporfin in PDT)
    v. *TAP* (Treatment of Age-Related Macular Degeneration with Photodynamic therapy)
    vi. *PIER* (A Phase IIIb, Multicenter, Randomized, Double-Masked Degeneration with photodynamic therapy)

20. **What is MARINA trial?**
    i. It is done for minimally classic and occult with no classic lesion
    ii. It is divided into three groups: (i) Sham injection, (ii) Ranibizumab 0.3 mg every 4 weeks for 24 months, and (iii) Ranibizumab 0.5 mg every 4 weeks for 24 months
    iii. After 2 years, mean VA was better in the ranibizumab group versus placebo

21. **What is ANCHOR trial?**
    i. This study was done for predominantly classic CNVM
    ii. Ranibizumab is superior to verteporfin in this condition
    iii. It is divided into three groups:
        - Verteporfin PDT + sham injection
        - Sham injection + Lucentis 0.3 mg every 4 weeks for 24 months
        - Sham + Verteporfin PDT + Lucentis 0.5 mg every 4 weeks for 24 months
    iv. Result—visual gain of 15 letters or more in:
        6% in group (I)
        36% in group (II)
        40% in group (III)

22. **What CATT trial?**
    i. It is a multicenter, prospective, noninferiority clinical trial that evaluated the safety and efficacy of ranibizumab and bevacizumab in the treatment of exudative ARMD
    ii. No statistical difference in VA between ranibizumab and bevacizumab therapy was found after 2 years
    iii. There was a trend toward a higher risk of venous thrombotic events among patients using bevacizumab. The percentage of patients with one or more serious systemic adverse events was higher in the bevacizumab group (39.9%) than in the ranibizumab group (31.7%).

6.14 VITRECTOMY

1. **What are the characteristic features of vitreous?**
   i. *Volume:* 4 mL
   ii. *Weight:* 4 g (two-thirds of eyeball)
   iii. *Viscosity:* Twice that of water
   iv. *Refractive index:* 1.3349 (same as aqueous)

2. **What are all the instruments used in vitrectomy?**
   i. Cutter
   ii. Intraocular illumination source
   iii. Infusion cannula
   iv. Accessory instruments such as scissors, forceps, flute needle, endodiathermy, and endolaser delivery system

3. **What is the number of oscillations in the guillotine blade?**
   i. Usually 1,500 times/min
   ii. Latest—over 2,500 times/min

4. **What is the normal length of the infusion cannula? In which circumstances is a longer cannula used?**
   The normal length is 4 mm. In special conditions such as choroidal detachment or eyes with opaque media, a 6 mm cannula is used.

5. **What are all the expanding agents? Why are they used?**
   i. Air
   ii. Sulfur hexafluoride which lasts for 10–14 days
   iii. Perfluoroethane which lasts for 30–35 days
   iv. Perfluoropropane which lasts for 55–65 days
   v. Expanding agents are used to achieve prolonged intraocular tamponade

6. **What are the indications for vitrectomy?**
   i. *Anterior segment indications*
      - Glaucoma—ghost cell glaucoma due to vitreous hemorrhage
      - Cataract
         a. Lensectomy in eyes which need vitrectomy
         b. Dislocated lens fragments
      - Pupillary membranes
   ii. *Posterior segment indications*
      - *Indications for vitrectomy in diabetic retinopathy*
         - *Vitreous hemorrhage, especially if*
            - Long-standing
            - Bilateral
            - Disabling because of frequent recurrences
            - Retinal neovascularization is inactive

- *Traction retinal detachment, especially if*
  - The macula is detached
  - It is of recent onset
- *Combined traction/rhegmatogenous detachment*
- *Macular heterotopia of recent onset*
- *Macular epiretinal membranes (ERMs)*
- *Florid retinal neovascularization—(controversial)*

iii. *Other posterior segment indications:*
- Retinal detachment with proliferative vitreoretinopathy
- Giant tears
- Opaque media
- Trauma
- Macular pucker
- Endophthalmitis
- Uveitis
- Acute retinal necrosis
- Massive suprachoroidal hemorrhage
- Macular hole
- Retinopathy of prematurity
- Sickle cell retinopathy
- Dislocated intraocular lenses
- Choroidal neovascular membrane
- Diagnostic vitrectomy and retinal biopsy

7. **What are the relevant anatomical factors with regard to vitrectomy?**
   i. Pars plicata of the ciliary body extends to a level of 2.5 mm beyond the limbus
   ii. Pars plana of the ciliary body extends about 3.5 mm behind from the level of pars plicata on the nasal side and 5 mm on the temporal side
   iii. Approximate distance from limbus to ora serrata is 5 mm on the nasal side and 7 mm on the temporal side
   iv. Medial rectus inserts 5.5 mm behind the limbus (nearest to the limbus) and superior rectus inserts 7 mm behind the limbus (farthest to the limbus)
   v. Distance from the limbus to the equator is 9–12 mm
   vi. Average thickness of sclera is 1 mm near the limbus, 0.7 mm over pars plana, 0.3 mm under the extraocular muscle insertion, 0.6 mm at the equator, and 1.2 mm near the optic disk

8. **What are the types of vitrectomy?**
   i. Open sky
   ii. Closed
      - Single port
      - Two port
      - Three port
      - Four port

9. **What are the advantages of pars plana vitrectomy over open sky vitrectomy?**
    i. Closed and controlled system of vitreous removal, avoiding collapse of the eye
    ii. Surgical quality improved by continuous infusion (using cannulas of 23 or 25 or 27 gauge), cutting (ocutome with 23 or 25 or 27 gauge), and aspiration
    iii. Enhanced visibility provided with an operating microscope with coaxial illumination with X and Y zoom movement
    iv. Visibility can be enhanced by wide-angle visualization systems such as Volk and BIOM
    v. Illumination enhanced by fiber-optic lighting system, which provides endoillumination
    vi. Endophotocoagulation possible using a diode laser
    vii. Use of miniature vitreoretinal scissors, internal tamponade using silicone oil, sulfur tetrafluoride (SF4), etc., is possible

10. **What is the technique of three-port pars plana vitrectomy?**
    i. A hand support is essential for intravitreal surgery. The surgeon rests both hands throughout the operation, avoiding fatigue and achieving fine control of the intravitreal manipulations
    ii. Under aseptic precautions, plastic drape is pushed down into the space between the patient's head and the hand support, forming a trough to collect fluid that would otherwise spill onto the floor
    iii. Small radial incisions through the conjunctiva and Tenon's capsule are made superonasally, superotemporally, and inferotemporally
    iv. The sclerotomy incisions in the standard three-port vitrectomy technique are typically placed at the 10 and 2 o'clock positions at the same distance from the limbus as the infusion cannula
    v. The entry incisions of size only to allow passage of instrument are parallel to the corneoscleral limbus and are 4 mm from it in phakic eyes and 3.5 mm in aphakic and pseudophakic eyes
    The first incision is for the infusion cannula, which is placed in the inferotemporal quadrant, just inferior to the lateral rectus.
    A mattress suture, which will secure the 4-mm diameter cannula infusion line, is preplaced prior to entering the eye.
    vi. After the infusion cannula is secured by its mattress suture, incisions are made in the superonasal and superotemporal quadrants for the vitrectomy instrument and the fiber-optics light pipe. Incisions made anterior to 2.5 mm from the limbus are likely to injure the pars plicata, resulting in intraocular bleeding. Incisions done farther than 5 mm from limbus are likely to injure the retina

Before entering the eye, the surgeon must be certain that the instrument is functioning properly

vii. If the pupil will not dilate, the iris must be retracted using pupillary stretching techniques or iris pins

viii. *Vitrectomy*

The safest removal of vitreous is achieved using low suction (100–150 mm Hg) and a high cutting rate (400 cpm). This permits removal of small quantities of vitreous with each "bite" and reduces the risk of pulling on the vitreous base and of suddenly aspirating and cutting a detached retina.

After the vitreous has been removed and blood on the retinal surface has been aspirated, supplementary panretinal photocoagulation is given with the endolaser or with the laser indirect ophthalmoscope to diabetics who require it.

ix. Once the media have been cleared and the intraocular portion of the surgery has been completed, the cornea is covered to prevent foveal burns by the operating microscope. The scleral incisions are closed with 8-0 nylon sutures and the conjunctival incisions with 6-0 plain catgut.

The surgeon must carefully examine the peripheral retina for iatrogenic breaks.

11. **Mention the intraoperative complications of vitrectomy.**
    i. Cornea
       - Avoid corneal trauma, especially in diabetic patients as they are vulnerable to recurrent erosion.
       - Do not perform corneal contact procedures such as tonometry, electroretinogram (ERG), and contact lens examinations.
       - Moisten cornea repeatedly throughout the procedure.
       - Endothelial damage during instrumentation and infusion; intraocular irrigating solutions are toxic to the corneal endothelium.
    ii. *Cataract:* Surgeon may inadvertently cause a break in the lens capsule with an instrument.
    iii. Choroidal hemorrhage
    iv. Choroidal detachment
    v. *Retina:*
       - Iatrogenic tears, the worst operative complication of vitrectomy, have been reported to occur in approximately 20–25% of cases
       - One-third of all iatrogenic breaks are in the region of the sclerostomies, which must be carefully inspected by indirect ophthalmoscopy and scleral depression at the end of the procedure

- If there is no vitreoretinal traction, cryotherapy of a peripheral tear with an intraocular gas tamponade will seal the tear

12. **What are all the postoperative complications?**
    i. *Cornea:*
       - Persistent stromal edema is twice as common in diabetics as in nondiabetics
       - Formerly, as many as 15% of diabetic patients had significant postoperative corneal decompensation, and as many as 3% required a corneal transplant. More recent studies show a marked decrease in corneal complications
    ii. *Glaucoma:*
       - Neovascular glaucoma—11-26% of diabetic eyes go on to neovascular glaucoma
       - Erythroclastic glaucoma
       - Chronic open-angle glaucoma: The incidence of chronic open-angle glaucoma after vitrectomy has been reported to be as high as 22% with most of the cases developing 5 or more years postoperatively
    iii. Hypotony
    iv. *Cataract:* Inadvertent touch by the vitrectomy instruments, toxicity of the intraocular irrigating solutions, and prolonged contact between the lens and long-lasting intraocular gases may all cause cataract
    v. Vitreous hemorrhage
    vi. Anterior hyaloid fibrovascular proliferation
    vii. *Retinal detachment:* Rhegmatogenous retinal detachment has been reported to occur in approximately 5-15% of cases
    viii. Endophthalmitis
    ix. Sympathetic ophthalmia
    x. In association with vitrectomy, therefore, the placement or alteration of buckling material or manipulation of the extraocular muscles may produce:
       - Strabismus
       - Anterior segment necrosis
       - Postoperative infection
    xi. Extrusion of scleral buckling materials

13. **What are the factors contributing to neovascular glaucoma?**
    i. *Preoperative factors:*
       - Neovascularization of the iris
       - Florid retinal neovascularization
       - Panretinal photocoagulation
       - Aphakia

ii. *Operative factors:*
      - Removal of the lens
      - Failure to reattach the retina (50% cases)
14. **What are the contraindications of vitrectomy?**
    i. If the eye has no light perception
    ii. In the presence of suspected or active retinoblastoma
    iii. Active choroidal melanoma
15. **What are the causes of ERM?**
    i. *Idiopathic*
    ii. *Secondary:*
       - Retinal vascular diseases
       - Vascular occlusion, e.g., branch retinal vein occlusion (BRVO), central retinal vein occlusion (CRVO) (12.5%)
       - Diabetic retinopathy
       - Telangiectasias
       - Macroaneurysm
       - Sickle cell retinopathy
       - Intraocular inflammation, tumors
       - *Trauma:* Retinal detachment and tears
       - Retinal angiomas
       - Hamartomas
       - Retinitis pigmentosa
    iii. *Iatrogenic:*
       - Retinal detachment surgery
       - Silicone oil
       - Retinopexy
       - Laser/cryotherapy
16. **What are the steps of macular hole surgery?**
    Surgery involves a pars plana vitrectomy procedure with tamponade. This can be done with or without peeling of the internal limiting membrane (ILM). In general, there is acceptance of improved success seen with peeling of the ILM.

    Surgical procedure:
    Standard three-port pars plana vitrectomy is performed. The posterior vitreous is detached and the vitreous base is debulked. The best place to initiate the separation is near the disk.
    i. *ILM peeling:*
       - ILM denuded area of the retina becomes slightly whitish and hence may aid in the identification of area with intact ILM, but staining the ILM definitely makes the removal easier by improving the visualization

- Agents used are triamcinolone acetonide, indocyanine green, trypan blue, and brilliant blue
- Use of VINCE (vitreoretinal internal limiting membrane color enhancer) enables selective painting of ILM that needs to be removed without unnecessarily staining perifoveal and peripheral retina
- Usually, the membrane is removed as a circular disk around the macular hole for at least two disk diameters in size

ii. *Internal tamponade:*
- A nonexpansile mixture of C3F8 and air of 12-14% is usually used, and the patients are encouraged to lie for 14-16 hours a day for the first 10 days
- Silicone oil tamponade has been used in lieu of gas in cases where the patient is unable to assume the prone position for prolonged periods.

6.15 CENTRAL SEROUS CHORIORETINOPATHY

1. **What is central serous chorioretinopathy (CSCR)?**
   CSCR is a disorder characterized by serous retinal detachment involving the macula and often associated with pigment epithelial detachment (PED). The primary pathology is due to choroidal vascular disturbance, leading to choroidal hyperpermeability, leakage from choriocapillaris, leading to retinal pigment epithelium (RPE) dysfunction and serous macular detachment.

2. **What are the risk factors of CSCR?**
   Numerous risk factors for CSCR have been reported, but the most consistent is the use of glucocorticoids for various systemic disorders. Others are:
   i. Type A personality
   ii. Emotional stress
   iii. Psychiatric disorders
   iv. Sleep disorders and sleep apnea
   v. Cushing's syndrome
   vi. Pregnancy
   vii. Gastroesophageal reflux disease (GERD)
   viii. Hypertension
   ix. Systemic lupus erythematosus
   x. Smoking

3. **At what age is CSCR common?**
   i. Common among young or middle-aged men, 30–50 years of age
   ii. Men typically outnumber women with a ratio of at least 6:1
   iii. In patients older than 50 years, the ratio is changed to 2:1

4. **Classify CSCR.**
   i. *Acute CSCR:* Duration of disease/symptoms <3 months
   ii. *Chronic CSCR:* Duration of disease/symptoms >3 months, previously known as diffuse retinal pigment epitheliopathy (DRPE)
   iii. Recurrent CSCR
   iv. Atypical CSCR—multifocal CSCR, bullous variant of CSCR

5. **Enumerate the typical clinical features of CSCR.**
   Symptoms:
   - Unilateral diminution of vision
   - Micropsia
   - Metamorphopsia
   - Contrast sensitivity loss
   - Color vision difficulty
   - Visual acuity in the range of 6/60–6/9

Signs:
- Serous PED
- Neurosensory detachment
- Focal or diffuse retinal pigment epithelial loss (gravitational tracts)
- Intraretinal fluid
- Cystoid macular edema (CME)
- Fibrin deposit in chronic CSCR cases

6. **What is the refractive error seen in CSCR?**

   CSCR results in hyperopic shift due to:
   i. Anterior displacement of neurosensory retina due to subretinal fluid
   ii. Mild choroidal thickening

   Other visual changes include:
   i. Micropsia due to an increase in distance between photoreceptors by subretinal fluid
   ii. Metamorphopsia due to irregular separation of photoreceptors by subretinal fluid

7. **What are the fundus fluorescein angiography (FFA) findings in CSCR?**

   In acute CSCR:
   i. *Ink blot:*
      - Is more common
      - Early phase—shows a hyperfluorescent spot
      - Late phase—spot gradually enlarges centrifugally until the area is filled with dye
   ii. *Smoke stack:*
      - Less common (10%)
      - Early phase—small hyperfluorescent spot due to leakage of dye through RPE
      - Late phase—fluorescein passes into the subretinal space and ascends vertically to the upper border of detachment, and then spreads laterally until the entire area is filled with dye

   In chronic CSCR:
   - Multiple leaks
   - Diffuse areas of leakage
   - Tear drop track can be seen.

8. **What are the typical optical coherence tomography (OCT) features of CSCR?**
   i. Neurosensory detachment
   ii. PEDs
   iii. Subretinal fibrin
   iv. CME

v. Ellipsoid zone discontinuity (in chronic cases)
vi. Foveal thinning and RPE degeneration (in chronic cases)

9. **When to treat CSCR?**
Acute CSCR usually resolves spontaneously within 3 months in the majority of patients.
Treatment is initiated only when the following guidelines are met:
   i. Unresolving CSCR of 3 months or more duration
   ii. If spontaneous recovery does not occur within a month in a patient with or without a history of recurrent CSCR in the same eye or if the other eye associated with visual loss due to previous episodes of CSCR
   iii. For patients with occupational needs for binocular vision (pilot, surgeons), immediate treatment can be initiated

10. **What are the treatment modalities of CSCR?**
   i. *Discontinuation of steroids or minimize the usage of steroids or use of steroid-sparing therapy, if the patient is on oral steroid for any systemic condition*
   ii. *Focal laser photocoagulation* (green/yellow/diode laser)
   Moderate-intensity burns are applied at the leak site (FFA) to produce mild graying of RPE. Spot size used is 100 μm and exposure time of 100 ms, with a power of 80–100 mW, to cause blanching of RPE
   iii. *Photodynamic therapy* (PDT) (half fluence or half dose)
   In conventional PDT, verteporfin is injected via elbow vein, and after 10–15 minutes of injection, a semiconductor laser at a wavelength of 689 nm, with a light energy density of 50 J/cm^2 and a power density of 600 mW/cm^2, is used to irradiate the region of interest in retina for 83 seconds. In CSCR, half dose of verteporfin or half fluence of light energy is used to avoid choroidal infarction
   iv. *Subthreshold micropulse laser*
   Duty cycle of 5% is used to produce micropulse laser. Either diode or yellow laser is used. The laser power used is 50% of the power used to produce a barely visible burn at a test spot, using a 5% duty cycle, 200 ms duration, and 100 μm spot size
   v. *Eplerenone*
   Eplerenone is an aldosterone antagonist used in the treatment of hypertension
   It has been shown to be beneficial in the treatment of CSCR as mineralocorticoid receptors have been implicated in the pathophysiology of CSCR. Eplerenone therapy is started after checking blood pressure, renal function tests, and serum electrolyte levels (sodium and potassium) at baseline. Initially, patients receive

25 mg tablet daily dose for 1 week and then 50 mg daily for 3 months. Patients are followed up monthly for potassium levels as it can cause hyperkalemia (potassium-sparing diuretic).

11. **What are the differential diagnoses of CSCR?**
    i. Multifocal choroiditis
    ii. Vogt-Koyanagi-Harada disease
    iii. Optic disk pit maculopathy
    iv. Posterior scleritis
    v. Exudative detachment (in cases of bullous CSCR)

12. **What are the complications of CSCR?**
    i. Choroidal neovascular membrane (natural history of disease or secondary to PDT)
    ii. Cystoid macular degeneration
    iii. Foveal thinning
    iv. Foveal RPE degeneration

13. **What are the recent treatment modalities for CSCR?**
    i. *Helicobacter pylori* treatment
    ii. Ketoconazole
    iii. Mifepristone
    iv. Finasteride
    v. Rifampicin
    vi. Antiadrenergics
    vii. Carbonic anhydrase inhibitors
    viii. Low-dose aspirin.

6.16 ANGIOGENESIS

1. **Name the angiogenic molecules.**
   i. VEGF (vascular endothelial growth factor)
   ii. Fibroblast growth factor
   iii. Integrins
   iv. Angiopoietin
   v. Protein kinase C
   vi. Ephrins

2. **Name antiangiogenic factors.**
   i. Pigment epithelial-derived factor
   ii. Matrix metalloproteinases
   iii. Angiostatin
   iv. Endostatin
   v. Thrombospondin
   vi. Steroids

3. **How many types of VEGF are present?**
   i. VEGF-A
   ii. VEGF-B
   iii. VEGF-C
   iv. VEGF-D
   v. VEGF-E

4. **How many isoforms of VEGF-A are present?**
   i. VEGF-206
   ii. VEGF-189
   iii. VEGF-165
   iv. VEGF-145
   v. VEGF-121

5. **Which is the main isoform of VEGF?**
   VEGF-A165 is the predominantly expressed isoform. It is critical for both developmental and pathological neovascularization.

6. **What is the role of other VEGFs?**
   i. VEGF-B, C, D play a role in tumor angiogenesis and development of the lymphatic system
   ii. VEGF-E has similar angiogenic activity to VEGF-A

7. **Where are the VEGF receptors found?**
   i. Endothelial cells
   ii. Retinal epithelial cells
   iii. Bone marrow-derived epithelial cells

8. **What are the factors upregulating VEGF?**
    i. Hypoxia
    ii. Hypoglycemia
    iii. β-estradiol
    iv. Epidermal growth factor
    v. Insulin-like growth factor
    vi. Pigment-derived growth factor
    vii. Fibroblast growth factor

9. **What is the source of VEGF?**
    i. Müller cell
    ii. Endothelial cells of vessels

10. **What are the properties of VEGF?**
    i. Stimulates angiogenesis
    ii. Increases vascular permeability
    iii. Proinflammatory action
    iv. Endothelial survival factor and fenestration factor
    v. Neuroprotective factor

11. **What are the pathological roles of VEGF?**
    i. Neovascular age-related macular degeneration (ARMD)
    ii. Diabetic retinopathy
    iii. Retinal vein occlusion
    iv. Retinopathy of prematurity
    v. Corneal neovascularization
    vi. Iris neovascularization
    vii. Systemically, it has a role in cancer, psoriasis, rheumatoid arthritis.

6.17 INTRAVITREAL INJECTIONS

1. **What is the need for intravitreal injections?**
   i. Poor ocular penetration of systemically administered drugs, especially posterior segment attributed to blood aqueous and retinal barrier
   ii. Higher efficacy of local treatment due to desired dose at the target site
   iii. Reduced systemic toxicity

2. **What are the common diseases treated by intravitreal injections?**
   i. Age-related macular degeneration (ARMD)
   ii. Clinically significant macular edema (CSME)/proliferative diabetic retinopathy (PDR)
   iii. Retinal vein occlusions
   iv. Endophthalmitis
   v. Uveitis
   vi. Cystoid macular edema (CME)
   vii. Choroidal neovascular membrane (CNVM) secondary to multiple retinal diseases

3. **What are the indications for intravitreal steroids?**
   i. Diabetic macular edema (DME)—diffuse/refractory CME
   ii. Venous occlusions with macular edema
   iii. Uveitic macular edema
   iv. Pseudophakic macular edema
   v. Adjunct to vitreoretinal surgery
   vi. Ocular hypotony
   vii. ARMD

4. **Classify vascular endothelial growth factor (VEGF) family. What are the isoforms of VEGF-A and their significance in management?**
   i. VEGF-A, -B, -C, -D, -E, and placental growth factor (PlGF)
   ii. VEGF-A isoforms 121, 145, 165, 189, and 206
   iii. 121—soluble, unbound to extracellular matrix (ECM)
   iv. 165—intermediately soluble, binds somewhat to ECM, critical for developmental and pathological retinal angiogenesis
   v. 189—sequestered to ECM
   vi. Pegaptanib—binds only to VEGF-A 165 isoform
   vii. Bevacizumab—binds to all VEGF-A isoforms
   viii. Ranibizumab (RBZ)—binds with higher affinity to VEGF-A than bevacizumab
   ix. Aflibercept—binds with maximum affinity to VEGF-A as well as VEGF-B and PlGF

5. **What is its mechanism of action?**
    i. Decrease expression of VEGF and VEGF receptor 2 (VEGFR-2)
    ii. Increase expression of decoy VEGFR-1
    iii. Decrease expression of intercellular adhesion molecule 1 (ICAM-1)
6. **What are the complications of intravitreal steroids?**
    i. Ocular hypertension (HTN)
    ii. Progression of cataract
    iii. Inflammation
        - Sterile endophthalmitis—idiosyncratic reaction to vehicle or contaminant
        - Pseudoendophthalmitis—white crystals enter the anterior chamber (AC) and appear as hypopyon. Seen in aphakic or pseudophakic patients with posterior capsular (PC) rent
        - Infectious endophthalmitis
    iv. Retinal detachment (RD)
    v. Glaucoma
    vi. Local subconjunctival hemorrhage (SCH)
7. **What are the indications for anti-VEGF?**
    i. Neovascular ARMD
    ii. Diabetic retinopathy (DR)
    iii. Retinal vein occlusion with CME
    iv. Iris neovascularization—intracameral
    v. Retinopathy of prematurity (ROP)
    vi. Corneal neovascularization—intracameral
8. **What are the indications for anti-VEGF in DR?**
    i. *Diffuse macular edema:*
        - Primary
        - Adjuvant with laser
        - Steroid responder
    ii. *PDR:*
        - Post-PRP (panretinal photocoagulation) refractory PDR
        - Vitreous hemorrhage
        - Preoperative injection—2–3 days prior to surgery to reduce the vascularity and intraoperative bleeding
        - Neovascular glaucoma (NVG)
9. **What are the contraindications of anti-VEGF?**
    i. *Systemic:*
        - Uncontrolled diabetes mellitus (DM)
        - Hypertension

ii. *Ocular:*
   - Blepharitis
   - Conjunctivitis
   - Inflammatory cause
iii. *Ischemic events:*
   - Transient ischemic attack (TIA), stroke, macular ischemia
   - Thromboembolic events
iv. *Any allergy to anti-VEGF*

Strategies in anti-VEGF therapy:
i. Inhibition of VEGF production
ii. Neutralization of free VEGF
iii. Blockage of VEGF receptors and intracellular signal transduction pathways
iv. Inhibition of endothelial cellular response to VEGF

9. **Provide some examples of anti-VEGF agents.**
   i. Bevacizumab—Avastin
   ii. RBZ—Lucentis
   iii. Pegaptanib—Macugen
   iv. VEGF trap—Eylea
   v. Squalamine lactate—Evizon
   vi. Sirna 027
   vii. SU 5416

10. **What is the half-life of various anti-VEGFs?**
    i. Lucentis—9 days
    ii. Macugen—10 days
    iii. Avastin—21 days

11. **Provide a comparison of different anti-VEGF agents.**

Intravitreal drug	Bevacizumab	Ranibizumab	Triamcinolone	Aflibercept
Intravitreal dose	1.25 mg	0.3 FDA 0.5 (commonly used)	2 mg, 4 mg	2 mg
Strength in vial	25 mg/mL	0.5 mg/0.05 mL	40 mg/mL	2 mg/0.05 mL
Amount to be injected	0.05 mL	0.05 mL	0.1 mL	0.05 mL
To be repeated after	1 month	1 month	3–4 months	2 months
No. of injections/vial	30–40	1	Up to 10	1

12. **What are the differences between Avastin and Lucentis?**

Avastin	Lucentis
• Full-length antibody	• Fragment antigen binding
• Designed for intravenous (IV) administration	• Ocular administration
• $t_{1/2}$ 20 days	• $t_{1/2}$ 9 days
• Less frequent injection	• Affinity matured—5–10 times more potent in binding to all isoforms
• Less potent in binding	• Penetrates full thickness of retina
• Less penetration	• Comparatively costlier
• More uveitis—as larger foreign protein	
• Comparatively cheaper	

13. **What are the complications of anti-VEGF?**
    i. *Ocular:*
        - Endophthalmitis
        - Intraocular pressure (IOP) rise
        - Uveitis
        - Vitreous hemorrhage
        - Retinal pigment epithelium (RPE) tear
        - Rhegmatogenous retinal detachment (RRD)
        - Cataract
        - SCH
    ii. *Systemic:*
        - Nonocular hemorrhage
        - Death
    iii. *Contraindications:*
        - Pregnancy
        - Active ocular infection/inflammation

14. **What are the guidelines for peri-injection management?**
    i. Informed written consent for intravitreal therapy
    ii. Confirmation of the patient identity, eye, and the medication to be injected
    iii. Pupillary dilation
    iv. Topical anesthetic
    v. 10% povidone iodine—skin and periocular area
    vi. 5% povidone iodine—conjunctival cul-de-sac
    vii. Sterile drape
    viii. Lid speculum—to isolate eye lashes

15. **What is the preparation process for different injections?**
    i. Drugs dispensed in a single-dose vial—RBZ and triamcinolone acetonide (TA)
        - Surface of the rubber cork is cleaned with alcohol swab
        - A drop of povidone iodine is placed for 2–3 minutes

ii. Drugs dispensed in a multidose vial—bevacizumab
      - Single-dose sterile injections dispensed by pharmacy
      - One vial distributed among many patients by the ophthalmologist (4 mL vial containing 100 mg)
16. **What are the recommended sites for injection?**
      i. Inferotemporal quadrant—preferred because of wide space, pars plana is wider here; if the patient has Bell's phenomenon, then its advantageous
         - Wide space to give an injection
         - Pars plana is wider
         - Advantages, especially in the presence of Bell's phenomena
      ii. 3.5 mm posterior to the limbus for a pseudophakic
      iii. 4 mm—phakic eye

Age	Distance of injection from limbus
1–6 months	1.5 mm
6 months–1 year	2 mm
1–2 years	2.5 mm
2–6 years	3 mm
7 years onward	• 4 mm phakic • 3.5 mm pseudophakic • 3 mm aphakic

17. **What are the recommended needle sizes?**
      i. Use a needle of 27-gauge or smaller with a length of 0.5–0.62 inches
      ii. Insert the needle at least 6 mm toward the center of the eye
      iii. Injections with crystalline TA are frequently applied with 27-gauge needles, while most liquid injections use 30-gauge needles
18. **What are the different methods used for anesthesia?**
      i. Topical anesthetic drops
      ii. Lignocaine-soaked cotton-tipped swabs
      iii. Lignocaine gel
      iv. Subconjunctival injection of anesthetic agents
19. **Discuss the procedure.**
      i. The patient is asked to look away from site of injection (superonasally)
      ii. Mark the injection site using the caliper
      iii. The needle is inserted perpendicular through sclera with the tip aimed toward the center of the globe (to avoid any contact with the posterior lens)
      iv. Remove the needle slowly and carefully
      v. A sterile cotton-tipped applicator is used to prevent reflux and to steady the eye

vi. Once the needle is withdrawn, any of the following can happen:
- Liquid vitreous coming out
- Spot of SCH
- Treatment—no special measures are required

20. **Discuss the injection procedure.**
The angle of the incision through the sclera may be directed in an oblique, tunneled fashion, as rectangular radial incisions should not be performed since it may remain open, inducing vitreous or drug reflux under the conjunctiva, as well as severe chemosis and even hypotony in vitrectomized eyes.

21. **Discuss the postinjection procedure.**
    i. Indirect ophthalmoscopy after any intravitreal injection
    ii. Normal disk perfusion as assessed by color of disk and venous pulsation
    iii. Vision should be grossly tested by show of fingers
    iv. Povidone iodine 5%—conjunctival cul-de-sac
    v. Eye patched for 4 hours
    vi. Antibiotic eyedrops for 1–2 weeks

22. **What are the various drugs and their doses?**

Therapeutic agent	Absolute indications	Relative indications	Standard dosage
Triamcinolone acetonide	Refractory CSME, refractory pseudophakic CME, central retinal vein occlusion (CRVO), branch retinal vein occlusion (BRVO)	–	2 mg in 0.05 mL/4 mg in 0.1 mL
Macugen (pegaptanib sodium)	CNVM • Wet ARMD • Non-ARMD	Refractory CSME, PDR, NVG, CRVO, BRVO	0.3 mg in 90 μL
Lucentis (RBZ)	CNVM • Wet ARMD • Non-ARMD	Refractory CSME, PDR, NVG, CRVO, BRVO	0.3 mg in 0.05 mL
Avastin (bevacizumab)	CNVM • Wet ARMD • Non-ARMD	Refractory CSME, PDR, NVG, CRVO, BRVO	1.25 mg in 0.05 mL

(ARMD: age-related macular degeneration; CME: cystoid macular edema; CNVM: choroidal neovascular membrane; CSME: clinically significant macular edema; NVG: neovascular glaucoma; PDR: proliferative diabetic retinopathy; RBZ: ranibizumab)

Drug	Indication	Dosage
Dexamethasone	Cystoids macular edema	400 µg in 0.1 mL
Vancomycin	Endophthalmitis	1 mg in 0.1 mL
Amikacin	Endophthalmitis	0.4 mg in 0.1 mL
Ceftazidime/cefazolin/cefotaxime	Endophthalmitis	2.25 mg in 0.1 mL
Amphotericin B	Endophthalmitis	5 µg in 0.1 mL
Air	Pneumatic retinopexy	0.5–0.8 cm^3
SF6 (100%)	Pneumatic retinopexy	0.5 mL
C3F8 (100%)	Pneumatic retinopexy	0.3 mL
Ganciclovir	CMV retinitis	2.5 mg in 0.05 mL
Avastin	ROP	0.675 mg in 0.03 mL

(CMV: cytomegalovirus; ROP: retinopathy of prematurity)

23. What are the studies in DR related to intravitreal injections?

Title	Purpose	Conclusion
RESOLVE (2005)	Safety and efficacy of RBZ in DME involving foveal center	RBZ is effective in improving best-corrected visual acuity (BCVA) and is well tolerated in DME
RIDE AND RISE (2007)	Efficacy and safety of intravitreal RBZ in DME	RBZ rapidly and sustainably improved vision, reduced the risk of further vision loss, and improved macular edema in patients with DME with low rates of ocular and nonocular harm
BOLT (2007)	Bevacizumab versus macular laser therapy (MLT) in CSME	The study supports the use of bevacizumab in patients with center involving CSME without advanced macular ischemia
DA VINCI (2008)	VEGF Trap-Eye versus LASER in DME	VEGF Trap-Eye produced a statistically significant and clinically relevant improvement in BCVA compared with macular LASER in DME at 24 and 52 weeks
Protocol I (2010)	Intravitreal RBZ for DME with prompt versus deferred laser treatment	5-year results suggest that focal or grid laser treatment at initiation of intravitreal RBZ is no better than deferring laser treatment for >24 weeks in eye with center involving DME with visual impairment
Protocol S (2015)	Panretinal photocoagulation versus intravitreous RBZ for PDR	Among eyes with PDR, treatment with RBZ resulted in visual acuity (VA) that was not inferior to PRP at 2 years. Although longer-term follow-up is needed, RBZ may be a reasonable treatment alternative for patients with PDR

Contd...

Contd...

Title	Purpose	Conclusion
Protocol T (2016)	To determine relative efficacy and safety of intravitreous aflibercept, bevacizumab, RBZ in the treatment of DME	All three anti-VEGF groups showed VA improvement from baseline to 2 years with a decreased number of injections in year 2. VA outcomes were similar for eyes with better baseline VA. Among eyes with worse baseline VA, aflibercept had superior 2-year VA outcomes compared with bevacizumab, but superiority of aflibercept over RBZ, noted at 1 year, was no longer identified
Protocol V (2019)	To determine relative efficacy and safety of aflibercept versus laser versus observation for patients with DME and very good vision	A 5-letter or more decrease in VA at 2 years was not significantly different between groups initially managed with aflibercept (16%), laser photocoagulation (17%), and observation (19%). Aflibercept was added for the laser photocoagulation and observation cohorts if vision worsened. For eyes with VA that worsened from baseline, aflibercept was started in 25% (60/240) and 34% (80/326) in the laser photocoagulation and observation groups, respectively

(CSME: clinically significant macular edema; DME: diabetic macular edema; PDR: proliferative diabetic retinopathy; PRP: panretinal photocoagulation; RBZ: ranibizumab; VEGF: vascular endothelial growth factor)

CHAPTER

Neuro-ophthalmology

7.1 NORMAL PUPIL

1. **Define pupil.**
   The pupil is an opening present in the center of the iris that controls the amount of light passing to the retina.

2. **What are the muscles involved in pupillary action, and where are they derived from?**
   i. Sphincter
   ii. Dilator
   Both are derived from neuroectoderm.

3. **What is the normal shape and size of the pupil, and how does it vary with age?**
   i. The normal pupil is approximately circular and usually placed slightly eccentrically toward the nasal side (inferonasal)
   ii. Average size (2.4-4 mm)
   iii. Larger in myopes
   iv. Smaller in hypermetropes
   v. Constantly smaller in very young and very aged because of decreasing sympathetic activity
   vi. Largest in adolescence

4. **What is the size of pupil when maximally dilated and maximally constricted?**
   i. *Dilated pupil:* 10 mm
   ii. *Constricted pupil:* 1-1.5 mm

5. **At what age does the pupillary light reaction start, and what is the range at birth?**
   i. Premature baby has no pupillary light reaction until 3 weeks of gestational age
   ii. Gradually increases up to 2 mm at birth

6. **Trace the light reflex pathway.**
   i.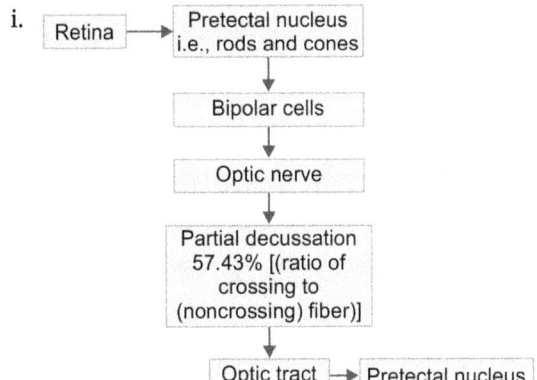
   ii. Intercalated neurons from the pretectal complex to the parasympathetic motor pool (Edinger-Westphal of oculomotor nuclear complex) Parasympathetic outflow from Edinger-Westphal nucleus

   ↓

   Ciliary ganglion

   ↓

   Pupillary sphincter

7. **How do you test the light reflex pathway?**
   i. *Direct response:*
      - The person testing should cover both eyes of the patient with the palms of his hands or with two cards
        - One eye is then uncovered. The pupil should contract briskly, and the contraction should be maintained
        - Similar response should be noted in the other eye
      - Patient should be asked to sit in a dimly lit room
        - Person testing should use a point light source or a pen torch. Patient should be asked to look into a distance approximately 6 meters (to avoid accommodation reflex)
        - Light should be brought from the temporal side, focusing onto the nasal side
   ii. *Indirect response:*
      - Criteria similar to that done in card test: It is obtained by uncovering one eye in such a way that it is not exposed to direct light while the other eye is alternately covered and exposed
      - Criteria are:
        - Dim light
        - Point light source

- Patient looking into distance
- Light should be brought from the temporal side, focusing onto the nasal side, so that it does not fall on the other eye, and the reflex is observed in the unstimulated eye

8. **Trace the near reflex pathway.**

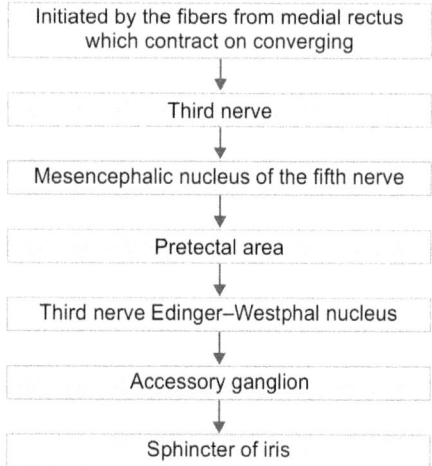

9. **How do you test pupillary reactions for accommodation?**
   Normal light:
   i. Ask the patient to look into the distance
   ii. Suddenly, ask the patient to fixate on a close object at 6 inches from the patient's nose
   Most accurately:
   i. Patient is facing a wall between two windows, and a small object is fixated for about half a minute 50 cm from his eye
   ii. This is gradually moved toward his eyes as it approaches a distance of 40 cm; slight contraction should be noted, which becomes stronger when the distance is 20–15 cm

10. **Describe other pupillary reactions.**
    i. *Hemianopic pupillary reaction of Wernicke's syndrome:* It is a crude method to estimate the function of nasal and temporal half of the retina. Point pencil of light is used
    ii. *Orbicularis (lid) reflex:* It is elicited by observing the pupillary contraction, which occurs when a forcible attempt is made to close the lids while they are held apart by fingers or speculum
    iii. *Oculosensory reflex:* It is elicited by touching the cornea or the conjunctiva lightly with cotton, and the pupil responds by dilating and then contracting. The reaction of the pupil will be sluggish when light is thrown on the nonfunctioning part of the retina

11. **How do you measure the size of the pupil?**
    Pupillometer

12. **Name some pupillometers.**
    i. *Haabs:* It is a rough method of examination of the pupil size measurement by direct comparison of the aperture of the pupil with a series of circular disks of graduated sizes
    ii. Similar method with ophthalmoscope is used in Morton's ophthalmoscope
    iii. *Projection pupillometer:* Depends on the projection of the scale on the eye of the subject:
       - Priestley Smith's keratometer and pupillometer
       - Bumke's
    iv. *Sanders:* It is a device attached to the corneal microscope of Zeiss. The light is reflected into the eye through a movable glass plate, which is graded in tint, in such a way that different parts transmit a different proportion of incident light. The degree of contraction can be accurately decided at different illumination, and the least intensity at which the pupillary reaction starts can be noted
    v. *Hemiakinesia meter:* This instrument is helpful in eliciting hemianopic pupillary response. This is possible because the illuminating system is duplicated. This provides for momentary stimulation of the peripheral retinal element, both in horizontal and oblique meridians

13. **What are the other methods of pupillometry?**
    i. Photographic
    ii. Cinematographic
    iii. Electronic

14. **What is the normal pupillary cycle time?**
    i. The normal pupillary cycle time is measured in slit lamp in dimly lit room
    ii. A stopwatch is needed; time taken from the time the light is on to the constant contraction of the pupil without any oscillation is noted. Normal 900 ms/cycle.

7.2 ABNORMAL PUPILS

1. **What are the characteristics of Marcus Gunn pupil?**
   Afferent pupillary defect
   Causes:
   i. Optic neuropathy
   ii. Extensive retinal damage
   iii. Amaurotic pupil

2. **What are the characteristics of Adie's tonic pupil?**
   i. Idiopathic
   ii. Female predilection
   iii. Dilated pupil with poor to absent light reaction
   iv. Slow constriction to prolonged near effort and slow redilatation after near effort
   v. Vermiform constriction of the iris sphincter on slit lamp examination
   vi. Demonstrates cholinergic supersensitivity to weak (0.125%) pilocarpine solution
   vii. It may be associated with diminished deep tendon reflexes

3. **What are the characteristics of Argyll Robertson pupil?**
   i. Miotic, irregular pupils
   ii. Light reflex absent
   iii. Accommodation reflex present
   iv. *Etiology:* Neurosyphilis, diabetes mellitus, chronic alcoholism, multiple sclerosis, sarcoidosis
   v. *Site of lesion:* Most likely in the region of sylvian aqueduct (dorsal midbrain)

4. **What is Parinaud syndrome?**
   Parinaud syndrome is dorsal midbrain syndrome caused due to compression of vertical gaze center at the rostral interstitial nucleus of the medial longitudinal fasciculus.
   i. Vertical gaze palsy, sunset sign
   ii. Eyelid retraction (Collier sign), pseudo-Argyll Robertson pupil

5. **What are the characteristics of Hutchinson pupil?**
   i. Hutchinson pupil is seen in comatose patient
   ii. Unilateral dilated poorly reactive pupil
   iii. *Etiology:* Due to expanding intracranial supratentorial mass that is causing downward displacement of the hippocampal gyrus and uncal herniation compressing the third cranial nerve

6. **What are the characteristics of Horner's pupil?**
    i. Miosis
    ii. Anhidrosis of the affected side of the face
    iii. Apparent enophthalmos due to narrow palpebral fissure
    iv. Ptosis of the upper lid

7. **What are the characteristics of Horner's syndrome?**
    i. Cocaine test
    ii. Paredrine test

    Causes of Horner's syndrome:
    i. First-order neuron lesion:
        - Cerebrovascular accident
        - Demyelinating disease
        - Neck trauma
        - Syringomyelia
        - Arnold–Chiari malformation
        - Neoplasm
    ii. Second-order neuron lesion (preganglionic):
        - Chest lesions—Pancoast tumor, mediastinal mass, cervical rib
        - Neck lesions—trauma, thyroid lesion
    iii. Third-order neuron lesion (postganglionic):
        - Migraine
        - Otitis media
        - Cavernous sinus lesion
        - Carotid-cavernous fistula

8. **Can midbrain lesions have relative afferent pupillary defect (RAPD)?**
   Yes. Since the efferent fibers are present up to the Edinger–Westphal nucleus. Beyond Edinger–Westphal nucleus, there will be no RAPD.
   Optic nerve lesion causes same eye RAPD, whereas optic tract lesions would produce fellow eye RAPD, since the nasal fibers have crossed over, and the nasal retina maintains eye and pupillary reactions.

9. **What are the causes of RAPD? How will you grade RAPD?**
    A. *Causes:*
        i. Optic neuritis
        ii. Anterior ischemic optic neuropathy
        iii. Compressive optic neuropathy
        iv. Optic nerve tumors
        v. Optic tract lesion
        vi. Glaucoma
        vii. Amblyopia
        viii. Central retinal vein occlusion (CRVO)
        ix. Retinal detachment (RD)
        x. Retinitis pigmentosa

B. *Grading:*
   i. Grade 1+—a weak initial papillary constriction followed by greater redilatation
   ii. Grade 2+—an initial papillary stall followed by greater redilatation
   iii. Grade 3+—an immediate papillary dilation
   iv. Grade 4+—no reaction to light or amaurotic pupil

Neutral density filters may be used to quantify the magnitude of RAPD. The 0.3 log unit filter may be used over each eye for identification of subtle RAPD.

10. **What is the reason for poor mydriasis in diabetes mellitus patients?**
Pupil in diabetics is less reactive, especially to mydriatics, due to neuropathy that affects autonomic nervous system.

7.3 OPTIC NERVE HEAD

1. **What are the dimensions of the optic nerve?**
   The optic nerve extends from the eyeball to the optic chiasma. It measures about 3.5–5.5 cm (35–55 mm) in length, with an average length of 50 mm. It comprises the following portions:
   i. *Intraocular portion:* It is the smallest portion and extends from the optic disk surface to the lamina cribrosa and is about 0.7–1 mm
   ii. *Intraorbital portion:* It is the longest portion about 33 mm long
   iii. *Intracanalicular portion:* It occupies the optic canal and is approximately 7–10 mm long
   iv. *Intracranial portion:* It extends to the cranial cavity and is about 10 mm long
   The diameter ranges from 3 mm in orbit to 7 mm near the chiasma.

2. **Define optic nerve head (ONH).**
   i. Optic nerve head is the part of the optic nerve that extends from the retinal surface to the myelinated portion of the optic nerve just behind sclera
   ii. In reference to glaucoma, the ONH is defined as the distal portion of optic nerve that is directly susceptible to elevated intraocular pressure (IOP)
   iii. The terms "disk" and "papilla" refer to the portion of the ONH that is clinically visible by ophthalmoscopy

3. **What are the dimensions of the ONH?**
   i. Optic nerve head is 1 mm long (anteroposterior)
   ii. Diameter—1.5 mm horizontally and 1.75 mm vertically
   iii. Mean area of disk—2.7 mm^2

4. **Describe the parts of ONH.**
   i. Superficial nerve fiber layer (NFL)—the prelaminar zone anterior to the level of Bruch's membrane (pars retinalis)
   ii. The prelaminar zone—level with the choroids (pars choroidalis)
   iii. The lamina cribrosa (pars sclerosis)
   iv. The retrolaminar portion—immediately behind the lamina

5. **What is physiological cup?**
   i. Central depression of the optic disk is known as the physiological cup
   ii. It is slightly pushed to the temporal side of the disk due to heaping of nasal fibers
   iii. From the center of this depression, vessels emerge, usually hugging the nasal side
   iv. Usually symmetrical in the two eyes

6. **What are the dimensions of the physiological cup?**
    i. *Median cup volume:* 0.28 mm^2
    ii. *Median cup depth:* 0.63 mm^2
    iii. *Mean cup area:* 0.72 mm^2
7. **What is neuroretinal rim (NRR)?**
    i. The tissue outside the cup is termed the NRR and contains the retinal nerve axons as they enter the ONH
    ii. Rim area ranges from 0.8 to 4.66 mm^2
    iii. It is widest inferotemporally
8. **What is the normal shape of cup?**
    i. Cup is 8% wider in the horizontal, so that NRR is wider above and below
    ii. Cup area correlates with disk area, and hence is large in large disks and small in small disks
9. **What is cup-to-disk ratio?**
    i. Ratio of the cup and disk width is measured in the same meridian. Its median value is 0.3
    ii. An asymmetry between both eyes of >0.2 has been taken to signify enlargement and to be of diagnostic importance in glaucoma
    iii. The vertical ratio is used as simple index of rim integrity in chronic glaucoma
10. **Why is the ONH considered a major zone of transition?**
    i. Nerve fibers pass from an area of high tissue pressure within the eye to a zone of low pressure that correlates with intracranial pressure
    ii. Transition from an area supplied by the central retinal artery alone to an area supplied by other branches of the ophthalmic artery
    iii. The axons become myelinated immediately at the posterior end of the ONH
11. **What is scleral ring?**
    The layers of the retina abruptly cease before the optic nerve is reached. The pigment epithelium and the underlying choroid may not extend right up to the nerve, thus leaving a white scleral ring surrounding disk.
12. **What is conus?**
    i. If the scleral ring is accentuated, it is termed conus—a crescent-shaped configuration usually seen on the temporal side
    ii. Large inferior conus is frequently associated with other abnormalities and approximately to a staphyloma
13. **What is crescent?**
    The pigment epithelium may stop short some distance from the disk, and the remaining space up to the margin of the optic nerve is covered

by the choroid. It is usually crescent shaped and situated temporally (also known as choroidal ring).

14. **What is parapapillary chorioretinal atrophy?**
    A crescent-shaped region of chorioretinal atrophy at temporal margin of normal disks and may be exaggerated in chronic glaucoma or high myopia. There are two types of zones:
    i. Zone alpha
    ii. Zone beta

15. **What are zone alpha and zone beta?**
    i. *Zone beta:*
       - Inner zone
       - It exhibits chorioretinal atrophy with visibility of sclera and large choroidal blood vessels
       - Seen more frequently in patients with primary open-angle glaucoma (POAG)
       - It contributes to absolute scotoma
    ii. *Zone alpha:*
       - More peripheral zone
       - It displays variable irregular hyper- and hypopigmentation of retinal pigment epithelium (RPE)
       - Larger in patients with POAG, but frequency is similar in glaucoma and normal subjects
       - It contributes to relative scotoma

16. **What is the site of emergence of retinal vessels?**
    The retinal vessels emerge on the medial side of the cup, slightly decentered superonasally

17. **What is the significance of venous pulsation?**
    i. Absence of spontaneous venous pulsation is an early sign of papilledema
    ii. 20% of normal population will not have spontaneous venous pulsation
    iii. Pulsations cease when intracranial pressure exceeds 200 mm of water

18. **What is the significance of retinal arterial pulsation?**
    Visible retinal arterial pulsations are rare and usually pathological, implying, for example:
    i. Aortic incompetence
    ii. High IOP

19. **What is microdisk and macrodisk?**
    i. Macrodisk, whose area lies >2 standard deviations above the mean (>4.09 mm^2):
        - *Primary macrodisk:* May be associated with optic nerve pit, morning glory syndrome
        - *Secondary macrodisk:* Seen with acquired globe enlargement such as high myopia and buphthalmos
    ii. Microdisk, whose area is <2 standard deviations below mean (<1.29 mm^2)

20. **What is the relationship between size of optic disk and certain ONH diseases?**
    Small optic disks have a smaller number of optic nerve fibers and a smaller anatomical reserve.
    i. Nonarteritic ischemic optic neuropathy (ION) is more common in small ONH due to problems of vascular perfusion and of limited space
    ii. Same is true for ONH drusen
    iii. Pseudopapilledema is also encountered with smaller ONH, particularly in highly hypermetropic eyes

21. **Are there any racial differences in the disk?**
    There is a racial difference in disk diameter. Blacks have larger disks and hence larger cups.

22. **What is the meniscus of Kuhnt?**
    Meniscus of Kuhnt refers to the central connective tissue that covers the nonmyelinated fibers of the optic disk on the vitreous side.

23. **What is the limiting tissue of Elschnig?**
    i. The limiting tissue of Elschnig is the border tissue or limiting tissue that separates the fibers of ONH from the retina and choroids
    ii. It is essentially a derivative of the connective tissue of the choroids and sclera

24. **How many nerve fibers converge to form the disk?**
    There are approximately 1.2 million retinal nerve fibers.

25. **Why is there a blind spot corresponding to the area of the ONH?**
    Because there are no rods or cones at the ONH, there is a physiological blind spot in the visual field.

26. **What is the arrangement of retinal fibers at the ONH?**
    i. Those from the peripheral part of the retina lie deep in the retina but occupy the most peripheral part of the optic disk, while fibers originating closer to the ONH lie superficially and occupy a more deeper portion of the disk

ii. The arcuate nerve fibers occupy the supero- and inferotemporal portion of the ONH and are most sensitive to glaucomatous damage, accounting for early loss in the corresponding region of the visual field

iii. The papillomacular fibers spread over approximately one-third of the distal optic nerve, primarily inferotemporally, where axonal density is higher. They intermingle with extramacular fibers, which might explain the retention of the central visual field

27. What do you mean by medullated nerve fibers at the ONH?
Normally, optic nerve fibers become medullated beyond the lamina cribrosa. Occasionally, myelin sheathing extends anterior to the lamina reaching a variable distance on the surface of the retina.

28. What is the composition of the ONH?
Four types of cells:
 i. Ganglion cell axons
 ii. Astrocytes
 iii. Capillary-associated cells
 iv. Fibroblasts

29. What type of glial element is present at the disk?
 i. The prominent glial element is astrocyte
 ii. It supports the bundles of nerve fibers
 iii. It provides cohesiveness to the neural compartments by arranging themselves to form an interface with all mesodermal structures (like vitreous, choroids, and sclera)
 iv. It also serves to moderate the conditions of neuronal functions. For example:
   - By absorbing extracellular potassium ions released by depolarizing axons
   - Storing glycogen for use during transient oligemia

30. What is the vascular supply of the ONH?
 i. Mainly posterior ciliary arterial circulations
 ii. Central retinal arterial circulations

31. Describe the vascular supply to the different parts of the ONH.
 i. Surface NFL—supplied by capillaries derived from retinal arterioles
 ii. Prelaminar region—supplied mainly from centripetal branches of peripapillary choroidal vessels
 iii. Lamina cribrosa region—supplied by centripetal branches of the short posterior ciliary arteries. Some is also delivered via the circle of Zinn–Haller, which encircles the prelaminar region and is fed via the short posterior ciliary arteries

iv. Retrolaminar region—supplied by centrifugal branches from the central retinal artery and centripetal branches from pial plexus formed by branches of the choroidal artery, circle of Zinn, central retinal artery, and ophthalmic artery

32. **What is the venous drainage of the ONH?**
    i. Primarily via the central retinal venous system
    ii. Under conditions of chronic compression or central retinal vein occlusion (CRVO), preexisting connections between superficial disk veins and choroidal veins—*optociliary veins*, enlarge and shunt blood to choroids

33. **What are the features of microvascular bed of the ONH?**
    i. It resembles the retinal and central nervous system (CNS) vessels anatomically
       - Pericytes (mural cells) engulf the capillaries
       - Nonfenestrated endothelium has tight junctions
    ii. The optic nerve vessels share with those of the retina and CNS the following physiological properties of:
       - Autoregulation
       - Presence of blood–brain barrier

34. **What is the significance of autoregulation?**
    i. Because of autoregulation, the rate of blood flow in the optic nerve is not much affected by IOP
    ii. In the optic nerve, the flow level is not affected by an increase in blood pressure (BP) because vascular tone is increased by autoregulation, thus increasing the resistance to flow

35. **What is the main control of flow in optic nerve vessels?**
    Anterior to lamina cribrosa, autoregulation controls flow.

36. **Why does fluorescein diffuse toward the center of the optic disk from its boundary during fundus fluorescein angiography (FFA)?**
    The choroid is not separated from the ONH by a cellular layer that has tight junctions. Hence, extracellular materials may diffuse into the extracellular space of the ONH.

37. **How do you examine the ONH?**
    i. *Direct ophthalmoscope:*
       - For disk examination
       - NFL through red-free filter
    ii. *Indirect ophthalmoscope:*
       - Young children
       - Uncooperative patients

- High myopes
- Substantial media opacities
  iii. Slit lamp using posterior pole lenses such as Hruby lens, 60, 78, and 90 diopter lens

38. **What is the location of ONH with respect to the foveola?**
    The center of ONH is approximately 4 mm superonasal to the foveolar.

39. **In what percentage of eyes is cilioretinal artery seen?**
    32%

40. **What is the difference between congenital and myopic crescents?**
    i. Most temporal crescents are myopic and are acquired during life due to continuous growth process
    ii. True congenital crescents are present at birth and remain unchanged throughout life

41. **What are the congenital anomalies of ONH?**
    i. *Coloboma of ONH:*
       - Results from a defective closure of fetal fistula
       - It may be confined to the ONH or may include choroids, retina, iris, and lens
       - Ophthalmoscopic appearance: The nerve is surrounded by peripapillary atrophy and shows extensive cupping and pallor
    ii. *Optic pit:* Usually located near the disk margin and often associated with serous detachment of the macula
    iii. *Situs inversus of the vessels:* The right eye's ONH vascular pattern appears like that of the left eye
    iv. *Situs inversus of the disk:* The scleral canal is directed nasally, and the vessel divisions sweep nasally for a considerable distance before assuming their usual course
    v. *Bergmeister's papilla:*
       - A large stalk-like vascularized tissue extending into the vitreous cavity from the ONH
       - It is due to the persistence of remnants of fetal vasculature extending from the ONH to the lens

42. **What are corpora amylacea?**
    i. Corpora amylacea are small hyaline masses of unknown pathologic significance, occurring more commonly with advancing age, and derived from degenerate cells
    ii. They are oval, highly refractile, either homogenous or showing concentric lamination, and enclosed in a definite capsule
    iii. They occur normally in the optic nerve as in other parts of the CNS

43. **Why in papilledema does the disk swell easily but not the adjacent retina?**

    This is because in the prelaminar region, loose glial tissue does not bind the axon bundle together as do the Muller cells of the retina.

44. **What are the ocular signs of head injury?**
    i. *Torchlight signs:* Subconjunctival hemorrhage (with no clear posterior demarcation)
    ii. *Fundus signs:*
        - Papilledema
        - Traumatic optic neuropathy (normal fundus with afferent pupillary defect)
        - Purtscher's retinopathy
    iii. *Field signs:*
        - Homonymous hemianopia
    iv. *Pupillary signs:*
        - Fixed dilated pupil due to:
            - Transtentorial herniation (Hutchinson's pupil)
            - Traumatic third nerve palsy
            - Traumatic mydriasis
            - Orbital blowout fracture
        - Small pupil:
            - Horner's syndrome
            - Pontine hemorrhage
    v. *Motor signs:*
        - Cranial nerve palsies
        - Internuclear ophthalmoplegia.

7.4 OPTIC NEURITIS

1. **Define optic neuritis.**
   Optic neuritis literally means "inflammation of the optic nerve," but it is defined as a demyelinating disorder of the optic nerve characterized by sudden monocular loss of vision, ipsilateral eye pain, and dyschromatopsia.

2. **Classification of optic nerve inflammation.**
   Ophthalmoscopically:
      i. Papillitis
      ii. Retrobulbar neuritis
      iii. Neuroretinitis
   Etiologically:
      i. Demyelinating
      ii. Parainfectious
      iii. Infectious
   Structurally:
      i. Perineuritis or peripheral optic neuritis
      ii. Inflammation of optic nerve substance

3. **What are the fibers affected in optic neuritis?**
   Based on topography, there are three types of optic neuritis:
      i. *Perineuritis or periaxial neuritis*: Affects the leptomeninges of optic nerve, spreading from the brain/orbit/sinuses. It extends along pial septa, *affecting extra macular fibers*
      ii. *Axial neuritis: Affects macular fibers*. Examples include multiple sclerosis (MS), toxic and nutritional neuropathies
      iii. *Transverse neuritis:* Both periaxial and axial neuritis progress to involve all fibers

4. **What are the causes of optic neuritis?**
      i. Etiology is numerous, and most cases are idiopathic
      ii. 90% cases are demyelinating diseases of the optic nerve
      iii. 20–40% cases develop signs and symptoms of MS in optic neuritis
         - *Infectious diseases:*
            - *Bacterial:* Bacterial endocarditis, syphilis, meningitis, chronic mastoiditis (lateral sinus thrombosis), brucellosis, endogenous septic foci
            - *Viral diseases:* Poliomyelitis, acute lymphocyte meningitis, coxsackie B virus encephalitis, recurrent polyneuritis, Guillain-Barré syndrome
            - *Parasitic diseases:* Sandfly fever, trypanosomiasis, neurocysticercosis

- *Ischemic diseases:*
  - Atherosclerosis
  - Diabetes mellitus
  - Takayasu's disease
  - Carotid vascular insufficiency
- *Inflammatory diseases:*
  - Collagen vascular diseases
  - Giant cell arteritis

5. **What are the triad of symptoms of optic neuritis?**
   i. Loss of vision
   ii. Ipsilateral eye pain
   iii. Dyschromatopsia

6. **What are the other symptoms of optic neuritis?**
   The associated visual symptoms are movement phosphenes, sound-induced phosphenes, visual obscurations in bright light, and Uhthoff's symptom.

7. **What is the cause of pain in optic neuritis?**
   According to Whitnall's hypothesis, the pain of optic nerve inflammation is caused by traction of the origins of the superior and medial recti on the optic nerve sheath at the orbital apex.

8. **Describe dyschromatopsia in optic neuritis.**
   Impaired color vision (dyschromatopsia) is always present in optic neuritis. In the absence of a macular lesion, color desaturation is a highly sensitive indicator of optic nerve disease. Color vision, a parvocellular ganglion cell function, is abnormal in patients with acute and recovered optic neuritis. The localized loss of red and green perception is the most sensitive test of interference with optic nerve function.

   Color vision defects are highly sensitive indicators of a previous attack of optic neuritis. Color vision defects can be detected clinically using Hardy-Rand-Ritter or Ishihara pseudoisochromatic plates. More sensitive testing can be achieved with the Farnsworth Munsell 100 Hue test. Typically, the patient observes a reduced vividness of saturated colors. In color terminology, saturation refers to the purity of color, and desaturation is the degree to which a color is mixed with white.

   Some patients who are shown a red target characterize the sensation as darker (i.e., red is shifted toward amber), whereas others say the color is bleached or lighter (i.e., red is shifted toward orange).

9. **Describe Uhthoff's phenomenon.**
   Uhthoff's symptom, episodic transient obscuration of vision with exertion, occurs in isolated optic neuritis and in MS.

However, exertion is not the only provoking factor for Uhthoff's symptom. Typically, the patient has blurring of vision in the affected eye after 5-20 minutes of exposure to the provoking factor. Color desaturation may also occur. After resting or moving away from heat, vision recovers to its previous level within 5-60 minutes.

In optic neuritis, Uhthoff's symptom correlates significantly with multifocal white matter lesions on brain magnetic resonance imaging (MRI) ($p < 025$).

Conversion to MS in patients followed for a mean of 3.5 years is significantly greater in patients with Uhthoff's symptom ($p < 01$).

Uhthoff's symptom also correlates with a higher incidence of recurrent optic neuritis.

Uhthoff's symptom in MS can be detected by Farnsworth Munsell 100 Hue testing and Octopus perimetry, as well as by fluctuations of visual evoked potential (VEP) amplitudes and contrast sensitivity.

10. **What are the clinical signs of optic neuritis?**
    The clinical signs of optic neuritis are those of optic nerve disease. They include:
    i. Visual acuity (distance and near)—reduced
    ii. Dyschromatopsia
    iii. Contrast sensitivity—impaired
    iv. Stereoacuity—reduced
    v. Visual field—generalized depression, particularly pronounced centrally
    vi. Afferent pupillary defect
    vii. Optic disk(s)—hyperemia and acute swelling

11. **What is the name of the chart used to test contrast sensitivity?**
    Pelli-Robson chart

12. **How is stereoacuity checked?**
    Titmus polaroid 3D vectograph stereoacuity test

13. **What is Pulfrich effect?**
    Patients notice reduced brightness and difficulty in depth perception. Because optic nerve damage results in delayed transmission of impulses to the visual cortex, patients with unilateral or markedly asymmetric optic neuritis will experience the Pulfrich effect, a stereo illusion.

14. **What are the visual field defects in optic neuritis?**
    i. Involvement of the visual field during an attack of optic neuritis, as well as following recovery, can be extremely variable
    ii. In acute optic neuritis, the cardinal field defect is a widespread depression of sensitivity, particularly pronounced centrally as a centrocecal scotoma

iii. When acuity is severely impaired, perimetric field charting is unreliable, and confrontation testing is recommended
iv. As vision improves, multiisopter kinetic Goldmann perimetry or computer-assisted automated static perimetry using a Humphrey Field Analyzer or Octopus perimeter are sensitive techniques for serial testing
v. A finding of generalized depression, paracentral scotomas, or scattered nerve fiber bundle-related defect(s) between 5 and 20° from fixation may indicate sequelae of prior demyelinating optic neuropathy

15. **What are the optic disk findings in optic neuritis?**
    i. The appearance of the optic disk may be normal
    ii. Swollen (papillitis) in 23%, blurred or hyperemic in 18%, and blurred with peripapillary hemorrhages around the disk in 2%
    iii. Temporal pallor suggests a preceding attack of optic neuritis
    iv. In recovered optic neuritis, 6 months after the first attack, a normal disk can be present in 42% of eyes; temporal pallor present in 28%; and total disk pallor evident in 18%
    v. In MS in remission, optic pallor is present in 38% of cases

16. **What are the retinal findings in optic neuritis?**
    Two retinal signs are associated with optic neuritis and MS:
    i. Retinal venous sheathing due to periphlebitis retinae
    ii. Defects in the retinal nerve fiber layer

17. **What are the investigations in optic neuritis?**
    There is usually no need for investigative studies in a healthy adult presenting with typical acute, monosymptomatic, unilateral optic neuritis and an unremarkable medical history. However, the following tests may be performed.
    i. Complete blood counts
    ii. Erythrocyte sedimentation rate (ESR)
    iii. Rule out diabetes
    iv. Rule out infectious disease etiology like:
        - Tuberculosis—chest X-ray, Mantoux (important as steroids will be used in the treatment of optic neuritis)
        - Syphilis
        - Human immunodeficiency virus (HIV) 1 and 2
        - Hepatitis B
    v. Any other suspected infectious disease serology
    vi. Rule out inflammatory disease conditions like:
        - Systemic lupus erythematosus (SLE), collagen vascular diseases—antinuclear antibody (ANA), rheumatoid arthritis

(RA), antineutrophil cytoplasmic antibody (ANCA), anti-double-stranded deoxyribonucleic acid (DNA)
- Giant cell arteritis—temporal artery biopsy

18. **What are the neuroimaging modalities in optic neuritis?**
Computed tomography (CT), MRI, VEP, and pattern electroretinogram are the neuroimaging modalities in optic neuritis.

19. **What are the MRI findings in optic neuritis?**
    i. Enhancing optic nerve on T1 contrast fat saturated:
       - Best seen on coronal images
       - On axial images, it may have "tram-track" enhancement pattern simulating optic nerve sheath meningioma
    ii. On T2 with fat saturation [or short tau inversion recovery (STIR) images]—mildly enlarged, hyperintense optic nerve
    iii. Acute and chronic MS lesions appear bright in T2 images
       - Lesions are round or ovoid in periventricular white matter, internal capsule, and corpus callosum (perpendicular to vente rides, at callososeptal interface)
       - They may also be linear with finger-like appearance (Dawson's fingers) on sagittal or coronal scaring periventricular region

20. **What are the VEP findings in optic neuritis?**
Prolongation of P100 latency is seen in optic neuritis.

21. **What are the differential diagnoses of optic neuritis?**
Unilateral optic neuritis:
    i. Ischemic optic neuropathy
    ii. Rhinogenous optic neuritis
    iii. Syphilis
    iv. HIV-associated optic neuropathies
    v. Infectious optic neuropathy
    vi. Nonorganic factitious visual loss

Simultaneous or sequential bilateral optic neuritis: When optic neuritis strikes both eyes, simultaneously or sequentially, the disorder must be distinguished from the following:
    i. Devic's disease
    ii. Immune-mediated optic neuropathy
    iii. Nutritional amblyopia
    iv. Jamaican optic neuropathy
    v. Leber's hereditary optic neuropathy
    vi. Functional blindness

22. **What is Devic's disease?**
Devic's disease (neuromyelitis optica) is an inflammatory CNS-demyelinating disease that is considered to be a variant of MS. It affects

both eyes simultaneously or sequentially in children, young adults, and the elderly and is accompanied by transverse myelitis within days or weeks.

Neuromyelitis optica has also been reported in association with SLE and pulmonary tuberculosis.

Familial cases of acute optic neuropathy and myelopathy may be linked to an inherited mutation in mitochondrial DNA (mtDNA), possibly a cytochromic oxidase subunit 2 mutation at nucleotide position 7706.

23. What are the treatment trials of optic neuritis?

Optic Neuritis Treatment Trial (ONTT) and Longitudinal Optic Neuritis Study (LONS)

Purpose:
  i. To assess the beneficial and adverse effects of corticosteroid treatment for optic neuritis
  ii. To determine the natural history of vision in patients who suffer optic neuritis
  iii. To identify risk factors for the development of MS in patients with optic neuritis

The treatment phase of the study was called the ONTT, whereas the current long-term follow-up phase is called the LONS.

Prior to the ONTT, well-established guidelines for treating optic neuritis did not exist. Although corticosteroids had been used to treat this disease, studies to demonstrate their effectiveness had not been satisfactory.

Patients were randomized to one of the three following treatment groups at 15 clinical centers:
  i. Oral prednisone (1 mg/kg/day) for 14 days
  ii. Intravenous methylprednisolone (250 mg every 6 hours) for 3 days, followed by oral prednisone (1 mg/kg/day) for 11 days
  iii. Oral placebo for 14 days

Each regimen was followed by a short oral taper. The oral prednisone and placebo groups were double masked, whereas the intravenous methylprednisolone group was single masked.

The rate of visual recovery and the long-term visual outcome were both assessed by measures of visual acuity, contrast sensitivity, color vision, and visual field at baseline, at seven follow-up visits during the first 6 months, and then yearly. A standardized neurologic examination with an assessment of MS status was made at baseline, after 6 months, and then yearly.

Patient eligibility:
The major eligibility criteria for enrollment into the ONTT included the following:
  i. Age range of 18–46 years
  ii. Acute unilateral optic neuritis with visual symptoms for 8 days or less
  iii. A relative afferent pupillary defect and a visual field defect in the affected eye
  iv. No previous episodes of optic neuritis in the affected eye
  v. No previous corticosteroid treatment for optic neuritis or MS
  vi. No systemic disease other than MS that might be the cause of the optic neuritis

Results:
The study has defined the value of baseline ancillary testing, the typical course of visual recovery with and without corticosteroid treatment, the risks and benefits of corticosteroid treatment, and the 5-year risk of the development of MS after optic neuritis.
These results are briefly summarized below:
  i. Routine blood tests, chest X-ray, brain MRI, and lumbar puncture are of limited value for diagnosing optic neuritis in a patient with typical features of optic neuritis
  ii. Brain MRI is a powerful predictor of the early risk of MS after optic neuritis
  iii. In optic neuritis patients with no brain MRI lesions, the following features of the optic neuritis are associated with a low 5-year risk of MS: Lack of pain, optic disk edema (particularly if severe), peripapillary hemorrhage, retinal exudates, and mild visual loss
  iv. Visual recovery begins rapidly (within 2 weeks) in most optic neuritis patients without any treatment, and then improvement continues for up to 1 year. Although most patients recover to 20/20 or near 20/20 acuity, many still have symptomatic deficits in vision
  v. The probability of recurrence of optic neuritis in either eye within 5 years is 28%. Visual recovery after a second episode in the same eye is generally very good
  vi. Treatment with high-dose intravenous corticosteroids followed by oral corticosteroids accelerated visual recovery but provided no long-term benefit to vision
  vii. Treatment with standard-dose oral prednisone alone did not improve the visual outcome and was associated with an increased rate of new attacks of optic neuritis
  viii. Treatment with the intravenous followed by oral corticosteroid regimen provided a short-term reduction in the rate of development

of MS, particularly in patients with brain MRI changes consistent with demyelination. However, by 3 years of follow-up, this treatment effect had subsided

The treatments were generally well-tolerated, and side effects during the treatment period were mild.

24. **What are the visual field defects noted in ONTT?**
    i. Generalized visual field depression was present in 48.2% of eyes
    ii. Altitudinal or other nerve-fiber bundle-type defects were present in 20.1% of eyes
    iii. Central or centrocecal scotoma was present in 8.3% of eyes
    iv. Other defects were present in 23.4% of eyes.

7.5 PAPILLEDEMA

CLINICAL FEATURES AND CAUSES

1. **Definition of papilledema.**
   Bilateral passive hydrostatic, noninflammatory edema of the optic disk or nerve head due to raised intracranial pressure.

2. **What is the place of production and pathway of cerebrospinal fluid (CSF)?**

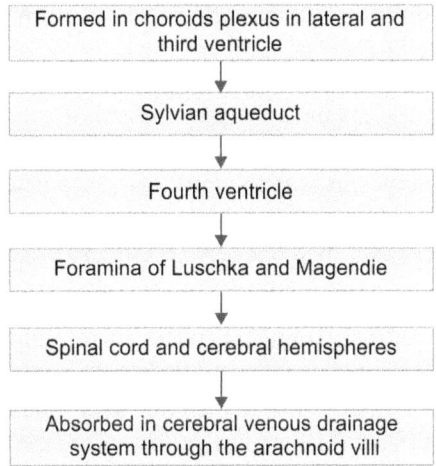

3. **What is normal CSF pressure?**
   Normal CSF pressure in adults = 80–200 mm H_2O
   Pressure >250 mm H_2O elevated

4. **What is meant by the term "axoplasmic transport"?**
   i. Optic nerve axoplasmic transport transports material (proteins and organelles) from the retinal ganglion cells to the entire axons and to its termination in the lateral geniculate body, where some of the material is degraded and returned to the cell body via the retrograde transport system
   ii. Orthograde axoplasmic transport (from eye to the brain) has a slow component (proteins and enzymes) that progresses at 0.5–3.0 mm/day, an intermediate component (mainly mitochondria), and a rapid component (subcellular organelles) that moves at 200–1,000 mm/day
   iii. Retrograde axoplasmic transport of lysosomes and mitochondria (from the brain to the eye) also occurs at an intermediate rate

5. **What is the relationship between intraocular pressure (IOP) and papilledema?**
   Normally, the IOP (14–20 mm Hg) is higher than the tissue pressure in the optic nerve (6–8 mm Hg). This pressure differential is the force driving the axoplasm in the region of the lamina cribrosa.
   Hence, a fall in the IOP or an increase in the optic nerve tissue pressure following a rise in the CSF pressure will interfere in the axoplasmic flow, leading to stasis and accumulation of the axoplasm.

6. **What are the theories of papilledema?**
   i. Inflammatory theory by Gowers and Leber—edematous inflammation was set up by toxic material associated with intracranial disease
   ii. Vasomotor theories by Korner—papilledema is caused by venous stasis, which is part of a generalized increase in systemic venous pressure due to an accentuated inhibitory action of vagus resulting from central stimulation of increased intracranial pressure
   iii. Axoplasmic stasis theory by Hayreh
   The most accepted theory is Hayreh's theory of axoplasmic stasis.

7. **What is Hayreh's theory of pathogenesis of papilledema?**
   i. Patency of the meningeal spaces surrounding the optic nerve and intracranial structures and transmission of increased CSF pressure to the region posterior to the optic nerve sheath is the first step
   ii. There is free diffusion of substances from the CSF to the optic nerve and thereby increases the optic nerve tissue pressure in the setting of increased intracranial tension (ICT)
   iii. Increased optic nerve tissue pressure causes alteration of pressure gradient across the lamina cribrosa, which causes blockage of axoplasmic flow from retinal ganglion cells to lateral geniculate body
   iv. Venous changes are secondary due to compression of fine vessels lying in the prelaminar region and in the surface layers by the swollen axons

8. **How frequent is the occurrence of papilledema in children?**
   i. *Infants:* Uncommon due to open fontanels
   ii. Children aged 2–10 years are commonly affected due to increased infratentorial tumors

9. **What are the causes of papilledema?**
   i. *Space-occupying lesions:*
      - Neoplasms—infratentorial tumors (common)
      - Abscess—temporal lobe
      - Inflammatory mass

- Subarachnoid hemorrhage
- Infarction
- A-V malformations
  ii. *Focal or diffuse cerebral edema:*
   - Trauma
   - Toxic
   - Anoxia
  iii. *Reduction in size of cranial vault:*
   - Craniosynostosis
  iv. *Blockage of CSF flow:*
   - Noncommunicating hydrocephalus
  v. *Vitamin A toxicity*
  vi. *Reduction in CSF resorption:*
   - Communicating hydrocephalus
   - Infectious meningitis
   - Elevated CSF proteins (meningitis)
   - Spinal cord tumor, Guillain-Barré syndrome (GBS)
  vii. *Increased CSF production*
  viii. *Idiopathic intracranial hypertension (IIH) [pseudotumor cerebri (PTC)]*

10. **Which tumors are more prone to develop papilledema and why?**
    Tumors of the midbrain, parietooccipital lobe, and cerebellum mostly cause papilledema.
    Tumors → Infratentorial (more common)
    → Supratentorial
    i. *Infratentorial tumors:* Produce papilledema by obstruction of the aqueduct or by compression of vein of Galen or the posterior superior sagittal sinus
    ii. *Supratentorial tumors:* Produce papilledema by deflection of the falx and pressure upon the great vein of Galen
    Others: Intracranial masses—metastatic tumors, brain tumors

11. **Which intracranial tumor is least likely to cause papilledema?**
    i. Medulla oblongata tumors
    ii. Tumor of the anterior fossa

12. **What are the common causes of papilledema in children?**
    Posterior fossa tumors—medulloblastoma

13. **What are the stages of papilledema?**
    i. Early
    ii. Established
    iii. Chronic
    iv. Atrophic
    (As suggested by Hughlings Jackson in 1871)

14. What are the clinical features of early papilledema?
   i. Visual symptoms are mild or absent
   ii. Optic disk shows hyperemia and blurring of superior and inferior margins and blurring of retinal nerve fiber layer
   iii. The physiological cup is normal

15. How does the edema progress?
The edema (blurring of the optic nerve) starts at the superior and inferior margins and extends around the nasal side, and finally the temporal side (SINT).

16. What are the pathological features of papilledema?
   i. Signs of passive edema without evidence of inflammation
   ii. Edematous changes are located in front of the lamina cribrosa
   iii. Axoplasmic stasis is seen
   iv. Nerve fibers become swollen and varicose and ultimately degenerate
   v. Proliferation of neuralgia and mesoblastic tissue around the vessels becomes thickened

17. What are the clinical features of established papilledema?
   i. Transient visual obscuration—5 seconds, rarely exceeds 30 seconds at irregular intervals
   ii. Visual acuity normal or decreased
   iii. Enlargement of blind spots
   iv. Gross elevation of the disk surface with blurred margins
   v. Obliteration of the cup
   vi. Venous pulsation absent
   vii. Microaneurysm formation and capillary dilatation on disk margin
   viii. Flame-shaped hemorrhages, cotton-wool spots
   ix. Circumferential retinal folds (Paton's lines)
   x. Hard exudates on hemorrhages and macula (macular fan)

18. Why do transient visual obscurations occur in papilledema?
Transient visual obscurations of vision may occur in one or both eyes simultaneously with rapid recovery, usually lasting seconds but sometimes lasting hours.

Patients may experience up to 20–30 attacks per day, with obscurations precipitated by change of posture or from lying down to sitting or standing position.

The cause of these transient obscurations is related to transient compression or ischemia of the optic nerve.

Spasms of the ophthalmic artery/posterior cerebral artery, ciliary aqueduct obstruction by a tumor producing a ball valve effect causing transient ophthalmology.

19. What is the usual duration of the transient obscuration of vision in papilledema and its precipitating factors?
   i. 5 seconds. It rarely exceeds 30 seconds at irregular interval
   ii. Precipitated by:
   - Standing up from a sitting position
   - Stooping
   - Turning the head abruptly

20. Name other conditions causing transient obscuration of vision.
   i. *Amaurosis fugax:*
   - Usual duration 5-15 minutes
   - Fundi may show emboli
   ii. *Retinal migraine:*
   - Duration 15-20 minutes
   - Frequently accompanied or followed by headache
   iii. *Acute glaucoma:*
   - Several hours
   iv. *Hemicrania:*
   - 15-45 minutes
   v. *Epileptic fits (partial):*
   - Few seconds

21. In what percentage of normal individuals can we see pulsations over the optic nerve head?
Absence of spontaneous venous pulsations—occurs when the intracranial pressure rises above 200 mmH$_2$O. If there is spontaneous venous pulsation, it strongly suggests that papilledema is absent. Absence of spontaneous venous pulsations may be a finding in 20% of normal population.

22. What is macular fan?
The nerve fibers in the macula are arranged in a radial fashion. Hence, hard exudates and hemorrhages are arranged in a radial manner in the macula, which are more prominent on the nasal side of the fovea due to the vascular compromise in and around the disk.

23. What are the clinical features of chronic (vintage) papilledema?
Visual acuity is variable with constricted visual field. Optic disk changes are:
   i. Champagne-cork appearance with no exudates and hemorrhages
   ii. Central cup obliterated but peripapillary retinal edema absorbs
   iii. Small white opacities on the disk—corpora amylacea
   iv. Pigmentary changes in the macula

24. **What are the clinical features of atrophic papilledema?**
    i. Visual acuity is severely impaired with constriction of visual field.
    ii. Optic disk grayish-white with indistinct margins as a result of gliosis
    iii. Narrow retinal vessels due to sheathing of vessels, which are extension of gliosis
    iv. Reduced disk elevation—flat disk

25. **What are the causes of optic atrophy in papilledema?**
    i. Increased intracranial pressure compromises the vascular supply (focal infarct, ischemia, axon damage), which causes nerve fiber atrophy. Decreased vascularity of the disk causes pale gray color leading to secondary optic atrophy
    ii. Appearance depends on the fact that absorption of exudates causes organization and formation of fibrous tissue on the disk. This fibrous tissue obscures the lamina cribrosa and fills in atrophic cup, then extends over the edges, which are thus ill-defined along vessels and perivascular sheath
    iii. Number of vessels also decreases (Kestenbaum's sign)

26. **What is the other staging system of papilledema?**
    Frisen's grading system:

    Stage 0:
    i. Mild nasal elevations of the nerve fiber layer
    ii. A portion of major vessels may be obscured in upper pole

    Stage 1: Very early papilledema
    i. Obscuration of the nasal border of the disk
    ii. No elevation
    iii. Disruption of normal retinal nerve fiber layer
    iv. Concentric or radial retinochoroidal folds

    Stage 2: Early papilledema
    i. Obscuration of all the borders
    ii. Elevation of nasal border
    iii. Complete peripapillary halo

    Stage 3: Moderate papilledema
    i. Obscuration of all the borders
    ii. Increased diameter of optic nerve head
    iii. Obscuration of one or more segments of major blood vessels leaving the disk
    iv. Peripapillary halo, irregular outer fringe with fingerlike extensions

    Stage 4: Marked papilledema
    i. Elevation of the entire nerve head
    ii. Obscuration of all the borders

iii. Peripapillary halo
iv. Total obscuration on the disk of a segment of major blood vessels

Stage 5: Severe papilledema
i. Dome-shaped protrusions representing anterior expansion of optic nerve head
ii. Peripapillary halo
iii. Total obscuration of a segment of major blood vessels
iv. Obliteration of optic cup
v. Obscuration of all the borders

27. **How does the blurring of disk margins appear in papilledema?**
The blurring of disk margins usually appears first in the upper and lower margins. Usually start at the upper nasal quadrant, spreading then round the nasal margin, and appearing last at the temporal margin (SINT).

28. **Why are the upper and lower quadrants affected first?**
The distribution depends on the density of capillaries, with the papillomacular bundle occupying the greater part of the outer aspect of the disk. The upper and lower quadrants are the most heavily crowded with nerve fibers.

29. **Why is there an enlargement of blind spot?**
An enlargement of blind spot is due to the separation of the retina around the disk by the edema.
i. Due to compression, detachment, and lateral displacement of the peripapillary retina and due to generalized decrease in sensitivity of the peripapillary retina. The outer layer of the neural retina may buckle, and rods and cones are displaced away from the end of the Bruch's membrane
ii. *Stiles–Crawford effect:* This phenomenon proposes that the wrinkles and the folds in the peripapillary retina cause light to fall obliquely on the photoreceptors, thus making the light a less effective stimulus

30. **List the differential diagnoses for the enlargement of blind spot.**
    i. Papilledema
    ii. Papillitis
    iii. Glaucoma
    iv. Progressive myopia
    v. Coloboma of optic nerve
    vi. Inferior conus
    vii. Juxtapapillary choroiditis
    viii. High alcohol consumption
    ix. Drugs:
    - Aldosterone
    - Betamethasone
    - Vitamin A
    - Prednisolone

31. What are the visual field defects common in cases of papilledema?
 i. Enlargement of blind spots
 ii. Concentric contractions more common
 iii. Relative scotoma first to green and red
 iv. Complete blindness
 v. Homonymous hemianopia
 vi. Central and arcuate scotomas
 vii. Most commonly involves inferior nasal quadrant

32. What are the systemic features of increased intracranial pressure?
 i. Headache—more severe in the morning, worsening progressively. Intensifies with head movement
 ii. Sudden nausea—projectile vomiting
 iii. Horizontal diplopia is caused by stretching of the sixth nerve over the petrous tip (false localizing sign). Sometimes fourth nerve palsy
 iv. Loss of consciousness/generalized motor rigidity
 v. Bilaterally dilated pupil (rare)

33. What are the causes of headache, loss of consciousness, and generalized motor rigidity?
Headache: It is associated with increased intracranial pressure due to stretching of the meninges, while sharply localized pains can be due to involvement of sensory nerve at the base of the skull or localized involvement of the meningeal nerves.

Loss of consciousness: It occurs from compression of the cerebral cortex and the reduction of its blood supply.

Generalized motor rigidity: Herniation of the hippocampal gyrus through the tentorium from increased intracranial pressure results in crowding of the temporal lobe into the incisura of each side.

Tentorial herniation thus places pressure on the crura cerebri, resulting in generalized motor rigidity. Finally, direct pressure on the nerves and dorsal midbrain produces bilaterally dilated pupils that do not respond to light stimulation.

34. How is the elevation of the disk seen on direct ophthalmoscopy?
First, with a direct ophthalmoscope, retinal vessels below the disk are focused, and then the vessels above the disk are seen.

A difference of 2-6 D may be found between the focus of the vessels on the top of the disk and those on the retina.

A difference of 3 D is equivalent to approximately 1 mm difference of level at the fundus.

35. **Which refractive error may mimic papilledema?**
    Astigmatism and hypermetropia (pseudoneuritis): It is a condition that usually occurs in hypermetropic eyes when the lamina is small, and the nerve fibers are heaped up as they debouch upon the retina.

36. **What are the earliest features of resolution in papilledema?**
    i. Retinal venous dilatation and disk capillary dilatation regression
    ii. Disappearance of disk hyperemia

37. **What are the last abnormalities that usually resolve after the treatment of papilledema?**
    i. Blurring of disk margins
    ii. Abnormalities of the peripapillary retinal nerve fiber layer

38. **What are the poor prognostic factors for papilledema?**
    i. *Rapidity:* The more rapid the onset, the greater the danger of permanent visual loss
    ii. Duration of papilledema
    iii. Papilledema of more than 5 D, extensive retinal hemorrhages and exudates, and macular scar
    iv. Early pallor of the disk and attenuated arterioles
    v. Gliosis of the disk
    vi. Obscurations of vision and presence of opticociliary shunts

39. **Mention the criteria for IIH.**
    (Modified from criteria established by WE Dandy)
    i. Signs and symptoms of increased intracranial pressure
    ii. Absence of localizing findings on neurologic examination
    iii. Absence of deformity, displacement, and obstruction of ventricular system and otherwise normal neurodiagnostic studies except for increased CSF pressure (>200 mmH$_2$O in nonobese patient and >250 mmH$_2$O in obese patient)
    iv. Awake and alert patient
    v. No other cause of increased intracranial pressure present

40. **What are the diagnostic criteria of PTC?**
    i. Symptoms and signs solely attributable to increased intracranial pressure
    ii. Elevated CSF pressure
    iii. Normal CSF composition
    iv. Normal neuroimaging studies
    v. No other etiology of intracranial hypertension identified
    vi. Treated with diuretics and lumbar puncture (LP)

41. **What are the drugs that may produce a secondary PTC?**
    i. Nalidixic acid
    ii. Penicillin
    iii. Tetracycline
    iv. Minocycline
    v. Ciprofloxacin
    vi. Nitrofurantoin

42. **Why are pupillary reactions normal in cases of early and established papilledema?**
    Pupillary reactions are normal because neuronal conduction is not dependent on axonal transport but rather on the myelin sheath.

43. **What is the differential diagnosis of papilledema?**
    i. Papillitis
    ii. *Pseudopapilledema due to:*
        - High hypermetropia
        - Anterior ischemic optic neuropathy (AION) (nonarteritic)
        - Drusen of optic nerve
    iii. Optic neuritis
    iv. Tilted optic disk
    v. Hypoplastic disk
    vi. Myelinated nerve fiber

44. **How can one differentiate between pseudopapilledema and papilledema?**
    Pseudopapilledema:
    i. Swelling never >2 D
    ii. No venous engorgement, edema, or exudates
    iii. Blind spot is not enlarged
    iv. Fundus fluorescein angiography (FFA)—no leaking. FFA is the most sensitive method to differentiate papilledema and pseudopapilledema

45. **How can one differentiate between optic neuritis (papillitis) and papilledema?**
    Optic neuritis:
    i. Relative apparent pupillary defect
    ii. Moderate swelling; 2-3 D shelving gradually into the surrounding retina
    iii. Central scotoma with field loss of color discrimination
    iv. Visual symptoms are marked
    v. Acute depression of central vision
    vi. Usually uniocular
    vii. Associated vitreous opacities

Papilledema:
   i. Normal pupil
   ii. Severe swelling of the optic disk
   iii. Enlargement of the blind spot
   iv. Visual symptoms are minimal
   v. Usually bilateral

46. **How can one differentiate crowded disk and tilted disk from papilledema?**
    i. Peripapillary nerve fiber layer and retinal vessels that traverse it remain normal
    ii. Venous pulsations are usually present
    iii. No vascular engorgement/hemorrhages
    iv. No cotton-wool spots
    v. An oval disk with one side displaced posteriorly, usually at the inferior margin and the other side elevated anteriorly, usually at the superior margin
    vi. Oblique direction of retinal vessels
    vii. High myopia/moderate oblique myopic astigmatism is usually present.

47. **Differentiate between nonarteritic AION from papilledema.**
    i. Associated with hypertension—40%, diabetes mellitus—24%
    ii. Visual acuity decreased >6/60
    iii. Color vision defective
    iv. Altitudinal field defects

48. **Differentiate between papilledema and optic disk drusen.**
    i. Drusen—common in children and young
    ii. Familial and very slow growing
    iii. Visual defects do not correspond to location of the drusen
    iv. Small optic nerve head
    v. Calcified laminated globular aggregates on the disk
    vi. FFA is normal

49. **Differentiate between hypertensive retinopathy and papilledema.**
    Hypertensive retinopathy: It is characterized by:
    i. Less venous dilatation
    ii. More marked arterial narrowing
    iii. Abnormalities of arteriovenous crossings with
    iv. Retinal hemorrhages and exudates more scattered than confined to the proximity of the disk

50. Differentiate between optic neuritis, papilledema, and ischemic neuropathy.

Features	Optic neuritis	Papilledema	Ischemic neuropathy
Symptoms			
Visual	Rapidly progressive loss of central vision	No visual loss ± transient obscuration	Acute field defect (common altitudinal)
Others	Tender globe, pain on motion, orbit or brow ache	Headache, nausea, vomiting	None (headache in cranial arteritis)
Bilaterality	Rare	Always	• Unilateral in acute stage • Second eye involved subsequently with picture of Foster–Kennedy syndrome
Signs			
Pupil	No anisocoria ↓ light reaction on side of neuritis	• No anisocoria • Normal reaction unless asymmetric atrophy	No anisocoria ↓ light reaction on side of disk infarct
Visual acuity	Decreased	Normal	Variable (severe loss common in arteritis)
Fundus	Variable degrees of disk swelling with few flame hemorrhages, cells in vitreous	Variable degrees of disk swelling, hemorrhages, cystoids infarcts	Usually segmental disk edema with few flame hemorrhages
Visual prognosis	Vision usually returns to normal or functional levels	Good	Poor prognosis

51. What are the causes of unilateral optic disk edema?

Oculo-orbital:
  i. Papillitis
  ii. Drusen
  iii. Ischemic optic neuropathy
  iv. Central retinal venous occlusion
  v. Optic nerve glioma/meningioma
  vi. Ocular hypotony

Mixed intracranial:
  i. Unilateral optic atrophy and true papilledema (Foster-Kennedy syndrome)
  ii. Preexisting atrophy before development of increased intracranial pressure (pseudo-Foster-Kennedy syndrome)
  iii. Unilateral high myopia and true papilledema
  iv. Cavernous sinus thrombosis
  v. Carotid-cavernous fistula

Pure intracranial:
  i. Posterior fossa tumor
  ii. Pseudotumor cerebri
  iii. Subarachnoid hemorrhage
  iv. Brain abscess
  v. Optochiasmatic arachnoiditis

52. **What are the causes of bilateral optic disk edema with normal visual function?**
    i. Hypertensive retinopathy
    ii. Spinal cord tumors
    iii. GBS
    iv. Hypoxemia and anemia
    v. Cyanotic congenital heart disease

53. **What is Foster-Kennedy syndrome?**
    Foster-Kennedy syndrome refers to specific clinical findings characteristically seen in frontal lobe/olfactory groove tumors, especially meningioma. The syndrome is believed to occur subsequent to increased ICT as a result of an asymmetrical frontal lobe mass, which compresses the optic nerve on one side leading to atrophy, while the other side demonstrates papilledema due to the increased ICT.

54. **What are the features associated with Foster-Kennedy syndrome?**
    The features associated with Foster-Kennedy syndrome include anosmia (if the olfactory nerve is affected), nausea, projectile vomiting (suggestive of increased ICT), emotional lability, and memory loss (suggestive of frontal lobe lesions).

55. **What is the treatment of Foster-Kennedy syndrome?**
    The treatment of the condition is symptomatic relief from the features of increased ICT and treatment of the etiology (tumor) of the condition.

56. **What is pseudo-Foster-Kennedy syndrome?**
    Pseudo-Foster-Kennedy syndrome is defined as preexisting optic atrophy in one eye, whereby the affected atrophied optic nerve cannot demonstrate changes of papilledema even in the presence of increased

ICT. The other eye manifests with disk edema. There is no intracranial mass that can be deemed to be the cause of an increase in ICT in such cases.

INVESTIGATIONS

1. **What is the investigation of choice in papilledema?**
    i. Magnetic resonance imaging (MRI) with or without contrast is the best investigation of choice
        - MRI angiography
        - MRI venography
            - To rule out arterial disease and venous obstruction (thrombosis)
            - Arnold-Chiari malformations
            - To see structured lesions (mainly posterior fossa lesions)
            - To see hydrocephalus
    ii. Fascial resolution is better in MRI, which provides three-dimensional image
    iii. Soft-tissue lesions are well appreciated

2. **What is the role of computed tomography (CT) scan in papilledema?**
    i. To rule out intracranial lesions that would produce increased intracranial pressure and rule out obstructive hydrocephalus
        - Acute vascular causes—like subarachnoid, epidural, subdural, intracranial hemorrhages, acute infarctions
        - After head injury—cerebral edema
    ii. Patient with contraindication to MRI like pacemaker, metallic clip, metallic foreign body

3. **What is the role of LP in papilledema?**
    i. Diagnostic—to evaluate for intracranial hypertension by recording the opening pressure
    ii. To send CSF for microbial/infectious studies like—total leukocyte count (TLC), differential count (DC), glucose, protein, cytology, venereal disease research laboratory (VDRL)
    iii. Therapeutic—PTC

4. **What is the main hazardous disadvantage of LP?**
    It is usually contraindicated because of the danger of herniation of the brain into the foramen magnum, which causes pressure on the medulla, leading to sudden death in cases with intracranial space-occupying lesions with midline shift.

5. **What are the complications of LP?**
    i. Poor compliance
    ii. Painful to the patient
    iii. Difficult in obese patients

iv. May produce a remission of PTC by creating a permanent fistula through the dura mater
v. Spinal epidermoid tumors
vi. Infection

6. **How does CT scan help in diagnostic of disk edema due to Graves' disease?**
It shows marked enlargement of extraocular muscle with compression of optic nerve, leading to disk edema.

7. **What are the X-ray findings of papilledema in children and adults?**
Adults:
   i. Demineralization of subcortical bone, leading to loss of "lamina dura" (white line) of sellar floor, followed by thinning of dorsum sella and the posterior clinoid process
   ii. In extreme cases, the sella becomes very shallow and flattened with its floor and anterior wall demineralized and the posterior clinoid process and dorsum sella destroyed
   iii. Increased ICT causes enlargement of the emissary veins in the occipital region
   iv. Congenital cyst or chronic subdural hematoma may show localized thinning or a bulge

Children:
   i. Presents with sutural diastasis, i.e., sutural widening
   ii. Increased convolutional markings with thinning of the bone
   iii. Any separation beyond 2 mm is suspicious of increased tension

8. **What are the FFA findings in papilledema?**
Early phase:
   i. Disk capillary dilatation
   ii. Dye leakage spots
   iii. Microaneurysm over the disk

Late phase:
   i. Leakage of dye beyond the disk margin
   ii. Pooling of dye around the disk as vertically oval pooling

TREATMENT OF PAPILLEDEMA

1. **What is the medical and surgical treatment for benign intracranial hypertension?**
   i. *Medical treatment:*
      - Acetazolamide 500 mg BD
      - Dehydrating agent—oral glycerol
      - Corticosteroids
      - Weight reduction

ii. *Surgical:*
   - Repeated LP
   - Decompression
   - Shunting procedure—lumboperitoneal shunt

2. **How many times LP can be done before subjecting the patient to decompression?**
   Multiple LPs can be done to relieve the increased ICT. LP needle creates a sieve that allows sufficient regress egress of CSF, so that ICT is normalized.

3. **How long does it take for regression of papilledema following treatment?**
   i. Fully developed papilledema may disappear completely within hours, days, or weeks, depending on the way in which ICT is lowered.
   ii. *Brain tumor*—papilledema can resolve 6-8 weeks after successful craniotomy to remove a brain tumor.
   iii. *PTC*—resolution of papilledema within 2-3 weeks after lumboperitoneal shunts in IIH and several days after optic nerve sheath fenestration.

4. **During treatment of papilledema, how is therapeutic success determined?**
   i. Relief of headache
   ii. Diminished frequency of transient visual obscuration
   iii. Regression of papilledema
   iv. Stability or improvement of field defects
   v. Weight reduction

5. **What are the indications of decompression?**
   i. Failure of medical treatment as evidenced by clinical signs:
      - Marked degree of swelling (>5 D)
      - Great engorgement of veins
      - Presence of extensive hemorrhage
      - Early appearance of exudate spots
   ii. Progressive headaches unrelieved with medical treatment
   iii. Progressive optic neuropathy evidenced by early contraction of visual field

6. **Which patient with PTC should be treated? And how?**
   i. *Those patients who develop:*
      - Signs of visual loss from chronic papilledema (optic neuropathy)
      - Intractable headaches
      - Persistent diplopia

ii. *Treatment:*
      - Repeated LP
      - Decompression
      - Shunting procedure

7. **How do you manage a case of pregnancy-induced hypertension (PIH) presenting with papilledema?**
   i. General—bed rest
   ii. Diet—only fluids
   iii. Sedative—phenobarbitone/diazepam
   iv. Control of blood pressure (BP)
   v. Control edema—proteinuria/diuretic/frusemide, hypertonic glucose
   vi. Finally, if the patient does not respond to treatment, pregnancy has to be terminated

8. **What are the operative disk decompressions done to relieve papilledema?**
   i. Subtemporal decompression
   ii. Suboccipital craniectomy
   iii. Direct fenestration of optic nerve sheath decompression (ONSD) via medial or lateral orbitotomy

9. **What is the procedure of ONSD?**
   The surgeon makes a window or multiple incisions in the normally bellowed anterior dural covering of the optic nerve sheath using either a lateral or a medial approach (the latter preferred).

10. **What are the features and treatment of fulminant IIH?**
    i. *Features:*
       - Rapid onset of symptoms
       - Significant visual loss
       - Macular edema
       - Cerebral venous thrombosis and meningeal process should be considered
       - Malignant cause requires rapid treatment
    ii. *Treatment:*
       - Intravenous (IV) corticosteroids and insertion of lumbar drain used while waiting for definitive treatment

11. **How do you manage a patient with PTC?**
    i. *No symptoms of papilledema:*
       - Periodic monthly review
       - If vision is normal for 3 months, then 2-monthly review

ii. *With transient obscuration of vision/signs of optic nerve dysfunction:*
   - T. acetazolamide-1 g daily depending on the patient's tolerance
   - Reexamine the patient every 2-3 weeks for signs of compromise
iii. *With progressive optic neuropathy:*
   - T. aacetazolamide corticosteroid (80-100 mg/day)
iv. *Other treatment modalities:*
   - Repeated LP
   - Lumboperitoneal shunt
   - Optic nerve sheath decompression

12. **If the patient has visual symptoms only, what is the treatment of choice?**
Bilateral optic nerve sheath decompression

13. **If the patient has headache only with no visual symptoms, what is the treatment of choice?**
Lumboperitoneal shunt.

Neuro-ophthalmology **601**

7.6 OPTIC ATROPHY

1. **Define optic atrophy.**
   Optic atrophy describes a group of clinical conditions that have abnormal pallor of the disk as a common physical sign. It is not a disease but a pathological endpoint of any disease that causes damage to the ganglion cells and axons with overall diminution of the optic nerve and visual acuity.

2. **What are the features of optic atrophy?**
   i. Loss of conducting function
   ii. Abnormal pallor of the disk
   iii. Proliferation of glial tissue
   iv. Reduction in number of capillaries
   v. Destruction of nerve fibers
   vi. Diminished volume of nerve fiber bundle
   vii. Increased excavation

3. **What are the clinical features of optic atrophy?**
   i. Reduced visual acuity
   ii. Relative afferent pupillary defect (RAPD)/afferent pupillary defect (APD)
   iii. Defective color vision
   iv. Visual field loss central, paracentral, altitudinal scotomas

4. **What is the normal color of disk, and why?**
   The disk is reddish pink in color with a mild pale physiological cup in the center.
   The normal color of the disk depends on the following factors:
   i. *Composition of the optic disk:*
      - Axons of retinal ganglion cells
      - Blood capillaries
      - Astrocytes
      - Connective tissue
   ii. Relationship of these structures to each other
   iii. Behavior of light falling on the disk
   iv. Vascularity of the disk

5. **What is the pathology of optic atrophy?**
   There are two main factors:
   i. Degeneration of optic nerve fibers
   ii. Proliferation of astrocytes and glial tissue

The disease may be focal, multifocal, or diffuse, causing axonal interruption and their destruction by:
   i. Direct effect
   ii. Investing glial tissue
   iii. Decreasing capillary blood supply—gross shrinkage and atrophy of the optic nerve

6. **What are the causes of pallor in optic atrophy?**
   Optic nerve degeneration causes:
   i. Reduced blood supply and disappearance of smaller vessels from view
   ii. Glial tissue formation occurs, which is opaque
   iii. Loss of tissue causes visibility of opaque scleral lamina

7. **What is Kestenbaum capillary number?**
   Capillaries on the normal disk were counted by Kestenbaum to be 10-12. In optic atrophy, it was reduced to 6 or less.

8. **What is Wallerian degeneration (ascending or antegrade optic atrophy)?**
   Primary lesion is in the optic nerve head, retina, or choroid, which proceeds toward the brain. Visual axons are severed, and their ascending segment disintegrates.
   There is swelling and degeneration of terminal buttons of axons within the lateral geniculate body (LGB).

9. **Which fibers are the first to be affected in ascending optic atrophy?**
   The rate of degeneration is proportional to the thickness of nerve fibers. Hence, larger axons degenerate faster than small-caliber axons.

10. **What are the causes of ascending optic atrophy?**
    i. Retinitis pigmentosa (RP)
    ii. Central retinal artery occlusion (CRAO)
    iii. Glaucoma
    iv. Papilledema
    v. Toxic amblyopia
    vi. Extensive panretinal photocoagulation (PRP)

11. **How soon can ascending optic atrophy set in and be completed?**
    The process can be identified within 24 hours and completed within 7 days.

12. **What pathological process occurs in the LGB in optic atrophy?**
    Transsynaptic changes occur in layers 1, 2, 3, and 5. Axons are reduced in size but not in number. Shrinkage and reduction of cytoplasm especially. Endoplasmic reticulum—reduced Nissl granule staining is seen.

13. **What are the examples of transsynaptic antegrade atrophy?**
    i. Glaucoma
    ii. After trauma
    iii. After enucleation

14. **What is the earliest sign of optic atrophy?**
    Retinal nerve fiber layer changes are seen even before the onset of disk pallor or field defect. This defect can be slit-like wedge shaped/diffuse loss.

15. **What is descending optic atrophy?**
    Descending optic atrophy refers to the retrograde degeneration of axons. The primary lesion is in the brain or optic nerve. The atrophic process proceeds toward the eye, leading to secondary effects on the optic disk and the retina.

16. **What is the time span for the completion of descending optic atrophy?**
    Approximately 6–8 weeks. The time course of this descending degeneration is independent of the distance of the injury from the ganglion cell body.

17. **What are the histopathological hallmarks of optic atrophy?**
    i. Loss of myelin and axon fibers
    ii. Loss of the parallel architecture of the glial columns
    iii. Gliosis
    iv. Widening of the space separating the optic nerve and meninges
    v. Thickening of the pial septa of the nerve to occupy space lost by nerve fiber loss

18. **Define primary optic atrophy (POA).**
    There is orderly degeneration of optic nerve fibers and is replaced by columns of glial tissue without any alteration in the architecture of the optic nerve head. This reflects a chronic process that has not been preceded by swelling or congestion of the optic disk.

19. **Describe the features of POA.**
    i. Chalky white disk
    ii. Sharply defined margins
    iii. Lamina cribrosa is well seen
    iv. Surrounding retina, retinal vessels, and periphery are normal
    v. Shallow, saucer-shaped cup is seen

20. **What are the common causes of POA?**
    i. *Retrobulbar neuritis*
    ii. *Compressive lesions of the optic nerve, e.g.:*
        – Pituitary tumors

- Meningiomas
- Gliomas

iii. *Traumatic optic atrophy*
iv. *Demyelinating diseases, e.g., tabes dorsalis, multiple sclerosis*

21. **What is secondary optic atrophy (SOA)?**
    Secondary optic atrophy is characterized by marked degeneration of optic nerve fibers with excessive proliferation of glial tissue, resulting in the loss of entire architecture of the optic nerve head.
    It is preceded by swelling or congestion of the optic nerve head.

22. **What are the causes of SOA?**
    i. Papillitis
    ii. Papilledema

23. **Describe the features of SOA.**
    i. Gray or dirty gray pallor of the disk
    ii. Poorly defined margins
    iii. Physiological cup is obliterated and filled with proliferating fibroglial tissue
    iv. Peripapillary sheathing and narrowing of arteries
    v. Veins are tortuous and sometimes narrowed
    vi. Hyaline bodies and drusen in and around the disk

24. **What is the most common cause of altitudinal pallor?**
    Acute ischemic optic neuropathy

25. **What is the most common cause of segmental optic atrophy?**
    Temporal pallor: This is due to the degeneration of axial fibers of the retrobulbar optic nerve, resulting in atrophy of the papillomacular bundle.

26. **What are the types of field defects occurring due to temporal pallor?**
    Centrocecal scotoma or central scotoma due to the loss of the papillomacular bundle

27. **How does wedge-shaped pallor occur?**
    Branch retinal artery occlusion leads to the degeneration of infarcted ganglion cells, causing atrophy of the corresponding wedge of the disk.

28. **What is the most common cause of consecutive optic atrophy (COA)?**
    Central retinal artery occlusion is the most common cause of COA. It is an ascending type of optic atrophy. Other causes are:
    i. Degenerative—RP, cerebromacular degeneration, myopia
    ii. Postinflammatory—choroiditis, chorioretinitis
    iii. Extensive PRP
    iv. Longstanding retinal detachment (RD)

29. What are the clinical features of COA?
   i. Disk has a waxy pallor
   ii. Normal disk margin
   iii. Marked attenuation of arteries
   iv. Associated retinal pathology may be seen
   v. Normal physiologic cup

30. What is cavernous optic atrophy?
Cavernous optic atrophy is nothing but glaucomatous optic atrophy (Schnabel's). This is characterized by axonal degeneration without any proliferation of glial tissue, resulting in formation of caverns with marked excavation of the optic disk. The caverns are filled with hyaluronic acid.

31. What is the mechanism of ischemic optic atrophy?
Ischemic optic atrophy occurs when the perfusion pressure of the ciliary system falls below the IOP.

32. What are the causes of ischemic optic atrophy?
   i. Systemic hypertension
   ii. Temporal arteritis
   iii. Atherosclerosis
   iv. Diabetes
   v. Collagen disorders

33. When does optic atrophy manifests in CRAO?
2–3 weeks

34. Name some chemicals causing optic atrophy.
   i. Arsenic
   ii. Lead
   iii. Benzene
   iv. Chromium
   v. Nitro and dinitrobenzene

35. What are the drugs that can cause optic atrophy?
   i. Quinine (total blindness in small doses in susceptible persons)
   ii. Ethambutol
   iii. Streptomycin
   iv. Isoniazid (INH)
   v. Chloroquine (Bull's eye maculopathy)
   vi. Oral contraceptives

36. What is the most common cause of toxic amblyopia?
Tobacco—in cigar and pipe smokers

37. **What are the pathogenesis and features of tobacco-induced optic atrophy?**

    Cyanide is the normal constituent of tobacco, which is detoxified by sulfur metabolism to harmless thiocyanate. In tobacco users, sulfur metabolism is deranged. There is degeneration of the axial portion of retrobulbar optic nerve due to demyelination. The resulting toxic degenerative neuritis leads to secondary fibrosis and gliosis within papillomacular bundle. It is associated with a deficiency of vitamin B12.

38. **What is the treatment of tobacco amblyopia?**
    i. Abstention from tobacco and alcohol
    ii. Injections of hydroxocobalamin 1,000 μg intramuscularly. The dose should be repeated five times at intervals of 4 days

39. **Name some metabolic disorders causing optic atrophy.**
    i. Diabetes
    ii. Thyroid ophthalmopathy
    iii. Cystic fibrosis
    iv. Nutritional amblyopia
    v. Hypophosphatasia
    vi. G6PD deficiency
    vii. Mucopolysaccharidosis
    viii. Acute intermittent porphyria—Menkes disease

40. **What is nutritional amblyopia?**

    It is due to atrophy of papillomacular nerve fibers caused by a deficiency of vitamin B12, B6, B1, B2, and niacin.

    Characterized by:
    i. Progressive bilateral visual loss
    ii. Centrocecal scotoma
    iii. Temporal pallor

41. **What is the pathogenesis of tropical amblyopia?**

    Tropical amblyopia is common in people eating cassava. It occurs due to reduced levels of serum cyanocobalamin and absence of sulfur-containing amino acids.

42. **What are the features of tropical amblyopia?**
    i. Bilateral blurred disk
    ii. Temporal pallor
    iii. General features such as ataxia, paresthesia of lower extremities, tinnitus, deafness, absence of deep tendon reflexes, and posterior column sensory loss

43. **Which variants of diabetes cause optic atrophy?**
    i. *Juvenile diabetes mellitus:*
       - Autosomal recessive
       - Pronounced rod and less severe cone dystrophy (Wolfram syndrome)
    ii. DIDMOAD syndrome—diabetes mellitus, diabetes insipidus, optic atrophy, and deafness

44. **Specify the types of mucopolysaccharidosis causing optic atrophy.**
    i. Hurler's syndrome
    ii. Sanfilippo's syndrome

45. **What is the mechanism of traumatic optic atrophy?**
    i. Tears in the nerve substance
    ii. Perforation of nerve by fractured bone spicules
    iii. Hemorrhage into nerve sheath
    iv. Contusion necrosis
    v. Avulsion of the optic nerve

46. **What is the most common site of injury leading to traumatic optic atrophy?**
    A blow to the lateral wall of the orbit.

47. **What is the time span after which the optic atrophic process manifest clinically first as temporal pallor in traumatic optic neuropathy?**
    2-4 weeks

48. **What could be the pathophysiology of reversible loss of vision in traumatic optic neuropathy?**
    Compression of the intracanalicular portion of the optic nerve due to edema.

49. **What is the cause of intermittent visual claudication?**
    Takayasu disease—loss of vision may occur during exercise and improves at rest.

50. **What percent of foveal fibers must be present for normal visual acuity?**
    44% of foveal fibers.

51. **Name some hereditary causes of optic atrophy.**
    i. Congenital/infantile optic atrophy—recessive and dominant form
    ii. Leber's optic atrophy
    iii. Behr's optic atrophy

52. **What are the differential diagnoses of optic atrophy?**
    i. Coloboma of disk
    ii. Optic pit

iii. Morning glory syndrome
iv. Medullated nerve fibers
v. Myopic disk
vi. Optic disk hypoplasia
vii. Drusen of the disk

53. **Name histopathological techniques to highlight demyelination of optic nerve.**
    i. Special myelinophilic stains:
       - Luxol fast blue
       - Weigert stain
    ii. Paraphenylenediamine—stains remnants of optic nerve myelin long after the degeneration/atrophy has occurred
    iii. Demyelination is indicated in a hematoxylin and eosin tissue section by the more compact nature of the nerve parenchyma

54. **What is the specific color vision loss in optic nerve disorders?**
    Optic nerve disorders manifest a relative red–green deficiency.

55. **How can color vision loss due to retinal and optic nerve pathology be differentiated?**
    Retinal diseases manifest a relative blue–yellow deficiency, whereas optic nerve disorders show a relative red–green deficiency.

56. **Name some causes of traction optic atrophy.**
    i. Glaucoma
    ii. Postpapilledema
    iii. Sclerosed calcified arteries
    iv. Aneurysm of internal carotid artery
    v. Bony pressure at the optic foramen
    vi. Tumors of the optic nerve sheath, pituitary, frontal temporal, or sphenoidal lobes
    vii. Swelling of the optic nerve, which may get strangulated at the optic foramen
    viii. Inflammatory adhesion in basal arachnoiditis

57. **What are the types of segmental or partial optic atrophy?**
    i. Temporal pallor
    ii. Altitudinal pallor
    iii. Wedge-shaped pallor

58. **Classify optic atrophy.**
    Pathological:
    i. Ascending
    ii. Descending

Ophthalmoscopical:
  i. POA
  ii. SOA
  iii. COA

Etiological:
  i. Consecutive
  ii. Postinflammatory
  iii. Pressure/traction
  iv. Toxic
  v. Metabolic
  vi. Traumatic
  vii. Hereditary
  viii. Circulatory

59. How is optic atrophy classified ophthalmoscopically?
  i. Primary
  ii. Secondary
  iii. Consecutive
  iv. Cavernous or glaucomatous
  v. Segmental or partial

60. How can methyl alcohol poisoning occur commonly?
Methanol (methyl alcohol) is found in cleaning materials, solvents, paints, varnishes, Sterno fuel, formaldehyde solutions, antifreeze, gasohol, "moonshine", windshield washer fluid (30–40% methanol), and duplicating fluids. It is consumed as local liquor (wood alcohol).

61. What are the features of methyl alcohol poisoning?
  i. Nonspecific symptoms such as headache, dizziness, nausea, lack of coordination, confusion, and drowsiness
  ii. Central nervous system (CNS) involvement in the form of unconsciousness, semiconsciousness, and giddiness
  iii. Visual symptoms are the predominant presenting features
  iv. Shock may occur as a late event
  v. Unconsciousness and death with sufficiently large doses

62. How does methyl alcohol poisoning affect the optic nerve?
The symptoms of methanol poisoning are nonspecific except for visual disturbances. Ocular changes consist of:
  i. Retinal edema
  ii. Blurring of the disk margins

iii. Hyperemia of the disks

iv. Optic atrophy as late sequelae

Metabolic acidosis is the most striking disturbance seen in methanol poisoning. It is probably due to the accumulation of formic acid and lactic acid. Formic acid inhibits cytochrome oxidase in the fundus of the eye.

Disruption of the axoplasm is due to impaired mitochondrial function and decreased adenosine triphosphate (ATP) production. Swelling of axons in the optic disk and edema result in visual impairment.

The ocular changes correlate to the degree of acidosis. Retinal damage is due to the inhibition of retinal hexokinase by formaldehyde, an intermediate metabolite of methanol.

63. What is the treatment of methyl alcohol poisoning?

The essential therapy of methanol poisoning is adequate alkalinization and ethanol administration. Ethanol competes with methanol for the enzyme alcohol dehydrogenase in the liver, thereby preventing the accumulation of toxic metabolites of methanol in the body. The recommended dose of ethanol is 0.6 g/kg body weight (a loading dose) followed by an infusion of 66 mg/kg/h in nondrinkers and 154 mg/kg/h in chronic drinkers.

Dialysis is recommended in those patients who have visual disturbances, blood methanol of 50 mg% or more, ingestion of >60 mL of methanol, and severe acidosis not corrected by sodium bicarbonate administration.

64. What are the features of excessive use of artificial sweeteners containing aspartame (NutraSweet)?

i. Decreased vision—including blindness in one or both eyes

ii. Blurring, "bright-flashes", tunnel vision, "black spots"

iii. Double vision

iv. Pain in one or both eyes

v. Decreased tears

vi. Difficulty in wearing contact lens

vii. Unexplained RD and bleeding

65. How do artificial sweetening agents affect the optic nerve?

Each of the components of aspartame—phenylalanine (50%) and aspartic acid (40%), the methyl ester, is converted to methyl alcohol or methanol (10%) and further to formaldehyde, which is toxic to the retina and optic nerves. Methanol causes swelling of the optic nerve and degeneration of ganglion cells in the retina.

66. Fundus portraits of different types of optic atrophy.

Primary disk	Secondary disk	Consecutive disk	Cavernous disk	Temporal disk
Chalky white in color	Gray dirty gray pallor	Waxy pallor of the disk	i. Vertical pallor of cup–notching of neuroretinal rim (NRR) ii. Pallor of rim	Disk is pale on the temporal side
Sharply defined margins	Poorly defined margins	Normal disk margin	i. Visibility of lamina pores–laminar dot sign ii. Backward bowing of lamina cribrosa	Clear disk margin
Lamina cribrosa well seen	Physiological cup obliterated and filled with fibroglial tissue obscuring view of lamina cribrosa	Normal physiological cup	i. Bayoneting and nasalization of retinal vessels ii. Splinter hemorrhages at the disk margin iii. Saucerization of optic disk	
Vessels	*Vessels*	*Vessels*	*Vessels*	*Vessels*
Retinal vessels normal	Peripapillary sheathing of arteries and narrowing of arteries		Baring of circumlinear vessels	
	Veins are tortuous and narrowed, occasionally sclerosed or hyaluronized	Marked attenuation of arteries	Peripapillary halo and atrophy	Vessels are normal
Surrounding retina normal	Hyaline bodies or drusen seen in and around the disk		Nerve fiber layer defect	

67. **How is optic atrophy treated?**

There is no real cure or treatment for optic atrophy. Therefore, it is important to have regular eye examination (especially if there is a family history of eye diseases) and to see an ophthalmologist immediately if any changes in vision are noted.

7.7 OPTIC DISK ANOMALIES

1. **What are the congenital optic disk anomalies?**

   Definition: Unusual configuration of the disk(s) typically present since birth.

   Key features: Small, pale, or unusual shaped disk may reflect mere curiosities or significant anomalies associated with visual field defects.

   Associated features: Abnormalities of the surrounding retina (e.g., in morning glory syndrome), anterior segment (e.g., in iris coloboma), face, or brain occasionally may be seen.

   Congenital optic nerve head (ONH) anomalies are important because:
   i. Relatively common
   ii. Some may be mistaken for papilledema
   iii. Some may give rise to visual field defects
   iv. Some are associated with central nervous system (CNS) malformation
   v. Some may be associated with other ocular abnormalities

2. **What are the features of congenital ONH anomalies?**

   The following are the general concepts useful in evaluating and managing children with congenital optic disk anomalies:
   i. Children with bilateral optic disk anomaly generally present in infancy with poor vision and nystagmus; those with unilateral anomaly present during the preschool years with sensory esotropia
   ii. CNS malformations are common in patients with malformed optic disks
      - Small optic disk is associated with malformations of cerebral hemisphere, pituitary infundibulum, and midline intracranial structures (septum pellucidum, corpus callosum)
      - Large optic disks of morning glory configuration are associated with the transsphenoidal form of basal encephalocele
      - Large optic disks of colobomatous configuration may be associated with systemic anomalies
      - Magnetic resonance imaging (MRI) is advisable in infants with small optic disks (unilateral or bilateral) and in infants with large optic disks who have either neurodevelopmental deficits or midfacial anomalies suggestive of basal encephalocele
   iii. Color vision is relatively preserved in an eye with a congenitally anomalous optic disk, in contrast to the severe dyschromatopsia in acquired optic neuropathies

iv. Any structural ocular abnormality that reduces visual acuity in infancy may lead to superimposed amblyopia. Occlusion therapy therefore should be tried in patients with unilateral optic disk anomalies and decreased vision

3. **What are the features of ONH?**

   The most common optic disk anomaly encountered in ophthalmologic practice.

   Incidence has increased in recent times because of maternal alcohol and drug abuse.

   Pathogenesis:
   Primary failure of retinal ganglion cell differentiation at the 13–15 mm stage of embryonic life.

   Ophthalmoscopic appearance:
   i. Abnormally small ONH
   ii. Gray in color and is often surrounded by a yellowish mottled peripapillary halo, bordered by a ring of increased or decreased pigmentation (double ring)
   iii. Major retinal blood vessels are tortuous
   iv. Histopathologically, a subnormal number of optic nerve axons with normal mesodermal elements and glial supporting tissue
   v. Double ring sign:
      – Outer ring—normal junction between the sclera and lamina cribrosa
      – Inner ring—abnormal extension of retina and retinal pigment epithelium (RPE) over the outer portion of lamina cribrosa

   Visual acuity:
   i. Ranges from 6/6 to no perception of light (PL)
   ii. Localized visual field defects
   iii. Generalized constriction of visual fields

   Systemic associations:
   i. Superior segmental ONH—type 1 diabetes mellitus (DM)
   ii. Growth hormone deficiency is the most common
   iii. Neonatal hypoglycemia or seizures with ONH—congenital panhypopituitarism

   Investigation:
   Magnetic resonance imaging demonstrates thinning and attenuation of prechiasmatic intracranial optic nerve.

4. **What are excavated optic disk anomalies?**
   i. Morning glory disk anomaly
   ii. Optic disk coloboma
   iii. Peripapillary staphyloma

5. **What are the features of morning glory disk anomaly?**
   It is a congenital, funnel-shaped excavation of the posterior fundus that incorporates the optic disk.
   Ophthalmoscopically:
   i. The disk is markedly enlarged, orange or pink in color, and it may appear to be recessed or elevated centrally within the confines of a funnel-shaped peripapillary excavation
   ii. A wide annulus of chorioretinal pigmentary disturbance surrounds the disk within the excavation
   iii. A white tuft of glial tissue overlies the central portion of the disk
   iv. Blood vessels appear increased in number and often arise from the disk periphery; they have a straight course
   v. Macula may be incorporated in the excavation (macular capture)

   Features:
   i. Morning glory anomaly is usually a unilateral condition
   ii. Visual acuity 6/60 to finger counting
   iii. Females > males
   iv. Rare in blacks
   v. Associated with transsphenoidal form of basal encephalocele
   vi. Patients with transsphenoidal encephalocele usually display a characteristic malformation complex consisting of midfacial anomalies, hypertelorism, widened bitemporal diameter, depressed nasal root, and V-shaped fusion line involving the upper lip
   vii. A transsphenoidal encephalocele may appear clinically as a pulsatile posterior nasal mass or a "nasal polyp" high in the nose
   viii. Morning glory disk anomaly patients are at risk of acquired visual loss
   ix. In 30%, serous retinal detachment starts in the peripapillary area and extends to the posterior pole

6. **What are the features of optic disk coloboma?**
   i. Coloboma means mutilated
   ii. Coloboma of the optic disk results from incomplete or abnormal coaptation of the proximal end of the embryonic fissure
   iii. In optic disk coloboma, a sharply defined, glistening white, bowl-shaped excavation occupies an enlarged optic disk
   iv. Excavation is decentered inferiorly, reflecting the position of the embryonic fissure
   v. Inferior neuroretinal rim is thin or absent, while the superior is spared
   vi. Iris and ciliary coloboma often coexist
   vii. Axial scans show crater-like excavation of the posterior globe at its junction with the optic nerve
   viii. Visual acuity may be decreased

ix. Optic disk coloboma may arise sporadically or be inherited in an autosomal dominant fashion
x. Eyes with isolated optic disk coloboma are prone to develop serous macular detachments

7. **What are the features of peripapillary staphyloma?**

   It is a rare, unilateral, deep fundus excavation that surrounds the disk.

Peripapillary staphyloma	Morning glory disk
Deep, cup-shaped excavation	Less deep, funnel-shaped excavation
Optic disk: Relatively normal and well defined	Optic disk: Grossly anomalous and poorly defined
Absence of glial and vascular anomalies	Central glial bouquet; anomalous vascular pattern

8. **How do you differentiate morning glory syndrome from optic disk coloboma?**

   Ophthalmoscopic findings:

Morning glory disk	Optic disk coloboma
Optic disk lies within the excavation	Excavation lies within the optic disk
Symmetrical defect	Asymmetrical defect
Central glial tuft	No central glial tuft
Severe peripapillary pigmentary disturbance	Minimal peripapillary pigmentary disturbance
Anomalous retinal vasculature	Normal retinal vasculature

   Systemic and ocular findings:

Morning glory disk	Optic disk coloboma
Females > males	No sex or racial predilection
Rarely familial	Often familial
Rarely bilateral	Often bilateral
No iris, ciliary body, or retinal colobomas	Iris, ciliary, and retinal colobomas are common
Rarely associated with multisystem genetic disorder	Often associated with multisystem genetic disorder
Basal encephalocele common	Rare

9. **What are the features of megalopapilla?**

   Features:

   Two phenotypic variants:
   i. First is a common variant in which abnormally large optic disk (>2.1 mm in diameter)

- Frequently bilateral with large cup-to-disk ratio, where the cup is round or horizontally oval with no vertical notching, differentiating it from normal tension glaucoma
ii. Second phenotypic variant, the normal optic cup is replaced by grossly anomalous noninferior excavation that obliterates the adjacent neuroretinal rim

10. **What are the features of optic pit?**
    i. Round or oval, gray, white, or yellowish depression in the optic disk
    ii. Commonly involve the temporal optic disk but may be situated in any sector
    iii. Temporally located pits are often accompanied by adjacent peripapillary pigment epithelial changes
    iv. One or two cilioretinal arteries are seen to emerge from the bottom or margin of the pit in 50% cases
    v. Typically unilateral; the disk is larger than in the fellow eye
    vi. Serous macular elevation develops in 25–75% cases
    vii. Maculopathy becomes symptomatic in third to fourth decade of life

11. **What are the sources of fluid in an optic disk pit?**
    i. Vitreous cavity via the pit
    ii. Subarachnoid space
    iii. Blood vessels at the base of pit
    iv. Orbital space surrounding the dura

12. **What are the features of congenital tilted disk syndrome?**
    Fairly common, nonhereditary, bilateral condition in which the superotemporal optic disk is elevated and the inferonasal disk is posteriorly displaced, resulting in an oval-appearing disk with its long axis obliquely oriented.

    Accompanying features:
    i. Situs inversus of retinal vessels
    ii. Congenital inferonasal conus
    iii. Thinning of inferonasal RPE and choroid
    iv. Bitemporal hemianopia
    v. Affected patient may have myopic astigmatism
    vi. Disk is small, oval, or D shaped with an axis oblique
    vii. Visual field defects involving the upper temporal quadrants may be present as a result of inferonasal fundus changes

13. **What are the features of Aicardi syndrome?**
    Cerebroretinal disorder of unknown etiology

    Clinical features:
    i. Infantile spasms
    ii. Agenesis of the corpus callosum

iii. A characteristic electroencephalogram (EEG) pattern termed "hypsarrhythmia"
iv. A pathognomonic optic disk appearance consisting of multiple depigmented "chorioretinal lacunae" clustered around the disk
v. Histopathologically, these lacunae are well circumscribed, full-thickness defects limited to the RPE and the choroids
vi. Other congenital optic disk anomalies may accompany the chorioretinal lacunae

Ocular associations:
i. Microphthalmos
ii. Retrobulbar cyst
iii. Pseudoglioma
iv. Retinal detachment, macular scars
v. Cataract
vi. Pupillary membrane, etc.

Systemic associations:
i. Vertebral malformations (fused vertebra, scoliosis, and spina bifida)
ii. Costal malformations (absent ribs, fused ribs, or bifurcated ribs)
iii. CNS anomalies include:
  - Agenesis of corpus callosum, cortical migration anomalies, and malformations

14. What are the features of optic disk drusen?
  i. Intrapapillary drusen are crystalloid, acellular refractile bodies that often appear in longstanding anomalously elevated disk
  ii. Incidence in general population is 0.3–2%
  iii. Bilateral and familial "emerge" over time
  iv. Patients with retinitis pigmentosa and angioid streak show increased incidence
  v. Thought to develop from stagnant axoplasm dammed up by a small disk, a tight cribriform plate, or a narrow scleral canal
  vi. May be small or large, superficial or deep
  vii. Produce field loss, sparing 10° of the visual field

Investigations:
  i. *Fluorescein angiography:* Drusen show late staining with fluorescein (hyperfluorescence), whereas in papilledema, the staining disk often shows feathery leakage into the adjacent nerve fiber layer
  ii. *Autofluorescence:* Drusen show autofluorescence when viewed with 430 nm wavelength (blue) light source using a yellow filter
  iii. *Computed tomography (CT) scan:* Drusen show mineralization
  iv. *Ultrasonography:* Drusen reflect sound waves

Differentiating drusen from early *papilledema* poses a diagnostic challenge.

Drusen have the following features:
  i. Absent optic cup
  ii. Disk has a pink/yellow color, and margin has a "lumpy" appearance.
  iii. Emerging vessels show anomalous premature branching
  iv. Autofluorescence

15. What are the features of myelinated nerve fibers?
  i. Myelination of the optic nerve begins in the fetus, approaching the optic chiasm by about 7 months of gestation
  ii. Myelination stops usually at lamina cribrosa at about 1 month of age and is complete by about 10 months after birth
  iii. In approximately 0.5% of population, myelination continues past the optic disk and into the nerve fiber layer of the retina
  iv. Characteristically, myelinated nerve fibers are white and feathered at the edges
  v. They do not have any effect on visual fields, but the blind spot may be enlarged.

7.8 ANTERIOR ISCHEMIC OPTIC NEUROPATHY

1. **Define anterior ischemic optic neuropathy (AION).**
   Anterior ischemic optic neuropathy is defined as the segmental or generalized infarction within the prelaminar or laminar portion of the optic nerve. It is caused by occlusion of the short posterior ciliary arteries.

2. **Give the clinical classification of AION.**
   i. Arteritic AION (AAION)
   ii. Nonarteritic AION (NAION)

3. **What are the risk factors for NAION?**
   Risk factors:
   i. Nicotine smokers
   ii. Diabetes (diabetic papillopathy—common in juvenile diabetics)
   iii. Hypertensives and patients with migraine—longstanding hypertension (HTN) is thought to affect the autoregulation of blood flow to the optic nerve head
   iv. Hypercholesterolemia
   v. Cerebrovascular disease
   vi. Carotid artery disease
   vii. Acute severe blood loss
   viii. Uremia
   ix. Favism resulting in an acute hemolytic anemia
   x. Nocturnal hypotension
   xi. Elevated intraocular pressure (IOP)
   xii. Uncomplicated cataract extraction
   xiii. Rarely associated with cavernous sinus thrombosis and radiation optic neuropathy

4. **What is the pathogenesis of NAION?**
   Nonarteritic anterior ischemic optic neuropathy is thought to be caused by vascular insufficiency. This hypothesis is supported by the following facts. Abrupt onset of visual loss, which is typical of a vascular disease:
   i. Common in older patients with systemic vasculopathies
   ii. Closure of small blood vessels in histopathology specimens
   iii. Lack of evidence of inflammation

   The prelaminar and laminar portions of the optic nerve are supplied by an elliptical arterial circle called Zinn's corona or Haller's circle, formed by the anastomosis around the optic nerve between medial and lateral paraoptic short posterior ciliary arteries. The ellipse is divided into superior and inferior parts by the entry points of the lateral and medial short posterior ciliary arteries, providing an attitudinal blood supply to the anterior optic nerve. Reduced perfusion pressure within the territory of the paraoptic branches of the short posterior ciliary arteries results in an altitudinal visual field loss.

Optic disks of patients with AION are usually small with little or no physiologic cupping. A small cup-to-disk ratio implies a small optic disk diameter and small scleral canal, resulting in crowding of nerve fibers through a restricted space in the lamina cribrosa. The ischemia in AION causes axoplasmic flow stasis, which causes compression of the capillaries within this crowded disk resulting in further ischemia.

Hence, the "disk at risk" is one with:
  i. Small physiologic cup
  ii. Elevation of disk margins by a thick nerve fiber layer
  iii. Anomalies of blood vessel branching
  iv. Crowded and small optic nerve head

Blood flow to the optic nerve head is directly proportional to the perfusion pressure and inversely proportional to the vascular resistance in the blood vessels. Vascular resistance is influenced by the blood vessel wall changes, which are affected in disease states such as HTN, diabetes mellitus, arteriosclerosis, and vasospasm.

5. **What are the clinical features of NAION?**
   i. Affects patients between 45 and 70 years of age
   ii. Patients present with monocular sudden painless visual loss. Two-thirds of cases have a moderate to severe impairment, and one-third of cases are spared or have minimal visual impairment
   iii. Diminished color perception. The degree of color vision loss is directly related to the amount of visual acuity loss (as opposed to patients with optic neuritis, where color vision is significantly impaired despite minimal loss of visual acuity)
   iv. Visual field defects are most often in the form of inferior altitudinal defects, which spare fixation. Other field defects such as central scotomas, arcuate defects, quadrantic defects, and generalized constriction may also occur
   v. Relative afferent pupillary defect
   vi. On ophthalmoscopic examination, there may be:
      – Focal or diffuse disk swelling
      – Disk may be pale or hyperemic
      – May have splinter hemorrhages at the disk margin

About 7% of cases have been associated with hard exudates in a star pattern at the macula, which may be misdiagnosed as neuroretinitis.

Focal hyperemic telangiectatic vessels may appear on the optic disk of an eye with NAION within days or weeks of onset of symptoms. This phenomenon is called luxury perfusion—a vascular autoregulatory response to ischemia.

Disk swelling resolves in 1-2 months with the development of optic atrophy but with no cupping and attenuated vessels.

6. **What are the investigations used in NAION?**
    i. Erythrocyte sedimentation rate (ESR)
    ii. C-reactive protein
    iii. Serum lipids
    iv. Blood glucose
    v. Packed cell volume and
    vi. Fibrinogen levels

7. **What is the treatment for NAION?**
    No therapy is of significant benefit.
    Medical therapy:
    i. Underlying systemic conditions should be treated
    ii. Patients should discontinue smoking
    iii. Antiplatelet agents and anticoagulants have been tried
    iv. Steroids–their role is controversial

    Surgical therapy:
    i. Stellate ganglion block
    ii. Optic nerve sheath decompression (ONSD)

    The Ischemic Optic Neuropathy Decompression Trial:
    i. It is a multicenter prospective study of NAION
    ii. The primary objective of this study was to assess the safety and efficacy of ONSD versus careful observation of patients with NAION. The secondary objectives were documentation of the natural history of the disease, identification of risk factors, and assessment of the contralateral eye risk as well as other nonocular vasoocclusive events
    iii. The study found that 42.7% of patients, on careful observation at 6 months, showed an improvement in visual acuity by three lines or more, while 45% experienced little or no change
    iv. In the patients who underwent ONSD, only 32.6% of patients had an improved visual acuity of three lines or more, while 43.5% experienced little or no change
    v. Hence, ONSD did not appear to be effective in the management of NAION
    vi. ONSD group also studied the role of aspirin in NAION and concluded that its role in the prevention of NAION is still unclear

8. **What are the causes of AAION?**
    i. Giant cell arteritis (GCA) or temporal arteritis (most common cause type of AAION)
    ii. Rheumatoid arthritis

iii. Herpes zoster virus (HZV) infection
iv. Relapsing polychondritis
v. Takayasu's arteritis
vi. Behcet's disease
vii. Polyarteritis nodosa
viii. Systemic lupus erythematosus
ix. Churg-Strauss angiitis

9. **What are the clinical features of AAION?**
    i. Sudden monocular profound loss of vision, which is preceded by transient visual obscurations and flashes of light
    ii. Bilateral involvement may occur
    iii. Periocular pain may or may not occur
    iv. Patients have pale swollen disks with splinter hemorrhages. The disks typically look chalky white. The disk edema resolves, leaving behind a markedly cupped disk

10. **What are the ocular features of GCA?**
    i. Amaurosis fugax
    ii. Central retinal artery occlusion (CRAO)
    iii. AION
    iv. Choroidal infarcts
    v. Cotton-wool spots
    vi. Anterior segment ischemia
    vii. Hypotony
    viii. Conjunctival and episcleral congestion
    ix. Corneal edema
    x. Extraocular muscle ischemia
    xi. Oculomotor nerve palsy
    xii. Ophthalmic artery occlusion
    xiii. Cortical blindness

11. **What are the systemic manifestations of GCA?**
    i. Malaise
    ii. Weight loss, depression, and fever
    iii. Polymyalgia rheumatica—stiffness and pain of proximal muscle groups in the morning and after exertion
    iv. Jaw claudication
    v. Headache
    vi. Palpable, nodular, and nonpulsatile temporal artery
    vii. Anemia
    viii. Myocardial infarction
    ix. Stroke
    x. Renal failure

12. **How do you diagnose AAION?**
    i. ESR—normal in 20% of cases, usually >50 mm/h (by Westergren's method). Age-related normal for males is age $\dfrac{mm/h}{2}$ and for females is age + $\dfrac{10\ mm/h}{2}$
    ii. C-reactive protein—raised
    iii. Fluorescein angiography—delayed or absent filling of the choroidal circulation
    iv. Alkaline phosphate level in serum—raised
    v. ANA—positive
    vi. Temporal artery biopsy:
        - Gives a definitive diagnosis
        - A 3 cm long specimen should be taken as skip lesions are evident.

    Occult GCA: Ocular involvement without associated signs and symptoms but with raised ESR and temporal artery biopsy positive for GCA.

13. **How do you treat AAION?**

    Systemic steroids are the mainstay of treatment. The treatment protocol is as follows:

    $$\left.\begin{array}{c} \text{IV methyl prednisolone 1 - 2g/day} \\ + \\ \text{Tab prednisolone 80 mg/day} \end{array}\right\} \text{for 3 day}$$

    Then,
    Tablet prednisolone   60 mg × 3 days
    　　　　　　　　　　　40 mg × 4 days

    Taper by 5 mg/week till 10 mg/day

    Maintenance dose of 10 mg/day for 12 months

    Throughout the treatment, the signs, symptoms, and ESR are monitored.

7.9 OCULOMOTOR NERVE

1. **Enumerate the salient features in the embryology of the third nerve.**
    i. The third nerve develops in the cranial portion of the neural tube from the most medial row of neuroblasts, the somatic efferent column
    ii. The third nerve nucleus becomes visible at the 8-9 mm stage

2. **What are the functional components of the third nerve?**
    i. Somatic efferent—fibers to extraocular muscles (EOM)
    ii. General somatic afferent—carries proprioceptive impulses from these muscles
    iii. General visceral efferent—parasympathetic supply to eye

3. **Describe the anatomy of the third nerve nucleus.**
    Location: Midbrain at the level of the superior colliculus.
    Dimension: Longitudinal column of large multipolar neurons, 10 mm in length, in the floor of cerebral aqueduct.
    Relations: Above, it extends as far as the floor of the third ventricle. Below, it is related to the nucleus of the trochlear nerve.
    Blood supply: The nuclei and the fascicles are supplied by the median group of arteries that arise from the bifurcation of basilar artery at the origin of superior cerebellar and posterior cerebral arteries.

4. **What are the components of the third nerve nucleus?**
    i. Principal nucleus
    ii. Edinger-Westphal (EW) nucleus dorsal to the principal nucleus

5. **What is Warwick's classification of principal nucleus?**

Nucleus	Muscle supplied
• Dorsolateral	• Inferior rectus
• Intermediate	• Inferior oblique
• Ventromedian	• Medial rectus
• Paramedian	• Superior rectus
• Caudal central	• Levator palpebrae superioris (LPS)

6. **Which nucleus has contralateral innervation, and what is its significance in diagnosis?**
    Fibers from paramedian group nucleus are partly crossed and supply the contralateral superior rectus. Therefore, a nuclear third nerve palsy of one side causes a paresis of contralateral superior rectus.

7. **Which nucleus is unpaired and has a bilateral supply?**
    Both LPS muscles are supplied by a single midline caudal subnucleus. Lesion that damages this region thus produces a bilateral symmetric ptosis.

Some lesions of the oculomotor nuclear complex may spare this region, causing a fixed dilated pupil and ophthalmoparesis but no ptosis.

8. **Describe the anatomy of EW nucleus.**
    i. The EW nucleus is made up of small multipolar neurons
    ii. It consists of two lateral components and a medial component united anteriorly
    iii. Anterior part of median component and lateral components are parasympathetic
    iv. Cranial half of this is concerned with light reflexes
    v. Caudal half is concerned with accommodation reflex
    vi. Posterior part of the EW nucleus is forked and was previously erroneously termed as convergence nucleus of Perlia

    The nucleus for the proprioceptive fibers is situated in the trigeminal nerve nuclear complex. They reach the nucleus either through communication to the ophthalmic nerve in the cavernous sinus or through connections between the oculomotor nucleus and the mesencephalic nucleus of the trigeminal nerve.

9. **Describe the blood supply of the third nerve.**
    i. In the subarachnoid space, the nerve receives vascular twigs from the posterior cerebral artery, superior cerebellar artery, and the tentorial and dorsal meningeal branches of the meningohypophyseal trunk of the internal carotid artery
    ii. In cavernous sinus, the tentorial, dorsal meningeal, and inferior hypophyseal branches of the meningohypophyseal trunk supply the nerve along with branches from the ophthalmic artery

10. **Describe the topographic arrangement of fibers within the third nerve.**
    i. Within the subarachnoid space, pupillomotor fibers appear to be located superficially in the superior portion of the nerve. The fibers in this portion of the third nerve are arranged in a superior and inferior division
    ii. Within the cavernous sinus and orbit, the pupillary fibers are located in the inferior division of the nerve. The position of the fibers going to the specific EOM is unknown

11. **What are the muscles supplied by the third nerve?**
    i. The superior division innervates the:
        - Superior rectus
        - LPS
    ii. The inferior division innervates the:
        - Inferior rectus
        - Medial rectus

- Inferior oblique
- Sphincter muscle of the iris (pupil)
- Ciliary muscle (accommodation)

12. **What is ciliary ganglion?**
    Ciliary ganglion is a peripheral parasympathetic pinhead size ganglion situated at the apex of the orbit, between the optic nerve medially and the lateral rectus laterally, in the central surgical space.

13. **What are the various roots of the ciliary ganglion?**
    i. Parasympathetic root is a branch from the nerve to the inferior oblique, carrying preganglionic fibers from EW nucleus
    ii. Sympathetic root carries postganglionic fibers from the superior cervical sympathetic ganglion
    iii. Sensory root is a twig from nasociliary nerve

14. **What are the types of third nerve palsies?**
    i. Congenital
    ii. Acquired

15. **What are the causes of congenital third nerve palsies?**
    i. *Aplasia* or hypoplasia of the third nerve nucleus
    ii. *Birth trauma:* It is due to the damage to the subarachnoid portion of the third nerve, either at its exit from the brainstem or just before it enters the cavernous sinus
    iii. *Syndromes associated with congenital third nerve palsy:*
        - *Congenital adduction palsy with synergistic divergence:* Patients with this syndrome have congenital unilateral paralysis of adduction associated with simultaneous bilateral adduction on attempted gaze into the field of action of the paretic medial rectus muscle
        - *Vertical retraction syndrome:* The main features are limitation of movement of the affected eye on elevation or depression associated with a retraction of the globe and narrowing of the palpebral fissure
        - Oculomotor nerve paresis with cyclic spasms

16. **What are the various levels at which third nerve can be affected in an acquired palsy?**
    At the level of:
    i. Oculomotor nucleus
    ii. Oculomotor nerve fascicle
    iii. In the subarachnoid space
    iv. At or near the entrance to the cavernous sinus

v. Within the cavernous sinus
vi. Within the supraorbital fissure
vii. Within the orbit
viii. Uncertain or variable location

17. **What are the causes of third nerve palsy?**
    Any focally destructive lesion along the course of the third cranial nerve can cause oculomotor nerve palsy or dysfunction. Some of the most frequent causes include the following:
    i. *Nuclear portion:*
       - Infarction
       - Hemorrhage
       - Neoplasm
       - Abscess
    ii. *Fascicular midbrain portion:*
       - Infarction
       - Hemorrhage
       - Neoplasm
       - Abscess
    iii. *Fascicular subarachnoid portion:*
       - Aneurysm
       - Infectious meningitis—bacterial, fungal/parasitic, and viral
       - Meningeal infiltrative
       - Carcinomatous/lymphomatous/leukemic infiltration, granulomatous inflammation (sarcoidosis, lymphomatoid granulomatosis, and Wegener granulomatosis)
    iv. *Fascicular cavernous sinus portion:*
       - Tumor—pituitary adenoma, meningioma, craniopharyngioma, and metastatic carcinoma
       - Vascular
       - Giant intracavernous aneurysm
       - Carotid artery—cavernous sinus fistula
       - Carotid dural branch—cavernous sinus fistula
       - Cavernous sinus thrombosis
       - Ischemia from microvascular disease in vasa nervosa
       - Inflammatory—Tolosa-Hunt syndrome (idiopathic or granulomatous inflammation)
    v. *Fascicular orbital portion:*
       - Inflammatory—orbital inflammatory pseudotumor, orbital myositis
       - Endocrine (thyroid orbitopathy)
       - Tumor (e.g., hemangioma, lymphangioma, and meningioma)

18. **What is the most common cause of isolated third nerve palsy with pupillary involvement?**
    Intracranial aneurysms

19. **What are the investigations for a third nerve palsy?**
    i. *Basic investigations:*
       - Blood sugar
       - Blood pressure
       - Lipid profile
       - Erythrocyte sedimentation rate (ESR)—to rule out giant cell arteritis
    ii. *X-ray skull lateral view*—to rule out sellar lesions involving the cavernous sinus
    iii. In complicated third nerve palsies where other neural structures are involved, have the patient undergo a magnetic resonance imaging (MRI)/magnetic resonance angiography (MRA)
    iv. In isolated third nerve palsies with no pupillary involvement where the patient is over 50 years, MRI scanning, an ischemic vascular evaluation, and daily pupil evaluation are indicated
    v. If the patient is under 50 years and has a nonpupillary involved isolated third nerve palsy, intracranial angiography is indicated since ischemic vasculopathy is less likely to occur in this age group than aneurysm. In the majority of cases, it can pick aneurysms >3 mm in size
    vi. Cerebral *angiography*—angiography is the definitive test for berry aneurysm in all intracranial locations. If the adult patient of any age presents with a complete or incomplete isolated third nerve palsy with pupillary involvement, consider this to be a medical emergency and have the patient undergo intracranial angiography immediately [computed tomography (CT) angiography or magnetic resonance angiography (MRA)]. In these cases, the cause is likely subarachnoid aneurysm, and the patient may die if the aneurysm ruptures
    vii. Children under the age of 14 rarely have aneurysms; the majority of third nerve palsies in this age group are traumatic or congenital
    viii. Lumbar puncture—the main purpose of lumbar puncture is to demonstrate the presence of blood in cerebrospinal fluid, an inflammatory reaction, neoplastic infiltration, or infection
    ix. Cytologic examination of cerebrospinal fluid is used to diagnose meningeal carcinomatosis and lymphomatous or leukemic infiltration

20. **How do aneurysms affect the third nerve, and what is the most common site?**
    i. Aneurysms usually arise from the junction of internal carotid and posterior communicating arteries
    ii. In its course toward the cavernous sinus, the third nerve travels lateral to the posterior communicating artery and may be injured by:
       - Direct compression
       - Hemorrhage
       - Major rupture
       - During aneurysm surgery

21. **Why are pupillary fibers spared in ischemic lesions and more commonly affected in compressive lesions?**
    The pupillomotor fibers are arranged in the outer layers of the third nerve and are therefore closer to the nutrient blood supply enveloping the nerve. So, they are spared in 80% of ischemic lesions, but being outer, they are affected in 95% of compressive lesions.

22. **Why is the third nerve more commonly affected in cavernous sinus lesions?**
    The third nerve is firmly attached to the dura adjacent to the posterior clinoid process just posterior to the cavernous sinus, so is more vulnerable to:
    i. Stretch
    ii. Contusion injuries
    iii. Frontal head trauma
    iv. Aneurysms
    v. Surgery in the perisellar region

23. **What are the causes of painful third nerve palsy with pupil involvement?**
    i. Posteriorly draining, low-flow carotid-cavernous fistula
    ii. Tumors
    iii. Compressive lesions—aneurysms of posterior cerebral and basilar vessels
    iv. Intrinsic lesions of the third nerve—schwannomas and cavernous angiomas

24. **How can you demonstrate whether the fourth nerve is involved in the situation of a third nerve palsy?**
    The patient is asked to abduct the eye and then look down. If the fourth nerve is functioning, the eye should intort.

25. **Localization of third nerve lesions and clinical manifestations.**

Structure involved	Clinical manifestations
Lesions affecting oculomotor nucleus:	
1. Oculomotor nucleus	• Ipsilateral complete third palsy. • Contralateral ptosis and superior rectus paresis
2. Oculomotor subnucleus	Isolated muscle palsy (inferior rectus)
3. Isolated levator subnucleus	Isolated bilateral ptosis
4. Paramedian mesencephalon	Plus minus syndrome (ipsilateral ptosis and contralateral eyelid retraction)
Lesions affecting oculomotor fascicles:	
1. Isolated fascicle	Partial or complete third nerve palsy with or without pupillary involvement
2. Fascicle and superior cerebellar peduncle	Ipsilateral third nerve palsy with contralateral ataxia and tremor (Claude's syndrome)
3. Fascicle and cerebral peduncle	Ipsilateral third nerve palsy with contralateral hemiparesis
4. Fascicle and red nucleus/substantia nigra	Ipsilateral third nerve palsy with contralateral choreiform movements (Benedict's syndrome)

26. **What are the features of nuclear third nerve palsy?**
    i. Ptosis—always bilateral
    ii. Mydriasis and cycloplegia—always bilateral
    iii. Contralateral superior rectus paresis or bilateral superior rectus paresis
    iv. Incomplete involvement of different subnuclei
    v. Bilateral total third nerve palsy can happen without ptosis

27. **How does fascicular third nerve palsy present?**
    Damage to fascicular or subarachnoid portion of the third nerve presents as:
    i. Isolated pupillary dilation with reduced light reaction
    ii. Ophthalmoplegia with or without pupillary involvement

28. **What are the factors responsible for third nerve palsy in hippocampal gyrus herniation?**
    i. Direct compression of the third nerve
    ii. Mechanical stretching of the third nerve
    iii. Shifting of basal arteries with herniating brainstem—posterior cerebral arteries drawn tightly across the dorsal surface of the third nerve

29. What is Hutchinson's pupil?

Dilation of one pupil when the other is contracted, resulting from compression of the third nerve due to:
 i. Meningeal hemorrhage at the base of the brain
 ii. Herniation of the uncus of the temporal lobe through the tentorial notch

The effect is caused by the pressure of the posterior cerebral artery on the superior surface of the oculomotor nerve where the pupillary fibers are concentrated.

30. What is sphenocavernous syndrome?

Sphenocavernous syndrome is characterized by paralysis or paresis of the third, fourth, and sixth nerves within the cavernous sinus or the superior orbital fissure.
 i. Associated with involvement of the first division of the fifth nerve
 ii. Optic nerve involvement can cause visual loss
 iii. Oculosympathetic paresis may lead to proptosis and edema of the eyelids and conjunctiva

31. What is pseudo-orbital apex syndrome?

Large intracranial masses may expand to such a degree that they compress the intracranial optic nerve or the cavernous portion of the third nerve and prevent adequate venous drainage from the orbit, resulting in pseudo-orbital apex syndrome.

32. Enumerate some common lesions causing sphenocavernous syndrome.

 i. Aneurysms
 ii. Meningiomas
 iii. Pituitary tumors
 iv. Craniopharyngiomas
 v. Nasopharyngeal tumors
 vi. Metastatic tumors
 vii. Infectious/inflammatory

33. What are the common causes of pupil-sparing third nerve palsy?

The most important cause is ischemia due to:
 i. Diabetes
 ii. Hypertension
 iii. *Atherosclerosis:*
   - Migraine
   - Systemic lupus erythematosus
   - Giant cell arteritis

34. **How can a pupil-sparing isolated third nerve palsy be investigated?**
    Ischemia laboratory workup:
    i. Blood pressure
    ii. Complete blood count
    iii. ESR
    iv. Blood sugar, glycosylated hemoglobin
    v. Venereal disease research laboratory (VDRL), fluorescent treponemal antibody absorption (FTA-ABS) [treponema pallidum hemagglutination assay (TPHA)]

35. **How long does it take for pupil-sparing palsy to recover?**
    Ischemic third nerve palsies resolve within 4–16 weeks without treatment, and the resolution is almost complete.

36. **What is aberrant regeneration of the third nerve or oculomotor synkinesis or misdirection syndrome?**
    Aberrant regeneration occurs as a consequence of complete third nerve palsy in which there is gross limitation of ocular movement amounting to virtual paralysis. The regenerating autonomic and voluntary nerve fibers grow along the wrong myelin tubes that contained functioning neurons before degeneration.

37. **Why is aberrant degeneration seen commonly in third nerve palsy?**
    The third nerve supplies a number of different muscles. The regenerating sprouts from axons that previously innervated one muscle group may ultimately innervate a different muscle group with a different function.

38. **What are the clinical presentations of aberrant regeneration of the third nerve?**
    i. *Lid-gaze dyskinesis:*
       - *Pseudo von Graefe sign:* Some of the nerve fibers to the interior rectus may end up innervating the elevator so that the lid retracts when the patient looks down
       - *Inverse Duane's syndrome:* Some of the medial rectus fibers may end up supplying some of the innervation to the levator so that the lid retracts when the patient adducts their eye
    ii. *Pupil-gaze dyskinesis:*
        Pseudo-Argyll Robertson pupil: Some of the medial rectus fibers may end up innervating the pupillary sphincter muscle so that there is more pupil constriction during convergence than as a response to light

39. **What are the two forms of aberrant regeneration?**
    i. *Primary:* No preceding third nerve palsy
    ii. *Secondary aberrant regeneration:* After third nerve palsy

40. What are the syndromes associated with third nerve palsy?

i. *Benedict's syndrome:* It involves the fasciculus as it passes through the red nucleus. It causes ipsilateral third nerve palsy and contralateral extrapyramidal signs

Level of lesion: Red nucleus

ii. *Weber's syndrome:* It involves the fasciculus as it passes through the cerebral peduncle. It causes ipsilateral third nerve palsy and contralateral hemiparesis

iii. *Nothnagel's syndrome:* It involves the fasciculus at the level of superior cerebellar peduncle. It causes ipsilateral third nerve palsy and cerebellar ataxia

iv. *Claude's syndrome*—combination of Benedict and Nothnagel's syndrome

v. *Uncal herniation syndrome*—a supratentorial space-occupying massive causes downward displacement and herniation of the uncus across the tentorial edge compressing the third nerve. A dilated and fixed pupil (Hutchinson's pupil) in a patient with altered consciousness may be the presenting feature

vi. *Orbital syndrome*—while crossing the superior orbital fissure any division of the third nerve may be affected causing paresis of structures innervated by them

vii. *Cavernous sinus syndrome*—occurs in association with fourth, fifth, and sixth nerves and oculosympathetic paralysis. Third nerve cavernous palsy is usually partial and pupil sparing

41. What is primary oculomotor nerve synkinesis?

Acquired oculomotor synkinesis may occur as a primary phenomenon without a preexisting acute third nerve palsy. The common causes are slowly growing tumors of:

i. Cavernous sinus meningioma, aneurysms, trigeminal schwannomas
ii. Subarachnoid space

42. What are the indications of neurological imaging in third nerve palsy?

i. All children <10 years irrespective of pupillary findings
ii. Children >10 years with pupil involvement
iii. If the pupil becomes dilated after 5-7 days of onset
iv. Multiple cranial nerves affected
v. No improvement is seen within 3 months.
vi. Signs of aberrant degeneration of the nerve develop
vii. Other neurological signs

43. How can third nerve palsy be managed?

Medical management:
   i. Medical management is watchful waiting since there is no direct medical treatment that alters the course of the disease. Nearly all patients undergo spontaneous remission of the palsy, usually within 6-8 weeks
   ii. Treatment during the symptomatic interval is directed at alleviating symptoms, mainly pain and diplopia
   iii. Nonsteroidal anti-inflammatory drugs (NSAIDs) are the first-line treatment of choice for the pain. Diplopia is not a problem when ptosis occludes the involved eye
   iv. When diplopia is from large-angle divergence of the visual axes, patching one eye is the only practical short-term solution
   v. When the angle of deviation is smaller, fusion in the primary position can often be achieved using horizontal or vertical prism, or both
   vi. Since the condition is expected to resolve spontaneously within a few weeks, most physicians would prescribe the Fresnel prism

Surgical management:
   i. For practical purposes, surgical care of third cranial nerve palsy includes clipping, gluing, coiling, or wrapping of the berry aneurysm by a neurosurgeon in the acute stage
   ii. Patients who do not recover from third cranial nerve palsy after 6-12 months may become candidates for eye muscle resection or recession to treat persistent and stable-angle diplopia
   iii. Some of these patients also may require some form of lid-lift surgery for persistent ptosis that restricts vision or is cosmetically unacceptable to the patient
   iv. *Neurosurgery:* Third cranial nerve palsy due to berry aneurysm, with or without concomitant subarachnoid hemorrhage, requires neurosurgical management in most cases
   v. *Ophthalmology:* The ophthalmologist provides symptomatic treatment for diplopia using:
      - Occlusion
      - Prism
      - Eye muscle surgery
      - Lid-lift procedures for ptosis
      - Botulinum toxin into the lateral rectus muscle
   vi. In treatment for nonresolving third nerve palsy due to diabetes mellitus (DM)—first correct the squint before correcting the ptosis (otherwise, there would be diplopia)

44. What are the indications of follow-up in third nerve palsy?
   i. Truly isolated palsy—which may be still evolving. Review within 2 weeks

ii. Age > 40 years
iii. History of diabetes or hypertension

45. For how long is surgical intervention deferred in third nerve palsy?
  i. Strabismus and lid surgeries can be considered after 6 months. Most ischemic palsies have complete recovery by 3 months (maximum 6 months)
  ii. In complete traumatic palsies, recovery is usually not complete, and surgical correction of squint is quite difficult

46. What are the differential diagnoses of third nerve palsy?
  i. Neuromuscular disease—myasthenia
  ii. Orbital diseases—myositis
  iii. Cavernous sinus lesions
  iv. Chronic meningitis
  v. Midbrain pathology

47. What are the differentiating features between concomitant/nonparalytic and nonconcomitant/paralytic squint?

Features	Paralytic squint	Nonparalytic squint
1. Onset	Usually sudden	Usually slow
2. Diplopia	Usually present	Usually absent
3. Ocular movements	Limited in the direction of paralyzed muscle	Full
4. False projection	*It is positive:* The patient cannot correctly locate the object in space when seeing in the direction of the paralyzed muscle in the early stages	Negative
5. Head posture	Particular head posture depending on the muscle paralyzed, may be present	Normal
6. Nausea and vertigo	Present	Absent
7. Secondary deviation	More than primary deviation	Equal to primary deviation
8. Pathological sequelae in muscles	Present	Absent

48. Daroff's rules for nuclear third nerve palsies
  i. Conditions that obligate nuclear involvement:
    - Bilateral third nerve palsy without ptosis (bilaterally spared LPS function)

- Unilateral third nerve palsy with contralateral superior rectus weakness and bilateral partial ptosis

ii. Conditions that exclude a nuclear lesion:
- Unilateral ptosis
- Unilateral internal ophthalmoplegia
- Unilateral external ophthalmoplegia associated with normal contralateral superior rectus function

iii. Conditions that neither exclude nor obligate a nuclear lesion:
- Bilateral total third nerve palsy
- Bilateral ptosis
- Bilateral internal ophthalmoplegia
- Bilateral medial rectus palsy.

7.10 FOURTH NERVE PALSY

1. **What are the peculiarities of the fourth nerve?**
   Trochlear nerve palsy is the most common cause of acquired vertical strabismus in the general population.
   i. It is the only cranial nerve to have a dorsal emergence
   ii. It has all the fibers crossed
   iii. It is the most slender cranial nerve
   iv. It has the longest intracranial course of all the cranial nerves (75 mm)

2. **Where is the nucleus of the fourth nerve located?**
   The nucleus of the fourth nerve is situated in the midbrain at the level of the inferior colliculus, anterolateral to cerebral aqueduct and dorsal to medial longitudinal bundle.

3. **What are the symptoms of fourth nerve palsy?**
   The symptoms of fourth nerve palsy are due to superior oblique palsy, which leads to:
   i. *Diplopia:* It can be vertical, some degree of horizontal and torsional. The last one is more pronounced on down gaze, i.e., in the field of action of the superior oblique muscle
   This, in turn, leads to symptoms like *asthenopia*, difficulty in walking down the stairs, and difficulty in reading
   ii. *Image tilting:* The image is tilted in the direction of the affected side. This symptom is rare in congenital palsy
   iii. *Anomalous head posture:* To prevent diplopia, the face is turned and the head is tilted toward uninvolved side, and the chin is depressed. This position places the eyes in a position where the cooperation of the affected muscle is not required

4. **How does one test involvement of the fourth nerve?**
   Bielschowsky's head tilt test: It is employed to diagnose paretic superior oblique as well as vertical rectus muscle in hypertropia.
   The three steps are:

   Step 1: Identify the type of hypertropia [right hypertropia (RHT) or left hypertropia (LHT)]

   Step 2: Identify whether vertical deviation increases on dextroversion or levoversion

   Step 3: Determine whether vertical deviation increases on tilting the head toward the right or left. If the hypertropia is due to weakness of one of the eighth vertically acting muscles, the paretic muscle is identified by answering these questions. Each step cuts possible number of muscles in half. After the last step, only one muscle remains

In a superior oblique paralysis, there is ipsilateral hypertropia, which increases on contralateral gaze and ipsilateral head tilt.

5. **How does one test involvement of the fourth nerve in the presence of third nerve palsy?**
    i. In presence of third nerve palsy, fourth nerve function is tested by asking the patient to depress the abducted eye and watching for intorsion
    ii. Isolated fourth nerve palsy can occur in ischemic conditions, e.g., diabetes mellitus and herpes zoster

6. **How does one test the torsional component of the fourth nerve?**
    i. *Double Maddox rod test:*
        - Done to quantify the torsional component of diplopia
        - >10° of torsion is suggestive of bilateral fourth nerve palsy
    ii. Landcaster's red-green test
    iii. Ophthalmoscopic examination
    iv. Hess's charting

7. **What are the differential diagnoses of vertical diplopia?**
    i. *Skew deviation:*
        - It is a vertical misalignment of visual axis
        - It may be transient, constant or alternating, concomitant or incomitant
        - It is due to imbalance of supranuclear inputs
        - It is associated with brainstem and cerebellar signs and symptoms
        - It is not associated with torsional diplopia or cyclodeviation
    ii. *Myasthenia gravis:*
        - It can involve isolated superior oblique and mimic fourth nerve palsy
        - It shows diurnal variation
        - It can involve other extraocular muscles
        - Tensilon test—positive
        - Electromyography (EMG) and acetylcholine (Ach) receptor antibodies—positive
    iii. *Thyroid ophthalmopathy:*
        - Other signs of hyperthyroidism are present
        - T_3 and T_4 levels—suggestive
        - In superior oblique palsy, the hypertropia is worse on *downgaze*, while in thyroid ophthalmopathy, it is worse on *upgaze*

8. **What are the causes of superior oblique paresis?**
    i. Fourth nerve palsy
    ii. Traumatic (may be bilateral)

iii. Vascular mononeuropathy
iv. Diabetic
v. Decompensated congenital paresis
vi. Posterior fossa tumor (rare)
vii. Cavernous sinus/superior orbital fissure syndromes
viii. Neurosurgical procedures
ix. Herpes zoster
x. Myasthenia gravis
xi. Graves' myopathy (fibrotic inferior oblique, superior rectus)
xii. Orbital inflammatory pseudotumor
xiii. Orbital injury to trochlea

9. **What are the syndromes associated with fourth nerve palsy?**
    i. *Nuclear-fascicular syndrome:* Distinguishing nuclear from fascicular lesions is virtually impossible due to the short course of fascicles within the midbrain
    Common etiologies are:
    - Hemorrhage
    - Infarction
    - Demyelination
    - Trauma
    ii. *Subarachnoid space syndrome:*
    Causes:
    - Trauma
    - Basal meningitis
    - Neoplasms like pinealomas and tentorial meningiomas and aneurysms
    - When bilateral-site-anterior medullary velum.
    - Associated signs and symptoms of the condition are present.
    iii. *Cavernous sinus syndrome:* Associated with other cranial nerve palsies like third, sixth, fifth, and ocular sympathetic paralysis
    iv. *Orbital syndrome:* It occurs due to trauma, inflammation, and tumors.
    It is seen in association with other cranial nerve palsies, e.g., third, fifth, and sixth. Associated orbital signs are proptosis, chemosis, and conjunctival injection.
    v. *Isolated fourth nerve palsy*
    - Congenital:
        - *Diagnostic keys:* Large vertical fusion amplitude (10–15 prism diopters)
        - Family album tomography (FAT) scan
    - Acquired:
        - In ischemic conditions, e.g., diabetes mellitus and herpes zoster

Neuro-ophthalmology

10. **Describe the management of superior oblique paresis.**

    Medical management:
    i. Primary aim is to *prevent diplopia* while waiting for spontaneous improvement
    ii. Occlusion of one eye with a patch or opaque contact lens can be done
    iii. Fresnel's prism can be used for vertical displacement
    iv. Treatment of diabetes and hypertension is done appropriately
    v. Evaluations at frequent intervals during waiting period
    vi. Role of botulinum toxin is controversial

    With this treatment, superior oblique function may:
    i. *Recover completely*, e.g., in cases of ischemia, closed injury, after relief of compression from tumor or aneurysm
    ii. *Recover incompletely*, leaving the patient with mild but persistent vertical diplopia, torsional diplopia, or both
    iii. *No recovery*, e.g., mesencephalic injury or transection of trochlear nerve

    Chances of further improvement after 6 months are rare.

    Surgical management:
    i. About 50% of patients require resurgery in future
    ii. The available options are:
    - Weaken the antagonist, i.e., weakening of ipsilateral inferior oblique
    - Weaken the yoke muscle, i.e., weakening of the contralateral inferior rectus
    - Weakening the ipsilateral superior rectus
    - Strengthening the superior oblique
    - More than one muscle surgery

11. **What is Knapp's classification?**

    The choice of surgery is decided by *Knapp's classification*. It depends on magnitude of hypertropia in the diagnostic positions of gaze. There are seven classes. For every class, a specific surgery is recommended.

    i. *Class 1:*
       - Hypertropia is greatest in adduction and elevation
       - Ipsilateral inferior oblique overaction is present. Treatment is inferior oblique myomectomy
    ii. *Class 2:*
       - Hypertropia is greatest in adduction and depression
       - Treatment is superior oblique tuck (8–12 mm) with recession of the contralateral inferior rectus as second procedure
    iii. *Class 3:*
       - Hypertropia is of equal magnitude in entire paralyzed field of gaze

- Treatment is ipsilateral inferior oblique myotomy
- If hypertropia is >25 prism diopters, it is combined with superior oblique tuck

iv. *Class 4:*
- Hypertropia is more in entire paralyzed field of gaze and in downgaze also
- Contracture of the ipsilateral superior rectus or contralateral inferior rectus
- Forced duction test is done
- Treatment is as in class 3 plus recession of ipsilateral superior rectus or contralateral inferior rectus

v. *Class 5:*
- Hypertropia is more in all downgazes
- Treatment is superior oblique tuck, recession of ipsilateral superior rectus, or contralateral inferior rectus

vi. *Class 6:*
- Bilateral fourth nerve palsy
- Treatment is as in classes 1–5, but bilateral surgery

vii. *Class 7:*
- Classic superior oblique paralysis associated with restriction of elevation in adduction (pseudo-Brown's syndrome)
- Cause is direct trochlear trauma.

7.11 ABDUCENS NERVE PALSY

1. **Location of the nucleus.**
   Its nucleus is located in the pons in the floor of the fourth ventricle, at the level of the facial colliculi.

2. **What are the causes of sixth nerve palsy?**
   Nonlocalizing:
   i. Increased intracranial pressure (ICP)
   ii. Intracranial hypotension
   iii. Head trauma
   iv. Lumbar puncture or spinal anesthesia
   v. Vascular, hypertension
   vi. Diabetes/microvascular
   vii. Parainfectious processes (postviral; middle ear infections in children)
   viii. Basal meningitis

   Localizing:
   i. Pontine syndromes (infarction, demyelination, tumor): Contralateral hemiplegia; ipsilateral facial palsy, ipsilateral horizontal gaze palsy (± ipsilateral internuclear ophthalmoplegia); ipsilateral facial analgesia
   ii. Cerebellopontine angle lesions (acoustic neuroma, meningioma): In combination with disorders of the eighth, seventh, and ophthalmic trigeminal nerves (especially corneal hypoesthesia), nystagmus, and cerebellar signs
   iii. Clivus lesions (nasopharyngeal carcinoma, clivus chordoma)
   iv. Middle fossa disorders (tumor, inflammation of medial aspect of petrous): Facial pain/numbness, ± facial palsy
   v. Cavernous sinus or superior orbital fissure (tumor, inflammation, aneurysm): In combination with disorders of the third, fourth, and ophthalmic trigeminal nerves (pain/numbness)
   vi. Carotid-cavernous or dural arteriovenous fistula

   Common causes of sixth nerve palsy:
   i. Collier's sphenoidal palsy
   ii. Superior orbital fissure syndrome
   iii. Arteriosclerosis
   iv. Hypertension
   v. Diabetes
   vi. Trauma and raised intracranial tension (ICT)

3. What are the clinical features of sixth nerve palsy?

Symptoms:

Horizontal diplopia—uniocular, painless, and increases on looking toward lateral side

An abnormality of the abducens nerve is the most likely cause of strictly horizontal double vision, especially if it is worse at a distance than near and worse on lateral gaze.

Signs:
  i. Limitation of abduction
  ii. Esotropia in primary position
  iii. Uncrossed diplopia
  iv. Slight face turns toward the side of diplopia

  All other ocular movements are normal.

  In early cases, secondary deviation is greater than primary deviation (nonconcomitant).

  Later, due to contractures developing in the ipsilateral antagonist, they become equal (concomitant).

  Still later, with the development of contractures in the contralateral synergist (with secondary underaction of antagonist of contralateral synergist), the primary deviation increases.

Uncrossed horizontal diplopia:
  i. Increases toward paralyzed side
  ii. Horizontal displacement of image
  iii. Vertical displacement also occurs due to increased effectiveness of obliques in adduction
  iv. Field of binocular vision constricted toward the affected side

4. What are the features seen on Hess charting?
  i. Enlargement toward the direction of action of ipsilateral antagonist medial rectus (MR) and opposite MR (contralateral synergist)
  ii. Contraction away from the direction of action of lateral rectus (LR) muscle of opposite eye (antagonist of contralateral synergist)
  iii. False projection outward toward the paralyzed side

5. What are the conditions that mimic the sixth nerve palsy?
  i. Thyroid ophthalmopathy
  ii. Myasthenia gravis
  iii. Medial wall orbital blowout fracture
  iv. Duane's syndrome (type 1)
  v. Mobius syndrome
  vi. Spasm of the near reflex
  vii. Essential infantile esotropia
  viii. Divergence paralysis
  ix. Post scleral buckling/squint surgery

6. **What are the syndromes associated with abducens nerve palsy?**
    i. *Brainstem syndrome:*
        - Brainstem lesion affecting the sixth nerve also affects the fifth, seventh, and eighth nerves
        - Structures in the lower pons affected by a lesion of the sixth nerve:
            - *Oculomotor sympathetic central neuron:* Ipsilateral Horner's syndrome
            - *Para pontine reticular fiber (PPRF):* Ipsilateral horizontal conjugate gaze palsy
            - *Medial longitudinal fascicle (MLF):* Ipsilateral internuclear ophthalmoplegia
            - *Pyramidal tract:* Contralateral hemiparesis
        - *Millard-Gubler syndrome:*
        Due to the lesion in the ventral paramedian pons. Clinical features:
            - Ipsilateral seventh nerve paresis
            - Ipsilateral sixth nerve paresis
            - Contralateral hemiparesis
        - *Raymond's syndrome:*
            - Ipsilateral sixth nerve paresis
            - Contralateral hemiparesis
        - *Foville's syndrome:*
        Due to the lesion in the pontine tegmentum
            - Horizontal conjugate gaze palsy
            - Ipsilateral Horner's syndrome
            - Ipsilateral fifth, sixth, seventh cranial nerve palsies
            - Ipsilateral paralysis of the abduction
    ii. *The subarachnoid space syndrome:*
        - *Vascular causes:* Compression of the nerve by atherosclerosis and aneurysm of the anterior inferior cerebellar artery, posterior inferior cerebellar artery, or the basilar artery
        - *Posterior fossa causes:* Space-occupying lesion (SOL) above the tentorium, posterior fossa tumors, structural anomalies, and head trauma
        Mechanism: All these causes lead to increased ICP, which leads to the downward displacement of the brainstem. This may cause stretching of the sixth nerve, which is tethered at its exit from the pons and in Dorello's canal. This gives rise to the "nonlocalizing" sixth nerve palsies of raised ICP
        - *Other causes:* Meningitis—often bilateral palsy
        Basal tumors: Like meningioma, chordoma, and Schwannoma
        After lumbar puncture—with or without raised ICP

iii. *Petrous apex syndromes:*
Contact with the petrous pyramid makes the portion of the sixth nerve within the Dorello's canal susceptible to pathologic processes affecting the petrous bone
- *Gradenigo's syndrome:*
At the Dorello's canal, the sixth nerve lies adjacent to mastoid air cells. So severe mastoiditis leading to inflammation of tip of the petrous bone causes inflammation of the sixth nerve. Mechanism is by the inflammatory involvement of the inferior petrosal sinus or pseudotumor cerebri leading to raised ICP with sixth nerve paresis.

In addition, the Gasserian ganglion and facial nerve are also nearby to the petrous apex, leading to the involvement of the fifth and seventh cranial nerves
Features:
  - Ipsilateral sixth nerve palsy
  - Ipsilateral decreased hearing
  - Ipsilateral facial pain in the distribution of the fifth nerve
  - Ipsilateral facial paralysis
- *Petrous bone fracture:*
Basal skull fractures following head trauma may involve the fifth, sixth, seventh, and eighth cranial nerves
Associated findings—hemotympanum, Battle's sign, cerebrospinal fluid (CSF) otorrhea
- *Pseudo-Gradenigo's syndrome:*
Lesions other than inflammation can involve petrous apex and produce symptoms suggestive of Gradenigo's syndrome
Causes:
  - Tumors/aneurysms of the intrapetrosal segment of the internal carotid artery (ICA)
  - Nasopharyngeal carcinoma
  - Cerebellopontine angle tumor-like acoustic neuroma
Mechanism:
The nasopharyngeal carcinoma extends through foramina at the base of the skull, spreading beneath the dura to damage the extradural portions of the fifth and sixth nerves.
The cerebellopontine angle tumor can cause:
  - Fifth, sixth, seventh, and eighth cranial nerves paralysis
  - Ataxia
  - Papilledema
- *Lateral sinus thrombosis or phlebitis:*
Leads to involvement of the inferior petrosal sinus causing sixth nerve palsy

iv. *The cavernous sinus syndrome:*
    The nerve runs within the body of the sinus, in close relation to the ICA. Some oculosympathetic fibers within the cavernous sinus leave the ICA and join briefly with the sixth nerve before joining the ophthalmic division of the fifth nerve
    This is responsible for the isolated sixth nerve palsy with ipsilateral Horner's syndrome
    Causes of the sixth nerve palsy in cavernous sinus lesion:
    - *Vascular:* ICA aneurysm, direct carotid-cavernous fistula, and dural carotid-cavernous fistula
    - *Neoplastic:* Meningioma, metastasis, pituitary adenoma, and Burkitt's lymphoma
    - *Inflammatory:* Granulomatous: Tuberculosis (TB), sarcoid Nongranulomatous: Sphenoid sinus abscess
v. *The orbital syndrome:*
    The nerve enters the orbit through the superior orbital fissure within the annulus of Zinn. The nerve supplies the LR muscle only a few millimeters from the superior orbital fissure. For this reason, isolated sixth nerve within the orbit is rare.
    Causes:
    - Intraorbital tumor
    - Orbital trauma
    - Inflammatory pseudotumor
    - Orbital cellulitis
vi. *Isolated sixth nerve palsy:*
    - *Benign transient isolated sixth nerve palsy:* It occurs rarely. In children, it is most often caused by viral illness and recent vaccination. In adults, it is most often caused by vascular lesions such as hypertension, diabetes mellitus (DM), and ischemic heart disease (IHD)
    - *Chronic isolated sixth nerve palsy:* Some patients do not recover spontaneously and have no obvious lesion despite an extensive evaluation

7. **How will you manage sixth nerve palsy?**
    i. Usually, it will recover spontaneously within 3-4 months, but sometimes recovery may take up to 1 year in case of traumatic etiology
    ii. If it does not recover, then some serious pathology like tumor, aneurysm, or stroke is often present. If the nerve palsy has not shown much improvement over 3-4 months, or if other cranial nerve involvement appears, then further evaluation is needed

iii. Correction of the strabismus—should not be considered until 8-10 months have passed without improvement unless it is known that the sixth nerve is no longer intact
iv. During this period, one can do occlusion of one eye either by patching or by using opaque contact lens. Children <8 years should undergo alternate patching of the eyes to prevent amblyopia
v. Prisms can be used for the correction of diplopia
vi. Chemodenervation of the antagonist MR muscle with botulinum toxin can be used. Strabismus surgery, whenever required, usually consists of either weakening of the ipsilateral MR combined with strengthening of the ipsilateral LR or some type of transposition procedure

8. **Which muscle is spared in retrobulbar block?**
Superior oblique as the trochlear nerve lies outside the muscle cone.

7.12 MYASTHENIA GRAVIS

1. **What is myasthenia gravis (MG)?**
   Myasthenia gravis is an acquired autoimmune disorder of neuromuscular transmission.

2. **What is the literal meaning of MG?**
   From Greek *Mys* = muscle and *asthenia* = weakness and Latin *gravis* = heavy or weighty

3. **What is the pathophysiology of MG?**
   Myasthenia gravis is an autoimmune disease in which antibodies are directed against postsynaptic acetylcholine receptors. There is a slight genetic predisposition: Particular human leukocyte antigen (HLA) types seem to be predisposed for MG (B8 and DR3 more specific for ocular myasthenia).

4. **What is the recent thought on the pathophysiology of MG?**
   It has recently been realized that a second category of gravis is due to autoantibodies against the MuSK (muscle-specific kinase) protein, a tyrosine kinase receptor that is required for the formation of the neuromuscular junction. Antibodies against MuSK inhibit the signaling of MuSK normally induced by its nerve-derived ligand, agrin. The result is a decrease in patency of the neuromuscular junction and the consequent symptoms of myasthenia.

5. **What is the source of antibody in myasthenia?**
   The antibodies are produced by plasma cells that have been derived from B cells. These plasma cells are activated by T helper cells. The thymus plays an important role in the development of T cells, which is why MG may be associated with thymoma.

6. **What is the role of the thymus gland in MG?**
   T helper cells, which have been activated in the thymus, probably stimulate the production of acetylcholine receptor autoantibodies. Up to 65-70% myasthenics have thymic hyperplasia with 5-20% incidence of thymoma.

7. **Does the level of acetylcholine receptor antibody titer correlate with the severity of the disease?**
   No. The level of the acetylcholine receptor antibody titer does not correlate well with the severity of the disorder.

8. **What are the symptoms of MG?**
   Ocular symptoms:
   i. Drooping of upper lid
   ii. Diplopia

Systemic symptoms:
  i. Weakness and fatigability of skeletal muscles
  ii. Mild generalized disease: Facial and bulbar muscles affected
  iii. Severe generalized disease: Impairment of respiration

9. **Classify MG.**
   The most widely followed classification of MG is that of Osserman, which is as follows:
   i. Ocular myasthenia
   ii. Generalized myasthenia:
     - *Mild generalized myasthenia:* Slow progression, no crisis, and responds well to drugs
     - *Moderately severe generalized myasthenia:* Severe skeletal or bulbar involvement but no crisis; response to drugs is less than satisfactory
   iii. *Acute fulminant myasthenia:* Rapid progression of clinical symptoms with respiratory crisis, poor response to drugs, high incidence of thymoma, and high mortality
   iv. *Late severe myasthenia:* Symptoms are same as in acute fulminating type. The difference is that the progression from class 1 to class 2 has occurred slowly, i.e., over 2 years

10. **What are the commonly involved muscles in myasthenia?**
    Muscles that control eye and eyelid movement, facial expression, chewing, talking, and swallowing are especially susceptible. The muscles that control breathing and neck and limb movements can also be affected. Often the physical examination is within normal limits.

11. **What is the reason for predilection for eye muscle?**
    There are several lines of thought:
    i. Slight weakness in a limb may be tolerated, but slight weakness in the extraocular muscles would lead to misalignment of the two eyes, even a small degree of which could lead to diplopia. Eyes may also be less able to adapt to variable weakness because extraocular muscles use visual rather than proprioceptive (body position sensing) cues for fine-tuning
    ii. Compared to extremity muscles, extraocular muscles are smaller, served by more nerve fibers, and are among the fastest-contracting muscles in the body. This higher level of activity may predispose them to fatigue in MG

12. **Which extraocular muscle is most commonly involved?**
    i. Medial recti are most commonly affected.
    ii. Myasthenic ophthalmoparesis can mimic any pupil-sparing ocular motility disorder.

13. **Why is the pupil and ciliary muscle unaffected?**
    Myasthenia involves skeletal and not visceral musculature, and therefore the pupil and ciliary muscles are unaffected.

14. **How do you examine a case of suspected ocular myasthenia?**
    Muscle fatigability can be tested for many muscles. A thorough investigation includes:
    i. *Looking upward and sideward for 30 seconds:* Ptosis and diplopia
    ii. *"Peek sign"*: After complete initial apposition of the lid margins, they quickly (within 30 seconds) start to separate, and the sclera starts to show

15. **What is ice pack test?**
    i. Cooling may improve neuromuscular transmission. In a patient with MG who has ptosis, placing ice (wrapped over a towel) over an eyelid will lead to cooling of the lid, which leads to improvement of the ptosis
    ii. A positive test is clear resolution of the ptosis, with at least >2 mm of improvement
    iii. The test is thought to be positive in about 80% of patients with ocular myasthenia

16. **What is lid fatigue test?**
    In this test, the patient is asked to keep looking up for several minutes and then observed for the appearance of worsening of ptosis.

17. **What is sleep test?**
    Resolution of ptosis or ophthalmoparesis after 30minute period of sleep, with reappearance of the sign 30 seconds to 5 minutes after awakening.

18. **What is enhanced ptosis?**
    With bilateral ptosis, enhanced ptosis may be seen, where one upper eyelid becomes more ptotic when the other upper eyelid is manually elevated. This phenomenon is explained by Hering's law of equal innervation to yoke muscles.

19. **What is Cogan's eyelid twitch?**
    When the patient looks down for at least 10-20 seconds and then makes an upward saccade back to primary gaze, a transient overshoot of the upper eyelid may be seen. This may be followed by nystagmoid twitches of the upper eyelid and then downward drifting of the eyelid to a normal or ptotic position. This is caused by rapid recovery on resting in downgaze and easy fatigability in upgaze of the myasthenic levator muscle.

20. **What are the blood tests done to diagnose MG?**
    If the diagnosis is suspected, serology can be performed in a blood test to identify antibodies against the acetylcholine receptor.

21. **What is repetitive nerve stimulation test?**
    i. Muscle fibers of patients with MG are easily fatigued. By repeatedly stimulating a muscle with electrical impulses, the fatigability of the muscle can be measured. This is called the repetitive nerve stimulation test
    ii. In single-fiber electromyography, which is considered to be the most sensitive (although not the most specific) test for myasthenia, a thin needle electrode is inserted into a muscle to record the electric potentials of individual muscle fibers. By finding two muscle fibers belonging to the same motor unit and measuring the temporal variability in their firing patterns (i.e., their "jitter"), the diagnosis can be made

22. **What is edrophonium test?**
    i. Edrophonium inhibits the enzyme acetylcholinesterase (which destroys acetylcholine in the neuromuscular junction), thereby increasing the available acetylcholine
    ii. Before the test, ptosis, ocular motility, and eye alignment should be assessed. Initially, atropine sulfate (0.6 mg) is given
    iii. *Dose of edrophonium:* 0.5-1.0 mg/kg
    iv. In adults—1-2 mg test dose is given, watch for positive response. If there is no improvement, the remaining 8-9 mg is given in increments of 0.1-0.2 cc and wait for 45-60 seconds between increments
    v. *Onset of action:* 30-60 seconds after IV injection
    vi. Effect resolves within 5 minutes.

23. **What is neostigmine test?**
    i. Neostigmine is a longer-acting antiacetylcholinesterase that can also be used similarly
    ii. *Dose:* 0.03 mg/kg or 1.0-1.5 mg intramuscularly, preceded by atropine 1 cc (0.6 mg) intramuscular (IM)

24. **What is the role of atropine in edrophonium test?**
    Atropine serves two purposes in the test:
    i. First, it counters the muscarinic side effects of edrophonium, especially cardiac arrhythmias
    ii. Second, placebo responders may improve with this alone

25. **What are the conditions that can give false positive responses in the edrophonium test?**
    i. Intracranial mass lesions
    ii. Orbital apex syndrome from metastasis
    iii. Multiple sclerosis
    iv. Amyotrophic lateral sclerosis
    v. Lambert-Eaton syndrome
    vi. Guillain-Barré syndrome

26. **What are the imaging tests done in MG?**
    i. Chest X-ray is frequently performed to diagnose:
       - Lambert-Eaton syndrome
       - Widening of the mediastinum suggestive of thymoma
    ii. Computed tomography (CT) or magnetic resonance imaging (MRI) are more sensitive ways to identify thymomas and are generally done for this reason

27. **How does the pulmonary function test help in monitoring of MG progression?**
    Spirometry (lung function testing) is done to assess respiratory function (FEV1), or the peak expiratory flow rate (PEFR) may be monitored at intervals in order not to miss a gradual worsening of muscular weakness.

28. **What is transient neonatal myasthenia?**
    In the long term, pregnancy does not affect MG. Up to 10% of infants with parents affected by the condition are born with transient (periodic) neonatal myasthenia (TNM), which generally produces feeding and respiratory difficulties. A child with TNM typically responds very well to acetylcholinesterase inhibitors. Immunosuppressive therapy should be maintained throughout pregnancy as this reduces the chance of neonatal muscle weakness, as well as controlling the mother's myasthenia.

29. **What are the myasthenic symptoms in children?**
    Three types of myasthenic symptoms in children can be distinguished:
    i. *Neonatal:* In 12% of pregnancies with a mother with MG, she passes the antibodies to the infant through the placenta, causing neonatal MG. The symptoms will start in the first 2 days and disappear within a few weeks after birth. With the mother, it is not uncommon for the symptoms to even improve during pregnancy, but they might worsen after labor
    ii. *Congenital:* Children of a healthy mother can, very rarely, develop myasthenic symptoms beginning at birth. This is called congenital myasthenic syndrome (CMS). CMS is not caused by an autoimmune process but due to synaptic malformation, which in turn is caused by genetic mutations. Thus, CMS is a hereditary disease. More than

11 different mutations have been identified, and the inheritance pattern is typically autosomal recessive

iii. *Juvenile:* Myasthenia occurring in childhood, but after the peripartum period.

The congenital myasthenia cause muscle weakness and fatigability similar to those of MG. The symptoms of CMS usually begin within the first 2 years of life, although in a few forms, patients can develop their first symptoms as late as the seventh decade of life. A diagnosis of CMS is suggested by the following:
- Onset of symptoms in infancy or childhood
- Weakness which increases as muscles tire
- A decremental electromyography (EMG) response, on low frequency, of the compound muscle action potential (CMAP)
- No anti-acetylcholine receptor (AChR) or MuSK antibodies
- No response to immunosuppressant therapy
- Family history of symptoms that resemble CMS

30. What are the various autoimmune diseases associated with MG?

Myasthenia gravis is associated with various autoimmune diseases, including:
  i. Thyroid diseases, including Hashimoto's thyroiditis and Graves' disease
  ii. Diabetes mellitus type 1
  iii. Rheumatoid arthritis
  iv. Lupus and demyelinating central nervous system (CNS) diseases

Seropositive and "double-seronegative" patients often have thymoma or thymic hyperplasia. However, anti-MuSK positive patients do not have evidence of thymus pathology.

31. What is the management of MG?

Symptomatic therapy:

Acetylcholinesterase inhibitors: Neostigmine and pyridostigmine can improve muscle function by slowing the natural enzyme cholinesterase that degrades acetylcholine in the motor end plate; the neurotransmitter is therefore around longer to stimulate its receptor. Usually, one can start with a low dose, e.g., 3 × 20 mg pyridostigmine, and increase until the desired result is achieved. If taken 30 minutes before a meal, symptoms will be mild during eating. Side effects, like perspiration and diarrhea, can be countered by adding atropine. Pyridostigmine is a short-lived drug with a half-life of about 4 hours.

Disease-modifying therapy:
  i. *Medical:*
      - *Immunosuppressive drugs:* Prednisone, cyclosporine, mycophenolate mofetil, and azathioprine may be used

- Treatments with some immunosuppressives take weeks to months before effects are noticed
 ii. *Surgical:*
    - Thymectomy, the surgical removal of the thymus, is essential in cases of thymoma in view of the potential neoplastic effects of the tumor
    - It is usually indicated in all patients with myasthenia

32. **What is the role of steroids in the treatment of MG?**
Steroids are useful in inducing remission. However, because of the possible side effects, the treatment with steroids is reserved for severe cases.

33. **What are the drugs exacerbating the symptoms of myasthenia?**
The adverse effects of many medications may provoke exacerbations; therefore, carefully obtaining a medication history is important. Some of the medications reported to cause exacerbations of myasthenia include the following:
 i. *Antibiotics:* Macrolides, fluoroquinolones, aminoglycosides, tetracycline, and chloroquine
 ii. *Antidysrhythmic agents:* β-blockers, calcium channel blockers, quinidine, lidocaine, procainamide, and trimethaphan
 iii. *Miscellaneous:* Diphenylhydantoin, lithium, chlorpromazine, muscle relaxants, levothyroxine, adrenocorticotropic hormone (ACTH), and paradoxically, corticosteroids

34. **What is cholinergic crisis?**
 i. One of the confusing factors in treating patients with MG is that insufficient medication (i.e., myasthenic crisis) and excessive medication (i.e., cholinergic crisis) can present in similar ways
 ii. Cholinergic crisis results from an excess of cholinesterase inhibitors (i.e., neostigmine, pyridostigmine, and physostigmine) and resembles organophosphate poisoning. In this case, excessive ACh stimulation of striated muscle at nicotinic junctions produces flaccid muscle paralysis that is clinically indistinguishable from weakness due to myasthenia
 iii. Myasthenic crisis or cholinergic crisis may cause bronchospasm with wheezing, bronchorrhea, respiratory failure, diaphoresis, and cyanosis
 iv. Miosis and the SLUDGE syndrome (i.e., salivation, lacrimation, urinary incontinence, diarrhea, gastrointestinal upset and hypermotility, emesis) may also mark cholinergic crisis. However, these findings are not inevitably present
 v. Despite muscle weakness, deep tendon reflexes are preserved

35. How is myasthenic crisis treated?

A myasthenic crisis occurs when the muscles that control breathing weaken to the point that ventilation is inadequate, creating a medical emergency and requiring a respirator for assisted ventilation. In patients whose respiratory muscles are weak, crises—which generally call for immediate medical attention—may be triggered by infection, fever, an adverse reaction to medication, or emotional stress.

If the myasthenia is serious (myasthenic crisis), plasmapheresis can be used to remove the putative antibody from the circulation. Also, intravenous immunoglobulins (IVIG) can be used to bind the circulating antibodies. Both of these treatments have relatively short-lived benefits, typically measured in weeks.

36. What are the complications in a patient with myasthenia?

i. Respiratory crisis
ii. Pulmonary aspiration
iii. Permanent muscle weakness
iv. Side effects related to medication used and surgery-related complications

37. What are the other ancillary treatment modalities for reducing ocular disabilities in other myasthenia?

i. *Ptosis:* It can be corrected with placement of crutches on eyeglasses, ptosis tape to elevate eyelid droop
ii. *Diplopia:* It can be addressed by occlusion with eye patching, frosted lens, occluding contact lens, or by simply placing opaque tape over a portion of eyeglasses, plastic prisms (Fresnel prisms)

38. What are the differences between MG and myopathy?

Features	MG	Myopathy
Ptosis	Asymmetrical	Symmetrical
Diplopia	Present	May or may not be present
Diurnal variation	Present	Absent
Fatigability	Present	Absent
Response to the stigmine	Positive	Negative
Clinical course	Variable characteristics	Slowly progressive
Other eye signs	Absent	Retinal pigment disturbance may be present
Age	Any age	Any age—under 20 suspect heart block

39. **Differential diagnosis of MG.**

    Prominent ocular signs:
    i. *Mitochondrial myopathy:* Progressive external ophthalmoplegia
    ii. Oculopharyngeal muscular dystrophy
    iii. Intracranial mass lesion
    iv. Senile ptosis

    Bulbar dysfunction:
    i. Motor neuron syndromes
    ii. Polymyositis
    iii. Thyroid disorders
    iv. Oculopharyngeal dystrophy

    Generalized MG:
    i. Lambert–Eaton syndrome
    ii. Botulism
    iii. Congenital myasthenic syndromes
    iv. Myopathies or muscular dystrophies.

7.13 NYSTAGMUS

1. **Define nystagmus.**
   Nystagmus is defined as a regular, rhythmic, involuntary, repetitive, to-and-fro movement of the eye.

2. **Classification of nystagmus.**
   Based on physiology and pathology:
   Physiological:
   i. End gaze
   ii. Optokinetic
   iii. Vestibulo-ocular reflexes (VOR)

   Pathological:
   i. Sensory deprivation (ocular)
   ii. Motor imbalance nystagmus
      - Congenital nystagmus
      - Spasmus nutans
      - Latent nystagmus
      - Ataxic nystagmus
      - Downbeat nystagmus
      - Upbeat nystagmus
      - Convergent refraction nystagmus
      - See-saw nystagmus of Maddox
      - Periodic alternating nystagmus

   Based on the type of nystagmus:
   i. Pendular
   ii. Jerk

   Based on direction of movement:
   i. Horizontal
   ii. Vertical
   iii. Rotatory

   Congenital/infantile:
   i. Acquired
   ii. Toxic/drug/metabolic
   iii. Neurological
   iv. Functional/voluntary

3. **What are the types of nystagmus?**
   There are different types depending upon:
   i. *Rate:* The number of to-and-fro movements in 1 second. It is described in hertz (Hz)
      - Slow (1–2 Hz)

- Medium (3-4 Hz)
- Fast (5 Hz or more)
ii. *Amplitude:*
- Fine (<5)
- Moderate (5-15°)
- Large (>15°)
iii. *Direction:*
- Horizontal
- Vertical
- Rotational
iv. *Movement:*
- Pendular
- Jerk

4. What is the anatomic basis of nystagmus?
The goal of the eye movement control system is to maintain images of objects steady on the retina to preserve visual acuity. The slow eye movement systems that provide this stability of images are:
i. Visual fixation
ii. Vestibular system
iii. Optokinetic system
iv. Neural integrator
v. Smooth pursuit system
vi. Vergence eye movement system

5. What are the main points in history-taking in nystagmus?
Following points should be asked in history-taking:
i. Present from birth or not
ii. Oscillopsia
iii. Vertigo
iv. Visual loss
v. Diplopia

6. What are the other movement disorders which can mimic nystagmus?
i. *Nystagmoid movements* are those that are not regular and rhythmic in nature
ii. *Ocular bobbing:* Fast downward movement of both eyes followed by a slow drift back toward mid position. It is usually seen in patients with severe brainstem dysfunction
iii. *Ocular dipping:* Slow downward movement of eyeball followed by delayed rapid upward movement and spontaneous roving horizontal eye movements

iv. *Ping pong gaze:* Slow roving horizontal conjugate movement from one extreme to the other occurring regularly or irregularly every few seconds. It is seen in acute diffused bilateral cerebral disease with intact brainstem
v. *Ocular dysmetria:* It is seen in cerebral disease
vi. *Ocular flutter:* Brief, horizontal, bilateral ocular oscillation occurring intermittently when the patient looks straight or changes his gaze. It is seen in certain cerebellar diseases
vii. *Opsoclonus:* It consists of large amplitude, involuntary, repetitive, unpredictable, conjugate, chaotic saccades in horizontal, vertical, and torsional planes. Its causes include organophosphorus poisoning, Epstein-Barr virus infection, and hypertension
viii. *Superior oblique/myokymia:* It consists of intermittent monocular torsional movement of one eyeball. It is associated with torsional diplopia. It responds to carbamazepine. It causes midbrain tectal tumors

7. **What are the two components of jerk nystagmus, and how is the direction defined?**
The two components are: a slow component in one direction and a fast one in the opposite direction. The direction is defined by the direction of the fast component as viewed by the patient.

8. **What is Alexander's law?**
Alexander's law states that the amplitude of jerk nystagmus is largest in the gaze of the direction of its fast component.

9. **What is null point?**
Null point is the position of gaze in which the nystagmus is lessened or totally absent.

10. **What are the causes of monocular nystagmus?**
    i. Strabismus
    ii. Amblyopia
    iii. Internuclear ophthalmoplegia

11. **What are the features of congenital nystagmus (manifest)?**
    i. Most common type (80%)
    ii. Present from birth
    iii. Binocular
    iv. Horizontal and pendular
    v. Remains horizontal even in vertical gaze
    vi. Disappears at one position—null point
    vii. Decreases on convergence, eye closure
    viii. Absent during sleep

ix. No oscillopsia, normal vision
x. Particular head posture
xi. Associated head oscillations may be there
xii. Inversion of optokinetic nystagmus

12. **What are the features of pendular nystagmus?**
    i. May have horizontal, vertical, and torsional component
    ii. May be congenital or acquired
    iii. Associated with visual problems
    iv. Most common cause being demyelination of the neural circuit known as the myoclonic triangle (the dentato-rubro-olivary pathways—associated with visual loss oscillopsia, palatal myoclonus)

13. **What are the features of gaze-evoked nystagmus?**
    i. Fast phase is toward the direction of gaze (up on looking up, down on looking down)
    ii. Amplitude may be greater toward the side of lesion
    iii. Drug-induced nystagmus tends to be minimal in downgaze

14. **What are the features of vestibular nystagmus?**
    i. Seen in primary position
    ii. Purely horizontal or horizontal rotatory
    iii. Fast component opposite to the side of lesion
    iv. Suppressed by visual fixation, increased when fixation is removed
    v. Intensity increases in the direction of fast phase (*Alexander's law*)
    vi. Associated vertigo, tinnitus

15. **What are the features of downbeat nystagmus?**
    i. Primary position nystagmus
    ii. Fast component downward
    iii. Oscillopsia often present and may precede
    iv. Best elicited by looking down and out
    v. Craniocervical junction lesions, e.g., Arnold-Chiari malformations and certain drugs

16. **What are the features of upbeat nystagmus?**
    i. Fast phase beats upward
    ii. Lesion in the posterior fossa—either brainstem or cerebellar vermis or some drugs

17. **What are the features of seesaw nystagmus (of Maddox)?**
    i. Primary position nystagmus worsens on downgaze
    ii. One eye elevates as well as intorts, while the other eye descends and extorts
    iii. Site of lesion is parasellar, parachiasmal

18. What are the features of Bruns nystagmus?
   i. A combination of large amplitude, low-frequency horizontal nystagmus on looking to the ipsilateral side (due to cerebellar component) and small amplitude, high-frequency nystagmus on looking contralaterally and in primary position (due to vestibular component)
   ii. Often seen in tumors of cerebellopontine angle

19. What are the features of optokinetic nystagmus?
It is a normal nystagmus that results when a person gazes at a succession of objects moving past in one direction; for example, gazing from a fast-moving train. The nystagmus is always in the direction opposite to the direction of movement of the object.

20. What is the significance of eliciting optokinetic nystagmus?
   i. To test the presence of some vision (in malingering and children)
   ii. To test the integrity of the horizontal and vertical gaze centers for saccadic and pursuit movements
   iii. To differentiate homonymous hemianopia of occipital cortical lesion from that of a lesion of optic radiation and adjacent opticomotor pathway (parietal lobe lesion). (In parietal lobe lesions, it will be lost due to disruption of the smooth pursuit pathways.)

21. How will you detect the side of the parietal lobe lesion by demonstrating optokinetic nystagmus?
Nystagmus will be absent or defective when the targets are moved toward the side of the lesion, i.e., away from hemianopia. This is called positive optokinetic nystagmus sign and suggests a parietal lobe lesion, usually a neoplasm.

22. What is latent nystagmus?
It is a type of congenital jerk nystagmus that occurs during fixation when one eye is covered. This is frequently associated with strabismus.

23. What is spasmus nutans?
   i. Spasmus nutans is a triad of nystagmus, head nodding, and torticollis
   ii. Onset is between 4 months and 1 year and lasts for 1–4 years
   iii. It indicates serious neurological problem
   iv. It has vertical and torsional components

24. How do you clinically differentiate congenital nystagmus from others?
A good rule is that horizontal nystagmus that remains horizontal even on vertical gaze is always congenital nystagmus until proved otherwise.

25. **How do you induce caloric nystagmus?**
   Cold or warm water is irrigated into the external auditory canal. With cold water, the fast phase will be in opposite direction, while with warm water, the fast phase will be in the same direction. *"COWS"* (Cold Opposite Warm Same).

26. **What should be the position of the patient to show caloric-induced nystagmus?**
   The patient should be supine with the head bent forward by 30° so that the horizontal semicircular canals are almost horizontal in position.

27. **What is the significance of demonstrating caloric nystagmus?**
   i. To test the integrity of vestibular ocular system
   ii. To induce eye movement in patients who are incapable of moving them in response to command—either because of their state of consciousness or because of their orientation

28. **What are the degrees of nystagmus?**
   i. *1st degree:* Nystagmus only in the direction of fast component
   ii. *2nd degree:* Nystagmus also in primary position gaze
   iii. *3rd degree:* Nystagmus, in addition to the above two gazes, is also present in the direction of slow component

29. **What is the role of perinatal history in nystagmus?**
   History of intrauterine infection (rubella, *Toxoplasma*), maternal alcohol abuse or anticonvulsant drugs (optic nerve hypoplasia), and neonatal asphyxia or neonatal seizures (cerebral damage) is very helpful in case of nystagmus.

30. **What is the role of family history in nystagmus?**
   i. Most common X-linked
   ii. Autosomal dominant is also likely, but autosomal recessive is rare

31. **What are the treatment modalities in nystagmus?**
   i. *Optical aids:*
      - Prisms—to shift gaze into the null point
      - Soft contact lens—helps probably by stimulating trigeminal afferent, especially in congenital nystagmus
   ii. *Biofeedback:*
      - Training mechanism to decrease nystagmus—visual and auditory
   iii. *Medical modalities:*
      - Baclofen in acquired periodic alternating nystagmus
      - Clonazepam and anticholinergic in downbeat nystagmus
      - Memantine and gabapentin help in acquired pendular nystagmus.

Botulinum toxin:

Injected into the retrobulbar space or into the extraocular muscles in the better eye, especially in pendular nystagmus. There may be transient improvement in the visual acuity and oscillopsia. However, the side effects override the small and transient improvements.

iv. *Surgery:*

This helps correct the head posture by shifting the null point from an eccentric location to a straight-ahead position in visually disabling nystagmus.
- Kestenbaum–Anderson procedure:
  - By recession of horizontal muscles, the versions are blocked
- Faden operation:
  - Acts like a recession by creation of a more posterior attachment, first reducing the area of contact.

7.14 VISUAL FIELDS IN NEURO-OPHTHALMOLOGY

1. **What is the purpose of perimetry in neuro-ophthalmology?**
    i. To detect generalized or focal defects in the island of vision that may identify the location of pathology affecting the visual pathways
    ii. To aid in differential diagnosis since different pathologies may produce different kinds of field defects
    iii. To quantitate the severity of defects in order to detect any progression, recovery, or response to therapy
    iv. To reveal hidden visual loss in patients who may be totally unaware of such defects

2. **What are the types of visual field testing?**
    i. Confrontation
    ii. Amsler grid
    iii. Tangent screen
    iv. Goldmann perimetry
    v. Static perimetry—octopus/Humphrey visual analyzer
    vi. Newer tests—swap, high pass resolution, flicker, motion, and displacement

3. **What are the chiasmal anatomical variations?**
    i. *Prefixed (10%):* Chiasm lies on the tuberculum sellae, and pituitary tumor can compress the posterior chiasm or optic tract
    ii. *Normally fixed (80%):* Chiasm lies on the diaphragm and projects backward onto the dorsum sellae, and pituitary tumor can compress the anterior chiasm
    iii. *Post fixed (10%):* Chiasm lies on the dorsum sellae, posterior to the fossa, and pituitary tumor compress the optic nerves

4. **What are the field defects in lesions of the optic chiasma?**
    i. Bitemporal (heteronymous) hemianopia
    ii. Traquair's junctional scotoma
    iii. Incongruous contralateral homonymous hemianopia (very rare)
    iv. Posterior involvement affects crossing macular fibers—bitemporal hemiscotomas

    Compression of chiasma:
    i. From below, e.g., pituitary adenoma—defects start superiorly and progress inferiorly in the temporal hemifields
    ii. From above, e.g., craniopharyngioma, suprasellar meningioma—defects start inferiorly and progress superiorly in the temporal hemifields
    iii. *Binasal hemianopia:* It is rare. A rare neuro-ophthalmic cause is aneurysm of the internal carotid artery producing compression of

temporal fibers ipsilaterally and also contralaterally by displacing the chiasma against the opposite internal carotid artery

5. **What is junctional scotoma?**
   Inferonasal retinal fibers cross into the chiasm and cross anteriorly approximately 4 mm in the contralateral optic nerve (Wilbrand's knee) before turning back to join uncrossed inferotemporal temporal fibers in the optic tract.

   Lesion in this region causes ipsilateral central scotoma and contralateral superotemporal defect. This is called junctional scotoma.

6. **What are the field defects in optic tract lesions?**
   Homonymous contralateral, incongruous hemianopia

7. **What are the pupillary abnormalities in optic tract lesion?**
   i. *Relative afferent pupillary defect (RAPD):* On the opposite side of the lesion (eye with temporal field loss)
   ii. *Behr's pupil:* Anisocoria with larger pupil on the side of hemianopia
   iii. *Wernicke's pupil:* Light stimulation of a "blind" retina causes no pupillary reaction, while light projected on an "intact" retina produces normal pupillary constriction

8. **What are the field defects in lesions of the lateral geniculate body?**
   Such defects are generally rare.
   i. Incongruous homonymous hemianopia
   ii. Quadruple sectoranopia
      - Homonymous hemianopia with sparing of a horizontal sector
      - Occurs with infarction of anterior choroidal artery
   iii. Relatively congruous, homonymous, horizontal sectoranopia
   iv. Only a horizontal sector involved
   v. Occurs with infarction of lateral choroidal artery

9. **What are the characteristics of internal capsule lesion?**
   Internal capsule lesion results in contralateral homonymous hemianopia with contralateral hemianesthesia due to damage of thalamocortical fibers.

10. **What are the field defects in temporal lobe lesions?**
    Mid peripheral/peripheral contralateral homonymous superior quadrantanopia (pie in the sky).

11. **What are the nonvisual manifestations of temporal lobe lesions?**
    i. Seizures
    ii. Formed hallucinations
    iii. If it affects uncinate gurus, it is called uncinate fits characterized by an aura of unusual taste or smell

12. **What are the field defects in parietal lobe lesions?**
    i. Contralateral inferior homonymous quadrantanopia (pie on the floor)
    ii. Homonymous hemianopia, denser inferiorly
13. **What are the nonvisual manifestations of parietal lobe lesions?**
    i. Word blindness and visual agnosia
    ii. Numbness on the contralateral side
    iii. Loss of tactile stimulation
    iv. Gerstmann syndrome (when dominant parietal lobe is affected), a combination of acalculia, agraphia, finger agnosia, and left-right confusion
14. **What is extinction phenomenon?**
    Extinction phenomenon is seen in parietal lobe lesions. Patients with this phenomenon may not have a true visual field defect but may not perceive objects on one half of the visual field when both sides are simultaneously stimulated.
15. **What are the field defects in occipital lobe lesions?**
    i. Exquisitely congruous contralateral, homonymous hemianopia
    ii. Macular "sparing"
    iii. Macular "splitting"
    iv. Central, macular homonymous hemianopia
    v. Temporal crescent sparing
16. **What are the reasons for macular sparing?**
    i. Dual blood supply, from the terminal branches of the middle cerebral artery and from the posterior cerebral artery
    ii. Bilateral representation of macula
    iii. Functional overlap of two sides of visual field
17. **What is cortical blindness?**
    It is seen in bilateral occipital lobe infarcts. Pupillary reflex is normal. Anton syndrome is denial of blindness and is classically associated with cortical blindness.

HOMONYMOUS HEMIANOPIA

1. **What are the characteristics of optic tract hemianopia?**
    i. Reduction in ipsilateral visual acuity, defects with both bitemporal and hemianopic character
    ii. Incongruity
    iii. Associated bow-tie optic atrophy (from selective involvement of decussated axons)
    iv. A contralateral RAPD

2. **What are the causes of homonymous hemianopia?**

   Optic tract lesions—visual conduction system posterior to the optic chiasma and anterior to the lateral geniculate body
   i. Saccular aneurysms of the internal carotid artery
   ii. Pituitary tumors—pituitary adenomas—chromophobe (the most common), basophil, acidophil, mixed, adenocarcinoma
   iii. Metastases
   iv. Demyelinating diseases
   v. Trauma
   vi. Migraine

   Temporoparietal lesions—temporal lobe lesions—pie in the sky and later pie on the floor if parietal lobe is involved.
   i. Vascular accidents—thromboembolism, vasospasm, subdural hematoma, and fracture skull
   ii. Tumors—meningioma, glioma, retinoblastoma, pinealoma, ependymoma, and metastases
   iii. Demyelinating diseases—Schilder's disease, Krabbe's leukodystrophy, polymorphic light eruption (PMLE), and migraine

   Occipital lesions:
   i. Vascular accidents—thromboembolism, vasospasm, subdural hematoma, fracture skull, and subclavian steal phenomenon
   ii. Vertebrobasilar insufficiency
   iii. Tumors—meningioma, glioma, retinoblastoma, pinealoma, ependymoma, and metastases
   iv. Demyelinating diseases—Schilder's disease, Krabbe's leukodystrophy, PMLE, and migraine
   v. Trauma
   vi. Poisons—digitalis, lysergic acid diethylamide (LSD), mescaline, opium, and carbon monoxide
   vii. Migraine

BITEMPORAL HEMIANOPIA

1. **What are the causes of bitemporal hemianopia?**

   Chiasmal lesions:
   i. Aneurysm of the internal carotid artery, intrasellar, syphilitic, and septic
   ii. Vascular—arteriosclerosis, arterial compression
   iii. Chiasmal basal arachnoiditis, chiasmal neuritis—tuberculosis, syphilis, and cysticercosis
   iv. Tumors—meningioma, glioma, retinoblastoma, pinealoma, and ependymoma

Pituitary lesions:
   i. Hyper-/hypopituitarism
   ii. Pituitary tumors
   iii. Pituitary adenomas—chromophobe (the most common), basophil, acidophil, mixed, and adenocarcinoma
   iv. Third ventricle enlargement
   v. Metastases

Perisellar lesions:
   i. *Suprasellar tumors:* Craniopharyngioma, meningioma, frontal lobe tumors, and ependymoma
   ii. Chordoma
   iii. *Presellar tumors:* Meningioma of olfactory groove, neuroblastoma
   iv. *Parasellar tumors:* Sphenoid bone meningioma, metastases, and disseminated sclerosis

Injury:
Most common causes include:
   i. *In children:* Craniopharyngioma and chiasmal glioma
   ii. *In 20–40 years age:* Pituitary tumors
   iii. *Above 40 years:* Meningioma, basal arachnoiditis, and aneurysms

2. **What are the clinical features of bitemporal hemianopia?**
   i. Monocular/binocular visual field defects that respect vertical meridian
   ii. Asymmetry of field loss is the rule, such that one eye may show advanced deficits, including reduced acuity, whereas only relative temporal field depression is found in the contralateral field
   iii. With few exceptions, these slow-growing tumors produce insidiously progressive visual deficits in the form of variations on a bitemporal theme
   iv. Most tumors are slow growing and so are the progress of visual symptoms
   v. Aneurysms may provoke sudden worsening or fluctuations in vision that mimic optic neuritis, at times with confounding improvement during corticosteroid therapy
   vi. Without temporal fields, objects beyond the point of binocular fixation fall on nonseeing nasal retina, so that a blind area exists, with extinction of objects beyond the fixation point
   vii. Suprasellar tumors of presumed prenatal origin, such as optic gliomas or craniopharyngiomas, may be associated with congenitally dysplastic optic disks

3. **What are the conditions that can mimic chiasmal field defects?**
   i. Tilted disks (inferior crescents, nasal fundus ectasia)
   ii. Nasal sector retinitis pigmentosa

iii. Bilateral cecocentral scotomas
iv. Papilledema with greatly enlarged blind spots
v. Overhanging redundant upper lid tissue
vi. Dominant optic atrophy
vii. Ethambutol toxic optic neuropathy

4. **What is the treatment of visual field defects?**
    i. Visual field defects, particularly of the homonymous variety or those present in one-eyed patients, frequently pose unique problems of eye movement. Such patients typically experience difficulty in moving the eye very far into a large "blind" area
    ii. A prism with the base oriented toward the blind area and covering only the portion of the spectacle lens corresponding to the blind area can produce a favorable result. For example, a patient with sight in only the left eye and a left hemianopia would be helped in "seeing" objects in his left field with a base-out Fresnel prism applied to the temporal portion of the left lens
    iii. With a small eye movement from the primary position (no prism) to the left (into the prism), the visual field would be shifted by the amount of the eye movement plus the power of the prism. Thus, a small flick of the eye to the left would provide the subject with a large view of the visual scene normally lying in his "blind" area

5. **What are the field defects in neurological diseases?**
    i. *Optic nerve head lesions:*
        – *Optic neuritis:* Central or centrocecal scotoma
        – *Papilledema:* Enlargement of blind spot
        – *Anterior ischemic optic neuropathy (AION):* Inferior/superior altitudinal field defects
    ii. *Lesions at the chiasm:* Bitemporal hemianopia
        Hemianopia or field defect in one eye when there is asymmetric compression by an enlarging tumor, e.g., pituitary macroadenoma
    iii. *Optic tract, lateral geniculate body (LGB)/retrochiasmatic lesions:* Contralateral incongruous homonymous hemianopia
        (*Note:* The more posterior the lesion, the more congruous the field defect)
    iv. *Temporal lobe lesions:* Contralateral homonymous superior quadrantanopia (pie in the sky)
    v. *Parietal lobe lesions:* Contralateral homonymous inferior quadrantanopia (pie in the floor)
    vi. *Occipital lobe:* Contralateral complete homonymous hemianopia with or without macular sparing
    vii. *Lesions affecting occipital lobe tip:* Central homonymous hemianopia.

7.15 CAVERNOUS SINUS THROMBOSIS

1. **Describe briefly anatomy of cavernous sinus.**
    i. The cavernous sinuses are irregularly shaped and trabeculated, and consist of incompletely fused venous channels located at the base of the skull in the middle cranial fossa
    ii. They lie on either side of the sella turcica, are just lateral and superior to the sphenoid sinus, and are immediately posterior to the optic chiasma
    iii. Each cavernous sinus is formed between layers of the dura mater, and multiple connections between the two sinuses exist
    iv. The cavernous sinuses receive venous blood from the facial veins (via the superior and inferior ophthalmic veins) as well as the sphenoid and middle cerebral veins. They, in turn, empty into the inferior petrosal sinuses, then into the internal jugular veins and the sigmoid sinuses via the superior petrosal sinuses
    v. There are no valves, however, in this complex web of veins, blood can flow in any direction depending on the prevailing pressure gradients
    vi. The internal carotid artery, with its surrounding sympathetic plexus, passes through the cavernous sinus
    vii. The third, fourth, and sixth cranial nerves are attached to the lateral wall of the sinus
    viii. The ophthalmic and maxillary divisions of the fifth cranial nerve are embedded in the wall
    This intimate juxtaposition of veins, arteries, nerves, meninges, and paranasal sinuses accounts for the characteristic etiology and presentation of cavernous sinus thrombosis

2. **What are the causes of cavernous sinus thrombosis?**
   Causes of cavernous sinus thrombosis can be divided into the following:
   Septic or infective:
    i. Most cases of septic cavernous sinus thrombosis are due to an acute infection in an otherwise normal individual. However, patients with chronic sinusitis or diabetes mellitus may be at a slightly higher risk
    ii. The causative agent is generally *Staphylococcus aureus*, although streptococci, pneumococci, and fungi may be implicated in rare cases
       – *Infection of the face:*
         - Especially the middle one-third
         - Causative organism: *Staphylococcus aureus*
         - Bacteria → facial vein and pterygoid plexus → ophthalmic vein → cavernous sinus

- *Sinusitis:*
  - It can involve the sphenoid or the ethmoid sinuses
  - It can be:
    - *Acute:* Caused by gram-positive organisms, namely *S. aureus*, pneumococci
    - *Chronic:* Caused by gram-negative organisms, coagulase-negative staphylococci, fungi, e.g., *Aspergillus* and *Mucoraceae*
- *Dental infections:* (10%)
  - Common with maxillary teeth
  - Common pathogens involved in odontogenic septic cavernous sinus thrombosis are:
    - Streptococci
    - *Fusobacterium*
    - *Bacteroides*
- Otitis media:
  - Cavernous sinus thrombosis is a rare complication
  - Seen in untreated, incompletely treated, incorrectly treated disease
- Orbital cellulitis:
  - Rare

Aseptic or noninfective:
  i. Polycythemia
  ii. Sickle cell disease or trait
  iii. Paroxysmal nocturnal hemoglobinuria
  iv. Arteriovenous malformations
  v. Trauma
  vi. Intracranial surgery
  vii. Vasculitis
  viii. Pregnancy
  ix. Oral contraceptive pills
  x. Congenital heart disease
  xi. Dehydration
  xii. Marasmus
  xiii. Compression or obstruction due to expanding mass (e.g., pituitary adenoma, meningioma) → sterile thrombosis part of the paraneoplastic hypercoagulability syndrome

3. **What are the clinical features of cavernous sinus thrombosis?**
   History:
   i. Patients generally have sinusitis or a midface infection (most commonly a furuncle) for 5–10 days. In up to 25% of cases where a furuncle is the precipitant, it will have been manipulated in some fashion (e.g., squeezing and surgical incision)

ii. Headache, fever, and malaise typically precede the development of ocular findings. As the infection tracks posteriorly, patients complain of orbital pain and fullness accompanied by periorbital edema and visual disturbances
iii. In some patients, periorbital findings will not develop early on, and the clinical picture is subtle
iv. Without effective therapy, signs will appear in the contralateral eye by spreading through the communicating veins to the contralateral cavernous sinus. This is pathognomonic for cavernous sinus thrombosis. The patient rapidly develops mental status changes from central nervous system (CNS) involvement and/or sepsis. Death will follow shortly thereafter

Ocular and physical examination:
Other than the findings associated with the primary infection, the following signs are typical:
  i. Initially, signs of venous congestion may present:
     - Chemosis
     - Eyelid edema
     - Periorbital edema
  ii. Manifestations of increased retrobulbar pressure follow:
     - Exophthalmos
     - Ophthalmoplegia
  iii. Increased intraocular pressure (IOP):
     - Sluggish pupillary responses
     - Decreased visual acuity is common due to increased IOP and traction on the optic nerve and central retinal artery
  iv. Cranial nerve palsies are found regularly:
     - Isolated sixth nerve dysfunction may be noted before there are obvious orbital findings
     - Impaired extraocular movements
  v. Depressed corneal reflex is possible
  vi. Appearance of signs and symptoms in the contralateral eye is diagnostic of cavernous sinus thrombosis, although the process may remain confined to one eye
  vii. Meningeal signs may be noted, including nuchal rigidity, Kernig's and Brudzinski's signs
  viii. Systemic signs indicative of sepsis are late findings. They include chills, fever, shock, delirium, and coma

Ocular features depend on the origin of the infection.
  i. Anterior infection (facial, dental, orbital) → acute presentation in the following order:
     - Deep-seated pain around the eye
     - Increased temperature

- Orbital congestion
- Lacrimation
- Conjunctival edema
- Eyelid swelling
- Ptosis
- Proptosis
- Ophthalmoparesis

Such patients are usually toxic with +ve blood cultures.

ii. Sphenoid sinusitis/pharyngitis →
  - Delayed presentation of signs
  - Subacute or chronic
  - Isolated abducens nerve paresis is the most consistent early neurologic sign

iii. Secondary to otitis media →
  - Signs and symptoms are slow
  - Protracted course

Visual loss is common, and causes are ischemic oculopathy, ischemic optic neuropathy, and neurotrophic keratopathy (corneal ulceration).

Aseptic: Signs and symptoms are similar to the septic type but without any laboratory or clinical evidence of infection.
- No fever, chills, leukocytosis, or signs and symptoms suggestive of meningitis
- Pain around and behind the eye
- Loss of corneal sensations, decreased facial sensations
- Ophthalmoparesis
- Proptosis and chemosis are less severe
- Sympathetic dysfunction
- Increased IOP
- Stasis retinopathy

Visual loss is usually uncommon regardless of the severity.

4. **What are the differential diagnoses of cavernous sinus thrombosis?**

Differential diagnoses of cavernous sinus thrombosis	
Diagnosis	Signs/symptoms
Traumatic retrobulbar hemorrhage	• Accumulation of blood within the orbit • History of trauma or surgery • Bullous subconjunctival hemorrhage • Pain, decreased vision, lid ecchymosis, increased IOP, and proptosis
Orbital cellulitis	• Lid edema, erythema, and tenderness • Pain and fever but normal vision

Contd...

Contd...

Differential diagnoses of cavernous sinus thrombosis	
Diagnosis	Signs/symptoms
Orbital fracture and ruptured globe	• History of trauma • Periocular bruising, enophthalmos • Pain, decreased vision, lid edema, and restricted eye movements
Conjunctivitis	• Conjunctival follicles and/or papillae • Red eye, decreased vision, lid edema, and discharge • Corneal neovascularization • Itching and/or pain
Thyroid-related orbitopathy	• Lid retraction, lid lag, and scleral show • Foreign body sensation, decreased tearing • Dyschromatopsia, diplopia, proptosis, and decreased vision
Cavernous sinus thrombosis	• Altered level of consciousness • Dilated and sluggish pupils; cranial nerve third, fourth, and/or sixth palsies • Fever, nausea, vomiting • Chemosis and lid edema, proptosis
Lacrimal gland neoplasia	• Temporal upper eyelid swelling • Inferonasal globe displacement • Tearing, pain, diplopia • Palpable mass under superotemporal orbital rim
Orbital inflammation–idiopathic (orbital pseudotumor)	• Acute onset of orbital pain, headaches • Binocular diplopia, decreased vision, proptosis, and lid edema • Induced hyperopia, decreased corneal sensation, and increased IOP
Orbital vasculitis	• Systemic signs and symptoms (sinus, renal, pulmonary, and skin) • Fever, increased erythrocyte sedimentation rate (ESR)

5. How do you investigate a case of cavernous sinus thrombosis?
   i. Cavernous sinus thrombosis is a clinical diagnosis, and laboratory studies are seldom specific
   ii. *Hematological investigation:*
   - Most patients exhibit a polymorphonuclear leukocytosis, often marked with a shift toward immature forms
   - Complete blood count is done to look for polycythemia as an etiologic factor
   - Decreased platelet count would support thrombotic thrombocytopenic purpura; leukocytosis might be seen in sepsis. In addition, if heparin is used as treatment, platelet counts should be monitored for thrombocytopenia
   - Blood cultures generally are positive for the offending organism

iii. *Immunological tests:*
- Antiphospholipid and anticardiolipin antibodies should be obtained to evaluate for antiphospholipid syndrome
- Tests that may indicate hypercoagulable states include protein S, protein C, antithrombin III, lupus anticoagulant, and Leiden factor V mutation. These evaluations should not be made while the patient is on anticoagulant therapy

iv. Electrophoresis—sickle cell preparation or hemoglobin electrophoresis

v. Cerebrospinal fluid examination—examination of the cerebrospinal fluid is consistent with either a parameningeal inflammation or Frank meningitis

6. **What are the imaging studies done in cavernous sinus thrombosis?**
Computed tomography (CT): It is the investigation of choice to confirm the diagnosis.
   i. On noncontrast study—thrombosis of the cavernous sinus can be appreciated as increased density
   ii. Contrast scan reveals filling defects within the cavernous sinus. Empty delta sign appears on contrast scans as enhancement of the collateral veins in the superior sagittal sinus walls surrounding a nonenhanced thrombus in the sinus
   iii. Negative CT cannot reliably rule out cavernous sinus thrombosis when the clinical suspicion is high
   iv. Useful in ruling out other conditions such as neoplasm and in evaluating coexistent lesions such as subdural empyema. CT of the sinuses is useful in evaluating sinusitis; CT of the mastoids may be helpful in lateral sinus thrombosis

Magnetic resonance imaging (MRI):
   i. MRI shows the pattern of an infarct that does not follow the distribution of an expected arterial occlusion. It may show absence of flow void in the normal venous channels
   ii. Magnetic resonance venography (MRV) is an excellent method of visualizing the dural venous sinuses and larger cerebral veins
   iii. Single-slice phase-contrast angiography (SSPCA) takes <30 seconds and provides rapid and reliable information
   iv. If magnetic resonance studies are not diagnostic, conventional angiography should be considered

Contrast studies:
   i. Carotid arteriography is an invasive procedure and is therefore associated with a small risk
   ii. Direct venography can be performed by passing a catheter from the jugular vein into the transverse sinus with injection outlining the venous sinuses

7. **How do you treat a case of cavernous sinus thrombosis?**

    Emergency department care:
    i. The mainstay of therapy is early and aggressive antibiotic administration. Although *S. aureus* is the usual cause, broad-spectrum coverage for gram-positive, gram-negative and anaerobic organisms should be instituted pending the outcome of cultures
    ii. Anticoagulation with heparin may be considered. The goal is to prevent further thrombosis and reduce the incidence of septic emboli. Heparin is contraindicated in the presence of intracerebral hemorrhage or other bleeding diathesis
    iii. Corticosteroids may help to reduce inflammation and edema and should be considered an adjunctive therapy. When the course of cavernous sinus thrombosis leads to pituitary insufficiency, however, corticosteroids definitely are indicated to prevent adrenal crisis
    iv. Surgery on the cavernous sinus is technically difficult. The primary source of infection should be drained, if feasible (e.g., sphenoid sinusitis and facial abscess)

    Medical treatment:
    Antibiotic therapy ideally is started after appropriate cultures but should not be delayed if there are difficulties in obtaining specimens. Antibiotics selected should be broad-spectrum, particularly active against *S. aureus*, and capable of achieving high levels in the cerebrospinal fluid.

    Drug categories:
    i. Antibiotics
    ii. Anticoagulants
    iii. Corticosteroids

    i. *Antibiotics*—empiric broad-spectrum coverage for gram-positive, gram-negative, and anaerobic organisms. Therapy must be comprehensive and should cover all likely pathogens in the context of the clinical setting

    The common antibiotics are:
    - Oxacillin [2 g intravenous (IV) q4h]
    - Ceftriaxone (2 g IV 112h)
    - Metronidazole (500 mg IV q6h)

    ii. *Anticoagulants:* Unfractionated IV heparin and fractionated low-molecular-weight subcutaneous heparins are the two options in anticoagulation therapy
    Dose: 80 mg/kg IV bolus; then 18 mg/kg IV infusion; titrate
    iii. *Corticosteroids:* These agents have anti-inflammatory properties and cause profound and varied metabolic effects. In addition, these agents modify the body's immune response to diverse stimuli

Complications of cavernous sinus thrombosis:
  i. Meningitis
  ii. Septic emboli
  iii. Blindness
  iv. Cranial nerve palsies
  v. Sepsis and shock

Prognosis

Septic cavernous sinus thrombosis:
  i. Mortality is up to 30%, with the majority of survivors suffering permanent sequelae and neurological deficits
  ii. Full recovery is seen in <40%
  iii. Rarely Fröhlich's syndrome has been reported

Aseptic cavernous sinus thrombosis:
  i. Variable
  ii. Depends on the underlying cause
  iii. Extent and severity of neurologic dysfunction
  iv. Mortality rate is much low
  v. Damage to the cranial nerves → persistent pareses, trigeminal neuralgia
  vi. Permanent visual loss is rare but can occur.

7.16 CAROTICOCAVERNOUS FISTULAS

1. **Define caroticocavernous fistula.**
   Caroticocavernous fistula is an abnormal communication between the cavernous sinus and dural veins and the carotid arterial system.

2. **Classify caroticocavernous fistula.**

Cause	Velocity of blood flow	Anatomy
Traumatic	High flow	Direct and dural
Spontaneous	Low flow	Internal carotid and external carotid, or both

   High flow: Carotid-cavernous fistulas, characterized by direct flow into the cavernous sinus from the intracavernous carotid artery

   Causes: These usually are traumatic and most often diagnosed in young men.

   Low flow: Spontaneous shunts occur between the cavernous sinus and one or more meningeal branches of the internal carotid artery (usually the meningohypophyseal trunk), the external carotid artery, or both. These shunts have a low amount of arterial flow and almost always produce signs and symptoms spontaneously.

   Causes:
   i. Spontaneously
   ii. In the setting of atherosclerosis, hypertension
   iii. Collagen vascular disease
   iv. During or after childbirth
   v. Elderly, especially women

3. **Describe dural shunts.**
   i. Dural shunts between the arterial and venous systems have lower flow
   ii. They may produce symptoms in younger patients spontaneously or in older patients due to hypertension, diabetes, atherosclerosis, or other vascular disorders
   iii. Anatomically, these shunts arise between the meningeal arterial branches and the dural veins
   iv. The meningohypophyseal trunk and the artery of the inferior cavernous sinus provide the arterial supply to most dural shunts
   v. Such shunts may be due to an expansion of congenital arteriovenous malformation or due to spontaneous rupture of one of the thin-walled dural arteries that transverse the sinus

4. **What are the ocular manifestations of caroticocavernous fistulas?**
   Ocular signs of caroticocavernous fistulas are related to venous congestion and reduced arterial blood flow to the orbit. These abnormalities usually are unilateral but can be bilateral or even contralateral to the fistula.

   Conjunctiva: Chemosis of the conjunctiva and arterialization of the episcleral vessels occurs in most patients. Arterialization of episcleral veins is the hallmark of all caroticocavernous fistulas or dural shunts.

   Glaucoma: Stasis of venous and arterial circulation within the eye and orbit may cause ocular ischemia, and increased episcleral venous pressure may cause glaucoma.

   Orbit:
   i. Exophthalmos is a common sign that occurs in almost all patients who have caroticocavernous fistulas. Rapid-flow fistulas may develop exophthalmos within hours or several days
   ii. The orbit can become "frozen," with no ocular motor function; usually, this is accompanied by conjunctival chemosis and hemorrhage. Vision may be reduced markedly as a result of optic nerve ischemia
   iii. "Pulsating exophthalmos" is uncommon in caroticocavernous fistula. Usually, the orbit is rigid from hemorrhage and edema and incapable of "pulsation"

   Bruits: Bruits associated with fistulas and dural shunts can be appreciated both subjectively and objectively. A bruit can be heard best when the examiner uses a "bell stethoscope" over the closed eye, over the superior orbital vein, or the temple. A subjective bruit (heard by the patient) almost always can be obtained from the history; however, an objective bruit heard over the orbit or temple by auscultation is relatively uncommon.

   A bruit is not pathognomonic of caroticocavernous fistula. It also can be heard in normal infants, in young children, and in severe anemia.

   Optic nerve: Immediate or delayed visual loss occurs frequently in direct caroticocavernous fistulas due to optic nerve ischemia from apical orbital compression.

   Longstanding fistulas can lead to loss of vision as a result of distention of the cavernous sinus or retrobulbar ischemia.

   Cranial nerve palsy:
   i. Diminished arterial flow to cranial nerves within the cavernous sinus may cause diplopia
   ii. The abducens nerve is affected most often as it lies in the cavernous sinus itself

iii. Since the third and fourth nerves are encased in the superior internal dural wall of the sinus, they may be protected from changes caused by the fistula
iv. Mechanical restriction from venous congestion and orbital edema also may contribute to limitation of eye movements

Fundus picture:
   i. Ophthalmoscopic findings due to venous stasis and impaired retinal blood flow include retinal venous engorgement and dot and blot retinal hemorrhages
  ii. Central retinal vein occlusion may be observed in high-velocity caroticocavernous fistulas with arterialized venous channels
 iii. High episcleral and intraocular pressures rarely result in damage to the optic nerve
  iv. In unusual cases of central vein occlusion, neovascular glaucoma can occur

5. **What is the investigation of choice in caroticocavernous fistula?**
   Digital subtraction angiography.

7.17 CAROTID ARTERY OCCLUSION

1. **What are the common modes of presentation of carotid artery occlusion to an ophthalmologist?**
   i. *Transient* ischemic *attack:* If the transient ischemic attack involves the carotid system, the symptoms include hemiparesis, hemisensory loss, aphasia, and transient monocular blindness (amaurosis fugax).
   ii. *Purely* ocular *symptoms,* such as:
      - Paratransient ischemic attack or complete visual loss due to an artery obstruction
      - Decreased visual acuity
      - Pain resulting from the ocular ischemic syndrome
   iii. Other patients are asymptomatic, and any ocular findings consistent with carotid artery disease are incidental

2. **What is amaurosis fugax?**
   Amaurosis fugax ("fleeting darkness or blindness"; ocular transient ischemic episode):
   i. Most common symptom of carotid artery disease
   ii. This phenomenon may be defined as a painless unilateral, transient loss of vision that usually progresses from the periphery toward the center of the field
   iii. Often, the visual deficit takes the pattern of a dark curtain descending from above or ascending from below
   iv. Complete or subtotal blindness follows in seconds and lasts from 1 to 5 minutes (rarely longer)
   v. Vision returns to normal within 10–20 minutes, at times by reversal of the pattern of progression
   vi. The return of vision can be sectorial or altitudinal and is occasionally described as a "curtain rising"
   vii. Generally, the vision returns to normal immediately after an attack. The frequency of these attacks varies from one or two attacks per month to 10 or 20 attacks per day
   viii. The retina—if observed during an amaurotic attack—may be normal, or it may show obstruction (such as in central retinal artery obstruction)
   ix. It may exhibit migratory white retinal emboli (within the retinal arterioles and in association with disruption of the arterial circulation), or it may show cholesterol emboli moving through the arterial system
   x. It is important to recognize amaurosis fugax as a transient ischemic attack because it is frequently caused by microembolization from an atheromatous ulcerative lesion in the ipsilateral extracranial carotid artery, at least in older patients

xi. About a third of all patients with an untreated transient ischemic attack can be expected to have a stroke; this rate is about four times greater than that of an age-matched population

3. **What are causes of amaurosis fugax?**
    i. Migraine
    ii. Hematology disorders
    iii. Ocular hypertension
    iv. Arterial hypotension
    v. Vasospasm
    vi. Temporal arteritis
    vii. Pseudotumor cerebri
    viii. Structural cardiac defects
    ix. Ophthalmic artery stenosis
    x. Ophthalmic artery aneurysms

4. **What is ocular ischemic syndrome?**
   Ocular ischemic syndrome refers to the constellation of ophthalmic features that result from chronic hypoperfusion of the entire arterial supply to the eye, including the central retinal, posterior ciliary, and anterior ciliary arteries.
   The occlusion is at the level of:
    i. Carotid artery
    ii. Proximal to the point where the central retinal and ciliary arteries branch from the ophthalmic artery

5. **What is the clinical presentation of ocular ischemic syndrome?**
    i. Patient, typically >50 years old, is more likely to be male than female
    ii. Patient reports having a loss of vision in one or both eyes over a period of weeks to months
    iii. Ocular or periocular pain here may or may not be associated; it is found in approximately 40% of persons with ocular ischemic syndrome. Typically, the pain is described as a dull ache over the eye or brow
    iv. Ischemia to the anterior segment structures or ocular angina is thought to be the cause of this pain in some cases
    v. History of difficulty adjusting from bright light to relative darkness represents inability of ocular circulation to supply enough oxygen to sustain increased retinal circulation
    vi. Similar complaints occur after exertion, change in posture, and postprandial period
    vii. Additionally, the patient may relate a history of transient focal neurologic deficits

Ocular symptoms and signs of carotid artery occlusion
Symptoms:
  i. Visual loss
  ii. Pain—"ocular angina" (40% case)
  iii. Prolonged recovery after light exposure
  vi. Amaurosis fugax (10% cases)
  v. Associated with transient focal neurologic deficits

Signs:
  i. Spontaneous retinal arterial pulsations
  ii. Midperipheral retinal hemorrhage
  iii. Cholesterol emboli
  iv. Disk edema—anterior ischemic optic neuropathy (AION)
  v. Neovascularization of disk, retina, and iris
  vi. Narrowed retinal arterioles
  vii. Dilated retinal veins
  viii. Arteriovenous communications

Other peculiar presentations:
  i. Ipsilateral Horner's syndrome
  ii. Carotid dissection
  iii. Ischemic anterior uveitis
  iv. Neovascular glaucoma

Systemic associations—most patients will have already been diagnosed with diabetes mellitus, hypertension, ischemic heart disease, and cerebrovascular disease.

Differential diagnosis:
  i. Diabetic retinopathy
  ii. Nonischemic central retinal vein occlusion (CRVO)

Diagnostic workup:
Prompt noninvasive vascular workup is mandatory:
  i. To confirm carotid vascular disease
  ii. Establish cause (atheroma, emboli, dissection, vasculitis, compression, etc.)
  iii. Ocular and cerebral tolerance of carotid occlusion

Investigations:
  i. Carotid color Doppler
  ii. Cerebral angiography and arteriography (gold standard)
  iii. Digital subtraction angiography
  iv. Ultrasonography
  v. Magnetic resonance imaging (MRI) angiography
  vi. Spiral computed tomography (CT) angiography
  vii. Fundus fluorescein angiography

6. **What are the features of ocular ischemic syndrome on fluorescein angiogram?**
   Characteristic fluorescein angiographic features reflect the chronic hypoperfusion of the retinal and choroidal circulations, as well as ischemic damage to the neurosensory retina and retinal vessels.
   i. Prolonged arteriovenous transit time
   ii. Prolonged arm-to-retina circulation times (over 20 seconds)
   iii. Retinal vascular staining
   iv. Retinal capillary nonperfusion
   v. Delayed or patchy choroidal filling
   vi. Macular edema

7. **What are the other tests that can be done for diagnosing ocular ischemic syndrome?**
   i. *Photopic stress test:*
   A marked difference in photopic stress recovery times between the two eyes is suggestive of macular disease, such as ocular ischemic syndrome; diseases of the optic nerve would be less affected.
   ii. *Electroretinography:*
   Eyes with ocular ischemic syndrome show a decreased amplitude of both A- and B-waves. The B-wave, which corresponds to the inner retinal layer, probably reflects the function of the bipolar and/or Müller cells, and it is diminished by compromised perfusion of the central retinal artery.
   The A-wave correlates with photoreceptor function and is affected by choroidal ischemia.
   iii. *Orbital color Doppler imaging:*
   Central retinal and posterior ciliary artery peak systolic velocities markedly reduced.
   iv. *Ophthalmodynamometry and oculoplethysmography:*
   The normal ophthalmic artery has a systolic pressure of approximately 100 mm Hg and a diastolic pressure of approximately 60 mm Hg.
   In ocular ischemic syndrome, the systolic pressure is often <40 mm Hg, and the diastolic pressure may be <10 mm Hg. It is often useful to measure an unaffected contralateral eye for comparison.
   v. *Carotid duplex (B-mode and Doppler) scanning:*
   Although safe and inexpensive, carotid duplex scanning has limitations and is less reliable than carotid angiography in distinguishing between a completely occluded artery and one that is nearly occluded; it is used as screening techniques for atherosclerotic disease.

vi. *Carotid angiography (digital subtraction aortogram):*
Despite its expense and low but definite morbidity rate, carotid angiography remains the most reliable method of assessing atherosclerotic carotid disease, and it serves as the "gold standard" in the evaluation of all other tests of the carotid arteries.

8. **What is the treatment of ocular ischemic syndrome?**
Treatment is directed primarily at:
 i. Treating ocular neovascularization and neovascular glaucoma
 ii. Restoring blood flow into the eye with surgery

Treatment of ocular neovascularization:
 i. Fundus fluorescein angiography to determine the cause of neovascularization of the disk/neovascularization elsewhere (NVD/NVE)
 ii. Retinal ablative procedures—panretinal photocoagulation (PRP)/anterior retinal cryoablation still remains the first modality of treatment

Systemic antiplatelet therapy:
 i. Aspirin
 ii. Ticlopidine
 iii. Pentoxifylline
 iv. Dipyridamole
 v. Clopidogrel

Indications for medical management:
 i. Inoperable carotid disease
 ii. Nonstenotic carotid disease
 iii. Medical contraindication to surgery

Surgical management: In most cases, carotid endarterectomy remains the treatment of choice for symptomatic patients with severe stenotic atherosclerotic disease of the internal carotid artery.

7.18 OPHTHALMOPLEGIA

1. **What are the types of ophthalmoplegia?**
   i. *Total ophthalmoplegia*—if all the extrinsic and intrinsic muscles of one or both eyes are paralyzed
   ii. *External ophthalmoplegia*—if only the extrinsic muscle of one or both eyes are paralyzed
   iii. *Internal ophthalmoplegia*—if only the intrinsic muscles (sphincter pupillae and ciliary muscle) of one or both eyes are paralyzed
   iv. *Painful ophthalmoplegia:* The syndrome of painful ophthalmoplegia consists of periorbital pain or hemicranial pain combined with ipsilateral ocular motor palsies, oculosympathetic paralysis, and sensory loss in the distribution of ophthalmic and occasionally maxillary division of trigeminal nerve. The etiology of painful ophthalmoplegia may be divided into those with the involvement of cavernous sinus/superior orbital fissure and those without the involvement of the same

2. **Describe briefly anatomy of the superior orbital fissure.**
   Superior orbital fissure connects the middle cranial fossa with the orbit. It lies between the roof and lateral wall of the orbit and is a gap between greater wing and lesser wing of sphenoid, and is bounded by:
   i. Body of sphenoid medially
   ii. Lesser wing of sphenoid above
   iii. Greater wing of sphenoid below
   iv. A part of frontal bone may complete the fissure laterally

   Subdivisions: A common tendinous ring (tendon of Zinn) encircles the optic foramen and middle of superior orbital fissure and gives origin to recti muscles of the eyeball. The central part of the fissure within the ring is called oculomotor foramen.

3. **What are the structures passing through the superior orbital fissure?**
   The various structures transmitted are:

   Above the common tendinous ring:
   i. Trochlear nerve medially
   ii. Frontal nerve laterally
   iii. Superior ophthalmic vein
   iv. Rarely recurrent lacrimal artery

   Through the oculomotor foramen:
   i. Superior division of third cranial nerve
   ii. Inferior division of the third cranial nerve
   iii. Nasociliary nerve

iv. Sympathetic root of ciliary ganglion
v. Abducent nerve inferonasally

Below the tendinous ring: Inferior ophthalmic vein

4. **What are the causes of parasellar syndrome producing painful ophthalmoplegia?**
    i. Trauma
    ii. Vascular:
        - Intracavernous sinus carotid artery aneurysm
        - Posterior carotid artery aneurysm
        - Carotid artery fistula
        - Cavernous sinus thrombosis
    iii. Neoplasm:
        - Primary intracranial neoplasm—pituitary adenoma, meningioma, sarcoma, craniopharyngioma, neurofibroma, Gasserian ganglion neuroma, and epidermoid
        - Primary cranial tumor—chondroma, chordoma, and giant cell tumor
        - Local metastasis—nasopharyngeal tumor, cylindroma, chordoma, and squamous cell carcinoma
        - Distant metastasis—lymphoma, multiple myeloma
        - Inflammation:
            - Bacterial—sinusitis, mucocele
            - Viral—herpes zoster
            - Fungal—mucormycosis
            - Spirochetal—Treponema pallidum
            - *Mycobacterium*
            - Unknown causes—sarcoidosis, Wegner's granulomatosis, and Tolosa-Hunt syndrome

5. **What are the causes of painful ophthalmoplegia with no involvement of the cavernous sinus/superior orbital fissure?**
    i. *Orbital disease:*
        - Idiopathic orbital inflammation (pseudotumor)
        - Contiguous sinusitis
        - Mucormycosis or other fungal infection
        - Metastatic tumor
        - Lymphoma/leukemia
    ii. *Diabetic ophthalmoplegia:*
        - Mononeuropathy
        - Multiple cranial nerve palsy
    iii. *Posterior fossa aneurysm:*
        - Posterior communicating artery
        - Basilar artery

    iv. Cranial arteritis
    v. Migrainous ophthalmoplegia
    vi. Gradenigo's syndrome
    vii. Reader's syndrome
    viii. Trauma

6. **What are the ways in which trauma can produce ophthalmoplegia?**
   Craniocerebral trauma may produce painful ophthalmoplegia in various ways, namely:
   i. Basilar skull fracture with ocular motor damage
   ii. Intracavernous carotid artery injury with subsequent aneurysm formation
   iii. Caroticocavernous fistula
   iv. Painful ophthalmoplegia may occur as an acute phenomenon or as delayed phenomenon
      - *Acute painful ophthalmoplegia:*
        - *Cranial nerve involvement*—immediate paralysis of third, fourth, and sixth cranial nerves is a well-known complication of closed head trauma
        - *Orbit involvement:* The direct injury to the orbit can cause immediate impairment of ocular motility due to trauma to the ocular muscles, orbital hemorrhage and edema, or entrapment of the muscle or fasciae in the fracture site
      - *Delayed painful ophthalmoplegia:* This may be due to various reasons:
        - Progression of the local edema after injury to the ocular motor nerve or to the orbit, which tends to produce maximal impairment within few days after injury and manifestation itself as a worsening of the immediate impairment
        - Progressive brainstem edema, which becomes maximal within few days after the injury and is generally accompanied by other brainstem signs. This may be due to the injury to the blood vessels outside the brainstem rather than direct brainstem injury
        - Sixth nerve and rarely fourth nerve paresis due to increased intracranial pressure without herniation and third nerve paresis due to transtentorial herniation can all result from verity of mass lesions secondary to head injury
        - Posttraumatic sphenoid mucocele can cause painful ophthalmoplegia, usually after delay of months or years
        - Sudden severe exophthalmos and painful ophthalmoplegia due to an orbital meningocele occurring 1 month after a frontal fracture has been reported

7. **What are the features of ophthalmoplegia due to intracavernous carotid artery aneurysm?**
    i. Compromise about 3% of all intracranial aneurysm
    ii. Most of these syndromes occur in middle-aged individuals without the history of incident head trauma
    iii. The onset of signs and symptoms may be abrupt but may be slow and insidious
    iv. Pain in and around the eye and face is the prominent symptom
    v. The sixth nerve, being the close relation to the internal carotid artery (ICA), is affected first, and in most cases, third and fourth nerve are involved subsequently
    vi. Trigeminal sensory loss is regarded the classical manifestation of this disease
    vii. Aneurysmal expansion can produce additional findings that vary with its directions
        - Anterior expansion—can produce exophthalmos and ipsilateral and ipsilateral visual failure due to optic nerve compression
        - Posterior expansion—may extend as far as petrous part of temporal bone and give rise to ipsilateral hearing loss
        - Inferior expansion—into the sphenoid sinus with subsequent rupture explains the massive and sometimes fatal epistaxis suffered by the patients
        - Medial erosion of the aneurysm into the sella turcica can produce signs and symptoms which mimic a pituitary tumor

8. **Why is pupil spared in intracavernous carotid artery aneurysm causing third cranial nerve paresis?**
    i. The small pupil may be due to simultaneous involvement of both the third nerve and the sympathetic fibers surrounding the ICA
    ii. The absence of large pupil in the cavernous sinus lesion may sometimes reflect sparing of the inferior division of the third nerves

9. **Where do you ligate the carotid artery?**
    i. Ligation of the carotid in the neck with or without intracranial clipping distal to the aneurysm
    ii. Occlusion of the carotid artery by the detachable balloon catheter

10. **What are the features of ophthalmoplegia due to caroticocavernous fistula?**
    i. This represents the direct communication between the intracavernous carotid artery and the surrounding cavernous sinus
    ii. The large majority arises traumatically
    iii. Spontaneous fistula may develop.
        Causes:
        a. Preexisting aneurysm
        b. Angiodysplasias, such as Ehler–Danlos or pseudoxanthoma elasticum

iv. The clinical features usually develop immediately, although there may be a delay. The degree of the external symptom depends on the amount of the anterior drainage of the shunted blood

11. **What are the clinical features of caroticocavernous fistula?**
    i. *Conjunctiva:* There is arterialization of the bulbar conjunctiva, often with marked proptosis and chemosis. Conjunctival prolapse with inversion of the fornix may occur
    ii. *Cornea:* Exposure keratitis and possible corneal anesthesia from the fifth nerve damage
    iii. *Orbit:* Severe proptosis with limitation of the eyelid closure
    iv. *Glaucoma* is usually due to increased episcleral venous pressure with open angles. Neovascular glaucoma may develop secondary to hypoxic retinopathy. Blood in the trabecular meshwork is the common finding on gonioscopy
    v. *Bruit* may accompany these findings
    vi. *Cranial nerves:* Any of the cranial nerves may be involved
    vii. *Vision:* Visual loss may be due to:
        - Traumatic optic neuropathy
        - Ocular steal phenomenon
        - Hypoxic retinopathy due to decreased ocular blood flow

    Management: The treatment of choice is balloon immobilization

12. **What are the features of ophthalmoplegia due to pituitary apoplexy?**
    i. Pituitary tumors frequently invade the cavernous sinus and cause cavernous sinus syndrome
    ii. Pituitary apoplexy, which occurs as a result of infarction of the pituitary adenoma, which has outgrown its blood supply
        - It can be precipitated by radiation therapy, trauma, and pregnancy
        - The condition is characterized by acute onset of headache, painful ophthalmoplegia, bilateral amaurosis, drowsiness or coma, and subarachnoid hemorrhage
        - Headache is usually of sudden onset, generalized or only retrobulbar
        - Unilateral or bilateral ophthalmoplegia is due to involvement of third, fourth, and sixth cranial nerves in the cavernous sinus
        - The cerebrospinal fluid (CSF) shows xanthochromia, pleocytosis, and elevated protein levels
        - Computed tomography (CT) scan often shows infarction of the tumor with hemorrhage in and above enlarged sella

    Treatment:
    It is a life-threatening condition and needs prompt treatment. Corticosteroids are the mainstay of treatment.

If there is no improvement, surgical transnasal decompression is done.

13. What is the classical triad of pituitary apoplexy?
   i. Headache
   ii. Diplopia
   iii. Subarachnoid hemorrhage

14. What are the features of cavernous sinus meningiomas?
   i. Cavernous sinus meningiomas manifest as slowly progressive, painless lesion occurring in older women, and they may occasionally present as sudden painful ophthalmoplegia
   ii. Presents with ptosis, diplopia, and parasympathetic pupillary involvement
   iii. The demonstration of primary aberrant regeneration of the third nerve without a preceding neuropathy is exceedingly suggestive of meningioma
   iv. Management includes observation, radiation, surgical therapy or combination of all the three. They are extremely radiosensitive

15. What are the features of nasopharyngeal tumors?

Ophthalmic signs and symptoms	Otolaryngeal symptoms
1. Proptosis	1. Nasal congestion
2. Facial pain	2. Facial discomfort
3. Eye pain	3. Sinusitis
4. Visual loss	4. Facial swelling
5. Epiphora	5. Erythema
6. Globe displacement	6. Headache
7. Limitation of extraocular movements	7. Epistaxis
8. Diplopia	8. Nasal mass
9. Photophobia	9. Difficulty in chewing
10. Conjunctival chemosis	10. Facial numbness
11. Palpebral mass within the orbit	
12. Bony erosion	
13. Dacryocystitis	
14. Horner's syndrome	

16. What are the features of Tolosa–Hunt syndrome?
This is a variant of acute inflammatory pseudotumor affecting the cavernous sinus or superior orbital fissure.

The diagnostic criteria are:
i. Steady boring retro-orbital pain which may precede ophthalmoplegia
ii. Second, third, or fourth cranial palsy with or without Horner's syndrome
iii. Symptoms lasting for days to weeks
iv. Occasional spontaneous remission, although neurological defect may persist
v. Recurrent attacks in the intervals of months to years
vi. No evidence of disease outside cavernous sinus

Pathology—orbital periostitis with granulomatous vasculitis in the cavernous sinus

Investigations:
i. Hematological tests are nonspecific
ii. CSF analysis is unremarkable
iii. Carotid angiography shows abnormalities in the configuration of intracavernous carotid artery in the form of irregular narrowing or constriction. These changes are resolved with steroid therapy
iv. Orbital venography shows occlusion of superior ophthalmic vein on the affected side. There may be partial or absent filling of cavernous sinus. Follow-up venography shows persistent filling defects suggestive of fibrosis in the involved areas

Treatment: Corticosteroids are the mainstay of the treatment.

7.19 MALINGERING

1. **What are the tests to detect malingering?**
    i. *Total binocular blindness:*
        - *Observation:*
            - Truly blind moves cautiously and bumps into things naturally; hysterics avoids objects, "seeing unconsciously", malingerer goes out of his or her way to bump into objects
            - Patients who are truly blind in both eyes tend to look directly at the person with whom they are speaking, whereas patients with nonorganic blindness, particularly patients who are malingering, often look in some other direction
            - Similarly, patients claiming complete or near complete blindness often wear sunglasses, even though they do not have photophobia, and external appearance of eyes is perfectly normal
        - *Pupillary response*—earliest and single most important test
            - Intact direct and consensual response excludes anterior visual pathway disease
            - In patients with better than NPL, there is no consistent relationship between amount of visual loss and pupillary deficit
        - *Menace reflex*—blinking to visual threat
        - *Reflex tearing*—sudden strong illumination thrown into eyes difficult to suppress reflex tearing in a patient with good visual acuity
        - *Signature*—truly blind patients have no difficulty in doing signature. While functionally blind patients sign their name with exaggerated illegibility
        - Another way to detect nonorganic visual loss in a patient who claims to be unable to see shapes and objects in one or both eyes is to ask patient to touch the tips of index fingers of both hands together. If the patient claims loss of vision in one eye only, opposite eye is patched before test is performed

        As physician knows, the ability to touch the fingers of both hands together is based not on vision but on proprioception. Thus, patients with organic blindness can easily bring the tips of the fingers of two hands together, whereas patients with nonorganic blindness, particularly malingerer, will not do so. As the patient's hand is held up in front of him and he is asked to look at his hand, the malingerer tends to look to the right or left, anywhere, but not at his hand.

- *Optokinetic nystagmus* (OKN)—if patient claims NPL, light perception only, or perception of hand movements in one or both eyes. Rotating optokinetic drum or horizontally moving tape can be used to produce a horizontal jerk nystagmus that indicates intact vision of at least 3/60. It is important in this regard that the images on the tape or drum be sufficiently large that the patient is not able to look around them. When testing a patient who claims complete loss of vision in one eye only, we begin test by rotating the drum or moving the tape in front of the patient while he/she has both eyes open. Once we elicit good OKN, cover the unaffected eye with palm of our hand or a handheld occluder. The patient with nonorganic loss of vision in one eye will continue to slow jerk nystagmus
- *Mirror test:* A large mirror is held in front of patient's face, and patient is asked to look directly ahead. Mirror is then rotated and twisted back and forth, causing image in mirror to move. Patients with vision better than NPL show nystagmoid movement of the eyes because they cannot avoid following the moving mirror
- *Visual-evoked potential (VEP):* Flash and pattern reversal stimuli correlation exist between check size and level of acuity. Although difficult, it is possible to consciously alter response to pattern reversal stimulation with convergence, meditation, and intense concentration. P300 component of VEP is suggestive of conscious stimulation of the cerebral tissue, even though the patient says that he does not view the pattern stimulus

ii. *Total monocular blindness:*
More common than binocular blindness, total monocular blindness tends to occur with malingering. It can use any of the above tests with unaffected eye occluded
- Diplopia tests:
  - Suspected eye occluded while strong prism held with apex bisecting pupil of good eye. Patient admits monocular diplopia. As suspected, eye is uncovered, the entire prism is placed before good eye, producing binocular diplopia. If patient still reports diplopia, functional blindness is revealed
  - Make patient walk up and down stairs with vertical prism over allegedly blind eye
- Prism dissociation tests:
  Prism dissociation tests can be used to detect mild degrees of nonorganic monocular visual loss. In these tests, patient is first asked if he or she has experienced double vision in addition to loss of vision in affected eye. If answer is negative, the patient is told that the examiner will test the alignment of both eyes and that test should produce vertical double vision.

A 4-prism diopter loose prism is then placed base down in front of unaffected eye at the same time that 0.5 prism diopter loose prism is simultaneously placed with base in any direction over the eye with decreased vision.

In this way, the patient does not become suspicious that examiner is paying specific attention to one or the other eye A 6/6 or larger letter projected at a distance, the patient is asked if he/she has double vision.

When patient admits diplopia, she/he is then asked whether the two letters are of equal quality or sharpness, and an assessment of visual acuity can be made.

- *Fixation tests:*
  - 10 prism base out test:
    • Relies upon refixation movement to avoid diplopia
    • 10 D base out prism in front of normal eye produces shift of both eyes with refixation movement of the other eye
  - Vertical bar (reading)
    A ruler is held 5 inches from nose in between eyes while patient reads at near. Overlap of visual fields allows a binocular person to read across the bar. If patient reads without interruption, functional blindness is confirmed. Can also use prism in front of suspect eye, resulting in diplopia, which should interrupt reading
- *Fogging tests:*
  - With both eyes open on the phoropter, patient starts reading eye chart. Examiner progressively adds more plus to the good eye while patient keeps reading
    Final line read is patient's visual acuity in suspected eye
  - *Crossed cylinder technique:*
    • A variation of this test is the use of paired cylinders. A plus cylinder and minus cylinder of same power (usually from 2 to 6 D) are placed at parallel axes in front of the normal eye in a trial frame. The patient's normal correction is placed in front of the affected eye. The patient is asked to read with both eyes open, a line that previously has been read with the normal eye but not with the affected eye
    • As patient begins to read, the axis of one of the cylinders rotated through 10–15°. The axes of two cylinders thus will no longer be parallel due to blurring of vision in normal eye
      If patient continues to read the line or can read it again when asked to do so, he/she must be using affected eye
  - Instill cycloplegic agent into unaffected eye and ask the patient to read at near

- *Color tests:*
  - Red/green duochrome in projector, red/green glasses worn such that red lens covers suspected eye. Eye behind red lens sees letters on red and not on green side of chart. And eye behind the green lens sees only letters on the green side
  If patient reads the entire line, the suspected eye is being used.
  - Red/green glasses and worth four dot test—patient should see appropriate number of dots
  - *Ishihara color testing:*
    - In this test, red and green filters are used in front of each eye, while subject views Ishihara's color plates. The numbers and lines on Ishihara plates are visible only through red filter while plates 1 and 36 are seen by all persons, even if color blind, and are more distinctly seen through this filter. Even with visual acuity of 3/60, all color plates can be seen through red filter
    - The test for detecting functionally impaired vision is performed as follows:
    - After testing visual acuity of each eye, the patient is given the red and green goggles with red filter over the eye with alleged impaired vision. With a sound eye, patient will not see plates through green filter. If the patient sees the plates, the visual acuity must be 3/60 or better. If there is no response, the goggles should be switched so that the red filter will be over the sound eye, and if the patient does not respond even 1 and 36, then test should be done without any goggles to prove wrong answers
  - *Polaroid glasses and vector graphic slides:*
    - Polarizing lenses can be used in several ways to detect nonorganic visual loss in patients with decreased vision in one eye only
    - In American Optical Polarizing Test, the patient wears polarizing glasses, and the test object, a project-O-chart slide, projects letters alternately so that one letter is seen by both eyes, the next by the left eye, the next by right eye and so on
    - Another test uses polarizing lens placed before a projector. The patient is asked to read the chart while wearing polarizing lenses, with one eye or the other being allowed to see the whole projected image at a time, with vertical polarizer in one eye and horizontal polarizer in the other eye

- *Red Amsler grid test:*
  - Using red-green filters, red Amsler grid test is useful in cases with unilateral field loss when the professed visual field defect extends to within 10° of fixation. A paracentral scotoma must be demonstrated monocularly with Amsler grid. The patient is then asked to look at red Amsler grid on black background, using red filter in front of eye with scotoma and green filter in front of normal eye. The red on black can be seen only through red filter
  - A positive response indicates a credibility problem and proves functional visual loss
- *Stereoscopic tests:*
  - Stereoacuity is directly proportional to Snellen's acuity. Test plates used are Titmus fly or Randot test
  - 40 seconds of arc stereoacuity is compatible with no worse than 20/20 or 6/6 Snellen's acuity OU

Relationship of visual acuity and stereopsis:

Visual acuity	Stereopsis
6/6	40 seconds
6/9	52 seconds
6/12	61 seconds
6/18	78 seconds
6/24	94 seconds
6/36	124 seconds
6/60	160 seconds

iii. *Diminished vision:*
   Simulation of visual acuity <6/6 is more difficult to detect. Binocular or monocular can use most of the tests above plus the following:
   - Doctor killing refraction (DKR) or toothpaste refraction
     Start with 6/5 line and express disbelief the patient could not see big letters on the 6/6 line then proceed up chart until patient reads
   - Visual angle—varying test distance with eye chart, Landolt's C rings or Tumbling E block such that patient sees a smaller visual angle or demonstrates inconsistencies. For example, reading 6/6 letter at 10 ft is equivalent to 6/12 acuity
   - Move patient back and forth slightly in the chair, helping them get into focus or place combinations of lenses adding up to plano in a trial frame to help magnify their image

iv. *Field defects:*
   - *Constricted field (on kinetic perimetry):*
     - These field defects show steep margins
     - Remains same regardless of size of object and test distance from screen (tunnel vision)
     - The degree of functional constriction may vary in the same patient from one examination to the next. This may be demonstrated in malingering using tangent screen
     - Marks used to outline the patient's visual field are moved to new positions closer to fixation when the patient is absent
     - When the test is repeated, the new field will confirm to new pin arrangement
   - *Monocular hemianopias:*
     Field testing monocularly and binocularly—fields overlap
   - *Paracentral field defect:*
     In this malingering can be detected with the help of red Amsler grid test.

CHAPTER

8

Orbit

8.1 ECTROPION

1. **What is ectropion?**
   Ectropion is an eyelid malposition characterized by an outward turning of the eyelid margin away from the globe accompanied by separation between the eyelid and the globe.

2. **What is the surgical anatomy of the eyelid?**
   The eyelid is a bilamellar structure.
   Anterior lamella consists of:
   i. Skin
   ii. Thin areolar subcutaneous connective tissue
   iii. *Orbicularis oculi:* It is a striated muscle, which is anatomically divided into three parts, namely orbital, preseptal, and pretarsal
   Posterior lamella consists of:
   i. Tarsal plate
      - Dense fibrous tissue
      - 25-29 mm long
      - 1-1.5 mm thick
      - Upper tarsus: 8-12 mm in height
      - Lower tarsus: 4-5 mm in height
   ii. Conjunctiva

3. **What are the upper lid and lower lid retractors?**
   i. The upper lid and lower lid retractors lie between the anterior and the posterior lamella
   ii. *Upper lid retractors:*
      - Levator palpebrae superioris
      - Muller's muscle
   iii. *Lower lid retractors:*
      - Capsulopalpebral fascia
      - Sympathetically innervated inferior tarsal muscle

4. **What is capsulopalpebral fascia?**
   i. *Origin:* As capsulopalpebral head from delicate attachments to inferior rectus muscle

ii. Extends anteriorly and splits into two and surrounds the inferior oblique muscle
iii. Again rejoins to form Lockwood's ligament and fascial tissue anterior to this forms the capsule palpebral fascia
iv. *Insertion:* On the inferior fornix along with the inferior tarsal muscle and on the inferior border of tarsus

5. **How are the eyelids attached to the bony orbit?**
   Eyelids are attached to the bony orbit via the medial and lateral tendons.
   Medial canthal tendon: Two limbs:
   i. Anterior (superficial)—attached to the anterior lacrimal crest
   ii. Posterior (deep)—attached to the posterior lacrimal crest
   iii. Lacrimal sac is enclosed between the two
   iv. Common canaliculus lies immediately posterior to the anterior limb

   Lateral canthal tendon:
   i. Laterally, the tarsal plate becomes fibrous strands that form the crura of lateral canthal tendon
   ii. The crura of upper and lower lids fuse to form the common lateral canthal tendon
   iii. It is about 1-3 mm thick and 5-7 mm long
   iv. Insertion is 1.5 mm inside the lateral orbital rim on Whitnall's tubercle as a part of the lateral retinaculum
      Laxity of lateral canthal tendon is due to stretching and redundancy of the free portion of tendon between the tarsal plate and the tubercle

6. **How is ectropion classified?**
   Classification:
   Upper lid ectropion
   Lower lid ectropion—more common
   i. Medial
   ii. Lateral
   iii. Total
   Etiologically
   i. Involutional
   ii. Cicatricial
   iii. Paralytic
   iv. Mechanical
   v. Congenital

7. **How do we stage the severity of ectropion?**
   Staging
   i. *Mild:* Posterior lid margin just falls away from contact with the globe
   ii. *Moderate:* Complete eversion of lid margin exposing the conjunctiva
   iii. *Severe:* Complete eversion of lid (tarsal ectropion)

8. **What are the clinical features of ectropion?**
   Clinical features:
   Can be asymptomatic:
   i. *Punctal eversion:* This leads to decreased tear drainage and disuse punctal atrophy → epiphora → constant wiping → eczematous changes in the skin → further aggravation of the ectropion
   ii. *Conjunctival exposure:* This leads to keratinization, hyperemia, xerosis → punctal stenosis, and chronic conjunctivitis → chronic irritation and foreign body sensation
   iii. *Corneal exposure:* It is due to improper closure of the lids → keratitis → pain, photophobia, and decreased vision

9. **How to clinically evaluate ectropion?**
   Clinical evaluation: Aim is → find type
   i. Underlying mechanism
   ii. Decide the appropriate treatment
   It is done in three parts:
   i. *Ocular*
   ii. *Local:* Look for:
      - Herpes zoster dermatitis
      - Surgical scars
      - Traumatic scars
      - Facial anatomy and symmetry
      - Facial function
   iii. *Systemic:* Look for:
      - Skin disorders, e.g., lamellar ichthyosis
      - Actinic dermatitis
      - Parkinsonism

10. **How do you test for the following?**
    i. *Lid laxity:* Two tests:
       - *Pinch/retraction/distraction test:* If the central portion of the lower lid can be pinched (between the index finger and the thumb) and is able to be pulled >6 mm from the globe, significant lid laxity is present
       - *Snap back test:* Central portion of the lid is pulled and released; failure to snap back in its original position indicates lid laxity
    ii. *Canthal tendon integrity:*
       - *Lateral tendon:*
         - Rounding of the lateral canthal angle
         - Horizontal shortening of the palpebral fissure
         - Decrease in distance between temporal limbus and lateral canthal angle
         - Direct palpation of inferior crus of the lateral canthal tendon with simultaneous medial traction

- Medial tendon:
  - Look for the position of the punctum during lateral traction of the lid. Movement of punctum lateral to nasal limbus or displacement of >3 mm indicates partial dehiscence
  - Rounding of the medial canthal angle
  - Direct palpation of the medial canthal tendon with simultaneous lateral traction
iii. *Orbicularis muscle tone:* Ask the patient to squeeze the eyes tightly and try and open the eyes against resistance
iv. *Lower lid retractor disinsertion:*
  - Inferior fornix deeper than the normal
  - Higher resting position of the lower lid
  - Diminished excursion of lower lid in the downgaze
  - Disinserted edge of the retractors may be seen as a whitish band in the inferior fornix below the inferior edge of the tarsus
v. *Lacrimal apparatus:* Look for:
  - Direction of the punctum
  - Stenosis of the punctum
  - Patency of the lacrimal drainage system
vi. *Cicatricial component:* Grasp the lower lid margin and pull superiorly; if it does not reach 2 mm above the inferior limbus → vertical deficiency is present
vii. *Inferior scleral show:* This is seen if associated with lid retraction. In such cases, mere lid shortening procedures will aggravate the retraction and have to be combined with free full-thickness skin graft
viii. *Orbitotarsal disparity:* When contact and thereby pressure are inadequate between orbital contents and eyelid, there is lid instability
ix. *Corneal sensations:* Decreased sensations, especially in case of paralytic ectropion, indicate early surgical intervention
x. *Lagophthalmos*

11. What is involutional ectropion and its mechanisms?
i. *Involutional ectropion:*
  - Most common
  - Gradual onset
  - Most common in the lower lid
  - Earliest symptom: tearing
  - Earliest sign: Inferior punctal eversion
ii. *Mechanisms:*
  - Laxity of both medial and lateral canthal tendons
  - Partial dehiscence of the canthal tendon

- Orbicularis muscle undergoes ischemic changes due to microinfarcts → laxity
- Fragmentation of elastic and collagenous tissue within the tarsus leads to thinning and instability
- Dehiscence of lower lid retractors

12. What is the management of involutional ectropion?

Medical management:
   i. To relieve tearing and inflammation, lubricating antibiotic ointment can be used
   ii. Antibiotic—steroid combination can be used preoperatively for 2-3 weeks to decrease eyelid edema and hyperemia

Punctal ectropion: Following procedures can be done:
   i. *Suture technique:*
      - Two double-armed 5-0 chromic sutures are taken
      - The first suture is taken at the inferior border of tarsus at the junction of nasal and medial one-third of lid
      - The second is taken at a similar position at the junction of medial and lateral one-third of lid
      - Both emerge through the skin at the level of infraorbital rim

      Advantage:
      It is useful in debilitated patients.
      Disadvantages:
      - Temporary method
      - Recurrence
      - Foreshortening of the inferior fornix
   ii. *Medial spindle procedure:* Also called the tarsoconjunctival excision
      - The lower punctum is inverted by vertically shortening the posterior lamella and tightening the lower lid retractors
      - Diamond-shaped area (6 mm × 3 mm) of tarsoconjunctiva is excised below the punctum. It is closed with absorbable sutures from upper apex to lower apex including the lower lid retractors
   iii. *Electrocautery:*
      - Several deep burns placed 2 mm apart along the entire lower lid at the junction of conjunctiva and the lower margin of the tarsus
      - The effect can be titrated by depth and duration of cauterization
      - Recurrence is common
   iv. *Punctoplasty:*
      - Done in combination with ectropion if associated with punctal stenosis
      - One-snip and two-snip procedures can be employed
   v. *Otis Lee procedure:*
      - Done in case of severe punctal ectropion or in atonic medial ectropion involving both upper and lower puncta

- Horizontal incision at the junction of skin and conjunctiva medial to the puncta
- Lids joined with nonabsorbable suture
- Excess skin is removed

vi. *Smith's lazy-T procedure:*
   - Done when medial ectropion is associated with horizontal lid laxity
   - Done when the medial canthal tendon is firm
   - Pentagonal wedge of excess horizontal eyelid tissue is resected 4 mm lateral to the punctum
   - This is coupled with excision of diamond of tarsoconjunctiva below the punctum to invert it
   - Conjunctiva is closed horizontally with interrupted catgut sutures
   - Eyelid is closed

vii. *Medial canthal tendon plication:*
   - Indicated in excess medial tendon laxity
   - Canalicular part of medial canthal tendon is shortened by suturing the medial end of the lower tarsal plate to the main part of medial canthal tendon with nonabsorbable suture

viii. *Pentagonal wedge resection:*
   - Generalized ectropion with horizontal lid laxity
   - No excess skin is seen
   - A full-thickness pentagon is resected to correct the excess horizontal lid laxity
   - Done usually 5 mm from the lateral canthus or at the maximum lid laxity
   - Lid defect is repaired

ix. *Smith's modification of Kuhnt–Szymanowski procedure:*
   - Done when the medial canthal tendon is firm
   - Associated with horizontal lid laxity and excess skin
   - Subciliary blepharoplasty incision is made
   - Pentagonal wedge resection is done to correct horizontal lid laxity
   - Excess skin is removed as a triangular flap
   - Both skin and lid are closed

x. *Lateral tarsal strip procedure:*
   - Done when the ectropion is associated with horizontal lid laxity and lateral tendon laxity
   - A subciliary incision is made from the lateral two-fifths of the eyelid up to the lateral canthus and extending posteriorly
   - Lateral canthotomy is done
   - Inferior crux of lateral tendon is incised

- Tarsal strip is made by excising the mucosa cilia orbicularis and skin at the lateral end
- Lid is shortened by removing the excess tarsus
- Tarsal strip is sutured to the lateral orbital tubercle
- Excess skin is removed

xi. *Edelstein–Dryden procedure:*
- Done when ectropion is associated with midfacial trauma involving the lacrimal system
- Associated with the detached posterior horn of the medial tendon
- Periosteal flap is made from nasal bone and everted and hinged medially to lacrimal sac fossa and sutured to nasal margin of the tendon
- Thus, a new posterior horn is created

13. What is cicatricial ectropion?

i. Seen in both upper and lower lids
ii. Associated with vertical shortening within the anterior lamella of the lid

Etiology:
i. Trauma—mechanical, thermal, chemical, radiation
ii. Actinic dermatitis
iii. Herpes zoster dermatitis
iv. Basal cell carcinoma
v. Lamellar ichthyosis
vi. Iatrogenic, e.g., postblepharoplasty

Management:

Medical: Ocular lubricants, soft contact lens, air humidification, digital massage of the scar

Steroids injection in the scar

Wait for 6 months post-trauma for the scar to soften before surgery.

Surgical:
i. *Z-plasty:*
   - Done for localized vertical scar crossing the skin tension lines
   - Initial incision is made along the scar and another incision at each end of the central line at an angle of 60°
   - Scar tissue is excised
   - Two flaps of skin are transposed which increase the length of the skin in the line of scar contraction at the expense of shortening the skin at right angles to it
   - It also alters the line of the scar
ii. *V-Y plasty:*
   - Done for localized vertical scar but with minimal skin shortening
   - V-shaped incision with apex of V at the base of the scar

- Scar tissue is excised and V is closed as Y, thereby lengthening the lid vertically

iii. *Skin replacement:*
- Indicated in generalized shortage of the skin
- Can be a transposition flap from the upper lid (if excess skin is present) or a thin full-thickness skin graft (in case of extensive scarring)
- Skin graft can be taken from the upper eyelid, retroauricular skin, and supraclavicular area

14. **What is paralytic ectropion?**
    i. Due to facial nerve palsy, a loss of orbicularis tone → tarsal instability and an ectropion
    ii. Preexisting involutional changes make the condition more pronounced
    iii. It is associated with failure of lacrimal pump function
    iv. Other features of facial nerve palsy are seen

15. **What is the management of paralytic ectropion?**
    Management: Primary goal is to protect the cornea.
    i. *Medical:* Apart from lubricants and moisture chambers, Donaldson's patch can be used
    ii. *Surgical:* Indications are:
       - Progressive corneal deterioration
       - Permanent facial paralysis
       - Corneal anesthesia
       - Dry eye
       - Lack of good Bell's phenomenon
       - Monocular vision on the paralytic side

    Medial canthoplasty:
    i. Indicated in paralytic medial ectropion
    ii. Eyelids are sutured together medial to lacrimal puncta to reduce the increased vertical interpalpebral distance at the medial canthus caused by the unopposed action of the lid retractors and to bring the lacrimal puncta into the tear film
    iii. Excess skin is cut

    Lateral canthal sling:
    i. Usually combined with medial canthoplasty
    ii. Indicated in generalized lid laxity

    Temporary suture tarsorrhaphy:

    Facial sling:
    Used to support the lid when large bulk of atonic midfacial tissue continues to drag down the lower lid. Commonly, fascia lata is used.

Temporalis transfer:
Reserved for most severe cases that have recurred after previous surgery and in permanent facial nerve damage.

16. **What is mechanical ectropion?**
    i. Secondary to mechanical factor which either displaces the lid or pulls the lid out of its normal position against the globe
    ii. For example, large lid tumors, conjunctival chemosis from orbital inflammatory conditions, and severe lid edema
    iii. *Management:* Treat the cause

17. **What is congenital ectropion?**
    i. Rare, familial, but no Mendelian inheritance
    ii. Due to deficiency of eyelid skin → vertical shortening → ectropion
    iii. Associated with blepharophimosis syndrome
    iv. At rest, the lids are apposed, but on an attempt to look up or close the lids → eversion
    v. Treatment is horizontal lid tightening with free full-thickness skin grafting

18. **What are the features of upper lid ectropion?**
    i. Rare, congenital, common in black male infants, associated with trisomy 21
    ii. Usually bilateral
    iii. Can also be seen in cicatricial conditions, e.g., lamellar ichthyosis
    iv. *Mechanisms:* Vertical shortening of anterior lamella, vertical lengthening of posterior lamella, failure of fusion between septum and levator aponeurosis, and spasm of orbicularis
    v. *Treatment:* Pressure patch over reinverted lids
       Lid reconstruction procedures.

8.2 ENTROPION

1. **Define entropion.**
   Entropion is defined as inward rotation of the eyelid margin such that the cilia brush against the globe.

2. **How do you classify entropion?**
   i. Involutional entropion (senile entropion)
   ii. Cicatricial entropion
   iii. Congenital entropion
   iv. Spastic

3. **What is the pathophysiology of involutional entropion?**
   Involutional entropion affects mainly the lower lid because the upper lid has a wider tarsus and is more stable.
   Pathogenesis:
   i. Horizontal lid laxity/medial and lateral tendon laxity
   ii. Overriding of preseptal over pretarsal orbicularis during lid closure
   iii. Lower lid retractor weakness (excursion decreased of lower lid in downgaze)

4. **What are the causes of cicatricial entropion?**
   Cicatricial entropion is caused by severe scarring of the palpebral conjunctiva which pulls the lid margin toward the globe.
   Causes:
   i. *Infection*
      - Trachoma
      - Chronic blepharoconjunctivitis
      - Herpes zoster ophthalmicus
   ii. *Trauma*
      - Chemical
      - Mechanical
      - Radiation
   iii. *Immunological*
      - Erythema multiforme
      - Ocular cicatricial pemphigoid
      - Cicatricial vernal conjunctivitis
      - Dysthyroid

5. **What is congenital entropion?**
   i. Congenital entropion is caused by the improper development of retractor aponeurosis insertion into the inferior border of the tarsal plate

ii. It is extremely rare.
iii. Inversion of entire tarsus and lid margin
iv. Epiblepharon and horizontal tarsal kink are to be differentiated

6. How is congenital entropion classified?
Classification of congenital entropion is based on severity.
Kemp and Collin classification:
i. *Minimal*
   - Apparent migration of meibomian glands
   - Conjunctivilization of the lid margin
   - Lash globe contact on upgaze
ii. *Moderate*
   Same features plus
   - Lid retraction
   - Thickening of tarsal plate
iii. *Severe*
   Lid retraction (incomplete closure)
   - Gross lid retraction
   - Metaplastic lashes
   - Presence of keratin plaques

7. What are the examinations to be done in a case of entropion?
i. *Lid margin and ocular surface*—look for signs of punctate keratopathy due to blepharitis, meibomianitis, trichiasis, foreign bodies, dry eyes, and corneal disease
ii. *Lid instability*—forceful lid closure
   Excursion of the lower lid in downgaze, usually 3-4 mm—loss of movement indicates retractor weakness/disinsertion
iii. *Lid laxity*—pinch test
iv. *Lid elasticity*—snap test
v. *Medial canthal tendon (MCT) laxity*
vi. *Cicatricial component*—see directly by everting the lids. It can also be ascertained by pulling the lid superiorly. If it does not reach 2 mm above the lower limbus, the lid is vertically deficient
vii. Syringing
viii. Jones dye test
ix. Schirmer's test

8. What are the preoperative evaluation tests to be done in a case of entropion?
Preoperative evaluation/testing
i. *Assessment of capsulopalpebral fascia*
   - Higher eyelid resting position in primary gaze
   - Presence of white infratarsal band

- Increased depth of inferior conjunctival fornix
- Reduction in vertical eyelid excursion from upgaze to downgaze
   ii. *Assessment of horizontal eyelid laxity*
   - Passive horizontal eyelid distraction
   - Hill's test—central eyelid pulled >6 mm between eyelid and cornea—abnormal
   iii. *Enophthalmos*
   - Assessment of relative enophthalmos—exophthalmometry
   iv. *Assessment of preseptal orbicularis muscle override*
   - Subjective assessment—done in primary gaze/forceful eyelid closure/spontaneous blink
   - Thick appearance of the eyelid
   v. *Assessment of posterior lamellar support*
   - Height of tarsal plate
   vi. *Presence of cicatrizing conjunctival disease*
   - Trachoma
   - Stevens-Johnson syndrome
   - Ocular cicatricial pemphigoid
   - Chronic meibomian gland dysfunction
   - Chemical injury/topical medication
   vii. *Corneal/conjunctival status*
   viii. *Lash position/lacrimal and meibomian gland function*

9. **What is the nonsurgical management of entropion?**
   i. Taping
   ii. Treatment of associated blepharitis, meibomianitis, and corneal disease
   iii. Lubricants
   iv. Botulinum toxin injection
   v. Bandage contact lenses

10. **What are the temporary surgical measures in involutional entropion?**
    i. *Transverse sutures* are placed through the lid to prevent the upward movement of the preseptal orbicularis muscle
    ii. *Everting sutures* are placed obliquely to shorten the lower lid retractors and transfer their pull to the upper border of the tarsus
    iii. *Transverse sutures*—three double-armed 4-0 catgut sutures are taken through the lid from the conjunctiva to the skin in the lateral two-thirds of the lid. Start below the tarsus and make each needle emerge through the skin about 2 mm apart, just below the level at which they entered the conjunctiva
    iv. *Everting sutures*—they are similar but start lower in the fornix and emerge nearer to the lashes
    v. Sutures are removed after 10-14 days

11. **What are the principles of permanent treatment in involutional entropion?**
    i. Strengthening the lid retractors as in Jones, Reeh, Wobigs and modified Jones procedure where the inferior lid retractors are plicated or attached to the tarsus
    ii. Shortening the anterior lamina by suturing the preseptal orbicularis to pretarsal orbicularis so as to prevent migration of orbicularis, forming a cicatrix between the two parts of orbicularis
    iii. Removal of horizontal lid laxity, if present, by tarsal strip procedure, where small strips of lid margin, conjunctiva, and skin are removed to create a free end of the tarsal plate that functions as the canthal ligament

12. **What is Wies procedure?**
    i. Transverse lid split + everting sutures
    ii. This is indicated in cases with minimum horizontal lid laxity when long-term results are required

13. **What is Quickert procedure?**
    i. Transverse lid split + everting sutures + horizontal lid shortening
    ii. This is a long-term procedure for cases where horizontal lid laxity also presents

14. **What is Jones procedure?**
    Plication of lower lid retractors
    Indication: Recurrence after Quickert procedure

15. **What are the steps of modified Jones procedure?**
    i. Mark a subciliary incision along the length of the lid. If there is lengthening, the amount of shortening required should be marked
    ii. Incision is made into the skin—muscle up to the tarsal plate. The tarsal plate is exposed
    iii. Blunt dissection is continued at the inferior margin of tarsus. The stretched is dehisced. Retractors will be visible
    iv. Three double-armed 6-0 Vicryl sutures are passed; the retractors may be plicated or simply reattached. The three sutures are tightened and correction observed. The straightening of the margin is immediately seen. The end point is when the posterior margin is just apposed to the globe
    v. The skin and muscle lamina usually need to be shortened and are excised in a spindle manner
    vi. Associated lengthening—by excising the lid in a full-thickness pentagonal shape (Bick's procedure)
    vii. Sutures are removed in 6–7 days

16. **What is the surgical procedure for congenital entropion?**
    Hotz procedure
    i. Minimal ellipse of skin and orbicularis is excised from medial two-thirds of the lower lid
    ii. Skin is fixed to the lower edge of the tarsus

17. **What is the management of cicatricial entropion?**
    i. Marginal incision and grafting
    ii. Tarsal fracture and margin rotation—Tenzel procedure—indicated when lid retraction is <1.5 mm from the limbus
    iii. *Posterior lamellar grafting* in cases of posterior lamellar shortening—indicated when lid retraction is >1.5 mm from the limbus
    iv. *Tarsal wedge resection*—a common procedure used in cases with trachomatous scarring (especially if tylosis is present)

18. **What are the various materials used as posterior lamellar grafts?**
    i. Conchal cartilage
    ii. Nasal chondromucosa
    iii. Palatal mucoperichondrium
    iv. Buccal mucosa
    v. Tarsoconjunctival composite graft
    vi. Mucous membrane graft
    vii. Amniotic membrane transplant—now becoming more popular

19. **What are the complications after surgery for entropion?**
    i. *Recurrence*—it is the most common complication of surgical correction of entropion
    ii. *Ectropion*—possible mechanisms include excessive skin removal, over advancement of the retractors onto the anterior face of the tarsal plate. Shortening of the septum, hematoma, and excessive scar formation
    iii. *Lagophthalmos*—shortened septum—warm compresses and massage with corticosteroid ointment may correct mild cases
    iv. *Lid necrosis*—margin rotation techniques are more common
    v. *Lid infection, wound dehiscence*
    vi. *Graft complications*—symblepharon, corneal injury induced by rough posterior eyelid surface.

8.3 PTOSIS

1. **What is the definition of blepharoptosis?**
   Blepharoptosis is the drooping or inferior displacement of the upper eyelid.

2. **How will you classify blepharoptosis?**
   Two classification systems:
   According to onset:
   i. Congenital
   ii. Acquired
   According to cause:
   i. Neurogenic
      - Third nerve palsy
      - Third nerve misdirection
      - Horner's syndrome
      - Marcus Gunn jaw-winking syndrome
   ii. Myogenic
      - Myasthenia gravis
      - Myotonic dystrophy
      - Ocular myopathies
      - Simple congenital
      - Blepharophimosis syndrome
   iii. Aponeurotic
      - Involutional attenuation
      - Repetitive traction like rigid contact lenses
   iv. Mechanical
      - Plexiform neuroma
      - Hemangioma
      - Acquired neoplasm

3. **What are the causes of unilateral ptosis?**
   i. *Myogenic:*
      - Dysfunction of levator palpebrae superioris (LPS)
   ii. *Neurogenic:*
      - Third cranial nerve palsy—upper division, complete
      - Cervical sympathetic—Horner's syndrome
   iii. *Aponeurotic:*
      - Congenital ptosis
      - Senile ptosis
      - Trauma to aponeurosis
      - Postoperative—cataract, squint, retinal detachment

4. **What are the components of ptosis workup?**
    i. Palpebral fissure height
    ii. Margin reflex distance (MRD)
    iii. Margin crease distance (MCD)
    iv. LPS action
    v. Lagophthalmos
    vi. Bell's phenomenon
    vii. Marcus Gunn phenomenon
    viii. Tarsal height
    ix. Pupillary reaction
    x. Corneal sensation
    xi. Ocular movements
    xii. Fatigability test
    xiii. Cogan's lid twitch sign
    xiv. Ice pack test

5. **How can we classify the amount of ptosis based on the relationship between upper lid level and pupil?**
    i. Mild—upper eyelid margin just above the upper border of pupil
    ii. Moderate—upper eyelid margin at the upper border of pupil or covering half of the pupil
    iii. Severe—upper eyelid margin at or below the lower border of pupil

6. **How to classify the amount of blepharoptosis?**
    The difference in MRD1 of the two sides in unilateral cases
    Or
    The difference from normal in bilateral cases gives the amount of ptosis.
    Amount of ptosis may be classified as:
    i. Mild ptosis   — 2 mm or less
    ii. Moderate ptosis — 3 mm
    iii. Severe ptosis — 4 mm or more

7. **What is the normal position of the upper lid?**
    The upper lid margin covers 1–2 mm of the superior cornea.

8. **What is Whitnall's ligament?**
    Whitnall's (superior transverse) ligament is a sleeve of elastic fibers around the levator muscle located in the area of transition from levator muscle to levator aponeurosis. It functions to convert the anterior-posterior vector force of the levator to a superior-inferior direction during eyelid movement.

9. **What is MRD1 and its significance?**
    Margin reflex distance
    The distance between the center of the lid margin of the upper lid and the light reflex on the cornea in the primary position would give MRD1.

i. If the margin is above the light reflex, the MRD1 has a *positive value*
ii. If the lid margin is below the corneal reflex in cases of very severe ptosis, the MRD1 would have a *negative value*. The latter would be calculated by keeping the scale at the middle of upper lid margin and elevating the lid till the corneal light reflex is visible. The distance between the reflex and the marked original upper lid margin would be the MRD1
iii. MRD1 is the single most effective measurement in describing the amount of ptosis

MRD1: Normal 4-5 mm. The mean measurement in Indian eyes is 4.1 ± 0.5.

It must be remembered that ptotic lid in unilateral congenital ptosis is usually higher in downgaze due to the failure of the levator to relax.

The ptotic lid in acquired ptosis is invariably lower than the normal lid in downgaze.

10. **What is marginal reflex distance 2 (MRD2)?**
    MRD2 is the distance from the corneal light reflex to the lower eyelid margin.

11. **What are the various methods to evaluate levator function?**
    i. *Berke's method (lid excursion):*
       This method measures the excursion of the upper lid from extreme downgaze to extreme upgaze with the action of frontalis muscle blocked.

       The patient is positioned against a wall while the surgeon's hands press the forehead above the eyebrows ensuring that there is no downward or upward push. The patient is then asked to look at extreme downgaze and then in extreme upgaze and the readings are recorded in millimeters. Crowell Beard reported normal eyelid excursion to be between 12 and 17 mm.
    ii. *The levator function is classified as:*
        8 mm or more — good
        5-7 mm — fair
        4 mm — poor
    iii. *Putterman's method:*
         This method is carried out by the measurement of the distance between the middle of upper lid margin and the 6 o'clock limbus in extreme upgaze. This is also known as the margin limbal distance (MLD).

         Normal is about 9.0 mm

         The difference in MLD of two sides in unilateral cases
             Or
         The difference with normal in bilateral cases multiplied by three would give the amount of levator resection required.

iv. *Assessment in children:*
   Measurement of levator function in small children is a difficult task. The presence of lid fold and increase or decrease in its size on movement of the eyelid gives us a clue to the levator action. Presence of anomalous head posture like the child throwing his head back suggests a poor levator action.

v. *Iliff test:*
   This test is another indicator of levator action. It is applicable in the first year of life. The upper eyelid of the child is everted as the child looks down. If the levator action is good, the eyelid reverts on its own.

12. What is palpebral fissure height?
i. Palpebral fissure height is the distance between the upper and lower lid margins, measured in pupillary plane
ii. The upper lid margin normally rests about 2 mm below the upper limbus and the lower lid margin rests 1 mm above or at the level of lower limbus
   Normal value: Males: 7-10 mm; Females: 8-12 mm
iii. It is measured after negating the frontalis action

13. What is MCD? What is its significance?
The MCD is the distance from the central eyelid margin to the central upper lid skin crease with the upper lid in the downgaze and skin fold slightly elevated to expose the crease.

Normal values: Varies with race and gender. In Indians, male = 5-7 mm and female = 7-9 mm

The insertion of the fibers from the levator muscle into the skin contributes to the formation of the upper eyelid crease. The significance is twofold:
i. The crease is usually elevated in patients with involutional ptosis and is often shallow or absent in patients with congenital ptosis
ii. MCD helps in marking the incision site on the eyelid

14. What is Bell's phenomenon?
Bell's phenomenon is the involuntary protective reflex producing upward rotation of eyeball on closure of the eye.

Confirmation of presence of Bell's phenomenon is important before undertaking any surgical procedure to avoid the risk of postoperative exposure keratopathy.

15. How do we grade Bell's phenomenon?
  i. Good—less than one-third of the inferior part of the cornea is visible
  ii. Fair—one-third to one-half of the inferior part of the cornea is visible
  iii. Poor—more than one-half of the inferior part of the cornea is visible

16. What are the different types of Bell's phenomenon?
  i. *Normal:* Upward and outward movement of eyeball
  ii. *Inverse:* Upward and inward movement of eyeball
  iii. *Reverse:* Downward movement of eyeball
  iv. *Perverse:* Lateral movement of eyeball

17. Define lagophthalmos?
Lagophthalmos is the incomplete or defective closure of the eyelids. The inability to blink and effectively close the eyes leads to corneal exposure and excessive evaporation of the tear film.

18. What are the causes of lagophthalmos?
  i. Paralytic lagophthalmos—facial nerve palsy
   - Bell's palsy
   - Trauma
   - Infection
   - Tumors
  ii. Cicatricial lagophthalmos—trauma and surgery
  iii. Nocturnal lagophthalmos—during sleep

19. How will you grade lagophthalmos?
House-Brackmann grade:
  i. Grade 1: Normal and eyelid closure
  ii. Grade 2: Full eyelid closure with minimal effort
  iii. Grade 3: Full eyelid closure with maximal effort
  iv. Grade 4: Incomplete closure with normal facial symmetry
  v. Grade 5: Incomplete closure with facial asymmetry
  vi. Grade 6: No eyelid movement

20. How is tarsal height measured and what is its significance?
The upper lid is everted and the vertical height of the tarsus is measured over the central portion of the lid with a caliper. This measurement is usually between 10 and 12 mm in Caucasians and between 6.5 and 7.5 mm in Asians. This is the range between low, medium, and high crease height.

The height of the tarsus determines the overall central position of the crease during blepharoplasty. The shaved-off tip of the wooden cotton tip applicator dipped with methylene blue is ideal for drawing a thin crease line. The crease height is carefully transcribed onto the external skin surface over the central part of the eyelid skin.

This point directly overlies the superior tarsal border and will serve as a reference point for the overall crease height along the central one-third of the eyelid, whether the crease shape is to be nasally tapered, parallel, or laterally flared.

For those patients who already have a crease, the tarsal height still has to be measured to confirm whether the apparent crease seen is indeed the correct crease line to use.

21. What is pseudoptosis?

Pseudoptosis is a false impression of eyelid drooping. It may be caused by:
  i. *Lack of support* of lids by the globe as in artificial eye, microphthalmos, phthisis bulbi, or enophthalmos
  ii. Contralateral lid retraction
  iii. *Ipsilateral hypotropia:* The pseudoptosis will disappear when hypotropic eye assumes fixation on covering the normal eye
  iv. *Brow ptosis* due to excessive skin on the brow or seventh nerve palsy
  v. *Dermatochalasis* in which excessive upper lid skin overhangs the eyelid margin

22. What is Marcus Gunn jaw-winking syndrome?

Marcus Gunn jaw-winking syndrome is the most common type of congenital synkinetic neurogenic ptosis. About 5% of congenital ptosis manifests this phenomenon.

This synkinesis is thought to be caused by an aberrant connection between the motor division of fifth cranial nerve and the levator muscle.

Signs:
Retraction of ptotic lid in conjunction with stimulation of the ipsilateral pterygoid muscles by chewing, sucking, opening the mouth, or contralateral jaw movement.

Jaw-winking does not improve with age, although patients may learn to mask it.

Treatment:
No surgical treatment is entirely satisfactory.

Management depends on the cosmetic significance of the jaw-winking, where jaw-winking is not significant; the choice of the procedure depends on the amount of ptosis and the levator action is carried out as in any case of congenital simple ptosis. A larger levator resection is necessary and undercorrection is common. In case of significant jaw-winking bilateral levator excision with a fascia lata, sling surgery is the procedure of choice.

23. How is Marcus Gunn phenomenon graded?

Elevation of the upper lid on jaw movement	Degree of Marcus Gunn phenomenon
Symmetrization with the opposite eye	Mild
To upper lid	Moderate
Beyond upper limbus	Severe

Retraction of lid	Degree of Marcus Gunn phenomenon
2 mm	Mild
2–5 mm	Moderate
>5 mm	Severe

24. How do you differentiate congenital ptosis from acquired ptosis?

Characteristics	Congenital ptosis	Acquired ptosis
Cause	Myogenic (poorly developed levator muscle)	Aponeurotic (stretching or even disinsertion of levator aponeurosis)
Palpebral fissure height	Mild-to-severe ptosis	Mild-to-severe ptosis
Upper lid crease	Weak or absent crease in normal position	Higher than normal crease
Levator function	Reduced	Near normal
Downgaze	Eyelid lag	Eyelid drop
Amblyopia	Commonly seen in 20%	Uncommon
Marcus Gunn jaw-winking phenomenon	May or may not be present	Absent

25. What is blepharophimosis–ptosis–epicanthus inversus syndrome (BPES)?

Blepharophimosis–ptosis–epicanthus inversus syndrome is an autosomal-dominant condition with marked hypoplasia of the tarsal plate. Blepharophimosis is a reduction in the maximum vertical distance between the upper and lower eyelids combined with a short palpebral fissure.

Two clinical types are as follows:
BPES 1: Transmission through males only. Associated menstrual irregularity and infertility due to ovarian failure
BPES 2: No associated infertility and transmitted through both sexes.

26. What are the precautions to be undertaken before administering local anesthesia for ptosis surgery?

After appropriate marking, the upper eyelid is typically infiltrated with a small volume of local anesthetic, typically 1–1.5 mL of 1–2% lidocaine mixed with epinephrine, in a subcutaneous plane. The anesthetic paralyzes the orbicularis oculi muscle and the epinephrine can stimulate Muller's muscle, rendering the intraoperative eyelid position higher than what is expected postoperatively. To avoid this, some surgeons will set the eyelid height 1-1.5 mm higher than the desired postoperative position. Care should be taken not to pierce the orbital septum while injecting local anesthesia as excess anesthesia can weaken the levator making intraoperative assessment difficult. Allowing the epinephrine 7-10 minutes to work increases its hemostatic effect allowing better visualization of tissue planes.

27. **What are the various options for ptosis repair?**

    Ptosis repair is a challenging oculoplastic surgical procedure.

    Nonsurgical treatment: It is unusual but may include devices called eyelid crutches that are attached to eyeglass frames. They are occasionally useful in patients with neurogenic or myogenic ptosis in whom surgical correction can lead to severe, exposure-related corneal problems.

    It is advisable to wait till 3-4 years of age for surgical correction when the tissues are mature enough to withstand the surgical trauma and a better assessment and postoperative care are possible due to improved patient cooperation. There should be no delay in surgical management in cases of severe ptosis where the pupil is obstructed and the possibility of the development of amblyopia is high.

    Surgical approach depends on:
    i. Whether ptosis is unilateral or bilateral
    ii. Severity of ptosis
    iii. Levator action
    iv. Presence of abnormal ocular movements, jaw-winking phenomena, or blepharophimosis syndrome

    The choice of the surgical procedure is as follows:

    Fasanella-Servat operation:
    i. Mild ptosis (<2 mm or less)
    ii. Levator action (>10 mm)
    iii. Well-defined lid fold—no excess skin

    Levator resection:
    i. Mild/moderate/severe ptosis
    ii. Levator action (≥4 mm)

    Brow suspension ptosis repair:
    i. Severe ptosis
    ii. Levator action (<4 mm)
    iii. Jaw-winking ptosis or blepharophimosis syndrome

    Bilateral ptosis:

    In cases of bilateral ptosis, simultaneous bilateral surgery is preferred to ensure a similar surgical intervention in the two eyes. However, in cases where gross asymmetry exists between the two eyes, the eye with a greater ptosis is operated first and the other eye is operated after 6–8 weeks.

28. **What are the indications and contraindications of various ptosis repair procedures?**

    Fasanella–Servat operation
    Indications:
    i. Ptosis (<2 mm)
    ii. Levator function (>10 mm)
    iii. Mild congenital ptosis
    iv. Horner's syndrome
    v. Senile (involutional) ptosis
    vi. Minor contour adjustment, after previous ptosis or other upper lid surgery
    vii. Well-defined lid fold—no excess skin

    Contraindications:
    i. Dry eye syndromes
    ii. Corneal diseases
    iii. Bleb

    Levator resection
    Indications:
    i. Mild/moderate/severe ptosis
    ii. Levator function (≥4 mm)

    Contraindications:
    i. Levator function (<4 mm)
    ii. Poor Bell's phenomenon
    iii. Decreased corneal sensation
    iv. Decreased tear production

    Brow suspension
    Indications:
    i. Severe ptosis
    ii. Levator function (<4 mm)
    iii. After levator excision surgery (done previously)
    iv. Blepharophimosis
    v. Jaw-winking
    vi. Infants where levator function is not assessable (to prevent amblyopia)

    Contraindications:
    i. Mild-to-moderate ptosis with good levator function
    ii. Absent Bell's phenomenon
    iii. Restricted elevation (do undercorrection)

    [e.g., chronic progressive external ophthalmoplegia (CPEO), ocular myopathies, long-standing third nerve palsy]

29. What are the various surgical steps in the different techniques for ptosis correction?

Modified Fasanella–Servat surgery:
It is done for:
 i. Mild ptosis (<2 mm or less)
 ii. Levator action (>10 mm)

It is the excision of tarsoconjunctiva, Muller's muscle, and levator.
Xylocaine with adrenaline is used for local anesthesia in adults but general anesthesia is necessary for children.

Surgical steps:
 i. Three sutures are passed close to the folded superior margin of the tarsal plate at the junction of middle, lateral, and medial one-third of the lid
 ii. Three corresponding sutures are placed close to the everted lid margin starting from the conjunctival aspect near the superior fornix in positions corresponding to the first three sutures
 iii. Proposed incision is marked on the tarsal plate such that a uniform piece of tarsus, decreasing gradually toward the periphery, is excised
 iv. A groove is made on the marked line of incision and the incision is completed with a scissor. The first set of sutures helps in lifting the tarsal plate for excision
 v. The tarsal plate not >3 mm in width is excised

Levator resection:
This is the most commonly practiced surgery for ptosis correction. It may be performed through the skin or conjunctival route.

Surgical steps:
 i. The proposed lid crease is marked to match the normal eye considering the margin crease
 ii. Incision through the skin and orbicularis is made along the crease marking
 iii. The inferior skin and orbicularis are dissected away from the tarsal plate
 iv. The upper edge is separated from the orbital septum
 v. The fibers of the aponeurosis are cut from their insertion in the inferior half of the anterior surface of the tarsus
 vi. The levator is freed from the adjoining structures
 vii. The lateral and the medial horns are cut whenever a large resection is planned
 viii. Care should be taken that Whitnall's ligament is not damaged
 ix. A double-armed 5-0 Vicryl is passed through the center of the tarsal plate by a partial thickness bite

x. It is then passed through the levator aponeurosis at a height judged by the preoperative evaluation. Intraoperative assessment is made
xi. Two more double-armed Vicryl 5-0 sutures are passed through the tarsus about 2 mm from the upper border in the center and at the junction of central third with the medial and lateral thirds
xii. These sutures are then placed in the levator and intraoperative assessment is made
xiii. Excess levator is excised
xiv. Four to five lid fold forming sutures are placed

Brow suspension repair:
This surgery is the procedure of choice in simple congenital ptosis with poor levator action. A number of materials such as nonabsorbable sutures, extended polytetrafluoroethylene (ePTFE), muscle strips, and banked or fresh fascia lata strips have been used for suspension.

Temporary sling:
Thread sling is carried out in very young children with severe ptosis where prevention of amblyopia and uncovering the pupil are the main aims.

The suture sling procedures have a relatively higher recurrence rate or may show formation of suture granuloma. Definitive surgery may be performed at a later date when a fascia lata sling is carried out.

Fascia lata sling:
Fascia lata sling is considered in children above 4 years of age having severe congenital simple ptosis with poor levator action. Even in cases of unilateral severe ptosis, a bilateral procedure is preferred because a unilateral surgery causes marked asymmetry in downgaze. The results of bilateral surgery are more acceptable.

30. **What are the types of materials used in sling surgery?**
    i. Autogenous fascia lata
    ii. Silk suture material
    iii. Prolene suture material
    iv. Gore-Tex
    v. Braided polyester
    vi. Silicone rods, etc.

31. **What are the needles used in sling surgery?**
    i. *WRIGHT needle* is a widely used instrument for the insertion of fascia lata; handling this instrument is very difficult
    ii. *18 gauge hypodermic needle 4/0 monofilament polypropylene suture*—less slippage, easy control of needle direction, and depth of penetration more accurate

32. **What are the complications of sling surgery?**
    i. *Most common:* Undercorrection
    ii. *Others:* Overcorrection
        - Unsatisfactory eyelid contour
        - Globe perforation
        - Increased dermatochalasis
        - Upper eyelid ectropion
        - Scarring
        - Wound dehiscence
        - Eyelid crease/fold asymmetry
        - Conjunctival prolapse
        - Tarsal eversion
        - Lagophthalmos with exposure keratitis (poor LPS)

33. **How will you estimate the amount of levator resection?**

Degree of ptosis	LPS function	Amount of levator resection needed	Ideal postoperative correction
Mild (<2 mm)	Good (>8 mm)	Small (10–13 mm) Moderate (14–17 mm)	Undercorrect by 1–3 mm
Moderate (3 mm)	Moderate (5–7 mm) Poor (<5 mm)	Large (18–22 mm) Maximum (23 mm or more)	Match the normal lid; fully correct the ptosis
Severe (>4 mm)	Poor (<5 mm)	Supramaximal (>27 mm)	Overcorrect by 1–2 mm

34. **How do we manage a patient with ptosis and strabismus?**
    Vertical strabismus—strabismus surgery first followed by ptosis correction after 3 months. For example, hypotropia can cause pseudoptosis. In such condition, correction of the squint corrects the ptosis also.
    Horizontal strabismus—can be done at the same sitting.

35. **What is the timing of surgery for congenital ptosis?**
    Correct ptosis by 5 years of age. If possible, it is advisable to wait till 3-4 years of age in cases of congenital ptosis. The following advantages are obtained:
    i. Better assessment is possible
    ii. Tissues are better developed to withstand surgical trauma
    iii. Better postoperative care is possible due to better cooperation

    However, an exception to this timing is bilateral or unilateral ptosis where there is complete obscuration of the visual axis.

36. **What are the two techniques of brow suspension surgery?**
    i. Crawford's technique
    ii. Fox's technique

37. **What are the points to present in a case of ptosis?**

	Normal
Vertical palpebral fissure height	9–10 mm
MRD1	4–5 mm
MRD2	4–5 mm
Levator function	12–17 mm
MCD	• Males: 5–7 mm • Females: 7–9 mm
Bell's phenomenon	
Lagophthalmos	
Marcus Gunn phenomenon	

8.4 EYELID RECONSTRUCTION

1. **What are the common causes of eyelid defects?**
   Eyelid tissue loss is usually the result of trauma or resection of a pathologic process such as tumor or segmental trichiasis.
   i. *Defects due to trauma:* Eyelid wounds, especially those resulting from trauma, tend to gape widely giving the unnerving appearance of a large amount of tissue loss. Fortunately, the eyelid is quite elastic and a large majority of these defects can be repaired with direct closure
   ii. *Defects due to surgical resection of tumor:* Reconstruction of the eyelid is simplified by the technique of resection. Resection of a lesion of the eyelid should be made with full-thickness incisions

2. **What are the principles of eyelid reconstruction?**
   i. The repair depends on its size and position and the state of surrounding tissues
   ii. Components which require consideration include the posterior lamella, the anterior lamella, both lamella or a full-thickness defect, the medial and lateral canthi, and the lacrimal drainage system
   iii. The approach should proceed by considering direct repair first, followed by lateral cantholysis and then a tissue transfer procedure using either a flap or a graft

3. **What is the anesthesia required?**
   i. Local anesthesia for repair of eyelid lacerations is best obtained by performing a regional block. Anesthesia of most of the lower eyelid can be obtained by injecting 1 cc of anesthetic into the infraorbital foramen
   ii. Anesthesia of the upper lid is obtained by blocking the supraorbital nerve. Again, additional anesthesia may be necessary laterally because of the lacrimal nerve. Anesthesia to the medial canthal area and the lacrimal sac is obtained by blocking the infratrochlear nerve

4. **What are the preoperative preparations?**
   i. The eye should be anesthetized with xylocaine eye drops. A corneal shield lubricated with antibiotic ointment is useful. The surrounding skin should be prepped with betadine, but the solution should not be used to cleanse the wound. The wound should be irrigated profusely with warmed saline. All dirt and foreign particles should be cleansed, especially embedded dirt which can cause permanent discoloration and tattooing

ii. Wound edges should be minimally debrided of all necrotic tissue. Irregular edges should be freshened to allow for straight surgical margins to suture together. Identifiable landmarks such as eyebrows or eyelid margins should be sutured first

5. **Classify common reconstruction options of periocular defects.**

Region and defect	Closure option	Indication
Eyelids		
Partial thickness (anterior lamellar)	• Primary closure • Local skin and myocutaneous flap • Full-thickness skin graft	
Full-thickness	Primary closure	Defects <15 mm or <25% of lid margin
	Primary closure + lateral canthotomy + cantholysis	Defects 25–50% of lid margin
	Tenzel semicircular flap	Defects of 50–75% of lid margin
	Hughes tarsoconjunctival flap, full-thickness skin graft, or local flap	Lower eyelid defects >75% of lid margin
	Cutler–Beard technique	Upper eyelid defects >75% of lid margin
	Free graft for posterior lamella local flap for anterior lamella	Defects > 75% of lid margin
	Mustarde rotating cheek and opposing lid flaps	Large lid defects >75%
	Composite lid grafts	Defects < 8 mm of lid margin
Medial canthus		
	Local flaps (e.g., nasoglabellar transposition flap)	
	Paramedian forehead flap	
	Full-thickness skin grafts	
	Combination of above	
Lateral canthus		
	Local flaps	
	Full-thickness skin grafts	

6. **What are the procedures for repairing anterior lamellar defects?**
    i. Direct skin closure
    ii. Skin flaps

iii. Skin graft:
   - Full thickness
   - Partial thickness

7. **How is direct skin repair done?**
   Wounds involving a small loss of partial thickness eyelid skin with an intact eyelid margin can usually be closed primarily. Skin can be closed with 6-0 or 7-0 silk in adults and 7-0 chromic gut in children. If tissue closure results in some tension, the wound should be closed with horizontal tension rather than vertical tension to try avoiding ectropion. Sutures can be removed at 5–7 days and scar massage beginning in 1 week after suture removal.

8. **What are the various types of skin flaps used?**
   i. *V-Y plasty*—to lengthen structures, e.g., telecanthus repair and close defects. Glabellar flap is its variant
   ii. *Rhomboid flap*—used in the closure of medial and lateral periorbital defects. The rhombic flap is useful for nonmarginal lesions where vertical tension on the eyelids can be avoided
   iii. *Z-plasty*—to increase the length of skin and to change the direction of scar

9. **What are the various types of skin grafts used for anterior lamellar repair?**
   i. *Full-thickness skin grafts:* A full-thickness skin graft contains both epidermal and dermal components. For eyelid reconstruction, the contralateral eyelid is the best donor site. If not enough tissue can be obtained from there, the postauricular region and supraclavicular region are also good choices. All donor sites should be hairless to avoid trichiasis

   After harvesting the full-thickness graft in the standard way, the graft is sewn into place. A standard bolster is then placed. The dressing may be removed in 5 days
   ii. *Split-thickness skin grafts (STSGs):* An STSG is composed of epidermal components only. STSGs have a poor texture and color match with eyelid skin and tend to contract more than full-thickness grafts. They, therefore, are not used very much in eyelid reconstruction unless there is no other alternative (e.g., a badly burned patient without full-thickness skin to harvest). It is usually taken from the inner arm or thigh

10. **What are the various procedures for posterior lamellar reconstruction?**
    Posterior lamellar graft:
    i. Tarsal rotation
    ii. Hughes procedure

iii. Ear cartilage graft
iv. Mucous membrane graft
v. Tarsoconjunctival graft

11. **What is the principle of posterior lamellar graft?**
    The posterior lamella consists of tarsus and conjunctiva. In cases of posterior lamellar shortening, grafts such as sclera, cartilage, or mucosa graft can be used to lengthen the posterior lamella. In the upper lid, grafts are placed between tarsus and LPS. In the lower lid, grafts are placed between tarsus and lower lid retractors.

12. **What is a free tarsoconjunctival graft?**
    For full-thickness defects that are too large to close primarily, a graft taken from the posterior surface of the ipsilateral or contralateral upper eyelid will provide both conjunctiva and tarsus to reconstruct the posterior lamella. The donor site is left to granulate. The graft is sutured to the residual tarsus or canthal tendons in the recipient site and then covered by a sliding myocutaneous flap to reconstruct the anterior lamella. This technique works equally well for the lower or upper eyelid.

13. **What are Hughes tarsoconjunctival flap and skin graft procedure?**
    The Hughes procedure is a two-staged operation for the reconstruction of total or near-total lower eyelid defects. As with the free tarsoconjunctival graft, a block of tarsus and conjunctiva is marked out on the ipsilateral upper lid. However, the upper border is left attached superiorly and a conjunctival flap is dissected off of the underlying Müller's muscle to the superior fornix. The tarsal flap is advanced down into the lower lid defect and sutured to residual tarsus or canthal tendons and the lower lid retractors. The anterior lamella is reconstructed with a skin graft or myocutaneous flap. After 3 weeks, the conjunctival flap is cut off along the new lower lid margin.

14. **How to repair eyelid defects with eyelid margin involvement?**
    i. The wound edges should be sharply trimmed (minimally). A 6-0 or 7-0 silk is first placed through a meibomian gland 3 mm from the eyelid margin to a depth of 3 mm. The suture is brought out of the laceration and into the other side 3 mm deep to the lid margin emerging 3 mm from the laceration. The second suture is placed in a similar fashion through the posterior lash line. The third is placed between these in the gray line. They are tied anteriorly and left long.
    ii. The tarsus is then closed by placing an absorbable suture through three-fourth to seven-eighth of the tarsal thickness. Full-thickness bites of the tarsus in the upper lid would expose to the conjunctival surface and most likely cause a corneal abrasion. A heavier suture

should be used for the lower lid tarsus (5-0 chromic) than the upper lid tarsus (6-0 chromic) because there is greater tension on the lower lid

iii. The skin can then be closed with 6-0 or 7-0 interrupted silks with the eyelid margin sutures tucked under the eyelash margin sutures to keep from touching the cornea. Skin sutures can be removed in 5–7 days, while the eyelid margin sutures should remain for 10–14 days

15. **What is lateral cantholysis?**
For full-thickness defects with moderate loss of tissue, closure may be obtained by performing a lateral canthotomy with cantholysis. The lateral canthotomy is performed by making a horizontal cut from the lateral canthus to the orbital margin using straight Stevens scissors. This maneuver splits the tendon into upper and lower limbs. An additional 3-5 mm of length can be obtained by cutting either limb (depending on which eyelid is involved). The eyelid margin can then be closed. The skin of the lateral canthotomy can be closed with 6-0 silk.

16. **How will you classify full-thickness lid defect repair?**
   i. *Horizontal extent of the defect*
      Can be classified as:
      - <30%
      - 30–50% defect
      - >50% defect
   ii. *Assess the vertical extent of the defect*
      - Vertically shallow (5–10 mm)
         - Skin mobilization and posterior lamellar reconstruction
      - Intermediate (10–15 mm)
         - Skin flap and posterior lamellar reconstruction
      - Large vertical (>15 mm)
         - Rotation flap + posterior lamellar reconstruction

17. **How is the procedure of the semicircular flap of Tenzel done?**
   i. This flap is a variation of lateral cantholysis. It adds rotation to the lateral advancement. A full-thickness semicircular flap of skin and orbicularis muscle which is high arched [i.e., vertical diameter (22 mm) is more than horizontal diameter (19 mm)] is fashioned superior to the lateral canthal angle for lower eyelid defects and inferior to the lateral canthal angle for upper eyelid defects
   ii. After cantholysis and wide undermining are performed, the flap is rotated to close the defect with minimal tension. Again, it is important to secure the deep orbicularis musculature to the periosteum to prevent drooping of the lateral canthal angle

18. **What are the various skin muscle flaps used for full-thickness eyelid reconstruction?**
    i. Temporal advancement flap
    ii. Semicircular flap of Tenzel
    iii. Mustarde cheek rotation flap
    iv. Median forehead flap
    v. Temporal forehead or Fricke flap
    vi. Cutler-Beard flap
    vii. Glabellar flap

19. **What is Cutler-Beard or bridge procedure?**
    i. The Cutler-Beard procedure is used for the repair of large full-thickness defects of the upper lid
    ii. The true width of the defect should be determined by grasping the cut tarsal edges with a forceps
    iii. The horizontal width of the defect is then marked on the lower lid 1-2 mm below the inferior tarsal border. This avoids compromising the marginal artery of the lower eyelid
    iv. The horizontal incision is placed through the skin and conjunctiva. Vertical incisions (usually 1-2 cm) are made full-thickness into the lower fornix until enough laxity exists to allow the flap to advance
    v. The flap is then brought beneath the bridge of the lower eyelid margin and tarsus to cover the globe. It is then sutured into the upper lid defect
    vi. The dressing is important for the success of this flap. It is important to avoid any pressure on the inferior margin bridge of tissue. A protective shield should be worn until the flap is taken down 6-8 weeks later. This is accomplished by severing the flap about 2 mm from the desired lid margin. Again, the conjunctival side should be longer than the skin side so that it can wrap around and create a new lid margin

20. **What is the Mustarde cheek rotation flap?**
    i. It is useful for the reconstruction of very large lower eyelid defects, especially if the defect extends into the cheek tissue
    ii. The flap is created by making an incision at the lateral canthus which extends superolaterally and then curves inferiorly to just in front of the ear. Wide undermining is then done (beware of facial nerve branches) to allow the flap to rotate
    iii. This flap is not used as much anymore because the thick cheek skin does not make a good match with the eyelid skin. Additionally, it has the potential for numerous complications including facial nerve paralysis, sagging of the lateral canthal angle, ectropion, pseudotrichiasis from facial skin hairs, and cheek flap necrosis

21. What is glabellar flap?
i. It is used for the repair of defects involving medial canthus and medial part of the upper lid. In it, a V-Y flap is advanced and rotated from the glabellar region
ii. An inverted V incision is made in the midline of the brow. The flap is undermined and sutured into the defect

22. What are the precautions to be employed before the closure of wounds?
i. Ensure complete hemostasis and remove all blood clots
ii. Eliminate tension in wound edges by adequate undermining
iii. There should be no dead space
iv. Meticulous wound closure in layers. Adequate closure of deeper tissues using inverted mattress suture
v. Ensure eversion of wound edges and no overlapping

23. What are the important points to be kept in mind while suturing nonmarginal lid defects?
i. Smaller defects can be sutured without undermining
ii. Round defects should be converted into an elliptical shape
iii. All vertical tension on lid margins should be eliminated by adequate undermining
iv. Incisions should be parallel to lines of tension/lid margin
v. Defects should be sutured in three layers
vi. For larger defects, local skin flaps/grafts should be indicated

24. What are the basic differences between upper and lower lid reconstruction?

Upper eyelid reconstruction	Lower eyelid reconstruction
More important than lower lid due to cornea closure	Less important for corneal protection
Should be done on priority if both lids are missing	Can wait
Incision should be parallel to lines of tension and lid margin, preferably at lid crease	Wound parallel to lines of tension and lid margin would result in scleral show/ectropion. Hence, wound should be converted perpendicular to lid margin
Gravitational effect and lid laxity do not cause adverse effects	Can cause ectropion, retraction, scleral show
Thinner skin	Thicker
Height of tarsus: 8–9 mm	Height: 5 mm
Less important for tear drainage	More important for tear drainage

25. **How are the full-thickness lid margin defects managed?**
    i. *Less than 30% defect*
        - Direct closure
        - Direct closure with canthotomy and cantholysis
    ii. *30–50% defect*
        - Direct closure with canthotomy and cantholysis
        - Rotational flaps like Tenzel semicircular flap
    iii. *Greater than 50% defect*
        - Cutler-Beard technique for upper lid
        - Reverse Cutler-Beard technique for lower lid
        - Hughes tarsoconjunctival flap
        - Mustarde cheek rotational flap
    iv. *Total loss of upper lid*
        - Mustarde switch flap
        - Transposition cheek flap
        - Fricke temporal forehead transposition flap
        - Posterior lamellar graft is necessary for lining all these flaps.
    v. *Total loss of upper lid and partial loss of lower lid*
        - *If the total loss of lower lid is associated with the presence of lateral part of lower lid*: This part of the lower lid is used as a switch flap for the upper lid (Mustarde operation). The remaining part of the lower lid is reconstructed with a temporal frontal pedicle flap lined by the mucous membrane
        - *If the total loss of upper lid is associated with the presence of the medial part of lower lid*: This need not be transferred to the upper lid. The upper lid is formed by supraorbital/forehead flap and the lower lid by cheek rotation flap is lined by mucous membrane
    vi. *Absence of both lids with intact eyeball*:
        Protection of cornea:
        - By suturing the remnants of conjunctiva over it
        - By free mucosal grafts

26. **What are the techniques for upper eyelid reconstruction?**
    i. Direct closure
    ii. Tenzel lateral semicircular rotation flap
    iii. Cutler-Beard bridge flap
    iv. Tarsoconjunctival flap
    v. Free tarsoconjunctival graft
    vi. Mustarde marginal pedicle rotation flap
    vii. Composite eyelid graft
    viii. Local myocutaneous flap with posterior lamellar graft
    ix. Periorbital flaps with posterior lamellar grafts
        Inclusion of few fibers of LPS while forming a lid crease is essential

27. **What are the techniques for lower eyelid reconstruction?**
    i. Direct closure
    ii. Lateral semicircular rotation flap
    iii. Reverse Cutler-Beard operation
    iv. Free tarsoconjunctival graft with myocutaneous advancement flap
    v. Hughes tarsoconjunctival advancement flap
    vi. Mustarde cheek rotation flap
    vii. Temporal forehead flap with posterior lamellar grafts
    viii. Composite eyelid graft.

8.5 BLEPHAROPHIMOSIS SYNDROME

1. **What is blepharophimosis syndrome?**

   Approximately 6% of children with congenital ptosis demonstrate the typical findings of blepharophimosis syndrome.

   Clinical features commonly seen are as follows:
   i. There is severe bilateral ptosis with poor levator function
   ii. The palpebral fissures are horizontally shortened (blepharophimosis)
   iii. Epicanthus inversus
   iv. Telecanthus—the intercanthal distance is more than half the interpupillary distance. It occurs due to an increase in the length of medial canthal tendons
   v. True hypertelorism is occasionally present
   vi. Lateral ectropion of lower lids
   vii. High arching of eyebrows

   Associated features may include tarsal plate hypoplasia and poorly developed nasal bridge. Some patients demonstrate low-set "lop" ears. Blepharophimosis is a dominantly inherited condition, although the severity of findings varies among affected family members. Sporadic cases also occur.

   Blepharophimosis is associated with primary amenorrhea in some family lines.

   Treatment of blepharophimosis usually requires a staged approach.

   Mustarde double "Z" plasty or Y-V plasty with transnasal wiring is done as a primary procedure. This gives a good surgical result in terms of both correction of telecanthus and deep placement of the medial canthus. The results are long-lasting.

   Brow suspension is carried out 6 months after the first procedure for correction of ptosis.

8.6 THYROID-RELATED ORBITOPATHY AND PROPTOSIS

1. **What is the volume of the orbit?**
   The volume of the orbit is 30 mL.

2. **Why is the new terminology of thyroid orbitopathy preferred over the older thyroid-related ophthalmopathy?**
   Thyroid orbitopathy is a disease in which orbit is the primary site of involvement in which the following changes take place:
   i. Increase in the volume of extraocular muscles
   ii. Increased fat synthesis
   iii. Associated primary lacrimal gland dysfunction
   iv. Compression of the orbital part of the optic nerve

3. **What is the difference in the terminologies of exophthalmos and proptosis?**
   i. *Exophthalmos* is an active or a dynamic disease characterized by the forward protrusion of the eyeball, classically seen in thyroid-related orbitopathy (TRO) and hence usually bilateral
   ii. *Proptosis* is a passive protrusion of the eyeball, classically seen in retro-orbital space-occupying lesions and hence usually unilateral

4. **What is physiological proptosis?**
   Physiological proptosis is seen in infants, owing to the fact that orbital cavities do not attain their full volume as rapidly as the eyeball. It is also seen in conditions such as bending forward or during straining/strangulation.

5. **What are the accepted exophthalmometry values to determine proptosis or enophthalmos?**
   i. Proptosis >21 mm
   ii. Enophthalmos <10–12 mm

6. **Mention a few causes of acute proptosis.**
   i. Orbital emphysema
   ii. Orbital hemorrhage
   iii. Orbital cellulitis

7. **Mention a few causes of intermittent proptosis.**
   i. Orbital varices (90%)
   ii. Highly vascular neoplasms such as hemangioma or lymphangioma
   iii. Recurrent orbital hemorrhages
   iv. Due to vascular congestions such as:
      - Strangulation, suffocation
      - Intense muscular efforts

- Constriction of jugular veins in cases of cavernous sinus thrombosis
v. Periodic orbital edema (particularly angioneurotic edema)
vi. Intermittent ethmoiditis
vii. Recurrent emphysema

8. **Mention causes of pulsating proptosis.**
   Pulsating proptosis may be vascular or cerebral in origin.
   Vascular pulsations:
   i. Aneurysm of carotid or ophthalmic artery
      - A-V aneurysms (most common—carotid-cavernous communications 90%)
      - Saccular aneurysms
      - Cirsoid aneurysm of orbit
   ii. Venous dilatations
      Orbital varix—rarely pulsates
   iii. Thrombosis of cavernous sinus
   iv. Vascular tumors in orbit—hemangioma, lymphangioma (rarely)

   Cerebral pulsations:
   Transmission pulsation presents when there is an orbital wall defect.
   i. Orbital root defect associated with meningocele or encephalocele
   ii. Neurofibromatosis associated with large dehiscence in the orbital wall
   iii. Traumatic hiatus

9. **What is the anatomical basis for the increase in proptosis with straining or internal jugular venous or carotid artery compression?**
   i. Acutely raised pulmonary artery pressure may be transmitted to the veins of the head and neck including the facial vein
   ii. The facial vein lacks valves, so that raised facial venous pressure may, in turn, be transmitted to the orbit through its anastomosis with the superior ophthalmic vein (principal venous drainage of orbit). This is the probable anatomical basis for congestive expansion of the orbit

10. **What are the causes of unilateral proptosis?**
    The causes can be divided as follows:
    i. TRO
    ii. Deformities of the cranium and asymmetric orbital size
    iii. Inflammatory lesions
       - Acute inflammations
         - Inflammation of orbital tissue
         - Lacrimal gland
         - Whole globe (panophthalmitis)

- Paranasal sinuses
- Eyelids
- Cavernous sinus
- Chronic inflammations
  - Granulomas
  - Tuberculoma
  - Gummas
  - Sarcoidosis
  - Chronic dacryoadenitis
iv. Circulatory disturbances
- Varicoceles
- Retrobulbar hemorrhage
  - Trauma
  - Hemophilia
- Aneurysms
v. Cysts
- Dermoid cyst
- Parasitic cyst
- Implantation cyst
- Cyst of optic nerve
- Cyst of lacrimal gland
- Congenital cystic eyeball
vi. Tumors
- Primary orbital tumors
- Lacrimal gland tumors
- Optic nerve tumors
- Secondaries
vii. Traumatic
- Retrobulbar hemorrhage
- Retained intraocular foreign body
- Emphysema
viii. Associated with general disorders
- Lymphatic deposits in leukemia
- Lipogranulomatous deposits as in histiocytosis
- Localized amyloidosis

11. What do you mean by orbitotonometry or piezometry?

The assessment of compressibility of orbital contents or the "tension of orbit" is called orbitotonometry or piezometry.

i. It is of diagnostic value
ii. It gives an idea of the effectivity of treatment. For example, orbitonometer of Cooper

12. **What are the different types of exophthalmometry?**
    The different types of exophthalmometry are:
    i. Clinical exophthalmometry
    ii. Stereophotographic method of exophthalmometry
    iii. Radiographic exophthalmometry

    Clinical methods are:
    i. Zehender's exophthalmometer
    ii. Gormaz exophthalmometer
    iii. Luedde exophthalmometer (used in children)
    iv. Hertel exophthalmometer (used for axial proptosis)
    v. Davenger's exophthalmometer
    vi. Watson's ocular topometer (in eccentric proptosis)
    vii. Measurement of displacement of the globe with perspex ruler

13. **What are the causes of bilateral proptosis?**
    i. Thyroid orbitopathy
    ii. Developmental anomalies of the skull
       - Craniofacial dysostosis
       - Generalized osteodysplasia
    iii. Osteopathies
       - Infantile cortical hyperostosis
       - Fibrous dysplasia
       - Osteoporosis
       - Rickets
       - Acromegaly
    iv. Encephalocele in the ethmoidal region
    v. Edema
       - Angioneurotic edema
       - Cavernous sinus thrombosis
    vi. Neoplasms
       - Symmetric lymphoma
       - Chloromas
       - Malignancy of nasopharynx
       - Metastatic neuroblastoma

14. **What is the most common cause of unilateral proptosis in adults?**
    Thyroid orbitopathy.

15. **What is the most common cause of bilateral proptosis in adults?**
    Thyroid orbitopathy.

16. **What is the most common cause of unilateral proptosis in children?**
    Orbital cellulitis.

17. **What do you mean by pseudoproptosis?**
    Pseudoproptosis is the clinical appearance of proptosis wherein no real forward displacement of the globe takes place.

18. **What are the causes of pseudoproptosis?**
    Pseudoproptosis can be classified as follows:
    i. *When the globe is enlarged*
        - Congenital buphthalmos/congenital cystic eyeball
        - High axial myopia
        - Staphyloma
        - Unilateral secondary glaucoma in childhood
    ii. *Retracting lids*
        - Microblepharon
        - Dermatosis or ichthyosis or from scarring
        - Sympathetic overaction such as Graves' disease or Parkinson's disease
    iii. *Lower lid sagging*
        - Facial palsy
        - Retraction of the inferior rectus
        - Following the recession of inferior oblique
    iv. *Deformation of orbit or facial asymmetry*
        - Asymmetry of the bony orbit
        - Progressive facial hemiatrophy (Parry–Romberg syndrome)
        - Harlequin orbit
        - Hypoplastic supraorbital ridges as in trisomy 18
        - Shallow orbit as in Crouzon disease (craniofacial dysostosis)
    v. *Opposite eye enophthalmos*

19. **What are the causes of enophthalmos?**
    The causes of enophthalmos are:
    i. Microphthalmos
    ii. Phthisis bulbi
    iii. Blowout fracture
    iv. Subluxation of the globe
    v. Age-related absorption of the fat

20. **Classify proptosis.**
    Proptosis can be classified based on different criteria:
    i. Unilateral or bilateral
    ii. Axial or eccentric
    iii. Acute, chronic, recurrent, intermittent
    iv. Pulsatile or nonpulsatile

21. What do you mean by axial proptosis?
Axial proptosis is caused by any space-occupying lesion in the muscle cone or any diffuse orbital inflammatory or neoplastic lesions. For example, optic nerve glioma, cavernous hemangioma, meningioma, schwannoma, and metastatic tumors from cancer—breast, lung, or prostate.

22. What do you mean by eccentric proptosis?
Proptosis caused by any extraconal lesion or fracture displacement of orbital bones protruding inwardly is eccentric proptosis.

23. Give a few causes of nonaxial proptosis.
  i. *Lateral displacement of globe/down and out:*
   - Ethmoidal mucocele
   - Frontal mucocele
   - Lacrimal sac tumors
   - Nasopharyngeal tumors
   - Rhabdomyosarcoma
  ii. *Down and in:*
   - Lacrimal gland tumors
   - Sphenoid wing meningioma
  iii. *Upward:*
   - Tumors of the floor of the orbit
   - Maxillary tumors
   - Lymphoma
   - Lacrimal sac tumors
  iv. *Downward:*
   - Fibrous dysplasia
   - Fibrous mucocele
   - Lymphoma
   - Neuroblastoma
   - Neurofibroma
   - Schwannoma
   - Subperiosteal hematoma

24. What is the differential diagnosis (DD) for a palpable mass in the superonasal quadrant?
  i. Mucocele
  ii. Mucopyocele
  iii. Encephalocele
  iv. Neurofibroma
  v. Dermoid cyst
  vi. Lymphoma

25. **What is the DD for a palpable mass in the superotemporal quadrant?**
    i. Prolapsed lacrimal gland
    ii. Dermoid cyst
    iii. Lacrimal gland tumor
    iv. Lymphoma
    v. Nonspecific orbital inflammation

26. **What are the important causes of proptosis in the following age groups?**
    Proptosis can be divided into the following categories:
    Newborn
    i. Orbital sepsis
    ii. Orbital neoplasm
    Neonates
    i. Osteomyelitis of maxilla
    Infants
    i. Dermoid cyst
    ii. Dermolipoma
    iii. Hemangioma
    iv. Histiocytosis X
    v. Orbital extension of retinoblastoma
    Children
    i. Dermoid cyst
    ii. Teratoma
    iii. Capillary hemangioma
    iv. Lymphangioma
    v. Orbital nerve glioma
    vi. Plexiform neurofibroma
    vii. Rhabdomyosarcoma
    viii. Acute myeloid leukemia
    ix. Histiocytosis
    x. Neuroblastoma
    xi. Wilms' tumor
    xii. Ewing's tumor
    Adults
    i. Thyroid orbitopathy
    ii. Cavernous hemangioma
    iii. Orbital varices
    iv. Optic nerve meningioma
    v. Schwannoma
    vi. Fibrous histiocytoma
    vii. Lymphoma
    viii. Secondaries from breast, lung, and prostate carcinoma

27. **What is proptometry?**
    Proptometry is the measurement of the distance between the apex of the cornea and the bony point usually taken as the deepest portion of the lateral orbital rim with the eye looking in primary gaze.

28. **Which instruments are used for measuring eccentric proptosis?**
    i. Topometer of Watson
    ii. Perspex ruler
    iii. Luedde exophthalmometer

29. **How to palpate in case of proptosis?**
    Insinuation of the orbital margins is done using the little finger and the patient is asked to look down to palate the orbital rim since the down position would relax the orbital septum.

30. **What are the types of exophthalmometry?**
    Types of exophthalmometry are:
    i. *Absolute exophthalmometry:* The amount of proptosis is compared with a known normal value
    ii. *Comparative exophthalmometry:* The reading is compared from time to time in the same eye
    iii. *Relative exophthalmometry:* The reading is compared between two eyes

31. **Which age group is commonly affected and what is the sex preponderance in TRO?**
    i. The average age of onset is in the 40s
    ii. Females are three to six times more affected than males

32. **What refractive errors are associated with TRO?**
    i. Astigmatism due to lid retraction
    ii. Induced hyperopia as a result of the flattening of posterior pole due to retrobulbar mass

33. **What is the reason of dilated vessels over muscles?**
    With increasing inflammation of muscles, the anterior radials of the muscular vessels become engorged, producing characteristic dilated and visible vessels subconjunctivally over the insertions.

34. **What is the sequence of muscle involvement in TRO?**
    i. Inferior rectus
    ii. Medial rectus
    iii. Superior rectus
    iv. Lateral rectus

35. **Why is inferior rectus most commonly involved in TRO?**
    i. Inferior rectus involvement occurs due to a well-developed connective tissue system around the inferior oblique and inferior

rectus muscles, which also have good septal connections with adjacent periorbita

ii. Also, inferior rectus contains a high concentration of macrophages ($CD4^+$ memory T cells, CD8 T cells) which may account for disease activity in muscles

36. **What are the reasons for restricted ocular movements in TRO?**
    The causes for restricted ocular movements can be divided into:
    i. Edematous muscle—this occurs in an active stage caused by imbibition of fluid into the muscle belly, which causes an increase in the size of the muscle. This causes restriction of contraction of the muscle
    ii. Fibrosed muscle—this occurs following chronic disease
    iii. Fibrosis causes contracture and restriction of muscle movements

37. **What are the causes of muscle enlargement in TRO?**
    i. Increased glycosaminoglycans (GAGs) with secondary water retention
    ii. Immunologic response meditated through antigen, target cells, and cytokines
    iii. Destruction of muscle fibers and infiltration by mature fat cells
    iv. Fibrosis of muscle

38. **What are the systemic associations of TRO?**
    Autoimmune or immunoregulatory diseases:
    i. Myasthenia gravis
    ii. Pernicious anemia
    iii. Vitiligo

39. **What is Braley's test?**
    i. Braley's test is also known as differential tonometry or positional tonometry
    ii. It refers to an increase in intraocular pressure (IOP) measured during upgaze
    iii. An increase in IOP of >6 mm Hg is significant
    iv. Normal—2 mm Hg
    v. An increase in IOP of >9–10 mm Hg suggests optic neuropathy

40. **What are the clinical signs in thyroid eye disease?**
    i. *Facial signs:*
       - Joffroy's sign: Absent crease on the upper forehead on upgaze
    ii. *Eyelid signs:*
       - Kocher's sign: Staring appearance
       - Vigoroux sign: Eyelid fullness or puffiness
       - Rosenbach's sign: Tremors of the eyelid (when closed)

- Riesman's sign: Bruit over the eyelids
- *Upper eyelid signs*:
  - von Graefe's sign: Upper lid lag on downgaze
  - Dalrymple's sign: Upper eyelid retraction
  - Stellwag's sign: Incomplete and infrequent blinking
  - Grove sign: Resistance to pulling the retracted upper lid
  - Boston's sign: Uneven jerky movements of the upper lid on inferior gaze
  - Gellinek's sign: Abnormal pigmentation on the upper lid
  - Gifford's sign: Difficulty in everting the upper lid
  - Mean sign: Increased superior scleral show on upgaze
- *Lower eyelid signs:*
  - Enroth's sign: Edema of the lower lid
  - Griffith's sign: Lower lid lag on upgaze

iii. *Extraocular movements sign:*
  - Möbius's sign: Inability to converge eyes
  - Ballet's sign: Restriction of one or more extraocular muscles
  - Suker's sign: Poor fixation on abduction
  - Jendrassik's sign: Paralysis of all extraocular muscles

iv. *Conjunctival signs:*
  - Goldzieher's sign: Conjunctival injection

v. *Pupillary involvement sign:*
  - Knies's sign: Uneven pupillary dilatation
  - Cowen's sign: Jerky contraction of the pupil to light

41. What is the reason for the increase in IOP in TRO?
  i. Enlargement of recti interferes with uveoscleral drainage in various positions of gaze
  ii. Increased tension due to resistance of inferior rectus opposing supraduction, provoking compression of eye and elevation in IOP in upgaze

42. What are the causes of the increase in IOP in upgaze?
  i. TRO
  ii. Fractures
  iii. Myositis
  iv. Irradiation
  v. Orbital metastasis

43. Are all patients with TRO hyperthyroid?

Approximately 80% of the patients with TRO are hyperthyroid at the time of diagnosis or develop hyperthyroid status within 6 months of the disease.

Ten percent are hypothyroid and the rest 10% are euthyroid.

44. What is the most significant environmental factor causing TRO?
Smoking: Smokers with TRO have more severe disease than nonsmokers.

45. What are the causes of upper lid retraction in TRO?
The causes of upper lid retraction in TRO are:
  i. Fibrotic contracture of the levator associated with adhesion with overlying orbital tissue
  ii. Sympathetic overstimulation of Muller's muscle
  iii. Secondary overaction of levator superior rectus complex in response to hypophoria produced by fibrosis of inferior rectus muscle

46. What is the cause of lower lid retraction?
The cause of lower lid retraction is fibrosis of the inferior lid retractors (capsulopalpebral head).

47. How do you grade lid retraction?
  i. Mild—intersection of the lid at superior limbus, 1-2 mm of superior scleral show, marginal reflex distance (MRD) 1: 6 mm
  ii. Moderate—2-4 mm of superior scleral show, MRD1: 6-10 mm
  iii. Severe—>4 mm of superior scleral show, MRD1: >10 mm

48. What is the importance of measuring lid retraction?
If surgical correction is mandatory for lid retraction, the size of spacer graft depends on the amount of lid retraction.

1 mm of lid retraction = 3 mm of spacer graft

49. When does one get ptosis instead of lid retraction in TRO?
  i. When there is apical compression and congestion of orbit as in tight orbit syndrome
  ii. Severe proptosis may cause disinsertion of aponeurosis of elevators of lids leading to ptosis
  iii. Ptosis may be associated with myasthenia gravis

50. What are the causes of vision loss in TRO?
  i. Exposure keratopathy
  ii. Diplopia due to involvement of extraocular muscles
  iii. Optic nerve traction
  iv. Optic nerve compression (by enlarged extraocular muscle)
  v. Macular edema
  vi. Macular scar
  vii. Glaucomatous optic neuropathy (systemic steroid induced)
  viii. Posterior subcapsular cataract secondary to steroids used in the treatment of TRO

51. Where is the site of compression of the optic nerve by enlarged extraocular muscles?
Orbital apex caused by the crowding of the enlarged muscles.

52. What is the earliest and most sensitive indicator of optic nerve damage and why?
  i. Color vision: Pseudoisochromatic plates and Farnsworth–Munsell Hue test
  ii. Color vision is affected earlier because axons that precede macula are most sensitive to damage
  iii. Pattern reversal visual evoked potential: Also sensitive for detecting early damage

53. What are the visual field defects seen in optic neuropathy due to TRO?
  i. Central scotoma
  ii. Inferior altitudinal defect

Less commonly:
  i. Enlarged blind spot
  ii. Paracentral scotoma
  iii. Nerve fiber bundle defect
  iv. Generalized constriction

54. What are the causes of exposure keratopathy in TRO?
  i. Severe proptosis preventing mechanical closure of eyelids
  ii. Retraction of the upper and lower eyelids
  iii. Decreased secretion of tears due to primary lacrimal gland dysfunction

55. What are Sallmann's folds?
Sallmann's folds are choroidal folds seen in the macula in case of retrobulbar mass. They are also seen in TRO.

Other conditions where choroidal folds may be seen are:
  i. Idiopathic
  ii. Retrobulbar tumors
  iii. Choroidal melanomas
  iv. Ocular hypotony
  v. Posterior scleritis
  vi. Postscleral buckling

56. What are raccoon eyes? Where is it seen in the context of orbit?
Raccoon eyes are dark purple discoloration/periorbital ecchymoses giving an appearance similar to that of a raccoon/panda.

They are seen in the following conditions:
  i. Bilateral proptosis due to metastatic neuroblastoma
  ii. Fracture of the base of skull
  iii. Amyloidosis
  iv. Kaposi's sarcoma
  v. Multiple myeloma

57. **What do you mean by temporal flare in a patient with TRO?**
    The upper eyelid retraction in Graves' disease has a characteristic temporal flare, with a greater amount of sclera visible laterally as compared with medially.

58. **What is the cause of temporal flare in TRO?**
    The results of inflammation, resultant adhesions, and fibrosis clearly affect the lateral horn of the levator aponeurosis.
    i. The lateral horn of the levator aponeurosis is much stronger than the medial horn, and its insertion through the lateral orbital retinaculum at the lateral orbital tubercle is much more defined than its medial insertion. The lateral fibers of the muscular portion of the levator muscle, proximal to Whitnall's ligament, blend with the superior transverse ligament as it courses to the lateral orbital attachment, exerting a strong pull on the lateral aspect of the eyelid through the aponeurosis, the suspensory ligament of the fornix, and the conjunctiva
    ii. Müller's muscle, an involuntary muscle, may develop overreaction or be enlarged secondary to a direct inflammatory infiltrate in TRO. An involved Müller's muscle, with its substantial lateral extensions, contributes to and may cause more temporal flare than in those patients with TRO but without this muscle involvement

59. **Which is the most common extraocular muscle involved in TRO and why?**
    Inferior rectus (second most common muscle involved is medial rectus): Inferior rectus involvement occurs due to a well-developed connective tissue system around it and also because it has the greatest number of septal connections with adjacent periorbita.

60. **Mention a few conditions which are associated with extraocular muscle enlargement.**
    Extraocular muscle enlargement can be classified as:
    Inflammatory:
    i. Graves' orbitopathy
    ii. Myositis
    iii. Orbital cellulitis
    iv. Sarcoidosis
    v. Vasculitides
    Neoplastic:
    i. Rhabdomyosarcoma
    ii. Metastasis
    iii. Lymphoid tumors

Vascular:
  i. Carotid-cavernous fistula
  ii. A-V malformation
  iii. Lymphoid tumors

Miscellaneous:
  i. Acromegaly
  ii. Amyloidosis
  iii. POEMS syndrome
  iv. Trichinosis
  v. Lithium therapy

61. **What is differential tonometry?**
    Differential tonometry refers to an increase in the IOP measured during upgaze. This is caused by the compression of the globe by fibrosed inferior rectus. An increase in IOP of >6 mm Hg is significant.

62. **What is the significance of retinoscopy in a case of proptosis?**
    i. To identify any high axial myopia which manifests as pseudoproptosis
    ii. Axial length may be decreased in a case of retrobulbar mass causing hyperopic shift due to compression of the posterior pole

63. **What is the difference between von Graefe's sign and pseudo-von Graefe's sign?**
    von Graefe's sign: It is seen in thyroid orbitopathy due to retarded descent of the globe on downgaze.
    Pseudo-von Graefe's sign: It is seen in third cranial nerve palsy with aberrant regeneration of the nerve where there is lid retraction on attempted downgaze.

64. **What is the cause of an increase in the volume of extraocular muscles?**
    In a patient with TRO, there is a 100-fold increase in the synthesis of GAGs by the preadipocyte fibroblasts, which causes imbibition of water into the muscles causing the thickness to increase.

65. **What is the type of hypersensitivity reaction in thyroid orbitopathy?**
    Type V hypersensitivity reaction.

66. **What is the significance of ultrasonography (USG) in a patient with suspected TRO?**
    USG can detect early thyroid disease in a case with unequivocal laboratory tests.
    i. It helps differentiate TRO from pseudotumor
    ii. It can predict whether the disease is active or inactive. The amount of internal reflectivity is less in a patient with active disease

67. What is the frequency of orbital USG?

The frequency of orbital USG is 8–15 MHz.

68. How do you differentiate between enlarged muscles in myositis from that of TRO on USG?

In myositis, there is a typical enlargement of the tendinous insertion of the muscles whereas in TRO there is a fusiform enlargement of the muscle belly.

69. How do you clinically differentiate active and inactive disease?

Features	Active disease	Inactive disease
Accompanying signs of inflammation such as chemosis and congestion	More	Less (usually eye will be quiet)
Amount of proptosis	Severe	Less
Restriction of extraocular movements	1 or 2 gazes	May be in all gazes

Inflammatory score (activity of the disease)	
1. Orbital pain	
No pain	0
At gaze	1
At rest	2
2. Chemosis	
Not beyond the gray line	1
Beyond the gray line	2
3. Eyelid edema	
Present but no overhanging of tissues	1
Roll in eyelid skin like festoons	2
4. Conjunctival injection	
Absent	1
Present	2
5. Eyelid injection	
Absent	1
Present	2
Total	0–8

If the score is <3/8 and there is no deterioration, then management is conservative with cool compresses, head elevation, and nonsteroidal anti-inflammatory drugs (NSAIDs).

If the score is >4/8 or if there is evidence of progression, then the management is oral or intravenous (IV) steroids, radiotherapy, or immunosuppressive agents.

70. What do you mean by VISA?
VISA is a new classification of TRO which helps in grading and planning management at all the levels of TRO, where VISA stands for:
V: Vision
I: Inflammation
S: Strabismus
A: Appearance

71. What is the best investigation for early diagnosis of compressive optic neuropathy in Graves' disease?
The best investigation for early diagnosis of compressive optic neuropathy in Graves' disease is magnetic resonance imaging (MRI).

72. What are the indications of orbital imaging in a patient with TRO?
 i. Suspicion of optic nerve compression
 ii. Evaluation before orbital decompression surgery
 iii. Orbital irradiation
 iv. To rule out pseudotumor

73. What is the significance of computed tomography (CT) scanning in a patient of TRO?
 i. CT scan allows reliable identification of even minimally enlarged recti muscles
 ii. In patients with unilateral proptosis, it can detect subclinical enlargement of extraocular muscles in the contralateral eye
 iii. It can detect patients with a risk of developing optic neuropathy as depicted by:
   - Severe apical crowding
   - Dilated superior ophthalmic vein

74. What are the characteristic findings of CT scan in TRO?
Fusiform enlargement of extraocular muscles which is usually bilateral and symmetric with sharply defined borders and sparing the tendinous insertions.

75. What is the best cross-sectional view in CT scan to visualize enlarged muscle?
Coronal section.

76. What are the laboratory tests done in TRO?
 i. Thyroid-stimulating hormone (TSH)
 ii. Thyroxine (total and free T4)
 iii. Triiodothyronine (T3)
 iv. Thyroid-stimulating immunoglobulin

77. How will you treat TRO?
The treatment has to be done in conjunction with the management of the underlying thyroid disease by an endocrinologist.
   i. Topical lubrication with artificial tears
   ii. Lid taping at bedtime
   iii. Cold compresses in the morning and head elevation in the night
   iv. Punctal occlusion for more severe dry eye symptoms
   v. Lateral tarsorrhaphy useful in cases of lateral chemosis or widened lateral palpebral fissure or to prevent exposure together
   vi. Surgical eyelid recession (lengthening) for eyelid retraction after 6 months
   vii. If diplopia is present, then oral steroids, Fresnel prism, or strabismus surgery as indicated.
   viii. For threatened optic nerve involvement, oral steroids and orbital decompression

78. Which wall should not be decompressed?
Removal of the inferior wall is avoided, if possible, due to a higher incidence of induced diplopia.

79. What are the indications of orbital decompression surgery?
   i. Compressive optic neuropathy
   ii. Exposure keratopathy
   iii. Cosmetically unacceptable proptosis

80. What is the most common site of orbital wall decompression?
Deep lateral wall.

81. What are the principles/goals of orbital decompression?
   i. Expanding orbital volume (bony expansion)
   ii. Reducing orbital soft tissue (fat decompression)

82. What is the approach for orbital decompression?
   i. For exophthalmometry, <22 mm
      Lateral wall + fat decompression
   ii. For exophthalmometry, 22–25 mm
      Lateral wall + fat + medial wall decompression
   iii. For exophthalmometry, >25 mm
      Lateral wall + fat + medial wall decompression + posterior orbital floor decompression + lateral rim advancement

83. What are the complications of orbital decompression?
   i. Most common is worsening of diplopia or new double vision
   ii. Infraorbital hyperesthesia
   iii. Risk of visual loss
   iv. Bleeding and infection

84. What are the indications of extraocular muscle surgery and which surgery is preferred for the same?

i. Diplopia in primary gaze
ii. Quiescent disease and stable angle of deviation for a minimum of 6 months

The preferred surgery to correct diplopia is recession of the inferior oblique muscle with adjustable sutures.

85. How long will you wait for strabismus surgery in TRO and why?

We wait for 6 months as diplopia tends to get resolved with prisms and/or systemic corticosteroids in the acute phase. Also, TRO tends to be progressive, and hence we wait for 6 months so that strabismus measurement stabilizes.

86. How does strabismus surgery affect eyelid retraction?

Recession of tight inferior rectus often improves upper eyelid retraction. Superior rectus had to work against tight inferior rectus; thus, associated levator muscles were overactive, causing eyelid retraction.

When inferior rectus is recessed, overactivity ends.

87. What should be the sequence of surgery in patients with thyroid orbitopathy?

The evaluation and treatment of TRO may require one or multiple stages of surgery, depending on the severity and manifestation of the disease process. Each stage will affect the decision-making for subsequent stages, and therefore the surgery should be staged in a specific sequence, with orbital decompression, then strabismus surgery if indicated, and finally eyelid repositioning and removal of excess fat and skin.

Any of the stages may be skipped when deemed unnecessary or not indicated, but maintaining the correct order reduces the number of procedures to a minimum.

Orbital decompression can result in a change in the extraocular muscle position and function relative to the globe, displacement of the muscle cone, and alteration of the muscle pulley system, which may result in postoperative phorias or diplopia.

Recession or resection of the vertical extraocular muscles for the correction of hypertrophies, especially large deviations, may increase the retraction of the eyelids secondary to alterations of the anatomical connectivity between the retractor complex and the vertical extraocular muscles. This is avoidable by careful and meticulous dissection of the extraocular muscles. Orbital decompression can also change the position of the eyelids.

88. Differentiate between orbital pseudotumor and Graves' orbitopathy.

Features	Idiopathic pseudotumor	Graves' orbitopathy
Sex—F:M ratio	Equal	3:1
Mode of onset	Acute, subacute, or chronic	Chronic
Pain	Often present. May be severe	Painless (unless keratitis or orbital congestion is present)
Laterality	Usually unilateral	Usually bilateral
Lid signs	Lid edema, lid erythema, ptosis	Lid and periorbital edema, lid retraction, lid lag, and lagophthalmos
Systemic symptoms	Malaise	Generally well. Associated symptoms of thyroid disease
Laboratory findings	Elevated erythrocyte sedimentation rate (ESR)	Abnormal thyroid functions
Radiography	• Infiltrate or a mass • Uveoscleral enhancement • Extraocular muscle enlargement including tendon	• Spindle-shaped extraocular muscle enlargement • Sparing tendon • Inferior and medial recti are most commonly involved
USG	• Uveoscleral thickening • Sub-Tenon's effusion	Extraocular muscle enlargement detected before CT scan

89. Which neuroimaging test is best to evaluate the etiology of proptosis?

CT scan is superior in most cases.

MRI may be desirable in certain cases when optic nerve dysfunction is present.

90. What are the indications for CT scan in proptosis?

i. Acute proptosis
ii. Progressive proptosis
iii. When there is relative afferent pupillary defect (RAPD)
iv. Orbital fracture
v. Orbital foreign body

91. What is a Coca-Cola sign?

A Coca-Cola sign is a CT scan finding seen in the coronal section where there is bilateral bowing of lamina papyracea/medial wall of the orbit due to bilateral medial rectus enlargement in TRO.

92. What are the indications of biopsy in proptosis?

i. Pseudotumor refractory to medical treatment
ii. Suspected lymphoma or other malignancies

93. How is orbital bruit best examined?

Place the stethoscope bell over the closed eyelids and ask the patient to gently open the eyelids.

94. What are the bones comprising the walls of the orbit?

　i. *Medial wall (weakest wall)*
　　(from front to back)
　　- Frontal process of maxilla
　　- Lacrimal bone
　　- Orbital plate of ethmoid
　　- Body of sphenoid
　ii. *Inferior wall*
　　- Orbital surface of maxilla (medially)
　　- Orbital surface of zygomatic (laterally)
　　- Palatine bone (posteriorly)
　iii. *Lateral wall (strongest wall)*
　　- Zygomatic bone (anteriorly)
　　- Greater wing of sphenoid (posteriorly)
　iv. *Roof*
　　- Orbital plate of frontal bone (anteriorly)
　　- Lesser wing of sphenoid (posteriorly)

95. What are the approaches to orbital surgery?

Surgical approaches can be:
　i. Superior orbitotomy
　ii. Medial orbitotomy
　iii. Lateral orbitotomy
　iv. Inferior orbitotomy
　v. Transcranial approach
　vi. Transnasal endoscopic approach
　vii. Transantral approach

Anterior can also be divided as:

Inferior orbitotomy:
　i. Extraperiosteal approach—subciliary incision
　ii. Conjunctival incision in inferior fornix for orbital floor fracture repair

Superior orbitotomy:
　i. Coronal approach
　ii. Conjunctival incision
　iii. Subbrow incision
　iv. Eyelid crease incision

Anterior orbitotomy—superomedial lesion-lid split incision

Medial orbitotomy:
　i. Inferomedial lesion—dacryocystorhinostomy (DCR) like incision
　ii. Medial orbitotomy—conjunctival approach for central and peripheral space
　iii. Endoscopic approach
　iv. Lateral orbitotomy
　v. Transfrontal orbitotomy

96. What is lateral orbitotomy?

Lateral approach is used for deeper orbital lesions that cannot be reached through an anterior incision. The type of skin incisions include:
  i. "S"-shaped (Stallard–Wright)
  ii. Horizontal canthal crease
  iii. Eyelid crease incision

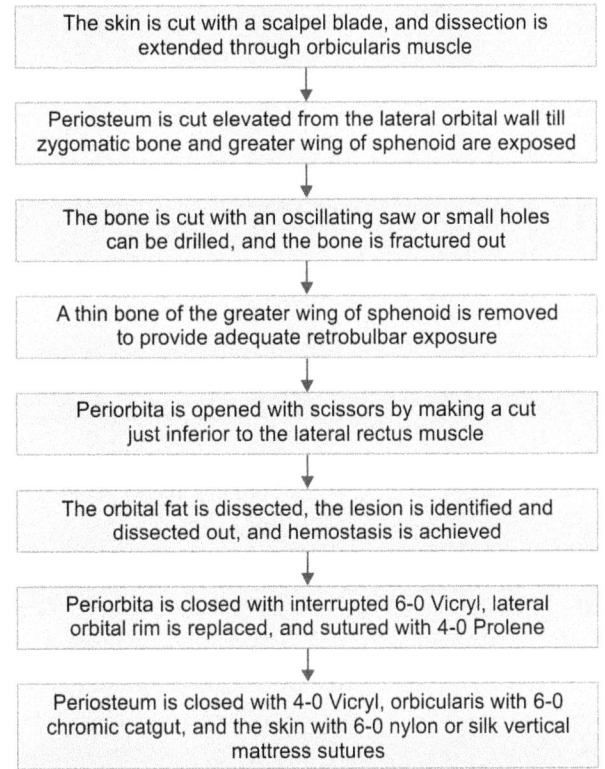

97. What are the surgical spaces of the orbit?

The surgical spaces of the orbit include:
  i. Central surgical space (intraconal space)
  ii. Peripheral surgical space (extraconal space)
  iii. Subperiosteal space
  iv. Preaponeurotic space
  v. Tenon's space
  vi. Periorbital tissues

98. What are the TRO signs?

The signs of TRO were given by Werner's classification and grading of thyroid orbitopathy.

Class	Grade	Mnemonic	Suggestions for grading
0		N	No physical signs or symptoms
1		O	Signs only
2		S	Soft-tissue involvement
	0		Absent
	A		Minimal
	B		Moderate
	C		Marked
3		P	Proptosis of 3 mm or more
	0		Absent
	A		3–4 mm
	B		5–7 mm
	C		8 mm or more
4		E	Extraocular muscle involvement
	0		Absent
	A		Limitation of motion at extremes of gaze
	B		Evident restriction of motion
	C		Fixation of globe
5		C	Corneal involvement
	0		Absent
	A		Punctate lesions
	B		Ulceration
	C		Necrosis or perforation
6		S	Sight loss (due to optic nerve)
	0		Absent
	A		20/20–20/60
	B		20/70–20/200
	C		Worse than 20/200

99. What are the differences between optic nerve glioma and optic nerve sheath meningioma?

Optic nerve glioma	Optic nerve sheath meningioma
i. Age: Children and young girls	i. Middle-aged adults, mostly women
ii. Arise from astrocytes of the optic nerve	ii. Arise from meningoendothelial cells of arachnoid villi
iii. Visual loss followed by proptosis	iii. Proptosis presents first followed by visual loss
iv. CT: Fusiform enlargement of the optic nerve	iv. Tubular thickening of the optic nerve ("tram-tracking")
v. X-ray shows regular enlargement of the optic foramen	v. Irregular enlargement

8.7 BLOWOUT FRACTURES OF THE ORBIT

1. **Who were the first to describe orbital blowout fractures?**
   Smith and Regan were the first to describe orbital blowout fractures in 1957.

2. **What is the mechanism of a blowout fracture?**
   A blowout fracture of the orbital floor is typically caused by a sudden increase in the orbital pressure by an impacting object which is greater in diameter than the orbital aperture (about 5 cm), such as a fist or tennis ball, so that the eyeball itself is displaced and transmits rather than absorbs the impact. Since the bones of the lateral wall and the roof are usually able to withstand such trauma, the fracture most frequently involves the floor of the orbit along the thin bone covering the infraorbital canal.

3. **What are the theories explaining the mechanism of the blowout fracture?**
   Two theories have been proposed to explain the mechanism of the blowout fracture:
   i. Hydraulic theory
   ii. Buckling theory

4. **What is hydraulic theory?**
   In hydraulic theory, the external injury is supposed to cause an increase in the intraorbital pressure which causes the thin orbital floor medial to the infraorbital groove and the medial wall to give way and help in absorbing the impact of the injury and thereby protect the globe from injury.

5. **What is buckling theory?**
   In buckling theory, the stress of the initial injury is transmitted directly from the orbital rim to the orbital floor and results in a fracture.

6. **How are blowout fractures classified?**
   Blowout fractures are classified into two types:
   i. Pure blowout fracture
   ii. Impure or complex blowout fracture
      - A *pure blowout* fracture is a fracture of the orbital wall without the involvement of the orbital rim
      - An *impure blowout* fracture is a variety in which the orbital rim and the adjacent facial bones are involved

7. **How are pure blowout fractures classified?**
   i. Trapdoor refers to cases in which either edge of the inferior orbital wall is attached to its original position (teardrop sign)

ii. Nontrapdoor refers to cases in which the inferior orbital wall is completely separated from its original position and the periorbital tissue has escaped into the maxillary sinus

8. **What are the symptoms in a blowout fracture?**
    i. Pain with vertical eye movement
    ii. Binocular diplopia
    iii. Eyelid edema
    iv. Crepitus, particularly after nose bleeding

9. **What are the clinical signs seen in a patient with blowout fracture?**
    Eyelid signs: Ecchymosis and edema of eyelids, occasionally subcutaneous emphysema

    Infraorbital nerve anesthesia involving the lower lid, cheek, side of the nose, upper lip, upper teeth, and gums is very common because the fracture frequently involves the infraorbital canal.

    Diplopia with limitation of upgaze, downgaze, or both:

    Diplopia may be caused by one of the following mechanisms:
    i. Hemorrhage and edema in the orbit may cause the septa connecting the inferior rectus and inferior oblique muscles to the periorbita to become taut and thus restrict movement of the globe. Ocular motility usually improves as the hemorrhage and edema resolve
    ii. Mechanical entrapment f the inferior rectus or inferior oblique or adjacent connective tissue and fat within the fracture. Diplopia typically occurs in both upgaze and downgaze (double diplopia)
    iii. In these cases, forced duction and differential intraocular pressure tests are positive. Diplopia may subsequently improve if it is mainly due to entrapment of connective tissue and fat, but usually persists if there is significant involvement of the muscles themselves
    iv. Direct injury to an extraocular muscle is associated with a negative forced duction test. The muscle fibers usually regenerate and normal function returns within about 2 months

    Enophthalmos may be present if the fracture is severe, although it tends to manifest only after a few days as the initial edema resolves. In the absence of surgical intervention, enophthalmos may continue to increase for about 6 months as post-traumatic orbital degeneration and fibrosis develop.

10. **What is the differential diagnosis of muscle entrapment in orbital fracture?**
    i. Orbital edema and hemorrhage
    ii. Cranial nerve palsy

11. **Why are pediatric patients particularly vulnerable to trapdoor fracture?**
    Pediatric patients are particularly vulnerable to trapdoor fracture since their bones tend to be cartilaginous and bendable.

12. **What is "white-eyed blowout fracture"?**
    White-eyed blowout fracture is a well-described entity, especially in the pediatric group, which presents with signs of entrapment of the extraocular muscles with a relatively white eye which reveals minimal signs of inflammation. These patients can also have symptoms suggestive of oculocardiac reflex with resultant bradycardia and nausea.

13. **What are the causes of vision loss following a blowout fracture?**
    In patients with orbital floor fractures, vision loss can result from injury to the optic nerve or increased orbital pressure causing a compartment syndrome.

14. **What is the initial management of blowout fractures?**
    The majority of blowout fractures do not require surgical intervention. Initial treatment is conservative with antibiotics; ice packs and nasal decongestants may be helpful. The patient should be instructed not to blow the nose because of the possibility of forcing infected sinus contents into the orbit. Systemic steroids are occasionally required for severe orbital edema, particularly if this is compromising the optic nerve.

15. **What are the indications of surgery in cases of blowout fracture?**
    i. Diplopia with limitation of upgaze and/or downgaze within 30° of the primary position with a positive traction test result 7–10 days after injury and with radiologic confirmation of a fracture of the orbital floor
    ii. Enophthalmos that exceeds 2 mm and that is cosmetically unacceptable to the patient
    iii. Large fractures involving at least half of the orbital floor, particularly when associated with large medial wall fractures

16. **When is surgery indicated as an emergency in blowout fracture?**
    Urgent surgery (<24 hours) is indicated in pediatric cases with entrapment.

17. **How do we manage white-eyed blowout fracture?**
    The "white-eyed" fracture requires urgent repair to avoid permanent neuromuscular damage. Release of the entrapped muscle should be done to avoid restriction and fibrosis.

18. **What are the preoperative investigations done?**
    i. Visual acuity testing, papillary reflex
    ii. Ocular motility evaluation using Hess chart/Lees screen

iii. Hertel exophthalmometry
iv. Slit-lamp biomicroscopy
v. Applanation tonometry
vi. Fundus ophthalmoscopy
vii. Evaluation of sensitivity in the distribution of infraorbital nerve
viii. Forced duction test (FDT)—to confirm mechanical restriction
ix. Imaging—computed tomography (CT) scan of the orbit (2 mm slice) in axial, coronal, and sagittal planes to identify the extent of fracture
x. Determining the nature of maxillary antral soft-tissue densities which may represent prolapsed orbital fat, extraocular muscles, hematoma, or unrelated antral polyps
CT scan is the imaging of choice in orbital fractures

19. **What are the various approaches to the orbital floor during surgical management?**
For orbital floor fractures, surgical procedures are routinely performed via:
    i. Transorbital approach
    ii. Transantral approach
    iii. Endoscopic endonasal approach

20. **Explain transorbital approach.**
Most anterior fractures are managed by the transorbital route which can be via:
    i. Transcutaneous incision
    ii. Transconjunctival incision
        – Inferior forniceal (to approach floor)
        – Transcaruncular (to approach medial wall)

21. **What are the approaches to posterior and medial fractures?**
The transantral approach is used to approach posteriorly placed fractures which might be difficult to approach through the anterior approach.
The endoscopic approach is in managing medial wall fractures.

22. **What are the steps done in the surgical management of blowout fractures?**
    i. Open reduction of the fracture
    ii. Release of entrapped tissues
    iii. Repositioning of the herniated orbital soft tissue within the orbit
    iv. Repair of the post-traumatic defect with an orbital implant as needed

Orbit 763

23. **Describe transcutaneous approach.**
    i. In transcutaneous approach, the skin incision is made in the lower eyelid at 3-4 mm below the subciliary fold following the natural curve of the lid
    ii. Dissection is then carried down until the periosteum is reached at the level of the orbital rim
    iii. The incision is then carried through the periosteum just below the orbital rim
    iv. The reflection of the periosteum is made over the rim using a periosteal elevator until the fracture is visualized
    v. To relieve any orbital structure entrapment and to restore the orbital contents to their original place, a forced traction of the globe is made
    vi. The implant is then cut to the appropriate size and then placed to bridge the fracture site and is anchored anteriorly with screws in case there is no posterior support
    vii. The periosteum is closed with 5-0 chromic catgut and the subcutaneous tissue is approximated
    viii. The 6-0 silk is used to close the skin

24. **What is transconjunctival approach?**
    In transconjunctival approach, the orbital rim periosteum is reached via the inferior fornix incision in case of floor fractures and transcaruncular incision for medial wall fractures.

25. **What are orbital implants?**
    The orbital implant restores the structural integrity of the orbital wall by bridging the defect and preventing orbital contents from herniating into the adjacent periorbital sinuses. The implant also prevents extraocular motility limitations by minimizing scar tissue adhesions with orbital contents. These implants can also serve to augment the orbital volume by compressing the intraorbital contents to correct enophthalmos.

26. **What are the current orbital implants?**
    The current orbital implants include:
    i. Autogenous bone grafts
    ii. Human donor grafts
    iii. Xenografts
    iv. Alloplastic implants

27. **What are the properties of an ideal alloplastic implant?**
    The ideal alloplastic implant should be readily sizable, sterilizable, strong, inert, nonallergenic, durable, noncarcinogenic, easily manipulated, shaped, and suitable for single-stage reconstruction.

Also, the implant should be accepted and well integrated into the surrounding tissues with minimal inflammatory response, foreign body reaction, or risk of infection.

The implant should provide mechanical support strong enough to hold up the orbital contents and have the stability to be easily anchored to the surrounding bone to prevent migration and extrusion.

Finally, it should be readily available in larger quantities, if necessary, at a reasonable cost.

28. **What are the various materials used as orbital implants?**
    i. Autogenous bone grafts (iliac crest/rib)
    ii. Silastic sheets
    iii. Porous polyethylene (MEDPOR)—porous polyethylene implants are available as sheets which can be cut, channel implants which have provisions for inserting a plate which can be fixed to the orbital rim with screws and with titanium sheets (TITAN)
    iv. Titanium implant—these are available as titanium sheets which can be cut or preshaped models

29. **What are the complications of blowout fracture surgery?**
    i. Decreased visual acuity
    ii. Diplopia
    iii. Undercorrection/overcorrection of enophthalmos
    iv. Lower eyelid retraction
    v. Infraorbital nerve hypoesthesia
    vi. Infection
    vii. Extrusion of implant
    viii. Chronic sinusitis
    ix. Dacryocystitis
    x. Chronic skin orbital floor fistulas/maxillary sinus orbital fistulas
    xi. Loss of lacrimal pump mechanism
    xii. Intraorbital hemorrhage.

8.8 ORBITOTOMIES

1. **What are the walls of the orbit?**
   i. Medial wall
   ii. Inferior wall (floor)
   iii. Lateral wall
   iv. Roof

2. **What are the contents of a medial wall?**
   A medial wall is quadrilateral in shape and the thinnest wall of the orbit and consists of:
   i. Frontal process of maxilla
   ii. Lacrimal bone
   iii. Orbital plate of ethmoid bone
   iv. Body of sphenoid

3. **What is the most common complication in these surgeries?**
   Hemorrhage is the most common due to injury of ethmoid vessels, medial-palpebral, frontal, and dorsal-nasal arteries.

4. **What are the contents of the floor of the orbit?**
   The floor of the orbit is triangular in shape; it consists of:
   i. Orbital surface of the maxillary bone medially
   ii. Orbital surface of the zygomatic bone laterally
   iii. Palatine bone posteriorly

5. **What are the contents passing through the infraorbital foramen?**
   Infraorbital nerve, artery, and vein.

6. **What are the contents of the lateral wall of the orbit?**
   The lateral wall of the orbit is triangular in shape and consists of:
   i. Zygomatic bone anteriorly
   ii. Greater wing of sphenoid posteriorly
   In the posterior part of the wall, there is a small projection called spina recti lateralis, which gives origin to a part of the lateral rectus muscle.

7. **What is the importance of the lateral wall?**
   i. The lateral wall protects the posterior part of the eyeball
   ii. Palpation of retro-orbital tumors is easier
   iii. Lateral orbital surgeries are more popular
   iv. It is devoid of foramina, so hemorrhage is less
   v. It is the strongest portion of the orbit
   vi. Once sawed open, it has direct access to superolateral, inferolateral, and retrobulbar contents

8. **What are the contents of the roof?**
   The roof is triangular and consists of:
   i. Orbital plate of frontal bone
   ii. Behind this is a lesser wing of sphenoid
   iii. The anterolateral part has a depression called the fossa for the lacrimal gland

9. **What are the surgical approaches?**
   i. Superior approach
   ii. Inferior approach
   iii. Medial approach
   iv. Lateral approach

10. **What are the incisions for the superior approach?**
    i. Transcutaneous
    ii. Transconjunctival
    iii. Vertical eyelid splitting

11. **How is a transcutaneous incision made?**
    i. An upper eyelid crease incision is made
    ii. Access to superior orbital rim by dissecting superiorly in the postorbicularisfascial plane anterior to the orbital septum
    iii. An incision is made in the arcus marginalis of the rim, and a periosteal elevator is then used to separate the periosteum from the frontal bone of the orbital roof
    iv. The periorbita is kept intact to prevent orbital fat from obscuring the vision

12. **How is transconjunctival incision made?**
    Incision in the superior conjunctiva can be used to reach the superonasal, episcleral, intra- or extraconal spaces, but dissection must be performed medial to the levator muscle to prevent postoperative ptosis.

13. **How is vertical eyelid splitting made?**
    Incise the eyelid and levator aponeurosis vertically to expose the superomedial intraconal spaces.
    It allows extended transconjunctival exposure for the removal of superomedial intraconal tumors.

14. **What are the types of inferior approach and how are they made?**
    Inferior approach is suitable for masses that are visible or palpable in the inferior conjunctival fornix of the lower eyelid, as well as for deeper inferior extraconal masses.
    Transcutaneous incision:
    i. Infraciliary blepharoplasty incision is made in the lower eyelid and dissection beneath the orbicularis muscle to expose the inferior orbital septum and inferior orbital rim

ii. For access to the inferior subperiosteal space, an extended subciliary incision or an incision in the lower eyelid crease with downward reflection of the skin and orbicularis muscle allows exposure of the rim

Transconjunctival incision:
  i. To reach the extraconal surgical space and the orbital floor, an incision is made through the inferior conjunctiva and the lower eyelid retractors
  ii. Exposure to the globe is optimized when this incision is combined with a lateral canthotomy and cantholysis
  iii. The intraconal space may be reached by opening the reflected periosteum and retracting the muscle and intraconal fat

15. **What are the types of medial approach and how are they made?**
   While dissecting the medial orbit, care should be taken to avoid damaging:
   i. Medial canthal tendon
   ii. Lacrimal canaliculi and sac
   iii. Trochlea
   iv. Superior oblique tendon
   v. Inferior oblique muscle
   vi. Sensory nerves and vessels

   Types of incision
   Transcutaneous incision (Lynch or frontoethmoidal incision)
   i. Tumors within or near the lacrimal sac, the frontal or ethmoidal sinus, and the medial rectus muscle can be approached
   ii. Skin incision is placed vertically just medial to the incision of the medial canthal tendon
   iii. Mainly used to enter the subperiosteal space

   Transconjunctival incision
   i. An incision in the bulbar conjunctiva allows entry into the extraconal or episcleral surgical space
   ii. If the medial rectus is detached, one can enter the intraconal surgical space to expose the region of the anterior optic nerve for examination biopsy or sheath fenestration
   iii. If the posterior optic nerve or muscle cone needs to be seen, combined lateral/medial orbitotomies can be performed
   iv. Lateral orbitotomy with removal of lateral orbital wall displaces the globe temporally, maximizing medial access to deeper orbit

   Transcaruncular incision
   i. An incision through the posterior third of the caruncle or the conjunctiva immediately lateral to it allows excellent exposure of the medial periosteum

ii. Medial dissection just posterior to the lacrimal sac allows access to the subperiosteal space along the medial orbital wall
iii. Incision and elevation of the medial periorbita have the advantage of providing better cosmetic results than the traditional Lynch incision
iv. The combination of transcaruncular route with an inferior transconjunctival incision allows extensive exposure of the inferior and medial orbit
v. This approach provides access for the repair of medial wall fractures, for medial orbital bone decompression, and for drainage of medial subperiosteal abscess

16. **How is lateral approach done?**
    i. Lateral approach is used when a lesion is located within the lateral intraconal space, behind the equator of the globe, or in the lacrimal gland fossa
    ii. The traditional "S"-shaped Stallard–Wright skin incision extending from beneath the eyebrow laterally and curving down along the zygomatic arch allows good exposure of the lateral rim
    iii. It has been replaced by an upper eyelid crease incision or a lateral canthotomy incision
    iv. Dissecting through the periorbita and then the intermuscular septum, either above or below the lateral rectus and posterior to the equator, provides access to retrobulbar space
    v. If the lesion is too big, the bone of the lateral rim is removed
    vi. Tumors can be prolapsed by the application of gentle pressure on the eyelid

17. **What are the complications?**
    i. Hemorrhage
    ii. Optic nerve injury
    iii. Damage to vessels and nerves
    iv. Damage to muscles and tendons
    v. Injury to lacrimal gland.

8.9 BOTULINUM TOXIN

1. **What is botulinum toxin (botox)?**
   Botulinum toxin is a protein produced by the bacterium *Clostridium botulinum* and is considered the most powerful neurotoxin.

2. **When was it discovered and by whom?**
   The German physician and poet *Justinus Kerner (1786–1862)* first developed the idea of a possible therapeutic use of botulinum toxin, which he called *"sausage poison".*

3. **What is the mechanism of action of botox?**
   Botulinum toxin acts by binding presynaptically to high-affinity recognition sites on the cholinergic nerve terminals and decreasing the release of acetylcholine, causing a neuromuscular blocking effect.

4. **What is the structure of botox?**
   i. Botox are proteins that are produced by several different clostridial bacterial species and are related to the tetanus toxin
   ii. The neurotoxin proteins are synthesized along with hemagglutinin and nontoxin hemagglutinin proteins that together form a protein complex progenitor toxin

5. **What is the concern with the use of botox?**
   The formation of blocking antibodies leading to nonresponse of subsequent botox injections, called *"secondary nonresponders",* is a concern with the use of botox.

6. **What are the preparations used?**
   i. Botox (Allergan Irvine, USA)
   ii. Dysport (Ipsen, France)
   iii. Myobloc (Elan Pharma, USA)

7. **What are the contents of 1 vial?**
   Each vial contains 100 Units (U) of *C. botulinum* neurotoxin complex.
   i. 0.5 mg human albumin
   ii. 0.9 mg sodium chloride
   All these in sterile vacuum dried solid without preservatives.

8. **What is the botulinum toxin concentration with various amounts of diluents used?**

Diluent added (0.9% NaCl) (mL)	Botox used (U/0.1 mL) (U)	Dysport dose (U/0.1 mL) (U)
1	10	50
2	5	25
4	2.5	12.5
8	1.25	6.25

9. **What are the dose recommendations for common therapeutic indications of botulinum toxin in ophthalmic plastic surgery?**

Clinical condition	Approximate dose of botox required (U)
Benign essential blepharospasm	30–40
Hemifacial spasm	15–20
Chemotarsorrhaphy	5–10
Upper eyelid retraction	5–25
Lower eyelid senile entropion	10–20
Injection to the lacrimal gland	2.5–5

10. **What are the common complications?**
    i. Upper eyelid ptosis
    ii. Lagophthalmos
    iii. Entropion
    iv. Ectropion
    v. Functional epiphora due to lacrimal pump failure
    vi. Diplopia
    vii. Eyelid hematoma.

8.10 LACRIMAL SECRETORY AND DRAINAGE SYSTEMS

1. **How is a tear produced from the lacrimal gland?**
   Afferent pathway: Ophthalmic branch of the trigeminal nerve
   Efferent pathway: Lacrimal fibers via the superior branch of the zygomatic nerve (VII nerve).

2. **What is the cause of the upper and lower canaliculi?**
   The upper and lower canaliculi run 2 mm vertically and then turn 90° and run 8–10 mm medially to connect with the lacrimal sac.

3. **Which structure prevents tear reflux from the sac back into the canaliculi?**
   Valve of Rosenmüller

4. **In any lacrimal sac distension, why does it distend more inferiorly than superiorly?**
   The lacrimal sac distends more inferiorly than superiorly because superiorly, the sac is lined with fibrous tissue.

5. **Where do the angular artery and vein lie?**
   7–8 mm, medial to the medial canthal angle

6. **What are the key points with regard to the nasolacrimal duct (NLD)?**
   i. NLD is 12 mm in length
   ii. It travels through bone within the nasolacrimal canal in an inferior, lateral, and posterior direction
   iii. It opens into the nose through an ostium under the inferior meatus
   iv. This ostium is 2.5 cm posterior to the naris

7. **What are the factors involved in normal tear drainage?**
   i. Action of the orbicularis muscle
   ii. Negative pressure produced in the lacrimal sac during eyelid opening
   iii. When the eyelids are fully open, the puncta open and the negative pressure draws a tear into the canaliculi

8. **What are the common symptoms in congenital lacrimal drainage obstruction?**
   i. *Constant tearing with minimal micropurulence:* Block is at the upper level caused by punctal or canalicular dysgenesis
   ii. *Constant tearing with frequent micropurulence and matting of lashes:* Complete obstruction of the NLD
   iii. *Intermittent tearing with micropurulence:* Intermittent obstruction of the NLD as a result of a swollen inferior nasal turbinate

9. **What are "soft stops" and "hard stops" during probing performed for congenital lacrimal duct obstruction?**
    i. *Soft stops:* This implies resistance to the passage of the probe along with the medial movement of the eyelid soft tissue and signifies canalicular obstruction
    ii. *Hard stops:* If the probe advances successfully through the common canalicular system and across the lacrimal sac, the medial wall of the lacrimal sac and adjacent lacrimal bone will be encountered as a hard stop

10. **What is the distance from the punctum to the level of inferior meatus in an infant?**
    20 mm.

11. **How is the syringing test interpreted?**
    i. Difficulty in advancing the irrigating cannula and an inability to irrigate fluid: Total canalicular obstruction
    ii. If saline can be irrigated successfully but it reflexes through the upper canalicular system with no distension of lacrimal sac: Complete blockage of the common canaliculus
    iii. If mucoid material reflexes through the opposite punctum with palpable lacrimal sac distension: Complete nasolacrimal duct obstruction (NLDO)
    iv. A combination of saline reflux through the opposite canaliculus: Partial NLD stenosis

12. **What are the different types of punctal plugs used for conserving tears?**
    i. *Temporary plugs:* Collagen (dissoluble)
    ii. *Permanent plugs:* Silicone

13. **What is dacryocystorhinostomy (DCR)?**
    DCR surgery consists of making a permanent opening from the lacrimal sac into the nasal space through which tears will drain freely, resulting in the relief of epiphora and discharge.

14. **What are the indications and contraindications of external DCR?**
    Indications:
    Obstruction of the lacrimal sac or the NLD distal to the internal opening of the common canaliculus.
    i. Primary congenital NLDO
    ii. Secondary NLDO, e.g., dacryolithiasis, endonasal surgery, inflammatory sinonasal disease, or prior midfacial injury
    iii. Persistent congenital NLDO (after unsuccessful probing or intubation)

iv. Recurrent dacryocystitis
v. Chronic dacryocystitis

Contraindications:
i. Tuberculosis of the sac
ii. Malignancies of the sac
iii. Unstable systemic condition
iv. Atrophic rhinitis (relative contraindication)
v. Presence of a canalicular block (conjunctival DCR indicated)

15. **What are the types of DCR?**
    i. Conventional
    ii. Endonasal

16. **What are the surgical steps of external DCR?**
    i. Done under local anesthesia (LA) or general anesthesia
    ii. In both cases, the nose is premedicated with a decongestant—naphazoline
    iii. Patient is placed in a reverse Trendelenburg position to reduce venous congestion
    iv. Lacrimal duct syringing and probing are repeated on the table to confirm NLDO
    v. Skin incision—a medial incision 8 mm medial to the medial canthus, 2 mm above the medial palpebral ligament tendon, or a tear trough incision along the lacrimal crest can be made
    vi. *Exposure of the medial canthal tendon and anterior lacrimal crest:* Skin separated from the underlying orbicularis muscle and blunt dissection is done until the medial canthal tendon and periosteum are identified and divided as far as the spine on the anterior lacrimal crest
    vii. *Dissection of the lacrimal sac:* The periosteum along with the sac is reflected with a periosteal elevator laterally as far as the posterior lacrimal crest exposing the floor of lacrimal fossa
    viii. *Exposure of the nasal mucosa:* Traquair's periosteal elevator is used to separate the suture between the lacrimal bone and the frontal process of maxilla or between the lacrimal bone and ethmoid, thus exposing the nasal mucosa. A bone trephine, drill, hammer, and chisel can also be used. The nasal mucosa is detached from the periosteal elevator
    ix. Kerrison's bone punches are used to enlarge the opening of the rhinostomy
    x. The anterior lacrimal crest along with the frontal process of maxilla is removed
    xi. Sac lumen is identified by passing a probe via the canaliculus and medial wall incised vertically extended upward up to the fundus

and downward into the NLD. Flaps are made by converting the vertical incision to H shape

xii. Nasal flaps are created by a similar vertical incision converted to H shape

xiii. The anterior nasal mucosal flap is sutured to that of the sac with the 6-0 Vicryl followed by suturing of posterior flaps

xiv. The skin is then closed with 6-0 silk/nylon

17. **What are the advantages of external DCR?**
    i. Direct visualization of the lacrimal sac abnormalities such as stones, foreign bodies, and tumors
    ii. Sutured apposition and primary intention healing of mucosal flaps
    iii. Large osteotomy facilitates future closed placement of glass canalicular bypass tubes if required
    iv. Ready access for management of canalicular disease such as canaliculo-DCR, intubation, and canalicular bypass tube

18. **What are the techniques helping vasoconstriction and hemostasis?**
    Local anesthesia:
    i. Nasal packing with paraffin soaked gauzes or nasal decongestants like naphazoline
    ii. Supplementary intramucosal injection of local anesthetic with 1:200,000 epinephrine

    General anesthesia:
    i. Three intranasal cotton tip buds moistened with 1:1,000 epinephrine placed at and above the anterior end of the middle turbinate
    ii. Infiltration with LA at the site of incision
    iii. Controlled systemic hypotension—BP maintained at 90/60 mm Hg

    General measures:
    i. Reverse Trendelenburg position to reduce venous congestion
    ii. Continuous suction device to help maintain a bloodless field
    iii. Gentle diathermy of cut edges and respect for surgical planes

19. **What are the indications for intubation in DCR?**
    Conditions predisposing to fibrosis or closure of the rhinostomy:
    i. Repeat DCR
    ii. Failed DCR
    iii. Traumatic NLDO
    iv. Chronic inflammatory mucosal conditions—sinonasal disease, Wegener's disease
    v. Absent mucosa/sac
    vi. Poor flap construction

20. What are the indications and contraindications of endonasal DCR?

Indications:
  i. When obstruction is in the lower drainage system and the canaliculi are anatomically normal
  ii. Chronic epiphora due to acquired dacryostenosis
  iii. Chronic dacryocystitis
  iv. Recurrent dacryostenosis in children despite probing and lacrimal intubation
  v. Functional NLDO

Contraindications:
  i. History of midfacial trauma
  ii. Lacrimal sac neoplasms
  iii. Septal anomalies, large middle turbinate, nasal polyps, tight nostrils
  iv. Granular inflamed nasal mucosa

21. What are the surgical steps of endonasal DCR?
  i. Preparation and anesthesia
  ii. Identification of sac area
  iii. The fiberoptic probe is passed through the canaliculus into the sac and visualized in the nasal cavity
  iv. A mucosal incision made in the lateral wall of nasal cavity, just anterior to the ridge formed by the frontal process of the maxilla called the "axilla". It is extended 10 mm vertically and inferiorly
  v. Posterior incisions made at the superior and inferior margins of the flap using Yasargil scissors and free periosteal elevator are used to reflect the nasal flaps medially exposing the lacrimal bone
  vi. Osteotomy is done with the help of Kerrison's rongeur removing the frontal process of the maxilla and lacrimal bone exposing the lacrimal sac
  vii. The sac is filled with methylcellulose and the medial wall is incised vertically. The sac is massaged at the inner canthus to view the fundus and aid in removal of any dacryolith
  viii. The nasal mucosal flaps are mobilized laterally so that the flaps stay in close apposition and form a mucosal-lined fistula from the sac to the nose
  ix. Bicanalicular intubation is done with silicone tubes

22. What is the postoperative care after endonasal DCR?
  i. Saline spraying of the nostrils—three or four times a day for 1 week
  ii. Antibiotic steroid combination eye drops—TDS or QID—1 week
  iii. Lacrimal system is irrigated at 1 week and 1 month postoperatively
  iv. Tube removal done at the end of 1 month

v. Endoscopy at 1 month to confirm adequate healing at the surgical site
vi. Final follow-up—at 3 months to confirm the patency of lacrimal passage

23. **What are the advantages and disadvantages of endoscopic surgery?**

    Advantages:
    i. No scar
    ii. Less bleed
    iii. Less chances of injury
    iv. Less time consuming
    v. Less postoperative morbidity

    Disadvantages:
    i. Less success rate
    ii. Experience required is more
    iii. Expensive equipment

24. **What are the complications of DCR surgery?**

    Early complications:
    i. Wound infection
    ii. Bleeding
    iii. Tube lateral displacement
    iv. Infranasal synechiae
    v. Delayed healing

    Intermediate complications:
    i. Rhinostomy fibrosis
    ii. Granulomas
    iii. Corneal erosions from the tube

    Late complications:
    i. Webbed facial scar
    ii. Chronic fistula
    iii. Persistent intranasal synechiae

25. **What is functional failure?**

    Instead of anatomical patency of the lacrimal drainage system, there occurs persistent epiphora after DCR surgery with the absence of any attributable problems in the eyelids and ocular surface. This is known as functional failure.

26. **What are the causes of functional failure?**
    i. Canalicular obstruction
    ii. Small lacrimal sac (mostly in primary NLDO)
    iii. Narrow nasal cavity

iv. Thick maxilla
   v. Severe anteriorization of ethmoid sinus
   vi. Absence of mucous dacryocystitis

27. **How does distal canalicular or canalicular block affect functional success?**
    Distal canaliculi or common canaliculi is the narrowest portion of the lacrimal drainage system after DCR. So, it may act as a bottleneck in the tear drainage pathway.

28. **How does lacrimal sac size cause functional failure?**
    Cicatrized and contracted sac impinges upon the transmission of hydrostatic pressure resulting in a decrease in lacrimal pump activity.

29. **What is sump syndrome?**
    The surgical opening in the lacrimal bone is too small and too high. Thus there is a dilated lacrimal sac lateral to and below the level of inferior margin of the ostium in which the secretions collect and are unable to gain access to the ostium and thence the nasal cavity. This is sump syndrome.

30. **What are the bones that are broken during DCR?**
    i. Lacrimal fossa
    ii. Lacrimal bone
    iii. Frontal process of the maxillary bone
    iv. Part of the ethmoid bone
    v. Part of the nasal bone.

8.11 CONTRACTED SOCKET

1. **Define contracted socket.**
   Contracted socket is defined as a decrease in the depth of fornices and orbital volume which results in an inability to retain a prosthesis.

2. **What important past history will you ask a patient with contracted socket?**
   i. Nature of assault that led to loss of sight (e.g., trauma, tumor, congenital)
   ii. Any history of pain, redness, or watering in the other eye [to rule out (R/O) sympathetic ophthalmia]
   iii. Any family history positive [to R/O cancers such as retinoblastoma (RB)]

3. **What are the morphological types of contracted socket?**
   Morphological types of contracted socket are of four types:
   i. *Anophthalmic:* Seen after evisceration and enucleation and is the most common type
   ii. *Microphthalmic:* Seen in the presence of a phthisical eye
   iii. *Ophthalmic:* Seen following chemical, thermal, and radiation injuries, leading to symblepharon and ankyloblepharon
   iv. *Hypoplastic:* Seen when there is congenital underdevelopment of the bony socket

4. **What are the features of contracted socket?**
   i. Volume reduction and redistribution leading to postenucleation syndrome comprising:
      - Contraction of Tenon's capsule and retraction of extraocular muscles leading to backshift of muscle cone and retrusion of posterior wall
      - Shifting and retraction of levator muscle leading to superior sulcus depression
      - Change in the axis of action of the levator muscle from vertically upward to horizontally backward
   ii. Conjunctival shortening with shallowing of fornices

5. **What are the underlying precipitating causes that lead to socket disorders?**
   i. *Congenital and developmental:*
      - Congenital anophthalmos
      - Microphthalmos with cyst
      - Facial and orbital hypoplasia

ii. *Aging:*
   - Deficiency of orbital volume
iii. *Iatrogenic:*
   - Poor enucleation
   - Multiple operations on socket
   - Alloplastic material in socket
iv. *Traumatic:*
   - Mechanical
   - Chemical
   - Thermal
   - Radiation-induced

6. **Classify contracted socket and brief the management of each class.**

Grade	Character of socket	Management
0	Normal socket with adequate roomy fornices lined by healthy conjunctiva and no lid abnormality	Prosthetic eye (custom fit prosthesis)
1	• Posterior lamina shortening leading to entropion • Shallowing or shelving of the lower fornix	Correction of entropion. Inferior fornix forming mattress sutures over a silastic stent (closed method) or undermining of conjunctiva with excision of prolapsed fat and inferior fornix forming sutures (open method)
2	Absence of the lower fornix and pulling down of the fundus of the socket. Superior fornix may show contracture	Mucous membrane grafting with fornix forming sutures
3	Grade 2 plus absence of medial and lateral fornices	Mucous membrane/amniotic membrane grafting
4	Grade 3 plus severe shrinkage due to scarring leading to reduction of palpebral aperture in all directions. Absence of conjunctival lining of the socket	Split-thickness skin grafting
5	Inoperable socket	Spectacle prosthesis

7. **What is the use of dermis fat graft in anophthalmic socket?**
   Dermis fat graft is used to replace volume.
   Indications are:
   i. As a primary implant after primary enucleation
   ii. As a secondary implant after orbital implant migration or extrusion
   iii. After evisceration, it may be placed within the scleral shell
   iv. For superior sulcus deformity

The preferred site is the upper and outer quadrant of the gluteal region because it is not a weight-bearing area and has less chance of injuring sciatic nerve.

8. **What are the problems associated with dermis fat graft?**
    i. Atrophy of the graft
    ii. Necrosis of the graft
    iii. Central ulceration of the graft
    iv. Growth of the fatty tissue leading to proptosis of the artificial eye
    v. Pyogenic granuloma

9. **What is the important problem in the outcome of anophthalmic socket of a child?**
   In the outcome of anophthalmic socket of a child, there is an increased chance of facial dysmorphism.

10. **What is the age when facial bone growth completes?**
    14 years.

8.12 ORBITAL IMPLANTS AND PROSTHESIS

1. **What are the requirements of a functionally and cosmetically acceptable anophthalmic socket?**
   i. An orbital implant of adequate volume centered within the orbit
   ii. Eyelids with adequate tone and normal appearance to support a prosthesis
   iii. A socket lined with conjunctiva or mucous membrane with fornices deep enough to hold a prosthesis
   iv. Good transmission of motility from the implant to the overlying prosthesis
   v. Comfortable prosthesis similar to the normal eye

2. **What are orbital implants?**
   Orbital implants:
   i. Replace the volume lost by the enucleated eye
   ii. Impart motility to the prosthesis
   iii. Maintain cosmetic symmetry with the fellow eye

3. **Classify orbital implants.**

Type	Definition	Example
Nonintegrated	No direct or indirect integration of the synthetic implant with the orbital structures or with the prosthesis	Polymethyl methacrylate (PMMA) or silicone implants
Semi-integrated	Indirect (mechanical) integration of the synthetic implant with the orbital structures but not with the prosthesis	Allens, Iowa, Universal, Castroviejo
Integrated	Indirect (mechanical) integration of the synthetic implant with orbital structures and with prosthesis	Cutler's implant
Biointegrated	Direct (biological) integration of a natural or a synthetic implant with the orbital structures with or without integration with the prosthesis	Hydroxyapatite (BioEye) Porous polyethylene (Medpore) Aluminum oxide (Bioceramic)
Biogenic	An autograft or allograft of a natural tissue with direct (biological) integration with orbital structures but not with the prosthesis	Dermis fat graft Cancellous bone

4. **What are the commonly used orbital implants in clinical practice?**
   Nonintegrated implants such as PMMA and silicone implants

5. **How will the implant motility be improved in case of nonintegrated implants?**
   Implant motility can be improved by wrapping it with a donor sclera and attaching the extraocular muscles of the host to the sclera.

6. **What are the advantages and disadvantages of nonintegrated implants?**
   Advantages:
   i. Cheaper, affordable, especially in developing countries
   ii. Easier to perform surgery

   Disadvantages:
   i. Implant motility is not good
   ii. Increased chance of extrusion

7. **What are the advantages and disadvantages of biointegrated implants?**
   Advantages:
   i. Better implant motility
   ii. Better stability

   Disadvantages:
   i. High cost factor
   ii. Implant exposure

8. **What is motility peg insertion?**
   Motility peg insertion is an indirect attachment of the implant to the prosthesis, enhancing prosthesis motility. Pegging of hydroxyl apatite implant can sometimes be performed as early as 6 months after surgery, pending confirmation of vascularization. Pegging may, however, increase the risk of implant exposure and infection.

9. **How is the implant size calculated?**
   i. Implants provide about 65-70% of volume replacement of anophthalmic socket and the rest 35-30% by the prosthesis
   ii. A smaller implant has a higher tendency to displace or migrate and develop superior sulcus deformity. A larger implant is known to improve both cosmesis and motility. However, an inappropriately large implant may result in wound gap and implant exposure
   iii. Implant sizing has mostly been empirical and is often decided in the operating room
   iv. Generally, a 16-18 mm implant is used for infants, 18-20 mm in older children, and 20-22 mm in adults
   v. There are implant sizers that help gauge the appropriate size
   vi. Axial length of the other eye can also be taken as a guide (axial length in mm−2 = implant diameter in mm). An additional 2 mm is deducted from the axial length if the implant is traditionally wrapped

10. **What are the advantages of implant wrapping?**
    Advantages:
    i. An additional barrier, so decreased chance of implant exposure
    ii. Enables easy attachment of extraocular muscles, thus providing better prosthesis motility
    iii. Entails a smooth external surface, thus making the process of implant insertion easier
    iv. Helps in volume augmentation by adding around 1.5 mm to the implant diameter

11. **What are the materials used for implant wrapping?**
    i. Donor sclera (most popular)
    ii. Donor-processed pericardium and fascia lata (commercially available)
    iii. Autologous sclera (if the cause of enucleation is other than the suspected tumor)
    iv. Synthetic materials (polyglactin 910 mesh, polytetrafluoroethylene sheet)

12. **What are the special steps to take when enucleation is done for children?**
    i. A large adult-size implant should be used to replace orbital volume
    ii. Autogenous dermis fat grafts are preferred as anophthalmic implants.

8.13 MISCELLANEOUS OCULAR SURGERIES

ENUCLEATION

1. **Define enucleation.**
   Enucleation is the removal of the eyeball with the covering sclera and cornea along with a stump of the optic nerve.

2. **What are the indications of enucleation?**
   i. *Absolute indications:*
      - Intraocular malignancy (nontreatable)
      - Possibility of sympathetic ophthalmia
   ii. *Relative indications:*
      - Extensively traumatized globes with uveal tissue loss, retinal damage, disorganization of the globe
      - Irritable painful, deformed, or disfigured globes with or without atrophy, secondary to retinal detachment (RD), absolute glaucoma, etc.
      - Phthisis bulbi, especially painful
      - Blind globes with staphyloma
      - Severe buphthalmos with a painful blind eye
      - Blind eyes with inextractable foreign bodies

3. **Name the various enucleation techniques.**
   i. Enucleation without insertion of an implant
   ii. Enucleation with an exposed integrated implant
   iii. Enucleation with an implant inserted within Tenon's capsule
   iv. Enucleation with a wrapped implant (with sclera, fascia lata graft, or synthetic material)
   v. Enucleation with incorporation of dermis fat graft

4. **What is the important step before enucleation surgery?**
   Identify the patient and confirm the eye to be enucleated. Also, check the signature of two senior doctors advising enucleation.

5. **What are the special steps to undertake when enucleation is performed for an intraocular tumor?**
   i. In case of retinoblastoma, a long segment of the optic nerve should be cut to increase the chance for the tumor to be completely removed
   ii. Avoid penetrating the globe and manipulate the globe gently to minimize the risk of tumor dissemination

6. **What are the differences between live and cadaver enucleation?**
   i. *Live enucleation:*
      - *Indications:* Blind painful eye, intraocular tumor, trauma, risk of sympathetic ophthalmitis

- In live enucleation, isolate the rectus muscle and tie each muscle with a double-armed 4-0 long-acting absorbable suture
- Proceed with an implant provided that there is no contraindication, e.g., visible extraocular tumor extension, orbital cellulitis
- Use of cautery to cut the muscles and a wire snare for the optic nerve reduces trauma, which is essential when enucleating an eye with a tumor, e.g., malignant melanoma
- It is preferable in this case not to use a traction suture, but the suture is very useful in other circumstances, e.g., when enucleating a soft eye after trauma
- If no implant is to be inserted, pass the long-acting absorbable sutures from the rectus muscles through Tenon's capsule and the conjunctiva in the superior, medial, inferior, and lateral fornices and tie them before closing the conjunctiva. This will improve the motility of the fornice and artificial eye

A conformer or shell should be retained in the socket to maintain the fornices

ii. *Cadaver enucleation:*
   - *Indication:* Eye donation
   - In this, rectus muscles are isolated and cut and sutures or cautery may not be required
   - Optic nerve stump length specifications are not required
   - Either tractional suture or enucleation scoop can be used for removal of the globe in cadaveric enucleation
   - Implant is not required to maintain forniceal motility

EVISCERATION

1. **Define evisceration.**
   Evisceration is defined as the complete removal of the ocular contents through an opening in the cornea or sclera, leaving the optic nerve and sclera intact along with the attached extraocular muscles.
   The procedure may be performed with or without the removal of cornea.

2. **What are the indications of evisceration?**
   i. Endophthalmitis, virulent enough and resistant to antibiotic therapy
   ii. Panophthalmitis
   iii. Expulsive choroidal hemorrhage
   iv. Bleeding anterior staphyloma
   v. Globe injury with intact sclera shell
   vi. Blind eye due to absolute glaucoma, uveitis, corneal scarring with or without pain
   vii. Chemical burn with severe disfigurement

3. **What are the contraindications of evisceration?**
    i. Intraocular tumor
    ii. Phthisis bulbi
    iii. Advanced degeneration of the globe
    iv. Pathological examination of ocular contents desired
    v. Chronically inflamed eye
    vi. Nystagmus in the eye planned for destructive surgery
4. **What are the advantages of evisceration over enucleation?**
    i. *Less disruption of orbital anatomy:* Thus, the chance of injury to extraocular muscles and nerves and atrophy of fat is reduced with less dissection within the orbit. Good motility of the prosthesis is obtained
    ii. *Prevention of orbital spread:* Evisceration is preferred in cases of endophthalmitis because extirpation and drainage of the ocular contents can occur without invasion of the orbit. The chance of contamination of the orbit with possible subsequent orbital cellulitis or intracranial extension is therefore theoretically reduced
    iii. *A technically simpler procedure:* Performing this less invasive procedure may be important when general anesthesia is contraindicated or when bleeding disorders increase the risk of orbital dissection
    iv. *Lower rate of migration, extrusion, and reoperation*
    v. *Good motility of the prosthesis*
5. **What are the disadvantages of evisceration?**
    i. Cannot be performed for intraocular tumors
    ii. Theoretical increased risk of sympathetic ophthalmia
    iii. Inadequate specimen for pathologic examinations

EXENTERATION

1. **Define exenteration.**
   Exenteration is defined as the removal of all the soft tissues of orbit, i.e., the globe, extraocular muscles, fat, and other orbital contents along with the periorbita lining the orbital cavity.

2. **What are indications of exenteration?**
    i. Destructive tumors extending into the orbit from the sinuses, face, eyelids, conjunctiva, or intracranial space
    ii. Intraocular melanomas or retinoblastomas that have extended outside the globe (if evidence of distant metastases is excluded). When local control of the tumor would benefit the nursing care of the patient, exenteration is indicated

    iii. Malignant epithelial tumors of the lacrimal gland. Although the procedure is somewhat controversial, these tumors may require extended exenteration with radical bone removal of the roof, lateral wall, and floor

    iv. Sarcomas and other primary orbital malignancies that do not respond to nonsurgical therapy. Some tumors such as rhabdomyosarcomas that were previously treated by exenteration are now initially treated by radiation and chemotherapy

    v. Fungal infection. Subtotal or total exenteration may be necessary for the management of orbital zygomycosis which occurs most commonly in patients who are diabetic or immunosuppressed. However, attention is now being focalized on achieving control through more limited debridement of involved orbital tissues

3. What are the types of exenteration surgeries?

Subtotal: The eye and adjacent intraorbital tissues are removed such that the lesion is locally excised (leaving the periorbita and part or all of the eyelids). This technique is used for some locally invasive tumors, for debulking of disseminated tumors, or for partial treatment in selected patients.

Total: All intraorbital soft tissues, including periorbita, are removed, with or without the skin of the eyelids.

Extended: All intraorbital soft tissues are removed, together with adjacent structures (usually bony walls and sinuses).

CHAPTER 9

Pediatric Ophthalmology and Strabismus

9.1 PEDIATRIC-OPHTHALMIC MANAGEMENT

1. **What is the visual acuity during infancy?**
   1 month of age: 6/120
   6 months: 6/30
   12-18 months: 6/48-6/12
   36 months: 6/12-6/6

2. **How can we estimate visual acuity by examining the fixation of a child?**
   i. Central steady fixation: 6/6-6/9
   ii. Central steady fixation with strong dominance to the other eye: 6/12-6/24
   iii. Central fixation but unsteady: 6/36-6/60
   iv. Unsteady fixation: <6/60
   v. Gross eccentric fixation to no fixation: Vision <6/60

3. **What are the causes of defective vision since birth?**
   A. *Congenital:*
      i. Optic nerve hypoplasia
      ii. Congenital cataract
      iii. Congenital glaucoma
      iv. Nystagmus
   B. *Inherited:*
      i. Retinitis pigmentosa
      ii. Optic atrophy
      iii. Stargardt's disease
      iv. Maculopathies
      v. Myopic macular degeneration
      vi. Oculocutaneous albinism
   C. *Acquired:*
      i. Glaucoma
      ii. Refractive error
      iii. Eye injury
      iv. Retinopathy of prematurity
      v. Cerebral/cortical visual impairment

4. **What are the drugs used in refraction for children?**
   i. Cyclopentolate (0.5-2%) combined with tropicamide
   ii. Combination of phenylephrine 2.5% with 0.5% cyclopentolate in premature babies up to 6 months
   iii. Homide 2% (preferred in children with history of seizures)
   iv. Atropine 1% in ointment form (used 1-2 times daily for 3 days prior to retinoscopy to produce complete cycloplegia)

5. **What is the amount to be subtracted from retinoscopy findings to take into account the working distance?**

Working distance (in meters)	Diopters to be subtracted
1.0	1.00
0.75	1.33
0.66	1.50

6. **What are the general principles with regard to the prescription of spectacles in various refractive errors?**
   In general, correction of refractive errors depends upon its association with strabismus
   i. *Hypermetropia:*
      - With strabismus—full correction if esotropia, under correct if exotropia
      - Without strabismus—subjective acceptance/optimum correction
   ii. *Myopia:*
      - With strabismus—full correction if exotropia, under correct if esotropia
      - Without strabismus: The weakest concave spherical lens giving good distance vision should be prescribed
   iii. *Astigmatism:* Under correction below 3 years of age; full correction in older children

7. **What is amblyopia?**
   Amblyopia is a reduction of best-corrected visual acuity that cannot be attributed directly to the structural abnormality of the eye. It is often unilateral but can also occur bilaterally.

8. **What are the types and causes of amblyopia?**
   i. Strabismic amblyopia—develops in a deviated eye
   ii. Refractive amblyopia
   iii. Anisometropic amblyopia—develops when there is a difference in refractive error between the two eyes of 1.5 D hyperopia, 3 D myopia, or 2 D astigmatism

iv. Ametropic amblyopia is bilateral and seen in hyperopia >4–5 D and myopia >5–6 D
v. Visual deprivation amblyopia—occurs due to lesions that obscure the visual axis, such as ptosis, corneal opacities, cataract, and vitreous hemorrhage

9. **Is amblyopia more common in unilateral or bilateral ptosis?**
   Unilateral ptosis:
   i. Constant unilateral ptotic eye will result in amblyopia
   ii. Unilateral/lateral (U/L) ptosis eye causes astigmatism in which anisometric amblyopia is more common
   iii. Retinal image blur in one eye inhibits cortical activity from one eye preventing visual development

   Bilateral ptosis:
   i. Patient will have a chin-up position, and hence amblyopia is very rare

10. **How do you manage a case of amblyopia?**
    i. Exclude other causes of poor vision by performing a comprehensive eye examination
    ii. Clear the media
    iii. Correct refractive errors fully
    iv. Occlusion of the better eye
    v. Penalization of the better eye (pharmacological penalization with atropine/optical penalization with high plus lens)
    vi. Visual stimulation of the amblyopic eye
    vii. Dichoptic stimulation (computer-based binocular stimulation)

11. **What is a horopter?**
    Horopter is an imaginary plane in space in which all corresponding retinal points are seen singly

12. **What are the factors which are required for the presence of binocular single vision (BSV)?**
    i. Clear visual axis in both eyes
    ii. Eyes in orthophoria
    iii. Ability of the cerebral cortex to fuse the images

13. **What are the three grades of BSV?**
    i. Simultaneous macular perception
    ii. Fusion
    iii. Stereopsis

14. **What are the compensatory mechanisms which happen when BSV is interrupted?**
    i. Abnormal head posture
    ii. Suppression

iii. Anomalous retinal correspondence
iv. Blind spot syndrome

15. **What are synergists?**
    i. Muscles that are paired to achieve movement in the same direction are called yoke muscles or synergists
    ii. *Ipsilateral synergists:* Synergist muscles in the same eye [e.g., right superior rectus (SR) and right inferior oblique (IO) in dextroelevation]
    iii. *Contralateral synergists:* Synergist muscles in the opposite eyes [e.g., right lateral rectus (LR) and left medial rectus (MR) in dextroversion]

16. **What are yoke muscles?**
    Yoke muscles are otherwise called contralateral synergists. They are pairs of muscles, one in each eye, that produce conjugate ocular movements. For example, left LR is the yoke muscle for right MR in levoversion.

17. **What is Sherrington's law?**
    Sherrington's law (also called the law of reciprocal innervation) states that the increased innervation and contraction of an extraocular muscle (e.g., right LR) is accompanied by a reciprocal decrease in innervation and contraction of its antagonist (right MR).

18. **What is Hering's law?**
    Hering's law (also called the law of motor correspondence) states that equal and simultaneous innervations flow to the yoke muscles concerned with the direction of gaze.

19. **What are the various supranuclear control systems for eye movement?**
    i. Saccadic system
    ii. Smooth pursuit system
    iii. Vergence system
    iv. Optokinetic nystagmus
    v. Vestibular ocular reflex

20. **What are the steps in the evaluation of strabismus?**
    i. History
    ii. Inspection
        - Head posture
        - Asymmetry of face/skull
        - Palpebral fissure and lids
        - Anterior segment
    iii. Vision assessment
    iv. Corneal reflex (Hirschberg test)
    v. Sensory tests
        - Binocular vision—Worth four-dot test, Bagolini
        - Stereopsis—TNO, Langs, Titmus fly test

vi. Cover test
   - Cover–uncover test
   - Alternate cover test
   - Prism cover test
   - Simultaneous prism cover test
vii. Modified Krimsky (when vision is low in one eye)
viii. Ocular movements
ix. Special tests
   - Four-prism test (to assess microtropia)
   - Patch test [for intermittent exotropia (IXT)]
   - Parks three-step test (in vertical deviations)
   - Accommodative convergence/accommodation (AC/A) ratio (in convergence excess esotropia)
   - Forced duction test (to differentiate muscle palsy and restriction)
   - Synoptophore (especially to measure the deviation in all cardinal gaze positions)
x. Tests for diplopia
   - Diplopia charting
   - Hess charting/Lees test
   - Goldmann perimetry—to assess field of binocular vision
xi. Tests for torsion
   - Double Maddox rod
   - Lancaster red green
xii. Cycloplegic refraction
xiii. Fundus evaluation (to assess retina and torsion)

21. **What are the causes of pseudosquint?**
    i. Flat, broad nasal bridge
    ii. Prominent epicanthal folds
    iii. Narrow or very wide interpupillary distance (IPD)
    iv. Positive/negative angle kappa
    v. Asymmetry of face
    vi. Deep-set eyes

22. **What are phorias and tropias?**
    i. *Phoria:* A latent deviation in which fusional control is always present
    ii. *Tropia:* A manifest deviation in which fusional control is not present

23. **What are the causes for abnormal head postures?**
    Nonocular causes:
    i. Torticollis
    ii. Deafness
    iii. Disorders of the cervical spine
    iv. Habitual

Ocular causes:
  i. Diplopia
  ii. Limitation of ocular movements
  iii. Nystagmus
  iv. One eyed (to expand field of vision)

24. **What are the components of a head posture?**
    i. Head tilt/turn to the right or left shoulder
    ii. Face turn to right or left side
    iii. Chin elevation or depression

25. **What are the reasons for a head tilt in a case of strabismus?**
    The head is tilted for two reasons:
    i. *Vertical deviation:* The head is tilted to the side of the lower eye to elevate the diplopic images and make fusion possible
    ii. *Torsional deviation:* Normally, if the head is tilted to the right shoulder, the right eye will intort, and the left eye will extort. However, in cases like a left fourth nerve palsy, where the left eye is already extorted, the head is tilted to the right to compensate the extorsion

26. **What is the reason for a face turn in a case of squint?**
    The face turns either to left or right to place the eyes away from the field of main action of the paralyzed muscle and into the position of least deviation. For example, in the case of right sixth nerve palsy, the face is turned to the right to place the eyes in left gaze.

27. **What are the reasons for change in chin position?**
    The chin is elevated or depressed in cases of vertical strabismus for the following reasons:
    i. To place the eyes away from the field of action of the paretic muscle
    ii. To place the eyes in a position in which the deviation can be controlled
    iii. To avoid discomfort

28. **What is angle kappa?**
    Angle kappa is the angle formed between the optical axis and the visual axis.

29. **What are the tests based on light reflex to test for ocular alignment?**
    i. *Hirschberg test:* This test is based on the principle of the corneal light reflex (Purkinje image 1). Normally, light reflex will fall just nasal to the center of the pupil. About 1 mm of decentration of the corneal light reflex corresponds to about 7° or 15 prism of ocular deviation. If the light reflex is seen at the border of the pupil, it is a 15° or a 30 prism D deviation. If the light reflex is seen in the mid-iris region,

which is about 4 mm from the center of the pupil, it corresponds to 30° or 60 prism of ocular deviation

ii. *Krimsky test:* It involves placing prisms before the deviated eye. The prisms are adjusted to center the corneal reflection in the deviated eye, and the amount of prism required is taken as a quantitative measure. Modified Krimsky test is commonly employed, wherein the prisms are placed in front of the normal eye to make the observation easier in the deviating eye

iii. *Bruckner test:* The direct ophthalmoscope is used from an arm's distance to obtain a red reflex simultaneously in both eyes. The deviated eye will have a brighter reflex

30. What are the various cover tests?

i. *Cover-uncover test:* The cover test is to detect tropia, while the uncover test is to detect phorias. The patient is asked to fix a distant target. The fixing eye is closed, and the eye suspected of deviation is observed. No movement indicates that the eye is orthotropic. Now, the cover is removed, and the movement of the eye behind the cover is looked for movement. No movement indicates that the eyes are orthophoric

ii. *Alternate cover test:* It is a test to assess the deviation suspending the fusion mechanisms by placing the cover alternately in front of both eyes and observe the movement in both eyes

iii. *Prism cover test:* It is a test to quantitatively measure the angle of deviation. After performing the alternate cover test, prisms of increasing strength are placed in front of an eye with the base opposite the direction of the deviation. The alternate cover test is performed with increase in prism strength until the deviation is neutralized and no movement is seen

31. How many types of cover tests are there?

There are three types of cover tests. They are:

i. Cover–uncover test

ii. Alternate cover test

iii. Simultaneous prism and cover test

All can be performed fixating at near and distance

32. What are the prerequisites for cover test?

i. Good visual acuity

ii. Should have central fixation which is maintained

iii. Should have reasonably good ocular movements

33. How do you perform the monocular cover-uncover test?

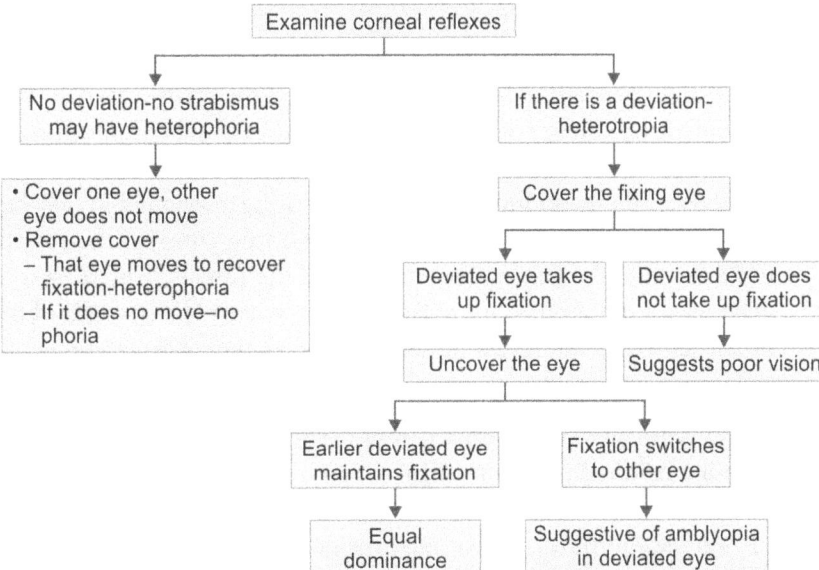

In this test, one eye is covered and then uncovered. During the process, the movement of the eye under cover is noted as the cover is taken away. In heterophoria, the eye behind the cover deviates and then straightens as the cover is removed. The phoria is graded as good, fair, or poor control depending upon the force at which the deviated eye takes up fixation.

34. What is alternate cover test?
   i. In alternate cover test, the cover is changed from one eye to the other and back several times. In cases of phoria, it gives information on the type of phoria
   ii. In case of tropia, it gives information on the type of deviation, whether it is constant/intermittent and unilateral/alternating

35. What do you mean by alternation of squint, and what does it imply?
   i. The deviation is seen in both eyes with equal dominance
   ii. On cover test, both eyes take up fixation equally well in presence of the other eye's deviation
   iii. It implies equal vision in both eyes (no amblyopia)

36. How do you place prisms in front of the eye to measure deviation?
   i. *Plastic prisms:* Placed in the frontal position, i.e., parallel to the infraorbital margin
   ii. *Glass prisms:* Prentice position—posterior face of the prism is perpendicular to the line of sight
   Plastic prisms are commonly used

iii. Apex of the prism is placed in direction of the deviation in front of the squinting eye, e.g., base out for esodeviation

37. How will you quantify the amount of deviation?

The patient is asked to fixate on a target, and the prisms are placed in front of the squinting eye. The prism is placed base-in for exodeviations, base-out for esodeviations, and base-down in hypertropia. An alternate cover test is then performed while observing the movement of each eye as the cover is changed. Sufficient time must be given for the patient to fix through the prism. The strength of the prisms is increased or decreased until there is no refixation movement. The strength of the prism achieving neutralization signifies the amount of deviation.

38. How do you assess ocular motility?

Versions are checked first binocularly, particularly paying attention to the nine cardinal positions of gaze. The nine positions of gaze are as follows:

i. Primary position—when the eyes are fixing straight ahead on an object at infinity (practically at 6 m)
ii. Cardinal positions are the six positions of gaze, the movement of which is made by yoke muscles
iii. Midline positions—straight up and straight down from the primary position (they do not isolate any one muscle as two elevators and two depressors are involved in the midline positions)

If versions are limited in any direction, duction (uniocular) movement should be assessed for each eye separately

39. How do you test for convergence?

The near point of convergence is tested by keeping the fixation object at 40 cm in the midsagittal plane of the patient's head. As the patient fixates, the target is moved closer, and the point at which one eye loses fixation and turns outwardly is tested. Royal Air Force (RAF) ruler is used for the same purpose. Normal value is 8–10 cm or less.

40. What is Parks–Bielschowsky three-step test used for?

Parks–Bielschowsky three-step test is an objective test used to know whether a cyclovertical muscle is involved in a patient with vertical deviation.

41. What are the principles on which the Parks–Bielschowsky three-step test is based on?

i. Torsional imbalance when a single cyclovertical muscle is paretic
ii. Vertical recti have the maximum vertical action in abduction and obliques in adduction

iii. Head tilt is based on vestibular stimulation, which produces a compensatory cyclorotation of the eyes. This is disrupted when a cyclovertical muscle is paralyzed and causes an increase in the vertical deviation

42. **How do you use Maddox rod?**
    i. Maddox rod is a device which consists of a series of parallelly arranged cylinders which convert a point source of light (spotlight) into a linear image at 90° to the axis of the cylinders. It is usually colored red and used at a 6 m distance. The rod is placed in a trial frame with the ridges horizontal, giving a vertical line. The patient fixes at a spotlight at the eye level and is asked where he sees the line. Fusion is impossible since the images are dissimilar; the eyes are therefore dissociated, making any latent squint to become manifest. In esophoria, the light will be on the same side as the line, and in exophoria, it will be on the opposite side
    ii. To detect the vertical phoria, the rod is placed with the ridges vertically so as to give a horizontal line. The other steps are the same as above

43. **What does the Maddox rod test do?**
    Maddox rod test dissociates both the eyes by employing two dissimilar images in front of both the eyes.

44. **What is double Maddox rod test?**
    Maddox rod test is a subjective test to detect and measure the amount of torsion associated with vertical deviation.

45. **How do you perform a double Maddox rod test?**
    Herein, two Maddox rods, preferably white and red, are placed one in front of each eye to produce two horizontal lines (ridges placed vertically). The patient is asked if both are straight and parallel or if one is tilted. A tilt toward the nose denotes extorsion, and a tilt toward the ear denotes intorsion. The side of the tilted line is identified, and its position is adjusted by rotating the concerned Maddox rod in the trial frame until two parallel lines are seen abolishing the tilt. The direction and degrees are read from the readings on the trial frame.

46. **What is the use of Maddox wing?**
    Maddox wing dissociates both the eyes for near fixation and is used to measure phorias.

47. **What is Worth four-dot test?**
    i. Worth four-dot test is a test used for estimating BSV
    ii. It dissociates both eyes by red and green goggles
    iii. It can be used at both near and distance

iv. The test consists of four round lights (in a box for distance, in a torch light for near), one red, two green, and one white. The patient is asked to view these round lights through red and green glasses. The colors being complimentary,; the red and white lights are seen through the red glass and green and white through the green glass (one red, one white, and two green)
v. The following is the interpretation:
   - *Normal fusion:* All four lights are seen
   - *Anomalous retinal correspondence:* All four lights are seen in the presence of a manifest squint
   - *Left suppression:* Two red lights are seen
   - *Right suppression:* Three green lights are seen
   - *Diplopia:* Five lights are seen, two red and three green indicating a manifest squint with normal correspondence

48. What are the uses of synoptophore?
Diagnostic:
i. To determine the grades of BSV and estimate the type of suppression, retinal correspondence, fusion range measurement, and measurement of angle kappa
ii. To measure the objective and subjective angles of deviation
iii. To measure the deviation in all nine positions
iv. To measure primary and secondary deviation

Therapeutic: Used to treat suppression and intermittent tropias and phorias

49. What are the types of exotropia?
i. *Concomitant exotropia:*
   - Infantile exotropia
   - IXT
   - Consecutive exotropia
   - Sensory exotropia
ii. *Incomitant exotropia:*
   - Paralytic—oculomotor nerve palsy
   - Myasthenia gravis
   - Duane's retraction syndrome (DRS)
   - Thyroid eye disease

50. What are the different types of esodeviation?
i. *Concomitant esotropia:*
   - Infantile esotropia
   - Accommodative esotropia:
     - Refractive accommodative esotropia
     - Nonrefractive accommodative esotropia
     - Partially accommodative esotropia

- Late onset or acquired esotropia
  - Basic esotropia
  - Convergence excess esotropia
  - Divergence insufficiency esotropia
- Cyclic esotropia
- Sensory esotropia
- Nystagmus blockade syndrome
- Consecutive esotropia

ii. *Incomitant esotropia:*
- Paralytic sixth nerve palsy
- Restrictive DRS, thyroid, trauma, etc.

51. What are the characteristic features of essential infantile esotropia?
  i. Presents by 4 months of age and persists
  ii. Large angle of deviation
  iii. Free alternation
  iv. Cross fixation
  v. No significant refractive error on cycloplegic refraction
  vi. No neurological defect
  vii. May be associated with inferior oblique overaction (IOOA), nystagmus, or dissociated vertical deviation (DVD)

52. What are the variants of essential infantile esotropia?
Ciancia syndrome and Lang's syndrome

53. What is the timing of surgery in cases of essential infantile esotropia?
Surgical correction is preferred by 6–18 months of age. Most surgeons operate at 12 months of age.
The requirement is:
  i. The deviation is constant with repeated measurements
  ii. Proper assessment of the associated oblique overactions

54. What are the surgical options for this condition?
  i. Monocular recess resect procedure
  ii. Bimedial recession with appropriate management of oblique overaction if present with strabismus

55. What are the special factors that have to be taken into account while operating in very small children?
  i. Exact measurement of squint is difficult as very young children may not be cooperative
     In small children, the results obtained per millimeter of surgery on a muscle are much more than in adults. Results may be less predictable due to this and the large angle in small eyeballs

ii. In children <6 months of age, posterior segment is still developing, so the results might be unpredictable due to growth of the eyeball
iii. Distance from the limbus to the rectus may be variable; hence measurements may be taken from the limbus

56. **What can be the postoperative outcomes when operating on a child with infantile esotropia?**
    i. Optimal outcome—subnormal binocular vision
    ii. Desirable outcome—microtropia
    iii. Acceptable—small residual angle
    iv. Unacceptable—large angle strabismus with suppression

57. **What are the characteristics of refractive accommodative esotropia?**
    i. Manifests at 2-3 years of age
    ii. Hypermetropia 2-6 D
    iii. Ocular deviation at near fixation more than distance fixation
    iv. Normal AC/A ratio

    The deviation gets corrected fully with refractive correction. If not treated promptly, it will result in amblyopia in one eye

58. **What is AC/A ratio?**
    AC/A ratio is the amount of convergence in prism diopter per unit change in accommodation in diopter. It can be measured by two methods:
    i. *Gradient method:*
    1st step: Patient wears the corrective spectacles and is made to fix at 6 m Snellen letter. Ocular deviation is measured by prism cover test
    2nd step: Three-dimensional (3D) lenses are added on both sides, and the deviation is again measured
    3rd step: The first measurement is subtracted from the second measurement and divided by 3D
    The measurement can also be done by making the patient fix for near and adding + 3D lenses in the trial frame
    ii. *Heterophoria method:* IPD + (deviation for near deviation for distance)/fixation distance in diopter

59. **When is AC/A ratio tested?**
    i. When there is a disparity in the near and distance deviation, especially if a patient is more exotropic or less esotropic for near, then a low AC/A ratio is suspected
    ii. If esotropia is more for near and less for distance, then a high ratio should be suspected
    iii. An abnormally high AC/A ration can be managed optically, medically or surgically

60. What is DRS?
i. DRS is a congenital restrictive strabismus, in which there is limitation of horizontal ocular movements and changes in height of palpebral fissure due to retraction of globe. Up/down shoots of the globe may be present during attempted adduction. DRS is now listed as a congenital cranial dysinnervation disorder
ii. Huber's classification:
   - *Type I:* Limitation in abduction
   - *Type II:* Limitation in adduction
   - *Type III:* Limitation in abduction and adduction

61. What are the disorders associated with DRS?
i. *Systemic association:*
   - Epilepsy
   - Deafness
   - Maldevelopment of the genitourinary system
   - Goldenhar's syndrome
   - Klippel–Feil syndrome
ii. *Ocular association:*
   - Ptosis
   - Dermoids
   - Nystagmus
   - Myelinated nerve fibers
   - Gustatory lacrimal reflex (crocodile tears)

62. What are the differential diagnoses of DRS?
i. Sixth nerve palsy
ii. Moebius syndrome
iii. Infantile esotropia
iv. Congenital oculomotor apraxia

63. How is DRS managed?
A. *Eso-DRS:*
   i. Unilateral with minimal co-contractions: MR recession or SR transposition
   ii. Unilateral with severe co-contraction: MR recession along with LR recession with or without Y split
   iii. Bilateral:
      - Bilateral MR recession with or without SR transposition
      - LR weakening with Y split in case of co-contractions
B. *Exo-DRS:*
   i. *With normal LR activity in abduction with absent overshoots:* LR recession
   ii. *With normal LR activity in abduction with presence of overshoots:* LR recession with Y split

iii. *Without normal LR activity in abduction:* LR periosteal fixation/supramaximal recession with or without partial vertical rectus transpositions

64. What is Brown syndrome?
Brown syndrome is also called superior oblique tendon sheath syndrome. The characteristic features are:
  i. Limitation of the active and passive elevation in adduction
  ii. Downdrift of the affected eye on contralateral version
  iii. Predominance of a V pattern
  iv. Positive forced-duction test
  v. Hess chart shows a limitation of movement but with a normal lower field

65. What are the types of Brown syndrome?
  i. Congenital
  ii. Acquired:
    - Trauma to the trochlea or superior oblique tendon
    - Inflammation of the tendon due to inflammatory conditions such as rheumatoid arthritis and scleritis

66. What is Mobius syndrome?
Mobius syndrome is a congenital disorder characterized by bilateral facial weakness, bilateral sixth nerve palsies, and horizontal gaze palsies (bilateral seventh and sixth nerve paralysis).

67. What are the indications for squint surgeries?
  i. To restore BSV
  ii. To correct abnormal head posture
  iii. To treat diplopia and confusion
  iv. For cosmetic purposes

68. What are the surgical procedures which cause weakening of the recti muscles?
  i. Recession
  ii. Retroequatorial myopexy (Faden's procedure)
  iii. Marginal myotomy
  iv. Myectomy
  v. Free tenotomy

69. What is the principle of recession?
In the recession procedure, the muscle is disinserted and reinserted to a point closer to its origin, inducing a laxity in the muscle action.

70. What are the maximal limits of recession?
  i. *Adults:* 6 mm for MR and 9 mm for LR
  ii. *Children:* 5.5 mm for MR and 8 mm for LR

71. **What is the principle of resection?**
    A resection strengthens the muscle function. Herein, a segment of the muscle near the insertion is removed, and the posterior end of the cut muscle is reattached to the insertion. The muscle is strengthened by making it shorter and taut.

72. **Why does surgery (recession or resection) performed on the inferior rectus muscle result in alteration of the palpebral fissure width?**
    Recession of the inferior rectus causes widening of the palpebral fissure, while resection causes narrowing. This is because the inferior rectus is bound to the lower eyelid by the inferior palpebral ligament.

73. **What is Faden's procedure?**
    Faden's procedure is a retroequatorial myopexy without disinsertion of the muscle. In this surgery, the muscle is sutured to the sclera well posterior to its insertion, thus considerably weakening the muscle in its field of action. The indications are:
    i. Nonrefractive accommodative esotropia
    ii. Nystagmus blockade syndrome
    iii. DVDs.

9.2 DIPLOPIA CHARTING

1. **What is diplopia charting?**
   Diplopia charting gives a pictorial record of diplopia in cases where there is separation of two images, changing with the position of gaze.

2. **What is the principle of diplopia charting?**
   Each retinal point has its own value of direction in gazes.

3. **What are the indications for diplopia charting?**
   In patients with incomitant deviation, diplopia charting can be an aid for diagnosis and for follow-up.

4. **What are the data derived from diplopia charting?**
   i. The areas of single vision and diplopia
   ii. The distance between the two images in the areas of diplopia
   iii. Whether the images are on the same level or not
   iv. Whether one image is tilted or both are erect
   v. Whether the diplopia is crossed or uncrossed

5. **What are the prerequisites for doing diplopia charting?**
   i. Patient should have binocular vision
   ii. Good visual acuity
   iii. Patient should be cooperative

6. **What are the materials required for diplopia charting?**
   i. A pair of red and green glasses
   ii. Linear light source

7. **Why linear light?**
   Linear light is preferable since it allows the patient to see a tilted image in the presence of cyclotropia.

8. **Explain the procedure.**
   i. The patient is seated comfortably
   ii. The procedure is explained to the patient in detail
   iii. It is made sure that the head is held straight for the whole procedure
   iv. Goggles are fitted such that the red glass is in front of the right eye
   v. The linear light is held vertically in the primary position at a distance of about 50 cm, and the patient is asked about the diplopia
   vi. Patient is asked which colored image appears straight in front of him and on which side does he see the second image
   vii. Ask if the image is higher/lower and if it is straight/tilted
   viii. If the patient is cooperative, he can be given two pencils and asked to hold them apart exactly as he sees the two lights in different gazes

9. **What are the precautions to be followed during the procedure?**
   i. Patient must not be allowed to turn his head to look in any position of gaze
   ii. The light source must be moved as far as possible in each direction of gaze, checking that it is visible to both the eyes
   iii. If the patient says that he sees only one light indicating possible binocular single vision, the examiner must make sure that the line image has not moved out of the visual field
10. **How do we record the results?**
    i. Patient's right and left sides are to be clearly labeled
    ii. Which eye projects the red image and green image is to be noted
    iii. Record the separation of images and tilted images as described by the patient using red and green colors
11. **How do we interpret the charting?**
    i. If two images are joined together—no diplopia
    ii. If images are separated—confirms diplopia
    iii. Maximum separation is in the quadrant in which the muscle is restricted/paralyzed
    iv. If horizontal separation with uncrossed images—esodeviation
    v. If horizontal separation with crossed images—exodeviation
    vi. If vertical separation with uncrossed images—oblique muscles involved
    vii. If vertical separation with crossed image—vertical recti muscle involved
12. **What are the disadvantages of diplopia charting?**
    i. It is mainly a subjective test
    ii. It needs a cooperative patient
    iii. Test is not reproducible
    iv. In many cases, the patients are uncooperative, or their intelligence is obscured by intracranial disease or contracture of the antagonistic muscles may have set in
    v. The test may give false interpretations if the paresis unmasks a latent squint or the patient starts fixing with the paralyzed eye, especially if this eye has greater visual acuity
13. **What are the causes of uniocular diplopia?**
    i. Light refraction—decentered intraocular lens (IOL), ectopia lentis, polycoria
    ii. Metamorphopsia—due to macular lesion
    iii. Cerebral polyopic—due to occipital lobe lesions.

9.3 HESS CHARTING

1. **What is the clinical significance of Hess charting?**
    i. The Hess screen test is an important diagnostic modality that helps in the diagnosis and prognostication of incomitant strabismus
    ii. It provides an accurate clinical method of determining the position of each visual axis in different directions of gaze
    iii. It provides a permanent and accurate record which may be compared with the results of subsequent examinations
    iv. It may help to differentiate recent-onset paralysis from long-standing one
    v. It may enable to differentiate paretic squint caused by neurological pathology from restrictive myopathy like thyroid eye disease or blowout fracture of the orbit

2. **Describe in detail about Hess chart.**
   The electrically operated Hess screen has largely replaced the original Hess screen.
   The Hess screen consists of a grayscale with a grid of intersecting lines at 15° and 30° with a controlled switch panel for illumination of red dots. The red dots form fixation points, and plotting is aided by a movable illuminated green indicator.
    i. A light source is present behind each red light aperture, the illumination of which is controlled from a control unit
    ii. Each of the red fixation spotlights can be switched on, in turn, by the insertion of a plug into the switchboard, the apertures of which correspond to the circular apertures of the Hess screen
    iii. The patient holds a green spotlight, the color of which is identical to that of the green eyepiece of red-green glasses
    iv. Each eye has to be tested separately. This can be done by changing the side of red and green glasses
    v. The eye behind the green glass is the testing eye. The patient tries to place a green light tip pointer on each of the red points in turns. The place indicated by the patient is recorded on a chart printed with similar markings. The recorded points are joined to form an inner and outer square
    vi. For interpreting the results of the Hess test, it is important to be aware of the muscle sequelae that follow paralytic strabismus and the laws that govern them

3. **What are the principles of Hess chart?**
    i. Foveal projection
    ii. Hering's law
    iii. Dissociation of eyes
    iv. Haploscopic principle

4. **What are the indications of Hess chart?**
    i. Patient with incomitant squint
    ii. Patients with divergence weakness type of esotropia to exclude mild sixth nerve palsy
    iii. To differentiate divergence palsy from sixth nerve palsy

5. **What are the stages in the development of muscle sequelae?**
    i. Overaction of contralateral synergist according to Hering's law
    ii. Overaction of ipsilateral antagonist as its action is unopposed by the parallel muscle
    iii. Secondary underaction of the contralateral antagonist. However, in long-standing palsies, there is the spread of comitance, and these stages cannot be easily discerned

6. **What are the prerequisites for Hess charting?**
    There are certain prerequisites required before conducting Hess charting:
    i. Full understanding of the procedure
    ii. Good vision in both eyes
    iii. Central fixation

7. **Describe the procedure.**
    i. The patient is seated at 50 cm facing the screen being plotted
    ii. Head erect and eyes in primary position with the head centered on the fixation spot
    iii. The patient wears red and green glasses
    iv. Patient is instructed to shine the green spotlight upon each red fixation light as it is illuminated
    v. With green glasses in front of left eye, he fixes red dots with his right eye; the indicator shows deviation of left eye and then glasses are reversed

8. **What are the features of the Hess chart used for interpretation?**
    A. *General guidelines*
        i. The central dot in each field indicates the deviation in the primary position
        ii. Smaller field belongs to the paretic eye
        iii. Inward displacement of the dots indicates underaction. The eye cannot move far enough to plot in normal position
        iv. Outward displacement of dot indicates overaction (or contracture). Excessive movement of eye causes dots to be plotted beyond the normal position
        v. Equal-sized fields indicate that muscle sequelae have developed. The features of muscle sequlae are the underaction of the affected muscle, overaction of the contralateral

synergist, contracture of ipsilateral antagonist of paretic muscle, secondary underaction of the contralateral synergist of contracted muscle. The paresis is therefore long-standing or congenital

vi. The outer fields should be examined for small under- and overactions, which may not be apparent on inner fields

vii. If the outer field is very close to the inner field, a mechanical cause for the limited movement is likely

viii. Each small square subtends 5°. The inner square, therefore, measures 15° movement from the primary position to each position of gaze. The outer square measures 30° of movement

ix. When the right eye fixes the red dots, the field of movement of the left eye is plotted and vice versa. The fixing eye determines the amount of innervation sent to nonfixing eye

x. The number of lights in the Hess chart is 24

B. *Interpretation of Hess chart*

i. Compare the size of the two fields

ii. Examine the smaller field (paretic eye) and note the position of maximum inward displacement, which will be in the direction of the main action of paretic muscle

iii. In the side with smaller field, note if there is outward displacement in the direction of action of the ipsilateral antagonist of the affected muscle. Outward displacement indicates contracture shown as overaction

iv. Examine the larger field and note the position of maximum outward displacement, indicating overaction of contralateral synergist of paretic muscle

v. In the side with larger field, note if there is inward displacement of the antagonist of the overacting muscle, indicating secondary underaction (this muscle is contralateral synergist of the contracted muscle)

vi. Look at the relationship between the inner and outer fields

vii. Look at the position of center dots (inward displacement indicates esotropia)

viii. Equal-sized fields indicate either symmetrical limitation of movement in both eyes or a concomitant strabismus

ix. Sloping fields denote A or V pattern

9. **What are the features of neurogenic defects?**

i. The smaller field has a proportional spacing between the outer and inner fields

    ii. Muscle sequelae are common
    iii. The Hess chart between the two eyes tends to become more similar in size with time
10. **What are the features of mechanical defects?**
    i. Compressed field either vertically or horizontally
    ii. The most obvious feature of a mechanical defect is normally the marked overaction of the contralateral synergist
    iii. Normally, there is no obvious overaction of the direct antagonist or underaction of the contralateral antagonist
11. **What are the uses of the Hess chart?**
    i. Diagnosis of a muscle palsy
    ii. Assessing progress
    iii. Planning muscle surgery
    iv. Evaluating results of incomitant strabismus
    v. Provides a permanent and accurate record which may be compared with the results of subsequent examinations

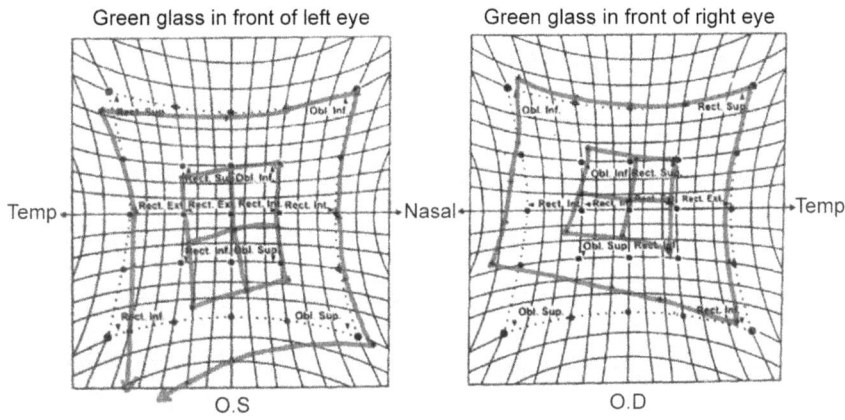

- Right eye has a smaller field—affected eye
- Right hypertropia of <5°
- Proportional spacing between inner and outer squares
- Limitation of right depression in adduction (right superior oblique underaction)
- Extorsion of field of the right eye
- Above point to right superior oblique palsy
- Overaction of right inferior oblique and left inferior rectus (muscle sequel)

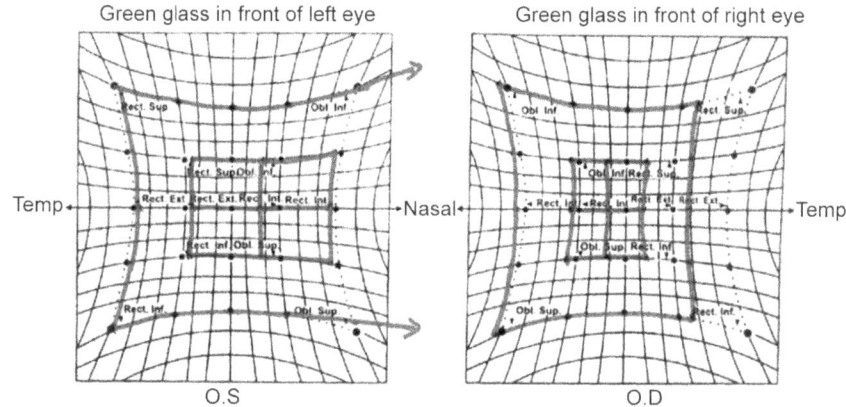

- Diagnosis–right lateral rectus palsy
- Right eye has a smaller field—affected eye
- Right esotropia of 5° in primary position (one small square)
- Right abduction restriction
- Proportional spacing between inner and outer squares
- Left medial rectus overaction (muscle sequalae).

CHAPTER 10

Optics and Refraction

1. **Classify the types of optical defects of the eye.**
   Optical defects can be classified as *physiological and pathological*.
   i. Physiological can be of the following types:
      - Diffraction of light
      - Chromatic aberration
      - Spherical aberration
      - Decentering
      - Peripheral aberrations
   ii. Pathological optical defects are of three main types. Subclassifications have been described later
      - Myopia
      - Hypermetropia
      - Astigmatism
         - *Diffraction of light:* The property of light waves is to deviate after passing through an aperture. The smaller the aperture (pupil), the more the diffraction
         - *Chromatic aberration:* Light of different wavelengths, i.e., different colors, get refracted differently. Shorter wavelengths (blue) are refracted more than longer wavelengths (red) light. More chromatic aberration takes place with a larger pupil size.

            Normally, the eye focuses light of the greatest intensity, yellow, which is in the middle of the spectrum. So, images formed by light of longer and shorter wavelengths are less intense and are neglected.

            The eye is hypermetropic for red and myopic for blue light.
         - *Spherical aberration:* The periphery of an optical lens has more refracting power than the center. So, the peripheral rays are brought to focus at a point earlier than the central rays. This is seen only when the pupil is widely dilated. A small pupil cuts off the peripheral rays
         - *Decentering:* The centering of the eye as an optical system is never exact. The various optical axes and center of lenses do not coincide with each other. But these variations are so small that they are functionally negligible

- *Peripheral aberrations:* There are several optical phenomena which combine to make the image formed at the peripheral retina less clear than the central image. The most important of these are oblique astigmatism and distortion of image. Most of these are neutralized by the peculiar shape of the eye

2. **What are the causes of pathological optical defects?**
    i. Positions of the elements of the system
        - Shorter anteroposterior (AP) diameter—axial hypermetropia
        - Longer AP diameter—axial myopia
        - Lenticular displacement—forward—myopia; backward—hypermetropia
    ii. Anomalies of the refractive surfaces
        - Decreased curvature of cornea—curvature hypermetropia
        - Increased curvature of cornea—curvature myopia
        - Irregular curvature—astigmatism
    iii. Obliquity of the elements of the system
        - Lenticular obliquity/subluxation—astigmatism
        - Retinal obliquity—irregular image formation (e.g., staphyloma)
    iv. Abnormalities of the refractive index (RI)
        - If RI of aqueous is too low or that of vitreous is too high—index hypermetropia
        - If RI of aqueous is too high or that of vitreous is too low—index myopia
        - RI of lens too low as a whole—index hypermetropia
        - RI of lens too high as a whole—index myopia
        - RI of cortex increases and equals the nucleus—index hypermetropia
        - RI of nucleus increases—index myopia
    v. Absence of lens—aphakia—extreme form of hypermetropia

3. **What are the important axes related to refraction?**
    i. *Optical axis:* The line passing through the center of curvature of the cornea and lens
    ii. *Visual axis:* The line joining the object or fixation point with the fovea and passing through the nodal point is called the visual axis
    iii. *Fixation axis:* The line joining the object and the center of rotation (which lies on the optical axis)
    iv. *Pupillary line:* Used as a substitute for the optical axis because, clinically, it is easier to determine the center of the pupil than the

center of the cornea. Pupillary center is determined by a light reflex and the line drawn perpendicular to it is the pupillary line

4. **What are the important angles in relation to refraction?**
    i. *Angle alpha:* This is the angle formed between the visual axis and the optical axis at the nodal point
        Normally, the visual axis cuts the cornea nasally; this is denoted as positive angle alpha. If it cuts temporally, it is negative alpha and if optical and visual axes coincide, the angle alpha is nil
    ii. *Angle gamma:* Angle formed between optical axis and fixation axis at the center of rotation
    iii. *Angle kappa:* Angle formed between the pupillary line and visual axis. Substituted for angle alpha as it can be measured clinically

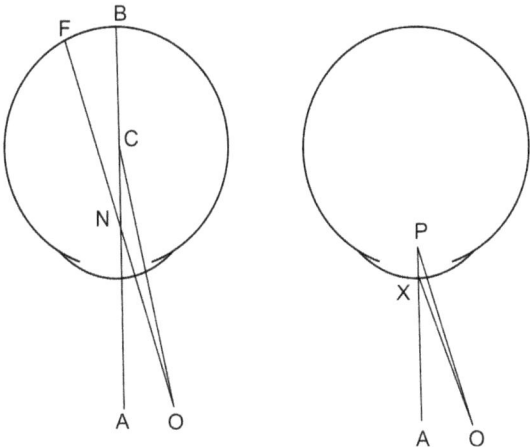

Definition of angles:
C—center of rotation; F—fovea; N—nodal point; O—point of fixation; P—center of pupil; X—point of the cornea that lies in the central pupillary line; AB—optical axis; AP—central pupillary line; OC—fixation axis; OF—visual axis; angle ONA—angle alpha;
angle OCA—angle gamma; angle OPA—angle kappa;
angle OPA—angle kappa, as measured clinically.

5. **Define nodal point and its importance.**
    i. *For thin lens:* The point at which the principal plane and principal axis intersect is called the principal point or nodal point
        Importance: Rays of light passing through the nodal point are undeviated
    ii. *For thick lens:* Nodal points correspond to the center of thin lens, rays directed toward the first nodal point leave as if from the second nodal point and parallel from with its original direction, i.e., undeviated

When the medium on both sides of a thick lens is same, the nodal points coincide with the principal points.

In the eye, since the refracting medium on two sides is different (air and vitreous), the nodal point and principal point do not coincide.

Importance: The nodal point straddles the posterior pole of the crystalline lens. Rays of light are refracted through the nodal point; thus, even a small posterior polar cataract can cause gross impairment in the vision.

In reduced eye: A single nodal point is postulated midway between the two nodal points and is located in the posterior part of the lens 7.08 mm behind the anterior corneal surface.

6. **Define hypermetropia.**

Hypermetropia is a form of refractive error in which parallel rays of light coming from infinity are brought to focus some distance behind the sentient layer of the retina when the accommodation is at rest.

The image formed is made up of circles of diffusion of considerable sizes and is blurred.

7. **What are the causes of hypermetropia?**
    i. *Axial hypermetropia*—1 mm shortening of AP diameter = 3 D of hypermetropia
        - As a part of growth and development of the eye, hypermetropia is the most common of all refractive anomalies
        - It is pathologically due to orbital tumor or inflammatory mass indenting the posterior pole
        - Intraocular neoplasm or edema may displace the retina forward
    ii. *Curvature hypermetropia*—1 mm increase in radius of curvature = 6 D of hypermetropia
        Cornea plana, flattening due to trauma or disease
    iii. *Index hypermetropia*—due to decrease in the effective refractivity of the lens. It is seen in old age and pathologically in diabetics under treatment
    iv. Backward displacement of lens, congenital or traumatic, leads to positional hypermetropia
    v. *Aphakia*—extreme form of hypermetropia in the absence of crystalline lens

8. **What are the optical changes of hypermetropia?**
    i. Image formed behind the retina
    ii. Image size smaller than in emmetropia
    iii. Rays emerging from the eye are divergent and tend to meet at a virtual point behind the eye

9. **What are the clinical features of hypermetropia?**
    i. Eyes are typically small—AP diameter, small cornea, shallow anterior chamber (AC)
    ii. At risk for angle closure glaucoma
    iii. Fundus shows a peculiar sheen or reflex effect called silk-shot retina
    iv. Pseudopapillitis of the optic disk—resembles optic neuritis. Hyperemic with irregular borders
    v. This leads to large positive angle kappa—apparent divergent squint
    vi. Accommodative convergent squint
    vii. Accommodative asthenopia and ciliary muscle spasm

10. **What are the components of hypermetropia?**
    i. Latent hypermetropia—is overcome physiologically by the tone of the ciliary muscles
    ii. Manifest hypermetropia—uncorrected at resting state of the eye
        - Facultative hypermetropia—can be overcome by increasing accommodation
        - Absolute hypermetropia—cannot be overcome by accommodation. Thus, total hypermetropia = Latent + Manifest = Latent + Facultative + Absolute

11. **Define myopia.**
    Myopia is that form of refractive error where parallel rays of light come to a focus in front of the sentient layer of the retina when accommodation is at rest.

12. **What are the types and causes of myopia?**
    i. Axial myopia occurs when the AP diameter is long. 1 mm lengthening corresponds to 3 D of myopia
    ii. Curvature myopia—associated with increased curvature of the cornea or both surfaces of the lens. 1 mm increased curvature induces 6 D of myopia. This is accompanied by astigmatism. For example, keratoconus, keratoglobus, lenticonus, and spasm of accommodation
    iii. Index myopia—seen in incipient cataract where the RI of the lens nucleus increases. Decreased RI of lens cortex may play a role in diabetic myopia
    Axial myopia may be divided as simple and pathological. Simple is further classified as physiological and intermediate.

13. **Describe the optical changes of myopia.**
    i. Parallel rays come to focus at a point in front of the retina
    ii. The farthest at which objects can be seen distinctly is called the far point or punctum remotum. The more the myopia, the closer the far point

iii. As the nodal point is further away from the retina, the image formed is larger than that of an emmetropic eye
iv. The negative angle kappa leads to an apparent convergent squint

14. **What are the clinical features of myopia?**
    i. AP elongation of the eye, limited to the posterior pole. The anterior part is relatively normal
    ii. Deep AC, sluggish pupil, atrophy of the circular ciliary muscles due to absence of any stimulus for accommodation
    iii. Fundus—generalized atrophy of the retina and choroid. Tessellated or tigroid retina with visible choroidal vessels
    iv. Temporal crescent and supertraction crescent nasally
    v. Posterior staphyloma
    vi. Cystoid degeneration at the ora serrata
    vii. Weiss reflex streak
    viii. Förster-Fuchs fleck—caused by proliferation of the pigmentary epithelium associated with an intrachoroidal hemorrhage or thrombosis. It is thought to be a precursor of choroidal neovascular membrane (CNVM)
    ix. Posterior vitreous detachment (PVD) and liquefaction of vitreous leading to muscae volitantes

15. **Why does the disk appear tilted in myopia?**
    The optic nerve appears to insert into the elongated globe at an angle. The tilted appearance is characterized by temporal flattening of the disk due in part to peripapillary scleral expansion. As a result, a hypopigmented myopic crescent or a myopic cone is seen where sclera is directly visible.

16. **What are the complications of high myopia?**
    i. Anisometropic amblyopia: If only one eye has high myopia
    ii. Retinal tears and retinal detachment
    iii. Complicated cataracts—probably due to aberrations of lenticular metabolism
    iv. Vitreous hemorrhage—accompanies a retinal tear. Choroidal hemorrhage may also leak into the vitreous
    v. Choroidal hemorrhage and thrombosis—quite common and may lead to severe visual loss involving foveal region
    vi. Choroidal neovascular membrane
    vii. Pigment epithelial detachments and macular or foveal detachments
    viii. Primary open-angle glaucoma—not a complication but common association with myopia

17. **What is astigmatism?**
    Astigmatism is the refractive error in which the refraction varies in different meridians of the eye.

18. Classify astigmatism.

Astigmatism can be classified based on:
i. Position and steepness of the principal meridians
ii. Position of the image formed on the retina/position of the principal foci
   - Based on the principal meridians, it is of the following types:
     - *Regular astigmatism:* Where the principal meridians (steepest and flattest axes) are perpendicular to each other
       * *With-the-rule astigmatism:* The vertical meridian is steepest (a rugby ball or American football lying on its side)
       * *Against-the-rule astigmatism:* The horizontal meridian is steepest. (A rugby ball or American football standing on its end.)
       * *Oblique astigmatism:* The steepest curve lies in between 120 and 150° and 30 and 60°
     - *Bioblique astigmatism:* Principal meridians are not at 90° to each other
     - *Irregular astigmatism:* No principal meridians can be determined
   - Based on principal focus, it is of the following types:
     - *Simple myopic:* One focus is in front and the other is on the retina
     - *Simple hypermetropic:* One focus is behind and the other is on the retina
     - *Compound myopic:* Both the foci are in front of the retina
     - *Compound hypermetropic:* Both the foci are behind the retina
     - *Mixed:* The foci are on either side of the retina

19. Define Sturm's conoid.

The configuration of the rays refracted through the toric surface is called Sturm's conoid. In this, one principal meridian is more curved than the other.

Unlike a point focus of spherical lens, it consists of two line foci which are at right angles to each other. The distance between them is known as the interval of Sturm.

20. What is circle of least diffusion?

The circle of least diffusion or the circle of least confusion is where the section between the two principal media is circular. In this, the divergence of vertical rays is exactly equal to the convergence of horizontal rays. It lies dioptrically midway between the two foci. For example, if the foci are D1 and D2, the circle of least confusion will be at $(D1 + D2)/2$ diopters or $2/(D1 + D2)$ meter away from the lens. The diameter of the circle of least confusion decreases as the two line foci come closer. The spherical equivalent (SE) represents the dioptrical midpoint and corresponds to the circle of least diffusion.

21. **What are the effects of lenses on the conoid of Sturm?**

    A plus or convex lens brings the line foci closer to the lens, decreasing the interval of Sturm. A minus or concave lens pushes the line foci away from the lens, increasing the interval of Sturm. In both cases, the distal focus moves more than the proximal focus. The cylindrical power, however, remains unchanged.

    A cross cylinder has the effect of contracting or expanding the interval of Sturm about the fixed circle of diffusion depending on the axis.

22. **What is presbyopia?**

    The amplitude of accommodation declines steadily with age. This is mainly due to sclerosis of the fibers of the crystalline lens and changes in its capsule. This inadequacy of accommodation is called presbyopia.

23. **How do you calculate for presbyopic correction?**

    The amount of presbyopic correction necessary for a given patient can be calculated if the remaining amplitude of accommodation is determined (from his near point) and the desired working distance is specified.

    In order to achieve comfortable near-vision, he must keep one-third to half of this in reserve. [Elkington says one-third in reserve and American Academy of Ophthalmology (AAO) Basic and Clinical Science Course (BCSC) advises half in reserve.]

    For example:
    i. Assume an emmetrope with near point = 50 cm. Therefore, amplitude of accommodation = 2 D
    ii. Target near distance = 33 cm. This needs 3 D of accommodation
    iii. If we give him +1 D of near correction, he will be able to read at 33 cm, but he will be using full accommodation to do so and this will lead to symptoms of eye strain
    iv. For comfortable near vision, he should have one-third (Elkington) or half (AAO BCSC) of accommodation in reserve
    v. So we should keep 0.67 D (one-third of 2 D) or 1.0 D (half of 2 D) in reserve and give correction accordingly
    vi. So an ideal correction would be +1 D + 0.67 D or +1 D + 1 D, i.e., +1.75 D (rounded to nearest practical value) or +2 D

24. **What are the prerequisites for prescribing presbyopic glasses?**
    i. Existing amplitude of accommodation
    ii. Reading distance or near work distance. Might be <33 cm, for example, with goldsmiths or watchmakers

iii. Purpose of near glasses. An executive bifocal or near vision alone is better suited for occupational work. People with desk jobs do better with progressive addition lenses (PALs)
iv. Age of patient
v. Preexisting refractive error
vi. Lens status—pseudophakic or phakic

25. **What are the various treatment options for myopia, hypermetropia, and presbyopia?**

Method	Myopia	Hyperopia	Presbyopia	Astigmatism
A: Noninvasive				
Spectacles	+	+	+	+
Contact lens	+	+	+	+
B: Invasive				
IA: Corneal—incisional				
a. Radial keratotomy	+	–	–	–
b. Astigmatic keratotomy	–	–	–	+
c. Hexagonal keratotomy	–	+	–	–
IB: Excimer laser				
a. PRK	+	+	+	+
b. LASEK	+	+	+	+
c. LASIK (includes femto)	+	+	+	+
d. Epi-LASIK	+	+	+	+
IC: Intrastromal corneal ring segments	+	–	–	–
ID: Conductive keratoplasty	–	+	–	+
IIA: Intraocular—phakic				
a. Phakic ACIOL	+	–	–	–
b. Phakic iris fixated IOL	+	–	–	–
c. Phakic PCIOL	+	–	–	–
IIB: Intraocular—pseudophakic				
Refractive lens exchange—multifocal/accommodating	+	+	+	–
Refractive lens exchange—toric	+	+	–	+

26. **Define keratomileusis and keratophakia.**
Keratomileusis—originally developed for myopia by Barraquer as "carving" of the anterior surface of cornea. Defined as a method to modify the spherical or meridional surface of a healthy cornea by tissue

subtraction. Microkeratome is used to remove lamella of anterior corneal stroma which is then shaped on a cryolathe before being replaced.

Keratophakia—developed as modification of keratomileusis in order to correct aphakia. Keratome is used to lift a lamella of anterior stroma and replaced over a shaped lenticule of donor corneal stroma to produce a new corneal surface contour.

27. Define accommodation.

The ability of the eye to focus the diverging rays from the near object on the retina is called accommodation.

28. What is far point?

The *far point* of distinct vision is the position of an object such that its image falls on the retina in the relaxed eye, i.e., in the absence of accommodation. The far point of the emmetropic eye is at infinity.

29. What is near point?

The *near point* of distinct vision is the nearest point at which an object can be clearly seen when maximum accommodation is used.

30. What is range of accommodation?

The *range of accommodation* is the distance between the far point and the near point.

31. What is amplitude of accommodation?

The *amplitude of accommodation* is the difference in dioptric power between the eye at rest and the fully accommodated eye.

32. What is schematic eye and its dimensions?

Schematic eye is a way to represent the complex refracting system of the human eye. It was given by Gullstrand. In the schematic eye, the refracting system is expressed in terms of its cardinal points in millimeter from the anterior corneal surface.

First principal point	P1	1.35
Second principal point	P2	1.60
First nodal point	N1	7.08
Second nodal point	N2	7.33
First focal point		−15.7
Second focal point		24.4
Refractive power		+58.64 D

33. What is reduced eye and its dimensions?

It is a simplified version of the schematic eye and was given by Listing. It assumes a single principal point and a single nodal point. The values are measured from the anterior corneal surface.

Principal point	P	1.35
Nodal point	N	7.08
First focal point		−15.7
Second focal point		24.13
Refractive power		+58.6 D

34. What is anisometropia?
Inequality of refractive status of both eyes.

35. What are the types of anisometropia?
  i. Simple
   - Myopic
   - Hypermetropic
  ii. Compound
   - Myopic
   - Hypermetropic
  iii. Mixed—antimetropia
  iv. Simple astigmatic
  v. Compound astigmatic

36. What is aniseikonia?
Inequality in the image sizes perceived in two eyes in presence of binocularity.

37. What is the etiology of aniseikonia?
  i. Optical aniseikonia
  ii. Retinal aniseikonia
  iii. Cortical aniseikonia

38. What are the clinical types?
  i. Symmetrical
   - Overall
   - Meridional
  ii. Asymmetrical
   - Regular
   - Irregular
   - Pin cushion

39. What are the symptoms of aniseikonia?
  i. Asthenopia
  ii. Depth perception difficulty
  iii. Obliquity
  iv. Watering
  v. Pain
  vi. Focusing difficulty

40. What is micropsia?
Micropsia is a condition affecting human visual perception in which objects appear smaller than they actually are.
Causes:
  i. Optical factors—wearing glass
  ii. Distortion of image in eyes—retinal edema, macular degeneration, central serous retinopathy
  iii. Brain lesion—traumatic brain injury, epilepsy, migraine

41. What is macropsia?
Macropsia is a condition affecting human visual perception in which the object within the affected section appears larger than normal.
Causes:
  i. Structural defects—epiretinal membrane, vitreomacular traction, retinoschisis
  ii. Drugs—zolpidem, citalopram, cocaine
  iii. Migraine
  iv. Epilepsy
  v. Hypoglycemia
  vi. Virus—Epstein-Barr virus, infectious mononucleosis

42. What is an eikonometer?
Instrument for measuring aniseikonia

43. What are the types of an eikonometer?
  i. Standard eikonometer
  ii. Space eikonometer

44. What are the treatment options for aniseikonia?
  i. Optical type:
    - Aniseikonic glasses
    - Contact lens
    - Lenticular surgeries
    - Corneal procedures
  ii. Retinal and cortical types
    - Treat cause

45. Which refractive error is more likely to cause amblyopia and why?
A disparity of >1 D in hypermetropic patients is enough to cause amblyopia of the more hypermetropic eye. This is because accommodation is a binocular function, i.e., individual eyes cannot accommodate by different amounts.

In myopic patients with anisometropia, amblyopia is less likely to develop as both eyes still have clear near vision. Although if one eye is highly myopic (a disparity of >4 D and not adequately corrected), it usually becomes amblyopic.

46. What are Purkinje-Sanson images?

Purkinje-Sanson images or catoptric images are formed by the partial reflection of light from the refracting interfaces of the eye.

The interfaces forming these images are anterior and posterior corneal surfaces and anterior and posterior lens surfaces.

47. What is the nature of these images?

Images 1, 2, and 3 are formed by a convex surface and are erect and virtual.

Image 4 is formed by a concave surface and is inverted and real.

48. What is a prism?

A prism is a transparent triangular piece of glass or plastic. It has two plane (flat) refracting sides, one apex (top) and a base (bottom). A ray of light incident to a prism always bends toward the base of the prism. The image formed appears displaced toward its apex.

49. What is the image formed in a prism?

The image formed by a prism is erect, virtual, and *displaced toward the apex of the prism.* In contrast, the rays are always displaced toward the base of the prism.

50. What are the positions for keeping a prism?

i. *Position of minimum deviation*—deviation is reduced to a minimum when light passes through the prism symmetrically
ii. *Prentice position*—in the Prentice position, one surface of the prism is normal to the ray of light so that all the deviation takes place at the other surface of the prism. The deviation of light in the Prentice position is greater than that in the position of minimum deviation because in the Prentice position, the angle of incidence does not equal the angle of emergence

51. Classify prisms based on the deviation they produce.

i. Right-angled prism—deviates by 90°
ii. Porro prism—deviates by 180°, image gets inverted but there is no right-left transposition
iii. Dove prism—no deviation, image is inverted but not transposed left to right

52. What are the ways of prism notation?

i. *The prism diopter:* A prism of one prism diopter power produces a linear apparent displacement of 1 cm, of an object situated at 1 m
ii. *Angle of apparent deviation:* The apparent displacement of the object O can also be measured in terms of the angle Q, the angle of apparent deviation. Under conditions of ophthalmic usage, a prism of 1 prism diopter power produces an angle of apparent deviation of 1/2°. Thus, 1 prism diopter = 1/2°

iii. *The centrad:* This unit differs from the prism diopter only in that the image displacement is measured along an arc 1 m from the prism
iv. *Refracting angle:* A prism may also be described by its refracting angle. However, unless the RI of the prism material is also known, the prism power cannot be deduced

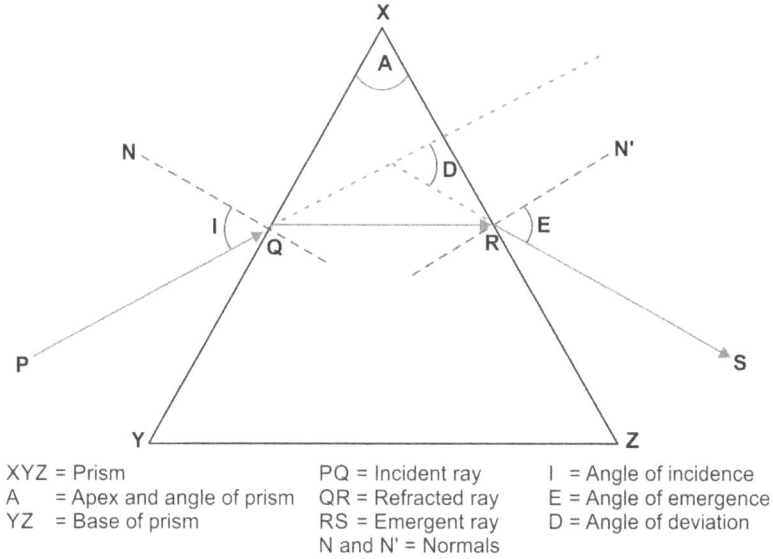

XYZ = Prism
A = Apex and angle of prism
YZ = Base of prism
PQ = Incident ray
QR = Refracted ray
RS = Emergent ray
N and N' = Normals
I = Angle of incidence
E = Angle of emergence
D = Angle of deviation

53. What are the uses of prism?

There are three main uses of prism in ophthalmology:
i. *Diagnostic prisms*
   - Assessment of squint and heterophoria
     - Measurement of angle objectively by prism cover test
     - Measurement of angle subjectively by Maddox rod and Risley prism
     - To assess likelihood of diplopia after proposed squint surgery in adults
     - Measurement of fusional reserve
     - The four-diopter prism test. This is a delicate test for small degrees of esotropia (microtropia)
   - Assessment of simulated blindness
   Forms of prism used in assessment include single prisms, the prisms from the trial lens set, and prism bars
ii. *Therapeutic prisms*
   - Convergence insufficiency. The most common therapeutic use of prisms in the orthoptic department is in building up the fusional reserve of patients with convergence insufficiency. The prisms are used base-out

- To relieve diplopia in certain cases of squint. These include decompensated heterophorias, small vertical squints, and some paralytic squints with diplopia in the primary position
- To reduce nystagmus and to improve near vision in a case of nystagmus with dampening on convergence
- Can also be used in small paretic deviations to improve the binocularity, thereby improving the head posture, e.g., superior oblique (SO) palsy, Brown's syndrome

Forms of therapeutic prism
- Temporary wear—used as clip-on spectacle prisms for trial wear. An improvement on these is Fresnel prisms which consist of a plastic sheet of parallel tiny prisms of identical refracting angle
- Permanent wear—permanent incorporation of a prism into a patient's spectacles

iii. *Prisms in optical instruments*

Instruments in which prisms are used include the slit-lamp microscope, operating microscope, applanation tonometer keratometer, ophthalmoscope, Gonio, synoptophore, etc.

54. What are the uses of curved mirror?

The theory of curved mirrors has a major clinical application. The anterior surface of the cornea acts as a convex mirror and is used as such by the standard instruments employed to measure corneal curvature, e.g., keratometer.

55. What is Prentice rule?

Prentice rule or formula is used to calculate the prismatic power induced by decentering a spherical lens.

It is given as $P = F \times D$

where P = prismatic power in prism diopters, F = lens power in diopters, and D = decentration in centimeters.

56. How do you do simple transposition of cylindrical lenses?

This is a change in the description of a toric astigmatic lens so that the cylinder is expressed in the opposite power.

Steps are:
i. *Sum:* Algebraic addition of sphere and cylinder gives new power of sphere
ii. *Sign:* Change sign of cylinder, retaining numerical power
iii. *Axis:* Rotate axis of cylinder through 90°. (Add 90° if the original axis is at or <90°. Subtract 90° from any axis value >90°.)

Examples of transposition:
i. +1.0 DS/+2.0 Dcyl × 75°
   New sphere = Sum = +1.0 + (+2.0) = +3.0 DS
   New cylinder = Reverse sign = −2.0 Dcyl

Axis = Rotate by 90° = 75 + 90 = 165°
Answer = +3.0 DS/–2.0 Dcyl × 165°
ii. –2.5 DS/–1.5 Dcyl × 90°
New sphere = Sum = –2.5 + (–1.5) = –4.0 DS
New cylinder = Reverse sign = +1.5 Dcyl
Axis = Rotate by 90° = 90 + 90 = 180°
Answer = –4.0 DS/+1.5 Dcyl × 180°
iii. +1.0 DS/–2.0 Dcyl × 150o
New sphere = Sum = +1.0 + (–2.0) = –1.0 DS
New cylinder = Reverse sign = +2.0 Dcyl
Axis = Rotate by 90° = 150 – 90 = 60°
Answer = –1.0 DS/+2.0 Dcyl × 60°
iv. +3.0 DS/–0.5 Dcyl × 60°
New sphere = Sum = +3.0 + (–0.5) = +2.5 DS
New cylinder = Reverse sign = +0.5 Dcyl
Axis = Rotate by 90° = 60 + 90 = 150°
Answer = +2.5 DS/+0.5 Dcyl × 150°
v. –2.5 DS/+1.0 Dcyl × 180°
New sphere = Sum = –2.5 + (+1.0) = –1.5 DS
New cylinder = Reverse sign = –1.0 Dcyl
Axis = Rotate by 90° = 180–90 = 90°
Answer = –1.5 DS/–1.0 Dcyl × 90°
vi. –1.0 DS/+3.0 Dcyl × 135°
New sphere = Sum = –1.0 + (+3.0) = +2.0 DS
New cylinder = Reverse sign = –3.0 Dcyl
Axis = Rotate by 90° = 135–90 = 45°
Answer = +2.0 DS/–3.0 Dcyl × 45°
vii. +2.5 Dcyl × 50°
New sphere = Sum = 0 + 2.5 = 2.5 DS
New cylinder = Reverse sign = –2.5 Dcyl
Axis = Rotate by 90° = 50 + 90 = 140°
Answer = +2.5 DS/–2.5 Dcyl × 140°
viii. –3.75 Dcyl × 160°
New sphere = Sum = 0 + (–3.75) = –3.75 DS
New cylinder = Reverse sign = +3.75 Dcyl
Axis = Rotate by 90° = 160–90 = 70°
Answer = –3.75 DS/+ 3.75 Dcyl × 70°

57. Why is cylinder power transposed?
  i. A minus cylinder (concave) makes the lens thinner, thereby making it lighter and more cosmetic
  ii. Also, it reduces some amount of aberrations

iii. It is difficult to manufacture a plus cylinder than a minus cylinder. Though now with the advent of machines, it is a lesser concern
iv. A plus cylinder is often difficult to adjust to for the wearer

58. **How do you calculate the spherical equivalent of a toric lens?**
Spherical equivalent (SE) gives the closest spherical power of a spherocylindrical lens. The *spherical equivalent* power is calculated from the toric lens prescription by algebraic addition of the spherical power and half the cylindrical power. The signs are left unchanged
SE = DS + (Dcyl/2)
For example, SE of +2.0 DS/–1.50 Dcyl × 90° = 2 + (–1.5/2) = 1.25 DS

59. **What is an achromatic lens?**
Lenses made with glasses of different refractive indices and different dispersions to form a compound lens to cancel out the effects are achromatic lenses. Flint ($u = 1.7$) has double the dispersion of crown glass ($u = 1.5$). Thus, an achromatic lens can be made by combining a convex crown lens with a concave flint lens of half power.

60. **What is an aplanatic or aspheric lens?**
If the lens is grinded in such a way that the curvature gradually decreases from the center to the periphery, the spherical aberration can be eliminated. These are aplanatic lenses. Another way of diminishing spherical aberration is by using meniscus or periscopic lenses where the anterior curvature is more than the posterior.

61. **What are the steps in refraction? (*marked ones are essential)**
    i. External examination in diffuse light*
    ii. Examination of motility of light
    iii. Cover test to detect squint and heterophoria
    iv. Uncorrected visual acuity—uniocularly and binocularly for near and distance*
    v. Vision with pinhole*
    vi. Visual acuity for near and distance with existing glasses*
    vii. Objective refraction: Autorefraction and retinoscopy*
    viii. Subjective refraction: Trial frame and lenses*
    ix. Refining of spheres with duochrome test and fogging*
    x. Refining of cylinder with Jackson's cross cylinder (JCC), astigmatic fan, or dial*
    xi. Testing of muscle balance for distance with full correction
    xii. Determination of near point of accommodation and convergence with full correction
    xiii. Addition for near work based on age and reading distance*
    xiv. Testing of muscle balance for near with full correction
    xv. Final glasses prescription*
    xvi. Cycloplegic refraction when indicated

62. Define retinoscopy.
Retinoscopy or skiascopy is an objective method of determining the refractive state of an eye based on the movement of shadow in the pupillary area.

63. What are the types of retinoscopes?
  i. Based on light source:
     - Reflecting retinoscope
     - Self-illuminating type
  ii. Based on type of beam:
     - Spot retinoscope
     - Streak retinoscope

64. What are the types of mirrors in a retinoscope?
A retinoscope uses a plane mirror and a concave mirror.

In newer retinoscopes, there is a plane mirror and a movable convex lens. The distance between them can be adjusted by pushing the handle up or down to convert it between a concave and a plane mirror.
  i. When the sleeve is moved to the lowest position, it acts as a plane mirror
  ii. At the highest position, it acts as a concave mirror

65. What are the stages of retinoscopy?
There are three stages of retinoscopy:
  i. *Illumination stage:* Patch of a subject's retina is illuminated
  ii. *Reflex stage:* The image of the retina is formed at the subject's far point
  iii. *Projection stage:* The observer locates this image by moving the illumination across the fundus and noting the behavior of the luminous reflex

66. What is the principal of retinoscopy?
The principal of retinoscopy is to convert the far point of the subject's eye to the nodal point of the observer's eye. At this point, the reflex is uniform and there is no change with movement of illumination. This is known as the point of neutrality or the point of reversal. Correcting lenses are placed in front of the subject till this point is reached.

67. What is the object in objective retinoscopy?
An area of fundus is illuminated by the light reflected into the patient's eye with the help of the retinoscope. This illuminated area is the object in retinoscopy.

68. What is working distance?
Working distance is the distance between the eyes of the subject and the observer. Theoretically, the further the distance, the more accurate the results are. But practically, it is difficult to see the reflex clearly on

Optics and Refraction

stretching one's arms. Usually, 2/3 m or 67 cm is taken as a comfortable working distance.

This corresponds to the far point of the subject's eye at neutrality. This induces a myopia of 3/2 = 1.5 D and that must be corrected from all the retinoscopic values obtained.

(All discussions here assume a working distance of 2/3 m.)

69. **What does direction of movement of reflex imply? (Working distance = 2/3 m)**
    i. With movement implies myopia of <1.5 D or emmetropia or hypermetropia
    ii. No movement of reflex means myopia of 1.5 D
    iii. Against movement of reflex means myopia of >1.5 D

70. **What are the characteristics of the retinoscopic reflex?**
    i. *Speed:* Large refractive errors have slow reflex whereas small refractive errors have faster reflex
    ii. *Brilliance:* Reflex is dull when far point is away from the observer and becomes clearer as it comes closer to neutrality. Against reflexes are usually dimmer than with reflexes
    iii. *Width:* Streak is narrow when the far point is away, becomes wider, and at neutrality, it fills the entire pupil. This holds true only for movement reflexes

71. **What are the characteristics of a cylindrical streak reflex?**
    i. Break—is seen when the streak is not oriented to the principal axes and disappears when it is rotated correctly
    ii. Width—varies with the angle of the streak. It is narrowest when the streak aligns with the axis
    iii. Intensity—brighter when oriented with the correct axis
    iv. Skew—is the oblique motion of the reflex. The intercept or streak moves slightly differently than the reflex when the axes are not aligned. It can be used to refine the axis in small cylinders

72. **What is the difference between static and dynamic refraction?**
    The dioptric power of the resting eye is called its *static* refraction. The dioptric power of the accommodated eye is called its *dynamic* refraction.

73. **What are the difficulties faced while performing retinoscopy?**
    i. Maintaining a steady working distance for all examinations
    ii. Subject accommodating during the examination. This can be addressed with fogging or by using cycloplegics
    iii. Bizarre reflex in dilated retinoscopy. Only the central reflex should be considered
    iv. Faint reflex due to hazy media or very high refractive errors
    v. Scissor reflex caused by aberrations or keratoconus

74. **What are the methods of refining the cylindrical refraction?**
    i. Astigmatic fan or dial
    ii. Jackson cross cylinder (JCC)
    iii. Stenopeic slit

75. **What is astigmatic dial?**
    Astigmatic dial is a test chart with radially arranged lines which is used to determine the axis of astigmatism. The spokes that are parallel to the principal meridian of the eye appear sharpest.

76. **What are the steps used in astigmatic dial refraction for refining cylinder?**
    i. Best visual acuity with spheres
    ii. Fog with plus sphere
    iii. Ask the patient to locate the sharpest line in the astigmatic dial
    iv. Add minus cylinder with axis parallel to this line until all lines appear equal
    v. Reduce the plus sphere till best visual acuity is obtained with Snellen chart

77. **What is Jackson's cross cylinder?**
    Jackson's cross cylinder is a type of toric lens used during refraction. It is a spherocylindrical lens in which the power of the cylinder is twice the power of the sphere and of the opposite sign. For example, +1 Dcyl combined with –0.50 Dsph.

    The net result is thus the same as superimposing two cylindrical lenses of equal power but opposite sign with their axes at right angles. The lens is mounted on a handle which is placed at 45° to the axes of the cylinders.

    Cross cylinders are named by the power of the cylinder, and this is marked on the handle.

78. **How is it used to check the correct axis?**
    To check the axis, the cross cylinder is held before the eye with its handle in line with the axis of the trial cylinder. The cross cylinder is turned over and the patient is asked which position gives a better visual result. The cross cylinder is held in the preferred position and the axis of the trial cylinder rotated slightly toward the axis of the same sign on the cross cylinder. This is repeated till there is no difference on flipping the JCC.

79. **How is it used to check correct power?**
    To check the power of the trial cylinder, the cross cylinder is held with first one axis and then the other overlying the trial cylinder. If the patient sees better at a certain orientation, cylinder power corresponding to the JCC axis is increased.

80. **What are the methods of refining spherical refraction?**
    i. Duochrome test
    ii. Fogging

81. **What is a duochrome test?**
    Duochrome or bichrome or red-green test is a subjective method of refining spherical power. A split red-green filter is used which makes the background appear as vertical red half and green half. Because of chromatic aberration, the shorter green wavelength is focused in front than the longer red wavelength. The eye normally focuses on yellow which is between red and green. Each eye is tested separately. As it is based on chromatic aberration, it can be used in color-blind individuals.
    i. If the power is accurate, the red and green halves should appear equally sharp
    ii. If the red side appears sharper, it implies that the eye is over-plused and minus power is added
    iii. If the green half appears sharper, the eye is over-minused and plus power is added
    (A useful mnemonic is RAM-GAP—red add minus, green add plus.)

82. **What are the uses for the different cells in a trial frame?**
    From behind to front, the four cells are used for:
    i. High power lenses
    ii. Spheres
    iii. Cylinders
    iv. Specials such as Maddox Rod, stenopic slit, prisms, and presbyopic adds

83. **What are the lenses in a trial set?**
    i. Spheres (both positive and negative)
       At 0.25 D, interval till 4 D
       At 0.50 D, interval till 6 D
       At 1.0 D, interval till 14 D
       At 2.0 D, interval till 20 D
    ii. Cylinders (both positive and negative)
        At 0.25, interval till 2 D
        At 0.50, interval till 6 D
    iii. Prisms ½, 1, 2, 3, 4, 5, 6, 8, 10, 12
    iv. Specials
        - Occluder
        - Pinhole
        - Stenopic slit
        - Maddox rod
        - Red-green lenses

84. **What is the principle of pinhole?**
    Theoretically, the pinhole allows only a single ray from each point of the object to pass through, and a clear image is formed irrespective of the

position of the screen. Similarly, when placed in front of an ametropic eye, a clear image is formed on the retina regardless of the refractive state.

85. What is the size of an ideal pinhole?
Clinically, the ideal pinhole is 1.2 mm in diameter (and is able to correct errors between +5.0 D and −5.0 D). If it is made any smaller, the blurring due to diffraction is more than the pinhole effect.

86. When do you use a multiple pinhole?
i. There are five pinhole sizes in the multipinhole from 0.8 to 1.5 mm
ii. The smaller pinholes provide routine acuity testing, while the larger pinholes provide testing for suspected reduced vision due to decreases in retinal illumination
iii. The multipinhole can also be used in visual acuity testing in mydriatic patients where the multipinhole compensates for the inability to contract the iris, thus assisting the eye in obtaining a retinal projection similar to that of a noncycloplegic eye
iv. Also, it can be used to see vision improvement in patients with central lens opacities or central retinal pathology

87. How do you measure interpupillary distance (IPD)?
Interpupillary distance can be measured in two ways:
i. A millimeter rule is rested across the bridge of the patient's nose and the patient is asked to look at the examiner's left eye. The zero of the rule is aligned with the nasal limbus of the patient's right eye. The patient is then instructed to look at the examiner's right eye and the position of the temporal limbus of the patient's left eye is noted, giving the anatomical interpupillary distance
(The limbus-to-limbus measurement excludes inaccuracy due to differences or changes in pupil size.)
ii. Alternatively, a fixation light may be held in front of each of the examiner's eyes in turn and a similar procedure followed, the distance between the corneal light reflexes on the patient's eyes being measured

88. Cycloplegics used in refraction along with some common properties.

Drug	Concentration	Onset of maximum cycloplegia	Duration of cycloplegia
Atropine sulfate	1.0	1–2 hours	7–14 days
Scopolamine HBr	0.25	30–60 minutes	3–4 days
Homatropine HBr	2.0; 5.0	30–60 minutes	1–2 days
Cyclopentolate HCl	0.5; 1.0; 2.0	20–60 minutes	1–2 days
Tropicamide	0.5; 1.0; 2.0	20–40 minutes	4–6 hours

89. **How much correction will you make for each?**
   1 D is deducted for atropine, 0.5 D for other cycloplegics.
   For phenylephrine and tropicamide, no correction is necessary.

90. **What are the indications for a cycloplegics refraction? (Duane's)**
   The indications for a cycloplegics refraction are:
   i. Accurate refraction in young children
   ii. Distinguish true myopia from pseudomyopia
   iii. Diagnose accommodative spasm
   iv. All forms of strabismus, particularly esotropia
   v. Pharmacologic occlusion therapy in amblyopia
   vi. Latent hyperopia
   vii. Mentally disabled or uncooperative patient
   viii. Visual acuity not consistent with manifest refraction
   ix. Suspected malingering or hysteria
   x. Opacities in the ocular media
   xi. Preoperative refractive laser patients

91. **What is postmydriatic test? When is it done?**
   Postmydriatic test refers to repeating the refraction after the effect of cycloplegia has worn off.
   Ideally, it should be done in all cases where a cycloplegics refraction was done.
   Practically, it is done when there is a difference in the correction in dry and cycloplegics refraction.
   The next visit depends on the cycloplegics agent used. For example, for atropine, it is done after 2 weeks, and for homatropine and cyclopentolate, it is done after 2-3 days.

92. **How will you reverse mydriasis?**
   Ideally, it should be allowed to reverse spontaneously depending on the action of the drug.
   Pharmacologically, it can be reversed by using:
   i. Pilocarpine—parasympathomimetic
   ii. Dapiprazole hydrochloride—alpha-adrenergic antagonist
   It is used to reverse mydriasis caused by an alpha agonist such as phenylephrine or by a sympatholytic such as tropicamide.

93. **What are some of the factors taken into account while prescribing glasses for children?**
   Prescribing spectacles for children has the following goals:
   i. Providing a focused retinal image
   ii. Achieving an optimal balance between accommodation and convergence
   iii. Allowing for normal growth and emmetropization of the eye

For myopia:
i. Cycloplegic refraction is mandatory
ii. Full refractive correction including cylinder should be given
iii. Intentional overcorrection may help with controlling intermittent exodeviations, but it leads to accommodative stress and asthenopic symptoms
iv. Contact lens may be tried in older children to avoid the problem of minification of images

For hypermetropia:
i. Minimal hyperopia may be left uncorrected if there is no esodeviation or complaints of reduced vision. This is physiological and usually corrects with growth of the eyeball
ii. In hyperopia with esotropia, give full cycloplegics correction

For anisometropia, give full cycloplegics correction for both eyes irrespective of age, presence of squint, and degree of anisometropia. This is to prevent the development of amblyopia.

94. **What are the properties commonly considered when choosing the lens material for spectacles?**
    i. RI—higher RI means thinner lenses
    ii. Specific gravity or density—lower specific gravity means lighter lenses
    iii. Abbe number—this value indicates the degree of chromatic aberration or distortion that occurs due to dispersion of light at the periphery. A higher Abbe number implies better-quality lenses
    iv. Impact resistance—indicates the durability/fragility of lenses

95. **What are the materials used commonly?**
    i. Standard glass—usually made of crown glass
        - Advantage—superior optics, scratch resistant
        - Disadvantage—low impact resistance, heavy, increased thickness
    ii. Standard plastic—made of hard resin or CR-39. Most common material
        - Advantage—light weight, ultraviolet (UV) absorption
        - Disadvantage—scratches easily, average thickness, average shatter resistance
    iii. Polycarbonate
        - Advantage—thinner, lighter lenses due to higher RI and lesser specific gravity, very high impact resistance
        - Disadvantage—high chromatic aberrations, scratches easily
    iv. Trivex
        - Advantage—high impact resistance, light weight, good optics, blocks UV
        - Disadvantage—not very thin lenses, scratches easily

v. High-index material—a lens with RI >1.60 is referred to as a high-index lens. Can be either glass or plastic. Plastics are made of thiourethanes
   - Advantage—thinner, more cosmetic lenses, good shatter resistance
   - Disadvantage—chromatic aberrations are more in high-index plastic

96. What is antireflection coating?
Antireflection coating is a thin layer added on the lenses to reduce glare and reflection of light from the surface. It uses the principle of destructive interference.

97. What are the materials used?
Commonly used materials are magnesium fluoride, silicon monoxide, and yttrium fluoride. Other metal oxides can also be used.

98. What are the materials used to make photochromatic lenses?
- Glass lenses—silver halides, usually silver chloride (A photochemical reaction changes silver halide salts to elemental silver.)
- Plastic lenses—organic photochromatic molecules such as oxazines and naphthopyrans (Photochemical reaction alters between cis- and trans-chemical structures.)

99. What are the types of bifocal glasses?
i. Split lens or Benjamin Franklin type
ii. Cemented bifocal
iii. Fused bifocals
   - Round top or kryptok
   - Flat top
   - Curved top
   - Ribbon segment
iv. Executive type
v. One piece type, e.g., Ultex-type

100. In bifocal spectacles, where is the center of near segment located?
The center of near segment is located 8–10 mm inferior and 1.5–3 mm nasal to the optical center of the distance lens. Commonly, 8 mm below and 2 mm nasal is used.

101. How do you apply Prentice rule in bifocal glasses?
The image displacement due to Prentice rule can be compensated by using certain types of bifocal designs:
i. With a plus lens, a round top bifocal segment is used
ii. With a minus lens, a flat top bifocal segment is used

102. What is PAL? What are its advantages and disadvantages?

PAL stands for progressive addition lenses. It is a type of multifocal lens where there is a gradual change of power from distance to near as one looks from top to bottom.

Advantages
  i. Gradual change of power
  ii. No abrupt image shifts
  iii. Clear vision at all focal distances
  iv. Cosmetically better—no visible demarcation line

Disadvantages
  i. Peripheral distortion. This aberration is caused by combined astigmatism resulting from the changing aspheric curves
  ii. Distortion is maximum in lower, inner, and outer quadrants
  iii. PAL spectacles take some time to get used to

103. What are the different parts of a PAL?

There are four parts of a PAL:
  i. Spherical distance zone
  ii. Reading zone
  iii. Transition zone or corridor
  iv. Zones of peripheral distortion

104. What are the types of PAL spectacles?

  i. Soft design—long progression and soft periphery
  ii. Hard design—short progression and hard periphery

105. What are the parts of a spectacles frame?

Rims, bridge, side-pieces, joints, nose-pads

106. What are the types of spectacle frames?

  i. Full-rim
  ii. Half-rim
  iii. Rimless
  iv. Nylon supra—half rim with a thin nylon thread supporting the lenses at the bottom

107. What materials are used?

  i. Metal—titanium, aluminum, nickel, stainless steel, gold
  ii. Plastic—perspex, cellulose nitrate, cellulose acetate, newer polymers
  iii. Tortoiseshell—made of hawkbill turtle shell

108. **What is the advantage of contact lens over spectacles in myopia?**
    i. Contact lens in high myopia avoids peripheral distortion and minification of images produced by strong concave spectacle lens
    ii. Aniseikonia is reduced with contact lens in cases of anisometropia
    iii. Cosmetically more acceptable

    (Note: Advantage of spectacles: Myopic spectacles have a base-in prismatic effect which reduces the amount of accommodation and convergence required for near work. Myopes using contact lens need greater convergence and accommodation for near and they tend to develop presbyopia relatively earlier.)

109. **What are the different types of refractive errors following various ocular surgery?**
    i. Post-LASIK—regression myopia, myopic astigmatism, hypermetropia
    ii. Corneal tear suturing—irregular astigmatism
    iii. Silicone oil
        - *Phakic eye:* Silicone oil forms a concave surface behind the lens which acts like minus lens inside the eye resulting in hyperopia
        - *Aphakic eye:* Silicone oil produces a convex surface which bulges through the pupillary aperture resulting in myopic shift. Myopic shift mainly depends on the pupillary diameter
    iv. *Buckle:* Indentation of scleral buckle causes axial elongation of eyeball resulting in myopic shift
    v. *Postpenetrating keratoplasty:* Inherent imprecision of penetrating keratoplasty (PKP) results in refractive unpredictability with mean postop astigmatism of 4–5 D

CASE SHEET WRITING
Optics and Refraction
Simple Myopia

i. Patient details—Mr ABC, 25 years, male
ii. Patient complaints—both eyes defective distance vision × 6 months
iii. Uncorrected visual acuity (UCVA)—right eye (RE) –6/60; left eye (LE) –6/36
iv. Vision with own spectacles—if present. Also, neutralize and determine spectacle power
v. Vision with pinhole RE –6/12; LE –6/9
vi. Check for phorias; mention if present

vii. Objective refraction with retinoscopy. Working distance = 2/3 m (66 cm) hence correction = –1.5 D

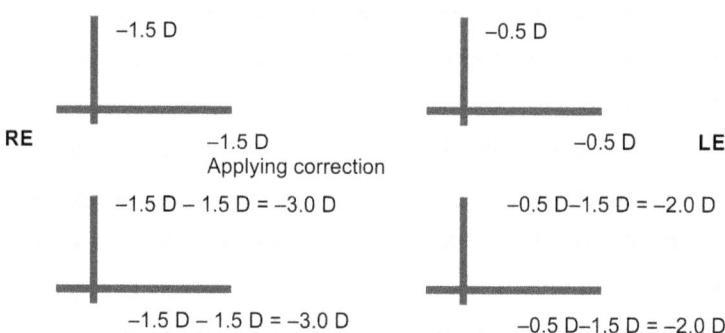

viii. Subjective refraction
- Confirming with trial frame and loose lens
  Start with the exact power obtained from retinoscopy
  - For myopes, decrease power till the patient can read clearly with minimum minus power, e.g., start with –3.0 D in RE and try with –2.75, –2.50, and so on
  - For hypermetropia, increase power till the patient reads clearly with maximum plus power
    RE 6/60 with –3.0 DS = 6/6
    LE 6/36 with –2.0 DS = 6/6
- Refining of power (optional)
  - Duochrome test—to avoid over- or undercorrection
  - Fogging with plus lenses

ix. Check for near vision (at 33 cm)
- RE N6 Nil glass
- LE N6 Nil glass

x. Optional, but mention these when asked in viva:
- Binocular balancing with four prism diopter kept base up and base down
- Back vertex distance for power more than ±5 D
- Cycloplegic correction factor based on the drug used for dilatation. In this case, 0.5 D is deducted from each value
- Muscle balance with full correction
- Decide to call for postmydriatic test (PMT) if pre- and postcycloplegic refraction is different

xi. Interpupillary distance or mean pupillary distance for each eye
RE 34 mm, LE 34 mm

xii. Will full correction, ask the patient to walk around and check the comfort level

xiii. Final prescription including lens type and design and frame type.
Comment: No drug correction for minus spheres

RE	Sph	Cyl	Axis	VA	LE	Sph	Cyl	Axis	VA
DV	−3.0 D	−	−	6/6	DV	−2.0 D	−	−	6/6
NV	−	−	−	N6	NV	−	−	−	N6

Distance vision only
Plastic lens, photochromatic monocular pupillary distance (MPD): RE 34 mm; LE 34 mm

Hypermetropia with Presbyopia

i. Patient details—Mr TGFBR, 45 years, male
ii. Patient complaints—both eyes defective vision for near and distance × 6 months
iii. UCVA—RE - 6/36; LE - 6/24 || RE - N18; LE - N12
iv. Vision with own spectacles—partly improving
   - Vision with own PG: RE = 6/9p; LE = 6/9 || BE N9
   - Existing PG power: RE = +1.0 DS; LE = +0.5 DS || BE Add +1.0
v. Vision with pinhole—RE −6/9; LE −6/6 p
vi. Check for phorias; mention if present
vii. Objective refraction with retinoscopy
   Working distance = 2/3 m (66 cm), hence correction = −1.5 D

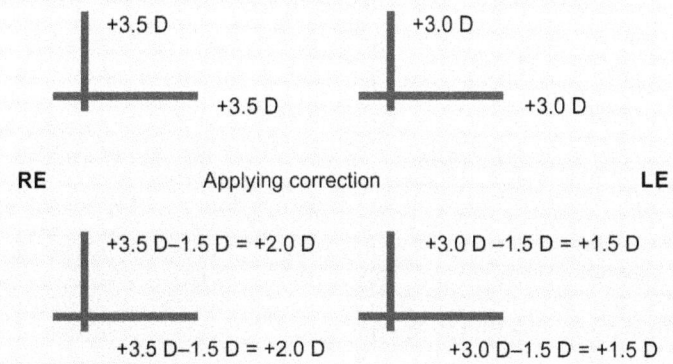

viii. Subjective refraction
   - Confirming with trial frame and loose lens
   Start with the exact power obtained from retinoscopy
      • For myopia, decrease power till the patient can read clearly with minimum minus power
      • For hypermetropia, increase power till the patient reads clearly with maximum plus power

For example, start with +2.0 D in RE and try with +2.25, +2.50, and so on RE 6/36 with +2.0 DS = 6/6
LE 6/24 with +1.75 DS = 6/6
- Refining of power (optional)
  - Duochrome test—to avoid over- or undercorrection
  - Fogging with plus lenses (In this case, put a plus lens greater than the correction, e.g., +4.0 D.)

ix. With distance correction in place, check for near vision at patient's reading/working distance.
- RE Add +1.5 D N6 at 33 cm
- LE Add +1.5 D N6 at 33 cm

x. Optional, but mention these when asked in viva:
- Binocular balancing with four prism diopter kept base up and base down
- Back vertex distance for power more than ±5 D
- Presbyopic correction is checked in an undilated pupil. Hence, cycloplegics correction is not required
- Muscle balance with full correction
- Decide to call for PMT if pre- and postcycloplegic refraction is different
- Interpupillary distance or mean pupillary distance for each eye
  - RE 32 mm; LE 32 mm
- Will full correction, ask the patient to walk around and check the comfort level

Final prescription including lens type and design, and frame type

RE	Sph	Cyl	Axis	VA	LE	Sph	Cyl	Axis	VA
DV	+2.0 DS	–	–	6/6	DV	+1.5 DS	–	–	6/6
NV (Add)	+1.5 DS	–	–	N6	NV (Add)	+1.5 DS	–	–	N6

RE	Sph	Cyl	Axis	VA	LE	Sph	Cyl	Axis	VA
DV	+2.0 DS	–	–	6/6	DV	+1.5 DS	–	–	6/6
NV	+3.5 DS	–	–	N6	NV	+3.0 DS	–	–	N6

Bifocal design—Kryptok or PAL
Plastic lens
MPD: RE 32 mm; LE 32 mm
Some examiners do not prefer the "Add" in prescription. In that case, write the sum of spheres in the NV section.

Compound Myopic Astigmatism

i. Patient details—Ms APMPPE, 30 years, female
ii. Patient complaints—both eyes defective vision for near and distance × 6 months

iii. UCVA—RE - 6/60; LE - 6/24
iv. Vision with own spectacles—partly improving
   - Vision with own PG: RE = 6/12; LE = 6/9
   - Existing PG power:
   RE = –1.0 DS/–0.5 Dcyl × 90°; LE = –0.5 DS/–0.5 Dcyl × 90°
v. Vision with pinhole—RE - 6/9; LE - 6/9
vi. Check for phorias; mention if present
vii. Objective refraction with retinoscopy
   Working distance = 2/3 m (66 cm), hence correction = –1.5 D

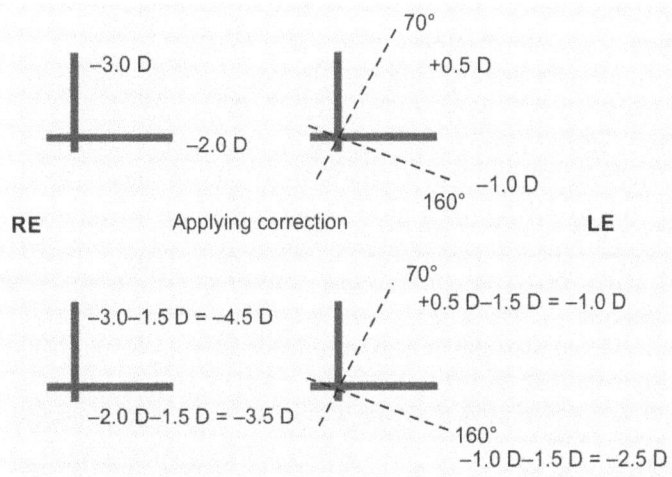

Power = –4.5 Dsp/+1.0 Dcyl × 90°   Power = –2.5 Dsp/+1.5 Dcyl × 160°
Transposing = –3.5 Dsp/–1.0 Dcyl × 180° Transposing = –1.0 Dsp/ –1.5 Dcyl × 70°

viii. Subjective refraction
   - Confirming with trial frame and loose lens:
     Start with the exact power obtained from retinoscopy
     - For myopia, decrease power till the patient can read clearly with minimum minus power
     - For hypermetropia, increase power till the patient reads clearly with maximum plus power
     - For astigmatism, correct sphere first to give the best vision and then correct cylinder
     In this case, after putting a –3.0 Dsph in RE for best corrected visual acuity (BCVA) of 6/9p, then start correcting the cylindrical power
   - Refining:
     In case of astigmatism, refining is done in the following order:
     - Cylinder axis with Jackson's cross cylinder (JCC) (align the cross cylinder axes 45° from the principal meridians)

- Cylinder power with JCC (align the cross cylinder axes with the principal meridians of the correcting cylinder)
  - Sphere power by fogging or duochrome
- For example, after subjective refraction and refining, the final power is as follows:
  RE = –3.5 Dsp/–1.0 Dcyl × 180°
  LE = –1.0 Dsp/–1.5 Dcyl × 70°
ix. With distance correction in place, check for near vision at the patient's reading/working distance
RE N6 Nil glass
LE N6 Nil glass
x. Optional, but mention these when asked in viva:
- Binocular balancing with four prism diopter kept base up and base down
- Back vertex distance for power more than ±5 D
- Cycloplegic correction factor based on the drug used for dilatation. In this case, 0.5 D is deducted from each value
- Muscle balance with full correction
- Decide to call for PMT if pre- and postcycloplegic refraction is different
xi. Interpupillary distance or mean pupillary distance for each eye
RE 32 mm; LE 32 mm
xii. Will full correction, ask the patient to walk around and check the comfort level. It is vitally important for spheres to confirm acceptance
xiii. Final prescription including lens type and design, and frame type. Comment: No drug correction for minus spheres

RE	Sph	Cyl	Axis	VA	LE	Sph	Cyl	Axis	VA
DV	–3.50	–1.0	180°	6/6	DV	–1.0	–1.5	70°	6/6
NV	–	–	–	N6	NV	–	–	–	N6

Distance vision only
Plastic lens, with antireflective coating (ARC)
MPD: RE 30 mm; LE 30 mm

Examples of Retinoscopy Problems

Example 1: 40 years/phenylephrine

$$\begin{array}{c|c} & +3.5 \\ \hline & +2.5 \end{array}$$

Eight steps for prescription
1. *Power cross*

$$\begin{array}{c|c} & +3.5 \\ \hline & +2.5 \end{array}$$

2. *Distance correction*

$$\frac{+2.5\ |}{\ \ \ \ \ |+1.5}$$

3. *Subjective*

$$\frac{+1.5\ \text{Dsph}}{+1\ \text{Dcyl} \times 180}$$

4. *Transposition*

$$\frac{+2.5\ \text{Dsph}}{-1\ \text{Dcyl} \times 90}$$

5. *Drug correction—nil*
6. *Near vision add +1*
7. *Glass prescription*

Sph	Cyl	Axis	Vn
+2.5	−1	90	6/6
+3.5	−1	90	N6

8. *Diagnosis:* Compound hypermetropic astigmatism against rule with presbyopia

Example 2: 25 years/homatropine

$$\frac{-1.5\ |}{\ \ \ \ \ |\pm}$$

Eight steps for prescription

1. *Power cross*

$$\frac{-1.5\ |}{\ \ \ \ \ |\pm}$$

2. *Distance correction*

$$\frac{-2.5\ |}{\ \ \ \ \ |-1}$$

3. *Subjective*

$$\frac{-1\ \text{Dsph}}{-1.5\ \text{Dcyl} \times 180}$$

4. *Transposition*

$$\frac{-2.5\ \text{Dsph}}{+1.5\ \text{Dcyl} \times 90}$$

5. *Drug correction—nil*
6. *Near vision—nil*

7. *Glass prescription*

Sph	Cyl	Axis	Vn
−1	−1.5	180	6/6
			N6

8. *Diagnosis:* Compound myopia astigmatism with rule

Donder's Rule for Near Vision

Reads @ 67 cm
Needs @ 25 cm
1. Available power NV @ 67 cm   −   1.5 D
2. Power needed at 25 cm   −   4 D
3. 1/3 reserve and remaining 1.5-1   −   1 D
4. Give required power 4-1   −   3 D

When Signs are Opposite in Sphere and Cylinders, How to Make a Diagnosis?

Diagnosis
1. +2.75 DS/−2.5 DC 180
2. +2.75 DS/−3.0 DC 180
3. +2.75 DS/−2.75 DC 180

Transpose
1. +0.25 DS/+2.5 DC 90   i. CHA
2. −0.25 DS/+3.0 DC 90   ii. MA
3. +0 DS/+2.75 DC 90   iii. SA

When spherical power is more than cylinder—compound astigmatism 0
When cylinder is more than sphered—mixed astigmatism
When sphere and cylinder are same—simple astigmatism

Astigmatism

1. **How can astigmatism be corrected?**
    i. Eyeglasses
    ii. Contact lenses, preferably rigid gas permeable (RGP)
    iii. Toric contact lenses
    iv. Refractive surgery
    v. Toric intraocular lenses

2. **What are the factors affecting the refractive outcomes following cataract surgery?**
    The factors affecting are:
    i. The accuracy of biometry measurements
    ii. Surgical techniques with respect to wound construction and placement

iii. Consistency of capsulotomy size
iv. Circularity and centration
v. Intraocular lens (IOL) type (especially with regard to a constant) and rotational stability (especially with toric IOL)
vi. Correlation between predicted and actual effective IOL position

3. **What are the surgical techniques of correcting astigmatism alongside cataract surgery?**
   i. Site of the incision (Incision on the steeper meridian is preferable.)
   ii. Size of the incision (A larger incision induces more astigmatism.)
   iii. Astigmatic keratotomy
   iv. Limbal relaxing incisions (LRIs)
   v. Toric IOLs

4. **What are the advantages of toric IOLs?**
   i. The lenses are introduced through a small incision and hence recovery is quick
   ii. The incision is unlikely to induce irregular astigmatism
   iii. There is potential for correcting high amounts of astigmatism even up to 5 D

5. **What are the disadvantages of toric IOLs?**
   i. They do not correct astigmatism at the source (cornea), so distortion may be induced, even if astigmatism is fully nullified
   ii. Residual astigmatism with toric lenses is usually oblique
   iii. They are not useful for correcting asymmetric bowtie astigmatism
   iv. The results also are dependent on the rotational stability of the lens

6. **What are the advantages of LRIs?**
   i. The technique is easy to learn and perform
   ii. LRIs can be quickly performed adding minimal time to cataract surgery
   iii. LRIs correct problem at the source (cornea)
   iv. There is no issue of rotation unlike toric IOLs
   v. LRIs can work well for asymmetric corneal astigmatism

7. **What are the disadvantages of LRIs?**
   i. The incisions are longer and possibly more irritating than a phako incision would be
   ii. Large incisions are less predictable, occasionally gape, can be difficult to hydrate, and sometimes require sutures
   iii. LRIs cannot be used in patients with keratoconus

8. **What is astigmatic keratotomy?**
   Astigmatic keratotomy refers to making transverse or arcuate cuts in the mid periphery perpendicular to the steepest meridian.

9. **What is the mechanism of astigmatic keratotomy?**
   The incised meridian flattens while the meridian 90° away steepens to nearly the same amount.

10. **How much astigmatism can be corrected by astigmatic keratotomy?**
    It can correct astigmatism up to 4-6 D.

11. **What are the risks involved in doing astigmatic keratotomy?**
    Irregular astigmatism, microperforations, and overcorrection

12. **How much astigmatism can be corrected by LRIs?**
    LRIs can correct up to –1.00 to –2.00 astigmatism.

13. **Describe the technique of astigmatic keratotomy?**
    i. Transverse incisions—done in pairs along the steepest meridian, and may extend for about 3 mm
    ii. Arcuate incisions—clear corneal incisions are made which remain at a constant distance from the center of the pupil

14. **How to place the toric IOL?**
    The toric IOL must be aligned with the appropriate steep meridian of astigmatism.

15. **How much astigmatism can clear corneal incisions correct?**
    i. A 3 mm temporal corneal curvature index (CCI) induces between 0.28 and 0.53 D of temporal flattening
    ii. A 3 mm superior or superotemporal CCI induces a flattening of up to 1.2 D
    iii. For correcting astigmatism >1.20 D, a wide incision or an additional opposite clear corneal incision is needed
    iv. Opposite clear corneal incisions are self-sealing, require no extra surgical equipment, and are reported to correct 0.50-2.0 D

16. **How much rotation of toric IOL is tolerated?**
    i. Rotation of 15° decreases the astigmatic correction to ≈50%
    ii. Rotation of 30° decreases astigmatic correction to close to zero with a large shift in the astigmatic axis
    iii. Rotation >30° can increase astigmatism and change its axis.

CHAPTER

Miscellaneous

11.1 VITAMIN A DEFICIENCY

1. **What is vitamin A?**
   Vitamin A is a fat-soluble vitamin stored in the liver. Vitamin A in the strictest sense refers to retinol. However, the oxidized metabolites, retinaldehyde, and retinoic acid are also biologically active compounds.

2. **What are available forms of vitamin A?**
   There are four forms of vitamin A:
   i. Acid—retinoic acid
   ii. Aldehyde—retinaldehyde
   iii. Alcohol—retinal
   iv. Ester—retinyl ester

3. **What is the role of retinaldehyde and retinoic acid in normal body?**
   Retinaldehyde is required for normal vision.
   Retinoic acid is necessary for normal morphogenesis, growth, and cell differentiation.

4. **What are the sources of vitamin A?**
   Vitamin A is available from both plant and animal sources as retinyl palmitate and carotene, respectively
   Animal sources—meat, milk, liver, fish, cod liver oil
   Plant sources—green leafy vegetables, carrots, fruits, especially yellow fruits (mango and papaya)

5. **What are the requirements of vitamin A?**
   Adults   300–750 µg/day
   Lactating female 1,150–4,600 µg/day

6. **What is the role of vitamin A in the body?**
   Role in general:
   i. Maintenance of mucus-secreting cells of epithelia of body
   ii. Normal morphogenesis, growth, and cell differentiation
   iii. Role in iron utilization
   iv. Role in humoral immunity, T-cell-mediated immunity, natural cell killer activity, and phagocytosis

Role in eye:
  i. Precursor of photosensitive visual pigment (rhodopsin)
  ii. Maintain conjunctival mucosa and corneal stroma
  iii. Outer segment turnover epithelium

7. **What is the blood level of vitamin A?**
   The blood level of vitamin A is made by measurement of serum retinol. Normal range—30–65 µg/dL or 150–300 IU/dL.

8. **What is the etiology of vitamin A deficiency?**
   i. *Primary vitamin A deficiency:* It is due to deficient dietary intake of vitamin A and other micronutrients
   ii. *Secondary vitamin A deficiency:* It is due to defects in absorptions and utilization. It occurs in the following conditions
   For example:
   - Malabsorption syndrome
   - Chronic liver disease
   - Severe infection
   - Chronic pancreatitis

9. **What are the risk factors of vitamin A deficiency?**
   i. *Age:* Preschool children (2–3 years of age)
   ii. *Sex:* males >females
   iii. *Social-economic status:* Low social class
   iv. *Physiological status:* Pregnant and lactating women are vulnerable to low vitamin A content in breast milk
   v. *Diet:* Rice-dependent communities in most tropics
   vi. *Seasons:* Dry summer
   vii. *Breastfeeding:* Highly protective, weaning diet highly crucial
   viii. *Cultural:* Dietary habits in some communities
   ix. *Infectious diseases:* Some diseases predispose to vitamin A deficiencies
   For example, diarrhea, intestinal parasites, acquired immunodeficiency syndrome (AIDS), measles.

10. **What is the World Health Organization (WHO) classification of xerophthalmia?**
    i. *XN:* Night blindness
    ii. *X1A:* Conjunctival xerosis
    iii. *X1B:* Conjunctival xerosis ± Bitot's spot
    iv. *X2:* Corneal xerosis
    v. *X3A:* Corneal ulceration/keratomalacia/involving less than one-third of corneal surface
    vi. *X3B:* Corneal ulceration/keratomalacia/involving more than one-third of corneal surface

vii. *XS:* Corneal scars
viii. *XF:* Xerophthalmia fundus

11. **What is xerophthalmia?**
    The term xerophthalmia is used to describe irregular, lusterless, and poorly wettable surface of the conjunctiva and cornea associated with vitamin A deficiency.

12. **Describe night blindness.**
    Night blindness is one of the most common and earliest manifestation. Its characteristics are as follows:
    i. It is reversible
    ii. It is due to inadequate or slow recovery of rhodopsin in retina after exposure to bright light
    iii. It occurs because retinol is essential for production of rhodopsin by rod photoreceptors
    iv. With oral replacement, night blindness may disappear in 48 hours

13. **Describe conjunctival xerosis.**
    The characteristic changes of conjunctival xerosis are usually confined to bulbar conjunctiva:
    i. Changes are dryness, lack of wettability, loss of transparency, thickening, wrinkling, and pigmentation
    ii. Histopathology
    – Metaplasia of normal columnar cells to stratified squamous
    – Prominent granular layer
    – Formation of metaplastic, keratinized surface

14. **What is Bitot's spot?**
    Bitot's spot is a classic sign of xerophthalmia.
    i. It is described as paralimbal grayish plaques of keratinized conjunctival debris, frothy foamy cheese in appearance, and not wetted by tear
    ii. Pathologically, it is a tangle of keratinizing epithelial cells mixed with saprophytic bacteria and sometimes fungi, fatty debris over edema of mucosa and submucosa

15. **What is the site of occurrence of Bitot's spot?**
    Site in decreasing order of frequency: Temporal → nasal → inferior → superior
    It is more significant diagnostically if nasal in position.

16. **Describe corneal xerosis.**
    Corneal xerosis is usually associated with conjunctival xerosis.
    Torchlight examination shows:
    i. Roughened and lusterless surface
    ii. Peau d'orange appearance

Slit-lamp examination shows:
  i. Stromal edema
  ii. Superficial punctate keratitis
  iii. Keratinization
  iv. Fluorescein shows pooling between plaques and keratinized epithelia—tree bark appearance

17. **What are the subclinical signs of vitamin A deficiency?**
    i. Dark adaptometry—abnormal rod threshold
    ii. Vision restoration test—delayed response after blanching
    iii. Pupil constriction—failure to constrict in low illumination
    iv. Conjunctival impression cytology—abnormal epithelial and goblet cell pattern

18. **Describe corneal ulceration in vitamin A deficiency.**
    Corneal ulcerations in vitamin A deficiency occur mostly in the inferior or nasal part.
    i. Ulcer has a very sharp margin as if cut with a trephine
    ii. More severe lesions result in frank necrosis or sloughing of stroma, known as keratomalacia
    iii. It is generally not reversed with treatment

19. **Describe xerophthalmic fundus.**
    i. Whitish yellow changes in pigment epithelium
    ii. Both eyes are affected
    iii. Corresponds to areas of temporary visual field loss
    iv. Appear to be window defect in fundus fluorescein angiogram (FFA)
    v. Known as Uyemura's syndrome

20. **How do you diagnose vitamin A deficiency?**
    Vitamin A deficiency diagnosis depends on:
    i. Clinical signs and symptoms
    ii. Serum vitamin A level
    iii. Conjunctival impression cytology for mucin-secreting cells, goblet cells, and epithelial cells

21. **How do you treat a patient with vitamin A deficiency?**

Children—<1 year of age	100,000 IU—immediately
<8 kg in wt	100,000 IU—next day
	100,000 IU—after 4 months
Children—1-6 years of age	200,000 IU—immediately
	—next day
	—after 4 months

i. It will take care of acute manifestation of vitamin A deficiency
ii. They should also be treated with both vitamin and protein-calorie supplements
iii. Maintenance of adequate corneal lubrication and prevention of infection and corneal melting is essential

22. What is prophylactic treatment for prevention of vitamin A deficiency?

Nutritional fortification:
i. Children—<1 year of age 100,000 IU every 6 months
        <8 kg of weight
ii. Children—1-6 years   200,000 IU every 6 months

23. What are the measures for eye care?

Immediate parenteral/oral supplementation of vitamin A is the first step. The ocular conditions can then be cotreated as follows:
i. For conjunctival xerosis—artificial tears every 3-4 hours
ii. For keratomalacia—broad-spectrum antibiotics

Atropine eye ointment two times a day.

    Subconjunctival injection of gentamicin with atropine can be given.

11.2 LOCALIZATION OF INTRAOCULAR FOREIGN BODIES

1. **Where does intraocular foreign body (IOFB) occur more commonly?**
   i. Males
   ii. Age 20–40 years
   iii. Work setting
   iv. Mostly a result of hammering metal on metal

2. **What history should be elicited from the patient having IOFB?**
   i. Circumstances and mechanism of injury
   ii. Nature of material
   iii. Any likelihood of contamination
   iv. Force with which it hits the eye

3. **Classify the different types of foreign bodies.**

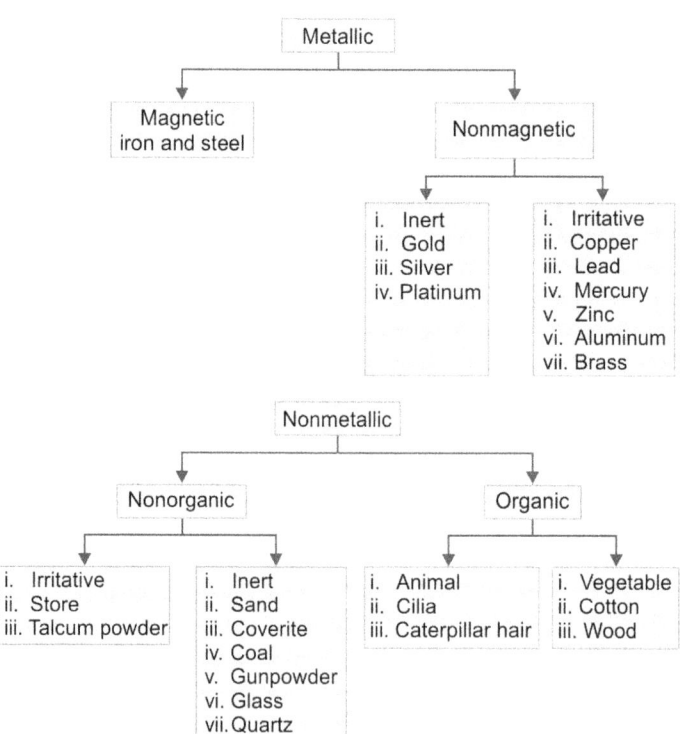

4. **How does the entrance of the foreign body into the eye cause damage?**
   i. By mechanical effects
   ii. By the introduction of infection
   iii. By specific action (chemical and otherwise) on the tissue

5. **Where can the foreign body be embedded in the anterior chamber (AC)?**
    i. The foreign body can fall to the floor of the anterior chamber or embedded in the angle
    ii. It can get embedded in the iris

6. **How can the foreign body pass into the vitreous?**
    i. Through the cornea, iris, and lens when there is a hole in the iris and traumatic cataract
    ii. Through the cornea, pupil, and lens
    iii. Through the cornea, iris, and zonule
    iv. Through the sclera directly

7. **What changes does the foreign body cause in the vitreous?**
    The foreign body may be suspended for some time and ultimately sink to the bottom of the vitreous cavity due to degenerative changes in the gel, which lead to liquefaction, partial or complete. The track of the foreign body through the vitreous is seen as a gray line.

8. **How can the foreign body penetrate the retina?**
    Mostly the particle has enough energy to carry it directly into the retina, where it may ricochet once or even twice before it comes to rest. Occasionally, it pierces the coats of the eye to rest in the orbital tissues (double perforation).

9. **How does the foreign body look if lodged in the sclera?**
    The foreign body often appears black with a metallic luster. It is surrounded by white exudates and red blood clot. Eventually, fibrous issue usually encapsulates it, and retina in the neighborhood becomes heavily pigmented.

10. **What degenerative changes does the foreign body cause in the posterior segment?**
    i. There may be widespread degeneration but, most frequently, fine pigmentary disturbances at the macula → often the result of concussion
    ii. Vitreous turns fluid usually
    iii. Bands of fibrous tissue may traverse along the path of the foreign body
    iv. Hemorrhage may be extensive
    v. Retinal detachment may follow

11. **What is the reaction of the ocular tissue to the nonorganic materials?**
    i. Nonorganic materials are inert
    ii. They excite a local irritative response, which leads to formation of fibrous tissue and results in encapsulation

iii. They produce a suppurative reaction
iv. They cause specific degenerative changes

12. What do organic materials produce?
Organic materials cause a proliferation reaction characterized by formation of granulation tissue.

13. What is siderosis?
Iron contamination of intraocular tissues causes a characteristic picture called siderosis (so does steel in proportion to its ferrous content). The condition is due to electrolytic dissociation of the metal, especially trivalent ion, by the current of rest in the eye, which disseminates the material throughout the tissues and enables it to combine with the cellular proteins, thus killing cell-causing atrophy.

14. What are the features of siderosis?
  i. A rusty staining of cornea—Coats' white ring when deposits are at the level of Bowman's membrane
  ii. Brown-colored iris, mid-dilated pupil, nonreactive due to damage to dilator muscle
  iii. Deposition of iron in the anterior capsules of the lens as a rusty deposit, arranged radially corresponding with the dilated pupil
  iv. The ring becomes stained first greenish and then reddish-brown
  v. Eventually, this leads to development of cataract
  vi. Retinal degeneration with attenuation of vessels
  vii. Secondary glaucoma of chronic type is a complication due to iron deposition in the trabecular meshwork
  viii. Powerful oxidants such as superoxide and hydrogen peroxide, which causes lipid peroxidation, leading to enzyme inactivation and cell membrane damage

15. How are the deposits of iron revealed pathologically?
The deposits of iron are revealed by the Prussian blue reaction with Perl's microchemical stain. The characteristic blue pigmentation is found particularly in the corneal corpuscles, in the trabecular meshwork, on the inner surface of the ciliary body, and in the retina, where the whole retinal vasculature system is clearly marked out.

16. What is the reaction of copper?
If the metal is pure, a profuse formation of fibrous tissue occurs, which is followed by a suppurative reaction and, eventually, shrinkage of globe. If the metal is alloyed (bronze/brass), a milder reaction occurs called chalcosis. It gets deposited where resistance to its migration is offered by a continuous membrane. So, it has a tendency to get deposited on basement membranes such as Descemet's membrane, anterior lens capsule, and internal limiting membrane. The typical sites are:

i. Deep parts of cornea more in the periphery, causing the appearance of a golden brown Kayser-Fleischer ring
ii. Under the lens capsule where it is deposited to form a brilliant golden green sheen aggregated in radiating formations like petals of a flower → sunflower cataract
iii. On the retina at the posterior pole where lustrous golden plaques reflect the light with a metallic sheen
iv. Greenish discoloration of iris
v. Impregnation on zonular fibers
vi. Brownish red vitreous opacities

17. Which metal is more toxic to the eye?
Iron is more toxic to retinal pigment epithelium (RPE). Iron from intraocular foreign bodies is mostly deposited in neuroepithelial tissues such as nonpigmented ciliary epithelium, retina, and RPE. Copper has an affinity for basement membranes.

18. What is the reaction of lead?
Lead is one of the most common forms of foreign body.

It is rapidly covered by a layer of insoluble carbonate, which prevents its diffusion. It produces few changes in the AC, and liquefaction and opacification of vitreous gel can occur. If the metal lies on retina or choroid, it causes an exudative reaction, partly purulent and partly fibrinous.

19. What is ophthalmia nodosa?
Caterpillar hair may penetrate the eye inciting a severe iridocyclitis characterized by the formation of granulomatous nodules.

20. What are the methods for localization of foreign body?
i. Clinical methods for direct visualization
ii. Special methods for indirect visualization

21. What will you look for in direct visualization?
i. Wound of entry
ii. Associated corneal, scleral, iris tear
iii. Penetrating tract in iris, vitreous
iv. Gonioscopy for angle recession
v. Any signs of siderosis or chalcosis

22. What are the clinical signs of importance?
i. Localized tenderness
ii. Mydriasis 3-6 weeks after an accident
iii. Undue persistence of irritation
iv. Delayed occurrence of unexplained uveitis

23. **What are the special methods for investigation?**
    i. Those depending on magnetic properties of the foreign body
    ii. Those depending on electrical conductivity and induction
    iii. Those depending on chemical analysis
    iv. Radiology including X-ray, computed tomography (CT), magnetic resonance imaging (MRI)
    v. Ultrasonography (USG)
    vi. Electroretinography (ERG)

24. **What are the instruments used for detection of foreign body based on electrical conduction?**
    i. *Berman's locator:* The detecting range for a magnetic foreign body is 10 times the diameter of the foreign body. For a nonmetallic foreign body, it ranges between 1 and 2 times. A nonmagnetic foreign body can be detected only if it is >3 mm in diameter
    ii. *Roper Hall's locator:* Also called electroacoustic foreign body detector, metallic foreign body is continuous while nonmetallic foreign body is intermittent
    iii. Carnay's locator
    iv. Ophthalmometalloscope of Hale

25. **What is the sensitivity for foreign body in radiographic methods?**
    i. 0.5 mm diameter will be evident in X-rays (all metals except aluminum, which has an equal bone density. So, the bone-free method is used.)
    ii. Only 40% are located with plain films, and they can be difficult to locate accurately

26. **What are the views most suitable for demonstration of foreign body?**
    i. *True lateral*—affected side toward the film
    ii. *Posteroanterior (PA)*—face against the film
        - Nose and chin in contact with film
        - Tube is centered to middle of orbit

27. **What are the different radiological methods used?**
    i. Direct methods
    ii. Methods depending on relational movements of eye
    iii. Methods on geometric projection
    iv. Bone-free methods
    v. Stereoscopic methods
    vi. Methods based on delineation of globe using contrast media

28. **What is the direct radiographic method?**
    i. Two exposures—PA and lateral are taken
    ii. The foreign body is located in relation to a marker bearing a known relation to the globe

29. **What are the limitations of the direct radiographic method?**
    i. Errors may arise from movement of marker
    ii. Markers cannot be kept in a badly damaged eye
    iii. Eyeball is thought to be 24 mm which is not always true

30. **What are the principles of methods depending on rotation of globe?**
    i. Head and X-ray tube remain fixed
    ii. Several exposures with eye moving in different directions
    iii. Three exposures in lateral view with eye looking straight upward and downward
    iv. Position of foreign body calculated with amount and direction of displacement with reference to center of rotation of globe

31. **What are its limitations?**
    i. There is no true center of rotation of the globe
    ii. The calculations are made in reference to a schematic eye—24 mm

32. **What is the principle of methods depending on geometric construction?**
    Sweet's method
    i. Eye and head remain fixed
    ii. Two X-rays are taken with X-ray tube in known position
    iii. Two metal indicators are used
    iv. Foreign body position localized with reference to fixed indicators

33. **What are the different methods based on geometric construction?**
    i. Mackenzie Davidson
    ii. Sweet's method (ingenious and very accurate)
       Indicators:
       – Center of cornea
       – Temporal side
    iii. Dixon's method
         ↓
         Modified by Bromley
         ↓
         Modified by McGregor

34. **What are its limitations?**
    i. Measurements are incorrect if the patient does not fix properly
    ii. Measurements on schematic eye of 24 mm axial length

35. **What is the principle in stereoscope methods?**
    i. Two X-rays are positioned at two fixed angles with markers attached to globe eye in different positions
    ii. Foreign body is calculated with reference to displacement of its shadow from the radiopaque marker

36. **How do you delineate the globe by using contrast media?**
    Injecting air or dye (thorotrast, lipiodol, diodrast) in Tenon's space

37. What are the disadvantages?
   i. Air embolism if air is used
   ii. Tissue reaction to eye

38. What is the principle in bone-free or Vogt's method?
Dental film is held over and perpendicular to the inner canthus of eye, and the rays are directed from the side so that a shadow of the profile of the anterior segment of the eye (8–12 mm) is recorded on the film.

39. What are the indicators for Vogt's method?
   i. Vogt's method is useful when a small foreign body is in the anterior segment of the eye
   ii. Foreign body density equals to that of bone

40. How is the limbal ring used to detect foreign body?
   i. Limbal ring was introduced by Stallard and Somerset
   ii. In this method, a metallic ring 11–14 mm in diameter, half the diameter of the schematic eye, is sutured to limbus and X-ray. PA view and lateral view are taken
   iii. Precaution:
      - Image of the ring on PA view should be circular
      - Image of ring on lateral view should be vertical
   iv. On PA view:
      - The center of the ring formed by the limbal ring is marked
      - A schematic eye of 24 mm is drawn from center
      - If the foreign body falls within the schematic eye, it is intraocular; otherwise, it is extraocular
      - A vertical corneal axis is drawn, passing through the center of the ring, and the distance of the foreign body nasal or temporal to this axis is noted and measured
   v. On lateral view:
      - A horizontal corneal axis is drawn
      - Distance of the foreign body above or below this axis is also noted, and the distance of foreign body from behind the limbal ring is also noted. To measure the anterior-posterior (AP) measurement from the front of cornea, 3 mm should be added to the measurement from the limbal ring
      - Finally, the position of the foreign body is charted on Bromley's chart or Cridland graticule

41. What are the limitations of the limbal ring test?
   i. Errors may arise from movement of ring and its inaccuracy of its fit
   ii. Inaccurate orientation of globe can occur
   iii. The ring cannot be sutured to a badly damaged eye
   iv. Standard eyeball size is taken as 24 mm which is not always true

42. **What is the contact lens method?**
    Comberg's method: It utilizes a contact lens with radiopaque markers (lead) in all four quadrants.
    A PA exposure is taken with the central ray focused on the anterior pole of the eye and lateral exposur, where the central ray passes through the limbus.
    From the frontal X-ray, the anterior pole of the eye is indicated by intersection of the diagonals joining the markers, and the distance of the foreign body from this point is determined. Its position in the sagittal plane is obtained from lateral view by measurement of the distance of the foreign body behind the markers.
    Worst Lovac contact lens: This contact lens is held in constant position during filming by a partial vacuum produced between the contact lens and cornea. It has a central opening which is connected to a metal tube attached to a rubber suction bulb. PA and lateral views are taken.

43. **What are the disadvantages of contact lens method?**
    i. It is assumed that the eyeball size is 24 mm
    ii. The marker may superimpose on the foreign body
    iii. It is an additional trauma to the eye
    iv. Improper positioning of lens can occur due to chemosis and AC deformation
    v. Sometimes, a poor contact lens fit will allow movement of lens, and so false limbal reference points may be identified

44. **What is the frequency of an ultrasonogram used to detect foreign bodies?**
    8–10 MHz. In the presence of severe inflammation, 5 MHz is used.

45. **What are the two modes used?**
    i. *A-scan:*
       - One-dimensional method
       - It may reveal orbital foreign body posterior to sclera
       - Foreign body appears as steeply rising echospike
    ii. *B-scan:*
       - Two-dimensional
       - More valuable than A-scan
       - Foreign body appears as acoustically white (opaque)

46. **What is quantitative echography used in the detection of a foreign body?**
    i. The reflectivity of a foreign body echospike is extremely high, reaching 100% with lowest gain
    ii. This allows a comparison with scleral signal

47. What are the advantages of USG?
   i. Can detect foreign body even in opaque medium
   ii. Can detect the presence of retinal detachment or vitreous hemorrhage
   iii. Gives axial length of eyeball
   iv. Can localize nonmetallic foreign body
   v. Can precisely localize intraocular or extraocular foreign body

48. What are the disadvantages of USG?
   i. Hazardous in open globe
   ii. Information only in two dimensions
   iii. More anterior part of globe may not be directed in USG

49. What is the relevance of ERG in the detection of foreign bodies?
   i. In siderosis bulbi, early ERG changes include an increased amplitude of the "a" wave and a normal "b" wave. Late changes include a diminished "b" wave and ultimately an extinguished ERG
   ii. In chalcosis, ERG shows initially a wave amplitude and later a decreased "a" and "b" wave amplitude

50. What are the advantages of CT scan?
   i. CT scan is extremely sensitive
   ii. No globe manipulation is required
   iii. Multiple foreign bodies can be localized
   iv. Little patient cooperation is required
   v. It allows detection of smaller foreign body 0.5 mm or more
   vi. It distinguishes metallic from nonmetallic and identifies composition of nonmetallic

51. What are the suggested cuts for CT scan?
Thin axial cuts (≥ 1.5 mm) and direct coronal cuts are used.

52. What are the limitations of MRI?
   i. If there is a magnetic foreign body, they have been shown to move on exposure to the magnetic field
   ii. Visual loss and vitreous hemorrhage have been attributed to movement of occult foreign body after MRI, and hence, they are contraindicated for magnetic foreign bodies

53. What is the management of intraocular foreign bodies?

Intravitreal	Well visualized	Poorly visualized
Magnetic	External magnet	Vitrectomy, forceps/retinal endoscopic microscope (REM)
Nonmagnetic	Vitrectomy/forceps	Vitrectomy/forceps

Contd...

Contd...

Intravitreal Intraretinal	Well visualized	Poorly visualized
Magnetic	Transcleral "trapdoor" or vitrectomy forceps/REM	Vitrectomy forceps/REM
Nonmagnetic	Transcleral "trapdoor" or vitrectomy forceps/REM	Vitrectomy forceps/REM

54. **What are the types of magnets?**
    i. *Hand-held magnet:*
       - It is small and low powered. It is applicable only when the foreign body is within 1 mm of its tip
    ii. *Giant magnet or Bronson's electromagnet:*
       - It has a strong magnetic field
       - It is of two types:
          - Haab's type of electromagnet
          - Ring method
    iii. *Intraocular magnet*

55. **What is the "Lancaster's working criteria for a magnet"?**
    The rule states that to be effective, a giant magnet should pull a steel bale of 1 mm diameter with a force of over 50 times its weight at a distance of 20 mm.

56. **What can be the associated complications with foreign bodies?**
    i. Vitreous hemorrhage
    ii. Retinal tears
    iii. Retinal detachment
    iv. Endophthalmitis
    v. Traumatic cataract
    vi. Iridocyclitis
    vii. Subluxated lens with zonular dialysis, etc.

57. **What is the treatment of siderosis?**
    i. First remove the foreign body
    ii. Galvanic deactivation
    iii. Administration of intravenous ethylenediaminetetraacetic acid (IV EDTA)
    iv. Subconjunctival injection of adenosine triphosphate
    v. Administration of desferrioxamine, which traps the free ions and converts them into nontoxic chelate

58. **What is the treatment of chalcosis?**
    i. Sodium thiosulfate
    ii. Sodium hyposulfate
    iii. British anti-Lewisite (BAL)

11.3 GENETICS

1. **What are genes?**
Genes are the basic units of inheritance, and they include the sequence of nucleotides that codes for a single trait or a single polypeptide chain and its associated regulatory regions. Approximately 20,000–25,000 genes are found among the 23 pairs of known chromosomes.

2. **What are chromosomes?**
Genes are located primarily in the cell nucleus, where they are assembled into chromosomes of varying sizes. Each normal human somatic cell has 46 chromosomes composed of 23 homologous pairs. Of the 46 chromosomes, 44 are called autosomes because they provide information on somatic characteristics; the remaining two chromosomes are X and Y.

   Females have two X chromosomes. Males have both an X and a Y chromosome. The male parent contributes his only X chromosome to all his daughters and his only Y chromosome to all his sons. Among these, Y chromosomal gene is the testis-determining factor (TDF) [also called sex-determining region Y (SRY)].

3. **What do you mean by the following terminologies: Hereditary, genetic, familial, congenital?**
Hereditary indicates that a disease or trait under consideration results directly from an individual's particular genetic composition (or genome), and it can be passed from one generation to another.

   Genetic denotes that the disorder is caused by a defect of genes, whether acquired or inherited.

   Familial: A condition is familial if it occurs in more than one member of a family. It can be caused by common exposure to infectious agents, excess food intake, or environmental agents.

   Congenital refers to characteristics present at birth. These characteristics may be hereditary or familial, or they may occur as an isolated event, often as the result of infection or a toxic agent.

4. **What are the characteristic features of an autosomal dominant disease?**
   i. Affected individuals usually have an affected parent
   ii. Disease does not usually skip a generation unless there are nonpenetrances
   iii. Affected individuals have a 50% risk of having affected offspring
   iv. Males and females are equally affected
   v. Males and females have an equal likelihood of transmitting the disorder to offspring

5. **Name some autosomal dominant disorders of eye.**
    i. Retinitis pigmentosa
    ii. All corneal dystrophies except three autosomal recessive (AR) types
    iii. Retinoblastoma
    iv. Von Hippel-Lindau disease
    v. Congenital fibrosis of extraocular muscles (CFEOM) types 1 and 3
    vi. Best disease
    vii. Neurofibromatosis 1 and 2
    viii. Familial exudative vitreoretinopathy (FEVR)
    ix. Cavernous hemangioma
    x. Wagner disease
    xi. Osteogenesis imperfecta
    xii. Tuberous sclerosis
    xiii. Aniridia
    xiv. Myotonic dystrophy
    xv. Familial radial drusen
    xvi. Marfan's syndrome
    xvii. Blepharophimosis syndrome
    xviii. CHARGE syndrome
    xix. Axenfeld-Rieger syndrome
    xx. Blepharophimosis syndrome
    xxi. Stickler syndrome
    xxii. Treacher-Collins syndrome
    xxiii. Waardenburg syndrome
    xxiv. Gorlin syndrome (nevoid basal cell carcinoma syndrome)

6. **What are the characteristic features of AR disease?**
    i. Affected individuals are born to unaffected parents
    ii. Offsprings are rarely affected unless there is consanguinity
    iii. Males and females are equally affected
    iv. There is a 25% risk to each subsequent child of parents with one affected child

7. **Name some AR disorders.**
    i. Retinitis pigmentosa
    ii. Macular dystrophy, lattice dystrophy type 3, congenital hereditary endothelial dystrophy (CHED) type 2
    iii. All sphingolipidoses except Fabry disease
    iv. All mucopolysaccharidosis except Hunter's syndrome
    v. CFEOM type 2 and unclassified type
    vi. Stargardt disease
    vii. Fundus albipunctatus
    viii. Leber congenital amourosis
    ix. Gyrate atrophy of choroid and retina

x. Oguchi disease
xi. Refsum disease
xii. Wilson disease
xiii. Congenital achromatopsia
xiv. Usher syndrome
xv. Bardet-Biedl syndrome
xvi. Weill-Marchesani syndrome
xvii. Wolfram syndrome (DIDMOAD)
xviii. Goldmann-Favre syndrome
xix. Homocystinuria
xx. Ectopia lentis et papillae

8. **What are the characteristic features of an X-linked recessive disease?**
   i. Affects males or males are generally more severely affected than females
   ii. Affected males have unaffected sons, but all daughters are carriers
   iii. A female carrier has a 50% risk of her son being affected or her daughter being a carrier

9. **What is the distinctive feature of X-linked inheritance?**
   The distinctive feature of X-linked inheritance, both dominant and recessive, is the absence of father-to-son transmission. Because the male X chromosome passes only to daughters, all daughters of an affected male will inherit the mutant gene.

10. **Name some X-linked recessive disorders.**
    i. Retinitis pigmentosa
    ii. Megalocornea
    iii. Fabry disease
    iv. Hunter's syndrome
    v. Lowe syndrome
    vi. Alport syndrome
    vii. Incontinentia pigmenti
    viii. Norrie disease (X-linked FEVR)
    ix. Choroideremia
    x. Congenital stationary night blindness
    xi. X-linked juvenile retinoschisis

11. **What are the characteristic features of mitochondrial inheritance?**
    i. Mitochondrial deoxyribonucleic acid (DNA) is derived exclusively from the ovum, and hence, the inheritance is maternal
    ii. Children of affected females all have the mutation but may not be affected due to nonpenetrance and variable expressivity

12. **Name some mitochondrial inheritance disorders of eye.**
    i. Neuropathy, ataxia, retinitis pigmentosa (NARP) syndrome
    ii. Chronic progressive external ophthalmoplegia (CPEO)
    iii. Kearns–Sayre syndrome
    iv. Leber's hereditary optic neuropathy (LHON)

13. **What are chromosomal disorders?**
    Chromosomal disorders result from an abnormal chromosome number or structure rearrangement. They can result from nondisjunction, deletions, or translocations. Aneuploidy denotes an abnormal number of chromosomes in cells. Trisomy 21 syndrome or Down syndrome is the most common chromosomal syndrome in humans with an overall incidence of 1:1,800 live births.

14. **What are the ocular findings in Down syndrome?**
    i. Almond-shaped palpebral fissures
    ii. Upslanting (mongoloid) palpebral fissures
    iii. Prominent epicanthal folds
    iv. Blepharitis, usually chronic, with cicatricial ectropion
    v. Nasolacrimal duct obstruction
    vi. Strabismus, usually esotropic
    vii. Nystagmus, typically horizontal
    viii. Keratoconus
    ix. Iris stromal hypoplasia
    x. Brushfield spots
    xi. Cataract
    xii. Aberrant retinal vessels (at disk)
    xiii. Optic atrophy
    xiv. Myopia

15. **What are the ophthalmically important chromosomal aberrations?**
    i. *Long arm 13 deletion (13q14) syndrome:* Retinoblastoma
    ii. *Short arm 11 deletion (11p13) syndrome:* Aniridia

16. **What is Knudson's two-hit hypothesis?**
    RB1 (retinoblastoma gene), a tumor suppressor gene, is located on long arm of chromosome 13. Both copies of the gene present on homologous loci on the two chromosomes must be abnormal to initiate oncogenesis. In the heritable forms, one copy is defective by birth. If the other copy is damaged by environmental factors, the tumor is formed. In the sporadic form, the hypothesis is that both copies of the gene are damaged due to environmental influences.

17. **What are the characteristic features of aniridia?**

    Aniridia is a panophthalmic disorder characterized by the following features:
    i. Subnormal visual acuity
    ii. Congenital nystagmus
    iii. Strabismus
    iv. Keratitis due to limbal stem cell failure
    v. Iris absence or severe hypoplasia
    vi. Cataracts (usually anterior polar)
    vii. Ectopia lentis
    viii. Glaucoma
    ix. Optic nerve hypoplasia
    x. Foveal or macular hypoplasia

18. **What is the significance of *PAX6* gene?**
    i. *PAX6* gene product is a transcription factor required for normal development of the eye. Mutations of *PAX6* have been reported in aniridia, Peter's anomaly, autosomal dominant keratitis, and dominant foveal hypoplasia
    ii. The genes responsible for these disorders participate in the development of periocular mesenchyme. These developmental disorders are inherited as autosomal dominant traits
    iii. *Axenfield-Reiger syndrome:* Mutations in *PITX2* gene and *FOXC1* gene
    iv. *Aniridia:* Mutation in *PAX6* gene
    v. *Nail-patella syndrome:* Mutation in *LMX1B* gene

19. **What are the genes associated with glaucoma?**

Disease	Gene
Juvenile open-angle glaucoma Adult open-angle glaucoma	*Myocilin (TIGR)* (1q25)
Congenital glaucoma	*CYP1B1* (2p16)
Normal-tension glaucoma	*Optineurin* (10p15)

20. **Name the genes associated with corneal disease.**

Disease	Gene
Dominant corneal dystrophies (lattice, macular, Avellino, Reis–Bucklers')	*Keratoepithelin* (5q31)
Meesmann's corneal dystrophy	*Keratin K3* (12q12–q13)
Fuch's endothelial dystrophy	*Collagen type VIII* (1q25)
Cornea plana (type 2 AR)	*KERA* (12q)

21. **Name the genes affected in congenital ocular genetic disorders.**

Disorder	Gene affected
Blepharophimosis syndrome	FOXL2X
Crouzon–Apert	FGFR2
Treacher–Collins	TCOF1
Marfan's syndrome	FBN1
Ataxia telangiectasia	ATM
Oculocutaneous albinism type 1	TYR
Oculocutaneous albinism type 2	OCA2
Stickler syndrome	COL9A1, COL11A1, COL11A2
Aniridia	PAX6, WT
Peter's anomaly	PAX6, PITX3, CYP1B1
Microphthalmos	PAX6
Cataract	PAX6, BMP4,7
Chédiak–Higashi syndrome	LYST
Retinitis pigmentosa	CRB1
X-linked retinoschisis	XLRS1
X-linked congenital idiopathic nystagmus	FRMD7

22. **What is pharmacogenetics?**

The study of heritable factors that determine how drugs are chemically metabolized in the body is called pharmacogenetics. This field addresses genetic differences among population segments that are responsible for variations in both the therapeutic and the adverse effects of drugs.

23. **What are the commonly used techniques for genetic testing?**
    i. Karyotyping analysis
    ii. Restriction fragment length polymorphism (RFLP)
    iii. Single-strand conformation polymorphism (SSCP)
    iv. Linkage analysis

24. **What is genetic counseling?**

Genetic counseling is a communication process which deals with human problems associated with the occurrence or risk of occurrence of a genetic disorder in a family. This process involves:
   i. Interpretation of family and medical histories to assess the chance of disease occurrence or recurrence
   ii. Education about inheritance, testing, management, prevention, resources, and research
   iii. Counseling to promote informed choices and adaptation to the risk or condition.

11.4 COMMUNITY OPHTHALMOLOGY

1. **What is the World Health Organization (WHO) definition of blindness?**
   i. *Based on visual acuity:* WHO defined blindness as visual acuity <3/60 or its equivalent in the better eye with best possible refractive correction [best-corrected visual acuity (BCVA) <3/60]
   ii. *Based on visual field:* Visual field <10° in the better eye, irrespective of the level of visual acuity

2. **How will you categorize visual impairment and blindness?**
   WHO classification (1992)

Category	BCVA
0—normal	6/6–6/18
1—visual impairment	6/24–6/60
2—severe visual impairment	<6/60–3/60 (economic blindness)
3—blind	<3/60–1/60 (social blindness)
4—blind	<1/60–perception of light (PL) + (legal blindness)
5—blind	No PL (complete/total blindness)

3. **What is the population of India?**
   As per the 2011 census, it is 1.21 billion and is estimated to grow at 1.6% annually.

4. **What is the percentage of pediatric patients?**
   <16 years: 29%

5. **What is the percentage of population above the age of 40 years?**
   30%

6. **What is the Indian definition of blindness?**
   Blindness is defined as BCVA <6/60 or its equivalent in the better eye or diminution of the field of vision to 20° or less in the better eye.

7. **What is avoidable blindness?**
   i. *Preventable* blindness which can be easily prevented by attacking the causative factor at an appropriate time, e.g., corneal blindness due to vitamin A deficiency and trachoma
   ii. *Curable* blindness in which vision can be restored by timely intervention, e.g., cataract blindness

8. **What is the magnitude of blindness?**
   Global—45 million blind and 180 million visually disabled
   India—9 million blind (one-fifth of the world)

Prevalence of blindness in India is 1.1% [National Programme for Control of Blindness (NPCB) 2001-2002]

9. **What are the causes of blindness in the Indian scenario?**
   The causes of blindness in the Indian scenario:
   NPCB survey (2001-2001), presenting vision <6/60
Cataract	— 62.6%
Refractive error	— 19.7%
Glaucoma	— 5.8%
Posterior segment pathology	— 4.7%
Corneal opacity	— 0.9%
Surgical complications	— 1.2%
Others	— 4.1%

10. **What is cataract surgery rate (CSR)?**
    CSR is the number of cataract surgeries performed per million population. According to 2005 statistics, CSR for India was 5,200 per million population. The highest is in Gujarat (13,108) and lowest in Sikkim (339).

11. **What is the management of ophthalmia neonatorum?**
    i. *Prophylaxis:* Antenatal—treat genital infection
       Intranatal—hygienic delivery
       Postnatal—1% tetracycline eye ointment or 1% silver nitrate (Crede's method) or 2.5% povidone-iodine immediately into the eyes of the babies after birth
    ii. *Curative:* Conjunctival swab for culture sensitivity and cytology is taken. Patient is started on broad-spectrum antibiotic such as topical fluoroquinolone till the reports arrive, following which specific treatment is started
    Neonatal conjunctivitis (ophthalmia neonatorum):

Infection	Treatment
Chlamydia trachomatis	Oral erythromycin 50 mg/kg in four divided doses for 14 days
Gram-positive bacteria	Erythromycin 0.5% e/o QID
Gram-negative bacteria (gonococcal)	• Systemic: Injection ceftriaxone 25–50 mg/kg intravenous (IV) or intramuscular (IM) single dose × 7 days or Injection cefotaxime 100 mg/kg IV or IM single dose × 7 days • Topical: Saline lavage hourly, bacitracin eye ointment QID, or penicillin drops 5,000–10,000 U/mL
Others	Topical gentamicin or tobramycin
Herpes simplex virus (HSV)	Topical and systemic antivirals

12. **What are the prophylaxis and treatment options in vitamin A deficiency?**
    A. *Prophylaxis:*
        i. Immunization (e.g., measles)
        ii. Vitamin A supplements
        iii. Nutritional education to mothers
        iv. Fortified foods

    These prophylactic measures can be observed under the following strategies.

    Short-term strategies:
    i. WHO recommendation: 6 monthly supplementation of high dose of vitamin A
       Children (age—1-6 years)—2 lakh IU orally every 6 months
       Infants 6-12 months old—1 lakh IU orally every 6 months
       Infants <6 months—50,000 IU orally
    ii. Indian recommendation: Child survival and safe motherhood (CSSM)
        First dose (1 lakh IU)—at 9 months along with measles vaccine.
        Second dose (2 lakh IU)—at 18 months along with booster dose of diphtheria, pertussis, tetanus/oral polio vaccine (DPT/OPV).
        Third dose (2 lakh IU)—at 2 years of age.

    Medium-term strategies:
    i. Food fortification (salt, *dalda*)
    ii. Food supplementation

    Long-term strategies:
    i. Improve intake of vitamin A in daily diet
    ii. Nutritional health education to school children

    B. *Treatment:* Keratomalacia reflects very severe vitamin A deficiency and should be treated as a medical emergency to reduce child mortality.
        i. *Systemic:*
           - Systemic treatment of xerophthalmia involves oral or intramuscular vitamin A
           - Multivitamin supplements and dietary sources of vitamin A are also administered
           - Vitamin A doses:
             Age >1 year—2 lakh IU on days 0, 1, and 14
             Age 6 months to 1 year—1 lakh IU on days 0, 1, and 14
             Age <6 months—50,000 IU on days 0, 1, and 14

ii. *Local:*
   - Intense lubrication
   - Topical retinoic acid may promote healing but is not sufficient without systemic supplements
   - Emergency surgery for corneal perforation may be necessary

13. **What are the objectives of Vision 2020? Which eye diseases covered under the same?**

    Vision 2020—The Right to Sight:
    Vision 2020 is a global initiative launched by WHO in Geneva on February 18, 1999, in a broad coalition with the international nongovernmental organizations (NGOs) to combat the problem of blindness.
    Objectives:
    To intensify and accelerate present prevention of blindness activities so as to achieve the goal of eliminating avoidable blindness by the year 2020 *Implementation:*
    Through four phases of 5-year plans, the first one started in 2000.
    Strategic approaches:
    The five basic strategies of this initiative are:
    i. Effective disease prevention and control
    ii. Training of eye health personnel
    iii. Strengthening of existing eye care infrastructure
    iv. Use of appropriate and affordable technology
    v. Mobilization of resources

    Priority diseases:
    Globally, five conditions have been identified for immediate attention for achieving goals of Vision 2020. They are:
    i. Cataract
    ii. Trachoma
    iii. Onchocerciasis
    iv. Childhood blindness
    v. Refractive error and low vision
       In the Indian scenario, in addition to aforementioned conditions, emphasis to be laid on:
       - Glaucoma
       - Diabetic retinopathy
       - Corneal blindness

14. **Comment briefly upon the NPCB.**

    NPCB was launched in the year 1976. It is a 100% centrally sponsored scheme with the goal of reducing the prevalence of blindness to 0.3% by 2020. Rapid Survey on Avoidable Blindness conducted under NPCB during 2006-2007 showed reduction in the prevalence rate of blindness from 1.1% (2001-2002) to 1% (2006-2007).

The main objectives of the program are to:
i. Reduce the backlog of blindness through identification and treatment of blind
ii. Develop comprehensive eye care facilities in every district
iii. Develop human resources for providing eye care services
iv. Improve quality of service delivery
v. Secure participation of voluntary organizations/private practitioners in eye care
vi. Enhance community awareness on eye care

The program objectives are to be achieved by adopting the following strategy:
i. Decentralized implementation of the scheme through District Health Societies (NPCB)
ii. Reduction in the backlog of blind persons by active screening of population above 50 years, organizing screening eye camps, and transporting operable cases to eye care facilities
iii. Involvement of voluntary organization in various eye care activities
iv. Participation of community and Panchayat Raj institutions in organizing services in rural areas
v. Development of eye care services and improvement in quality of eye care by training of personnel, supply of high-tech ophthalmic equipment, strengthening follow-up services, and regular monitoring of services
vi. Screening of school-age group children for identification and treatment of refractive errors with special attention in underserved areas
vii. Public awareness about prevention and timely treatment of eye ailments
viii. Special focus on illiterate women in rural areas. For this purpose, there should be convergence with various ongoing schemes for development of women and children
ix. To make eye care comprehensive, besides cataract surgery, provision of assistance for other eye diseases such as diabetic retinopathy, glaucoma management, laser techniques, corneal transplantation, vitreoretinal surgery, and treatment of childhood blindness
x. Construction of dedicated eye wards and eye operating theaters (OTs) in district hospitals in the northeastern (NE) states and few other states as per need
xi. Development of mobile ophthalmic units in NE states and other hilly states linked with teleophthalmic network and few fixed models

xii. Involvement of private practitioners in subdistrict, block, and village levels

15. **What is the prevalence of corneal blindness? How much is the requirement of cornea?**

    In India, there are around 120,000 corneally blind. This number is increasing by 25,000–30,000 each year.

    Total number of corneal tissues procured in India per year: 50,000

    Total number of corneal tissues utilized in India per year: 22,000 (roughly 45% utilization rate)

    Best performing states in India in corneal donation: Tamil Nadu and Gujarat.

    Causes of corneal blindness
    i. *Infective:*
       - Trachoma
       - Infective keratitis
       - Onchocerciasis
       - Ophthalmia neonatorum
       - Leprosy
    ii. *Nutritional:*
       - Vitamin A deficiency
    iii. *Trauma:*
       - Penetrating trauma
       - Chemical injury
    iv. *Inflammatory:*
       - Mooren's ulcer
       - Sjögren's syndrome
    v. *Inherited:*
       - Stromal dystrophies
       - Fuch's endothelial dystrophy
       - CHED
    vi. *Degenerative:*
       - Keratoconus
    vii. *Traditional eye medicines:*
       - Milk, blood, saliva, dried plant powder

16. **How many eye banks are there in India?**
    Approximately 800

17. **What are the prevalence and causes of childhood blindness?**
    It is estimated that 1.5 million children suffer from severe visual impairment and blindness, and of these, 1 million live in Asia.

    Causes of childhood blindness:
    - Hereditary—chromosomal disorders, single-gene defects
    - Intrauterine—congenital rubella, fetal alcohol syndrome

- Perinatal—ophthalmia neonatorum, retinopathy of prematurity, birth trauma
- Childhood—vitamin A deficiency, measles, trauma
- Unclassified—impossible to determine the underlying cause

18. **What are the recommendations for screening of children for eye diseases?**
    i. *At birth:*
       - Buphthalmos
       - Cataract
       - Ophthalmia neonatorum
       - Microphthalmia or anophthalmos
       - Nystagmus
       - Squint
       - Retinopathy of prematurity
    ii. *Preschool:*
       - Squint and amblyopia
       - Retinoblastoma
       - Vitamin A deficiency
    iii. *School:*
       - Refractive error

19. **What is trachoma? How does it cause blindness?**
    Trachoma is a leading cause for blindness in developing countries in Africa. Six million people are blind.

    Trachoma is caused by *Chlamydia trachomatis* and spread by fomites, houseflies, and flies.

    It results in conjunctival scarring leading to entropion, trichiasis, secondary corneal infections, and scarring.

    Treatment:
    i. Tetracycline eye ointment BD for 6 weeks
    ii. Oral erythromycin, azithromycin
    iii. Prophylaxis in endemic areas: Blanket therapy—1% tetracycline eye ointment BD for 5 days in a month for 6 months

    Prevention:
    SAFE strategy:
    i. Surgery to correct lid deformity and prevent blindness
    ii. Antibiotics to acute infections and community control
    iii. Facial hygiene
    iv. Environmental change

20. **How does onchocerciasis spread and what is its treatment?**
    Onchocerciasis is a parasitic infestation by *Onchocerca volvulus*, a filarial worm endemic in Africa, Central America, and Yemen.

Definitive host—man
Intermediate host—blackfly *Simulium*
Blindness results from corneal scar, glaucoma, retinopathy, and optic atrophy.
Treatment: Oral ivermectin 150 mg/kg body weight Available as Mectizan 6 mg per tablet in market.

21. **What are the functions of an eye bank?**
    i. Promotion of eye donation
    ii. Registration of the pledger for eye donation
    iii. Collection of the donated eyes from the deceased
    iv. Receiving and processing the donor's eyes
    v. Preservation of the tissue for short, intermediate, long, or very long term
    vi. Distribution of the donor tissue to the corneal surgeons
    vii. Research activities

22. **What are the contraindications to the use of donor cornea?**
    i. *Systemic* conditions potentially hazardous to eye bank personnel and fatal if transmitted:
        - Acquired immunodeficiency syndrome (AIDS) or human immunodeficiency virus (HIV) seropositivity
        - Rabies
        - Active viral hepatitis
        - Creutzfeldt-Jakob disease

        Other contraindications:
        - Subacute sclerosing panencephalitis
        - Progressive multifocal leukoencephalopathy
        - Reye's syndrome
        - Death from an unknown cause, including unknown encephalitis
        - Congenital rubella
        - Active septicemia, including endocarditis
        - Intravenous drug abusers
        - Leukemia
        - Lymphoma and lymphosarcoma
    ii. *Ocular:*
        - Intrinsic eye disease
            - Retinoblastoma
            - Active inflammatory diseases
            - Congenital abnormalities
            - Central opacities
            - Pterygium

- Prior refractive procedures
  - Radial keratotomy scars
  - Lamellar inserts
  - Laser photoablation
- Anterior segment surgical procedures

23. **What is the utilization percentage of donor corneas for optical keratoplasty?**

    50%

24. **How many corneas are retrieved per year in India?**
    - 50,000 corneas
    - Number of corneas required per year to meet the demand—2 lakh corneas per year (as per Vision 2020)

25. **How many eye banks are there in India?**

    252

26. **How many keratoplasties are performed in India?**

    In the year 2013–2014 (compiled data of top 10 eye banks)
    - Optical penetrating keratoplasty—4,737
    - Therapeutic keratoplasty—3,209
    - Descemet's stripping endothelial keratoplasty (DSEK)—1,245
    - Deep anterior lamellar keratoplasty (DALK)—436.

11.5 TRAUMATIC HYPHEMA AND GLAUCOMA

1. **How does hyphema cause raised intraocular pressure (IOP)?**
   Hyphema causes a secondary glaucoma which can be either open-angle or closed-angle glaucoma
   i. Open-angle glaucoma causes:
      - Obstruction of a trabecular meshwork by red blood cells, fibrin, debris, or inflammatory cells
      - Obstruction of a trabecular meshwork by melanin, which is released into the anterior chamber (AC) during trauma
      - Associated injury to the trabecular meshwork
      - Recurrent hemorrhage
      - Angle recession
      - Ghost cell glaucoma
   ii. Closed-angle glaucoma causes:
      - Pupillary block—due to clot formation of eight-ball hyphema
      - Peripheral anterior synechiae
      - Posterior synechiae with iris bombe

2. **What is an eight-ball hyphema?**
   Eight-ball hyphema is the formation of a big blood clot in AC along with degenerated red blood cells from an associated vitreous hemorrhage which impedes aqueous outflow.

3. **What is the frequency of rebleed after a traumatic hyphema?**
   4–35%

4. **When is rebleed common?**
   Rebleed is common during the first week after initial injury, usually the fourth day, because normal lysis and retraction of clot occur during that time. Hence, it is essential to follow up with these patients till that time post injury.

5. **How do you evaluate a patient with hyphema due to trauma?**
   i. Vision
   ii. Examine for other associated ocular injuries
   iii. Size of hyphema
      - Height in millimeters
      - Percentage of AC filled with blood
      - Number of clock hours of involvement
      - Presence of clot

      (Any increase in the size of hyphema which is suggestive of a rebleed)
   iv. Intraocular pressure

v. Corneal blood staining
vi. Gonioscopy (if possible in a case of trauma)
- To look for anterior synechiae
- Angle recession (in follow-up cases of traumatic glaucoma)
vii. Fundus evaluation—for signs of preexisting optic nerve head damage
viii. Examination of the other eye—specifically for fundus evaluation. If media is not clear for fundus examination in traumatized eye

6. **What are the laboratory investigations performed in traumatic hyphema cases?**
    i. Hemoglobin (Hb) electrophoresis
    ii. Liver function test (LFT)
    iii. Prothrombin time (PT), clotting time (CT), bleeding time (BT)
    iv. Platelet count
    v. Renal function test (RFT)

7. **What are the complications of traumatic hyphema?**
    i. Rebleeding
    ii. Glaucoma
    iii. Corneal blood staining

8. **What are the risk factors for rebleeding?**
    i. Initial size of hyphema—if total hyphema occurs
    ii. Degree of reduced visual acuity
    iii. Delayed medical attention
    iv. Use of drugs such as aspirin which inhibit platelet clotting action
    v. Increased IOP
    vi. Hypotony
    vii. Sickle cell trait/anemia

9. **How do you manage a case of traumatic hyphema?**
    i. Investigations—mentioned above
    ii. Aim of management
    - To resorb existing hyphema
    - To prevent rebleeding
    Resorption of hyphema:
        i. Conservative management
        - Bed rest
        - Patch
        - Avoid use of aspirin/nonsteroidal anti-inflammatory drugs (NSAIDs)
        ii. Medical treatment if IOP is elevated—to prevent optic nerve damage
        - Aqueous suppressant—topical beta-blockers
        - Topical steroids—1% prednisolone acetate QID

- Atropine 1% e/o BD
- To avoid: Aspirin (which has propensity to cause rebleed)

Miotics

Adrenergics

(Miotics and adrenergics are associated with increased intraocular inflammation)

Antifibrinolytic agents
- Tranexamic acid
- Aminocaproic acid
  - Used when clot is present
  - Systemic or topical
  - Help in preventing rebleeding

iii. Surgical:
- AC washout

Evaluation of suspended AC cells and debris through corneal paracentesis
- Clot removal by
  - Cryoextraction
  - Ultrasonic emulsification and extraction
  - Removal with vitrectomy cutting—aspiration instrument
    Clot removal is usually done between 4 and 7 days post trauma because clot reaches maximum consolidation and retraction at this time so it can be expressed out easily
- Trabeculectomy and iridectomy with irrigation of AC in recalcitrant cause of increased IOP

10. **Mention the surgical indications in a case of traumatic hyphema.**
    i. Corneal blood stain
    ii. Raised IOP:
       - >50 mm Hg for 5 days
       - >35 mm Hg for 7 days
       - Total or near total hyphema with IOP >25 mm Hg for 5 days
    iii. Total hyphema not resolving by day 5
    iv. Clots persisting for >10 days

11. **In a comparison between aminocaproic acid and tranexamic acid, which is better for preventing rebleeding?**
    i. According to studies, there is no difference between the two antifibrinolytic agents for preventing chances of a rebleed
    ii. However, side effects of systemic aminocaproic acid limit its use:
       - Light-headedness
       - Nausea, vomiting
       - Systemic hypotension
       - Increased IOP with accelerated clot dissolution

12. What is the mechanism of action of antifibrinolytic agents?

Antifibrinolytic agents competitively inhibit conversion of plasminogen to plasmin which degrades the fibrin in the clot.

There is a reduction in the rate of clot lysis, thereby giving the injured vessel more time to heal.

13. What are the side effects and contraindications of aminocaproic acid?

i. Side effects are:
   - Nausea, vomiting
   - Postural hypotension
   - Light-headedness
ii. Contraindicated in:
   - Active intravascular clotting disorders
   - Pregnancy
   - Hepatitis patients
   - Renal disease

Hence, there is a need to check for LFT and RFT in a case of traumatic hyphema if antifibrinolytic drugs have to be administered.

14. Why is it important to treat a patient of sickle cell trait/anemia having traumatic hyphema/glaucoma aggressively?

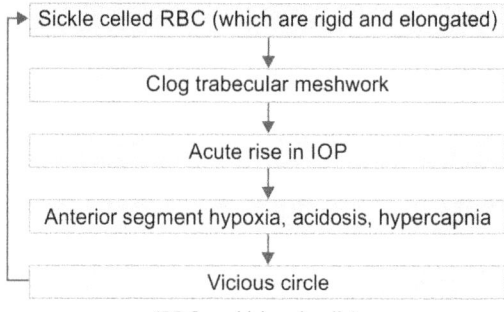

(RBC: red blood cells)

In these patients, the vascular system is already sludged with elongated, rigid sickled RBCs leading to ischemia and vaso-occlusion.

Further, if IOP rises (even if to a minimal extent of 25 mm Hg), it would lead to development of central retinal artery occlusion (CRAO) and rapid optic nerve damage.

Hence, there is a need to monitor closely and treat aggressively.

15. What special care is given to sickle cell anemic patients with a traumatic hyphema?

Aggressive treatment is provided with close monitoring to prevent rise in IOP:

i. Hospitalize the patient
ii. Manage with medical treatment first
iii. If IOP is >25 mm Hg for >24 hours, surgery is done
iv. Other modalities for sickle cell anemia patient—use of hyperbaric
v. Oxygen—intracameral or transcorneal (humidified O_2—1-3 L/min)

16. **Which antiglaucoma agent is contraindicated in sickle cell anemia and why?**

    Carbonic anhydrase inhibitor is contraindicated in sickle cell anemia because these agents increase the concentration of ascorbic acid in the aqueous humor leading to more sickling of RBCs in the AC.

17. **What are the various mechanisms by which traumatic glaucoma occurs?**

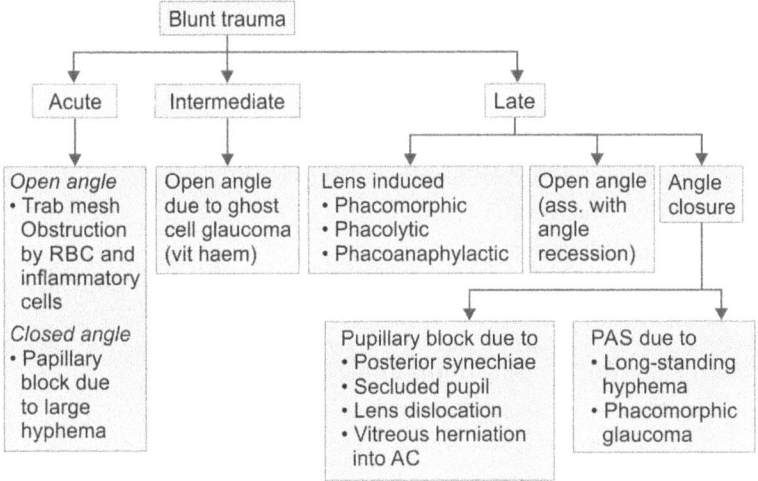

18. **What is ghost cell glaucoma?**

    Ghost cell glaucoma is a form of glaucoma in which degenerated RBCs (ghost cells) develop in the vitreous cavity and then subsequently enter the AC through a disrupted anterior hyaloid and obstructs aqueous outflow.

19. **What are ghost cells?**

    In the vitreous cavity, fresh RBCs get degenerated and are transformed from typical biconcave, pliable nature to tan or khaki-colored, spherical less pliable structures called ghost cells.

20. **How do ghost cells in AC cause glaucoma?**

    Ghost cells are nonpliable, spherical RBCs having thin walls and contain only denatured Hb called Heinz bodies within them. These nonpliable cells are unable to pass through the trabecular meshwork readily, thereby causing an obstruction in the outflow.

21. What is "candy-stripe sign"?

Large quantities of ghost cells in AC layer out inferiorly, creating pseudohypopyon, which is occasionally associated with a layer of fresh RBC—called candy-stripe sign when seen in slit-lamp biomicroscope.

22. What are the differential diagnoses for ghost cell glaucoma?
  i. Hemolytic glaucoma
  ii. Hemosideric glaucoma
  iii. Neovascular glaucoma

23. How do you confirm the presence of ghost cells in AC?

The presence of ghost cells in AC is confirmed by examination of aqueous aspirate under either phase contrast microscopy or routine light microscopy of a paraffin-embedded specimen stained with hematoxylin and eosin, which will reveal the presence of cells.

24. What is the mechanism of glaucoma postpenetrating injury?
  i. Inflammation
  ii. Hemorrhage
  iii. Intumescent/swollen lens—angle closure
  iv. Cyclitic membrane
  v. Lens subluxation
  vi. Forward displacement of lens iris diaphragm with pupillary block and iris bombe

25. How can a penetrating trauma cause hypotony?

A decrease in IOP postpenetrating injury could be due to:
  i. An open wound
  ii. Associated iridocyclitis

26. How do you manage glaucoma postpenetrating trauma?
  i. Treatment of penetrating wound is important—mostly surgical
  ii. Removal of the incarcerated portion of uveal tissue
  iii. Aspiration of lens matter
  iv. Anterior vitrectomy
  v. Removal of foreign body
  vi. Meticulous closure of any corneal—scleral wound
  vii. AC formation

Post initial wound management, glaucoma can be controlled by steroids (for reducing inflammation) and antiglaucoma medications.

27. What is angle recession?

Angle recession is an irregular widening of ciliary body band seen on gonioscopy. Histologically, it is a tear present between longitudinal and circular muscles of ciliary body.

11.6 STERILIZATION

1. Define sterilization and disinfection?

Sterilization is defined as the complete absence of any viable microorganisms, including spores.

Disinfection is reducing the number of viable microorganisms but not inactivating all viruses and bacterial spores.

2. What are the steps in sterilization?
  i. Cleaning
  ii. Packaging
  iii. Sterilization
  iv. Storage
  v. Indicators of sterilization

3. What are the types of cleaning?
  i. Manual cleaning with running water followed by drying
  ii. Mechanical cleaning using ultrasonicator

4. What are the different methods of sterilization?
  i. Autoclaving (steam under pressure)
  ii. Hot air oven (dry heat)
  iii. Chemical sterilization such as ethylene oxide gas or glutaraldehyde 2% solution

5. What are the usual components of handwash disinfectants?
  i. Iodophor
  ii. Chlorhexidine fluconate

6. What is the preferred autoclaving parameter?
  i. Pressure 15 pounds
  ii. Temperature: 121° C
  iii. Time: 30 minutes

7. What are the uses of various sterilization techniques?
  i. Dry heat (hot air oven): For bulk power, petroleum products, reusable glass, metal instruments, oil, and ointments
  ii. Autoclaving:
   - Do not load liquids with instruments because sterilization time is different
   - Instruments are placed in a perforated tray to allow steam penetration
   - Sharp and delicate instruments are kept at the top of the tray
   - Loose packing and space between items are very important for easy circulation and penetration of stream

- All detachable items in the instruments are disassembled. Oil and lubricants are to be wiped well
  iii. Ethylene oxide sterilization (ETO): Used for virophage, cryoprobe, fiber-optic light, intraocular lens' (IOL's) sutures, plastics
      Timing:
      - At 5 psi—12 hours
      - At 10 psi—6 hours

8. **What is the mechanism of action of each method?**
   i. *Steam:* It kills organisms by coagulation of the cell protein
   ii. *ETO:* It is a very effective alkylating agent which reacts with deoxyribonucleic acid (DNA) and destroys the ability of microorganisms to metabolize or reproduce it

9. **What are the different agents used as a chemical disinfectant?**
   i. ETO
   ii. Glutaraldehyde
   iii. Formalin for operating theater (OT) sterilization
   iv. 70% isopropyl alcohol
   v. 10% povidone-iodine

10. **How will you monitor the effectiveness of sterilization?**
    i. *Mechanical indicators:* Time, temperature, and pressure-recording devices
    ii. *Chemical indicators:* For testing ETO, dry heat, and steam processes
    iii. *Biological indicators:* Use heat-resistant bacterial endospores to demonstrate whether or not sterilization has been achieved.

11.7 LANDMARK STUDIES IN OPHTHALMOLOGY

CORNEA
1. **HEDS (Herpetic Eye Disease Study)**
   A. HEDS I
      Questions asked
      i. What is the role of topical steroids in treating herpes simplex stromal keratitis in conjunction with topical antivirals?
      ii. What is the role of oral acyclovir in treating herpes simplex stromal keratitis in patients receiving concomitant topical corticosteroids and antivirals?
      iii. What is the efficacy of oral acyclovir in treating herpes simplex iridocyclitis in combination with topical steroids and antivirals?

      Results
      The study conducted three randomized controlled trials wherein patients were examined for a 16-week period. A treatment failure was defined as worsening of stromal keratitis or uveitis at any scheduled visit, no change in stromal inflammation in the first 2 weeks or 3 later consecutive weeks, or occurrence of an adverse event.
      i. The patients who received prednisolone phosphate 1% drops had faster resolution of the stromal keratitis and fewer treatment failures. Delaying the initiation of corticosteroid treatment did not affect the eventual outcome of the disease.
      ii. On adding oral acyclovir 400 mg five times a day for 10 weeks to topical corticosteroids and trifluridine, no benefit was noted in stromal keratitis and a mild benefit was noted in iridocyclitis.

      Conclusion
      Topical steroids are useful in the treatment of herpes simplex virus (HSV) viral stromal keratitis. Systemic acyclovir is not useful in stromal keratitis.
   B. HEDS II
      Questions asked
      i. Does early treatment with oral acyclovir for HSV epithelial keratitis prevent progression to the complications of stromal keratitis and iridocyclitis?
      ii. What is the efficacy of oral acyclovir in preventing recurrences in patients with previous episodes of herpetic eye disease?
      iii. Is there any role of external or behavioral factors in the induction of ocular recurrences of HSV infections?

Results

    i. There was no benefit from the addition of oral acyclovir to topical trifluridine in preventing the development of stromal keratitis or iritis. Also, the study found that the risk of stromal keratitis or iridocyclitis was quite low in the year following an episode of epithelial keratitis treated with topical trifluridine alone.

    ii. There are no statistically significant external or behavioral factors leading to recurrence.

Conclusion

Oral acyclovir is not recommended during an active episode of epithelial keratitis.

C. HEDS III

The HEDS III study (HEDS-IRT), a randomized clinical trial to evaluate the addition of oral acyclovir to a regimen of topical prednisolone phosphate and trifluridine for the treatment of iridocyclitis, showed a trend in the results suggestive of a benefit of oral acyclovir. A treatment failure occurred in 11 (50%) of the 22 patients in the acyclovir-treated group and in 19 (68%) of the 28 patients in the placebo group.

2. **MUTT (Mycotic Ulcer Treatment Trial)**

  A. MUTT I

    Questions asked

      i. To compare the safety and efficacy of topical 5% natamycin and topical 1% voriconazole in filamentous fungal keratitis

      ii. What role do the above-mentioned drugs play in *Fusarium* and *Aspergillus* keratitis?

    Results

    MUTT was a randomized controlled trial for smear-positive filamentary fungal keratitis comparing natamycin 5% and voriconazole 1%, with the primary outcome being best spectacle-corrected visual acuity (BSCVA) at 3 months; secondary outcomes included corneal perforation and/or therapeutic penetrating keratoplasty.

      i. Natamycin treatment was associated with significantly better clinical and microbiological outcomes than voriconazole.

      ii. Voriconazole-treated cases were more likely to have a perforation.

      iii. Fusarium cases fared much better with natamycin than with voriconazole.

Conclusion
Natamycin is superior to voriconazole in the treatment of filamentary fungal keratitis. This difference is even more pronounced in keratitis caused by *Fusarium*. Voriconazole is not recommended as a monotherapy in filamentous keratitis.

B. MUTT II
Questions asked
What is the role of oral voriconazole in fungal keratitis?

Results
There was no difference in the rate of corneal perforation or the need for therapeutic penetrating keratoplasty (TPK) between oral voriconazole versus placebo, and patients who received oral voriconazole experienced a lot of adverse events.

Conclusion
Oral voriconazole is not found to be useful in the treatment of severe filamentous fungal keratitis.

3. **SCUT (Steroids in Corneal Ulcer Trial)**
Questions asked
Does the addition of topical corticosteroids to antibacterials as an adjunctive therapy for bacterial keratitis improve clinical outcomes?

Results
SCUT was a randomized controlled trial comparing 1.0% prednisolone sodium phosphate to placebo in the treatment of bacterial keratitis with culture-positive ulcers receiving 48 hours of moxifloxacin eye drops before randomization.

Although the steroid-treated group had a significant delay in reepithelialization and steroids were not associated with a statistically significant difference in BSCVA or infiltrate/scar size.

Conclusion
It is left to the discretion of the treating ophthalmologist to add steroids as per the case. Central large ulcers caused by *Pseudomonas* may benefit from adjunctive topical steroid therapy along with moxifloxacin. Ulcers caused by *Nocardia* should not be treated with steroids.

4. **CCTS (Collaborative Corneal Transplantation Studies)**
Questions asked
Is there a role of histocompatibility matching [human leukocyte antigen (HLA) matching] of corneal transplant donors and recipients in reducing the incidence of graft rejection in high-risk patients?

Results
It conducted two studies—the Crossmatch Study and the Antigen Matching Study—to assess the effectiveness of crossmatching and

HLA-A, -B, and -DR donor-recipient matching in preventing graft rejection among high-risk patients with and without lymphocytotoxic antibodies, respectively.

HLA matching or crossmatching does not reduce or increase the likelihood of corneal graft failure. Instead, ABO blood group matching may be effective in reducing the risk of graft failure.

Conclusion
HLA matching does not change the prognosis.

5. **CORTES (CORneal Transplant Epidemiological Study)**

Questions asked
Mention the changing trends for indications, patient demographics, and surgical techniques from the CORTES study.

Results
This study aimed to examine evolving indications and changing trends for corneal transplantation in Italy. Keratoconus, regraft, and pseudophakic bullous keratopathy were the leading indications for penetrating keratoplasty (PK), with keratoconus and regraft showing higher indications for anterior lamellar keratoplasty (ALK), whereas pseudophakic bullous keratopathy and regraft were the major indications for endothelial keratoplasty (EK).

Conclusion
There is an important shift in managing corneal diseases toward more conservative surgeries and changes in indications in corneal transplantation.

6. **DEWS (Dry Eye Workshop Study)**
   A. DEWS (2007)

   Questions asked
   What is DEWS, and what changes did it bring about in ocular surface disease?

   Results
   A new definition of dry eye was developed by the DEWS committee to reflect current understanding of the disease and recommended a three-part classification system. The first part is etiopathogenic and illustrates the multiple causes of dry eye. The second is mechanistic and shows how each cause of dry eye may act through a common pathway. Finally, a scheme is presented based on the severity of the dry eye disease (DED), which is expected to provide a rational basis for therapy. Risk factors for dry eye and morbidity of the disease are identified, and the impact on quality of life and visual function is outlined.

Conclusion
It recognizes the multifactorial nature of the dry eye.

B. DEWS II (2017)

Questions asked
Give a brief note on tear-film ocular surface (TFOS) DEWS II.

Results
There is a revised definition of the dry eye with addition of the phrase "loss of homeostasis and neurosensory abnormalities". Tear film instability, hyperosmolarity, and ocular surface inflammation and damage were determined to be important etiologies. It also takes neurotrophic conditions and neuropathic pain into consideration.

Conclusion
Loss of homeostasis of the tear film is the central pathophysiological concept, and differentiating between aqueous-deficient and evaporative DED was critical in selecting the most appropriate management strategy.

7. **CDS (Corneal Donor Study)**

    Question asked
    What role does the age of donor cornea play in the success of penetrating keratoplasty done for corneal endothelial disorders?

    Results
    This study was undertaken over a period of 10 years to assess the success rate of penetrating keratoplasty for endothelial disorders such as Fuchs and pseudophakic corneal edema. There was no significant difference in success rates comparing donors aged 12–65 years with those aged 66–75 years.

    Conclusion
    The age of donor cornea is not related to the long-term success rate of penetrating keratoplasty for endothelial disorders.

RETINA

Retinal Detachment Studies

1. **Silicone Oil Study (1985–1991)**

    Purpose
    Evaluate and compare silicone oil versus long-acting gas in retinal detachment (RD) with proliferative vitreoretinopathy (PVR).

    Inclusion criteria
    PVR of Grade C-3 or greater according to the Retina Society Classification and visual acuity of light perception or better

Outcome measure

Visual acuity of 5/200 or greater and macular reattachment for 6 months

Result/conclusion

No significant differences in the rates of complete retinal attachment, visual acuity (VA), and corneal abnormalities or glaucoma were found between treatment groups. Gas-treated eyes had more hypotony. Anterior PVR was more prevalent than posterior PVR and had a worse prognosis.

2. **SPR (Scleral buckling vs. Primary Vitrectomy in RRD)—Phakic Subtrial (1998–2003)**

Purpose

Scleral buckling (SB) versus primary vitrectomy in rhegmatogenous retinal detachment (RRD)

Inclusion criteria

Phakic patient with clear break situation

Outcome measure

Change in VA, postoperative development of PVR and cataract, and retinal reattachment rate at 1 year

Result/conclusion

SB achieved greater improvement in final VA than those who underwent primary pars plana vitrectomy (PPV).

Cataract progression was more with PPV. There is a benefit of SB in phakic eyes with respect to BCVA improvement.

3. **SPR (Scleral buckling vs. Primary vitrectomy in RRD)—Pseudophakic Subtrial: (1998–2003)**

Purpose

SB versus primary vitrectomy in RRD

Inclusion criteria

Medium–severe RRD not treatable with a single 7.5 × 2.75 mm silastic sponge, aphakic/pseudophakic patients with an unclear whole situation

Outcome measure

Change in VA, postoperative development of PVR and cataract and retinal reattachment rate at 1 year

Result/conclusion

No significant difference between the groups in terms of functional outcome. Primary anatomical success rate was significantly higher in the primary PPV group compared to the SB group. Primary vitrectomy is recommended in these patients.

11.8 DIABETIC RETINOPATHY

EPIDEMIOLOGICAL STUDIES

1. **WESDR (Wisconsin Epidemiological Study of Diabetic Retinopathy) (1979)**

   Purpose
   Prevalence, incidence, and progression of diabetic retinopathy and its component lesions along with visual loss

   Inclusion criteria
   Patients with diabetes diagnosed before 30 years of age and diabetics diagnosed at 30 years of age or older.

   Results/conclusion
   71% of younger-onset persons had retinopathy. In the older-onset group, 50% had retinopathy and 6% of the younger and 5% of the older-onset subjects had clinically significant macular edema (CSME). Both the frequency and severity of retinopathy and CSME increased with increasing duration of diabetes.

2. **DCCT (Diabetes Control and Complications Trial) (1983)**

   Purpose
   Effect of tight glycemic control on complications of diabetes for persons with type 1 diabetes

   Inclusion criteria
   Insulin-dependent diabetes mellitus (IDDM), age 13–39 years, absence of hypertension, hypercholesterolemia, and severe diabetic complications

   Outcome measures
   Appearance and progression of retinopathy and other complications over 6.5 years

   Results/conclusion
   Intensive therapy delays the onset and slows the progression of microvascular complications of diabetes (diabetic retinopathy, nephropathy, and neuropathy) in IDDM.

3. **EDIC (Epidemiology of Diabetes Interventions and Complications)**

   Purpose
   To examine the persistence of the original treatment effects 10 years after the DCCT (Diabetes Control and Complications Trial)

   Inclusion criteria
   Patients aged 19–45 years who were participants of the DCCT

Outcome measures
Appearance of micro- and macrovascular complications (presently in 13th year follow-up)

Results/conclusion
The persistent difference in diabetic retinopathy between former intensive and conventional therapy continues for at least 10 years but may be waning.

4. UKPDS (United Kingdom Prospective Diabetes Study) (1977)
Purpose
Improved blood glucose and blood pressure (BP) control in type 2 diabetes for preventing the complications of diabetes

Inclusion criteria
Newly diagnosed type 2 diabetes patients

Outcome measures
Follow-up of patients to major fatal and nonfatal clinical endpoints

Results/conclusion
Intensive blood-glucose control and tight BP control reduce the risk of diabetic complications, the greatest effect being on microvascular complications.

5. ABCD (Appropriate Blood Pressure Control in NIDDM) (1993)
Purpose
Intensive BP control versus moderate control in the prevention and progression of nephropathy, retinopathy, cardiovascular disease, and neuropathy in noninsulin-dependent diabetes mellitus (NIDDM)

Inclusion criteria
Hypertensive subjects with NIDDM were included.

Outcome measures
Glomerular filtration rate as assessed by 24 hours' creatinine clearance

Result/conclusion
The more intensive BP control decreased all-cause mortality.

LANDMARK STUDIES

1. DRS (Diabetic Retinopathy Study) (1971)
Purpose
Photocoagulation in preventing severe visual loss from proliferative diabetic retinopathy (PDR) efficacy and safety of argon versus xenon

Inclusion criteria
Best-corrected visual acuity (BCVA) of 20/100 or better in each eye and the presence of PDR in at least one eye or severe nonproliferative diabetic retinopathy (NPDR) in both eyes

Results/conclusions
   i. Photocoagulation reduced the risk of severe visual loss by 50% compared with no treatment
   ii. Xenon laser resulted in more harmful effects than argon laser
   iii. Defined high-risk PDR. Eyes with high-risk PDR should receive prompt pan-retinal photocoagulation (PRP)

2. **ETDRS (Early Treatment Diabetic Retinopathy Study) (1979)**
   Purpose
   Determine the best time to initiate PRP in diabetic retinopathy (DR) efficacy of photocoagulation in diabetic macular edema (DME) effectiveness of aspirin in altering course of DR

   Inclusion criteria
   Patients with moderate or severe NPDR or mild PDR in both eyes and with visual acuity (VA) of 20/40 or better [20/200 or better if macular edema (ME) was present]

   Results/conclusions
      i. Focal laser is useful for CSME
      ii. Scatter treatment is not indicated for eyes with mild-to-moderate NPDR and should be considered in severe NPDR or early PDR
      iii. Aspirin had no effect on DR

3. **DRVS (Diabetic Retinopathy Vitrectomy Study) (1976)**
   Purpose
   Early vitrectomy versus conventional management for recent severe vitreous hemorrhage.

   Inclusion criteria
      i. At least one eye with recent severe vitreous hemorrhage and VA of 5/200 or less
      ii. Extensive active neovascular or fibrovascular proliferations and VA of 10/200 or better

   Outcome measures
   VA was the main outcome measure. VA of 10/20 or better was considered "good vision", while <5/200 was considered "poor vision".

   Results/conclusion
   Early vitrectomy provided a greater chance of prompt recovery of VA, especially in type 1 diabetics and if vision is poor in the fellow eye. Early vitrectomy is of benefit, especially in those with both fibrous proliferations and at least moderately severe new vessels, in which extensive scatter photocoagulation has been carried out or is precluded by vitreous hemorrhage.

ANTI-VASCULAR ENDOTHELIAL GROWTH FACTORS FOR DIABETIC MACULAR EDEMA

1. **READ-2 (Ranibizumab for Edema of the Macula in Diabetes: A phase 2 study) (2006)**

   Purpose
   Compare ranibizumab (RBZ) with focal/grid laser or combination of both in DME

   Inclusion criteria
   DME with central foveal thickness (CFT) ≥ 250 µ, VA ≤ 20/40 but ≥20/320

   Outcome measures
   Change from baseline in BCVA

   Results/conclusions
   At 6 months, RBZ injections had a better visual outcome than focal/grid laser and provided benefits in DME for atleast 2 years. A combination of this treatment with focal/grid laser was even more beneficial in clearing the amount of residual edema and reducing the frequency of injections needed.

2. **RIDE and RISE (A Study of Ranibizumab Injection in Subjects with Clinically Significant Macular Edema with Center Involvement Secondary to Diabetes Mellitus) (2007)**

   Purpose
   Efficacy and safety of intravitreal RBZ in DME patients

   Inclusion criteria
   Adults with DME with CFT ≥275 µm, BCVA of 20/40–20/320 and glycated hemoglobin (HbA1c) ≤12%

   Results/conclusion
   RBZ rapidly and sustainably improved vision, reduced the risk of further vision loss, and improved ME in patients with DME, with low rates of ocular and nonocular harm.

3. **RESOLVE (Safety and Efficacy of Ranibizumab in Diabetic Macular Edema with Center Involvement) (2005)**

   Purpose
   Safety and efficacy of RBZ in DME involving the foveal center

   Inclusion criteria
   Adults, type 1 or 2 diabetes, CFT ≥300 µm, and BCVA of 73–39 ETDRS letters

   Outcome measures
   Efficacy in terms of BCVA and CFT and safety at 12 months

   Results/conclusions
   RBZ is effective in improving BCVA and is well tolerated in DME

4. **RESTORE (Ranibizumab monotherapy or combined with laser versus laser monotherapy for diabetic macular edema) (2008)**

   Purpose
   Superiority of RBZ 0.5 mg monotherapy or combined with laser over laser alone in DME

   Inclusion criteria
   Adults with type 1 or 2 diabetes mellitus (DM) and visual impairment due to DME

   Outcome measures
   Mean average change in BCVA from baseline to month 1 through month 12 safety

   Results/conclusion
   RBZ monotherapy and combined with laser provided superior VA over laser in patients with DME

5. **BOLT (a prospective randomized trial of intravitreal bevacizumab or laser therapy in the management of diabetic macular edema) (2007)**

   Purpose
   Bevacizumab versus macular laser therapy (MLT) in CSME

   Inclusion criteria
   Patients with center-involving CSME, at least 1 prior MLT, BCVA 20/40 to 20/320

   Outcome measures
   Difference in BCVA at 12 months between the bevacizumab (BVZ) and laser arms

   Results/conclusion
   The study supports the use of BVZ in patients with center-involving CSME without advanced macular ischemia.

6. **DA VINCI (DME and VEGF Trap-Eye: Investigation of Clinical Impact) (2008)**

   Purpose
   VEGF Trap-Eye versus laser in DME

   Inclusion criteria
   Adults > 18 years, CSME with central involvement, BCVA 20/40 to 20/320

   Outcome measures
   Change in BCVA at 24 and 52 weeks

   Results/conclusion
   VEGF Trap-Eye produced a statistically significant and clinically relevant improvement in BCVA compared with a macular laser in DME at 24 and 52 weeks.

7. **VISTA (VEGF Trap-Eye in Vision Impairment Due to DME) and VIVID DME (2011)**
   Purpose
   Efficacy of VEGF Trap-Eye on BCVA in DME with central involvement
   Inclusion criteria
   Adults >18 years, DME and BCVA 20/40 to 20/320
   Outcome measures
   Mean change in VA from baseline (ETDRS)
   Results/conclusion
   In both VISTA and VIVID, VEGF Trap-Eye was superior to macular laser photocoagulation for BCVA and anatomical outcomes.

8. **FAME (Fluocinolone Acetonide in diabetic Macular Edema) (2011)**
   Purpose
   To assess the efficacy of low-dose and high-dose fluocinolone acetonide (FA) implant in DME
   Inclusion criteria
   Persistent DME despite at least 1 macular laser treatment
   Outcome measures
   Percentage of patients with improvement from baseline BCVA in ETDRS letter score of ≥15 at 36 months
   Results/conclusion
   FA inserts improved BCVA over 2 years, and the risk-to-benefit ratio was superior for the low-dose insert. Almost all phakic patients in the FA groups developed cataracts. The incidence of incisional glaucoma surgery at month 36 was 4.8% in the low-dose group and 8.1% in the high-dose insert group.

9. **RETAIN (ranibizumab 0.5 mg treat-and-extend regimen for diabetic macular edema) (2013).**
   Purpose
   To demonstrate the noninferiority of RBZ treatment and extent with/without laser to RBZ (PRN) for BCVA in patients with DME
   Inclusion criteria
   DME with VA between 20/32 and 20/160
   Outcome measures
   i. Mean average change in BCVA from baseline to months 1–12 (primary)
   ii. Mean BCVA change from baseline to months 12 and 24, treatment exposure, and safety profile
   Results/conclusion
   Both treatments and extent regimens (with/without laser) were noninferior to PRN based on BCVA.

STEROIDS FOR DIABETIC MACULAR EDEMA

1. **MEAD (dexamethasone intravitreal implant in patients with diabetic macular edema) (2012)**

   Purpose
   To evaluate the safety and efficacy of dexamethasone implant 0.7 and 0.35 mg for DME

   Inclusion criteria
   Patients with DME, BCVA 20/50–20/200 central retinal thickness (CRT) ≥300 μm

   Outcome measures
   Improvement of >15 letters in BCVA from baseline, study of adverse events

   Results/conclusion
   Dexamethasone implant 0.7 and 0.35 mg resulted in ≥15-letter gain in BCVA, and side effects were acceptable.

2. **OZLASE Study (comparison of a combination of repeated intravitreal Ozurdex and macular laser therapy vs. macular laser only in center-involving diabetic macular edema) (2015)**

   Purpose
   To evaluate the efficacy and safety of combined repeated Ozurdex and MLT compared with MLT monotherapy in center involving DME.

   Inclusion criteria
   Patients with center involving DME

   Outcome measures
   Mean change in BCVA at week 56

   Results/conclusion
   Visual outcome following combination therapy did not differ from MLT alone in the center involving DME despite a significant decrease in central subfield thickness (CST) likely due to an entry-level ceiling effect and cataract development.

3. **OZDRY Study (comparison of fixed vs. pro-re-nata dosing of Ozurdex in refractory diabetic macular edema) (2015)**

   Purpose
   To compare the clinical effectiveness and safety of 5 monthly fixed dosing versus PRN Ozurdex treatment in patients with refractory DME

   Inclusion criteria
   Refractory DME, BCVA 20/40–20/200, CRT ≥300 μm

   Outcome measures
   Primary outcome measures—change in BCVA (noninferiority margin of five letters).

Secondary outcome measures—change in patient-reported outcome measures (PROMs), macular thickness, morphology, retinopathy, and safety profile.

Results/conclusion
The mean change in BCVA in 5-monthly fixed dosing of Ozurdex was noninferior to optical coherence tomography (OCT)-guided PRN dosing.

4. **PLACID STUDY (dexamethasone intravitreal implant in combination with laser photocoagulation for the treatment of diffuse diabetic macular edema) (2013)**

Purpose
To evaluate Ozurdex [dexamethasone intravitreal implant (DEX implant); Allergan, Inc., Irvine, CA] 0.7 mg combined with laser photocoagulation compared with laser alone for treatment of diffuse DME.

Inclusion criteria
Patients with DME

Outcome measures
Change in BCVA of >10 letters

Results/conclusion
Equal percentage of patients gained >10 letters between the two groups; however, greater improvement in BCVA occurred in DEX with laser group than in laser alone.

ANTI-VASCULAR ENDOTHELIAL GROWTH FACTOR AND STEROIDS FOR DIABETIC MACULAR EDEMA

1. **BEVORDEX: Efficacy of dexamethasone versus bevacizumab on regression of hard exudates in diabetic maculopathy: data from the BEVORDEX randomized clinical trial**

Purpose
To report the effect of BVZ versus dexamethasone on hard exudates (HEX) in DME

Inclusion criteria
Eyes with center-involving DME resistant to or unlikely to benefit from MLT were included.

Outcome measures
Change in area of HEX and distance of closest HEX to center of fovea

Results/conclusion
Bevacizumab and DEX were effective in reducing area of HEX in eyes with DME. DEX provided more rapid regression of HEX from the foveal center, although BVZ-treated eyes started to catch up by 24 months.

ANTI-VASCULAR ENDOTHELIAL GROWTH FACTOR FOR PROLIFERATIVE DIABETIC RETINOPATHY

1. **CLARITY Study (clinical efficacy of intravitreal aflibercept vs. panretinal photocoagulation for best corrected visual acuity in patients with proliferative diabetic retinopathy at 52 weeks) 2017**

   Purpose
   To report the safety and efficacy of intravitreal Aflibercept for PDR

   Inclusion criteria
   Type 1 or type 2 DM patients with PDR (untreated or previously laser treated active)

   Outcome measures
   Change in best-corrected near visual acuity (BNCVA) at week 52

   Results/conclusion
   Aflibercept was superior to PRP

2. **PROTEUS study**
   PROTEUS study compared the efficacy of RBZ (0.5 mg) plus PRP versus PRP alone in regression of neovascularization (NV) area in high-risk proliferative diabetic retinopathy (HR-PDR) over a 12-month period and found that combination treatment delivered better VA and anatomical outcomes with significant regression of NV.

DIABETIC RETINOPATHY CLINICAL RESEARCH NETWORK

1. **Protocol-I: Laser-Ranibizumab-Triamcinolone Study for DME**

   Purpose
   To evaluate intravitreal 0.5 mg RBZ or 4 mg triamcinolone combined with focal/grid laser compared with focal/grid laser alone for treatment of DME

   Inclusion criteria
   VA of 20/32 to 20/320 and DME involving the fovea

   Outcome measures
   BCVA and safety at 2 years

   Results/conclusion
   Intravitreal ranibizumab (IVR) with prompt or deferred laser is more effective at 2 years compared with prompt laser alone for the treatment of DME involving the central macula. In pseudophakic eyes, intravitreal triamcinolone + prompt laser seem more effective than laser alone but frequently increase the risk of intraocular pressure (IOP) elevation.

2. **Protocol-S: Panretinal Photocoagulation versus Intravitreous Ranibizumab for Proliferative Diabetic Retinopathy: A Randomized Clinical Trial**

   Purpose
   Compare RBZ versus PRP for PDR

   Inclusion criteria
   Patients with PDR

   Outcome measures
   Primary: Mean VA change at 2 years (five-letter noninferiority margin; intention-to-treat analysis)

   Secondary: VA area under the curve, peripheral visual field loss, DME development, NV, vitrectomy, and safety.

   Results/conclusion
   Among eyes with PDR, treatment with RBZ resulted in VA that was noninferior to (not worse than) PRP treatment at 2 years.

   Conclusions from 5-year results: VA was similar in both groups. Severe vision loss or serious PDR complications were uncommon in both groups; however, the RBZ group had lower rates of vision impairing ME and less visual field loss. Patient-specific factors such as cost, frequency of visits, and compliance should be considered when choosing treatment for patients with PDR. These findings support either anti-VEGF or PRP as viable treatments for PDR.

3. **Protocol-T Aflibercept, Bevacizumab, or Ranibizumab for Diabetic Macular Edema; 2-Year Results from a Comparative Effectiveness Randomized Clinical Trial**

   Purpose
   To provide 2-year results comparing anti-vascular endothelial growth factor (VEGF) agents for center-involved DME using a standardized follow-up and retreatment regimen

   Inclusion criteria
   Patients with DME

   Methods
   Randomization to 2.0-mg aflibercept, 1.25-mg repackaged (compounded) BVZ, or 0.3-mg RBZ intravitreous injections performed up to monthly using a protocol-specific follow-up and retreatment regimen. Focal/grid laser photocoagulation was added after 6 months if DME persisted. Visits occurred every 4 weeks during year 1 and were extended up to every 4 months thereafter when VA and macular thickness were stable.

   Main outcome measures
   Change in VA, adverse events, and retreatment frequency

Conclusion
All three anti-VEGF groups showed VA improvement from baseline to 2 years, with a decreased number of injections in year 2. VA outcomes were similar for eyes with better baseline VA. Among eyes with worse baseline VA, aflibercept had superior 2-year VA outcomes compared with BVZ, but superiority of aflibercept over RBZ, noted at 1 year, was no longer identified. Higher AntiPlatelet Trialists' Collaboration (APTC) event rates with RBZ over 2 years warrants continued evaluation in future trials.

4. **KESTREL and KITE: 52 weeks' results from two phase 3 pivotal trials of brolucizumab for DME**

Purpose
To compare the efficacy and safety of brolucizumab with aflibercept in patients with DME

Method
Patients were randomized into 1:1:1 to brolucizumab 3/6 mg or aflibercept 2 mg in KESTREL and 1:1 to brolucizumab 6 mg or aflibercept 2 mg in KITE. Brolucizumab group received 5 loading doses every 6 weeks followed by 12-week dosing or with optional dosing every 8 weeks if disease activity was identified at predefined assessment visits. Aflibercept group received five doses every 4 weeks, followed by fixed 8-weekly dosing.

Outcome measures
BCVA changed from baseline at 52 weeks. Proportion of patients maintained at 12-weekly dosing, anatomical and safety outcomes.

Results/conclusion
Brolucizumab 6 mg showed robust visual gains and anatomical improvements with an overall favorable benefit/risk profile in patients with DME.

RETINAL VEIN OCCLUSION STUDIES

1. **BVOS (Branch Vein Occlusion Study) (1984)**

Purpose
To assess the efficacy of scatter argon photocoagulation for prevention of NV and vitreous hemorrhage and improving VA in eyes with ME reducing vision to 20/40 or worse

Inclusion criteria
  i. Major BRVO without neovascularization
  ii. Major BRVO with neovascularization
  iii. BRVO with macular oedema and reduced vision

Outcome measures
Visual acuity and development of NV or vitreous hemorrhage

Result/conclusion

Scatter argon photocoagulation prevents the development of NV and vitreous hemorrhage but should be applied after the development of NV. Argon laser improved visual outcome in eyes with BRVO, and VA reduced from ME to 6/12 or worse.

2. **CVOS (Central Vein Occlusion Study) (1988)**

   Purpose
   i. To study the effects of early PRP for prevention of iris neovascularization (INV) in ischemic central retinal vein occlusion (CRVO)
   ii. To compare early PRP versus PRP at first identification of INV grid-pattern photocoagulation for loss of central VA due to ME

   Inclusion criteria
   Patients of CRVO, age 21 years or older, VA of light perception or better, IOP <30 mm Hg and sufficient clarity of the ocular media

   Outcome measures
   VA, fundus evaluation, fluorescein angiography, and INV

   Result/conclusion
   i. Prophylactic PRP did not prevent the development of INV. It is safe to wait for the development of early INV and then apply PRP
   ii. Macular grid photocoagulation was effective in reducing angiographic evidence of ME but did not improve VA
   iii. Patients with CRVO are recommended to have frequent follow-up examinations every 1 month for the first 6 months to look for INV

3. **SCORE (Standard care vs. COrticosteroid for REtinalvein occlusion) study (2004)**

   Purpose
   Standard care versus intravitreal injection(s) of triamcinolone acetonide for ME of CRVO and BRVO

   Inclusion criteria
   Center-involving ME secondary to either CRVO or BRVO, <24 months old, VA ≥19 letters and ≤73 letters, retinal thickness >250 μm in the central subfield

   Outcome measures
   Improvement by 15 or more letters from baseline in best-corrected ETDRS VA score at the 12-month visit

   Result/conclusion
   Intravitreal triamcinolone is superior to observation for treating vision loss associated with ME secondary to CRVO but not in BRVO. The 1 mg dose has a safety profile superior to that of the 4 mg dose.

4. **BRAVO (ranibizumab for the treatment of macular edema following branch retinal vein occlusion: evaluation of efficacy and safety) (2007)**

   Purpose

   Intravitreal RBZ versus sham injections in patients with ME due to BRVO.

   Inclusion criteria

   ME involving foveal center due to BRVO, CFT ≥250 μm on OCT and BCVA of 20/40 to 20/400

   Outcome measures

   Mean change in BCVA letter score at month 6 from baseline

   Result/conclusion

   RBZ provided rapid and effective treatment for ME following BRVO with low rates of ocular and nonocular safety events.

5. **CRUISE (Central Retinal Vein Occlusion Study: Evaluation of Efficacy and Safety) (2007)**

   Purpose

   Intravitreal RBZ versus sham injections in patients with ME due to CRVO.

   Inclusion criteria

   ME involving foveal center due to CRVO, CFT ≥250 μm on OCT, and BCVA of 20/40 to 20/320

   Outcome measures

   Mean change in BCVA letter score at month 6 from baseline

   Result/conclusion

   RBZ provided rapid improvement in 6-month VA and ME following CRVO, with low rates of ocular and nonocular safety events.

6. **GENEVA (Global Evaluation of implaNtable dExamethasone in retinal Vein occlusion with macular edemA) (2004)**

   Purpose

   Dexamethasone intravitreal implant versus sham in vision loss due to ME due to BRVO or CRVO

   Inclusion criteria

   Decreased VA due to ME associated with either CRVO or BRVO, BCVA of between 34 and 68 letters, central subfield ≥300 μm on OCT

   Outcome measures

   Time to achieve a ≥15-letter improvement in BCVA

   Result/conclusion

   Dexamethasone intravitreal implant can both reduce the risk of vision loss and improve the speed and incidence of visual improvement in eyes with ME secondary to BRVO or CRVO.

7. **COPERNICUS (Controlled Phase 3 Evaluation of Repeated Intravitreal Administration of VEGF Trap-Eye In Central Retinal Vein Occlusion: Utility and Safety)**

   Purpose

   Intravitreal VEGF Trap-Eye in eyes with ME secondary to CRVO

   Inclusion criteria

   Center-involved ME secondary to CRVO for no longer than 9 months, CST ≥250 µm, BCVA of 20/40–20/320

   Outcome measures

   Proportion of eyes with a ≥15-letter gain BCVA at week 24

   Result/conclusion

   Intravitreal VEGF Trap-Eye for ME secondary to CRVO resulted in a significant improvement in VA.

8. **GALILEO (General Assessment Limiting Infiltration of Exudates in Central Retinal Vein Occlusion with VEGF Trap-Eye)**

   Purpose

   Intravitreal VEGF Trap-Eye in patients with ME secondary to CRVO

   Inclusion criteria

   Center-involved ME secondary to CRVO for no longer than 9 months, CST ≥ 250 µm, BCVA of 20/40–20/320

   Outcome measures

   Percentage of eyes which gained ≥15 letters at week 24

   Result/conclusion

   Intravitreal VEGF Trap-Eye was efficacious in CRVO with an acceptable safety profile.

9. **VIBRANT (Intravitreal Aflibercept for Macular Edema Following Branch Retinal Vein Occlusion) (2016)**

   Purpose

   To determine efficacy and safety outcomes in eyes with ME after BRVO treated with 2 mg intravitreal aflibercept injection (IAI) compared with grid laser

   Inclusion criteria

   Treatment-naïve eyes with ME after BRVO if the occlusion occurred within 12 months and BCVA was between 20/40 and 20/320

   Outcome measures

   Percentage of eyes with improvement from BCVA letter score ≥15 at weeks 24 and 52

Results/conclusion

After 6 monthly IAI, injections every 8 weeks maintained control of ME and visual benefits through week 52. In the laser group, rescue IAI given from week 24 onward resulted in substantial visual improvements at week 52.

10. **MARVEL (Study of the Efficacy and Safety of Intravitreal Bevacizumab vs Ranibizumab in the Treatment of Macular Edema due to Branch Retinal Vein Occlusion) – Report 1: 2015**

    Purpose

    To assess the efficacy and safety of intravitreal bevacizumab (IVB) compared with ranibizumab (IVR) in the treatment of ME due to BRVO

    Inclusion criteria

    BRVO with ME

    Outcome measures

    The primary outcome measure was the difference in mean changes in BCVA at 6 months. Secondary outcome measures included mean change in CRT, the proportion of patients improving by >15 letters and the proportion of patients developing neovascularization.

    Results/conclusion

    This study demonstrated significant gain in VA in eyes with BRVO treated with either BVZ or RBZ.

11. **SCORE-2 (Study of Comparative Treatments for Retinal Vein Occlusion 2) Effect of Bevacizumab vs Aflibercept on Visual Acuity Among Patients With Macular Edema due to Central Retinal Vein Occlusion (2017)**

    Purpose

    To study whether BVZ is noninferior to aflibercept for VA in eyes with ME due to central retinal (CR) or hemiretinal vein occlusion

    Inclusion criteria

    Patients with ME due to CR or hemiretinal vein occlusion

    Main outcomes and measures

    The primary outcome was mean change in VA letter score (VALS) from the randomization visit to the 6-month follow-up visit, based on the best-corrected electronic ETDRS VALS (scores range from 0 to 100; higher scores indicate better VA).

    Conclusion and relevance

    Among patients with ME due to CR or hemiretinal vein occlusion, IVB was noninferior to aflibercept with respect to VA after 6 months of treatment.

RETINOPATHY OF PREMATURITY STUDIES

1. **CRYO-ROP (Cryotherapy for Retinopathy of Prematurity Cryotherapy for Retinopathy of Prematurity) (1986)**

   Purpose
   To assess the safety and efficacy of transscleral cryotherapy in infants with retinopathy of prematurity (ROP)

   Inclusion criteria
   Premature infants weighing <1,251 g at birth and had survived the first 28 days of life with threshold ROP

   Outcome measures
   Fundus photo and VA at 1 year of age

   Result/conclusion
   Cryotherapy reduces the risk of unfavorable retinal and functional outcome (by half) from threshold ROP. The benefit was maintained across 15 years of follow-up.

2. **ET-ROP (Early Treatment for Retinopathy of Prematurity) Study (2000)**

   Purpose
   To compare the early versus conventional timing of treatment in ROP

   Inclusion criteria
   Infants <1,251 g birth weight, examined by 42 days of life and with prethreshold ROP

   Outcome measures
   Functional (primary) and structural (secondary) outcome at 9 months

   Result/conclusion
   Early treatment significantly reduced unfavorable outcomes in both primary and secondary measures. Retinal ablative therapy is recommended for type I ROP; observation is recommended for type II ROP.

3. **BEAT-ROP (Bevacizumab Eliminates the Angiogenic Threat of Retinopathy of Prematurity) (2008)**

   Purpose
   Efficacy of IVB in ROP and compare it with conventional laser in ROP

   Inclusion criteria
   Infants ≤1,500 g at birth and ≤30 weeks' gestation who develop stage 3 + ROP in zone I or posterior zone II

   Result/conclusion
   IVB monotherapy, compared with conventional laser therapy, showed a benefit for zone I but not zone II disease. Trial was too small to assess safety.

4. **STOP-ROP (Supplemental Therapeutic Oxygen for Prethreshold Retinopathy of Prematurity) (1994)**

   Purpose
   To assess the supplemental oxygen in moderately severe ROP (prethreshold ROP)

   Inclusion criteria
   Newborns with prethreshold ROP in one or both eyes

   Outcome measures
   Adverse endpoint was progression to threshold ROP. Favorable endpoint was regression of the ROP into zone 3 or complete retinal vascularization.

   Result/conclusion
   Supplemental oxygen did not cause additional progression of prethreshold ROP but also did not significantly reduce the need of peripheral retinal ablative surgery. Supplemental oxygen increased the risk of adverse pulmonary events.

5. **HOPE-ROP (High Oxygen Percentage in Retinopathy of Prematurity) Study (1996)**

   Purpose
   Rate of progression from prethreshold to threshold ROP in infants excluded from STOP-ROP

   Inclusion criteria
   Newborns with prethreshold ROP in one or both eyes

   Outcome measures
   Adverse endpoint was progression to threshold ROP. Favorable endpoint was regression of the ROP into zone 3 or complete retinal vascularization.

   Result/conclusion
   HOPE-ROP infants progressed from prethreshold to threshold ROP less often than STOP-ROP infants.

6. **LIGHT-ROP (Effects of Light Reduction on Retinopathy of Prematurity (LIGHT-ROP) (1995)**

   Purpose
   To study the effect of ambient light reduction on the incidence of ROP

   Inclusion criteria
   Premature infants weighing <1,251 g at birth and having a gestational age of <31 weeks

   Outcome measures
   Development of ROP or full vascularization

   Result/conclusion
   Reduction in the ambient-light exposure does not alter the incidence of ROP.

7. PHOTO-ROP (Photographic Screening for Retinopathy of Prematurity Study) (2000)

Purpose

Digital fundus imaging compared to indirect ophthalmoscopy to screen for ROP

Inclusion criteria

Premature infants <31 weeks' postmenstrual age at birth and <1,000 g birth weight

Outcome measures

Sensitivity, specificity, positive, and negative predictive values of reading center image interpretations compared to clinical impressions based on bedside indirect ophthalmoscopy

Result/conclusion

Remote digital fundus imaging is unlikely to supplant bedside ophthalmoscopy due to limitations in diagnostic sensitivity, specificity, and accuracy when image quality is poor. However, fundus imaging is a useful adjunct to indirect ophthalmoscopy, especially when image quality is good.

8. RAINBOW Study (RAnibizumab Compared with Laser Therapy for the Treatment of INfants BOrn Prematurely with Retinopathy of Prematurity)

Purpose

To determine if IVR is superior to laser ablation therapy in the treatment of ROP

Inclusion criteria

Birth weight (BW) <1,500 g
Bilateral ROP with one of the following retinal findings in each eye:
  i. Zone I, stage 1+, 2+, 3 or 3+ disease
  ii. Zone II, stage 3+ disease
  iii. Aggressive posterior ROP

Primary outcome measures

Absence of active ROP and unfavorable structural outcome (time frame: 24 weeks after starting investigational treatment)

To achieve this outcome, patients must fulfill all the following criteria:
  i. Survival
  ii. No intervention with a second modality for ROP
  iii. Absence of active ROP
  iv. Absence of unfavorable structural outcome

Secondary outcome measures

  i. Requirement for intervention with a second modality for ROP (time frame: 24 weeks after starting investigational treatment)

ii. Time to intervention with a second modality for ROP or development of unfavorable structural outcome or death (time frame: 24 weeks after starting investigational treatment)
iii. Recurrence of ROP (time frame: 24 weeks after starting investigational treatment)
iv. Number of patients having any ocular adverse event (time frame: 24 weeks after starting investigational treatment)
v. Systemic RBZ levels (time frame: Within 24 hours, 14 days, and 28 days after RBZ treatment)
vi. Systemic VEGF levels (time frame: Before investigational treatment, 14 days, and 28 days after investigational treatment)
vii. Number of RBZ administrations (time frame: 24 weeks after starting investigational treatment)
viii. Number of patients having any systemic adverse event (time frame: 24 weeks after starting investigational treatment)

LASER PHOTOCOAGULATION IN CHOROIDAL NEOVASCULARIZATION

1. **MPS (Macular Photocoagulation Study)—Argon study (1979)**

   Purpose
   To evaluate laser treatment of choroidal neovascularization (CNV) (well-demarcated classic)

   Inclusion criteria
   Extrafoveal CNV in age-related macular degeneration (AMD), presumed ocular histoplasmosis (POH), idiopathic neovascular membranes (INVM) with VA ≥ 20/100

   Outcome measures
   Change in BCVA from baseline

   Conclusion
   Laser is beneficial in extrafoveal and juxtafoveal well-demarcated classic CNV.

2. **MPS (Macular Photocoagulation Study)—Krypton study (1979)**

   Purpose
   To evaluate laser treatment of CNV (well-demarcated classic)

   Inclusion criteria
   Juxtafoveal CNV in AMD, POH, INVM with VA ≥20/400

   Outcome measures
   Change in BCVA from baseline

   Conclusion
   Laser is beneficial in extrafoveal and juxtafoveal well-demarcated classic CNV.

3. **MPS (Macular Photocoagulation Study)—Foveal Study (1979)**
   Purpose
   To evaluate laser treatment of CNV (well-demarcated classic)

   Inclusion criteria
   Subfoveal new (<4 disk areas) or recurrent (<6 disk areas) CNV in AMD with VA 20/320 to 20/40

   Outcome measures
   Change in BCVA from baseline

   Conclusion
   Laser is beneficial in subfoveal classic CNV (especially if small) and in conditions with worse initial VA

PHOTODYNAMIC THERAPY IN CHOROIDAL NEOVASCULARIZATION

1. **TAP (Treatment of ARMD with Photodynamic Therapy) (1998)**
   Purpose
   To evaluate photodynamic therapy (PDT) in subfoveal CNV in AMD

   Inclusion criteria
   Subfoveal classic CNV, size ≤5,400 µ, VA ≥20/100

   Outcome measures
   Eyes with <15 letters VA loss at 2 years

   Conclusion
   PDT is beneficial in predominantly classic subfoveal CNV.

2. **VIP (Verteporfin in Photodynamic Therapy)—Myopic CNV (1998)**
   Purpose
   To evaluate PDT in subfoveal CNV in myopia

   Inclusion criteria
   Subfoveal CNV, size ≤5,400 µ, VA ≥20/100

   Outcome measures
   Eyes with <8 letters VA loss

   Conclusion
   PDT is beneficial in subfoveal CNV in myopia.

3. **VIP (Verteporfin in Photodynamic Therapy)—CNV in AMD (1998)**
   Purpose
   To evaluate PDT in subfoveal CNV in AMD, occult or classic with good VA

   Inclusion criteria
   Subfoveal CNV, size ≤5,400 µ, occult—VA ≥20/100 with recent progression; classic—VA >20/40

Outcome measures
Loss of 15 letters, that is, moderate vision loss

Conclusion
Occult CNV should be treated with PDT if <4 disk areas, VA <20/50 or if classic features develop.

4. **VIM (Visudyne in minimally classic choroidal neovascularisation) (2001)**

   Purpose
   To evaluate standard fluence (SF)/reduced fluence (RF) PDT in subfoveal minimally classic CNV in AMD

   Inclusion criteria
   Subfoveal, minimally classic, VA ≥20/250, lesion size <6 MPS disk areas

   Outcome measures
   Loss of 15 letters

   Conclusion
   PDT is beneficial in small subfoveal minimally classic CNV in AMD.

SUBMACULAR SURGERY TRIALS

1. **SST (Submacular Surgery Trial)—H (1997)**

   Purpose
   To compare surgical removal of subfoveal CNV in ocular histoplasmosis syndrome (OHS) or INVM versus observation

   Inclusion criteria
   Subfoveal CNV (new or recurrent after laser), <9 MPS disk areas, VA 20/50 to 20/800

   Outcome measures
   Improvement in VA or retention of VA

   Conclusion
   There is no benefit of performing surgery.

2. **SST (Submacular Surgery Trial)—B (1997)**

   Purpose
   To compare surgical removal of subfoveal CNV in AMD versus observation

   Inclusion criteria
   Large hemorrhages from subfoveal CNV (area of hemorrhage >CNV on FA), VA of 20/100 to light perception

   Outcome measures
   Improvement in VA or retention of VA

Conclusion
Submacular surgery did not improve VA but reduced the risk of severe VA loss compared to observation.

3. SST (Submacular Surgery Trial)—N (1997)
Purpose
To compare surgical removal of subfoveal CNV in AMD versus observation

Inclusion criteria
New subfoveal CNV due to AMD, <9 MPS disk areas, with poorly demarcated boundaries, VA of 20/100 to 20/800

Outcome measures
Improvement in VA or retention of VA

Conclusion
Submacular surgery did not improve or preserve VA is not recommended.

4. VISION (VEGF Inhibition Study in Ocular Neovascularisation)
Purpose
To assess the efficacy of pegaptanib sodium in early subfoveal CNV secondary to AMD

Inclusion criteria
All angiographic CNV lesion compositions of AMD

Outcome measures
Proportion of patients avoiding three lines of vision loss at 1 year

Result/conclusion
There is a benefit in receiving therapy with pegaptanib in year 2. The safety profile was favorable.

5. ANCHOR (Anti-VEGF Antibody for the Treatment of Predominantly Classic Choroidal Neovascularization in AMD)
Purpose
To compare RBZ versus PDT in predominantly classic neovascular AMD

Inclusion criteria
Predominantly classic, subfoveal CNV not previously treated with PDT or antiangiogenic drugs, total size <5,400 µm, BCVA of 20/40 to 20/320

Outcome measures
Percentage losing <15 letters and percentage gaining ≥15 letters from baseline

Result/conclusion
RBZ over a 24-month period was effective and superior to PDT treatment in maintaining or improving VA and lesion characteristics.

6. **MARINA (Minimally Classic/Occult Trial of the Anti-VEGF Antibody Ranibizumab in the Treatment of Neovascular ARMD)**

   Purpose
   To assess the efficacy of RBZ in minimally classic/occult neovascular AMD

   Inclusion criteria
   BCVA 20/40 to 20/320; primary or recurrent subfoveal CNV due to AMD, minimally classic or occult with no classic CNV; maximum lesion size of 12 disk areas, and presumed recent progression

   Result/conclusion
   RBZ for nonclassic neovascular AMD had substantially better VA outcomes compared to sham injections. RBZ treatment showed stabilization of lesion size.

7. **PIER [Phase IIIb, Multicenter, Randomized, Double-Masked, Sham Injection-Controlled Study of Efficacy and Safety of Ranibizumab (RBZ) in Subjects with Subfoveal CNV with or without Classic CNV secondary to AMD]**

   Purpose
   To assess the efficacy of RBZ given monthly for 3 months and then quarterly in patients with subfoveal CNV due to AMD

   Inclusion criteria
   All lesion types due to AMD if the active CNV accounted for at least 50% of the total lesion.

   Outcome measure
   Mean change from baseline VA at month 12th and 24th

   Result/conclusion
   RBZ provided significant VA benefit. With quarterly dosing, there was a steady decline in VA during months 4 through 24 in PIER compared to the VA stabilization achieved in ANCHOR and MARINA with monthly injections.

8. **EXCITE (Efficacy and Safety of Ranibizumab Inpatients with Subfoveal CNV Secondary to AMD)**

   Purpose
   To assess the quarterly versus monthly regimen of RBZ in subfoveal CNV secondary to AMD (PIER vs. MARINA/ANCHOR) regimen

   Inclusion criteria
   Classic and nonclassic subfoveal neovascular AMD

   Outcome measures
   Mean change in BCVA CRT from baseline to month 12

Result/conclusion
At month 12, BCVA gain in the monthly regimen was higher than the quarterly regimens.

9. **PrONTO (Prospective Optical Coherence Tomography Imaging of Patients with Neovascular AMD Treated with intra-Ocular Ranibizumab)**

Purpose
OCT-guided, variable dosing regimen RBZ for patients with neovascular AMD

Inclusion criteria
AMD patients with subfoveal CNV and a CRT of at least 300 µm

Outcome measures
Change in VA scores and OCT measurements from baseline at 24 months

Result/conclusion
OCT-guided variable-dosing regimen with RBZ resulted in VA outcomes similar to results from the phase III MARINA and ANCHOR studies.

10. **SUSTAIN (Study of Ranibizumab in Patients with Subfoveal CNV Secondary to AMD)**

Purpose
To assess the individualized RBZ (PRN regime) in patients with neovascular AMD

Inclusion criteria
AMD patients with subfoveal CNV naïve to RBZ treatment

Outcome measures
Frequency of adverse events, monthly change of BCVA and CRT from baseline

Result/conclusion
Like PrONTO, results from the SUSTAIN trial showed a rapid increase in VA in the first 3 months, which deteriorates slightly, but not nearly as much as in PIER, over the 9 months of PRN dosing.

11. **HARBOR [Phase III, double-masked, multicenter, randomized, Active treatment-controlled study of the efficacy and safety of 0.5 mg and 2.0 mg Ranibizumab administered monthly or on an as-needed Basis (PRN) in patients with subfoveal neOvasculaR age-related macular degeneration]**

Purpose
RBZ 0.5 and 2.0 mg monthly versus on PRN basis in treatment-naïve subfoveal neovascular AMD

Inclusion criteria
Subfoveal CNV due to AMD, lesions <12 disk areas and BCVA 20/40–20/320

Outcome measures
Mean change from baseline in BCVA at month 12th

Result/conclusion
RBZ 0.5 mg dosed monthly provides optimum results in patients with wet AMD. There is no additional benefit from the high dose in treatment-naïve wet AMD.

12. **SAILOR (Safety Assessment of Intravitreal Lucentis for AMD)**

    Purpose
    RBZ in a large population of subjects with neovascular AMD

    Inclusion criteria
    Angiographically determined subfoveal CNV secondary to AMD

    Outcome measures
    Safety outcomes included the incidence of ocular and nonocular adverse events; efficacy outcomes included changes in BCVA.

    Result/conclusion
    Intravitreal RBZ was safe and well tolerated in a large population with neovascular AMD. Although the risks of arterial thrombotic events related to RBZ are low, they are similar to those observed in previous RBZ studies, and ophthalmologists should be aware of these risks.

13. **HORIZON (Extension Trial of Ranibizumab for Neovascular Age-Related Macular Degeneration)**

    Purpose
    Long-term safety and efficacy of RBZ injections in patients with CNV secondary to AMD

    Inclusion criteria
    Patients who completed the controlled treatment phase of 1 of 3, 2-year clinical trials (ANCHOR, MARINA, or FOCUS) were randomized to receive RBZ or placebo.

    Outcome measures
    Incidence and severity of ocular and nonocular adverse events

    Result/conclusion
    The incidence of serious ocular and nonocular adverse effects during the 2-year study period of HORIZON trial was low and consistent with those observed during the 24 months of treatment in the prior phase III trials.

14. **SANA [Systemic bevacizumab (Avastin) Therapy for Neovascular Age-related macular degeneration]**

    Purpose
    Systemic BVZ for the treatment of subfoveal CNV in neovascular AMD

Inclusion criteria

AMD with subfoveal CNV, BCVA letter scores of 70-20, and a CRT of 300 μm

Outcome measures

Safety assessments, changes from baseline in VA scores, OCT measurements, and angiographic lesion characteristics

Result/conclusion

Systemic BVZ for neovascular AMD was well tolerated and effective for all 18 patients through 24 weeks, with an improvement in VA, OCT, and angiographic outcomes.

15. **ABC [Avastin (R) (Bevacizumab) for Choroidal neovascularisation trial]**

Purpose

To compare intravitreal BVZ versus PDT (for classic) or pegaptanib (for occult/minimally classic) for the treatment of neovascular AMD

Inclusion criteria

Predominantly classic or occult or minimally classic type neovascular AMD

Outcome measures

Proportion of patients gaining ≥15 letters of VA at 1 year

Result/conclusion

BVZ retreatment regimen is superior to standard care (pegaptanib sodium, verteporfin, sham), with low rates of serious ocular adverse events. Treatment improved VA on average at 54 weeks.

16. **CATT (Comparison of Age-related Macular Degeneration Treatments Trials)**

Purpose

To compare RBZ versus BVZ administered monthly or as needed for 2 years in neovascular AMD

Inclusion criteria

Active, subfoveal CNV, fibrosis <50% of total lesion area, VA 20/25-20/320 and at least 1 drusen in either eye or late AMD in fellow eye

Outcome measures

Mean change in VA at 1 year

Result/conclusion

RBZ and BVZ had similar effects on VA over a 2-year period. Treatment, as needed, resulted in less gain in VA. There were no differences between drugs in rates of death or arteriothrombotic events.

17. **IVAN (Inhibit VEGF in Age-related Choroidal Neovascularisation)**
    Purpose
    To compare RBZ versus BVZ intravitreal injections to treat neovascular AMD
    Inclusion criteria
    Untreated subfoveal neovascular AMD in the study eye with VA ≥25 letters
    Outcome measures
    Distance VA (efficacy) and arteriothrombotic events or heart failure (safety)
    Result/conclusion
    The comparison of VA at 1 year between BVZ and RBZ was inconclusive. Visual acuities with continuous and discontinuous treatment were equivalent. Macular atrophy frequently develops within a neovascular AMD in eyes receiving anti-VEGF therapy over 2 years.

18. **CLEAR—IT 2 (Phase 2, Randomized, Controlled Dose-and Interval-Ranging Study of Intravitreal VEGF Trap Eye in Patients with Neovascular Age-Related Macular Degeneration)**
    Purpose
    VEGF Trap-Eye for neovascular AMD
    Inclusion criteria
    Subfoveal CNV secondary to wet AMD
    Outcome measures
    Change in CR/lesion thickness (LT), change in total lesion and CNV size, mean change in BCVA, proportion of patients with 15-letter loss or gain, time to first PRN injection, reinjection frequency, and safety at week 52nd.
    Result/conclusion
    PRN dosing with VEGF Trap-Eye at weeks 16–52 maintained the significant anatomic and vision improvements established during the 12-week fixed-dosing phase with a low frequency of reinjections.

19. **VIEW 1 and 2 (VEGF Trap-Eye: Investigation of Efficacy and Safety in Wet AMD)**
    Purpose
    Monthly and every-2-month dosing of intravitreal VEGF Trap-Eye versus monthly RBZ in subfoveal CNV secondary to AMD.
    Inclusion criteria
    Subfoveal CNV secondary to AMD.
    Outcome measures
    Noninferiority (margin of 10%) of the VEGF Trap-Eye regimens to RBZ in the proportion of patients maintaining vision at week 52nd.

Result/conclusion

VEGF Trap-Eye dosed monthly or every 2 months after 3 initial monthly doses produced similar efficacy and safety outcomes as monthly RBZ.

20. HAWK and HARRIER (phase 3 trial of brolucizumab for neovascular ARMD)

Purpose

Two similarly designed phase 3 trials comparing brolucizumab 3 mg or 6 mg with aflibercept 2 mg to treat neovascular age-related macular degeneration (nAMD).

Intervention

After a loading dose of 3 monthly injections, brolucizumab-treated eyes received an injection every 12 weeks or every 8 weeks; if disease activity was present, aflibercept eyes received every 8 weeks dosing.

Outcome measures

Noninferiority in mean BCVA change from baseline to 48 weeks (margin: 4 letters); percentage of patients maintaining 12-week dosing throughout 48 weeks and anatomic outcomes.

Results/conclusion

Brolucizumab was noninferior to aflibercept in visual function at 48 weeks, and >50% of brolucizumab 6 mg treated eyes maintained 12 weekly dosing through 48 weeks. Anatomical outcomes favored brolucizumab over aflibercept. The overall safety with brolucizumab was similar to aflibercept.

21. FOCUS (RhuFab V2 Ocular Treatment Combining the Use of Visudyne to Evaluate Safety)

Purpose

RBZ combined with verteporfin PDT in predominantly classic CNV in AMD.

Inclusion criteria

Predominantly classic CNV in AMD (PDT was performed 7 days before initial RBZ or sham treatment).

Outcome measures

Proportion of patients losing fewer than 15 letters from baseline VA at 12 months.

Result/conclusion

A combination of RBZ and PDT was more efficacious than PDT alone for treating neovascular AMD, though RBZ treatment increased the risk of serious intraocular inflammation.

22. PROTECT

Purpose

To assess the safety of the same-day administration of verteporfin PDT (SF) and RBZ.

Inclusion criteria

Predominantly classic or occult CNV secondary to AMD.

Outcome measures

Incidence of severe vision loss (BCVA loss ≥30 letters).

Result/conclusion

Same-day verteporfin and RBZ were safe and not associated with severe vision loss or severe ocular inflammation.

23. TORPEDO

Purpose

To assess the efficacy of one-time RF-PDT followed by RBZ on a variable dosing regimen in neovascular AMD.

Inclusion criteria

Previously untreated, active neovascular AMD.

Outcome measures

Improvement in BCVA over 2 years.

Result/conclusion

Combined PDT and RBZ injection on the same day was well tolerated in all patients. 84% of patients had stable or improved vision at month 24th.

24. DENALI (Verteporfin plus ranibizumab for choroidal neovascularization in age-related macular degeneration)

Purpose

To compare RBZ in combination with verteporfin PDT versus RBZ monotherapy in subfoveal CNV in AMD.

Inclusion criteria

Subfoveal CNV in AMD, lesion size <9 disk areas, naïve to AMD treatment, and a BCVA letter score of 73–24.

Outcome measures

Mean change in BCVA from baseline at month 12th.

Result/conclusion

RBZ monotherapy or combined with verteporfin PDT improved BCVA at month 12. Verteporfin RF did not confer clinical benefits over verteporfin SF.

25. **MONT BLANC (verteporfin plus ranibizumab for choroidal neovascularization in Age-related macular degeneration)**

    Purpose
    To compare same-day verteporfin PDT and intravitreal RBZ versus RBZ monotherapy in neovascular AMD.

    Inclusion criteria
    Subfoveal CNV secondary to AMD, lesion size <9 disk areas, naïve to AMD treatment, and a BCVA letter score of 73-24.

    Outcome measures
    Mean change in BCVA from baseline to month 12th.

    Result/conclusion
    The combination was effective in achieving BCVA gain comparable with RBZ monotherapy. The study did not show benefits with respect to reducing the number of RBZ retreatment over 12 months.

26. **EVEREST (efficacy and safety of verteporfin photodynamic therapy in combination with ranibizumab or alone vs. ranibizumab monotherapy in patients with symptomatic macular polypoidal choroidal vasculopathy)**

    Purpose
    To compare verteporfin PDT combined with RBZ or alone versus RBZ monotherapy in symptomatic macular polypoidal choroidal vasculopathy (PCV).

    Inclusion criteria
    PCV with BCVA letter score between 73 and 24, greatest linear dimension (GLD) of the total lesion area <5,400 μm.

    Outcome measures
    Proportion of patients with indocyanine green angiography (ICGA) assessed complete regression of polyps at month 6th.

    Result/conclusion
    At month 6th, verteporfin combined with RBZ or alone was superior to RBZ monotherapy in achieving complete polyp regression.

27. **RADICAL (Reduced Fluence Visudyne-Anti-VEGF-Dexamethasone in Combination for AMD Lesions)**

    Purpose
    To compare RF PDT + RBZ versus either of two regimens of RF PDT + RBZ + dexamethasone versus RBZ monotherapy.

    Inclusion criteria
    Treatment-naïve subfoveal CNV due to AMD, GLD <9 disk areas, BCVA score of 25-73 letters.

Outcome measures
Mean number of retreatments and the mean change in BCVA from baseline at 24 months.

Result/conclusion
Significantly fewer retreatment visits were required with combination therapies than with RBZ monotherapy. Mean VA change from baseline was not statistically different among the treatment groups.

28. **CABERNET (The Choroidal Neovascularisation Secondary to AMD Treated with Beta Radiation Epiretinal Therapy)**
Purpose
To estimate the safety and efficacy of epimacular brachytherapy (EMBT) for the treatment of CNV in neovascular AMD.

Inclusion criteria
Predominantly classic, minimally classic, or occult with no classic lesions, secondary to AMD, with a total lesion size of <12 disk areas, and a GLD ≤5.4 mm.

Outcome measure
Proportion of patients losing <15 letters from baseline and the proportion gaining >15 letters.

Result/conclusion
The 2-year efficacy data do not support the routine use of EMBT for treatment-naïve wet AMD, despite an acceptable safety profile.

29. **AREDS (Age-Related Eye Disease Study) (1992)**
Purpose
Determine clinical course, prognosis, and risk factors of AMD and cataract. Evaluate effects of high doses of antioxidants and zinc on the progression of AMD, cataract, and vision loss.

Inclusion criteria
Extensive small drusen, intermediate drusen, large drusen, noncentral geographic atrophy (GA), pigment abnormalities in one or both eyes, or advanced AMD or vision loss due to AMD in one eye. At least one eye had best-corrected VA of 20/32 or better.

Outcome measures
Increase from baseline in nuclear, cortical, or posterior subcapsular opacity grades or cataract surgery moderate VA loss from baseline.

Result/conclusion
Patients with extensive intermediate-sized drusen, at least one large drusen, noncentral GA in one or both eyes, or advanced AMD or vision loss due to AMD in one eye should consider taking a supplement of antioxidants plus zinc. Use of a high-dose formulation of vitamin C, E,

and beta carotene in well-nourished older adult cohort had no apparent effect on the 7-year risk of development or progression of age-related lens opacities.

30. AREDS (Age-Related Eye Disease Study)-2 (2006)

Purpose
Evaluate the effect of the two dietary xanthophylls and two omega-3 fatty acids [long-chain polyunsaturated fatty acids (LCPUFAs)] on progression to AMD and/or moderate vision loss in people at moderate-to-high risk for progression.

Inclusion criteria
Persons aged 50–85 years with bilateral intermediate AMD or advanced AMD in one eye.

Outcome measure
Progression to advanced AMD.

Result/conclusion
Awaited.

31. CAPT (Complications of Age-related Macular Degeneration Prevention Trial) (1999)

Purpose
Low-intensity laser of eyes with drusen in the macula for preventing later complications of AMD.

Inclusion criteria
Male or female, aged at least 50 years, vision in each eye 20/40 or better with at least 10 large (>125 µm) drusen in each eye.

Result/conclusion
Low-intensity laser treatment did not demonstrate a clinically significant benefit for vision. Risk factors for CNV and GA stated.

ENDOPHTHALMITIS VITRECTOMY STUDY

1. EVS (Endophthalmitis Vitrectomy Study) (1990–1995)

Purpose
To assess the role of early PPV versus intravitreal antibiotics and intravenous antibiotics in postoperative endophthalmitis.

Inclusion criteria
Patients with endophthalmitis following cataract surgery or intraocular lens (IOL) implantation with VA <20/50 and > light perception (LP)

Outcome measures
VA by ETDRS chart and media clarity.

Follow-up
3 and 9 months.

Results follow-up
VA was better with PPV in patients with LP vision results were comparable when initial vision was HM or better. Intravenous antibiotics did not affect outcome.

Conclusion
Immediate vitrectomy is not necessary in patients with better than light perception vision at presentation, while results are better with PPV in patients in whom VA is light perception only.

11.9 CLINICAL TRIALS IN GLAUCOMA

1. **OHTS (Ocular Hypertension Treatment Study)**
   Questions asked
   i. Does medical reduction of intraocular pressure (IOP) prevent or delay the onset of optic nerve damage and visual field (VF) loss in patients with ocular hypertension?
   ii. Who are the people more likely to develop glaucoma and therefore perhaps benefit from treatment and which people with increased IOP are unlikely to develop glaucoma and therefore could probably be followed without treatment?

   Results
   i. The results of OHTS proved that topical antiglaucoma medication reduces the incidence of glaucoma.
   ii. The cumulative probability of developing primary open-angle glaucoma (POAG) was 4.4% in the medication group and 9.5% in the observation group.
   iii. Medical treatment reduced the development of glaucoma by >50% at the end of 5 years.
   iv. The predictive factors found included increasing age, increasing IOP, decreased thickness of the cornea, and increased cup/disk ratio.
   v. The risk of developing glaucoma is variable. It may be as low as 1-2% in some ocular hypertensive patients and as high as 25-35% in some patients over 5 years.

   Conclusion
   Patients receiving topical antiglaucoma medications had a lower risk of developing POAG than patients receiving no medication. The risk can be determined by analyzing parameters such as increasing patient's age, IOP, corneal thickness, cup/disk ratio, and higher pattern standard deviation.

2. **EMGT (Early Manifest Glaucoma Trial)**
   Questions asked
   i. What is the effect of immediate therapy to lower the IOP versus late or no treatment on the progression of early, newly detected OAG?
   ii. What is the extent of IOP reduction attained by treatment and what are the factors that influence glaucoma progression?

   Results
   i. Multicenter randomized controlled clinical trial comparing observation with betaxolol and laser trabeculoplasty for OAG.
   ii. Early signs of advancing disease were detected earlier in the untreated group when compared to the treated group.

iii. No factors, aside from exfoliation glaucoma, were related to longitudinal changes in IOP.
iv. A 25% decrease in IOP from baseline reduced the risk of progression by 50%.
v. Risk of progression decreased by 10% with each 1 mm Hg IOP reduction from baseline to the first follow-up visit.

Conclusion
Untreated patients had twice the glaucoma progression risk of patients who received treatment and those with the greatest IOP lowering enjoyed the most benefit.

3. **CNTGS (Collaborative Normal-Tension Glaucoma Study)**
   Question asked
   What is the role of IOP control in preventing the progression in normal-tension glaucoma (NTG)?

   Results
   i. One eye of each eligible subject was randomized either not to be treated (control group) or to have IOP lowered by 30% from baseline by surgical and/or medical means.
   ii. Mean IOP in the treatment group was 10.6 mm Hg, and that in the untreated group was 16.0 mm Hg.
   iii. Survival analysis showed statistically significant difference in disease progression in the two groups when examining for specifically defined endpoint criteria of optic disk appearances and field loss.
   iv. The incidence of cataract was higher in the treated arm, with the highest incidence in those whose treatment included filtration surgery.

   Conclusion
   A slower rate of incidence of VF loss was seen in cases with 30% or more lowering of IOP in NTG. Progression of VF loss was faster in women, in patients with migraine headaches, and in the presence of disk hemorrhages.

4. **EGPS (European Glaucoma Preventing Study)**
   Question asked
   How effective is the reduction of IOP by dorzolamide in preventing or delaying POAG in patients affected by ocular hypertension (OHT)?

   Results
   i. Patients were randomized to treatment with dorzolamide or placebo (excipients of dorzolamide).
   ii. Dorzolamide reduced IOP by 15–22% throughout the 5 years of the trial.

iii. Same predictors for the development of POAG in OHTS and EGPS: Baseline older age, higher IOP, thinner central corneal thickness, larger vertical cup-to-disk ratio, and higher Humphrey VF pattern standard deviation.

Conclusion

EGPS failed to detect statistical differences between the chosen medical therapy and placebo, either in IOP lowering effect or in the rate of progression to POAG.

5. **CIGTS (Collaborative Initial Glaucoma Treatment Study)**

   Question asked

   Are patients with OAG best managed with initial topical medication or by initial filtration surgery?

   Results
   i. Newly diagnosed OAG was randomized to either medication or trabeculectomy [with or without 5-fluorouracil (5-FU)].
   ii. There was no significant difference in VF loss between the two groups.
   iii. Patients randomized to surgery had initially poorer quality of life and underwent cataract surgery more than twice as often as patients in the medically treated group.
   iv. The average visual acuity in the two groups after 4 years was about equal.
   v. IOP reduction was greater with surgery than with medical therapy (48 vs. 35%).

   Conclusion

   Initial medical treatment and initial filtering surgery were both effective at preserving vision; there was a slight advantage for the medication arm in terms of comfort.

6. **AGIS (Advanced Glaucoma Intervention Study)**

   Question asked

   How are outcomes in OAG affected by the sequence of treatment with argon laser trabeculoplasty (ALT) and trabeculectomy?

   Results
   i. Eyes were randomized to receive either ALT followed by trabeculectomy 1 and trabeculectomy 2 (ATT sequence) or trabeculectomy 1 followed by ALT and then trabeculectomy 2 (TAT sequence).
   ii. Younger age and higher preoperative IOP were associated with increased failure rates for both groups.

iii. In black patients, the average percentage of eyes with VF loss was less in ATT sequence than in TAT sequence.
iv. In white patients, the average percentage of eyes with VF loss was less in TAT sequence.

Conclusion
Long-term visual function outcomes were better for the ATT sequence in black patients and better for the TAT sequence in white patients.

7. **TVT (Tube Vs. Trabeculectomy Study)**
Question asked
Trabeculectomy or tube shunt surgery: Which is safer and effective in lowering the IOP in eyes with previous intraocular surgery?

Results
  i. Patients with previous cataract and/or failed glaucoma surgery and uncontrolled glaucoma on maximum tolerated medical therapy were randomized to receive either nonvalved tube shunt surgery (Baerveldt implant) or trabeculectomy with application of mitomycin C for 4 minutes.
  ii. After 3 months, both procedures produced sustained pressure reduction to the low teens throughout the 5-year duration of the study.
  iii. Trabeculectomy had a higher long-term failure rate (47 vs. 30% after 5 years).
  iv. The tube shunt surgery group had a lower rate of early postoperative complications.
  v. The rates of visual loss and of late or serious complications were similar between the two groups.

Conclusion
Tube shunt had a higher success rate compared to trabeculectomy with mitomycin C (MMC) during 5 years of follow-up. Both procedures were associated with similar IOP reduction and use of supplemental medical therapy at 5 years. Additional glaucoma surgery was needed more frequently after trabeculectomy with MMC than tube shunt placement.

8. **GLT (Glaucoma Laser Trial)**
Question asked
How safe and effective is ALT as an alternative to treatment with topical antiglaucoma medication for controlling IOP in patients with newly diagnosed, previously untreated POAG?

Results
  i. Each patient had one eye randomly assigned to ALT [laser first (LF) eye] and the other eye assigned to timolol maleate 0.5% [medication first (MF) eye].

ii. LF eyes had lower mean IOPs than MF eyes.
iii. Fewer LF eyes than MF eyes required simultaneous prescription of two or more medications to control IOP.

Conclusion

There were no major differences between the two treatment approaches with respect to changes in visual acuity or VF over the 2 years of follow-up.

9. **GLTFS (Glaucoma Laser Trial Follow-up Study)**

    Question asked

    What are the differences between the two treatment groups of the Glaucoma Laser Trial with respect to IOP, VFs, optic disk cupping, and therapy for POAG?

    Results
    i. This was a follow-up study of patients who enrolled in the Glaucoma Laser Trial, and the median duration of follow-up was 7 years (maximum 9 years).
    ii. Eyes initially treated with laser trabeculoplasty had 1.2 mm Hg greater reduction in IOP and 0.6 dB greater improvements in the VF when compared to eyes initially treated with antiglaucoma medications.
    iii. The overall difference between eyes with regard to change in ratio of optic cup area to optic disk area indicated slightly more deterioration for eyes initially treated with medication.

    Conclusion

    Initial treatment efficacy with ALT was comparable to initial treatment with topical antiglaucoma medication.

10. **FFSS (Fluorouracil Filtering Surgery Study)**

    Questions asked
    i. Do postoperative subconjunctival injections of 5-FU increase the success of trabeculectomy in patients at risk for trabeculectomy failure?
    ii. What are the risk factors for failure of surgery?

    Results
    i. Patients with medically uncontrolled glaucoma after previous cataract extraction or unsuccessful filtering surgery, or both, were randomized to a trabeculectomy alone (standard treatment) or to trabeculectomy with adjunctive 5-FU injections.
    ii. The study demonstrated improved surgical control of glaucoma using 5-FU in patients at high risk for trabeculectomy failure.
    iii. After 5 years, 51% of eyes that received 5-FU and 74% of the eyes that did not receive 5-FU had failed trabeculectomies.

iv. Risk factors other than treatment that clearly affect success are preoperative IOP, number of previous ocular procedures with conjunctival incision, the number of procedures with conjunctival incisions, and Hispanic ethnicity.
v. The development of late-onset bleb leak was more likely to occur in the 5-FU group than in the standard therapy group.

Conclusion
Adjuvant 5-FU improved the success rates of trabeculectomy when followed up for 5 years, especially in eyes with poor prognosis.

11. **AVB (Ahmed vs. Baerveldt Study)**
Purpose
To compare two frequently used aqueous shunts for the treatment of glaucoma.

Results
i. Both implants were effective in lowering IOP. The Ahmed group had a lower mean IOP in the early postoperative period. The Baerveldt group had a greater IOP reduction than the Ahmed group at all follow-up visits beginning at 1 year and continuing to 5 years.
ii. After 5 years of follow-up, the Ahmed group had a higher failure rate of 53% compared with 40% in the Baerveldt group.
iii. The two groups had similar complication rates (Ahmed 63%, Baerveldt 69%) and intervention rates.
iv. Hypotony resulted in failure in five patients in the Baerveldt group compared with none in the Ahmed group.

Conclusion
Both implants were effective in reducing IOP and the need for glaucoma medications. The Baerveldt group had a lower failure rate and a lower IOP on fewer medications than the Ahmed group but had a small risk of hypotony that was not seen in the Ahmed group.

12. **ABC (Ahmed Baerveldt Comparison Study)**
Question asked
What are the relative efficacy and complications of the Ahmed glaucoma valve (AGV) and the Baerveldt glaucoma implant (BGI) in refractory glaucoma?

Results
i. The BGI group had a statistically significant lower mean IOP than the AGV group at most of the annual study visits, including at 5 years.
ii. The mean number of medications in the AGV and BGI groups did not vary significantly at any of the annual follow-up visits.

iii. Similar rates of surgical success were observed with both implants during 5 years of follow-up, but the reasons for treatment failure were different.
   iv. Failure after AGV was usually due to high IOP endpoints, while failure with the BGI was most commonly related to safety endpoints (hypotony, implant explantation, and loss of light perception).

   Conclusion
   Similar rates of surgical success were observed with both implants at 5 years. BGI implantation produced greater IOP reduction and a lower rate of glaucoma reoperation than AGV implantation, but BGI implantation was associated with twice as many failures.

13. **UKGTS (United Kingdom Glaucoma Treatment Study)**
    Question asked
    Does treatment with a topical prostaglandin analog, compared with placebo, reduce the frequency of VF deterioration events in patients with OAG?

    Results
      i. Patients were randomly assigned to treatment with latanoprost 0.005% or placebo.
      ii. Visual field preservation was significantly longer in the latanoprost group than in the placebo group.
      iii. The intraocular-pressure reduction compared with baseline was 3.8 mm Hg in the latanoprost group and 0.9 mm Hg in the placebo group.
      iv. A VF endpoint was reached by 24 months in 34% of participants in the untreated group versus in 20% of participants in the treated group.

    Conclusion
    The study provides evidence of the vision-preserving benefits of topical prostaglandin analogs.

14. **HORIZON study**
    Purpose
    To compare cataract surgery with implantation of a Schlemm canal microstent with cataract surgery alone for the reduction of IOP and medication use.

    Conclusion
    This 2-year study demonstrated a superior reduction in IOP and medicine use in the cataract surgery along with the Schlemm canal microstent group, compared to the cataract surgery alone group.

11.10 UVEITIS STUDIES

1. **SITE (Systemic Immunosuppressive Therapy for Eye diseases) Study**

   Purpose

   To compare the occurrence of malignancy in patients with severe ocular inflammatory disease treated with systemic corticosteroids alone or with systemic immunosuppressive drugs with or without systemic corticosteroids.

   Result

   It was a retrospective cohort study comparing ocular inflammatory disease treated with systemic steroids or immunosuppressive chemotherapy. The rate of malignancy in the immunosuppressant group was not significantly different from the rate in the corticosteroids alone group ($p > 0.90$).

   Conclusion

   These findings do not support the hypothesis of an increased risk of malignancy in patients with severe ocular inflammatory disease who are treated with systemic immunosuppressive agents compared with patients treated with systemic corticosteroids.

2. **MUST (The Multicenter Uveitis Steroid Treatment Trial) Study**

   Question asked

   Whether systemic corticosteroids plus immunosuppression when indicated (systemic therapy) is relatively more effective than fluocinolone acetonide (FA) implant (implant therapy) for noninfectious intermediate, posterior, or pan uveitis?

   Result

   This was a randomized controlled parallel superiority trial for 24 months.

   In each treatment group, mean visual acuity (VA) improved over 24 months, with neither approach superior to a degree detectable with the study's power.

   Implant-assigned eyes had a higher risk of cataract surgery, treatment for elevated intraocular pressure, and glaucoma.

   Systemic-assigned patients had more prescription-requiring infections without notable long-term consequences.

   Conclusion

   The specific advantages and disadvantages identified should dictate selection between the alternative treatments in consideration of individual patient's particular circumstances. Systemic therapy with aggressive use of corticosteroid-sparing immunosuppression was well tolerated, suggesting that this approach is reasonably safe for local and systemic inflammatory disorders.

3. **SAVE (Sirolimus as a Therapeutic Approach Uveitis) Study**

   Purpose

   To determine the efficacy and safety of repeated intravitreal and subconjunctival administrations of sirolimus in patients with noninfectious uveitis—1 year

   Result

   Open-label, prospective, and randomized interventional clinical trials in which patients with noninfectious intermediate, posterior, or panuveitis were randomized 1:1 to receive sirolimus intravitreal or subconjunctival injection. Sirolimus was administered at days 0, 60, and 120. At month 6, all subjects were allowed to receive sirolimus at intervals ≥2 months and until month 12. Changes in vitreous haze (VH), VA, and retinal thickness at month 12 were compared with baseline.

   At the end of 1 year, no statistical differences in efficacy were found between intravitreal and subconjunctival groups. No serious adverse events were determined to be secondary to sirolimus.

   Conclusion

   Repeated subconjunctival/intravitreal injections of sirolimus appear to be tolerated by patients with noninfectious uveitis over 12 months. The intravitreal route, however, was better tolerated.

4. **Shield, Insure, Endure Study**

   Purpose

   To determine the efficacy and safety of different doses of secukinumab, a fully human monoclonal antibody for targeted interleukin-17A blockade, in patients with noninfectious uveitis

   Result

   Three multicenter, randomized, double-masked, placebo-controlled, dose-ranging phase III studies: SHIELD, INSURE, and ENDURE.

   A total of 118 patients with Behçet's uveitis (SHIELD study); 31 patients with active, noninfectious, non-Behçet's uveitis (INSURE study); and 125 patients with quiescent, noninfectious, non-Behçet's uveitis (ENDURE study) were enrolled.

   The main endpoint is reduction of uveitis recurrence or VH score during withdrawal of concomitant immunosuppressive medication (ISM). Other endpoints included best-corrected VA, ISM use, and safety outcomes.

   Conclusion

   The primary efficacy endpoints of the three studies were not met. The secondary efficacy data from these studies suggest a beneficial effect of secukinumab in reducing the use of concomitant ISM.

5. **HURON Study**

    Purpose

    To evaluate the safety and effectiveness of an intravitreal implant of dexamethasone (DEX) for the treatment of noninfectious intermediate or posterior uveitis.

    Result

    In this 26-week trial, eyes with noninfectious intermediate or posterior uveitis were randomized to a single treatment with a 0.7-mg/0.35-mg DEX implant or sham procedure.

    The main outcome measure was the proportion of eyes with a VH score of 0 at week 8.
    i. The proportion of eyes with a VH score of 0 at week 8 was better with the 0.7-mg DEX implant, followed by 0.35-mg DEX implant, and less with the sham; this benefit persisted through week 26.
    ii. A gain of 15 or more letters from baseline best-corrected visual acuity (BCVA) was seen in significantly more eyes in the DEX implant groups than the sham group at all study visits.

    Conclusion

    In patients with noninfectious intermediate or posterior uveitis, a single DEX implant significantly improved intraocular inflammation and VA, persisting for 6 months. Dexamethasone intravitreal implant may be used safely and effectively for treatment of intermediate and posterior uveitis.

6. **MACRT (Monoclonal Antibody CMV Retinitis Trial) Study**

    Question asked

    Whether intravenous human monoclonal antibody to cytomegalovirus (CMV), MSL-109, is effective and safe as an adjuvant treatment for CMV retinitis?

    Result

    Two hundred nine patients with acquired immunodeficiency syndrome and active CMV retinitis were enrolled in a multicenter, randomized, placebo-controlled clinical trial. Patients received adjuvant treatment with MSL-109, 60 mg intravenously every 2 weeks, or placebo.

    Conclusion

    Intravenous MSL-109, every 2 weeks, appeared to be an ineffective adjuvant therapy for CMV retinitis, and the mortality rate was higher in the MSL-109-treated group.

7. **HPCRT (HPMPC Peripheral CMV Retinitis Trial) Study**

    Question asked

    Whether two doses of intravenous cidofovir (HPMPC) is effective and safe in short- and long-term treatment of small peripheral CMV retinitis lesions?

Result

It was a multicenter, randomized, controlled clinical trial.

Patients were randomly assigned to one of three groups: The deferral group, in which treatment was deferred until retinitis progressed; the low-dose cidofovir group (5 mg/kg once weekly for 2 weeks), then maintenance therapy once every 2 weeks; or the high-dose cidofovir group, which received cidofovir (5 mg/kg once weekly for 2 weeks), then maintenance therapy once every 2 weeks.

Progression of retinitis, the amount of retinal area involved by CMV, and the loss of VA were evaluated.

Conclusion

Intravenous cidofovir, high or low dose, effectively slowed the progression of CMV retinitis.

8. **CRRT (CMV Retinitis Retreatment Trial) Study**

Purpose

To assess the safety and efficacy of three therapeutic regimens (foscarnet, ganciclovir, or the combination) for recurrent or persistent acquired immunodeficiency syndrome (AIDS)-related CMV retinitis

Result

Patients were randomized to receive foscarnet, ganciclovir, or a combination of the two drugs.

Initially, patients undergo single or multiple cycles of induction therapy for 14 days, followed by maintenance therapy. Patients in whom the retinitis continues to progress or who are intolerant of the initial treatment switch to the alternative drug for further cycles of induction and maintenance.

Patients on the combination arm in whom retinitis continues to progress were given further cycles of the combination at an increased dose, or if one drug is causing toxicity, they were given further cycles with the alternative drug. Patients were followed up monthly for 6 months and then every 3 months thereafter.

Although no difference could be detected in VA outcomes, visual field loss and retinal area involvement on fundus photographs, both paralleled the progression results, with the most favorable results in the combination therapy group.

Conclusion

For patients with AIDS and CMV retinitis whose retinitis has relapsed and who can tolerate both drugs, combination therapy appears to be the most effective therapy for controlling CMV retinitis.

9. FGCRT (Foscarnet-Ganciclovir CMV Retinitis Trial) Study

Purpose

To evaluate the relative safety and efficacy of ganciclovir and foscarnet as the initial treatment of patients with CMV retinitis.

Result

The FGCRT was a multicenter, randomized, controlled clinical trial comparing foscarnet and ganciclovir as initial therapy for CMV retinitis.

Patients with previously untreated CMV retinitis were randomized to therapy with either intravenous ganciclovir or intravenous foscarnet. The outcome measures of this trial were survival and retinitis progression.

i. Excess mortality in the ganciclovir group (as compared with the foscarnet group) led the Policy and Data Monitoring Board to recommend suspension of the treatment protocol 19 months after the trial started.

ii. There was no difference between the two treatment groups in the rate of progression of retinitis.

Conclusion

These results suggest that for patients with AIDS, and CMV retinitis, treatment with foscarnet offers a survival advantage over treatment with ganciclovir.

10. COMA (Collaborative Ocular Melanoma) Study

Purpose

To compare the effectiveness of brachytherapy to enucleation for treatment of medium-sized choroidal melanomas.

Result

The COMS (Collaborative Ocular Melanoma Study) is a three-arm study that includes two multicenter randomized clinical trials designed to compare the effectiveness of brachytherapy to enucleation for the treatment of medium-sized choroidal melanomas and the effectiveness of enucleation with and without preoperative external-beam radiotherapy for large choroidal melanomas. The third arm is an observational study of small choroidal melanomas.

Conclusion

Similar rates of mortality after treatment with enucleation and brachytherapy shift the emphasis of selection of therapy to secondary outcomes such as preservation of vision.

11. FAUS (Fluocinolone Acetonide Uveitis Study)

Purpose

The purpose of this study was to evaluate the safety and efficacy of a 0.59- and 2.1-mg FA intravitreal implant in patients with noninfectious posterior uveitis.

Result

A prospective, multicenter, randomized, double-masked, dose-controlled study was performed. Patients were randomized to the 0.59- or 2.1-mg FA intravitreal implant and were evaluated at visits through 3 years. Outcomes included uveitis recurrence rate, BCVA, use of adjunctive therapy, and safety.

Conclusion

The FA intravitreal implant significantly reduced uveitis recurrence rates and led to improvements in visual acuity and reductions in adjunctive therapy. Lens clarity and intraocular pressure require monitoring.

12. **POINT study (PeriOcular vs. INTravitreal corticosteroids for uveitic macular oedema trial)**

Purpose

To evaluate the comparative effectiveness of three regional corticosteroid injections for uveitic macular edema: Periocular triamcinolone acetonide (PTA), intravitreal triamcinolone acetonide (ITA), and intravitreal dexamethasone implant (IDI).

Conclusion

Intravitreal triamcinolone acetonide and the IDI were superior to PTA for treating uveitic macular edema.

11.11 PEDIATRIC OPHTHALMOLOGY

1. **ATS (Amblyopia Treatment Study)**
   Questions asked
   i. What is more effective, patching or atropine, as treatment for moderate amblyopia in children <7 years of age?
   ii. How many hours of patching should be given for severe amblyopia (vision—6/60 to 6/120)?
   iii. How many hours of patching should be given for moderate amblyopia (vision—6/24 or better)?
   iv. Should amblyopia be treated after 7 years of age?
   v. Can amblyopia recur once the treatment has been stopped?
   vi. Do near activities enhance the effect of patching on visual acuity (VA) improvement in amblyopia?
   vii. Is levodopa/carbidopa therapy effective in amblyopia treatment?

   Results
   The Pediatric Eye Disease Investigator Group (PEDIG) is a collaborative network dedicated to facilitating multicenter clinical research in strabismus, amblyopia, and other eye disorders that affect children. It has conducted 20 amblyopia treatment studies since 1997.

   In ATS 01, 419 children <7 years with amblyopia and visual acuity (VA) in the range of 6/12 to 6/60 were assigned to receive either patching or atropine. VA improved in both groups by 3.16 lines in patching and 2.84 lines in atropine group, which was statistically not significant.

   In ATS 2A, 175 children <7 years with amblyopia in the range of 6/60 to 6/120 (severe amblyopia) were recruited and were assigned to full-time patching (all hours) or 6 hours of patching per day, and VA in the amblyopic eye after 4 months was noted. There was an improvement in the amblyopic eye VA from baseline to 4 months averaged 4.8 lines in the 6-hour group and 4.7 lines in the full-time group.

   In ATS 2B, 189 children <7 years with amblyopia in the range of 6/12 to 6/24 (moderate amblyopia) were assigned to 2 hours or 6 hours of daily patching, and VA in the amblyopic eye after 4 months was noted. The improvement in the VA of the amblyopic eye from baseline to 4 months averaged 2.40 lines in each group.

   ATS 06 recruited 425 children aged 3 to <7 years with amblyopia (6/12 to 6/120) and found that performing common near activities does not improve VA outcome when treating anisometropic, strabismic, or combined amblyopia with 2 hours of daily patching.

   ATS 14 enrolled amblyopic patients and added levodopa in one of two doses randomly assigned with equal probability (0.51 or 0.76 mg/kg/TID, referred to as lower dose and higher dose, respectively) and it showed promising results with improvement in VA with both doses.

Conclusions
i. Atropine treatment is as effective as patching in the initial active treatment of amblyopia.
ii. There was no demonstrable advantage to a greater number of hours of prescribed patching (>2 hours in moderate and 6 hours in severe amblyopia) either in the magnitude of improvement or in the rate of improvement.
iii. For patients aged 7-12 years, prescribing 2-6 hours per day of patching with near visual activities and atropine can improve VA even if the amblyopia has been previously treated.
iv. For patients 13-17 years, prescribing patching 2-6 hours per day with near visual activities may improve VA when amblyopia has not been previously treated.
v. Performing common near activities does not improve VA when treating anisometropic, strabismic, or combined amblyopia with 2 hours of daily patching.
vi. Approximately one-fourth of successfully treated amblyopic children experience a recurrence within the first year of treatment. For patients treated with 6 or more hours of daily patching, the risk of recurrence is greater when patching is stopped abruptly rather than when it is reduced to 2 hours per day prior to cessation.
vii. Levodopa/carbidopa therapy for residual amblyopia in older children and teenagers is well tolerated and may improve VA.

2. **Botulinum A toxin injection into extraocular muscles as an alternative to strabismus surgery**
Question asked
Is injection of botulinum A toxin into the extraocular muscles an effective, safe alternative treatment for strabismus?

Results
The maximum time of paralysis occurred 4-5 days following the injection. The maximum correction of strabismus was 40 prism diopters.

The paralytic effect correlated with the dose of toxin injected. At the 6.25×10^{-5} µg dose, all patients required retreatment, and concentrations $<6.25 \times 10^{-5}$ µg produced no effect on strabismus.

No systemic side effects were noted in any patient. There was only one case that had involvement of the adjacent extraocular muscles that resolved following day 2, otherwise, there were no unwanted ocular side effects documented.

Conclusion
Injection of botulinum A toxin into extraocular muscle to weaken the muscle appears to be a practical adjunct or an alternative to surgical correction.

3. **Botulinum A toxin injection as a treatment for blepharospasm**

   Question asked
   Is injection of botulinum A toxin into the orbicularis oculi muscle a safe and effective treatment for symptomatic relief in patients with essential blepharospasm?

   Results
   All patients injected with botulinum A toxin into the orbicularis oculi experienced some relief from their symptoms of blepharospasm. The duration of beneficial response varied, increasing with increasing doses of the drug.

   Patients who were administered doses >20 units per eye were less likely to return within 8 weeks compared with those patients who received smaller doses.

   If the spasm-free interval after injection is <3 months, then dosage is increased by 50% on subsequent injections, usually until ptosis begins to occur as a limiting side effect.

   By trial and error, the optimum regimen was found to comprise multiple, subcutaneous injections, using a solution of 5 units/0.1 mL, avoiding the center of the upper lid (to reduce the risk of ptosis and hypotropia) and the central or medial part of the lower lid (to avoid entropion and sagging of the lower lid).

   Conclusion
   Botulinum A toxin injection into the orbicularis oculi muscle is a safe, simple, repeatable, and symptomatically helpful treatment for blepharospasm.

4. **IATS (Infant Aphakia Treatment Study)**

   Questions asked
   i. To compare the visual outcomes of patients optically corrected with contact lenses versus intraocular lenses (IOLs) following unilateral cataract surgery during early infancy.
   ii. After what age IOL placement in pediatric patients is recommended?

   Results
   A multicenter randomized clinical trial of 114 infants with unilateral congenital cataract in referral centers who were between ages 1 and 6 months at surgery. Cataract surgery with or without primary IOL implantation was performed. Contact lenses were used to correct aphakia in patients who did not receive IOLs.

   At 4.5 years of age, the median logMAR VA was not significantly different between the treated eyes in the two treatment groups. However, since the initial cataract surgery, significantly more patients in the IOL group have had at least one additional intraocular surgery (contact lens, 21%; IOL, 72%; $p < 0.001$).

Conclusions
i. There was no significant difference between the median VA of operated eyes in children who underwent primary IOL implantation and those left aphakic. However, there were significantly more adverse events and additional intraoperative procedures in the IOL group.
ii. When operating on an infant younger than 7 months of age with a unilateral cataract, leaving the eye aphakic and focusing the eye with a contact lens was recommended.

5. **ATOM (Atropine for the Treatment of Myopia) Study**
Questions asked
i. Is atropine 1% eye drops effective in controlling myopic progression? (ATOM 1).
ii. What concentrations of atropine can be used to treat myopia, and which one is most efficacious with least side effects? (ATOM 2).

Results
In ATOM 1, 400 children 6–12 years old with myopia of at least −2 D and astigmatism of −1.5 D or less were recruited. One eye was administered 1% atropine once at night, and the other eye was untreated.

In ATOM 2, 400 children aged 6–12 years with myopia of at least −2 D and astigmatism of −1.5 D or less were recruited and randomly assigned in a 2:2:1 ratio to 0.5%, 0.1%, and 0.01% atropine to be administered once nightly for 2 years.

ATOM 1 showed a 77% reduction in mean progression of myopia in 2 years with atropine 1% eye drops. However, side effects such as pupil dilation, glare, and loss of accommodation were noted. Also, there was a significant rebound of myopia progression upon cessation of atropine 1% eye drops.

ATOM 2 compared the efficacy and visual side effects of three lower doses of atropine: 0.5%, 0.1%, and 0.01% and found that 0.01% atropine is clinically similar to 0.1%, 0.5%, and 1.0% in efficacy, as compared to placebo, and had a negligible effect on accommodation and pupil size and no effect on near visual acuity.

Conclusions
i. Atropine eye drops reduce myopia progression and axial elongation in children in a dose-related manner, but a rebound phenomenon occurs with the higher doses of atropine.
ii. Atropine eye drops are safe, with no serious adverse events, but in the higher doses, the side effects of pupil dilatation, loss of accommodation, and near vision limit practical use.
iii. Atropine 0.01% has the best therapeutic index, with clinically insignificant amounts of pupil dilatation, near vision and accommodation loss, and yet is as effective as the higher doses.

iv. Atropine 0.01% appears to retard myopia progression by 50%, and retreatment after a period of treatment cessation still appears to be equally effective.

6. **COMET (Correction of Myopia Evaluation Trial)**

   Question asked
   Do progressive addition lenses (PALs) reduce the rate of myopia progression by reducing retinal blur in myopic children?

   Results
   After 5 years of follow-up, the adjusted progression of myopia (mean ± se) was −1.97 ± 0.09 D in children wearing PALs and −2.10 ± 0.09 D in children wearing single-vision lenses (SVLs), resulting in a difference of 0.13 ± 0.10 D, which was not statistically significant.

   Conclusion
   The progression of myopia is similar between children wearing PALs and single-vision lenses.

7. **LAMP (Low-concentration Atropine for Myopia Progression) study**

   Purpose
   To evaluate the efficacy and safety of low-concentration atropine eye drops at 0.05%, 0.025% and 0.01% compared with placebo with regard to myopia progression

   Conclusion
   All three concentrations of atropine eye drops reduced myopia progression along a concentration-dependent response. Of these, 0.05% atropine was most effective in controlling spherical equivalent progression and axial length elongation over a period of 1 year.

11.12 STUDIES IN NEURO-OPHTHALMOLOGY

1. ONTT (Optic Neuritis Treatment Trial)

Purpose
  i. To assess the beneficial and adverse effects of corticosteroid treatment for optic neuritis.
  ii. To determine the natural history of vision in patients who suffer optic neuritis.
  iii. To investigate the relationship between optic neuritis and multiple sclerosis (MS).

Methodology
Patients were randomized to one of the three following treatment groups at 15 clinical centers:
  i. Oral prednisone (1 mg/kg/day) for 14 days.
  ii. Intravenous methylprednisolone (250 mg every 6 hours) for 3 days, followed by oral prednisone (1 mg/kg/day) for 11 days.
  iii. Oral placebo for 14 days.

Results
  i. Intravenous methylprednisolone followed by oral prednisone accelerated the recovery of vision. However, at 6 months, there was no significant difference in visual acuity, visual fields, color vision, or contrast sensitivity when compared with placebo.
  ii. Oral prednisone alone was found to increase the risk of recurrent optic neuritis.
  iii. Treatment with intravenous (IV) steroids followed by oral steroids reduced the rate of development of MS during the first 2 years.
  iv. By 3 years, the treatment effects subsided.

Conclusion
  i. There is no role for oral prednisolone alone as a treatment modality for optic neuritis.
  ii. IV methylprednisolone followed by oral prednisone accelerates the visual recovery, but the long-term visual outcome is the same as placebo.
  iii. IV steroid regimen reduced the risk of MS in the first 2 years, but the efficacy is lost by the third year.
  iv. MRI should be obtained in all cases of optic neuritis to assess the risk of MS.
  v. Chest X-rays, blood tests, and lumbar punctures are not necessary to evaluate patients with typical clinical features of acute optic neuritis.

2. **LONS (Longitudinal Optic Neuritis Study)**

   Questions asked
   i. What is the risk of developing MS after optic neuritis?
   ii. What are the factors predictive of high and low risk of developing MS?

   Results
   i. The probability of developing MS by 15 years was 50%.
   ii. Development of MS has a strong relation to the presence of lesions on a noncontrast enhanced baseline brain magnetic resonance imaging (MRI). A higher number of lesions do not appreciably increase the risk.
   iii. After 10 years, the risk of developing MS was very low for patients without baseline lesions but remained substantial for those with lesions.
   iv. The factors with a lower risk for developing MS were male gender, optic disk swelling, and certain atypical features of optic neuritis like:
       - No light perception
       - Absence of pain
       - Ophthalmoscopic findings of severe optic disk edema, peripapillary hemorrhages, or retinal exudates.

   Conclusion
   i. The presence of brain MRI abnormalities at the time of an optic neuritis attack is a strong predictor of the 15-year risk of MS.
   ii. In the absence of MRI lesions, male gender, optic disk swelling, and atypical clinical features of optic neuritis are associated with a low likelihood of developing MS.

3. **Idiopathic Intracranial Hypertension (IIH) Treatment Trial. (multicenter, randomized, double-masked, placebo-controlled study)**

   Questions asked
   i. Whether acetazolamide (ACZ) is beneficial in improving vision when added to a low-sodium weight reduction diet in patients with IIH and mild visual loss?
   ii. Does vitamin A play a role in the development of idiopathic intracranial hypertension (IIH)?
   iii. Do optic disk hemorrhages have any correlation with visual outcome in IIH?

   Results
   i. There was significant improvement in Frisén papilledema grade associated with ACZ treatment in the study eye and in the fellow eye.

ii. Acetazolamide-treated participants also experienced significant improvement in quality-of-life measures, including the VFQ-25 total score.
   iii. No significant treatment effects were noted with respect to headache disability or visual acuity.
   iv. At the study entry of the vitamin A metabolites, only serum all-trans retinoic acid (ATRA) was significantly different in IIHTT subjects and controls. Except for alpha-carotene and cerebrospinal fluid (CSF) ATRA, no other vitamin A measures were significantly altered over 6 months in either the ACZ or the placebo group.
   v. 71% of subjects that met the criteria for treatment failure had nerve fiber layer hemorrhages in at least one eye. Subjects with nerve fiber layer hemorrhages had a higher CSF pressure.

   Conclusion
   i. In patients with IIH and mild visual loss, the use of ACZ with a low-sodium weight-reduction diet resulted in modest improvement in visual field function.
   ii. Acetazolamide appears to have an acceptable safety profile at dosages up to 4 g/day in the treatment of IIH.
   iii. Vitamin A toxicity is unlikely a contributory factor in the causation of IIH.
   iv. Nerve fiber layer hemorrhages are common in patients with IIH with mild visual loss and correlate with the severity of the papilledema. They occur more frequently in treatment failure subjects and, therefore, may be associated with poor visual outcomes.

4. **The Longitudinal Idiopathic Hypertension Trial**
   Purpose
   To determine whether the beneficial effects of ACZ in improving vision at 6 months continues to month 12 in participants of the IIHTT (Idiopathic Intracranial Hypertension Treatment Trial)

   Results
   i. In the IIHTT, subjects were randomly assigned to placebo-plus-diet or maximally tolerated dosage of ACZ-plus-diet. At 6 months, some subjects from the placebo group were transitioned from placebo to ACZ.
   ii. At 12 months, papilledema grade, quality of life (QoL), and headache disability scores showed significant improvements in the group and transitioned from placebo to ACZ.

   Conclusion and Inference
   Improvements in papilledema grade, headache, and QoL measures continued from month 6 to 12 of the IIHTT in all treatment groups, most marked in the placebo group transitioned to ACZ.

5. **International Optic Nerve Trauma Study**

   Purpose
   i. To compare the visual outcome of patients of traumatic optic neuropathy treated with:
      - Corticosteroids
      - Optic canal decompression surgery
      - Observed without treatment.

   Results
   Visual acuity by ≥3 lines in 32% of the surgery group, 57% of the untreated group, and 52% of the steroid group.

   Conclusion
   There is no clear benefit for either corticosteroid therapy or optic canal decompression surgery in traumatic optic neuropathy.

6. **Champs Study (The Controlled High-Risk Avonex Multiple Sclerosis Trial)**

   Purpose
   To determine whether interferon beta (Avonex) treatment would benefit patients who had experienced a first acute demyelinating event involving the optic nerve, brain stem/cerebellum, or spinal cord and who displayed MRI brain signal abnormalities that have previously predicted a high likelihood of future MS-like events

   Results
   i. The Avonex-treated group demonstrated a 44% reduction in the 3-year cumulative probability of developing clinically definite MS.
   ii. Among placebo-treated patients, 82% had developed a new subclinical MRI signal abnormality by the 18th month after study entry.

   Conclusion
   This study supports the efficacy of Avonex therapy in significantly reducing the 3-year likelihood of future neurologic events and worsening of the brain MRI in patients with a first acute central nervous system (CNS) demyelinating event.

7. **A Randomized Placebo-Controlled Trial of Idebenone in Leber's Hereditary Optic Neuropathy (LHON) (multicenter double-blind, randomized, placebo-controlled trial)**

   Purpose
   To determine the efficacy and safety of idebenone in LHON (idebenone is a potent antioxidant and inhibitor of lipid peroxidation, interacting with the mitochondrial electron transport chain and facilitating mitochondrial electron flux in bypassing complex I)

Results
i. The primary endpoint was the best recovery in visual acuity. The main secondary endpoint was the change in best visual acuity. Other secondary endpoints were changes in visual acuity of the best eye at baseline and changes in visual acuity for both eyes in each patient.
ii. The primary endpoint did not reach statistical significance in the intention to treat population. However, post hoc interaction analysis showed a different response to idebenone in patients with discordant visual acuities at baseline; in these patients, all secondary endpoints were significantly different between the idebenone and placebo groups.

Conclusion
This trial provides evidence that patients with discordant visual acuities are the most likely to benefit from idebenone treatment, which is safe and well tolerated.

11.13 CATARACT SURGERY

1. **Beaver Dam Eye Study**

    Question asked

    What is the prevalence and severity of lens opacities in a rural community in the United States?

    Endpoints

    Frequency (%) of lens opacities by type, age group, and sex.

    Results
    i. NS more severe than level 3 in a five-step scale of severity was found in 17.3% of right eyes.
    ii. Cortical opacities involving at least 5% of the lens were found in 16.3% of the population.
    iii. Posterior subcapsular cataract (PSC) opacities occurred in 6.0% of the population, most commonly in the central circle.
    iv. In the 75+ year age group, visually significant cataract [defined as any cataract, early or late, in the presence of best-corrected visual acuity (BCVA) of 20/32 or worse in the affected eye] was found in 45.9% (worse eye) in women and 38.8% (worse eye) in men.
    v. In the 43–54-year age group, visually significant cataract was found in 2.6% (worse eye) in women and 0.4% (worse eye) in men.

    Criticisms and limitations

    Whether these prevalence estimates can be generalized to the entire US adult population depends on whether the adult population of Beaver Dam, Wisconsin, is representative of the general US adult population. This cannot be determined as no sociodemographic or health information is given.

2. **Intracameral antibiotics and barriers during cataract surgery—evidence and barriers**

    Questions asked
    i. Is intracameral (IC) moxifloxacin prophylaxis effective in decreasing the rate of endophthalmitis in cataract surgery?
    ii. Does polymerase chain reaction (PCR) increase rate of endophthalmitis in patients?
    iii. Is IC moxifloxacin prophylaxis effective in decreasing the rate of endophthalmitis in cataract surgery complicated by PCR?
    iv. What are the barriers and concerns in the prophylactic IC use of antibiotics during cataract surgery?

    Results

    Approximately half of the eyes did not receive IC moxifloxacin and half of the eyes did, and approximately half of the eyes that had PCR received IC moxifloxacin, and half did not.

i. There was a significant decline in the endophthalmitis rate with IC moxifloxacin as compared to without IC moxifloxacin prophylaxis
  ii. PCR increased the endophthalmitis rate nearly sevenfold
  iii. IC moxifloxacin reduced the endophthalmitis rate with PCR
  iv. Barriers and concerns are:
     - Lack of a commercially approved preparation in most countries
     - Using pharmacies to compound antibiotics raises the theoretical risk of introducing intraocular contaminants or adjuvants that can cause toxic anterior segment syndrome (TASS)
     - Concerns that routine intraocular antibiotic prophylaxis can lead to increasing bacterial drug resistance

Conclusion
Routine IC moxifloxacin prophylaxis reduced the overall endophthalmitis rate. There was also a statistical benefit for eyes complicated by PCR, and IC antibiotic prophylaxis should be strongly considered for this high-risk population. Considering the association of hemorrhagic occlusive retinal vasculitis with vancomycin and the commercial unavailability of IC cefuroxime in many countries, moxifloxacin appears to be an effective option for surgeons electing IC antibiotic prophylaxis.

3. **Long-Term Posterior Capsule Opacification Reduction with Square-Edge Polymethylmethacrylate Intraocular Lens**
   Questions asked
   i. Is there any difference in long-term posterior capsule opacification (PCO) formation and Nd:YAG capsulotomy rate of a square-edge (SE) polymethylmethacrylate (PMMA) intraocular lens (IOL) modification in comparison with a round-edge (RE) PMMA IOL?
   ii. Is there any difference in long-term PCO formation and Nd:YAG capsulotomy rate of an SE PMMA IOL in comparison with SE hydrophobic acrylic IOL (SE-Acrylic)?

   Results
   The patients were randomized into two groups—one with SE single-piece PMMA IOL in one eye and an RE single-piece PMMA IOL in the fellow eye, and the other group received an SE single-piece PMMA in one eye and an SE single-piece hydrophobic acrylic IOL in the fellow eye. 9-year follow-up was achieved.
   i. The mean PCO score was significantly lower in the SE-PMMA IOL eyes compared with the contralateral RE-PMMA eyes at all follow-up visits
   ii. The mean PCO score was statistically lower in the SE-PMMA IOL eyes compared with the contralateral SE-acrylic IOL eyes
   iii. 9-year Nd:YAG capsulotomy rates were less for SE-PMMA IOLs as compared to RE-PMMA IOLs, and they were also less for SE-PMMA IOL as compared to SE-acrylic IOLs

iv. The RE-PMMA PCO rate did not plateau and continued to increase throughout the 9-year study period

Conclusion

This prospective, 9-year fellow eye comparison study suggests that an inexpensive PMMA IOL design modification—a squared optic edged—could significantly reduce the burden of vision-impairing secondary membranes in developing countries.

4. **Accuracy of Intraocular Lens Power Calculation Formulas for Highly Myopic Eyes**

Question asked

Which is the most accurate IOL power calculation formulas for eyes with an axial length (AL) >26.00 mm?

Results
  i. The Barrett Universal II formula had the lowest mean absolute error (MAE), and SRK/T and Haigis had similar MAE, and the statistical highest MAE was seen with the Holladay and Hoffer Q formulas
  ii. The Barrett Universal II formulas yielded the highest percentage of eyes within ±1.0 D and ±0.5 D of the target refraction in this study

Conclusion

Barrett Universal II formula produced the lowest predictive error and the least variable predictive error compared with the SRK/T, Haigis, Holladay, and Hoffer Q formulas. For high myopic eyes, the Barrett Universal II formula may be a more suitable choice.

5. **Combination of toric and multifocal intraocular lens implantation in bilateral cataract patients with unilateral astigmatism**

Question asked

What is the quality of binocular visual function in bilateral cataract patients with unilateral astigmatism after combined implantations of toric with multifocal IOL as compared to toric and monofocal IOL implantation?

Results
  i. Mean near vision for patient satisfaction was statistically significantly higher in toric/multifocal IOL group patients versus than that in toric/monofocal group
  ii. The stereopsis of toric/multifocal IOL eyes decreased slightly in the monofocal IOL group. Visual disturbance was not noticed in either group

Conclusion

Although the combination of toric and multifocal IOL implantation results in compromising stereoacuity, it can still provide patients with high levels of spectacle freedom and good overall binocular visual acuity.

6. **Phacoemulsification versus manual small-incision cataract surgery (SICS) for white cataract**

   Question asked

   What is the safety and efficacy of phacoemulsification as compared to manual SICS to treat white cataracts?

   Results

   Approximately half of the patients were randomized to the phacoemulsification group and half to the manual SICS group.
   i. On the first postoperative day, the manual SICS group had less corneal edema than the phacoemulsification group
   ii. The mean time was statistically significantly shorter in the manual SICS group than in the phacoemulsification group

   Conclusion

   Both techniques achieved excellent visual outcomes with low complication rates. Because manual SICS is significantly faster, less expensive, and less technology dependent than phacoemulsification, it may be a more appropriate technique in eyes with mature cataract in the developing world.

7. **Double-flanged-haptic and capsular tension ring or segment for sutureless fixation in zonular instability**

   Question asked

   Is sutureless management of zonular dialysis >120° using a capsular tension segment (CTS) or a modified capsular tension ring (m-CTR) possible?

   Result

   A successful sutureless IOL implantation with a double-flanged m-CTR/CTS technique.

   Conclusion

   This double-flanged m-CTR/CTS technique allows suture-free options for managing zonular weakness or dialysis while performing cataract surgery.

8. **Safety, efficacy, and intraoperative characteristics of DisCoVisc and Healon ophthalmic viscosurgical devices (OVD) for cataract surgery**

   Question asked

   What is the safety and efficacy of DisCoVisc ophthalmic viscosurgical device as compared to Healon OVD?

   Results
   i. DisCoVisc OVD group and Healon OVD group had statistically similar outcomes for IOP and endothelial cell loss
   ii. Viscosity of Healon OVD was most often rated "cohesive" and DisCoVisc OVD most often rated "both dispersive and cohesive"

iii. Workspace most frequently rated "full chamber maintained" when using DisCoVisc OVD and most frequently rated "workspace maintained" when using Healon OVD. "Flat" or "shallow" workspace ratings occurred only in the Healon OVD group

Conclusion
DisCoVisc OVD had both cohesive and dispersive properties and was safe and effective for every stage of cataract surgery.

9. **Advanced Phaco Systems: Developments such as high-tech fluidics improve outcomes and safety for microincision cataract surgery**
Question asked
What are the advances made in phaco machines to facilitate smaller incisions and raise the bar for safety and efficiency?

Results
Centurion Vision System:
   i. The Centurion's Intrepid Balanced Tip provides a uniquely efficient tip motion. Because of that, movement at the shaft is relatively reduced so the chance for thermal effect at the incision is reduced
   ii. The fluidics capabilities of the Centurion give less concern about complications, such as intraoperative floppy iris syndrome (IFIS), and it is also easy to operate on small pupils. Turbulence is reduced and pupils do not come down
   iii. Two computer-controlled plates squeeze the balanced salt solution (BSS) bag gently to provide a constant IOP rather than relying on gravity and a hanging bottle

WHITESTAR Signature System:
   i. The system has the ability to sequentially use true peristaltic and true venturi pumps for different steps. The design allows us to utilize the holding power of the peristaltic pump during lens disassembly and then switch over to venturi fluidics to draw the pieces safely to the phaco tip
   ii. Uses elliptical phacoemulsification technology. The longitudinal and lateral energies blend into a smooth elliptical movement. There is less repulsion at the tip, so we can use lower fluidic parameters

Vision Stellaris Enhancement System:
   i. It has high-performance vacuum-based pump technology
   ii. It has forced infusion pressure, rather than a gravity-based hanging bag, which gives very precise pressure control

Conclusion
Phaco tip design is enabling surgeons to give patients all the benefits of microincision surgery. Elliptical phacoemulsification permits them to use lower pressure, which is, in turn, supported by advances in fluidics. Fluidics based on pumps, rather than gravity, give physicians

greater control for easier removal of both soft and hard cataracts. They experience complications, such as IFIS or rupture of the posterior capsule, less often.

10. **What are the types of IOL used in iris coloboma/aniridia patients?**

    Iris-reconstruction lenses are a combination of artificial iris devices and lenses by Morcher. The optics may vary in their diameters.

    i. *67B model:* 12.5-mm aniridia implant with a 3-mm optic meant for sulcus placement or scleral suturing
    ii. *50F:* 10-mm aniridia ring with occluder panels all the way around, meant to be dialed into the capsular bag against another one
    iii. *96F:* 11-mm partial aniridia ring with an occluder paddle that covers up to three clock hours.

CHAPTER 12

Management Summary of Commonly Kept Examination Cases

12.1 NONPROLIFERATIVE DIABETIC RETINOPATHY WITH CLINICALLY SIGNIFICANT MACULAR EDEMA

AIM
The aim of my treatment is to improve vision by reducing macular edema and prevent further progression of retinopathy.

MANAGEMENT
The treatment of macular edema has to be in conjunction with the physician to have good glycemic control and control of associated systemic factors such as hypertension and dyslipidemia.

Apart from the abovementioned measures, I would like to do *fluorescein angiography (FFA) for identifying:*
1. Areas of focal and diffuse leakage
2. Pathologic enlargement of foveal avascular zone (FAZ) since the management differs based on the above factors

I would like to do optical coherence tomography (OCT):
1. To detect subtle edema
2. To look for serous macular detachment
3. For the purpose of follow-up after treatment

There are various options to treat clinically significant macular edema (CSME):
1. Laser photocoagulation
2. Intravitreal/sub-Tenon's steroids
   Triamcinolone acetonide: 2 mg in 0.05 mL/4 mg in 0.1 mL
3. Intravitreal anti-vascular endothelial growth factor (anti-VEGF):
   - Bevacizumab (Avastin): 1.25 mg in 0.05 mL
   - Ranibizumab (Lucentis): 0.3 mg in 0.05 mL
   - Pegaptanib sodium: 0.3 mg in 90 µL
4. Pars plana vitrectomy (PPV)

What to look for in FFA:
1. Look for the type of leakage: Discrete or diffuse
2. Look for macular ischemia since laser photocoagulation is harmful in ischemic maculopathy.

What to look for in OCT:
1. Vitreomacular interface abnormality
2. Thickness of macula
3. Subclinical serous macular detachment
4. Foveal contour

First-line therapy includes either laser photocoagulation [focal modified Early Treatment Diabetic Retinopathy Study (ETDRS) grid].
Or
Intravitreal pharmacotherapy ± laser photocoagulation. The decision is made based on FFA and OCT findings.

1. *I would like to do laser photocoagulation in cases of:*
   - Parafoveal edema
   - Discrete areas of leakage in FFA
   - Mild-to-moderate retinal thickening on OCT
   - No vitreomacular interface abnormalities
2. *I would prefer intravitreal injections in cases of:*
   - Foveal edema (where foveal contour is altered)
   - Diffuse leakage on FFA
   - Moderate-to-severe retinal thickening in OCT
   - Serous macular detachment on OCT

   Anti-VEGF agents are preferred over steroids. Patients might require three to four anti-VEGF injections, one every month, to dry out the macula.
3. *I would like to do PPV in cases of:*
   - Taut posterior hyaloid face
   - Vitreomacular traction

COMBINATION THERAPY

Combination therapy is an alternative therapy where first an intravitreal injection is given to bring down the edema and then it is followed by grid laser.

FOLLOW-UP

Patients are reevaluated 3 months after laser treatment. If the patient is given intravitreal anti-VEGF therapy, then the patient is reviewed after 1 month.

Management Summary of Commonly Kept Examination Cases

During follow-up,
If CSME is persistent or in cases of recurrent CSME:
I would like to:
1. Repeat photocoagulation
2. Give intravitreal triamcinolone acetonide or intravitreal anti-VEGF agent
   If CSME is refractory to photocoagulation and pharmacotherapies, then I would like to do PPV.
1. *No vitreomacular traction:* PPV with internal limiting membrane (ILM) peeling is done
2. *Taut posterior hyaloid face or vitreomacular traction syndrome (VMT):* PPV.

12.2 PROLIFERATIVE DIABETIC RETINOPATHY

AIM

The aim of my management is essentially threefold:
1. I would like to retard and stop the proliferation of new vessels (*neovascularization*), so that complications such as vitreous hemorrhage and retinal detachment could be prevented
2. I would like to use adjuvant pharmacological agents, if indicated, to treat associated macular edema
3. I would also like to work closely with the general physician to achieve good metabolic control and also to sensitize him about the necessity for regular screening for diabetic nephropathy, since both these conditions have a high frequency of occurrence in the same individuals

After confirmation of my diagnosis, I would aim and advise for systemic control of diabetes mellitus followed by ocular management of proliferative diabetic retinopathy (PDR), which involves:

1. *Medical management:* Intravitreal anti-vascular endothelial growth factor (anti-VEGF) agents, triamcinolone acetonide, dexamethasone implants (Ozurdex)
2. *Laser treatment:* Scatter panretinal photocoagulation (PRP) focal grid laser
3. *Surgical management:* Pars plana vitrectomy (PPV) with endolaser PRP

My mainstay of the treatment for PDR involves the use of thermal laser photocoagulation in a panretinal pattern to induce regression of new vessel formation, i.e., neovascularization of disk (NVD) or neovascularization elsewhere (NVE), and to avoid its complications.

Also, I would perform PRP in PDR in any of the following associated findings:
1. NVD or NVE of any degree if associated with preretinal or vitreous hemorrhage
2. Rubeosis with or without neovascular glaucoma
3. Moderate-to-severe NVE alone, particularly in juvenile diabetic patients
4. Widespread retinal ischemia and capillary dropout on fluorescein angiography
5. PDR developing in pregnancy, particularly with the institution of tight metabolic control
6. Preproliferative retinopathy in the second eye of a juvenile diabetic patient with severe PDR in the other eye

And I would do a focal grid laser in case of associated diabetic macular edema (DME)/clinically significant macular edema (CSME) in the presence of the following criteria:
1. Retinal edema located at or within 500 μm of the center of the macula
2. Hard exudates at or within 500 μm of the center of the macula if associated with thickening of the adjacent retina

3. A zone of thickening larger than one disk area if located within one disk diameter of the center of the macula

I would do an urgent PRP along with intravitreal anti-VEGF therapy if the PDR is at the high-risk stage (i.e., if NVD is extensive or vitreous/preretinal hemorrhage has occurred recently).

I would start intravitreal anti-VEGF therapy such as *ranibizumab* (*Lucentis*) *0.3–0.5 mg/0.05 mL* or *bevacizumab* (*Avastin*) *1.25 mg/0.05 mL*, or *pegaptanib* (*Macugen*) *0.3 mg/0.09 mL*, or *aflibercept* (*Eylea*) *2 mg /0.05 mL* to temporarily decrease leakage and cause regression of diabetic neovascularization and also as an adjunct to vitrectomy for diabetic traction retinal detachment by reducing intraoperative bleeding and allowing for easier dissection when administered preoperatively.

Also, in the presence of associated macular edema, I would administer triamcinolone acetate *1 or 4 mg* intravitreal injection (IVTA) or dexamethasone intravitreal implant (Ozurdex) which contains dexamethasone *350 or 700 µL* available as a biodegradable slow-release implant.

I would advise surgical management with PPV in case of:
1. Development of sequelae of advanced PDR like dense, nonclearing persistent vitreous hemorrhage despite maximal PRP
2. Tractional retinal detachment (macula-threatening)
3. Combined traction-rhegmatogenous retinal detachment
4. Vitreous hemorrhage with coexisting rubeosis iridis
5. Presence of diffuse DME associated with posterior hyaloidal traction
6. Severe progressive fibrovascular proliferation
7. Anterior segment neovascularization with media opacities preventing photocoagulation
8. Dense premacular (subhyaloid) hemorrhage

I would follow up with the patients according to the type of PDR as follows:

Severity of PDR	Follow-up (months)	PRP scatter laser	Focal/ grid laser	Intravitreal anti-VEGF therapy/IVTA	Surgery (PPV)
Nonhigh-risk PDR	4	If needed	No	No	Not always
High-risk PDR	4	Highly recommended	No	Beneficial	Recommended
DME	4	Recommended	If needed, yes	If needed, yes	If needed in chronic DME
CSME	1	Recommended	If needed, yes	If needed, yes	If needed, in vitreomacular traction

12.3 RHEGMATOGENOUS RETINAL DETACHMENT

AIM

The main aim of my management is to achieve the anatomical restoration of the detached retina with the choroid with the ultimate aim being to restore the maximum possible visual acuity. In addition, I would also like to treat the other eye prophylactically for any predisposing lesions.

STEPS

1. The definitive treatment is surgery, but before intervening we should determine visual potential and explain the prognosis very clearly to the patient. (The patient should understand that in some cases, there may not be any improvement in vision postoperatively. And in even rarer cases, there is a drop in existing vision.)
2. The most important step is to do a thorough indirect ophthalmoscopic examination of the affected eye to find the extent of the retinal detachment (RD) and locate the breaks and predisposing lesions. The fellow eye should also be examined to search for such predisposing lesions.
3. The choice of procedure is based on certain factors:
    i. Location and extent of the RD and breaks
    ii. Presence or absence of proliferative vitreoretinopathy (PVR) changes
    iii. Age of the patient
    iv. Lens status
4. The principles of surgery are as follows:
    i. Find all breaks (see the lesion)
    ii. Create chorioretinal adhesion around each break (seal the lesion)
    iii. Bring the retina and choroid close together for a sufficient duration so that a chorioretinal adhesion is formed which will close the subretinal space permanently. This is done from the outside by scleral buckling and inside by intraocular gases or silicon oil

The procedures done are as follows:
1. *Laser demarcation:* It is indicated in small peripheral RDs with no risk of progression. It is usually found in young myopes with clear media.
    The aim is to create a band of effective chorioretinal adhesion which surrounds the detached area completely.
2. *Pneumatic retinopexy:* It is done in rhegmatogenous retinal detachments (RRDs) in phakic eyes with superior breaks, not extending beyond 2 clock hours and without any PVR changes.
    An expanding gas (C_3F_8 or SF_6) is injected into the retina. Cryo or laser is done to induce chorioretinal adhesion once the retina is reattached. The patient should be compliant and willing to maintain a specific head position postoperatively.

3. *Scleral buckling:* It is indicated in RRDs with breaks which are close together without any PVR changes.

   The aim of buckling is to create an indentation of the sclera beneath the retinal break.
4. *Vitrectomy:* It is indicated in eyes with extensive detachment, multiple breaks, breaks inaccessible to buckling (like posterior breaks), media opacities, PVR changes, and vitreous traction.

   It is usually combined with cataract surgery in phakic eyes because the chance of postoperative cataract development is very high.

   The aim of primary vitrectomy is to remove vitreous attachments to the retinal breaks, drain the subretinal fluid, tamponade the breaks with air, gas, or silicon oil, and create chorioretinal adhesion using endolaser photocoagulation or cryopexy.

   A supplemental scleral buckle can be combined along with primary vitrectomy in very extensive RDs, where complete clearance of vitreous is not possible, or in cases with a risk of PVR changes in the future.

12.4 RETINITIS PIGMENTOSA

AIM

The main aim of my management is to provide visual rehabilitation by appropriate management of comorbid ocular conditions and providing low-vision devices with the ultimate aim of achieving the maximum possible visual acuity.

In addition, I would like to exclude/manage systemic associations by a multidisciplinary approach and also provide genetic counseling, updated information of treatment options, psychological support, and counseling.

TREATMENT MODALITIES

Although retinitis pigmentosa (RP) is currently incurable, the morbidity associated can be reduced by a multidisciplinary approach. These patients require annual ophthalmic evaluation which includes visual acuity assessment, ocular examination, and color vision. Periodic electroretinography (ERG) may be considered for prognostic value.

A systemic examination is important to rule out syndromes associated with RP such as Usher syndrome, Waardenburg syndrome, Refsum disease, abetalipoproteinemia, mucopolysaccharidosis, Bardet-Biedl syndrome, Alport syndrome, Alström syndrome, Kearns–Sayre syndrome, and essential gyrate atrophy.

Counseling the patient regarding the prognosis and progressive nature of the disease is important.

MEDICAL TREATMENT

Considering the neurodegenerative etiopathogenesis, various antioxidant formulations may be prescribed on an empirical basis like:
- Vitamin A: 15,000 IU/day, beta-carotene: 25,000 IU/day
- Docosahexaenoic acid: 400 mg/day
- Lutein/zeaxanthin: 6–20 mg/day (increases macular pigment)

These nutritional supplements may help in preventing further retinal damage and in slowing down the progression of the disease.

CATARACT IN RETINITIS PIGMENTOSA

Many RP patients develop visually significant cataract at younger ages. If the patients have a recent-onset gross defective vision in daylight as well and if there is a significant central cataract, I would like to perform the cataract extraction after explaining the guarded visual prognosis. The patient needs continuous monitoring for the development of cystoid macular edema (CME) and posterior capsule opacification (PCO). These patients are at a higher risk of developing anterior capsular phimosis.

CYSTOID MACULAR EDEMA IN RETINITIS PIGMENTOSA

In cases of RP with macular edema, I would like to start topical carbonic anhydrase inhibitors such as dorzolamide (2%) e/d tds. If the patient does not respond, I would like to proceed to oral acetazolamide, an induction dose of 500 mg/day, followed by a maintenance dose of 250 mg/day.

If the patient is not responsive to carbonic anhydrase inhibitors, I would like to give an intravitreal injection of triamcinolone acetonide 2 mg in 0.05 mL/4 mg in 0.1 mL. Ozurdex (dexamethasone intravitreal implant) 0.7 mg can also be tried.

LOW-VISION AIDS

I would like to provide low-vision devices by:
1. Best refraction and simple magnification—magnifiers and closed-circuit television for near work
2. Control of glare by using dark glasses during outdoor activities—corning photochromatic filters (CPF)
3. Use of night vision scopes and high-intensity lanterns for night vision
4. Use of field enhancement procedures such as:
    i. Mirrors and prisms mounted on spectacles
    ii. Reverse Galilean telescopes
    iii. Image intensifiers

COUNSELING

The aim of *genetic counseling* is to educate patients about the hereditary nature of the disease. I would like to examine other family members to know the extent of manifestation and expected rate of progression and to establish the mode of inheritance.

I would like to provide *psychological and vocational counseling* to the patient for functional and emotional well-being.

Recent advances in the treatment of RP include:

Retinal transplantation: It involves transplanting fetal retinal cells along with attached retinal pigment epithelium (RPE) which provides nourishment to the photoreceptor cells of the patient.

Photoreceptor transplantation: It involves using adult human cadaver allogenic photoreceptor sheets harvested with the excimer laser within 24 hours of death.

Neuroprosthetic devices: Controlled electrical stimulation of the retina releases growth factors which may delay the degeneration of the retina from RP.

Pharmacologic agents: Neurotrophic factors such as basic fibroblast growth factor, ciliary neurotrophic factor, and anti-Parkinson drugs have been tried based on their antiapoptotic properties.

RETINAL PROSTHESIS

- *ARGUS II:* Artificial silicone retina of 2 mm diameter silicone chip implanted in subretinal space which stimulates the contacting retinal cells upon exposure to light.
- *EPI-RET 3 implants:* An extraocular camera fitted to spectacle lenses transmits images wirelessly to a receiver placed in the anterior vitreous. This receiver, in turn, stimulates an epiretinal implant via a connecting microcable.

Intravitreal or subretinal gene therapy: Adenoviral or lentiviral vector is used to replace the defect in identified forms of RP.

12.5 CENTRAL RETINAL VEIN OCCLUSION

AIM
The aims of my treatment would be:
1. To identify and treat the underlying systemic disorders to prevent recurrence
2. To identify and differentiate ischemic and nonischemic types of central retinal vein occlusion (CRVO) to predict the progression and treatment
3. To identify and treat the vision-threatening conditions, such as macular edema and neovascular glaucoma (NVG), promptly

TREATMENT SCHEDULE
1. The first step is to do a complete ophthalmic examination including slit-lamp examination for neovascularization of the iris, fundus examination for the severity of hemorrhage, and to look for macular edema, gonioscopy for neovascularization of the angles, and intraocular pressure for NVG. Poor presenting visual acuity and relative afferent pupillary defect (RAPD) are simple tools in predicting ischemic type.
2. The second step is to diagnose and treat underlying systemic disorders such as diabetes, hypertension, cardiovascular disorders, and dyslipidemia. In the younger age group, hypercoagulable diseases such as sickle cell anemia, leukemia, and polycythemia by doing complete blood count, prothrombin time, partial thromboplastin time, erythrocyte sedimentation rate (ESR), and antinuclear antibodies have to be ruled out. It is important to instruct the patient to avoid smoking and use of drugs such as oral contraceptive agents.
3. Optical coherence tomography (OCT) is done to quantify and monitor macular edema.
4. Fluorescein angiography (FFA) is not done routinely, but it can be done to confirm the ischemic type with capillary nonperfusion areas. If it has to be done, it has to be performed after 6 weeks after the resolution of the blood. Electroretinography (ERG) can also help in diagnosing the ischemic type in doubtful cases (b-wave amplitude reduction).
5. Macular edema, if present, can be treated with intravitreal anti-vascular endothelial growth factor (VEGF) agent, such as bevacizumab (Avastin)—1.25 mg in 0.05 mL, ranibizumab (Lucentis)—0.5 mg in 0.05 mL, aflibercept (Eylea)—2 mg in 0.05 mL, or intravitreal steroids such as triamcinolone acetonide—4 mg in 0.1 mL, or steroid implants such as Ozurdex (dexamethasone 0.7 mg).
6. Neovascularization, if present, should be treated with prompt panretinal photocoagulation (PRP). Intravitreal anti-VEGF agents can also be tried for NVG along with topical and systemic antiglaucoma therapy.

Medically unmanageable NVG cases are candidates for glaucoma drainage devices, trabeculectomy with mitomycin C (MMC), or in poor visual prognosis eyes with cyclodestructive procedures such as diode laser cyclophotocoagulation (DLCP) and cyclocryotherapy.
7. Radial optic neurotomy is a surgical mode of treatment with varying results, not commonly done.

Follow-up: The patient should be reviewed every month for the first 6 months, every 2 months up to 1 year after diagnosis, and every 4 months for 2 years.

12.6 OPTIC ATROPHY

AIM
My aim is to treat the underlying cause, preserve the existing vision, and rehabilitate the patient for daily activities.

TREATMENT
Optic atrophy is irreversible. Early diagnosis and appropriate treatment of the underlying cause can prevent further damage and the development of optic atrophy and vision loss.
1. *Primary optic atrophy:*
    i. *Retrobulbar optic neuritis:*
        - Injection methylprednisolone 1 g intravenously (IV) × 3 days followed by tapering doses of oral prednisolone
    ii. *Compressive lesions of the optic nerve:*
        Pituitary tumors
        Meningiomas } Surgical removal of the tumors
        Gliomas
    iii. *Traumatic optic atrophy:*
        - Optic atrophy occurs 3–6 weeks after injury
        - IV methylprednisolone given within 8 days of injury causes improvement in vision
        - Optic nerve decompression
    iv. *Toxic optic neuropathy:*
        Alcohols: Methanol, ethylene glycol
        The essential therapy of methanol poisoning is adequate alkalinization and methanol administration. Ethanol competes with methanol for the enzyme alcohol dehydrogenase in the liver, thereby preventing the accumulation of toxic metabolites in the body. Ethanol is given as 10% solution in 5% dextrose solution intravenously. A loading dose of 0.6 g/kg followed by an IV infusion of 0.007–0.16 g/kg/hr is recommended. Dialysis is recommended in those patients who have visual disturbances, blood methanol of 50 mg% or more, ingestion of >60 mL of methanol, and severe acidosis not corrected by sodium bicarbonate administration.

        The following drugs can cause optic neuropathy. Patients need to stop the drugs and use multivitamin supplementation.
        Antibiotics: Chloramphenicol, sulfonamides, linezolid
        Antimalarials: Chloroquine, quinine
        Antitubercular drugs: Isoniazid, ethambutol, streptomycin
        Antiarrhythmic agents: Digitalis, amiodarone
        Heavy metals: Lead, mercury
        Others: Carbon monoxide, tobacco

2. *Secondary optic atrophy:*
   i. *Papillitis:* IV methylprednisolone 1 g od × 3 days followed by tapering doses of oral prednisolone
   ii. *Papilledema*: Find out the cause for raised intracranial pressure by doing neuroimaging and treatment of the cause

   In case of idiopathic intracranial hypertension-weight reduction, T. acetazolamide 500 mg bd oral glycerol, corticosteroids

   Optic nerve decompression, repeated lumbar puncture, lumboperitoneal shunt
3. *Consecutive optic atrophy:*
   i. *Central retinal artery occlusion (CRAO)*: If the patient presents early as soon as the loss of vision occurs and if immediate treatment is done to reperfuse the retina, optic atrophy can be prevented. The treatment options include:
      - Ocular massage: Digital gonio massage
      - Anterior chamber paracentesis
      - Intraocular pressure (IOP) lowering drugs: Acetazolamide 500 mg, 20% IV mannitol, 50% oral glycerol
      - Carbogen inhalation
      - Retrobulbar or systemic vasodilators such as papaverine or tolazoline
      - Sublingual nitroglycerine
      - Fibrinolytic agents
      - Injection urokinase into internal carotid artery by femoral artery catheterization
      - Systemic thrombolysis using plasminogen
      - Systemic pentoxifylline
   ii. *Retinitis pigmentosa*
      - Treatment of allied conditions
      - Low-vision aids
      - Genetic counseling
      - Psychological and vocational counseling
4. *Cavernous optic atrophy:*
   Glaucoma
   i. IOP-lowering drugs
   ii. Filtering surgeries
   iii. Treating the cause of secondary glaucoma
   iv. Regular follow-up
   v. Screening of patients with a family history of glaucoma

5. *Segmental optic atrophy:*
    i. *Temporal pallor*
        • *Toxic amblyopia* (tobacco, ethyl alcohol): Stop smoking, abstinence from alcohol
        Injections of hydroxycobalamin 1,000 µg intramuscularly. The dose should be repeated five times at an interval of 4 days.
        • Nutritional amblyopia
        It is due to atrophy of papillomacular nerve fibers caused by deficiency of vitamins B12, B6, B1, B2, and niacin.
        Treatment-balanced diet, multivitamin supplements
    ii. *Altitudinal pallor*
        Acute ischemic optic neuropathy—IV methylprednisolone 1 g × 3 days followed by tapering doses of oral prednisolone
    iii. *Wedge-shaped pallor*
        Branch retinal artery occlusion—same as CRAO
6. *Hereditary optic atrophy:*
    i. Congenital optic atrophy ⎫
    ii. Leber's optic atrophy   ⎬ Genetic counseling
    iii. Behr's optic atrophy   ⎭

REHABILITATION

Generally, magnification and illumination control are used to enhance visual function.
1. *Reading:*
    i. Strong reading glasses
    ii. Optical and electronic magnifiers
    iii. Software to enlarge text on computer screens
2. *Illumination control:*
    Tinted wraparound sunglasses—reduce brightness but increase contrast
3. *Distance vision:*
    Handheld or spectacle-mounted telescopic devices

PROGNOSIS

Prognosis depends on many features. They are as follows:
1. *Pallor and optic atrophy:*
    Pallor does not signify optic atrophy unless there is a demonstrable defect in visual acuity, color vision, and field.
2. *Attenuation of arteries:*
    It is always a sign of poor prognosis.
3. *Papilledema combined with pallor:*
    Poor visual prognosis.

RECENT TRIAL

Intravitreal Stem Cell Transplantation

Neural progenitor cells delivered to the vitreous can integrate into the ganglion cell layer of the retina, turn on neurofilament genes, and migrate into the host optic nerve.

Stem Beads

Activation of endogenous stem cells that remains dormant within the optic nerve by implantation of biodegradable beads that release cell-activating growth factor.

12.7 PAPILLEDEMA

AIM

My primary aim would be to look for and treat the cause of increased intracranial pressure by either medical management or surgical management.

Papilledema is the result of raised intracranial pressure, which, in turn, could be caused by various etiologies such as:
  i. Idiopathic intracranial hypertension (IIH) (most common)
  ii. Mass lesions or tumors
  iii. Drugs
  iv. Cavernous sinus thrombosis and arteriovenous malformations

I would do an urgent neurologic evaluation and neuroimaging [magnetic resonance imaging (MRI) or computed tomography (CT) with contrast] to rule out:
  i. Intracranial mass lesion, hemorrhage, hydrocephalus, or venous thrombosis
  ii. Magnetic resonance (MR) venography—if a venous clot is suspected
  iii. MR angiography—if dural arteriovenous malformation is considered
   If the neuroimaging turns out to be normal, I would do a lumbar puncture to:
   - Rule out infections
   - Document for cerebrospinal fluid (CSF) opening pressure
   - Look for normal CSF composition

TREATMENT

I would treat the patient depending on the etiology causing the raised intracranial pressure.

Mass Lesions

If the raised intracranial pressure is due to a mass lesion blocking either the ventricular system or the venous outflow, I would refer the patient to a neurosurgeon to manage the condition by the removal of the lesion or if the mass lesion cannot be removed, a ventriculoperitoneal shunt or a lumboperitoneal shunt can be done.

IIH

If the neuroimaging is normal, then a diagnosis of IIH has to be made and the following treatment given:
  i. *General measures:*
   - If there is a presence of inciting factors such as drugs, I would advise the patient to discontinue those medications

- If the patient is obese, reduction in weight of the patient, as well as control of cholesterol, as a general measure yields good progress in the treatment of IIH

ii. *Medical treatment:*
I would start the patient on carbonic anhydrase inhibitors such as acetazolamide 250 mg bd and slowly increase it to 1 g so as to bring down the raised intracranial pressure

iii. *Surgical treatment:*
- Indications
  - Progressive loss of vision despite maximal medical therapy
  - Severe or rapid vision loss at onset including the development of an afferent pupillary defect or signs of advanced optic nerve dysfunction
  - Severe papilledema causing macular edema or exudates
- Surgical options
  - Optic nerve sheath decompression
  - Shunt procedures

iv. *Other causes:*
If any thrombus, hematoma (which could be secondary to trauma), or arteriovenous malformations are found out as a causative factor, I would promptly refer the patient to a neurosurgeon as it is a medical emergency.

Conditions such as sarcoid (which can give rise to a granuloma which can, in turn, obstruct the CSF outflow), tuberculosis, and syphilis need to be addressed with a combined approach of the ophthalmologist, rheumatologist (for sarcoid), and neurologist.

12.8 THIRD NERVE PALSY

AIMS

1. *Identifying the cause and treating them:*
   i. *Pupil involving the third nerve palsy* is a surgical emergency.

      The most common cause of pupil involving the third nerve palsy is an intracranial aneurysm and it requires immediate referral to neurosurgery for the relevant surgical rehabilitation such as clipping, gluing, coiling, or wrapping of the aneurysm.
   ii. In case of *pupil sparing the third nerve palsy*, ischemia is the most common cause. The cause for the ischemia is usually a vascular disorder, such as diabetes, and hence it should be looked for and controlled. With good metabolic control, the palsy will resolve spontaneously in 6–8 weeks.
2. *To relieve the patient's discomfort and treat symptomatically conservative treatment:*

   Treatment during a symptomatic interval is directed at alleviating symptoms, mainly pain and diplopia.

   Nonsteroidal anti-inflammatory drugs are the first line of treatment of choice for pain. Diplopia is not a problem when ptosis occludes the involved eye.

   When diplopia is from a large angle divergence of the visual axes, patching one eye is the only practical short-term solution.

   When the angle of deviation is smaller, fusion in the primary position often can be achieved by using a horizontal or vertical prism or both.

   Since the condition is expected to resolve spontaneously within a few weeks, most physicians would prescribe the Fresnel prism.

SURGICAL TREATMENT

It is ideal to wait for at least 6–8 months before contemplating any surgery.

Patients who do not recover from third cranial nerve palsy after 6–8 months may become candidates for surgical treatment.

Goals of Surgery

1. To improve alignment in the primary gaze
2. To produce or enlarge some degree of binocular single vision

Surgical Procedures

1. Eye muscle (*medial rectus*) resection or (*lateral rectus*) recession to treat persistent and stable angle diplopia
2. Some of these patients also may require some form of lid lift surgery like a frontalis sling for persistent ptosis that restricts vision or is cosmetically unacceptable to the patient
3. Botulinum toxin injection to the lateral rectus muscle can relieve the eye for better fusion in some patients with mild involvement.

12.9 SIXTH NERVE PALSY

AIM
The aim of my treatment is to identify and treat the primary cause of this problem. Till that time, to provide symptomatic relief for the patient and to avoid accidental injuries, I would give monocular occlusion of the affected eye or use prisms.

TREATMENT OPTIONS
1. *Isolated sixth nerve palsy in patients >50 years of age:* In such instances, the most common cause is vascular ischemia. I would like to work closely with the patient's physician to control their systemic condition such as diabetes and hypertension. I will explain to the patient that there is a high chance for spontaneous recovery within 3–4 months and also explain to them in advance that in case the recovery does not happen, then we would have to proceed with further investigations such as neuroimaging.
2. *Isolated sixth nerve palsy in patients <50 years of age (young patients):* Since the patient is young, I would like to look for varied causes. I would like to do neuroimaging apart from the blood investigations such as total count (TC), differential count (DC), erythrocyte sedimentation rate (ESR), fasting blood sugar (FBS), and postprandial blood sugar (PPBS). I will also rule out systemic hypertension. If all these parameters are normal, then I will reassure the patient that this condition will be self-limiting in around 3 months and would review the patient periodically.
3. If the sixth nerve palsy is associated with other neurologic involvement or other cranial nerve involvement, then a routine neuroimaging of the brain [magnetic resonance imaging (MRI)] is performed.
4. Surgical: In case the strabismus does not improve, then surgery can be considered, after waiting for at least 8–10 months. The surgeries performed will be ipsilateral weakening of the medial rectus and strengthening of the ipsilateral lateral rectus.
5. Botulinum toxin injection can be considered as a chemodenervation of the antagonist medial rectus to provide transient symptomatic relief. However, it may mask the progression of the lesion and the involvement of the other extraocular muscles.

12.10 MYASTHENIA GRAVIS

AIM

The aim of my treatment is to provide symptomatic relief to the patient from ptosis and diplopia and achieve remission of the disease by treating the underlying etiology, which is autoimmunity.

TREATMENT PROTOCOL

Management can be divided into:
1. Symptomatic therapy
2. Disease-modifying agents

First, for symptomatic therapy, I will start the patient on acetylcholinesterase inhibitors, pyridostigmine bromide or neostigmine bromide, thereby increasing the availability of acetylcholine at the neuromuscular junction. Pyridostigmine being the preferred agent due to its longer duration of action is started at a low dose: *30 mg tds* (onset of action occurs within 30 minutes and peaks at 1-2 hours).

He is then observed for the improvement of ptosis and relief from diplopia.

If improvement is seen, he can be maintained with the same dose. If there is no symptomatic relief, the dose can be increased until the desired result is achieved.

If the patient is not showing any improvement even with an increased dose of pyridostigmine, the next line of management, i.e., corticosteroids, is added at the lowest possible dose (T. prednisolone 10 mg/day).

This is slowly increased by 10 mg every 4 days to a dose of 1 mg/kg/day (60 mg/day) as a morning dose.

Once remission is achieved, the dose can be tapered slowly. If during tapering, exacerbation is seen, the patient is started with the previous high dose.

In situations where steroids are avoided/side effects are not tolerated by the patient, immunosuppressive drugs can be given. The most common, T. azathioprine, is initiated as a dose of 50 mg/day and increased by 50 mg every week to 150–200 mg/day.

12.11 THYROID-RELATED ORBITOPATHY

AIM

The aim of my treatment is to halt disease progression and to reduce disease activity:

The decision on whether thyroid-related ophthalmopathy (TRO) must be treated and requires what type of treatment relies on the activity and severity of the disease. Active disease is defined as the progression of any of the VISA parameters or Clinical Activity Score (CAS) of 4 or more (max score = 8). The level of activity can be further divided into mild (CAS 4 or less without deterioration), moderate to severe (CAS 5 or more, or progressive disease), or vision threatening. From the endocrine perspective, the goal of the treatment for patients with Graves' disease is the achievement of a euthyroid state. Patients should be counseled regarding the risks of smoking and the benefits of smoking cessation.

The order of treatment follows the sequence in the *V-I-S-A* grading system.

1. *V*ision-threatening TRO—due to dysthyroid optic neuropathy or corneal ulceration; it is treated first.
2. *I*nflammation is the next priority treated with conservative measures, corticosteroids, steroid-sparing immunosuppressives, and/or radiotherapy.
3. *S*trabismus is managed medically (e.g., Fresnel prisms) until the inflammation subsides. Later, strabismus surgery can be planned if required.
4. *A*ppearance—proptosis, eyelid retraction, dermatochalasis, and fat prolapse can be managed surgically.

MILD TRO (CAS <3)

The main aim of my treatment would be to alleviate the patient of his dry eye symptoms and to closely observe him for worsening of the disease. I would prescribe ocular lubricants and advise him to wear glasses for wind avoidance and to elevate the head end of the bed to reduce the periorbital swelling.

MODERATE/SEVERE TRO (CAS >4)

The aim of my treatment is to halt disease progression and to reduce disease activity. My first choice would be:

Intravenous (IV) dosage: 500 mg of IV methylprednisolone given weekly for 6 weeks followed by 250 mg of IV methylprednisolone weekly for 6 more weeks.

CAUTION: HEPATIC DYSFUNCTION

Alternatively, oral corticosteroids, T. prednisolone, at a dose of 1-1.5 mg/kg and tapered slowly depending on the response. Usually, the dose is tapered at 10 mg/week until 20 mg/day is reached and then reduced by 5 mg/week.

CAUTION: BLOOD SUGAR LEVELS, OSTEOPOROSIS
Pulse-steroid Therapy in Dysthyroid Optic Neuropathy

Adults: IV methylprednisolone 1 g od 3 days (or) 500 mg bd 3 days.

This is followed by rapid tapering of oral steroids.

Rituximab is a new promising drug with comparable results in active thyroid ophthalmopathy.

Cyclosporine is rarely useful individually but can be used along with steroids.

RADIOTHERAPY

Radiotherapy is beneficial only for moderate or worse active disease or with confirmed disease progression. The standard dosing regimen is 20 Gy/orbit in 10 fractions administered over 2 weeks. A temporary worsening of inflammation often occurs after orbital radiation (OR) and can be prevented with concurrent glucocorticoid use. OR is relatively contraindicated in diabetic patients and those with concurrent vascular disease due to the risk of worsening retinal microvascular function and should be used with caution in patients under 35 years of age due to the theoretic risk of secondary malignancy.

Surgery for Thyroid-related Orbitopathy

In Active Disease

Urgent indication: Prompt orbital decompression in dysthyroid optic neuropathy is usually done if the response to IV steroids is poor. Postdecompression patients may require steroid therapy. Medial wall decompression is more preferred, but balanced medial plus lateral wall decompression can be done.

In Inactive Disease

1. Inactive disease: Defined as no activity or progression over 6-12 months
2. The sequence of surgery for inactive TRO, if necessary, is typically decompression, followed by strabismus surgery, and finally eyelid repair

3. Medial wall removal (especially posteriorly) is most effective in relieving orbital apex crowding
4. Strabismus surgery is aimed at correcting diplopia in the primary position and downgaze by recessing the restricted muscles, frequently with adjustable sutures to improve postoperative alignment
5. Eyelid surgery may involve recession of the upper eyelid retractors, recession of the lower eyelid retractors with or without a spacer graft, and conservative blepharoplasty.

12.12 ENTROPION

AIM

The aim of the treatment is to relieve the symptoms, preserve the cornea, and maintain lid integrity.

The patients are started on medical management first with lubricants, ideally without preservatives. Bandage contact lenses may be used as a temporary measure, especially to protect the cornea. Botulinum toxin may be used in spastic entropion.

SURGICAL TREATMENT

Congenital Entropion (Epiblepharon, Tarsal Kink Syndrome)

The principle is to hold the two lamellae together by full-thickness eyelid eversion sutures.

Upper eyelid entropion (Kemp and Collin classification)

Degree of entropion	Procedure
Minimal	Anterior lamellar ± lid split at gray line
Moderate	Anterior lamellar reposition + lid split + tarsal wedge resection or lamellar division
Severe	Lamellar advance or rotation of terminal tarsoconjunctiva and posterior lamellar graft

Acquired Entropion

The principles are to:
1. Create a scar tissue between preseptal and pretarsal muscles
2. Tighten or shorten the lower lid retractors
3. Shorten lid tendons. All the described surgeries use either one or more principles.
    i. *Involutional entropion:*
        • No horizontal laxity: Wies-type procedure (transverse lid split and everting suture)
        • With horizontal laxity: Quickert procedure (Wies procedure + horizontal lid shortening)
        • Jones procedures: Lower lid retractor reinsertion
    ii. *Cicatricial entropion:*
        • Needs to be treated without delay to prevent corneal complications
        • Mild to moderate—tarsal wedge resection/tarsal fracture procedures
        • Severe—scar tissue excision + posterior lamellar graft
    iii. *Spastic entropion:*
        • Immediate treatment: Quickert–Rathbun sutures
        • Botulinum toxin injection relieves the spasm of orbicularis oculi, but action is delayed.

12.13 ECTROPION

AIM
The aim of the treatment is to relieve the symptoms, preserve the cornea, and maintain lid integrity.

CONGENITAL ECTROPION
1. Mild cases—topical lubricants
2. Severe cases—skin grafting to avoid permanent corneal scarring

ACQUIRED ECTROPION
Medical Treatment
1. Lubricant drops and ointment
2. Taping, goggles, bandage contact lens to protect the ocular surface

Surgical Treatment
1. *Involutional ectropion:*
   Treatment depends on:
   i. Degree and location
   ii. Degree of horizontal laxity
   iii. Laxity of medial and lateral tendon
   iv. Tone of orbicularis oculi
      - Generalized lid laxity with normal skin: Full-thickness resection; with excess skin: Kuhnt–Syzmanowksi procedure (horizontal shortening and blepharoplasty)
      - Lateral laxity: Lateral canthal suture, lateral tarsal strip
      - Medial laxity: Medial canthal suture, medial canthal resection
2. *Paralytic ectropion:*
   Depends on:
   i. Location
      i. Generalized—full-thickness resection or lateral canthoplasty
      ii. Lateral—lateral canthal elevation for mild and lateral tarsorrhaphy for severe types
      iii. Medial—Lee medial canthoplasty for mild and medial tarsorrhaphy for severe types
3. *Cicatricial ectropion:*
   i. Mild cases—simple lid tightening procedure like Z-plasty
   ii. Severe cases—scar excision and lengthening of anterior lamella by skin grafting/flaps
4. *Mechanical ectropion:*
   Elimination of specific cause like excision of lid mass/treating lid edema

12.14 LAGOPHTHALMOS

AIMS

The aims of the treatment are to:
1. Prevent exposure keratopathy
2. Protect the ocular surface
3. Reestablish eyelid function
4. Ensure a cosmetically acceptable appearance

TREATMENT

If the lagophthalmos is mild with good Bell's phenomenon and if the patient is asymptomatic, then I would like to offer reassurance and monitor the patient with frequent observational schedules.

The treatment of the symptomatic patient can be medical or surgical, depending on the severity and the longevity of the lesion.

I would like to start the patient on preservative-free artificial tear supplements, four times a day. Ointments can be applied to the cornea at bedtime. Protective goggles have to be worn throughout the day. At nighttime, it is better to tape the lids or patch the eye closed to prevent accidental rubbing of the cornea during sleep.

If the patient does not improve with time, then the following surgeries can be considered. A temporary lateral tarsorrhaphy can be done to narrow the interpalpebral fissure and to protect the cornea. Gold weights have been suggested to be implanted in the upper lid for paralytic lagophthalmos. Recession of the upper eyelid retractors (levator and Müller's muscle) can be done in lagophthalmos caused by thyroid-related ophthalmopathy (TRO) due to upper lid retraction.

If there is a *cicatricial/postsurgical lid shortening*, then a combination of full-thickness skin grafts, advancement flaps, tarsal-sharing procedures, and release of scar bands can be performed.

In cases of facial nerve palsy and floppy eyelid syndrome, the presence of lagophthalmos due to laxity can be corrected by lateral tarsal strip, which will improve the apposition of the lower lid to the globe and decrease tearing.

If the patients continue to have exposure of the cornea, then the lower eyelid retractor muscles recession and an additional spacing graft may be sutured in the lid to achieve further elevation. Autologous ear cartilage, nasal cartilage, or hard palate grafts are often used.

In cases of severe lagophthalmos, facial reanimation procedures include temporalis muscle transposition/transfer, nerve grafts and anastomoses, palpebral springs, soft-tissue repositioning, and suborbicularis oculi fat lifts can be done.

12.15 PTOSIS

AIM

The primary aim of the treatment is to improve the superior visual field and prevent amblyopia while obtaining a cosmetically appealing and symmetrical eyelid height and contour.

FUNCTIONAL POINT OF VIEW

The goals of the surgery are to elevate the eyelid margin above the pupillary axis for improvement in the superior visual field and to prevent amblyopia. There should also be adequate mobility of the lid when blinking, a normal lid fold, and no diplopia.

COSMETIC POINT OF VIEW

The goals of the surgery are to achieve a smooth curvature of the eyelid margin (normal contour), symmetry in the eyelid margin height, and symmetry in the soft tissues of the eyelid and eyebrow, particularly the amount of tarsal platform show (TPS).

MANAGEMENT OF PTOSIS

Nonsurgical Treatment

1. Lid crutches may be used to support a drooping lid mechanically. The type used is a wire support in the form of a semilunar soldered to the upper part of the rims of a pair of spectacles
2. Haptic contact lens with a shelf on which the margin of upper lid rests may be used
3. Elevation of the lid by a mechanical force: A strip of highly magnetic metal is implanted in the upper lid and a magnet is placed behind the upper rim of the frame

WHEN TO CORRECT PTOSIS SURGICALLY

1. Correction of mild-to-moderate ptosis in a child can often be delayed until the patient is several years old, although consistent chin-up positioning/complete ptosis may justify early surgery
2. In general, congenital ptosis should be repaired when accurate measurements are obtainable and before the child begins school. Most children can undergo repair around 4–5 years of age
3. Severe ptosis, which may cause amblyopia, must be surgically repaired as soon as possible to preserve normal vision

4. An acquired ptosis from a traumatic injury or a third nerve palsy should not be operated on before 6 months of age because often some levator function will return
5. Any other acquired ptosis may be repaired when the cause has been determined. In particular, myasthenia gravis must be ruled out

INDICATIONS FOR SURGERY IN CONGENITAL PTOSIS

In most instances, the primary reason for correcting congenital ptosis is cosmetic. In case of unilateral congenital ptosis of such severity that normal visual development is compromised by total occlusion of the visual axis, surgical intervention may be indicated shortly after birth.

In cases of severe bilateral ptosis that interferes with the child's learning walk, surgery may be indicated early. The levator action in these children is always so poor that a frontalis sling procedure is necessary. In general, ptosis causing significant stimulus deprivation or head posturing must be surgically treated without fail. Milder degrees of ptosis need to be corrected only if the patient desires good cosmesis.

CONTRAINDICATIONS FOR SURGERY

1. Poor orbicularis muscle function may produce lagophthalmos and corneal exposure
2. Loss of blink reflex or corneal sensitivity, paralysis of orbicularis, or significant keratitis sicca are definite contraindications for ptosis surgery
3. Total ophthalmoplegia may also result in postoperative corneal exposure as the cornea is exposed during sleep

CHOICE OF SURGERY FOR PTOSIS

In general, there are three major types of ptosis surgery:
1. External levator resection (including aponeurotic repair) for >4 mm for levator function
2. Posterior tarso Müller's muscle resection (not generally used in congenital ptosis unless due to congenital Horner's syndrome)
3. Frontalis suspension: For unilateral ptosis with poor levator function, a unilateral frontalis sling is a good option
4. Beard's technique (Chicken Beard technique): In this procedure, a bilateral frontalis sling procedure is performed, but the unaffected levator is not disinserted. This technique has the advantage of maintaining better symmetry in downgaze than a unilateral sling

PRINCIPLES OF SURGICAL CORRECTION

1. One inherent drawback to all ptosis procedures is that perfect cosmetic and functional results cannot be expected in every case

2. In general, the final result depends on the nature of ptosis, the type of operation selected, and the skill with which the operation is performed
3. Levator resection is performed on all levator maldevelopment (congenital dysmyogenic) ptosis cases with levator action of four or more whereas a frontalis sling is performed when the levator action is 3 mm or less

Surgical approach depends on:
1. Ptosis is unilateral or bilateral
2. Severity of ptosis
3. Levator action
4. Presence of abnormal ocular movements, jaw-winking phenomenon, or blepharophimosis syndrome

Fasanella–Servat Operation
1. Mild ptosis (<2 mm or less)
2. Levator action >10 mm
3. Well-defined lid fold—no excess skin

Levator Resection
1. Mild/moderate/severe ptosis
2. Levator action ≥4 mm

Brow Suspension Ptosis Repair
1. Severe ptosis
2. Levator action <4 mm
3. Jaw-winking ptosis or blepharophimosis syndrome

Bilateral Ptosis
In cases of bilateral ptosis, simultaneous bilateral surgery is preferred to ensure a similar surgical intervention in the two eyes. However, in cases where gross asymmetry exists between the two eyes, the eye with greater ptosis is operated on first and the other eye is operated on after 6–8 weeks.

Modified Fasanella–Servat Surgery
It is done for:
1. Mild ptosis (<2 mm or less)
2. Levator action >10 mm

It is the excision of tarsoconjunctiva, Müller's muscle, and levator. Xylocaine with adrenaline is used for local anesthesia in adults, but general anesthesia is necessary for children.

Surgical Steps

1. Three sutures are passed close to the folded superior margin of the tarsal plate at the junction of the middle, lateral, and medial one-third of the lid.
2. Three corresponding sutures are placed close to the everted lid margin starting from the conjunctival aspect near the superior fornix in positions corresponding to the first three sutures.
3. A proposed incision is marked on the tarsal plate such that a uniform piece of tarsus, decreasing gradually toward the periphery, is excised.
4. A groove is made on the marked line of the incision and the incision is completed with a scissor. The first set of sutures helps in lifting the tarsal plate for excision.
5. The tarsal plate not more than 3 mm in width is excised.

Levator Resection

This is the most commonly practiced surgery for ptosis correction. This technique involves shortening of the levator–aponeurosis complex through a lid crease incision. It may be performed through the skin or conjunctival route.

Surgical Steps

1. The proposed lid crease is marked to match the normal eye considering the margin crease.
2. Incision through the skin and orbicularis is made along the crease marking.
3. The inferior skin and orbicularis are dissected away from the tarsal plate.
4. The upper edge is separated from the orbital septum.
5. The fibers of the aponeurosis are cut from their insertion in the inferior half of the anterior surface of the tarsus.
6. The levator is freed from the adjoining structures.
7. The lateral and the medial horn are cut whenever a large resection is planned.
8. Care should be taken that Whitnall's ligament is not damaged.
9. A double-armed 5-0 Vicryl is passed through the center of the tarsal plate by a partial thickness bite.
10. It is then passed through the levator aponeurosis at a height judged by the preoperative evaluation. Intraoperative assessment is made.
11. Two more double-armed 5-0 Vicryl sutures are passed through the tarsus about 2 mm from the upper border in the center and at the junction of the central third with the medial and lateral thirds.
12. These sutures are then placed in the levator and an intraoperative assessment is made.
13. Excess levator is excised.
14. Four to five lid fold forming sutures are placed.

Brow Suspension Repair

This surgery is the procedure of choice in simple congenital ptosis with poor levator action. A number of materials such as nonabsorbable sutures, extended polytetrafluoroethylene (ePTFE), muscle strips, banked, or fresh fascia lata strips have been used for suspension.

Temporalis Sling Repair

1. Thread sling is carried out in very young children with severe ptosis where prevention of amblyopia and uncovering the pupil are the main aims.
2. The suture sling procedures have a relatively higher recurrence rate of or may show formation of suture granuloma.
3. Definitive surgery may be performed at a later date when a fascia lata sling is carried out.

Fascia Lata Sling

1. This procedure is designed to augment the patient's lid elevation through brow elevation.
2. It is considered in children above 4 years of age having severe congenital simple ptosis with poor levator action.
3. Even in cases of unilateral severe ptosis, a bilateral procedure is preferred because a unilateral surgery causes marked asymmetry in downgaze.
4. The results of bilateral surgery are more acceptable.
5. This procedure produces lagophthalmos in most cases.

12.16 BLEPHAROPHIMOSIS PTOSIS EPICANTHUS SYNDROME

AIMS

The aims of the treatment are to correct:
1. Ptosis to improve superior visual field and prevent amblyopia while obtaining a cosmetically appealing and symmetrical eyelid height and contour
2. Telecanthus to reduce the intercanthal distance, thus reducing the pseudosquinting
3. Epicanthus to achieve good cosmesis and reduce pseudoesotropia

INDICATIONS FOR SURGERY

1. Cosmetic
2. Ptosis causing significant stimulus deprivation or head posturing
3. Severe ptosis, which may cause deprivational amblyopia

MANAGEMENT

1. Management of blepharophimosis ptosis epicanthus syndrome (BPES) is primarily surgical, if indicated.
2. Care should be given to treat associated amblyopia.
3. The usual sequence of surgical treatment is correction of the epicanthic folds at about the age of 3-4 years and correction of the ptosis about 9-12 months later.
4. However, when ptosis is severe, surgical repair is recommended before the age of 3 years.
5. Frontalis sling is the procedure of choice for ptosis correction as BPES is usually associated with poor levator function.
6. Correction of lateral ectropion of the lower lids, if necessary, with a full-thickness skin graft in the teenage years.
7. Early surgery may be necessary for amblyopia.
8. The treatment of blepharophimosis syndrome requires coordination among oculoplastic surgeons, pediatric ophthalmologists, pediatric endocrinologists, gynecologists, and genetic counselors.
9. Systemic treatment of associated primary ovarian failure and hormone replacement therapy.
10. Optometric management:
    Detailed evaluation of ptosis and amblyopia and correction of associated refractive errors are essential.
11. Genetic counseling is an essential component in the management of BPES.

SURGICAL MANAGEMENT
Epicanthus Fold and Telecanthus
Medial canthoplasty by double Z or Y-Z plasties, transnasal wiring of the medial canthal tendons.

Ptosis
Generally, it is corrected with brow suspension procedure—frontalis sling.

12.17 MEDIAL CANTHOPLASTY

DOUBLE Z-PLASTY (MUSTARDE)

Principle

A double Z and a Y-V plasties are combined. The double Z lengthens and changes the position of the epicanthic fold and the Y-V plasty, by shortening the medial canthal tendon, corrects the telecanthus.

Indication

A marked epicanthic fold is associated with telecanthus, especially if there is entropion caused by traction from the fold.

Method

1. Make a mark on the skin at the site of the present medial canthus and at the site of the proposed medial canthus.
2. Join these lines and from center, draw two lines extending laterally at an angle of approximately 60°. These form the main limbs of Z-plasty.
3. From the end of each limb, draw a nearly horizontal line which angles slightly toward the proposed new medial canthus at approximately 45° to the main limb of the Z-plasty.
4. Draw a line laterally from the present medial canthus close to the upper and lower lid margin. This completes the skin marks in the figure of a "flying man".
5. Cut through the skin along these marks.
6. Excise the underlying subcutaneous tissue until the medial canthal tendon is exposed. In blepharophimosis syndrome, the tendon is usually elongated, thin, and buried under abnormal tissue.
7. Shorten the medial canthal tendon, if required.
8. Suture the subcutaneous tissues in the region of the old medial canthus to the subcutaneous and deep tissues in the region of the new medial canthus.
9. Transpose the skin flaps.
10. Suture the skin flaps with 6 "0" nylon.

12.18 MEDIAL CANTHAL TENDON SHORTENING WITH TRANSNASAL WIRE

PRINCIPLE
The intercanthal distance is reduced by removing the bone and wiring the two medial canthal tendons together across the nose.

INDICATIONS
Severe telecanthus and hypertelorism associated with blepharophimosis ptosis epicanthus syndrome (BPES) when the bone must be removed bilaterally to reduce the intercanthal distance.

METHODS
1. Expose and resect the medial canthal tendons.
2. Reduce the bone of the anterior lamellar crest and reflect the lacrimal sac laterally.
3. Pass a Mustarde awl (name of the instrument used in transnasal wiring) across the nose with a wire and a 4 "0" nylon suture.
4. Leave a loop of wire across the nose and one 4 "0" nylon suture.
5. Withdraw the awl with another 4 "0" nylon suture and the end of the wire leaving a loop behind.
6. Suture the resected medial canthal tendons to the transnasal wire loop.
7. Twist the wire to tighten it and correct the telecanthus.
8. Pass the 4 "0" nylon sutures through the medial canthoplasty flaps. Tie them together over bolsters to keep pressure on the wound.
9. Remove the sutures after 5 days.

12.19 BROW SUSPENSION/FRONTALIS SLING

PRINCIPLES
1. The frontalis normally lifts the eyebrow and contributes to eyelid elevation
2. This action of lifting the lid is enhanced by connecting the frontalis muscle and eyebrow to the lid with a subcutaneous "sling"
3. For a definitive cosmetic procedure, it is preferable to do a bilateral suspension

INDICATIONS
1. Ptosis with <4 mm of levator function
2. Prevention of amblyopia in an infant with severe ptosis in whom an assessment of levator function is not possible
3. Following a levator excision

METHODS
1. Make a medial, central, and lateral horizontal skin mark on the eyelid about 2-3 mm from the lash line. The skin crease will form here. Make two marks just above the eyebrow, one vertically above and a little lateral to the lateral eyelid mark, and the other vertically above and a little medial to the medial eye mark. Make a forehead mark above and between these two brow marks to complete an isosceles triangle. Preferably mark and operate on both the lids at the same time to ensure symmetry.
2. Make stab incisions through all the marks, widening the three forehead incisions a little.
3. Use a Wright fascia needle to pass each strip of fascia.
4. Pull up the two triangles of fascia to give a symmetrical lid curve. If there is a normal Bell's phenomenon, raise the lid level as high as possible but stop if it reaches the limbus or if the lid starts to leave the globe. Tie the fascia and reinforce the knot with a 6 "0" absorbable suture.
5. Pull one fascial strip from each eyebrow incision through the forehead incision. Tie the strips together and reinforce the knot with a 6 "0" absorbable suture.
6. Close the forehead and eyebrow incisions with 6 "0" nylon sutures. Leave the eyelid incisions open.
7. If required, tape a lower lid traction suture on top of the brow. Remove it at the first dressing 12–48 hours postoperatively. Remove the skin sutures at 5 days.
8. Use lubricant and antibiotic drops and ointment.

12.20 TRAUMATIC CATARACT

AIM

The management of traumatic cataract is essentially surgical; however, I would like to first control intraocular inflammation, maintain integrity of the eyeball, and then try to restore maximum useful vision and prevent infection.

I would like to classify it into preoperative, intraoperative, and postoperative management.

I would like to first evaluate the patient for the type of ocular injury, look carefully for zonular dehiscence in a dilated pupil, subluxation of the lens in a supine position, associated complications of trauma, intraocular inflammation, and intraocular pressure and also evaluate the other eye for sympathetic ophthalmia in penetrating trauma. Also, I would like to explain the guarded visual prognosis associated with traumatic cataract.

INTRAOPERATIVE MANAGEMENT

Blunt Injury with Traumatic Cataract

1. *Traumatic cataract without associated complications:* Choice of surgery: Phacoemulsification or manual small incision cataract surgery (SICS) intraocular lens (IOL): Three-piece acrylic, *in-the-bag* implantation
2. *Traumatic cataract with zonular dehiscence:*
   i. *Choice of surgery:* Phaco or manual SICS
   ii. *Grading of zonular dialysis (ZD)*
      - *<3 clock hours of ZD:* In the bag implantation of IOL, with haptics stabilizing the weak zones
      - *3–5 clock hours:* Cataract extraction with capsular tension ring (CTR), IOL implantation in the bag
      - *5–7 clock hours:* Cataract extraction with CTR/Cionni ring, IOL implantation in the bag
      - *>7 clock hours:* Cataract extraction with CTR/Cionni ring/CTS/iris or scleral fixated IOL
   iii. *Subluxation of lens*
      i. Anterior subluxation: Limbal approach, cataract extraction with sulcus implantation/scleral fixated three-piece acrylic IOL
      ii. Posterior subluxation: Pars plana approach with vitrectomy, lensectomy, scleral fixated IOL
3. *Traumatic cataract with vitreous disturbance:*
   i. *Minimal:* Manual/automated anterior vitrectomy, sulcus implantation of three-piece IOL
   ii. *Gross:* Pars plana approach with vitrectomy, lensectomy, scleral fixated IOL.

12.21 PENETRATING INJURY WITH TRAUMATIC CATARACT

INDICATIONS FOR PRIMARY CATARACT EXTRACTION

Corneal tear repair with cataract extraction with or without intraocular lens (IOL) implantation

Hyphema (<50%): Anterior chamber wash with cataract extraction with IOL implantation

Intraocular foreign body (IOFB)-induced cataract, especially iron, requires an early intervention due to the risk of ocular siderosis.

Advantages: Early visual rehabilitation, better visual outcome, single procedure

INDICATIONS FOR SECONDARY CATARACT EXTRACTION

Severe corneal edema with tear

High intraocular pressure (IOP) with hyphema (>50%)

Disadvantages: Poorer visual outcome, repeated manipulation, increased risk of infection.

12.22 MARFAN SYNDROME WITH SUBLUXATION OF LENS

AIM
The aim of my management is to give the best possible visual acuity by surgical and nonsurgical means and to prevent amblyopia in young patients.

STEPS OF MANAGEMENT
The choice of treatment depends on the following factors:
1. Severity or extent of subluxation with respect to visual axis and undilated pupil
2. Age of the patient

PREOPERATIVE EVALUATION
1. Undilated examination to see if the lens margin is crossing the pupillary region
2. Prone position or head tilt to rule out posterior subluxation
3. Examination of the retina and cornea as Marfan syndrome is associated with a higher incidence of retinal detachment and keratoconus

Spectacle correction is given in two situations:
1. Minimal subluxation with the pupillary area being phakic
2. Severe subluxation with the pupillary area being aphakic

INDICATIONS FOR SURGERY
1. Lens margin in the pupillary region
2. Risk of amblyopia
3. Anterior or posterior displacement of subluxated lens

SURGICAL OPTIONS
1. *Intracapsular lens extraction with anterior vitrectomy followed by spectacles or contact lens correction:* This is preferred in younger children. Intraocular lens (IOL) power prediction is difficult because of varying refraction. Since Marfan patients are usually myopic, aphakic correction is not very high and well tolerated.
2. *Intracapsular lens extraction with anterior vitrectomy and IOL implantation:* Scleral fixation with glue or haptic tucked in pockets is preferred over sutured scleral-fixated intraocular lens (SFIOL) or sutured iris-fixated intraocular lens (IFIOL). Surgeries are done in younger people and the life span results of sutures are not known. (If sutured, 9-0 Prolene or 8-0 Gore-tex is preferred.)

3. *Lens aspiration with bag preservation using capsular tension ring (CTR)/ capsular tension segment (CTS)/Cionni ring with PCIOL implantation:* This can be done in adults or older children with moderate subluxation. Since the subluxation may progress, CTS or Cionni ring is preferred over CTR to stabilize the bag. A three-piece posterior chamber intraocular lens (PCIOL) is kept in the bag. The three-piece gives the option of future scleral fixation or iris fixation should the need arise.
4. *If the lens is displaced posteriorly, pars plana lensectomy with vitrectomy is done.* Followed by silicone fixation IOL with glue or with haptics tucked in pockets.
5. *Other eye surgeries:* Most patients will require second eye surgery. The timing is based on the severity of subluxation and risk of amblyopia development. In children, we should wait till GA fitness is allowed for the second time.

SYSTEMIC CONSIDERATION

We should also ask for a cardiologist's opinion because Marfan syndrome is associated with mitral valve prolapse, aortic dissection, and aortic aneurysms.

12.23 ACTIVE UVEITIS IN RIGHT EYE AND UVEITIS WITH COMPLICATED CATARACT IN LEFT EYE

AIMS
The aims of my treatment would be to:
1. Effectively control inflammation
2. Relieve pain
3. Prevent complications
4. Treat the causative etiology, if possible

RIGHT EYE (ACTIVE UVEITIS)
Treatment of Uveitis
I would like to start the patient on topical 1% prednisolone acetate six to eight times a day at regular intervals along with a short-acting cycloplegic drug like 1% homatropine twice a day. I would review the patient periodically and titrate the dose of the topical steroids depending on the response. If there is a documented reduction of inflammation, I would taper the dosage to four times, three times, two times, and one time at weekly intervals.

If there is no adequate improvement, I would like to add oral prednisolone acetate 1 mg/kg body weight, after ascertaining that the patient does not have systemic contraindications such as diabetes mellitus or gastritis. The patient is examined periodically and if good improvement is seen, the systemic steroids are tapered and the patient is continued only on topical steroids.

Posterior sub-Tenon triamcinolone acetonide (40 mg) can be considered in cases of chronic uveitis with posterior segment involvement.

If the patient does not respond to oral and topical steroids or develops steroid-induced ocular or systemic complications, I would like to switch over to immunosuppressive therapy. Considering the cost of the treatment and also the better compliance to the drug due to the once-a-week regimen, my first choice would be tablet methotrexate. Dose: 7.5–25 mg/week in a single dose (15 mg/week), folate (1 mg/day) is administered concurrently to minimize nausea. Considering the bone marrow and hepatic toxicity of the drug, I would like to monitor the patient's blood counts and liver function tests every 1–2 months.

Indications for Immunosuppressive Use
1. Severe, sight-threatening steroid-resistant uveitis
2. Patients with steroid-induced complications
3. As a first-line drug in patients where long-term remission or cure has been shown to be achieved with immunosuppressants, e.g., Behçet's and Wegener's diseases.

LEFT EYE (UVEITIS WITH COMPLICATED CATARACT)

If the eye has been quiet for at least 3 months, I would like to go ahead with performing a cataract extraction with intraocular lens (IOL) implantation after taking proper preoperative and intraoperative precautions. I would also explain the guarded visual prognosis and consequences to the patient. Preoperatively depending on the chronicity and severity of the inflammation, I would like to start the patient on topical 1% prednisolone acetate six times a day at least 1 week before the surgery and, if needed, I would add oral prednisolone 20 mg/day which can be tapered according to the severity of the postoperative inflammation. Intraoperatively, I would be prepared to handle poor view due to band-shaped keratopathy, small pupil, and posterior synechiae and would also expect zonular weakness. I would use intracameral adrenaline (1.5%) to facilitate pupillary dilatation. Alternatively, I will perform multiple small sphincterotomies or use an iris hook to get adequate pupillary dilatation. I would prefer "in-the-bag" implantation of a three-piece monofocal acrylic IOL or, if available, a heparin-coated IOL. Care would be taken to take out the cortex and the residual viscoelastics completely. At the end of the surgery, I would give a subconjunctival injection of dexamethasone (0.4 mL of 4 mg/mL) or preservative-free intracameral dexamethasone (0.1 mL of 4 mg/mL). Postoperatively, I would continue the topical prednisolone and taper it depending on the response. I would also like to add a short-acting cycloplegic like 1% homatropine twice a day for at least 15 days and nonsteroidal anti-inflammatory drugs (NSAIDs) like 0.5% ketorolac three times a day for at least 6 weeks to prevent cystoid macular edema. I would also review the patient more often than normal to look for reactivation of the uveitis and also look for early occurrence of posterior capsular opacification.

12.24 PTERYGIUM

Why is pterygium more common nasally?
  i. Chronic exposure to ultraviolet (UV) light. As rays fall on the temporal side, due to internal reflection, they get reflected to the nasal side
  ii. The nasal bridge at the center prevents the rays directly
  iii. Dust and tear secretions accumulate more commonly in the nasal part

AIM

The aim of the treatment is to relieve the patient of the symptoms caused by pterygium by either medical therapy or surgical excision with tissue supplementation with an intention to prevent further recurrence.

Management

1. *Medical therapy:*
   - To manage mild irritation, topical lubricants or a mild topical antihistamine vasoconstrictor like 0.1% naphazoline qid are used
   - In case of inflammation of pterygium, mild topical corticosteroid like 0.1% fluorometholone or loteprednol qid is used for a short period of time
   - Secondary dellen is treated using preservative-free lubricating ointments and temporary patching for 24 hours
2. *Surgical management:*
   i. Surgical intervention is indicated in the following cases:
      - Reduced visual acuity due to induced astigmatism or encroachment onto the visual axis
      - Marked discomfort and irritation not relieved by medical management
      - Limitation of ocular motility secondary to restriction
      - Cosmetic reasons
   ii. The various surgical approaches are:
      - Pterygium excision
      - Conjunctival flaps and conjunctival autografts
      - Lamellar keratoplasty and penetrating keratoplasty in case of significant corneal thinning
      - Mucous membrane grafts and amniotic membrane grafts

My ideal treatment of choice would be the surgical excision of pterygium and supplementing the raw area with autologous conjunctival transplantation. This can be performed with local infiltration anesthesia. I would like to specifically remove as much subconjunctival tissue as possible, beneath the head of the pterygium, with minimal removal of the conjunctival tissue. The surface of the cornea can be smoothed by a mechanical burr or by using a 15 blade with short superficial shaving movements. I will prepare the conjunctival graft, as thin as possible, by clearing off the underlying Tenon's capsule. The conjunctival graft is secured with proper orientation, either by sutures or by fibrin glue. If the sutures are used, then the limbal side of the conjunctival graft is anchored with the peripheral cornea using a 10-0 nylon interrupted suture and the conjunctival side is attached with 8-0 Vicryl sutures. If the glue is used, care is taken to dry the bed before the application of the glue. If enough conjunctiva is not available, then amniotic membrane supplementation can be considered, but the recurrence rate with amniotic membrane is higher.

12.25 KERATOCONUS

■ AIM

The aim of the treatment is to try and arrest the progression of keratoconus and try to achieve the best possible visual acuity for the patient.

Toward this, I will prescribe spectacles or soft toric contact lenses for the patient. If this visual rehabilitation is inadequate, then I will prescribe rigid gas permeable (RGP) contact lenses to correct irregular astigmatism.

If there is a documented progression of keratoconus, as seen by serial topography, then corneal collagen cross-linking (C3R) can be done with the aim to prevent or slow down further progression and the residual refractive error may be corrected with RGP contact lenses, 3 months after the C3R procedure.

Intracorneal ring segments (INTACS) are sometimes used in mild or moderate cases to improve tolerance to contact lens wear.

In patients in whom there is corneal scarring or complete contact lens intolerance or not being able to be fitted with contact lenses, then corneal transplantation should be considered. Deep anterior lamellar keratoplasty (DALK) is the preferred surgical option. However, in cases of severe deep stromal scarring, penetrating keratoplasty (PKP) is performed.

12.26 MACULAR CORNEAL DYSTROPHY

Macular corneal dystrophy is also known as Groenouw type II dystrophy.

The definitive treatment is corneal transplantation in both eyes. However, in milder cases, initial symptomatic treatment is given to provide relief of symptoms.

The management includes the following:
1. I will recommend the use of tinted glasses to minimize photophobia
2. If there are recurrent erosions, I will treat them in the following manner
   i. *Acute episode:*
      - Use of antibiotic drops to reduce the risk of infection
      - Control of pain with the use of cycloplegic agents, topical nonsteroidal anti-inflammatory drugs, and oral analgesics
      - Promote epithelial healing by patching of eye and using therapeutic soft contact lenses

      Usually heals in 2-3 days, but I would like to follow up with the patient closely to ensure that erosions are healing
   ii. *Prevention of subsequent erosions:*
      - Use of hypertonic solutions such as 5% sodium chloride, especially in the form of eye ointment at bedtime. The patient is asked to continue them for several months
      - Instillation of lubricating eye drops
      - Bandage soft contact lenses protect the epithelial surface from further damage
      - Control of concomitant ocular surface conditions, if present, e.g., dry eye syndrome
3. *Surgical therapy:* The choice of procedure depends on the extent of corneal involvement.
   i. For dystrophies involving the anterior third of the stroma, phototherapeutic keratoplasty can be done.

      Phototherapeutic keratoplasty (PTK) uses an excimer laser. The goal is to aim for a central clearing of the opacities and thereby postpone or avoid lamellar/penetrating keratoplasty (PKP) rather than achieve a totally clear cornea. It removes superficial corneal opacities, smoothens corneal surface, and allows epithelium to adhere more tightly. The procedure produces significant visual improvement in these patients. The dystrophy may recur after PTK, in case of which a repeat PTK or a PKP may be necessary.
   ii. For dystrophies involving the anterior half of the stroma, deep anterior lamellar keratoplasty (DALK) is preferred.

iii. If visual acuity worsens and opacities are deep, a full-thickness corneal transplant (PKP) has to be performed. Most patients require a PKP by the fourth decade of their life. The eye which is more affected is operated first followed by the second eye after a time gap of 6 months.

Although the success rate is high, macular dystrophy recurs in the graft over years and regraft is necessary in such cases.

Genetic counseling: I would also like to educate the patients about the hereditary nature of the disease. Patients are less likely to have an affected child due to its autosomal recessive inheritance.

12.27 BACTERIAL CORNEAL ULCER

AIM

My aim of treatment is rapid cessation of replication and elimination of the infecting organism and thereby preventing structural damage to the cornea with the selection of appropriate therapy with minimal toxicity.

Initially, I would like to start with broad-spectrum antibiotics monotherapy (gatifloxacin 0.3% or moxifloxacin) on an hourly basis during waking hours for 3 days, which later can be modified according to culture results, antibiotics susceptibility, and clinical response.

I would also like to add mydriatics like homatropine 2% (cyclopentolate 1% or atropine 1%) in the affected eye twice daily to prevent ciliary spasm and dangerous results of iritis, e.g., posterior synechiae. I would like to give oral pain relievers such as paracetamol to relieve the pain and make the patient comfortable.

There is no need to change the initial therapy if this has induced a favorable clinical response, even if the cultures show a resistant organism.

If there is evidence of a gram-positive organism, I would like to start with topical chloramphenicol 5 mg/mL or cefazolin 5% initially hourly for 2 days as a loading dose and then I will modify the regimen depending on the therapeutic responses.

In case of gram-negative organisms, I would like to start with topical gentamicin 1.5% hourly or fluoroquinolones like 0.3% ciprofloxacin or ofloxacin for 2 days and then modify the regimen depending on the therapeutic responses.

In severe cases, I would like to start with combination therapy with fortified preparations such as duotherapy.

The most common combination used is cephalosporin and aminoglycoside to cover both gram-positive and gram-negative bacteria.

POSITIVE SIGNS OF CLINICAL IMPROVEMENT

1. Decreased pain
2. Decreased discharge
3. Decreased consolidation of corneal infiltrate
4. Decreased anterior chamber reaction
5. Decreased in hypopyon size
6. Corneal reepithelialization
7. Blunting of edges of the perimeter of stromal infiltrate
8. Cessation in corneal thinning

    Subconjunctival antibiotics are only indicated if there is poor compliance with topical treatment.

GENERAL PRINCIPLES
1. If inflammation is severe and persists after the infection is controlled, then topical steroids prednisolone 0.5-1% four times a day will help to promote healing and prevent vascularization.
2. If there is still no improvement after further 48 hours, then suspend the treatment for 24 hours; rescraping is performed with inoculation on a broader range of media and additional staining techniques are requested.
3. If the culture remains negative, it may be necessary to perform a corneal biopsy for histology and culture.
4. If still no improvement is seen and the ulcer progresses, I would like to do therapeutic keratoplasty with a plan to perform a later optical keratoplasty, if possible.
5. If the ulcer heals with a residual scar, it may cause surface irregularity and irregular astigmatism. I will proceed depending on the situation:
    i. In case of nebular opacity, vision can be improved with rigid gas-permeable contact lens
    ii. If the scar is dense and visual potential is present, corneal graft (optical keratoplasty) can be done
    iii. If the scar is present and has no visual potential, then I will advise for cosmetic contact lens or tattooing
6. If perforation occurs and if it is small over the iris, adhesions to the cornea will occur by the formation of pseudocornea by laying down of fibrin and collagenase and the defect will heal as adherent leukoma.
7. If the perforation fails to heal, I would like to proceed according to the size of the ulcer.
8. If the size is <2 mm, tissue adhesive n-butyl-2-ethyl-cyanoacrylate to seal the gap can be used.
9. If the size is 2-4, mm then either corneal patch graft or tenoplasty can be done.
10. If the size is >4 mm, then we have to do tectonic.
11. If severe ulcer with opaque media, I would like to do ultrasonography to look for exudates in the vitreous, which suggest endophthalmitis.

MANAGEMENT OF FUNGAL CORNEAL ULCER
In case of filamentous fungi, I would like to start the patient with 5% topical natamycin hourly initially, during the waking hours for at least 48 hours.

If no improvement is seen, topical azole (fluconazole 2% or miconazole 1%) can be added.

Or

Topical itraconazole 1% can be added as it is effective against a broad range of filamentous fungi.

Or

Topical voriconazole can be added.

In case of deep invasion of the cornea or anterior chamber involvement, I would like to start oral voriconazole 200 mg bd (after performing a baseline liver function test). I would also like to add oral doxycycline 100 mg bd if significant thinning is seen.

I would also like to check intraocular pressure digitally.

If the ulcer progresses despite pharmacological treatment, therapeutic keratoplasty is considered as an alternative.

Injection voriconazole 50 µg/0.1 mL intrastromal can also be tried.

INDICATIONS FOR THERAPEUTIC KERATOPLASTY IN THE ACUTE PHASE OF INFECTION IN CASE OF FUNGAL ULCER

1. Progression of infection despite appropriate and adequate pharmacological treatment
2. Impending orbital radiation (OR) actual perforation
3. Progression of infection to involve limbus and adjacent sclera

Technique of Keratoplasty

1. The size of trephination should include all the infected areas and at least 1-1.5 mm of the surrounding clear zone as well.
2. Interrupted sutures with slightly longer bites to avoid cheese wiring of the suture.
3. Anterior chamber irrigation to flush out all the septic materials.
4. Excise affected intraocular structure and try to preserve the lens, if possible.

If intraocular structure involvement/endophthalmitis is suspected, intracameral antifungals should be injected at the time of keratoplasty—amphotericin 5 µg/0.1 mL

Miconazole 25 µg/0.1 mL

After penetrating keratoplasty, continue topical antifungals to prevent recurrence. Do not use topical steroids in the postoperative period.

If the ulcer progresses toward limbus involves sclera (fungal keratoscleritis)

Then I would like to start oral antifungals and oral analgesic (to relieve pain and inflammation) and cryotherapy (retinal cryoprobe) to ulcer edges with excision of the sclera.

Or

Corneoscleral graft

SYSTEMIC ANTIFUNGAL INDICATIONS

1. Severe deep keratitis
2. When the lesion is near the limbus

3. Scleritis
4. Endophthalmitis

VARIOUS SYSTEMIC ANTIFUNGALS

T. voriconazole 400 mg bd for 1 day, then 200 mg bd

Or

T. itraconazole 200 mg daily and then reduce to 100 mg daily

Or

T. fluconazole 200 mg bd

Or

Tetracycline (doxycycline) for its collagenase activity.

12.28 HERPES SIMPLEX VIRUS KERATITIS

AIM
The aims of the treatment are to:
1. Control and eliminate the infection
2. Relieve the pain
3. Promote reepithelialization
4. Prevent the recurrence of infection with minimal drugs with minimal toxicity

EPITHELIAL KERATITIS
Initially, I would like to debride the epithelial lesion under topical anesthesia. I would like to start the patient with topical antivirals 3% acyclovir ointment five times a day for 2 weeks with:
1. Topical lubricants to relieve discomfort
2. Topical cycloplegic if required
3. Topical antivirals should not be continued after 2 weeks
4. Debridement can be used for dendritic ulcer to reduce the viral load but not in geographic ulcer
5. In case of slow healing or frequent recurrence or resistant case, I would like to add oral acyclovir 400 mg five times a day for 10 days
6. If frequent recurrence is seen, I would like to prescribe oral acyclovir 400 mg 12 hourly for 6 months to a year or longer

STROMAL KERATITIS (INCLUDING DISKIFORM KERATITIS, ENDOTHELITIS, AND IRIDOCYCLITIS)
Initially, I would like to start with topical steroids with antiviral cover four times a day [Herpetic Eye Disease Study (HEDS)].

As improvement occurs, I would like to taper, and subsequently, prednisolone 0.5–1% may be used at a once-daily safe dose at which antiviral cover can be stopped.

Topical cyclosporine 0.05% can be used to facilitate tapering of steroid such as in steroid-related raised intraocular pressure.

Necrotizing Stromal Keratitis
I would like to add oral acyclovir 400 mg bd for 10 days.

HERPES ZOSTER OPHTHALMICUS
I would like to start with oral acyclovir 800 mg five times a day for 10 days as soon as possible, preferably no longer than 4 days after the onset of the rash.

I will advise cold compress and strong analgesics.

Patients with shingles can transmit the disease to immunodeficient individuals and patients not immune (pregnancy) should be asked to avoid contact.

Other oral antivirals:
1. Valacyclovir 1 g tid
2. Famciclovir 500 mg tid
3. Brivudine 125 mg bd

Postherpetic neuralgia
I will advise cold compress and topical capsaicin 0.025% or 0.075% cream for 3 weeks.

Or

Local anesthesia
If not relieved, I will add oral drugs:
1. Simple analgesics paracetamol up to 4 g daily
2. Stronger analgesics codeine 250 mg daily
3. Amitriptyline 10–25 mg at night can be increased up to 75 mg
4. Carbamazepine 400 mg daily for lancinating pain

Acute eye disease
1. Skin and eyelid involvement: 3% acyclovir + 5% acyclovir ointment for the skin lesions
2. Acute epithelial keratitis: Topical antivirals
3. Episcleritis: Mild nonsteroidal anti-inflammatory drugs
4. Scleritis: Oral flurbiprofen 100 mg three times a day

Or

5. Topical dexamethasone 0.1% hourly and antiviral ointment 3% acyclovir five times a day and steroid ointment at night.

12.29 ACANTHAMOEBA KERATITIS

AIMS

The aims of the treatment are to:
1. Not to misdiagnose the ulcer
2. Eradicate the cyst as well as trophozoites
3. Prevent the recurrence
4. Use minimal drugs with minimal toxicity

The treatment is a prolonged one and it would take months for the ulcer to heal. I would like to start the patient on topical polyhexamethyl biguanide 0.02% as first-line therapy 6–24 times a day (no corneal toxicity) (it is available as 20% parent solution, which is diluted 1,000 times with saline/sterile water).

If needed, I would like to do debridement of the ulcer so better penetration of drugs can be facilitated.

I also would like to add analgesic flurbiprofen 100 mg three times a day. If the ulcer fails to heal, I would like to do keratoplasty.

If limbitis or scleritis develops, I will start prednisolone 1 mg/kg/day or cyclosporine 3.5–7.5 mg/kg/day which can be tapered.

INDICATIONS OF KERATOPLASTY

1. Nonhealing ulcer in spite of appropriate antiamebicidal therapy
2. Fulminant corneal abscess
3. Intumescent cataract

The rationale to eliminate the recurrence of acanthamoeba in recipient corneal graft:
- Cryotherapy/rapidly freeze cornea used either with or without penetrating keratoplasty
- The sterile pentamidine isethionate powder can be mixed with artificial tears and applied topically as recommended for brolene solution
- 0.15% dibrompropamidine (brolene ointment), 0.1% propamidine isethionate (brolene solution), miconazole (10 mg/mL)
- Clotrimazole (1.0%)
- Oral administration of ketoconazole 200–600 mg/day.

12.30 PRIMARY OPEN-ANGLE GLAUCOMA

TREATMENT PROTOCOL

My goal would be to set a target intraocular pressure (IOP) to achieve it with the least possible medication so that any further progression of the glaucoma is arrested. My first drug of choice would be latanoprost 0.005% eye drops, once a day, preferably at nighttime to blunt the early morning spike of the IOP. In case this drug is contraindicated, then my second choice would be to use 0.5% timolol maleate, twice a day, as a monotherapy.

If the target IOP is not achieved in a month by either of these medications in their individual capacity, then I will use both these drugs as a combination therapy. If the target IOP is still not achieved with these two drugs, then I will add a third drug. The choice of the third drug can be either brimonidine tartrate 0.2%, three times a day, or dorzolamide 2%, three times a day.

Since some studies have shown that adding a second medication decreased adherence to glaucoma treatment, I will advise a fixed combination therapy (combining two or more antiglaucoma drugs into a single preparation) in order to improve compliance. The commonly available fixed combination drugs are:
1. Timolol + brimonidine
2. Timolol + prostaglandin (PG) analog
3. Brimonidine + PG analog
4. Topical carbonic anhydrase inhibitors + PG analog
5. Topical carbonic anhydrase inhibitors + timolol

I will avoid using PG analog with pilocarpine because while PGs relax the ciliary muscle and increase the uveoscleral outflow, pilocarpine contracts and decreases the trabecular outflow.

If the target IOP is still not achieved after the usage of all three medications, then I will advise the patient to undergo trabeculectomy with or without mitomycin C. If there is a high chance for the trabeculectomy to fail, then I would consider performing shunt surgeries using aqueous drainage devices.

The most important thing is to make the patient comply with the treatment protocol. I will counsel the patient about the nature of the disease, the importance of routine follow-up, the necessity to adhere to medication in order to stop the disease progression, and also the need to screen family members.

12.31 POSTFILTER CASE: BEST EYE, RIGHT EYE (FUNCTIONING FILTER), AND LEFT EYE (NONFUNCTIONING FILTER)

AIM
The aim of my management will be to achieve and maintain the *target intraocular pressure (IOP)* in both eyes so as to preserve vision and thereby the quality of life of my patient.

MANAGEMENT
Right Eye (Functioning Filter)
1. I will check whether the target IOP is reached with the functioning filter (extent of optic nerve damage, progression of field defects, along with the age of the patient and central corneal thickness will decide the target IOP).
2. If the target IOP is achieved, then I will ask the patient to follow up every 3-6 months (depending on the stage).
3. If the target IOP is not achieved with the functioning filter, I will add a topical antiglaucoma medication such as timolol maleate 0.5% bd dosage to aid in achieving the *target IOP* and I will review the patient after a month and decide about the need for Humphrey field analyzer (HFA)-glaucoma progression analysis (GPA) as per the stage of his disease.

Left Eye (Nonfunctioning Filter)
1. The type of glaucoma and the conjunctival status are the two most important factors in determining the success of filtering surgery.
2. IOP and bleb morphology are the important things to be looked at after trabeculectomy surgery.
3. Blebs can be graded based on their size, elevation, vascularity, and structure.

Size (in mm):
Grade I: 1–3 mm
Grade II: 3–4 mm
Grade III: >4 mm

Elevation from scleral surface:
Nil, mild to moderate, and large

Vascularity:
Grade 0: Nil
Grade I: Few small vessels
Grade II: Normal conjunctival vascularity

Grade III: Locally congested
Grade IV: Large vessels on bleb site

Structure:
Type I: Localized encysted
Type II: Diffuse microcysts
Type III: Loculated thin bleb

1. *Early failure (immediate post-trabeculectomy):*
    i. I will check the IOP (management is different for too high or too low)
    ii. If it is too high, I will start topical antiglaucoma medications and, if needed, oral antiglaucoma medications (carbonic anhydrase inhibitors)
    iii. I will do a *gonioscopy* to check whether:
      * The ostium is patent
      * The peripheral iridectomy is larger than the ostium

      If there is a clot at the ostium, I would observe if the clot is small for it will resolve in a few days; if the clot is large and threatening the optic nerve, I would do an anterior chamber (AC) wash.

      If the iris is occluding the ostium, a low-energy argon laser or Nd:YAG laser can be used to disrupt the iris tissue at the ostium.
      * Other important steps include:
        - Hourly steroids topically
        - Digital pressure/massage: Constant and firm digital compression is applied over the inferior aspect of the globe through the patient's lower lid while the eye is upturned. The duration of each compression should not last for more than 10 seconds
        - Laser suturolysis/releasing sutures
        - Bleb needling [with lignocaine, 5-fluorouracil (5-FU), viscoelastics] in cases of subconjunctival adhesions and fibrosis
        - Regular IOP check along with fields (HFA-GPA) are mandatory during this period
        - Repeat filtering procedure with antimetabolites (success rates 50% if done in primary glaucomas)—higher dose (mitomycin C 0.4%) for a longer duration (up to 3 minutes)
        - Glaucoma drainage devices to be considered for patients with secondary glaucoma where the chances of failure of repeat trabeculectomy are very high [e.g., neovascular glaucoma (NVG), uveitic glaucoma, Sturge–Weber syndrome]
2. *Late failure:*
    i. Repeat filtering procedure with antimetabolites (success rates 50% if done in primary glaucomas)
      * Higher dose (mitomycin C 0.4%) for a longer duration (up to 3 minutes)
    ii. Glaucoma drainage devices to be considered

If the secondary trabeculectomy also fails or the patient is a poor candidate
   i. Young <40 years of age
   ii. Previous scleral buckle
   iii. Chronic conjunctival inflammation
   iv. Previous penetrating keratoplasty
   v. Aphakia
   vi. Pseudophakia
   vii. Postsclera buckle for retinal detachment
   viii. Previous conjunctival surgery

Postoperatively, *atropine 1% and scopolamine 0.25%* are to be given to relax the ciliary muscle and tighten the zonular–lens–iris diaphragm and, in turn, to deepen the AC.

Postoperative evaluation of the eye for the following should be done after repeat trabeculectomy:
   i. Extent and height of the bleb
   ii. Presence or absence of microcysts
   iii. Presence or absence of bleb leak
   iv. Visibility of scleral flap sutures
   v. IOP
   vi. Clarity of cornea
   vii. AC depth
   viii. AC inflammation
   ix. Hyphema
   x. Optic disk and macular appearance

CONCLUSION

1. IOP and bleb morphology give valuable information about the functionality of the filter; if needed, topical antiglaucoma medications are to be started to achieve target IOP, and regular follow-up with HFA-GPA is essential.
2. So, achieving target IOP is the primary goal to improve the quality of life and to preserve vision.

12.32 PSEUDOEXFOLIATION GLAUCOMA RIGHT EYE WITH IMC

In a patient with pseudoexfoliation (PXF) and IMC, I would like to manage the glaucoma very carefully because the glaucoma in pseudoexfoliation glaucoma (PXFG) tends to be more aggressive in terms of optic nerve head damage and they also have poor response to antiglaucoma medications. I would also like to measure the intraocular pressure (IOP) at various time points since the diurnal variations in PXF tend to be significantly more.

Before planning the treatment, I would first like to evaluate whether it is a case of:
1. PXFG with open angles
2. PXFG with narrow/occludable angles (by doing a gonioscopy)

PXFG with closed/narrow angles: I would like to first do a YAG peripheral iridotomy, control the pressures medically, and then treat it like a case of PXFG with open angles.

In PXFG (open angles) with IMC, one can do either of the three procedures depending on the clinical condition:
1. Cataract extraction with intraocular lens (IOL) implantation
2. Trabeculectomy
3. Combined cataract extraction with IOL implantation and trabeculectomy (glaucoma triple procedure)

The choice of the procedure depends on:
1. Severity of glaucoma in terms of optic neuropathy and visual field defect
2. IOP control
3. Number of glaucoma medications needed for IOP control

Before surgery, I would like to get an automated visual field analysis done to explain the visual prognosis following the surgery.

CATARACT SURGERY ALONE

This can be performed if the IOP is well under control with medications and there is no progressive optic neuropathy. The temporal section is preferred and the superior conjunctiva is preserved for future filtering surgery, if necessary. Since the pupillary dilation may be sluggish, intracameral adrenaline or sphincterotomies or iris hooks are used to dilate the pupil. Also, anterior capsular staining with trypan blue may be useful to delineate the difference between the anterior capsule and the PXF deposition. Zonular dialysis is very common in this group and hence we need to be ready to handle this with a capsular tension ring, if necessary.

TRABECULECTOMY ALONE

In conditions of early cataract and when the glaucoma is uncontrolled despite maximum tolerable medical therapy and advanced glaucomatous optic disk changes, the surgical procedure of choice is trabeculectomy (which has the highest chance of providing immediate and long-term IOP control).

Temporal clear corneal phacoemulsification can be done after 3–6 months after the control of IOP.

COMBINED PROCEDURE

1. It is done in cases with moderate glaucoma and visually significant cataract.
2. Long-term IOP control is greater with combined procedures than with cataract extraction alone.
3. Phacotrabeculectomy single site or twin site (superior trabeculectomy with temporal phacoemulsification) can be performed.

12.33 NEOVASCULAR GLAUCOMA

AIM
My aim of management is to:
1. Treat the underlying disease that initiated the anterior segment neovascularization
2. Reduce the intraocular pressure (IOP)
3. Reduce the inflammation
4. Give rest to the ciliary body and relieve pain

First of all, I would like to obtain a detailed systemic history from the patient.

In comprehensive ocular examination, I would like to carefully examine pupillary reaction and pupillary margin under high magnification to rule out neovascularization of the iris (NVI) and undilated gonioscopy to look for the presence or absence of neovascularization angle (NVA).

MANAGEMENT

In all cases of neovascular glaucoma (NVG), systemic diseases (e.g., hypertension, diabetes mellitus) have to be controlled and I will work in conjunction with the physician to ensure the same.

Before planning the treatment, I would first like to evaluate whether it is a case of:
1. *NVG with NORMAL IOP and ocular media clear/hazy:* In case where NVI/NVA has already developed but the IOP is still normal, the primary goal of the treatment is to reduce the retinal/ocular ischemia causing regression and involution of anterior segment neovascularization.
    i. *If media clear:* Panretinal photocoagulation (PRP) (number of burns 1,200–1,500 burns, spot size 200–500 µm, one burn width apart applied to the retina) with or without anti-vascular endothelial growth factor (anti-VEGF) (bevacizumab, intravitreally 1.25 mg/mL or intracamerally 0.25 mg/0.02 mL, after ruling out systemic contraindications) is the procedure of choice
    ii. *In patients with hazy media:* Anti-VEGF (bevacizumab) intravitreal 1.25 mg/0.05 mL or intracameral 0.25 mg/0.02 mL alone is given
2. *NVG with RAISED IOP and ocular media clear/hazy:*
    i. Osmotic agents [intravenous (IV) mannitol 1–2 mg/kg or isosorbide orally 1.5 g/kg] may provide acute but transient lowering of IOP by reducing vitreous volume
    ii. Further control of elevated IOP is usually accomplished with aqueous suppressants such as beta-blockers (timolol 0.5%), carbonic anhydrase inhibitors (dorzolamide 2%), and alpha-2 agonist (brimonidine 0.1%)

iii. Inflammation is controlled by topical prednisolone acetate 1% suspension and is titrated accordingly based on the therapeutic response
iv. Atropine 1% to decrease ocular pain and topical corticosteroids (prednisolone suspension 1%) can be used for inflammation

After the corneal edema resolves and inflammation subsides, adjunct combination of intravitreal bevacizumab and PRP should be done in case of clear media.

When media is hazy, intravitreal 1.25 mg/0.05 mL or intracameral 0.25 mg/0.02 mL alone is given.

Surgical management: In cases of late stages of NVG where medical management often fails to control IOP and with extensive synechial angle closure, surgical intervention is usually required.

1. *Trabeculectomy:* This procedure is reserved in eyes that have the potential for useful vision and when the extent of peripheral anterior synechiae (PAS) >180° and performed when the inflammation has been adequately controlled.

   Use of antimetabolites [mitomycin C (MMC) 0.2 mg/mL applied under the sclera flap for 3 minutes or 5-fluorouracil (5-FU) 50 mg/mL for 5 minutes or subconjunctivally 5 mg, 180° away from the trabeculectomy site, twice daily, injected in the first postoperative week and once daily in the second postoperative week] may improve the outcome.

   Preoperative PRP treatment, with anti-VEGF, should be done wherever possible to cause regression of NVI.

2. *Aqueous drainage implants:* These are indicated when conventional trabeculectomy fails or is not possible because of excessive conjunctival scarring.

   Molteno, Baerveldt, and Ahmed implants and Aurolab aqueous drainage implant (AADI) can be used.

   Use of anti-VEGF intravitreally or intracamerally is recommended at least 24 hours prior to surgery.

3. *Cyclodestruction:* It is reserved for the end-stage NVG with poor visual prognosis or when all methods have failed to control IOP and when control of pain becomes the primary therapeutic aim.

   These procedures can be done by cyclocryotherapy or direct laser cyclophotocoagulation or transscleral photocoagulation to destroy the ciliary body to reduce aqueous humor production.

4. *Retrobulbar alcohol injection 3 mL:* Patients with painful blind eyes who do not respond to medical/surgical treatment can be considered for this option.

5. *Enucleation:* If all the above surgical modalities fail to control pain, enucleation may be considered as the last resort.

12.34 ACUTE ATTACK OF ANGLE CLOSURE GLAUCOMA

(This narrative is given intentionally in active tense to familiarize the resident in the art of presentation in a viva.)

Management of angle closure glaucoma is essentially surgical. However, I would like to control the intraocular pressure (IOP) as much as possible by medical means before planning surgery.

If the IOP is very high (above 50 mm Hg), pressure-induced ischemia of the iris leads to paralysis of the sphincter muscle and hence miotic therapy does not help. For this reason, the first line of defense is to administer drugs which will promptly reduce the IOP.

I will start him on 20% intravenous mannitol in a dose of 1-2 g/kg/body weight over a period of 20-30 minutes.

In the absence of nausea or vomiting, I would like to use oral acetazolamide tablets, 250 mg, four times a day or oral hyperosmotic agents such as 50% oral glycerol in a dose of 1-1.5 g/kg/body weight, after ruling out diabetes mellitus. Apraclonidine 0.5% can be used to reduce the IOP quickly.

After bringing the IOP below 40 mm Hg, I will start my patient on 2% topical pilocarpine hydrochloride four times over 30 minutes and then once every 6 hours (which, by causing pupillary miosis, tightens the peripheral iris and pulls it away from the trabecular meshwork and relieves the pupillary block). Additionally, I will also use a combination therapy of topical beta-blockers such as 0.5% timolol maleate, twice a day, with alpha-2 adrenergic agonist such as 0.2% brimonidine tartrate, thrice a day, with a time interval of 10 minutes.

I would like to use topical steroids such as 1% prednisolone acetate, four times a day, to control the associated intraocular inflammation. Additionally, I would like to give analgesics such as oral ibuprofen 500 mg twice a day to control the pain.

I shall review the patient on an hourly basis. I will record the IOP and if the cornea is clear, I will do gonioscopy of both the affected eye and fellow eye.

Besides the medications, I will perform some maneuvers such as axially depressing the central cornea with a goniolens, which may force open the angle temporarily breaking the acute attack.

If the eye is uninflamed and the cornea is clear with reduced IOP, I will do primary peripheral iridotomies using Nd:YAG in both the affected and the fellow eye prophylactically.

If the cornea is not clear and if the gonioscopy reveals angle closure of less than two-third, I will perform a surgical iridectomy for the affected eye and do a YAG iridotomy for the fellow eye.

If the angle closure is more than two-third or if there is persistent inflammation with the edematous cornea and high IOP, then I will contemplate primary trabeculectomy.

Repeat or serial gonioscopy is essential for follow-up of the patient to be certain that the angle has adequately opened.

CHAPTER

Case Sheet Writing

The following description attempts to train a resident in describing various abnormalities of the fundus in a case of diabetic retinopathy.

Fundus of Mr C aged 70 years.

HIGH-RISK PROLIFERATIVE DIABETIC RETINOPATHY WITH CLINICALLY SIGNIFICANT MACULAR EDEMA (RIGHT EYE)

Fundus examination of the right eye:
1. Distant direct ophthalmoscopy at one arm's distance showed a good red glow. Direct ophthalmoscopy close to face revealed a clear media
2. Disk was vertically oval, normal in size, pink in color, with well-defined margins, and having a cup–disk ratio of 0.3 with a healthy neuroretinal rim
3. Vessels arise from the center of the disk, branching dichotomously, maintaining an arteriovenous ratio of 2:3
4. Fine, lacy frond of vessels occupying 1 o'clock hour area of the disk superiorly and 3 o'clock hours inferonasally suggestive of neovascularization of the disk are noted
5. A whitish, elevated semilunar-shaped fibrous band about 1 disk diameter (DD) inferonasal to the disk containing fine tufts of vessels suggestive of neovascularization elsewhere is seen
6. Background retina shows numerous red pinhead-shaped lesions not continuous with the blood vessels, suggestive of dot hemorrhages in all four quadrants
7. A single streak-shaped red lesion at the inferotemporal margin of the disk suggestive of a flame-shaped hemorrhage is seen
8. A tortuosity of the vein in the superotemporal arcade suggestive of venous looping is seen
9. Dilatation of the veins with focal narrowing in the superonasal and superotemporal arcades suggestive of venous beading is seen
10. Yellowish, waxy lesions with distinct margins suggestive of hard exudates arranged in clumps at the posterior pole, inferior, nasal, and temporal to the fovea with adjacent retinal thickening suggestive of clinically significant macular edema are seen

11. A dark red, well-defined accumulation of blood in the inferior retina obscuring the view of the underlying retinal vasculature suggestive of a vitreous hemorrhage is seen
12. On slit-lamp biomicroscopy with a +90 D lens, retinal thickening is seen at the macular area, and the above findings are confirmed. Indirect ophthalmoscopy showed the peripheries to be normal

FUNDUS EXAMINATION OF THE LEFT EYE

Diagnosis: Severe Nonproliferative Diabetic Retinopathy with Clinically Significant Macular Edema

1. Distant direct ophthalmoscopy at one arm's distance showed a good red glow. Direct ophthalmoscopy close to face revealed a clear media
2. Disk was normal in size, vertically oval, pink in color, with well-defined margins and having a cup–disk ratio of 0.3 with a healthy neuroretinal rim
3. Vessels arise from the center of the disk, branching dichotomously, maintaining an arteriovenous ratio of 2:3
4. Background retina shows numerous pinhead-shaped red lesions suggestive of dot and blot hemorrhages in all four quadrants
5. A streak-shaped red lesion inferior to the fovea suggestive of a flame-shaped hemorrhage is seen
6. Yellowish, waxy lesions with distinct margins arranged in clumps along the superior and inferior temporal arcades suggestive of hard exudates are seen
7. A yellowish lesion with distinct margins, 2 DD from the temporal disk margin, surrounded by an area of retinal thickening, suggestive of a hard exudate plaque, is seen
8. A yellowish fluffy lesion with indistinct margins inferior to the disk suggestive of a cotton wool spot is seen
9. A few atrophic hypopigmented chorioretinal scars along the inferotemporal arcade suggestive of old laser marks are seen
10. On slit-lamp biomicroscopy with a +90 D lens, the above findings are confirmed. Indirect ophthalmoscopy showed the peripheries to be normal

CENTRAL RETINAL VEIN OCCLUSION

Fundus examination of the right eye:
1. Distant direct ophthalmoscopy at one arm's distance showed a good red glow. Direct ophthalmoscopy close to face revealed a clear media
2. Disk was enlarged and hyperemic with obscured margins, an obliterated cup, and edematous neuroretinal rim. The disk and cup shape were not assessable due to the edema. Multiple streak-shaped superficial red

lesions oriented perpendicular to the disk margin within 1 DD of the optic disk were seen, suggestive of splinter hemorrhages
3. Vessels arise from the center of the disk, branching dichotomously with an arteriovenous ratio of 2:4. The veins were dilated and tortuous
4. Background retina shows multiple streak-shaped superficial red lesions suggestive of flame-shaped hemorrhages in all four quadrants of the posterior pole. Numerous fluffy, superficial yellowish lesions with indistinct margins suggestive of cotton wool spots are seen
5. Multiple hemorrhages and retinal thickening within 1 DD from the macula are seen, suggestive of macular edema
6. On slit-lamp biomicroscopy with a +90 D lens, the above findings are confirmed. Indirect ophthalmoscopy showed the peripheries to be normal

EXAMINATION OF A LONG CASE: PROPTOSIS

Guidelines
1. Duration of the complaints should be in a chronological order
2. Elaboration of the complaint should have an onset (insidious, sudden, etc.) and a progress mode (rapid, slow, etc.) and any relieving nature (e.g., pain relieved with closing the eyes)

Mr M, a 57-year-old male, farmer by occupation, hailing from Madurai, presented to us with complaints of:
1. Prominence of right eye of 4 months' duration
2. Swelling and pain of right eye of 1 month duration

History of Present Illness

The patient was asymptomatic till 4 months back when he noticed prominence of right eye, which was insidious in onset, progressive in nature, and more worse in the morning. The prominence was associated with mild discomfort and dryness of the right eye. He consulted a local ophthalmologist and was prescribed some eye drops, which provided some symptomatic relief.

The patient then developed swelling of the right eye of both upper and lower lids associated with pain and redness of the right eye, which was progressive in nature and worse in the morning. The pain was dull, aching in nature, more of retrobulbar discomfort, typically described by the patient as something pushing behind the eye. The pain was nonradiating, present both at rest and with movements of the eye.

The above symptoms were associated with gritty foreign body sensation of both eyes.
1. History of (H/o) loss of weight with good appetite associated with increased sweating, tremors, and palpitations since past 2 years
2. H/o swelling in the neck for the past 2 years
3. No h/o diplopia

4. No h/o defective vision or blackouts or transient loss of vision, or defective color perception
5. No h/o hyperpigmentation of lids/eyes
6. No h/o postural variation (bending forward)
7. No h/o variation with sneezing or coughing, or straining
8. No h/o photophobia, discharge, or colored halos
9. No h/o any other swelling in the body
10. No h/o dysphagia, dysphonia, easy fatigability, drooping of eyelids
11. No h/o radiation therapy or chemotherapy in the past
12. No h/o skin discoloration in the past
13. No h/o fever, headache, nausea, or vomiting
14. No h/o nasal block, frequent respiratory tract infection, epistaxis
15. No h/o trauma

Past History
1. H/o taking tablet carbimazole 5 mg BD for the past 2 years
2. No h/o diabetes mellitus, hypertension, or cardiac disease

Personal History
1. Patient consumes mixed diet
2. He is a chronic smoker, consumes an average of six to seven cigarettes per day
3. He occasionally consumes alcohol

Family History
1. No h/o similar complaints in the family

General Examination
1. Patient is averagely built and nourished
2. Pulse—90/min, regular in rhythm and volume
3. Respiratory rate was 18/min.
4. Blood pressure was 130/80 mm Hg taken in the left upper arm in the supine position
5. Higher functions are normal
6. No pallor, cyanosis, icterus, and clubbing
7. No evidence of any regional or generalized lymphadenopathy
8. No evidence of any skin changes or dryness
9. Examination of the neck revealed small midline swelling of 3 × 5 cm which moved with deglutition and did not move with protrusion of the tongue suggestive of a thyroid swelling
10. Fine tremors were noted when the patient was asked to stretch his arms and spread out his fingers

11. Tremors were not present at rest
12. There was no evidence of dysdiadochokinesia and finger
13. Nose past pointing test was negative
14. Central nervous system was within normal limits. There was no sign of confusion or dementia or lethargy
15. Cardiovascular system was normal without any murmurs
16. Respiratory system examination revealed normal vesicular breath sounds in both lungs on auscultation
17. Per abdominal examination was normal, with no evidence of any palpable intra-abdominal mass
18. Ears, nose, and throat (ENT) examination—anterior rhinoscopy was normal with no evidence of sinus tenderness

Ocular Examination

Visual acuity in both eyes is 6/12p, improving to 6/6 with +1.50 D sphere with 2.50 D sphere for near vision

Parameter	Right eye	Left eye
	Axial proptosis	Normal
Lids	Periorbital edema	Normal
Conjunctiva	Congestion nasally and temporally, mild chemosis, decreased tear film height, decreased tear film breakup height (<10 seconds)	Normal
Cornea	Few punctate epithelial erosions	Clear
Anterior chamber	Normal depth	Normal depth
Iris	Normal color and pattern	Normal color and pattern
Pupil	4 mm, briskly reacting to both direct and consensual light reflex	4 mm, briskly reacting to both direct and consensual light reflex
Lens	Clear	Clear
Extraocular movements (EOM)	Full	Full
Fundus	Normal	Normal

The above findings were confirmed with slit-lamp biomicroscopy, and fundus examination with 90 D examination revealed normal findings with no evidence of Sallmann macular folds.

Evaluation of Proptosis

1. Head posture is normal
2. Facial asymmetry is present

3. *Corneal reflex:* Eyes are orthophoric
4. To mention any signs of thyroid eye disease if present

Inspection

1. Axial proptosis of the right eye is noted
2. Nafziger's sign (protrusion of the eye beyond the orbital rim when examined from above and behind the patient) was positive on the right side
3. On inspection, eyebrows were normal with no evidence of madarosis
4. Lids revealed periorbital edema of both upper and lower lids

Right Eye

Inspection
1. In the right eye, lid margins were 3 mm from the superior and inferior limbus, suggestive of moderate lid retraction
2. Temporal flare was present
3. Elevation (−1) and adduction (−1) were mildly restricted
4. Lid lag was present on downgaze
5. There was minimal lagophthalmos with good Bell's phenomenon in the right eye
6. No variation of proptosis was observed in the right eye with posture, especially on bending forward and with Valsalva maneuver
7. The proptosis was nonpulsatile
8. There was no evidence of engorged veins/corkscrew vessels in the right eye

Palpation
1. Orbital margins were intact
2. Insinuation with fingers was possible in all four margins
3. No palpable mass was felt
4. Resistance to retropulsion was present
5. Proptosis was noncompressible and nonreducible
6. No thrills or pulsations were felt
7. There was no evidence of warmth or tenderness over the right eye
8. There was no change in the size of the proptosis with jugular vein compression or carotid artery compression

Left Eye

Inspection
1. Temporal flare was present
2. Lid margins were 1 mm from superior limbus and 2 mm from inferior limbus, respectively, suggestive of mild lid retraction

3. Lid lag was present on downgaze
4. There was minimal lagophthalmos with good Bell's phenomenon

Palpation

1. Orbital margins were intact
2. Resistance to retropulsion was present

Auscultation

1. No bruits were heard in both eyes

Measurements

Hertel's Exophthalmometry (Base at 105)

1. Right eye—22 mm
2. Left eye—18 mm

Applanation Tonometry

1. Tension by applanation tonometry was 16 mm Hg in the right eye and 18 mm Hg in the left eye in primary gaze
2. Tension by applanation tonometry was 26 mm Hg in the right eye and 24 mm Hg in the left eye in upgaze
3. *Schirmer's test:* At the end of 5 minutes, it revealed 12 mm of Whatman's strip wetting in the right eye and 15 mm in the left eye, suggestive of mild dry eye
4. Color vision testing with Ishihara's pseudoisochromatic plate was normal in both eyes
5. Central fields testing with Bjerrum's screen was normal in both eyes
6. Anterior rhinoscopy was within normal limits. Sinus examination was normal

Provisional Diagnosis

Right eye unilateral axial proptosis due to an acute inflammatory stage of thyroid-related orbitopathy

Differential Diagnosis

1. Thyroid-related orbitopathy
2. Cavernous hemangioma
3. Idiopathic inflammatory pseudotumor
4. Orbital cellulitis

FREQUENTLY ASKED QUESTIONS DURING PRESENTATION

1. **What is the rationale for asking history of radiation therapy or chemotherapy in the past?**
   To rule out any neoplasm elsewhere in the body which might have metastasized to the orbit
2. **What is the rationale for asking history of skin discoloration in the past?**
   To rule out thyroid-related skin changes (thyroid myxedema) and also neurofibromatosis (pigmented birthmarks)
3. **What is the rationale for asking history of hyperpigmentation of lids/eyes?**
   To rule out metastatic neuroblastoma (raccoon eyes)
4. **What is the rationale for asking history of fever, headache, nausea, and vomiting?**
   To rule out orbital cellulitis, cavernous sinus thrombosis
5. **What is the rationale for asking history of nasal block, frequent respiratory tract infection, and epistaxis?**
   To rule out sinusitis and nasopharyngeal carcinoma
6. **What is the rationale for asking history of trauma?**
   To rule out orbital hematoma and retrobulbar hemorrhage in cases of acute proptosis
7. **What is the rationale for asking history of dysphonia, dysphasia, and easy fatigability in a patient with proptosis?**
   To rule out associated myasthenia gravis

EXAMINATION OF A LONG CASE: PTOSIS

Mr P, a 65-year-old male, a shopkeeper by occupation, hailing from Chennai, presented to us with complaint of:
1. Drooping of the right upper lid since the past 3 months

History of Present Illness

The patient was apparently alright 3 months back when he noticed drooping of his right upper lid, which was insidious in onset, gradually progressive, and painless in nature. There were no aggravating or relieving factors.
   1. No h/o trauma (to rule out traumatic ptosis)
   2. No h/o diplopia (to rule out myogenic and neurogenic cases, e.g., myasthenia gravis, third nerve palsy)
   3. No h/o pain (presence of pain essentially rules out myasthenia)
   4. No h/o defective vision (to rule out orbital apex syndrome)
   5. No h/o any lid swellings or masses (to rule out mechanical ptosis)

6. No h/o previous ocular surgery (mild ptosis can occur after ocular surgeries)
7. No h/o diurnal variation (for myasthenia)
8. No h/o dysphagia, dysphonia, easy fatigability, difficulty in walking (for myasthenia)
9. No h/o heat intolerance, palpitations, weight loss, insomnia (to rule out thyroid eye disease)
10. No h/o fever, headache, nausea, vomiting

Past History
1. No h/o similar complaints in the past
2. No h/o diabetes mellitus, hypertension, cardiac disease

Personal History
1. Patient consumes a mixed diet
2. He is a nonsmoker
3. He occasionally consumes alcohol

Family History
1. No h/o similar complaints in the family

General Examination
1. Patient is averagely built and nourished
2. Pulse—80/min, regular in rhythm and volume
3. Respiratory rate was 15/min
4. Blood pressure was 110/80 mm Hg taken in the left upper arm in the supine position
5. Higher functions are normal
6. No pallor, cyanosis, icterus, and clubbing
7. No evidence of any regional or generalized lymphadenopathy
8. No evidence of any skin changes or dryness
9. Central nervous system was within normal limits
10. Cardiovascular system was normal without any murmurs
11. Respiratory system examination revealed normal vesicular breath sounds in both lungs on auscultation
12. Per abdominal examination was normal, with no evidence of any palpable intra-abdominal mass

Ocular Examination
Visual acuity in both eyes is 6/12 improving to 6/6 with +1.00 D sphere with 2.50 D sphere for near vision.

Parameter	Right eye	Left eye
Lids	Moderate ptosis	Normal
Conjunctiva	Normal	Normal
Cornea	Clear	Clear
Anterior chamber	Normal depth	Normal depth
Iris	Normal color and pattern	Normal color and pattern
Pupil	4 mm, briskly reacting to both direct and consensual light reflex	4 mm, briskly reacting to both direct and consensual light reflex
Lens	Clear	Clear
EOM	Full	Full
Fundus	Normal	Normal

The above findings were confirmed with slit-lamp biomicroscopy, and fundus examination with 90 D examination revealed normal findings.

Evaluation of Ptosis

Right Eye

1. Head posture—normal
2. Frontalis overaction—present
3. Margin reflex distance 1 (without blocking frontalis)—1 mm
4. Margin reflex distance 1 (with blocking frontalis)—0 mm
5. Margin reflex distance 2—4 mm
6. Palpebral fissure height—5 mm
7. Amount of ptosis—3 mm
8. Levator function—10 mm (fair)
9. Margin crease distance—10 mm
10. Lagophthalmos—absent
11. Bell's phenomenon—good
12. Jaw wink—absent
13. Lid lag—absent
14. Fatigability—absent
15. Ice pack test—negative
16. Ocular movements—no restriction
17. Pupil—normal

Provisional Diagnosis

1. Right eye senile aponeurotic ptosis

ECTROPION

Mr G, a 76-year-old farmer, came with complaints of watering and redness in his left eye for the past 3 months.

Evaluation:
1. *Pinch test*—approximately 10 mm (positive)
2. *Snap-back test*—returns to original position after 4 seconds (grade 2)
3. *Medial canthal laxity*—present—punctum stretched up to limbus
4. *Lateral canthus laxity*—present—lateral canthal angle moves 3 mm
5. *Inferior lid retractor laxity*—reduced movement of lower lid on downgaze present
6. *Lacrimal punctum eversion*—present—punctum directed away from the globe
7. *Orbicularis tone*—good
8. *Cicatricial skin changes*—absent
9. *Conjunctival exposure changes*—mild congestion over inferior conjunctiva
10. *Corneal exposure changes*—absent
11. *Corneal sensation*—present
12. *Lagophthalmos*—1 mm
13. *Grade of ectropion*—posterior lid margin everted (grade 2)

Diagnosis: Left eye involutional ectropion

ENTROPION

Mr F, a 66-year-old shopkeeper, came with complaints of watering and foreign body sensation in his right eye for the past 6 months.

Evaluation:
1. *Pinch test*—approximately 8 mm (positive)
2. *Snap-back test*—returns to original position after 3 seconds (grade 1)
3. *Medial canthal laxity*—present—punctum stretched beyond limbus
4. *Lateral canthus laxity*—present—lateral canthal angle moves 4 mm
5. *Inferior lid retractor laxity*—reduced movement of lower lid on downgaze present
6. *Trichiasis*—present
7. *Orbicularis tone*—fair
8. *Cicatricial skin changes/digital eversion test*—absent—lid can be everted easily (no cicatricial component)
9. *Conjunctival exposure changes*—congestion over inferior conjunctiva
10. *Corneal exposure changes*—nebular scar over the inferior part of cornea
11. *Grade of entropion*—lid in turning up to intermarginal strip (grade 2)

Diagnosis: Right eye involutional entropion.

13.1 THIRD NERVE PALSY—MODEL CASE SHEET

Mr G, a 52-year-old male, came with chief complaints of double vision for the past 5 days.

HISTORY OF PRESENT ILLNESS
1. He was asymptomatic till 5 days ago when he experienced sudden double vision as he was leaving for work. It was acute in onset, present binocularly, with progressive and horizontal separation of images
2. There was no diurnal variation and not increasing in any particular gaze
3. He noticed some restricted movement of the right eye, but it was not associated with pain
4. He was also able to appreciate that while occluding either eye, the diplopia subsided

No drooping of eyelids/defective vision or any history suggestive of defective field of vision.
1. No h/o headache/vomiting
2. No h/o fever/trauma/surgery
3. No h/o diurnal variation
4. No h/o weakness of one side of face/limb weakness/tremors
5. No h/o mental/sleep disturbances
6. No h/o anosmia/hard of hearing/nasal regurgitation/nasal twang
7. No h/o altered bowel/bladder habit
8. No h/o scalp tenderness/jaw claudication
9. In children—rule out postvaccination

Past History
1. No similar episodes in the past

Medical Treatment History
1. He gives h/o diabetes mellitus (DM) for the past 8 years and is on irregular medications
2. He also gives h/o systemic hypertension for the past 5 years and is on irregular medications
3. He has no h/o surgeries in the past

Personal History
1. Nonsmoker/nonalcoholic
2. Normal bowel and bladder habits
3. Consuming a balanced diet

General Examination

1. Conscious, oriented to place and time
2. Moderately built and nourished
3. No pallor
4. Icterus
5. Cyanosis
6. Clubbing
7. Lymphadenopathy
8. Pedal edema

Vitals

1. Afebrile
2. Pulse—80 beats/min—regular rhythm, with normal volume and character
3. Blood pressure—140/90 mm Hg recorded in supine position over the left arm
4. Respiratory rate—18 times/minute

Systemic Examination

1. Cardiovascular system (CVS)—S1 S2 + heard. No murmurs
2. Respiratory system (RS)—normal vesicular breath sounds are heard. No added sounds
3. Abdomen—soft. No organomegaly

Ocular Examination

1. Best corrected visual acuity 6/9 in both eyes (BE) (distance) (Near) N6 at 33 cm with +2.0 diopter sphere (DS)
2. No characteristic head posture noted
3. Hirschberg's test revealed 30' exotropia in the right eye
4. On torchlight examination:

Parameter	Right eye	Left eye
Lids/adnexa	Normal	Normal
Conjunctiva	Normal	Normal
Cornea	Clear	Clear
Anterior chamber	Normal depth	Normal depth
Iris	Normal color pattern	Normal color pattern
Pupil	3 mm round-D+-C+	3 mm round-D+-C+
Accommodation reflex present		
Lens	Early lens changes	Early lens changes

5. Extraocular movements: Right eye
   i. Restricted adduction, elevation, and depression
   ii. Abduction is present
   iii. Intorsion is present
   iv. The movements of the left eye are normal
6. The above findings were confirmed using a slit-lamp biomicroscopy with additional inference of
   i. (BE) - lens—grade I nuclear sclerosis
7. Fundus examination: Using a direct ophthalmoscope:
   i. Revealed a clear media, with normal disk and vessels, with a healthy macula foveal reflex (FR)±
   ii. The above findings were confirmed using a slit-lamp biomicroscopy and 90 D lens
   iii. The peripheries were examined using an indirect ophthalmoscope, and 20 D lens was found to be normal
8. Corneal sensations (BE)—normal
9. Color vision (BE)—normal (using Ishihara's chart)
10. Tension (BE) by noncontact tonometer—16 mm Hg
11. No signs of aberrant regeneration
12. Examination of other cranial nerves:
    i. Olfactory nerve
    ii. Optic nerve
    iii. Trigeminal nerve
    iv. Facial nerve
    v. Vestibule cochlear nerve
    vi. Glossopharyngeal nerve
    vii. Vagus nerve
    viii. Accessory nerve
    ix. Hypoglossal nerve
13. Motor system examination—normal
14. Sensory system examination—normal
15. Reflexes
    i. Superficial
    ii. Deep normal
16. Gait—normal
17. Cerebellar function tests—normal

Diagnosis

Right eye, pupil sparing, infranuclear incomplete third nerve palsy, due to an ischemic microangiopathy with probable etiology being DM/HM.

Explanation to the History Taking and Examination of the Model Case Sheet

1. **Diplopia**
    i. Onset—acute, subacute, insidious in onset
    ii. Progression—progressive or regressive
        - *Progressive*—all neoplasms, myasthenia, thyroid-related ophthalmopathy (TRO)
        - *Regressive*—inflammatory infection causes
    iii. Horizontal/vertical
        - *Horizontal diplopia*—lateral rectus/medial rectus involved
        - *Vertical diplopia*—elevators/depressors involved
    iv. Diplopia for near or far
        - *Near:* Trochlear nerve is involved
        - *Far:* Abducent nerve is involved
    v. Increases in which gaze—diplopia increases on looking toward the side of paralyzed muscle
    vi. Diurnal variation—to rule out myasthenia gravis
    vii. Diplopia worsens in the evening: Myasthenia gravis
    viii. Diplopia worsens in the morning: Thyroid orbitopathy due to venous stasis and accumulation of glycosaminoglycans

2. **Conditions causing ophthalmoplegia + pain**
    i. Tolosa-Hunt syndrome
    ii. Giant cell arteritis
    iii. Retrobulbar neuritis
    iv. Migraine
    v. Caroticocavernous fistula
    vi. Intrinsic lesions of the third nerve—schwannomas/cavernous hemangiomas

3. **History of drooping of lids**
    To know the involvement of levator palpebrae superioris (LPS)—to differentiate a nuclear from an infranuclear palsy

4. **History of defective vision**
    Orbital apex syndrome—optic nerve is affected

5. **History of defective field of vision**
    To know the status of cortical function

6. **Negative history**
    i. H/o headache/vomiting signs of raised intracranial tension
    ii. H/o fever/fits to rule out typhoid/tick fever/glandular fever
    iii. H/o trauma/surgery lumbar puncture can predispose to uncal herniation syndrome/other functional endoscopic sinus surgery (FESS) and neurosurgeries too

iv. H/o diurnal variation myasthenia/TRO
v. H/o weakness at one side of face/limb weakness/tremors (to rule out involvement of other cranial nerves and the syndromes associated with third nerve palsy)
vi. H/o epistaxis (raised blood pressure)
vii H/o vesicular eruption on one side of face—herpetic ophthalmoplegia can predispose to third nerve palsy
viii H/o anosmia/nasal regurgitation/nasal twang—to rule out involvement of other cranial nerves
ix. H/o altered bowel/bladder habits—involvement of the autonomic nervous system
x. H/o scalp tenderness/jaw claudication—giant cell arteritis
xi. For children—can cause postvaccination neuritis
xii. Rules out past vaccination

7. **Significance of medical treatment history**
DM and systemic hypertension are the most common causes of pupil-sparing third nerve palsy.

8. **History of smoking and alcoholism**
Smoker—predisposed to thromboembolism
Alcoholic—Wernicke's encephalopathy/trauma

9. **Importance of contact to tuberculosis**
Tuberculous meningitis can predispose to third nerve palsy

10. **Relevance of fundus examination**
Look for papilledema

11. **Causes of decreased corneal sensations**
    i. Herpes simplex keratitis
    ii. Neuroparalytic keratitis
    iii. Leprosy
    iv. Herpes zoster ophthalmicus
    v. Absolute glaucoma
    vi. Acoustic neuroma
    vii. Neurofibroma

12. **Examination of other cranial nerves**
    i. *Olfactory*—using asafetida and coffee beans, check each nostril separately
    Optic nerve:
    - Visual acuity
    - Pupil examination
    - Visual fields
    - Color vision

ii. *Trigeminal nerve*—motor muscles of mastication/jaw deviate toward the paralyzed side
Sensory—corneal sensations
Sensations over face
iii. *Facial nerve*—motor-orbicularis oculi
Wrinkling of forehead orbicularis oris (whistling) smile and dense (mouth deviated to healthy side) inflate mouth with air
Sensory—test in anterior two-thirds of tongue
iv. *Vestibule cochlear:*
For cochlear function, use 512 Hz because higher frequency—less accurate in finding difference between air and bone conduction
 - Lower frequency—vibrations produced may be misinterpreted as sound
 - Rinne's test: Normal sensory neural hearing loss—lateralized to normal ear conductive loss—lateralized to deaf ear
 - For vestibular functions, we check:
   - Nystagmus
   - Positional vertigo
   - Romberg's test
v. *Glossopharyngeal nerve*—taste in posterior one-third of tongue palatal reflex
vi. *Vagus*—gag reflex
vii. *Spinal accessory nerve*—sternomastoid/trapezius muscle
viii. *Hypoglossal nerve*—tongue deviates to paralyzed side.

13.2 GLAUCOMA—MODEL CASE SHEET

A 56-year-old gentleman came to us with complaints of defective vision of the right eye of 1 year duration and left eye of 6 months duration.

HISTORY OF PRESENT ILLNESS

On elaboration, he revealed that he had been suffering from defective vision for the past 1 year. He had consulted an ophthalmologist at his place who said he had raised pressures in both his eyes and put him on topical medications, twice-a-day regimen for both his eyes. He was not compliant to his medicines, and on his follow-up visit, his doctor had advised surgery for his right eye. He underwent the surgery to reduce his eye pressures. He feels that vision is unsatisfactory in both his eyes and has come for a second opinion.

1. No h/o night blindness
2. No h/o frequent change of glasses
3. No h/o headache
4. No h/o colored haloes
5. No h/o redness/watering/pain
6. No h/o injury/trauma

PAST HISTORY

He was a known diabetic for the past 15 years who was on oral hypoglycemic agents and an asthmatic on inhalational therapy whenever symptomatic.

Apart from the medications which he has been using for both his eyes, twice daily for the past 1 year and surgery to lower pressure in his right eye 6 months back, there is no other medical or surgical history.

PERSONAL HISTORY

Smoker, smokes 2–3 *beedis* per day for the past 30 years
   Not an alcoholic

FAMILY HISTORY

No h/o diabetes or ocular diseases among the family members

GENERAL EXAMINATION

Well-built and nourished
   Pulse rate—76/min, regular in rhythm and volume
   Blood pressure—130/70 mm Hg
   Cardiovascular, respiratory, and central nervous system examination within normal limits

OCULAR EXAMINATION

Parameter	Right eye	Left eye
Unaided vision	6/60	6/24
With pinhole	6/12	6/9
Near vision	N8 at 33 cm with +2 D	N6 at 33 cm with +2 D

No Facial Asymmetry

Parameter	Right eye	Left eye
Lids and adnexa	Normal	Normal
Conjunctiva	A flat, diffuse translucent bleb, extending from 11 to 2 o'clock position superiorly above the limbus, with dilated tortuous vessels over its surface, no microcysts and subconjunctival fibrosis obscuring the underlying details was seen, suggestive of a failing bleb	Normal
Cornea	Clear	Clear
Anterior chamber	Using a slit 1 mm in thickness inside the temporal limbus at an angle of 60°, the ratio of the corneal thickness to the gap between the posterior surface of cornea and the anterior surface of iris was 1:1, suggestive of an open angle with Van Herick's grading of grade 4	Using a slit 1 mm in thickness inside the temporal limbus at an angle of 60°, the ratio of the corneal thickness to the gap between the posterior surface of cornea and the anterior surface of iris was 1:1, suggestive of an open angle with Van Herick's grading of grade 4
Iris	A single, peripheral triangular defect measuring 2 mm in size with sharp well-defined edges seen superiorly at the 12 o'clock position close to the limbus, suggestive of a surgical iridectomy, is seen. Retroillumination was positive indicating patency	Normal in color and pattern
Pupil	4 mm, round and reacting sluggishly to light, with grade 3 relative afferent pupillary defect (RAPD)	Normal in size and shape, reacting well to direct, indirect being slightly sluggish
Lens	Nuclear sclerosis, grade 2	Nuclear sclerosis, grade 2
Extraocular movements (EOM)	Full	Full

FUNDUS EXAMINATION

Parameter	Right eye	Left eye
Media	Clear	Clear
Disk	A normal-sized pale vertically oval disk with a vertically oval cup with well-defined margins was seen with a cup–disk ratio of 0.9 with a concentric thinning of the neuroretinal rim. Bayonetting of vessels and laminar dot sign was present. Surrounding nerve fiber layer, seen with the help of a red free filter, showed a diffuse loss of retinal nerve fiber layer (RNFL). The vessels were arising centrally branching dichotomously with an arteriovenous (AV) ratio of 2:3. There was presence of associated peripapillary atrophy	A normal-sized pink vertically oval disk with a vertically oval cup with well-defined margins was seen with a cup–disk ratio of 0.75 with a focal notching superior and corresponding thinning of neuroretinal rim. An arcuate defect was seen superiorly in the nerve fiber layer with the help of a red-free filter corresponding to the superior notch. The vessels were arising centrally branching dichotomously with an AV ratio of 2:3. No peripapillary atrophy was observed
Posterior pole	Foveal reflex was present and background retina was normal	Foveal reflex was present and background retina was normal

GONIOSCOPY

Right eye	Left eye
Trabecular meshwork seen in all four quadrants with a patent ostium and peripheral iridectomy seen superiorly	Trabecular meshwork seen in all four quadrants

Intraocular Pressures

Intraocular pressures were recorded with Goldmann's applanation tonometer, which showed:

Right eye	Left eye
26 mm Hg	24 mm Hg

Diagnosis

Right eye: Primary open-angle glaucoma status post-trabeculectomy with failed bleb and grade 2 nuclear sclerosis

Left eye: Primary open-angle glaucoma and grade 2 nuclear sclerosis

1. **Why do we ask for history of night blindness?**
    i. Defective dark adaptation is a feature of open-angle glaucoma
    ii. Use of miotics will accentuate night blindness

2. **What is the cause for frequent change of glasses?**
   i. Patients experience more difficulty for near vision since constant high pressure over zonules and ciliary body impairs accommodation
   ii. Patients tend to confuse defective field of vision with defective vision and hence repeatedly change glasses

3. **What can cause sudden loss of vision in a glaucoma patient?**
   i. Acute intraocular pressure (IOP) rise resulting in corneal edema
   ii. Central retinal vein occlusion
   iii. Post-trabeculectomy in advanced glaucoma—snuff-out phenomena

4. **What are the structural abnormalities you will look for in a case of glaucoma?**
   i. *Lids and adnexa:*
      - Hemangioma (Sturge-Weber)
      - Hypertrichosis (use of latanoprost)
      - Periocular pigmentation (use of epinephrine)
   ii. *Conjunctiva:*
      - Dilated tortuous episcleral vessels (Sturge-Weber)
      - Bleb (location, extent, presence of microcysts, vascularity, visibility of scleral flaps, infection, presence of aqueous leak, subconjunctival fibrosis)
      - Circumcorneal congestion (in acute congestive glaucoma)
   iii. *Cornea:*
      - Edema
      - Descemet's folds
      - Keratic precipitates
      - Pigments on the endothelium (Krukenberg's spindle in pigmentary glaucoma)
      - Pseudoexfoliation on the endothelium
      - Prominent Schwalbe's line—congenital glaucoma
      - Peripheral anterior synechiae
      - Megalocornea
      - Cornea plana
      - Sclerocornea
      - Congenital corneal opacity (Peter's anomaly)
      - Prominent corneal nerves (neurofibromatosis)
   iv. *Anterior chamber:*
      - Depth—peripheral and central
      - Reactions—flare and cells
      - Hyphema
      - Hypopyon
   v. *Iris:*
      - Aniridia
      - Atrophic patches (following acute attack)

- Nodules
- Holes
- Pseudoexfoliation material
- Transillumination defects
- Peripheral iridectomy (number, position, patency, surgical/laser)
- Iris cysts
- Nevus
- Ectropion uvea

vi. *Pupil:*
- Size
- Shape
- Number
- Reaction to light—direct and indirect
- Resistant to dilatation
- Seclusion or occlusion papillae

vii. *Lens:*
- Pseudoexfoliation on anterior lens capsule
- Glaucomflecken
- Cataract—intumescent/dislocated/subluxated
- Zonular dialysis
- Spherophakia

5. **What are the management strategies for the following scenarios?**
    i. Primary open-angle suspect
    Baseline investigations:
    - Tension applanation
    - Central corneal thickness
    - Baseline fundus photo
    - Nerve fiber analysis—GDx
    - HFA-SITA SWAP (Humphrey field analyzer-Swedish interactive threshold algorithm short wavelength automated perimetry)—glaucoma progression analysis
    - Optical coherence tomography (OCT)—macular thickness analysis, i.e., ganglion cell complex

    Treatment:
    - Observe the patient if no risk factors
    - Follow-up after 2 months. If progression is documented, start antiglaucoma therapy

    ii. Established primary open-angle glaucoma
    Baseline investigations:
    - Tension applanation
    - Central corneal thickness

- Baseline fundus photo
- Nerve fiber analysis—GDx (role controversial in established glaucoma)
- HFA-24-2
- OCT—macular thickness analysis, i.e., ganglion cell complex

Treatment:
- Calculate the target pressure: This is done using the following formula:

$TP = IP(1-IP/100) - Z \pm 2$

where: TP = *target pressure*
IP = *initial pressure*
Z = *functional status*
(disk damage/field changes)

Z-0 Glaucoma suspect (low risk)
Z-0 Glaucoma suspect (high risk)
Z-1 Early glaucoma
Z-3 Moderate glaucoma
Z-5 Severe glaucoma
Z-7 End-stage glaucoma

- Start on single drug therapy (prostaglandin analogs are the first choice or else beta-blockers and alpha-adrenergic agonists can be started.)
- Review after 2 months and see if target pressure is maintained. If not, consider substituting or adding another drug
- Follow-up, and in spite of maximal tolerated medical therapy, if the pressures are still not under control, then consider trabeculectomy

iii. *Primary open-angle glaucoma (POAG) with significant cataract*
The following considerations should be taken into account while performing surgery in a glaucoma patient:
- Miotic pupils
- Posterior synechiae
- Exfoliation—zonular weakness
- Congested eyes—bleeding
- Prior surgery—scarring/filtering bleb
- Systemic diseases—diabetes, hypertension
- Ocular conditions—myopia, shallow chamber
- Increased incidence of postoperative IOP rise
- Suprachoroidal hemorrhage
    - *Cataract alone can be performed in the following scenario:*
        • Acceptable IOP control with one or two medications
        • No significant visual field loss or disk damage

- Older age
- Conditions where compliance and drug intolerance are not an issue
- Higher target IOP

Advantages of doing cataract alone:
- Single procedure
- Technically easier
- Short surgical time
- Reduced operative and postoperative complications
- Temporal clear corneal approach enables preserving viable conjunctiva

Disadvantages of doing cataract alone:
- Early postoperative spike of IOP
- Long-term IOP control questionable
- Subsequent filtering surgery prone for failure

- Combined surgery (cataract and filtering surgery) can be performed in the following scenario:
  - Multiple medications required to control IOP
  - Use of glaucoma medications restricted by cost, intolerance, compliance issues
  - Significant glaucomatous visual loss
  - Presence of ocular risk factors—exfoliation, pigment dispersion, angle recession
  - Monocular status—earlier visual recovery
  - Two separate procedures not feasible

  Advantages of combined surgery:
  - Restore vision promptly
  - Single procedure
  - Reduced glaucoma medications
  - Early postoperative IOP control
  - Long-term IOP control
  - Antimetabolite use possible to enhance success
  - Facilitate assessment of disk and visual fields

  Disadvantages of combined surgery:
  - More complications—shallow chamber, bleb leak, choroidal effusion/hemorrhage, hypotony, infection, astigmatism
  - Visual recovery longer than in cataract alone
  - Intensive postoperative care requirements than cataract alone
  - Less IOP control than filtering surgery alone—success of filtering compromised by filtering surgery
  - Glaucoma medications postoperative

A CASE OF UNILATERAL OLD RHEGMATOGENOUS RETINAL DETACHMENT

Right eye—subtotal rhegmatogenous retinal detachment (RRD)
Left eye—lattice with hole S/P barrage laser

Right Eye

Distant direct ophthalmoscopy: Shows a gray reflex

Direct ophthalmoscopy close to face
1. Media is clear
2. Disk appears normal in size, vertically oval, pink in color, having a cup–disk ratio of 0.3 with a healthy neuroretinal rim. The margins are well defined
3. The vessels are seen arising from the center of the disk, branching dichotomously and tortuous in nature
4. A convex shallow smooth membrane is seen superonasal, inferonasal, and inferotemporal to the optic disk involving the macula, suggestive of retinal detachment with macula off (focused using high plus power)

On Slit-lamp Examination

1. Posterior chamber intraocular lens (PCIOL) with posterior capsule rupture (PCR) present
2. Arteriovenous fistula (AVF) examination shows pigments or tobacco dust

On Indirect Ophthalmoscopy

1. Media is clear
2. Disk appears normal in size, vertically oval, pink in color, having a cup–disk ratio of 0.3 with a healthy neuroretinal rim
3. The vessels are seen arising from the center of the disk, branching dichotomously and tortuous in nature
4. A convex shallow smooth elevation of the retina with loss of an underlying choroidal pattern is seen. This undulating membrane in the vitreous cavity extends from 2 to 9 o'clock involving the macula, suggestive of subtotal RRD with macula off. Minimal shifting fluid is present
5. A wedge-shaped area of retina superotemporal to the optic disk appears to be attached
6. A retinal tear with the ends pointing toward ora, suggestive of horseshoe tear, is seen at 2 o'clock position in the equatorial zone. Rolled edges and wrinkling of surface are noted
7. Full-thickness fixed puckering of the detached retina with overlying preretinal membrane spanning 2 o'clock hours at the end of inferotemporal arcade is suggestive of star folds

8. Intraretinal cyst is seen 1 disk diameter away from the disk at 3 o'clock
9. Linear yellow areas beneath the surface of retinal detachment suggestive of subretinal bands with demarcation lines are present in the inferotemporal area

Left Eye

Distant direct ophthalmoscopy: Shows red glow

Direct ophthalmoscopy close to face
1. Media is clear
2. Disk appears normal in size, vertically oval, pink in color, having a cup–disk ratio of 0.3 with healthy neuroretinal rim
3. The vessels are seen arising from the center of the disk, branching dichotomously, maintaining an AV ratio of 2:3
4. Macula appears normal, and the foveal reflex is seen
5. The background retina appears normal

On slit-lamp examination: The above findings are confirmed.

On indirect ophthalmoscopy: On sclera indentation
1. The peripheral retina shows a sharply demarcated spindle-shaped area of retinal thinning spanning 3 o'clock hours, parallel to the ora, in the periphery of inferotemporal quadrant with vitreous condensation at the margin, suggestive of lattice degeneration
2. A full-thickness defect in the retina surrounded by two rows of regular, equally spaced pigmented lesions indicative of a lasered retinal hole is seen adjacent to the lattice

RHEGMATOGENOUS RETINAL DETACHMENT (FRESH)

Fundus Examination of Right Eye

1. Distant direct ophthalmoscopy at one arm distance showed a dull glow/gray reflex
2. Direct ophthalmoscopy close to face revealed a clear media
3. Retina could be seen with high "plus" power of the direct ophthalmoscope
4. Upon further examination with slit-lamp biomicroscopy with 90 D and indirect ophthalmoscopy with scleral indentation, the following findings were seen
5. Brown pigmented tobacco dust-like pigments were seen dispersed in the anterior vitreous suggestive of the Shafer sign
6. A bullous, translucent, grayish, convex elevation of the retina with corrugated appearance and convexity facing toward the disk with loss of an underlying choroidal pattern was seen from 1 to 10 o'clock hours

position suggestive of subtotal retinal detachment, which was extending from ora serrata toward disk area
7. The disk could be visualized amidst the detached retinal folds, and it was vertically oval, larger in size, pink in color with a tilted conformation, and well-defined margins having a cup–disk ratio of 0.4 with healthy neuroretinal rim
8. Peripapillary chorioretinal atrophy was seen
9. The vessels over the detached retina appeared darker than in the flat retina, and hence the venules and arterioles could not be differentiated
10. The detached retina was seen undulating with eye movements
11. The highest point of the detached retina was noted superonasally near 1 o'clock position
12. Macula was off
13. A superior wedge of attached retina was seen from 10 to 1 o'clock hour
14. A red-colored horseshoe-shaped tear with the ends pointing toward the ora was seen in the equatorial zone of the retinal surface superiorly between 1 and 2 o'clock positions

Fundus Examination of the Other Eye (Left Eye)

1. Indirect ophthalmoscopy with scleral indentation of the left eye showed the following findings
2. The disk was vertically oval, larger in size, pink in color with a tilted conformation and well-defined margins having a cup–disk ratio of 0.4 with healthy neuroretinal rim
3. Peripapillary chorioretinal atrophy was seen
4. Vessels arise from the center of the disk, branching dichotomously, maintaining an AV ratio of 2:3
5. Background retina showed a pale tessellated tigroid appearance with visibility of large choroidal vessels
6. Foveal reflex was dull due to retinal pigment degeneration at the macular region
7. An island of sharply demarcated, circumferentially oriented, spindle-shaped area of retinal thinning suggestive of lattice degeneration was seen from 12 to 2 o'clock hours zone between the equator and ora serrata with some condensed vitreous at the margin
8. No holes were found within the lattice

Diagnosis

1. Right eye fresh subtotal rhegmatogenous retinal detachment-macula off in myopic phakic eye
2. Left eye myopic fundus with lattice degeneration in phakic eye

BILATERAL RETINITIS PIGMENTOSA WITH CONSECUTIVE OPTIC ATROPHY

Fundus Examination of Both Eyes

1. Distant direct ophthalmoscopy at one arm's distance showed a faint red glow
2. Direct ophthalmoscopy close to face revealed a clear media
3. On direct ophthalmoscopy close to the face, the following findings were seen
4. Fine dust-like pigmented cells, cotton balls, and spindle-shaped opacities suggestive of vitreous condensations (not in all cases) were seen
5. Disk was normal in size, vertically oval-shaped, and cup–disk ratio was 0.3 with well-defined golden ring or yellowish halo with waxy pallor suggestive of consecutive optic atrophy
6. Vessel arising from the center of the disk and branching dichotomously. There is marked arteriolar attenuation, and the ratio is altered to 1:3
7. Background retina showed multiple scattered star-shaped pigment deposits in all the four quadrants, more in the superotemporal quadrant. In addition, there were multiple hypopigmented patches along the major vascular arcades, more in the midperiphery. The vessels could be traced over the lesion characteristic of intraretinal bony spicules suggesting retinal pigment epithelial (RPE) atrophy and intraretinal migration of RPE
8. Upon indentation using the indirect ophthalmoscope, similar bony spicules could also be seen close to ora serrata
9. There was diffuse mottling and granularity of retinal pigment epithelium
10. Overall gray fundus appearance (advanced stage) with greater visibility of underlying choroidal vessels

Macular Findings (any of the signs could be seen)

1. Healthy macula with a good foveal reflex (early disease)
2. Increased luster with whitish-wavy lines suggestive of preretinal fibrosis
3. Tapetal-like reflex (bright sheen) seen in the foveal or parafoveal region [classical of X-linked retinitis pigmentosa (RP)]
4. Loss of foveal reflex with diffuse thickening of the surrounding retina with cyst-like spaces (seen with red-free filter), suggestive of cystoid macular edema.

13.3 A CASE OF RIGHT EYE—MACULAR DYSTROPHY—AND LEFT EYE—ACUTE CORNEAL GRAFT REJECTION

A 35-year-old female patient presented to us with complaints of:
1. *Redness, pain in left eye × 10 days*
2. *Defective vision in left eye × 1 week*

HISTORY OF PRESENTING ILLNESS

The redness and pain started in her left eye around 10 days back. Initially, the redness was limited only to the lower part of the right eye, but it slowly involved the entire eye. The pain was pricking in nature, constant throughout the waking hours and relieved while keeping the eye closed. After 3 days of pain and redness, she noticed gradual defective vision in her left eye. The defective vision is more in the early morning hours, especially after getting up from sleep, which gets slightly better as the day progresses. The defective vision is the same for both distance and near.
1. No h/o trauma
2. H/o photophobia present
3. No h/o discharge from the eyes
4. H/o of an eye surgery performed in her left eye, around 2 years back, for defective vision and had reasonably good vision until the present episode

PAST HISTORY

The patient gives a history of mild defective vision of both her eyes from the adolescent age of around 17 years in both her eyes. She used to get constant irritation and watering, which used to subside on its own. After around 2 years, these episodes became more and more regular, and the visual acuity deteriorated significantly. She consulted her local ophthalmologist, who advised her to use lubricant eye drops and protective eyewear and advised her to consider surgery whenever she could not do her normal day-to-day activities.

The patient persisted with this regimen until around 2 years back when she underwent surgery for her left eye because of profound defective vision. She mentions this surgery as an "eye transplantation" and was hospitalized for a period of 10 days.

Subsequently, she was regular with her follow-up treatment. She felt that her visual acuity in her operated eye significantly improved over a period of 12 months. She used to get irritation on and off in her left eye and visited the hospital regularly. In some of these follow-up visits, some sutures were

removed in her left eye. Since her visual acuity in her left eye had improved and since she did not develop any irritation or pain, she has discontinued all medications for the past 3 months.
1. N/K/C/O diabetes mellitus (DM), hypertension, ischemic heart disease (IHD), bronchial asthma (BA)
2. No other systemic illness

PERSONAL HISTORY

Veg, nonsmoker, and nonalcoholic

FAMILY HISTORY

Mother and elder sister had similar complaints. The mother had undergone two eye surgeries, one in each eye, while the sister had undergone surgery for her left eye.

GENERAL EXAMINATION

1. Well-built and nourished
2. Pulse rate (PR): 78 BPM, regular in rhythm and volume
3. Blood pressure (BP): 120/80 mm Hg
4. Cardiovascular system (CVS): S1 and S2 heard. No murmurs
5. Respiratory system (RS): NVBS
6. Abdomen: Soft. No organomegaly
7. Central nervous system (CNS): No abnormality detected (NAD)

OCULAR EXAMINATION

Features	Right eye	Left eye
Best-corrected visual acuity (BCVA)	6/24	1/60
With pinhole (PH)	6/18p	Nip

No facial asymmetry is noted.

Features	Right eye	Left eye
Lids and adnexa	Normal	Normal
No distichiasis—predisposes to graft rejection due to constant irritation
Conjunctiva	Normal	Circumciliary congestion present, more in the inferior half
Cornea		• A centrally placed edematous full-thickness corneal graft of about 8 mm present secured to the recipient cornea which has numerous deposits with interrupted sutures

Contd...

Contd...

Features	Right eye	Left eye
		• Eight 10-0 nylon *sutures present. Of these*, three are loose and are seen in the 3, 5, and 7 o'clock positions
		• Three other sutures (at 8, 10, and 11 o'clock positions) have *sutural infiltrates* seen predominantly in the donor part. Around 10 suture marks are seen in other areas from where sutures would have been removed earlier.
		• *Graft host junction edematous* between 9–12 o'clock position and 5–7 o'clock position
		• *Superficial blood vessels* seen extending from 2 to 8 o'clock position. They are loosely branched
		• *Two areas of deep vascularization* seen, one at 10 o'clock position extending about 4 mm toward the center of the donor graft and the second at 4 o'clock position extending up to 6 mm toward the center of the graft
Epithelium	Few tiny *epithelial erosions*—Two centrally, three along the periphery at around 7 o'clock position, 3 mm away from the temporal limbus seen	*Epithelial edema* present No epithelial rejection line and epithelial defect seen
Stroma	• Diffusely hazy from the center to the periphery. In this generalized haziness, there are some areas of irregular, raised grayish-white deposits with irregular borders, seen more in the central part of the cornea. Majority of the lesions lie in the midstroma with few lesions extending to Descemet's membrane • There are no intervening clear spaces, and there is a diffuse stromal haze. On retro-illumination, the opacities appear opaque. These findings are suggestive of macular corneal dystrophy	• *Diffuse stromal edema* extending throughout the graft, more prominently seen at the central 360° extending up to 5 mm toward the graft host junction and peripherally between 9–12 and 5–7 o'clock positions • *Full-thickness stromal haze* seen peripherally in and around 10 o'clock position, adjacent to the *deep corneal vascularization*

Contd...

Contd...

Features	Right eye	Left eye
Descemet's membrane		Multiple *Descemet's membrane folds* seen on the donor graft
Endothelium	Multiple *guttas* are seen temporally, 4 mm away from the limbus, extending between 7 and 9 o'clock	• Multiple *keratic precipitates* arranged linearly, starting peripherally at around 4 o'clock position and extending up to the center, accompanied by corneal vascularization (Suggestive of the pathognomonic *"Endothelial Rejection Line of Khodadoust"*) • Few scattered keratic precipitates are seen on the endothelium • The peripheral cornea of the recipient reveals a similar picture of hazy cornea to that of the fellow eye
Anterior chamber	Normal depth, quiet	• 2 plus *flare* • 2 plus *cells* seen
Iris	Noncontact tonometry (NCP)	Hazy view
Pupil	3 mm, round, reacting to light	Hazy view
Lens	Clear	Hazy view
Extraocular movements (EOM)	Full	Full
Fundus Distant direct ophthalmoscopy	Revealed red glow	Revealed a dull glow

DIAGNOSIS

Right eye: Macular dystrophy
Left eye: Post-PKP acute endothelial Graft rejection

CORNEA PROFORMA FOR A CASE OF KERATOCONUS IN ONE EYE AND A CLEAR CORNEAL GRAFT IN THE OTHER EYE

A 25-year-old male patient came to us with complaints of defective vision in the right eye for the past 7 years.

History of Presenting Illness

He was apparently normal, 7 years back, when he started noticing defective vision in both his eyes. This was insidious in onset and gradual in progression. It was painless and more for distant vision than for near.

He was prescribed spectacles for the same. While he was satisfied for the first 6 months, his distant vision once again deteriorated, and he was once again prescribed a change of prescription. This did not improve his vision, and thereafter, he was advised to wear contact lenses. He wore the same for 2 years and after some time, became intolerant to contact lenses in his left eye. He was then advised surgery for the left eye, and following surgery, his vision improved in the left eye.

1. H/o frequent change of glasses for his right eye
2. H/o irritation and pain on and off in the right eye after even 4 hours of contact lens use
3. No h/o itching and frequent rubbing of the eyes [rules out ocular allergy and vernal keratoconjunctivitis (VKC)]
4. No h/o episodes of ocular pain associated with redness and sudden decrease in vision (rules out acute hydrops)
5. No h/o double vision (rules out monocular diplopia)

Past History

1. H/o ocular surgery in the left eye 4 years back, following which he was on regular medication for 2 years
2. He gives h/o repeated suture removals in the left eye on and off for the past 4 years. The last episode was around 3 months back

Systemic History

No h/o systemic disorders such as atrophy or asthma or joint deformities (rules out syndromic associations)

Family History

No h/o similar complaints among parents or siblings (keratoconus has an autosomal dominant mode of inheritance)

Personal History

1. Takes mixed diet
2. Nonsmoker and nonalcoholic

General Examination

Height and weight (rules out malformations associated with syndromes)

Vitals
PR, BP

Systemic Examination
CVS; S1S2, presence of cardiac murmurs (rules out cardiac abnormalities associated with syndromes)

Ocular Examination
1. Vision with PH in right eye—6/60 and 6/9 in the left eye
2. Scissoring reflex on retinoscopic examination

Torchlight Examination

Features	Right eye	Left eye
Facial symmetry	Normal	Normal
Lids	"V"-shaped configuration of the lower lid on downgaze suggestive of Munson sign. Look for ptosis [to rule out levator palpebrae superioris (LPS) disinsertion due to rigid gas permeable (RGP) wear]. edema, excoriations, congestion (rules out allergy)	Normal Evidence of trichiasis, entropion, lagophthalmos (predispose to graft rejection) Evidence of lid edema, congestion
Sclera	Normal (rules out blue sclera)	Normal
Conjunctiva	Evidence of bulbar and palpebral congestion (rules out allergy and hydrops)	Evidence of congestion or chemosis (rules out signs of rejection, graft infection)
Cornea	Conical reflection on the nasal cornea on shining the torch from temporal aspect suggestive of Rizzuti sign	A full-thickness central clear corneal graft present secured to the recipient peripheral cornea by interrupted sutures
Anterior chamber	Normal depth	Normal depth
Iris	Normal in color and pattern (no evidence of aniridia)	Iris normal in color and pattern
Pupil	3 mm size, circular in shape, brisk, regular, sustained reaction to direct and consensual light reflex	3 mm size, circular in shape, brisk, regular, sustained reaction to direct and consensual light reflex
Lens	Clear	Clear
Extraocular movements (EOM)	Full and free	Full and free

Slit-lamp examination: The above findings on torchlight examination were confirmed on slit-lamp evaluation.

Ocular findings	Right eye	Left eye
Lids	Normal	Normal
Sclera	Normal	Normal
Conjunctiva	Normal evidence of papillae	• Normal • Tear film height appears normal
Cornea	Epithelium: 1. Deposition of iron pigments in a semicircular pattern in the midperipheral area 2. On examining with a cobalt blue filter, it was better delineated, well defined inferiorly, nasally, and temporally deficient superiorly signs of Fleischer's ring 3. Evidence of subepithelial scarring (rules out previous hydrops) *Bowman's membrane:* Evidence of prominent corneal nerves *Stroma:* Conical protrusion of the cornea is noted along the central and inferior midperipheral aspects, of around 7 mm diameter, suggestive of corneal steepening 4. Stromal thickness reduced by around one-third in the central area of the corneal steepening compared to the adjacent areas, suggestive of corneal thinning. The area of thinning is similar to the area of steepening-fine, vertical lines present at the level of deep stroma in the central aspect of the corneal steepening and disappear on gentle pressure over the lids suggestive of Vogt's striae *Endothelium:* Appears normal	1. A full-thickness central clear disk of donor corneal tissue of around 8 mm in diameter, round in shape, is seen anchored to the peripheral recipient host cornea. 10-0 nylon interrupted sutures with their knots buried in the donor side are seen. None of it is loose. There are no areas of infiltration or vascularization. Additionally, 10 other areas of old suture marks are also seen 2. The graft host junction appears well secure with good wound apposition. The stroma, Descemet's membrane, and endothelium are normal. There is no evidence of any keratic precipitates
Anterior chamber	Normal depth. No evidence of cells or flare	Normal depth. No evidence of cells or flare
Iris	Normal color and pattern	Normal
Pupil	Normal	Normal
Lens	Clear	Clear

Contd...

Contd...

Ocular findings	Right eye	Left eye
Fundus	Distant direct ophthalmoscopy revealed an oil droplet sign Close-to-face examination showed: • Optic disk size, shape, margins, cup–disk ratio, neuroretinal rim, and vessels • Foveal reflex and background retina (rule out Leber's and retinitis pigmentosa)	Distant direct ophthalmoscopy revealed a red glow Close-to-face examination showed: • Optic disk size, shape, margins, cup–disk ratio, neuroretinal rim, and vessels • Foveal reflex and background retina

Diagnosis

Right eye—keratoconus
Left eye—a full-thickness clear corneal graft s/p optical keratoplasty

■ PAPILLEDEMA—CASE PRESENTATION PROFORMA

Fundus right eye	Fundus left eye
Distant direct ophthalmoscopy at one arm's distance showed a good red glow	Distant direct ophthalmoscopy at one arm's distance showed a good red glow
Direct ophthalmoscopy close to face revealed a clear media	Direct ophthalmoscopy close to face revealed a clear media
Size and shape of the disk could not be assessed due to blurring of disk margins and elevation of disk	Size and shape of the disk could not be assessed due to blurring of disk margins and elevation of disk
Disk was markedly hyperemic	Disk was markedly hyperemic
Margins were ill defined throughout, blurred, and obscured	Margins were ill defined throughout, blurred, and obscured
Gross elevation of the optic nerve head measuring +6 D equivalent in the direct ophthalmoscopic evaluation corresponding to about 2 mm elevation from the retinal surface	Gross elevation of the optic nerve head measuring +6 D equivalent in the direct ophthalmoscopic evaluation corresponding to about 2 mm elevation from the retinal surface
Physiological cup was obliterated	Physiological cup was obliterated
Vessels were arising from the center of the disk with an arteriovenous ratio of 2:4. The normal dichotomous branching was not appreciated	Vessels were arising from the center of the disk with an arteriovenous ratio of 2:4. The normal dichotomous branching was not appreciated

Contd...

Contd...

Fundus right eye	Fundus left eye
Retinal veins were congested, dilated, tortuous, and engorged. The engorgement was more marked adjacent to the disk. The arteries appeared normal	Retinal veins were congested, dilated, tortuous, and engorged. The engorgement was more marked adjacent to the disk. The arteries appeared normal
Areas of apparent venous discontinuity were noted, more in the temporal aspect of the disk	Areas of apparent venous discontinuity were noted
Spontaneous venous pulsation over the optic nerve head was absent	Spontaneous venous pulsation over the optic nerve head was absent
Segments of the major blood vessels seemed obscured as they crossed the disk margin	Segments of the major blood vessels seemed obscured as they crossed the disk margin
A peripapillary halo was seen	A peripapillary halo was seen
Blurring, edema, and opacification of the peripapillary retinal nerve fiber layer were seen	Blurring, edema, and opacification of the peripapillary retinal nerve fiber layer were seen
Reflexes from the peripapillary retinal nerve fiber layer were distorted	Reflexes from the peripapillary retinal nerve fiber layer were distorted
Numerous flame-shaped hemorrhages were seen adjacent to the disk margins more marked superiorly from 10 to 12 o'clock position and at 6 o'clock position	Numerous flame-shaped hemorrhages were seen adjacent to the disk margins more marked superiorly from 10 to 12 o'clock position and at 6 o'clock position
Numerous grayish-white fluffy lesions with indistinct margins were seen adjacent to the disk margins, suggestive of cotton wool spots	Numerous grayish-white fluffy lesions with indistinct margins were seen adjacent to the disk margins, suggestive of cotton wool spots
Circumferential retinochoroidal folds were seen for 360° around the disk, more marked nasally suggestive of Paton's lines	Circumferential retinochoroidal folds were seen for 360° around the disk, more marked nasally suggestive of Paton's lines
Foveal reflex was dull	Foveal reflex was dull
No hemorrhages/hard exudates/macular fan/macular star seen at the macula	No hemorrhages/hard exudates/macular fan/macular star seen at the macula

On slit-lamp biomicroscopy with a 90 D lens, the above findings were confirmed. The elevation of the optic nerve head was clearly demonstrated using this method.

On indirect ophthalmoscopy, the retinal peripheries were normal.

Diagnosis

In both eyes: Established papilledema.

13.4 UVEA: MODEL CASE SHEET

Mr X, a 40-year-old male, tailor by occupation, presented to us with chief complaints of pain, redness, and watering in his right eye for 1 week.

HISTORY OF PRESENTING ILLNESS

He had complaints of pain, redness, and watering in his right eye for 1 week, which was sudden in onset and progressive in nature. The pain was dull aching, nonradiating, and continuous in nature. There were no aggravating or relieving factors. It was associated with blurring of vision.

1. H/o difficulty in seeing bright light for 5 days
2. H/o defective vision in right eye for 1 year
3. Insidious in onset
4. Progressive in nature
5. No h/o discharge
6. No h/o headache
7. No h/o floaters
8. No h/o trauma
9. No h/o fever/chronic cough/loss of weight
10. H/o low backache on and off for 1 year
11. No h/o joint pain
12. No h/o skin problems/hair problems
13. No h/o mouth ulcers
14. No h/o genital ulcers
15. No h/o ringing in ears/hearing loss

PAST HISTORY

He gives history of similar pain and redness in his right eye—three episodes in the past 1 year. The last episode was around 4 months back. All episodes were resolved with some topical medications. Details were not available.

1. No h/o eye surgeries
2. No h/o diabetes/hypertension
3. No h/o any other systemic disorders

PERSONAL HISTORY

1. Takes mixed diet
2. Nonsmoker/nonalcoholic
3. No h/o bladder/bowel disturbances
4. No h/o bath in river/pond/pool
5. No h/o contact with pet animals/livestock

FAMILY HISTORY

1. No h/o similar complaints among family members
2. No h/o tuberculosis/diabetes/other autoimmune disorders among family members

GENERAL EXAMINATION

1. Patient well-built and nourished
2. Conscious and oriented
3. No pallor/icterus/cyanosis/clubbing
4. No lymphadenopathy/pedal edema

VITAL SIGNS

1. Afebrile
2. Pulse rate–80/min; respiratory rate–18/min
3. Blood pressure–110/80 mm Hg
4. Cardiovascular, respiratory, and central nervous system examinations were within normal limits

OCULAR EXAMINATION

1. Best-corrected visual acuity
2. Right eye 6/24 with pinhole (PH) 6/12
3. Left eye 6/6
4. No abnormal head posture
5. No facial asymmetry
6. Corneal reflex: Appears orthophoric by Hirschberg's test
7. Extraocular movements: Full range

On torchlight examination:

Parameter	Right eye	Left eye
Lids and adnexa	Normal	Normal
Conjunctiva	Circumciliary congestion	Normal
Cornea	Clear	Clear
Anterior chamber	Normal depth	Normal depth
Iris	Normal in color and pattern	Normal in color and pattern
Pupil	4 mm, irregular, sluggishly reacting to light	4 mm, round, reacting to light
Lens	Cataractous lens	Clear

On slit-lamp examination:

Parameter	Right eye	Left eye
Lids and adnexa	• Normal • No poliosis • No madarosis	Normal
Conjunctiva	Pale red, dilated, congested vessels showing no branching arranged radially around the limbus, associated with a serous discharge. The vessels cannot be moved by moving the conjunctiva and by applying pressure fill from the limbus, which is suggestive of circumcorneal congestion	Normal
Cornea	Around 20–25, flat small-sized, round, white, nonconfluent, nonpigmented deposits with round edges were seen on the inferior aspect of corneal endothelium in base down triangular pattern suggestive of fresh nongranulomatous keratic precipitates	Clear
Anterior chamber	• Normal depth, on using a $1 \times 1 \text{ mm}^2$ wide beam with maximum illumination oriented at 45° on high magnification around 10–20 cells were seen per field corresponding to SUN grade 2+ • There was associated misty appearance of the aqueous due to which the iris and lens details were hazy corresponding to flare of SUN grade 3+	Normal depth
Iris	• Normal color • But the pattern was lost • No iris atrophic patches. No iris nodules seen	Normal color and pattern
Pupil	4 mm, irregular, sluggishly reacting to light. Adherence of the iris to the anterior lens capsule suggestive of posterior synechiae was seen from 3 to 5 o'clock	4 mm, round, reacting to light
Lens	Opacification of the posterior part of the lens (posterior subcapsular cataract) with a polychromatic luster was seen suggestive of complicated cataract	Clear
Anterior vitreous face	Quiet	Quiet

FUNDUS EXAMINATION

Direct ophthalmoscopy	Right eye	Left eye
At arm's distance	Central dark shadow with peripheral red glow due to central posterior subcapsular cataract (PSCC)	Good red glow

Contd...

Contd...

Direct ophthalmoscopy	Right eye	Left eye
Close to face	• Media hazy due to anterior chamber reaction and posterior subcapsular cataract. Vertically oval disk • Normal in size and shape cup–disk ratio of 0.3 Vessels arising from the center of disk branching dichotomously maintaining arteriovenous (AV) ratio of 2:3 • Foveal reflex (+) • Background retina appears normal	• Media clear. Vertically oval disk • Normal in size and shape. Margins well defined. Cup–disk ratio of 0.3. Vessels arising from the center of disk branching dichotomously maintaining AV ratio of 2:3 • Foveal reflex (+) • Background retina normal

The above findings were confirmed using slit-lamp biomicroscopy and 90 D lens.

The peripheries examined using an indirect ophthalmoscope and 20 D lens were found to be normal.

INTRAOCULAR PRESSURE

Intraocular pressure was recorded with Goldmann's applanation tonometer (at 9:00 AM) which showed.

Right eye	Left eye
19 mm Hg	18 mm Hg

CLINICAL SUMMARY

Mr X, a 40-year-old male, came with complaints of pain, redness, watering, and photophobia in the right eye for 1 week. He had history of defective vision in the same eye for 1 year.

On examination, the right eye showed circumciliary congestion with nongranulomatous keratic precipitates on endothelium. Anterior chamber showed 2+ cells with 3+ flare along with posterior synechiae and posterior subcapsular cataract. The left eye was within normal limits.

Fundus examination of both eyes was within normal limits.

ANATOMICAL DIAGNOSIS

1. Right eye—acute on chronic nongranulomatous anterior uveitis with complicated cataract
2. Left eye—normal

DIFFERENTIAL DIAGNOSIS
1. Human leukocyte antigen (HLA) B27 associated uveitis
2. Tuberculosis
3. Syphilis
4. Viral

What are the various rings in ophthalmology?
1. *Ring keratitis:* The hallmark of *Acanthamoeba* keratitis
2. *Kayser-Fleischer's ring:* Wilson's disease
3. *Corneal rust ring:* A small reddish-brown, circular opacity remains in the cornea after the removal of an iron foreign body
4. *Coats' white ring:* Remnants of a foreign body
5. *Fleischer's ring:* Visible all around the base of cone in keratoconus
6. *Pseudo-Fleischer's ring:* Iron deposition can be seen in hyperoxia
7. *Soemmering's ring:* Early opacification of posterior lens capsule after cataract surgery
8. *Vossius' ring:* Iron pigment on anterior lens capsule in concussion injury to eye
9. *Weiss ring:* Epipapillary glial tissue torn from the optic disk in posterior vitreous detachment
10. *Double ring sign:* With the peripheral margin of the encircling ring corresponding to the border of a normal-sized optic disk. Seen in hypoplasia of the optic disk
11. *Golden ring:* A golden ring within the lens is evidence of successful delineation during hydrodissection and delineation
12. *Intrastromal corneal ring segments* are implanted in deep corneal stroma to modify the corneal curvature
13. *Capsular tension rings* (CTR) were used for zonular reinforcements in eyes with a weak zonular apparatus such as in pseudoexfoliation and Marfan syndrome, and when zonular rupture or dehiscence occurs after trauma or surgical trauma
14. *Flieringa ring:* A stainless steel ring sutured to the sclera to support the globe during difficult eye operation. It is usually used in corneal transplant surgeries
15. *Wessely immune ring:* It refers to formation of a ring-shaped infiltrate in the corneal stroma that arises from a type 3 immune response involving antigen–antibody complex formation
16. *Elschnig's scleral ring:* It is a normal anatomic variation whereby a thin white ring, known as the scleral lip, is seen immediately adjacent to the optic disk margin.

CHAPTER 14

Ophthalmology Question Bank

14.1 OPHTHALMOLOGY QUESTION BANK (MS EXAM)

ANATOMY
1. Describe the development and anatomy of vitreous*
2. Describe the course of sixth cranial nerve*
3. Describe the anatomy of the angle of anterior chamber*** and developmental anomalies associated with it
4. Describe the anatomy of the visual pathways and visual cortex. Mention localizing signs of visual pathway
5. Blood supply of visual cortex*
6. Muscles of iris
7. Levator palpebrae superioris**
8. Development of retina
9. Circle of Willis*
10. Superior oblique muscle
11. Optic chiasm*
12. Ciliary body*
13. Blood supply of lacrimal gland
14. Orbital walls*
15. Development of lens
16. Eyelid—upper eyelid**
17. Anatomy of fovea
18. Cavernous sinus*
19. Blood supply of optic nerve*
20. Peripheral fundus
21. Surgical spaces of orbit**
22. Limbus*
23. Ophthalmic artery
24. Suspensory ligaments
25. Blood–retinal barrier
26. Limbal stem cells
27. Optic nerve head*
28. Anatomy of macula
29. Intraocular muscles

30. Vitreous attachments
31. Trochlear nerve
32. Orbicularis oculi*
33. Superior orbital fissure
34. Anatomy of trigeminal nerve
35. Craniosynostosis
36. Nasociliary nerve

PHYSIOLOGY

1. Describe the theories of accommodation** and its anomalies
2. Discuss the factors maintaining intraocular pressure*
3. Discuss binocular vision**
4. Describe the corneal physiology and mechanism of its transparency***
5. Factors responsible for corneal avascularity
6. Theories of color vision*
7. Blood-retinal barrier
8. Formation and circulation of aqueous humor**
9. Precorneal tear film and functions of tear fluid*
10. Electroretinogram*
11. Scotopic vision*
12. Visually evoked potential**
13. Mechanism of lacrimal tear drainage
14. Physiological nystagmus
15. Electrooculography**
16. Macular function tests*
17. Protective mechanism of ocular surface
18. Blood-aqueous barrier*
19. Grades of binocular vision
20. Reduced eye
21. Panum's area
22. Entoptic phenomenon
23. Corneal endothelium
24. Tonometry
25. Convergence insufficiency
26. Color vision tests
27. Abnormal pupillary reflex
28. Light-near dissociation
29. Factors affecting ocular rigidity
30. Metabolism of lens
31. Physiology of accommodation
32. Tests for binocular single vision
33. Vitreous degeneration
34. Pupil and its reactions

BIOCHEMISTRY

1. Metabolism of vitreous***
2. Lipid profile and its significance in ophthalmology
3. Glycosylated hemoglobin and its importance
4. Sorbitol pathway**
5. Composition and drainage of aqueous humor***
6. Photochemistry of vision
7. Metabolism of cornea*
8. Biochemical changes leading to cataract
9. Wald's visual cycle**
10. Biosynthesis of prostaglandins
11. Anaerobic glycolysis*
12. Compare the composition of normal and cataractous lens
13. Homocystinuria*
14. Biochemical composition of tears*
15. Lipoproteins
16. Vitamin A
17. Aerobic glycolysis*
18. Mechanism of diabetic cataract
19. Lipid metabolism
20. Vascular endothelial growth factor (VEGF)
21. Lens proteins
22. Composition of tear film*
23. Axoplasmic flow in optic nerve
24. Corneal transparency
25. Metabolism of lens
26. Metabolic defect in albinism

PHARMACOLOGY

1. Local anesthetics in ophthalmic practice*
2. Drugs used in herpes zoster ophthalmicus
3. Tear substitutes***
4. Mitomycin C
5. Botulinum toxin in ophthalmology*
6. Fluorescein dye
7. Latanoprost
8. Antiviral drugs
9. Cyclosporine***
10. Viscoelastic*
11. Natamycin***
12. Albendazole
13. Brimonidine

14. Idoxuridine
15. Drug therapy for toxoplasmosis
16. Carbonic anhydrase inhibitors
17. Antimetabolites
18. Mast cell stabilizer
19. Mydriatics
20. Acetazolamide
21. Cycloplegics
22. Neuroprotectors
23. Ganciclovir
24. Anti-VEGFs
25. Intraocular drug implants
26. Immune modulators in ocular disorders
27. Hyperosmotic agents
28. Adhesives in ophthalmology
29. Infliximab
30. Carbonic anhydrase inhibitors
31. Antifungal agents**
32. Beta blockers*
33. Acyclovir**
34. Intravitreal antibiotics
35. Parasympathomimetic drugs used in ophthalmology

PATHOLOGY

1. Pathology of uveitis
2. Histopathology of malignant melanoma**
3. Pathology of trachoma
4. Sebaceous gland carcinoma
5. Hypertensive retinopathy
6. Keratoconus
7. Dalen-Fuchs nodules*
8. Pathogenesis of sympathetic ophthalmia
9. Retinoblastoma**
10. Pathogenesis of diabetic microangiopathy
11. Koeppe's nodules
12. Meningioma
13. Tumors of lacrimal gland
14. Bullous keratopathy
15. Metabolic cataract
16. Rhabdomyosarcoma
17. Nodules in the eye
18. Fine needle aspiration biopsy*
19. Glioma

20. Vogt-Koyanagi-Harada (VKH) disease
21. Horner Trantas spots*
22. Mooren's ulcer
23. Premalignant lesions of lid
24. Pathology of corneal dystrophies***
25. Sympathetic ophthalmia
26. Tumors of lacrimal sac
27. Asteroid hyalosis
28. Premalignant lesions of conjunctiva
29. Panophthalmitis
30. Vascular changes in diabetic retinopathy
31. Dyes used in ophthalmology
32. Pathogenesis of diabetic retinopathy

MICROBIOLOGY

1. Laboratory diagnosis of cytomegalovirus (CMV)
2. Polymerase chain reaction and its uses in ophthalmology***
3. Sterilization of operation theater
4. Mycobacterium
5. Laboratory diagnosis of trachoma*
6. Human leukocyte antigen (HLA)
7. *Neisseria*
8. Laboratory diagnosis of fungus
9. Enzyme-linked immunosorbent assay (ELISA)*
10. Acquired immunodeficiency syndrome (AIDS) virus
11. Gram's stain
12. Pseudomonas*
13. *Trichinella spiralis*
14. McCoy cell culture—chlamydial infection
15. CMV
16. Laboratory diagnosis for ocular tuberculosis
17. Sterilization of sharp instruments
18. Herpes zoster virus*
19. Cysticercosis and its ocular manifestations*
20. Trachoma-inclusion conjunctivitis (TRIC) organisms
21. Stains in fungal corneal ulcer
22. Acanthamoeba*
23. Antigen-antibody reaction
24. Graft versus host response
25. Fungi in ocular infection
26. *Corynebacterium diphtheriae*
27. Ocular immune response

28. Morax–Axenfeld bacillus*
29. Rhinosporidiosis
30. Microorganisms causing postoperative endophthalmitis
31. *Mycobacterium leprae*
32. Culture media for corneal scrapings
33. River blindness

REFRACTION AND COMMUNITY OPHTHALMOLOGY
Essay
1. Discuss the causes of blindness and rehabilitation of the blind*
2. Discuss in detail global blindness and role of National Programme for Control of Blindness (NPCB)
3. What is NPCB? Discuss its goals and strategies**
4. Discuss etiology, classification, clinical features, investigation, and management of hypermetropia
5. Classification, pathogenesis, ocular manifestations, diagnosis, and recent trends in treatment of amblyopia*
6. Causes and management of sudden loss of vision
7. Describe in detail about optics of ophthalmoscopes
8. Discuss the various intraocular lens (IOLs) power calculations, their merits, and demerits
9. Describe the optics of slit lamp. Discuss in detail the various types of illuminations in slit-lamp and mention the various uses of slit lamp*
10. Discuss in detail teleophthalmology, its uses, merits, and demerits in community eye care
11. Definition, optics, methods, and stages of retinoscopy
12. Describe with the help of a diagram the principles of retinoscopy. Discuss glass prescription
13. Ocular morbidity in school-going children
14. Discuss the refractive surgeries for myopia
15. Evolution of corneal refractive surgeries
16. Discuss the different types of refractive surgeries. Discuss merits and demerits of each surgery

Short Notes
1. Explain the principle and clinical utility of an autorefractometer
2. Importance of diabetic retinopathy screening in rural areas*
3. Importance of school survey in the prevention of childhood blindness
4. Tests for malingering and their importance
5. Discuss the classification of accommodation. How will you manage presbyopia?
6. Contrast sensitivity—tests and its importance**

7. Vision 2020**
8. Amblyopia and its management*
9. Low vision aids***
10. Ocular myiasis
11. Duochrome test**
12. Tests for color vision
13. Organization of eye camps
14. Anomalous retinal correspondence*
15. IOL power calculation after keratorefractive surgery
16. NPCB—objectives and functions
17. Prophylactic laser treatment in myopia
18. Glaucoma screening at primary eye care level
19. Parinaud oculoglandular syndrome
20. Management of postoperative astigmatism following cataract surgeries**
21. Anomalies of accommodation
22. Binocular single vision
23. Convergence insufficiency*
24. School screening program***
25. Jackson cross cylinder**
26. Fogging technique
27. Surgical management of presbyopia
28. Principles of retinoscopy*
29. Irregular astigmatism
30. Role of prisms in ophthalmology**
31. Aniridia
32. Optics of eye
33. Aberrations
34. Preventable blindness—causes and incidence
35. Microtropia
36. District blindness control society*
37. Compound astigmatism
38. Back vertex distance
39. Cover tests for strabismus
40. Properties of laser used in ophthalmology
41. Role of district program manager
42. Worth four dot test
43. Evaluation of patient undergoing refractive corneal surgery
44. Epikeratophakia
45. Surgeries for astigmatism
46. Femtosecond lasers
47. Discuss the indications, advantages, and disadvantages of conductive keratoplasty

48. Unilateral aphakia—management
49. Recent concepts in low vision aids
50. Autorefractometer
51. Refractive index of the media and its importance in the eye
52. Orthoptic exercise

CONJUNCTIVA, EPISCLERA, AND SCLERA
Short Notes
1. Management of ophthalmia neonatorum
2. Vernal keratoconjunctivitis (VKC)*
3. Giant papillary conjunctivitis
4. Membranous conjunctivitis
5. Ligneous conjunctivitis
6. Necrotizing scleritis
7. Scleromalacia perforans
8. Differential diagnosis of a limbal nodule
9. Ocular surface squamous neoplasia
10. Clinical features and management of epidemic keratoconjunctivitis

CORNEA
Essay
1. Discuss the etiology, clinical features, complications, and management of dry eye*
2. Discuss the causes and prevalence of corneal blindness in India. What are the prerequisites for arranging an eye bank?
3. Discuss peripheral ulcerative keratitis and its clinical features and management
4. Discuss the indications, types, and complications of penetrating keratoplasty
5. Discuss the types, indications, and complications of lamellar keratoplasty

Short Notes
1. Discuss the indications and uses of therapeutic contact lens**
2. Types of contact lenses and indications
3. Rigid contact lens
4. Causes, clinical features, and management of interstitial keratitis**
5. Organization of eye banks
6. Media used for donor eyes
7. Storage and preservation of donor cornea**
8. Grading of donor cornea
9. Graft rejection*

10. Bullous keratopathy*
11. Contact lens materials
12. Keratoprosthesis*
13. Eye bank legislation
14. Extended wear contact lens
15. Keratoconus
16. Bandage contact lens
17. Toric contact lens
18. Recurrent pterygium
19. Recurrent herpes simplex virus infection
20. Confocal laser microscopy
21. Viral infections of the eye
22. Optical keratoplasty
23. Mooren's ulcer—different types, differential diagnosis, and management
24. Schirmer's test
25. Neuroparalytic keratitis
26. Ocular surface squamous neoplasia
27. Filamentary keratitis
28. Lamellar keratoplasty*
29. Acanthamoeba keratitis
30. Herpes zoster ophthalmicus*
31. Trachoma
32. Principles of corneal tear repair
33. Management of keratomalacia
34. Chemical injury
35. Investigation for keratoconus
36. Corneal topography
37. Corneal collagen cross-linking (C3R)
38. Management of pterygium
39. Recent trends in the management of dry eye
40. Pachymetry and its uses
41. Corneal vascularization
42. Deep anterior lamellar keratoplasty
43. Specular microscopy
44. INTACS (implantable intracorneal ring segment)
45. Uses of amniotic membrane in ophthalmology
46. Terrien marginal degeneration
47. Corneal scrapping
48. Hypotonic riboflavin
49. Endothelial keratoplasty
50. Cornea plana

GLAUCOMA

Essay
1. Discuss in detail childhood glaucomas and their management
2. Discuss lasers in ophthalmology and their applications
3. Define and classify glaucoma. Discuss in detail the recent procedures in antiglaucoma surgeries
4. Complications of trabeculectomy and its management
5. Factors predisposing to narrow angle, discuss in detail acute congestive glaucoma
6. Describe the etiopathogenesis, clinical features, complications, and management of neovascular glaucoma
7. Differential diagnosis and management of shallow anterior chamber following intraocular surgery

Short Notes
1. Clinical features and management of Posner-Schlossman syndrome*
2. Mitomycin in eye
3. Rubeosis iridis
4. Pseudoexfoliative glaucoma—problems associated with management*
5. Buphthalmos
6. Inflammatory glaucoma
7. Discuss in detail the etiopathogenesis, clinical features, and management of neovascular glaucoma**
8. Noncontact tonometers
9. Tonometry
10. Laser trabeculoplasty*—argon laser trabeculoplasty (ALT) and selective laser trabeculoplasty (SLT)
11. Pigmentary glaucoma—clinical features and management
12. Von Hippel-Lindau's disease—ocular and systemic features
13. Tuberous sclerosis
14. Management of unilateral congenital glaucoma
15. Ocular hypertension
16. Laser surgeries to treat glaucoma*
17. Automated perimetry*
18. Ocular and systemic risk factors for primary angle-closure glaucoma
19. Sturge-Weber syndrome*
20. Pigmentary glaucoma
21. Gonioscopy—goniolens*
22. Angle recession glaucoma
23. Nonpenetrating glaucoma surgeries
24. Steroid-induced glaucoma
25. Iridocorneal endothelial (ICE) syndrome*

26. Preperimetric syndrome
27. Ultrasound biomicroscopy
28. Laser polarimetry
29. Glaucoma implants
30. Anterior segment imaging techniques
31. Bleb failure
32. Neuroprotection in glaucoma**
33. YAG peripheral iridotomy (YAG PI)
34. Pharmacologic modulations of glaucoma filtration surgery
35. Recent advances in imaging of optic disk in glaucoma
36. Minimally invasive glaucoma surgery

LENS
Short Notes
1. Accommodative IOLs
2. Pharmacological agents used in cataract treatment
3. Pseudoexfoliation
4. Current concepts in IOLs
5. Floppy iris syndrome
6. Phakic IOL**
7. Phacodynamics
8. Presenile cataract
9. Difference between hydrophilic and hydrophobic IOLs
10. Multifocal IOLs
11. Ectopia lentis*
12. Management of subluxated lens
13. Ocular viscoelastic devices (OVDs)
14. Secondary IOLs in the management of aphakia
15. IOLs power estimation in post-LASIK (laser-assisted in situ keratomileusis) eyes
16. Trypan blue dye
17. Capsular tension ring
18. Phaconit
19. Evolution of IOLs implantation
20. Management of intraoperative posterior capsular rupture
21. Ideal IOL—features and its importance

PEDIATRIC OPHTHALMOLOGY
Essay
1. Nystagmus—various etiology, types, clinical characteristics, and management in detail*
2. How will you manage a case of 5-year-old boy with esotropia?

Short Notes
1. Vision recording in infants and children*
2. Management of pediatric aphakia
3. Management of nystagmus
4. Accommodative esotropia**
5. Types and management of esotropia
6. Accommodative convergence to accommodation (AC/A) ratio*—definition and its importance
7. Double elevator palsy—management
8. A-V phenomenon
9. Tests for suppression
10. Prism bar test*
11. IOL power calculation in children
12. Complications of strabismus surgeries
13. Congenital esotropia*
14. Duane's retraction syndrome
15. Principles of strabismus surgery
16. Brown's syndrome**
17. Microtropia
18. Optokinetic nystagmus—importance in localizing the lesion
19. Principles of management of pediatric cataract
20. Adjustable sutures in strabismus surgery
21. Faden procedure

UVEA
Essay
1. Describe etiology, clinical features, investigations, complications, and management of intermediate uveitis
2. Discuss melanoma of choroid, its pathology, investigations, and principles of treatment
3. Describe etiology, clinical features, complications, and management of posterior scleritis

Short Notes
1. Sequelae of chronic iridocyclitis and management options in different stages
2. Ocular manifestations of leptospirosis
3. Management of recurrent anterior uveitis
4. Toxoplasmosis*
5. Sympathetic ophthalmitis—clinical features, pathology, and management*
6. Pars planitis

7. Masquerade syndrome**
8. Clinical phases, systemic association, and complications of VKH syndrome
9. Toxocariasis
10. Congenital anomalies of uveal tract
11. White dot syndrome
12. Bilateral panuveitis
13. Eales disease
14. Biologics in uveitis
15. CMV retinitis
16. Chronic iridocyclitis—complications and management
17. Immunosuppression in uveitis
18. Etiology and management of uveitis in children

RETINA

Essay

1. Discuss the differential diagnosis of sudden loss of vision and management of central retinal artery occlusion
2. Discuss the etiology, classification, clinical features, and differential diagnosis of retinal detachment (RD). Describe the management of rhegmatogenous RD
3. Describe various surgical procedures for treating RD
4. Discuss retinopathy of prematurity and its management*
5. Pathological myopia**
6. Clinical features, syndromes associated, and treatment of retinitis pigmentosa
7. Discuss branch retinal vein occlusion*, its classification, investigation, and management*
8. Causes, complications, and management of dropped nucleus***
9. Classify and discuss central retinal vein occlusion. Discuss its management
10. Discuss the procedure of fundus fluorescein angiography and its usefulness in diagnosis, management, and assessing prognosis of retinal problems
11. (a) Causes of hyperfluorescence and blocked fluorescence in fluorescein angiography. (b) Fluorescein angiography features in central serous retinopathy (CSR)
12. Discuss the recent advances in RD surgery
13. Localization, complication, and removal of intraocular foreign body*
14. Diagnosis, treatment, and follow-up of age-related macular degeneration (AMD)
15. Pars plana vitrectomy, indications, procedure, and its complications in detail

16. Describe in detail the peripheral retinal degenerations. Discuss the management of tractional RD
17. Etiopathogenesis, clinical features, and recent management of macular hole
18. Causes and management of subretinal neovascular membrane
19. Causes and management of exudative RD
20. Discuss the exudative (wet type) AMD and the recent trends in its management
21. Classification and management of diabetic retinopathy

Short Notes
1. Toxic maculopathies
2. Acquired maculopathies
3. Bull's eye maculopathy
4. AMD. Stargardt's dystrophy
5. Macular hole—recent trends in management
6. Vitreous substitutes*
7. Management of postoperative endophthalmitis
8. Chloroquine maculopathy
9. CSR*
10. Intravitreal antibiotics
11. Lattice degeneration in retina
12. Vitrectomy*
13. B scan—interpretation*
14. Cryopexy
15. Choroidal folds*
16. Coloboma
17. Choroidal detachment
18. Intravitreal therapy
19. Ocular ischemic syndrome
20. Photodynamic therapy
21. Macular dystrophies
22. Optical coherence tomography (OCT)—principle and types*
23. Indications and utility of B-scan
24. Role of oils and gases in RD surgery
25. Principles of photocoagulation
26. Fundus camera
27. Classification of hypertensive retinopathy
28. Ultrasound in ophthalmology
29. Indocyanine green (ICG) angiogram
30. Amsler grid
31. Intravitreal injections

32. Recent advances in prevention of acute infectious postoperative endophthalmitis
33. Management of vitreous hemorrhage
34. Surgical management of giant tears
35. Surgical management of high myopia
36. Indications and complications of scleral buckling
37. Delivery systems, parameters of laser treatment in ophthalmology
38. Wide field fundus fluorescein angiography
39. Advanced diabetic eye disease
40. Ocular coherence tomography angiography
41. Microinvasive vitreoretinal surgery
42. Advances in visualization system used in transconjunctival vitrectomy
43. Retinal implants
44. Anti-VEGF agents
45. Diabetic macular edema—current practice pattern
46. OCT angiography
47. Retinoblastoma—current practice pattern
48. Bevacizumab
49. Grid LASER
50. Fluorescein in ophthalmology
51. Sulfur hexafluoride (SF6)

NEURO-OPHTHALMOLOGY

Essay

1. Trace the course and relations of fourth nerve. Mention the peculiarities and diagnosis of its palsy
2. Discuss the etiology, classification, clinical features, differential diagnosis, and management of optic neuritis.** Add a note on the relationship with multiple sclerosis
3. Causes, clinical manifestations, and management of papilledema*
4. Clinical features, types, syndromes associated, and treatment of oculomotor nerve palsy*
5. Trace the pathway of sixth nerve. Discuss sixth nerve palsy and management*
6. Causes, diagnosis, and treatment of papillitis
7. Describe the pupillary pathway and discuss in detail abnormal pupillary reactions
8. Discuss the etiopathogenesis, clinical features, and investigations of myasthenia gravis
9. Discuss in detail the etiopathogenesis, classification, and clinical features of optic atrophy. How will you manage a case of optic nerve injury?

10. Etiology, clinical features, differential diagnosis, and management of anterior ischemic optic neuropathy
11. *Visual pathway:* Discuss with suitable diagrams about field defects caused by lesions along the pathway

Short Notes
1. Causes of isolated fourth nerve palsy*
2. Visual field defects in pituitary lesions
3. Visual fields in chiasmal lesions
4. Cortical blindness
5. Horner's syndrome***—types and diagnostic features
6. Toxic amblyopia—causes, clinical features, and management
7. Hess chart
8. Myasthenia gravis**
9. Anterior ischemic optic neuropathy*
10. Papilledema
11. Migraine*
12. Morning glory syndrome
13. Aberrant third nerve
14. Optic atrophy
15. Craniopharyngioma
16. Diplopia
17. Neuroretinitis
18. Chronic progressive external ophthalmoplegia
19. Internuclear ophthalmoplegia**
20. Aberrant regeneration of cranial nerves
21. Foster Kennedy syndrome
22. Pseudopapillitis
23. Botulinum toxin
24. Multiple sclerosis
25. Bell's phenomenon
26. Cavernous sinus thrombosis
27. Tolosa–Hunt syndrome
28. Hemifacial spasm
29. Motor evaluation of motor strabismus
30. Electroretinogram

LIDS AND ADNEXA
Essay
1. Discuss the examination of a case of ptosis, its investigations, and management**
2. Discuss the various types and management of ectropion

Short Notes

1. Pathogenesis and treatment of blepharitis*
2. Examination of a case of ptosis*
3. Acquired ptosis—causes and management*
4. Ectropion*
5. Entropion*
6. Essential blepharospasm
7. Xeroderma pigmentosum
8. Causes of trichiasis and its management
9. Senile ptosis

LACRIMAL APPARATUS

Essay

1. Discuss the etiology, investigation, and management of epiphora*
2. *Chronic dacryocystitis:* Discuss briefly the etiology, pathogenesis, and management of congenital dacryocystitis

Short Notes

1. Differential diagnosis of watering in newborn
2. Sjogren's syndrome
3. Endonasal dacryocystorhinostomy (DCR)
4. Endoscopic DCR*
5. Congenital dacryocystitis
6. Surgical management of obstruction of lacrimal drainage apparatus

ORBIT AND OCULOPLASTY

Essay

1. Define and classify pseudotumor of the orbit. Discuss the types, clinical features, differential diagnosis, and management in detail
2. Etiopathogenesis, clinical features, investigations, and management of unilateral proptosis**
3. Describe procedure, indications, and complications of exenteration
4. Clinical features, investigations, and surgical management of dysthyroid ophthalmopathy

Short Notes

1. Superior orbital fissure syndrome*
2. Orbital floor fracture*
3. Orbital implants**
4. Ocular prosthesis*
5. Orbital pseudotumor—differential diagnosis and management

6. Crouzon's syndrome
7. Luxation of globe
8. Lateral orbitotomy*
9. Blowout fracture of orbit**
10. Enophthalmos
11. Orbital cellulitis*
12. Optic nerve decompression
13. Cavernous sinus thrombosis
14. Anophthalmic socket
15. Orbital decompression*
16. Pseudohypopyon

MISCELLANEOUS
Essay
1. Describe normal and abnormal flora and discuss its clinical significance
2. Sterilization of operation theater and ophthalmic instruments

Short Notes
1. Ocular manifestations of leukemia
2. Siderosis bulbi—cause and clinical features
3. Ocular manifestation of connective tissue disorders
4. Chalcosis
5. Magnetic resonance imaging in ocular disorders
6. Positron emission tomography (PET) scan
7. Onchocerciasis
8. Role of genetics in retinitis pigmentosa
9. Nutritional factors causing ocular morbidity
10. Genetics of glaucoma
11. Ocular manifestations of blood disorders
12. Gene therapy
13. Nanotechnology-based drug delivery system in ophthalmology
14. Stem cells in ophthalmology
15. Fine needle aspiration cytology (FNAC)
16. How is autoclaving done? What are sterilized in it?

14.2 OPHTHALMOLOGY QUESTION BANK (DNB EXAM)

CONJUNCTIVA, EPISCLERA, AND SCLERA
1. Describe the etiopathogenesis and histopathology of ocular surface squamous neoplasia (OSSN). Write briefly on the use of antimetabolites in the management of OSSN*
2. Enumerate two immunosuppressive drugs used in the treatment of allergic eye diseases. Elaborate on their mechanism of action and side effects
3. How do you diagnose severe ocular surface disease? Discuss the causes and management of these entities when existing in a unilateral and bilateral manner
4. Classify allergic conjunctivitis. Describe clinical features, pathology, and treatment of vernal conjunctivitis**
5. Clinical features, pathogenesis, differential diagnosis, and management of a case of viral conjunctivitis
6. Clinical features, differential diagnosis, and management of ophthalmia neonatorum
7. Clinical features and management of adenoviral keratoconjunctivitis
8. A 10-year-old child with complaints of blurring of vision and whitish opacities in both eyes is brought to the outpatient department (OPD). Discuss differentiation diagnosis and management of this case
9. (a) What is a dermoid cyst? (b) Systemic associations of dermoid cyst. (c) Differential diagnosis of epibulbar swelling

CORNEA
1. Classify fungal infections of the eye. Discuss in brief the presentation, diagnosis, and specific management of fungal keratitis
2. Describe clinical features, laboratory diagnosis, prevention, and management of acanthamoeba keratitis*
3. Give the principle of keratometry. What are the types of keratometers and basic difference between them? Give typical keratometric features in keratoconus
4. Discuss the etiology, diagnostic clinical signs, and investigations in a suspected case of keratoconus. How will you manage the case?
5. Contact lens options in keratoconus and irregular corneas with high astigmatism
6. Discuss in detail the interventional modalities to halt progression of keratoconus. Discuss in detail the various refractive surgeries that can be done to provide visual rehabilitation in nonprogressive keratoconus
7. Enumerate the conditions associated with corneal neovascularization. Briefly discuss the mechanism and various treatment modalities with their rationale of treatment in the management of this condition

8. Describe the corneal topography findings in keratoconus. How do you grade the severity of keratoconus?*
9. A 25-year-old man complaining of itching and redness of both eyes since childhood presents with gradually increasing refractive error and photophobia. Outline the workup and management
10. (a) Clinical features and causative organisms of a case of bacterial corneal ulcer. (b) How will you investigate such a case?
11. Discuss in detail the surgical management of corneal ulcers. What is the role of confocal microscopy in diagnosis and management of corneal ulcers?
12. Anatomy and physiology of corneal endothelium
13. Describe microscopic structure of cornea. Factors responsible for transparency of cornea.** Clinical features, etiology, and management of corneal edema
14. Clinical features, evaluation, and management of alkali ocular injury*
15. (a) Development of cornea. (b) What is megalocornea? (c) Difference between megalocornea and buphthalmos
16. Discuss the causes and presentation of pterygium. How will you manage it?
17. Current techniques for management of recurrent pterygium. PERFECT technique for pterygium management
18. Discuss indications, surgical procedures, complications, and advances in endothelial keratoplasty
19. Indications, advantages, disadvantages and long-term results of Descemet's stripping endothelial keratoplasty (DSEK)
20. Critically evaluate DSEK/Descemet's stripping automated endothelial keratoplasty (DSAEK) and Descemet's membrane endothelial keratoplasty (DMEK)
21. Types, indications, advantages, disadvantages, and complications of anterior lamellar keratoplasty**
22. Describe in detail complications of blade-based LASIK (laser-assisted in situ keratomileusis). Classify them as vision threatening and nonvision threatening in your description
23. (a) How will you work up a case for LASIK surgery? (b) What are the modalities available and which one is preferred and why?
24. Enumerate keratorefractive surgeries. Intraoperative and postoperative complications of LASIK and their management
25. Differentiate between regression, progression, and ectasia post-LASIK with respect to refractive errors. What is wavefront-guided (WF)-guided, WF-optimized, and Contoura procedure?
26. Enumerate the stromal corneal dystrophies, their pathology, clinical features, and management*

27. Describe different types of recurrent corneal erosions. Give an outline of their treatment
28. A 30-year-old female got up at night with severe pain and watering in her left eye. She gave a history of a nail injury to her eye 1 year back. How would you approach and manage such a case?
29. Etiopathogenesis, clinical features, and management of chronic, nonhealing peripheral corneal ulcer*
30. Clinical presentation, differential diagnosis, and management of recurrent herpes simplex keratitis
31. A 30-year-old male reports with acute-onset unilateral red eye and diminished vision of 3 days' duration with watery discharge, a corneal epithelial lesion, stromal infiltration, and an immune ring on the endothelium. He gives a history of previous episodes of red eye in the same eye and has lesions suggestive of previous corneal disease. Make a flowchart describing how you would arrive at a diagnosis and how you would manage the case
32. What is Dua's classification of chemical injuries? How is it better than Roper-Hall classification? Discuss the management strategies of grade 3 and grade 4 chemical injuries*
33. Describe healing of epithelial defect. What are the causes of persistent epithelial defect? How will you manage such cases of persistent epithelial defect?
34. What are the indications of amniotic membrane use in ophthalmic surgery? What is the mechanism of action and side effects of its use?
35. A 60-year-old male underwent penetrating keratoplasty in the right eye and was later diagnosed as a case of graft failure. What are the preoperative examinations that were mandatory for this patient? What are the causes of graft failure? How will you manage a case of graft failure?
36. Write immunological aspect, clinical features, risk factors, and management of corneal graft rejection
37. A 12-year-old child sustained injury to right eye while playing with bow and arrow. Discuss management of corneoscleral perforation with iris tissue prolapse in this patient
38. (a) Enumerate the various consequences of a closed globe injury by a blunt object. (b) How would you distinguish between open globe and closed globe injury?
39. Give ideal requirements for setting of eye bank. What are the functions of eye bank? Mention the various medias with their constituents for cornea preservation. What are their advantages and disadvantages?*
40. Causes, clinical presentation, and treatment modalities for pseudophakic bullous keratopathy*

41. Keratoprosthesis: (a) Types and (b) indications
42. Confocal microscopy in corneal lesions
43. Limbal anatomy—clinical significance
44. Discuss the newly available options for the management of limbal stem cell deficiency
45. A 34-year-old lady presents with chronic inflammation and irritation of superior limbus. What is the most likely diagnosis, pathogenesis, and management of the disease?
46. Describe the barriers to drug penetration in the cornea. What is partition coefficient? Describe various factors affecting drug penetration with respect to drug formulation and corneal anatomy
47. Tissue adhesives in ophthalmology

GLAUCOMA

1. Discuss clinical features, pathogenesis, differential diagnosis, and management of primary congenital glaucoma
2. Discuss etiopathogenesis, diagnosis, and management of acute angle-closure glaucoma
3. What is Sturge-Weber syndrome? Give its classification, clinical signs, investigations, and principles of management of associated glaucoma*
4. What are the various types of tonometers? Describe the optics and methods of sterilization of Goldmann's applanation tonometer. What are its sources of error, and how to overcome them?
5. Principles, technique, advantages, and possible sources of error in performing Goldmann's applanation tonometry
6. Anatomy and development of angle of anterior chamber (AC) of eye.* Developmental anomalies of angle of AC
7. (a) What are mechanisms of aqueous formation? (b) Detailed anatomy of the angle of anterior chamber** with special mention to trabecular meshwork and Schlemm's canal. (c) Optical principle to see the angle structures—gonioscopy and its types**
8. (a) Classify pharmacological agents available to treat glaucoma. (b) Mechanism of action of topical agents. (c) Adverse effects and contraindications of systemic agents
9. Discuss aqueous humor dynamics and pharmacokinetics of drugs that increase uveoscleral outflow
10. What are artificial drainage shunts? Write briefly about various drainage devices. Give indications and complications of these devices**
11. Indications and adverse effects of Ahmed glaucoma valve surgery
12. Discuss the investigations and management of a 55-year-old diabetic patient presenting with neovascular glaucoma and cataract with visual acuity of 3/60 and intraocular pressure (IOP) of 46 mm Hg

13. Pathogenesis, causes, presentation, complications, and management of neovascular glaucoma****
14. Define open-angle glaucoma suspect. Discuss the management options and follow-up. What are the global indices in automated perimetry?
15. What are the minimum diagnostic criteria for primary open-angle glaucoma (POAG)? Give the severity classification of POAG with the concept of target pressure*
16. Write about diagnostic features of glaucoma field defect on automated perimetry
17. Newer perimetry techniques
18. What is advanced glaucoma? Give the pathogenesis of glaucomatous ocular damage* How will you follow up a case of advanced glaucoma? What are the various treatment options?
19. Pathogenesis, diagnosis, and management of a case of angle recession glaucoma
20. (a) Etiopathogenesis of flat anterior chamber after glaucoma surgery. (b) How would you critically evaluate and manage such a case?**
21. (a) Etiopathogenesis, clinical features, and diagnosis of pseudo-exfoliative glaucoma. (b) Give specific features of true exfoliation in eye
22. Discuss the pathology, clinical features, and management of pseudoexfoliation syndrome (PXF)
23. Differentiate between: (a) Spaeth and Shaffer classification angle, (b) iris processes and PAS (peripheral anterior synechiae), and (c) pigmentary and PXF glaucoma
24. Ocular hypertension—clinical features, evaluation, and management*
25. An 8-year-old female child had accidental blunt trauma to the eye with a tennis ball and presented to the emergency with total hyphema. Outline the steps of evaluation and management
26. Grading, investigations, complications, and management of traumatic hyphema*
27. What is ocular perfusion pressure? Describe briefly the role of ocular perfusion pressure in glaucoma
28. Describe the mechanism of action, technique, indications, and effects of laser iridotomy and selective laser trabeculoplasty (SLT). Briefly compare SLT with argon laser trabeculoplasty*
29. Cycloablation techniques in management of glaucoma
30. Management of a painful blind eye with medically uncontrollable IOP of 50 mm Hg
31. Classify the various nonpenetrating glaucoma surgeries. What are their indications, advantages, and disadvantages over conventional glaucoma surgeries?
32. (a) Rho-kinase inhibitors in ophthalmology. (b) Microinvasive glaucoma surgery (MIGS). (c) Neuroprotectors

33. List the various prostaglandin analogs available in the management of glaucoma. Give their mechanism of action, dose schedule, and side effects
34. Define and enumerate the iridocorneal endothelial (ICE) syndrome. Describe their salient features and management
35. Describe the indications, technique, and complications of laser peripheral iridoplasty and laser peripheral iridotomy
36. (a) What is normal tension glaucoma? (b) Etiopathogenesis, clinical characteristics, and management of a case of normal tension glaucoma
37. Causes and management of glaucoma associated with ocular trauma
38. (a) Use of mitomycin C in ophthalmology. (b) Mention its side effects
39. Criteria for early glaucomatous visual field changes
40. Recent advances in trabeculectomy
41. Management of intractable glaucoma or multiple failed glaucoma surgeries
42. What is canaloplasty? Discuss indications, technique, IOP lowering efficacy, and adverse effects
43. A 32-year-old lady presents in her second trimester for management of glaucoma. How will you treat her? What is the difference in management of glaucoma in first, second, and third trimesters and postpartum?
44. Releasable sutures in glaucoma surgery
45. What are the types of lens-induced glaucoma? Describe the medical and surgical treatment

UVEA

1. A patient who sustained corneoscleral perforation in a road traffic accident was admitted, and repair was done. Three days after the surgery, he complained of photophobia and blurry vision in the other eye. What is your diagnosis? How will you manage it? What are the histopathological findings expected in this case?
2. Uvea anatomy, blood flow, and anomalies
3. Describe the pathology of "malignant melanoma of choroid". How does the pathology influence the prognosis?
4. Classification, pathology, clinical features, differential diagnosis, adverse prognostic factors, and nonsurgical management of a case of choroidal melanoma*
5. Discuss in detail the differential diagnosis and management of a choroidal mass in a 50-year-old patient
6. What are the common causes of anterior uveitis in children? What are the common clinical presentations and management of juvenile spondyloarthropathy?
7. Various presentations of uveitis in spondyloarthropathies

8. Write the ocular manifestations, systemic associations, and management of Behçet's disease including recent drugs available for treatment
9. (a) Production, circulation, and drainage of aqueous humor.* (b) Describe components of blood–ocular barrier and its clinical importance
10. (a) Describe the anatomy of ciliary body. (b) What are its functions and how will you assess them?
11. Discuss the pathogenesis, clinical features, diagnosis, differential diagnosis, and management of intermediate uveitis
12. Classify scleritis. Discuss the clinical manifestations, investigations, and management of scleritis and its complications***
13. Discuss the clinical features, diagnosis complications, and management of uveitis associated with juvenile rheumatoid arthritis*
14. Discuss the clinical features, differential diagnosis, and management of metastatic endophthalmitis in a 15-year-old boy
15. Clinical features, laboratory investigations, and management of postcataract surgery endophthalmitis
16. Differential diagnosis and management of a 10-year-old boy presenting with bilateral diminution of vision and swelling of the right knee
17. Clinical features, diagnostic investigations, and management of ocular tuberculosis*
18. Clinical features, investigations, and management of ocular sarcoidosis
19. (a) Enumerate causes of iris cysts. (b) Discuss briefly the management of different types of iris cysts
20. Give the differential diagnosis of white dot syndrome. Discuss the clinical features and management of serpiginous choroiditis*
21. A 30-year-old lady presented with features of bilateral panuveitis. Discuss the differential diagnosis and management of the case
22. What are different classifications of uveitis? Discuss briefly about granulomatous uveitis and its management
23. What are the various clinical features and complications of an acute attack of acute uveitis? Discuss its management
24. Discuss pathophysiology and management of ocular toxoplasmosis
25. Describe the clinical features, treatment, and prognosis in a case of cytomegalovirus retinitis
26. Presentation, systemic features, investigations, and treatment of primary intraocular lymphoma
27. Immunomodulators—uses and side effects
28. What are the antimetabolites used in ophthalmology? Discuss their clinical uses and side effects
29. Choroidal multifocal choroiditis—clinical manifestations, evaluation, management
30. What are cytokines? Enumerate important pro-inflammatory cytokines. What role do they play in ocular inflammation?

31. What is the pharmacological mechanism of action of cyclosporine? What are its clinical uses in ophthalmology?
32. (a) Differential diagnosis of heterochromia iridis. (b) Features, complications, and management of a case of Fuch's uveitis syndrome

CATARACT AND LENS

1. Write short note on lens development,* anatomy, lens sutures, its metabolism, and factors affecting lens transparency.** What metabolic abnormalities cause diabetic and galactosemic cataract?
2. Define in relation to phacoemulsification:* (a) Flow rate and vacuum, (b) pulse mode and burst mode, (c) rise time, effective phaco time, and duty cycle, and (d) surge (causes and prevention)
3. What is ectopia lentis?* Discuss the clinical features and complete management of spherophakia and associated problems in a patient with Weill–Marchesani syndrome*
4. Briefly write about the development of crystalline lens and zonules. Enlist the biochemical mechanisms of cataractogenesis.** Briefly write about various congenital* and developmental anomalies of lens***
5. (a) What are multifocal intraocular lens (IOLs) and its principle**? (b) What are their types,* patient selection criteria, and their advantages? (c) What special surgical considerations will be utilized when implanting a multifocal IOL/premium IOLs?
6. What is capsular block syndrome? Classify capsular block syndrome with respect to early, intraoperative, and late causes. How are they avoided and/or managed?
7. Broadly classify viscoelastic substances used in ophthalmic surgery. What is soft-shell technique in cataract surgery and enlist important precautions while performing phacoemulsification in cases with low corneal endothelial counts
8. (a) Describe various surgical difficulties encountered when doing a phacoemulsification in a small pupil.* (b) How do you manage a case of nondilating pupil for phacoemulsification?* How will you manage a case of white cataract?
9. (a) Define and list out causes of complicated cataract.* (b) Principles of management of cataract associated with chronic anterior uveitis*
10. (a) Effect of blunt trauma on normal lens. (b) Causes and management of subluxated lens*
11. Grade the posterior capsular opacification. What are the types of capsulotomy done for posterior capsular opacification? Describe the intraoperative and postoperative methods to reduce posterior capsular opacification

12. Discuss the causes, preoperative, and intraoperative management of floppy iris syndrome
13. What are the causes of posterior capsular rupture, and how will you manage it in phacoemulsification surgery?
14. What is femto-assisted cataract surgery? Describe the procedure of toric IOL surgery
15. A 70-year-old male with a normal phakic contralateral eye had posterior capsular tear in the center during a phacoemulsification procedure after removal of the cortex. Make a flowchart describing your subsequent actions, explaining why you performed each step
16. What is the nature of biochemical abnormality in homocystinuria? Discuss its ocular and systemic manifestations, genetics, and management
17. Discuss various IOL power calculation formulae and how will you calculate IOL power in a postrefractive surgery patient?
18. A 76-year-old individual underwent phacoemulsification for grade 4 cataract. He received incompletely and developed diminution of vision 6 weeks after surgery. Discuss the causes of diminished vision and their management in brief
19. Principle, utility, and advantages of (a) square-edged optics, (b) aspheric optics, and (c) heparin-coated optics
20. Surface modifications of IOLs
21. How will you evaluate and discuss the important surgical steps involved in the management of a 35-year-old with posterior polar cataract?
22. What is blade free cataract surgery? What are its advantages over conventional phacoemulsification? What are its disadvantages?
23. Indications, advantages, disadvantages, and complications of a toric multifocal IOL implantation following cataract extraction
24. What is the concept and its applications in various full-range IOLs such as multifocal, accommodative, pseudoaccommodative, and extended depth of focus IOLs (EDOF IOLs)*
25. (a) What are the sources of aerosol generation in cataract surgery? (b) Mention the methods to decrease the sources of aerosol generation during surgery. (c) What are the precautions to be taken by an ophthalmic surgeon during COVID era while operating under a microscope?
26. (a) Mention the types of anterior capsulotomy in cataract surgery. (b) Compare the advantages and disadvantages of capsulotomy and capsulorhexis. (c) Discuss the uses, advantages, and disadvantages of Zepto in cataract surgery
27. Diagnosis, prophylaxis, and management of toxic anterior segment syndrome (TASS)

PEDIATRIC OPHTHALMOLOGY

1. Give various milestones in vision development in a child. Enumerate four important tests for visual activity testing in preverbal children and children between 3 and 6 years with one merit and demerit of each test.
2. Discuss the techniques for evaluating visual acuity from birth to 3 years of age
3. Define essential infantile esotropia. Give at least four differential diagnoses of essential infantile esotropia and give at least two differentiating features among them*
4. (a) Define and classify esotropia. (b) Management of a 6-year-old patient with esotropia***
5. (a) Classify esotropia. (b) How would you plan the management of convergence excess esotropia in a 5-year-old child? (c) Describe the choice of procedure and surgical planning in detail
6. Describe the clinical features and management of partially accommodative esotropia
7. Describe AV pattern deviations. Discuss etiology, clinical features, and management of the deviations
8. (a) Classify nystagmus.* (b) How will you investigate a case of nystagmus?* (c) What are the clinical conditions in which nystagmus is seen? (d) Management of nystagmus*
9. (a) How do you assess a case of congenital nystagmus? (b) What are the surgical options available to manage a case of nystagmus?
10. (a) Difference between a Horopter and Panum's area. (b) Sensory and motor adaptations of strabismus
11. (a) What is the accommodative convergence to accommodation (AC:A) ratio for convergence? (b) What are the methods of measuring it? (c) Briefly discuss the disorders resulting from an altered AC:A ratio
12. What is microtropia? Discuss the types and clinical features of microtropia
13. What is suppression in relation to strabismus? Discuss diagnosis and management strategies of suppression
14. Describe Faden's operation as applied in management of strabismus
15. Give indications of surgery for pediatric cataract. Outline complete management and specific surgical challenges in a 2-year-old child with unilateral cataract
16. Classify congenital cranial dysinnervation disorders (CCDDs). Describe Duane's retraction syndrome, classification, and management of a case of Duane's retraction syndrome with abnormal head posture
17. Discuss the diagnosis and management of dissociated vertical divergence. How will you differentiate it from inferior oblique overaction?
18. Indications and principles of inferior oblique weakening procedures

19. Discuss the causes, evaluation, and management of unilateral congenital cataract in a 2-year-old child*
20. A 2-year-old child presents with cataract in both eyes. Discuss the possible causative factors and their management
21. What are the types of pediatric cataract? Describe modification of IOL power calculation and visual rehabilitation after pediatric cataract surgery
22. A 7-year-old child presented with intermittent exotropia. Discuss its evaluation and treatment
23. Classify exotropia in children. Discuss its management
24. Describe the clinical features and management of intermittent divergent squint
25. What is amblyopia? Explain the concept of critical period in development of vision. Outline the principles of treating strabismus amblyopia
26. (a) What are the differences between an adult and pediatric eye? (b) What are the precautions to be observed in doing pediatric cataract surgery and why? (c) What is the relationship between pediatric cataract surgery and glaucoma? (d) Outline complete management of unilateral congenital cataract
27. A 6-year-old boy presents with unilateral leukocoria. What is the differential diagnosis, and describe management of its most common cause?
28. Superior oblique overaction—clinical features and management
29. Adjustable sutures in squint surgery

RETINA

1. Describe briefly the anatomy of choroid. Discuss the developmental basis of choroidal coloboma. Classify types of choroidal colobomas
2. Enumerate the routes of drug delivery in the eye. Mention four commonly used intravitreal drugs with their dosages and indications
3. Discuss clinical features, investigations, sequelae, and management of an intraocular metallic foreign body. What are the ophthalmological effects if it is not removed?
4. Describe clinical features, etiology, investigations, and various modalities of management in branch retinal vein occlusion
5. Etiopathogenesis, clinical features, investigation, and management of central retinal vein occlusion
6. What is the role of intraocular corticosteroids in retinal vein occlusions? Discuss the findings of SCORE and Posurdex trial in venous occlusions
7. Etiopathogenesis, clinical features, investigations, and management of central retinal arterial occlusion

8. What are the three landmark studies in establishing management protocols in diabetic retinopathy? What are the conclusions of each of them?
9. What is the principle of optical coherence tomography (OCT)? What are the types of OCTs available? What are the diagnostic and therapeutic issues of OCT in management of macular pathology and corneal diseases?*
10. Discuss clinical features, classification, investigations, and management of diabetic macular edema.** Write a note on VEGFs
11. Diagnosis and management of a nonresolving macular edema
12. Discuss the role of lasers in diabetic macular edema. Outline a complete plan of management in severe diabetic macular edema. What is the role of newer lasers in management of diabetic macular edema?
13. Discuss all possible ocular injuries with a cricket ball to the eye in a 20-year-old male. Give the management of traumatic retinal disorders
14. Describe the causes, investigations, and management in a case of tractional retinal detachment*
15. (a) Describe in brief the embryological evolution of retina. (b) What are the differences between rods and cones? (c) What is the importance of inner segment (IS)/outer segment (OS) junctions?
16. (a) Anatomy and development of the macula.** (b) Different zones of macula and their clinical importance. (c) Enumerate the Macular function tests***
17. Macro- and microanatomy of vitreous and its role in pathogenesis of retinal detachment
18. (a) Discuss vitreous substitutes in detail. (b) Eales disease
19. Anatomy, biochemical composition, and physiological role of retinal pigment epithelium*
20. (a) Detailed structure of retinal rods and cones. (b) Their distribution over the retina. (c) Implications in vision quality with rod and cone dysfunction
21. Etiology and classification of myopia. Clinical features of pathological myopia
22. Electrophysiological basis of electroretinogram (ERG) and electrooculogram (EOG) and their clinical applications*
23. Describe the surgical anatomy of pars plana. Enumerate the indications of pars plana vitrectomy.* Discuss the indications and dose of various pharmacological agents used through an intravitreal route
24. Describe the properties of various intraocular gases used in vitro-retinal surgery. What are their indications and complications?*
25. Define clinically significant macular edema, high-risk proliferative diabetic retinopathy (PDR), and management of these conditions

26. Discuss endophthalmitis vitrectomy study with respect to aim, design, and outcomes
27. Discuss the molecular genetics, clinical features, and tests of visual functions in typical retinitis pigmentosa
28. Write clinical features and management of retinal detachment with giant retinal tear in a 22-year-old boy with Marfan's syndrome
29. (a) What are the various types of anti-VEGF (anti-vascular endothelial growth factor) agents available? (b) What are their pharmacological features? (c) What is their role in retinal disorders? (d) What are their complications and limitations?
30. (a) What is Terson's syndrome? (b) What are its clinical features? (c) Discuss its differential diagnosis. (d) Describe the complications and their management
31. (a) Enumerate the causes of unilateral profound painless loss of vision. (b) How will you manage such a case in a 65-year-old male patient?
32. Investigations, diagnosis, and management of a 40-year-old male patient presenting with unilateral central scotoma
33. (a) Investigations and assessment of a case of long-standing diabetes with moderate non-PDR with clinically significant macular edema. (b) How will you manage such a case?
34. Ocular management of a 50-year-old diabetic patient, including medical, surgical, and laser treatment, who has 3/60 vision and PDR in both eyes
35. Pathology of various age-related macular lesions
36. Write the causes, clinical features, diagnosis, and surgical management of macular holes**
37. (a) Pathogenesis and sequelae of cotton wool spots and hard exudates on retina in diabetic retinopathy. (b) Diagnostic features of human immunodeficiency virus (HIV) retinopathy relationship to CD4 counts
38. (a) Clinical features and differential diagnosis of various types of retinal detachment. (b) Management of giant retinal tear
39. Describe the clinical features and clinicopathologic correlation of age-related macular degeneration (ARMD). Describe the role of various modalities in the management of ARMD*
40. Etiology, evaluation, classification, and management of retinopathy of prematurity*
41. What are the differential diagnoses and features to differentiate them from each other, in a patient with pigmented lesion on fundus examination? What are the indications for biopsy with management strategies in a case of primary acquired melanosis (PAM)?
42. (a) Define pachychoroid spectrum. (b) Polypoidal choroidal vasculopathy
43. Acute posterior multifocal placoid pigment epitheliopathy (APMPPE)—etiology, clinical features, investigations, management, and prognosis

44. What are the methods of localization, management, and complications of retained intraocular copper foreign body?
45. Ophthalmic consequences of hydroxychloroquine (HCQ) therapy, risk factors, evaluation, and management
46. Vitreous hemorrhage—causes, evaluation, and management
47. Principles, uses, and complications of silicone oil and their management**
48. Intravitreal aflibercept injection: Mechanism of action, indications, dosage, and adverse events. Add a note on comparative effectiveness with other drugs of the same drug group
49. (a) Diabetic retinopathy clinical research network (DRCR.net) protocols for macular edema. (b) VEGF-trap*—its advantages over current anti-VEGF agents
50. Discuss the immediate management of a 60-year-old diabetic patient who has collapsed after injection of dye during fluorescein angiography (FFA)
51. What is the difference between retinoschisis and retinal detachment? Discuss the various types of retinoschisis and their management
52. Discuss the CATT trial. What were the objectives, design conclusions, and implications of the trial in respect of anti-VEGF agents?
53. A 21-year-old myope (-2.5D) presented with sudden profound unilateral diminution of vision. Discuss the differential diagnosis, investigation, and management
54. Clinical features, differential diagnosis, and management of a case of Coat's diseases
55. Indications, advantages, and disadvantages of internal limiting membrane (ILM) peeling in vitreoretinal surgery
56. Etiopathogenesis and management of exudative retinal detachment
57. A 21-year-old myopic male presented with a total retinal detachment in the right eye, a single causative break at 11 o'clock anterior to the equator and no proliferative vitreoretinopathy (PVR). What are the surgical options for the management of retinal detachment? Explain clearly why you would recommend your chosen surgical option and outline the surgical steps
58. OCT angiography—principle and uses. Difference from FFA
59. Optic disk pit maculopathy—clinical features, evaluation, and treatment
60. Massive submacular hemorrhage—causes, clinical features, evaluation, and treatment
61. Myopic macular degeneration—clinical features, evaluation, and treatment
62. Recent advances in management of floaters and pupilloplasty
63. (a) What is an epiretinal membrane (ERM)? (b) Causes of ERM and its management

64. (a) What are the principles, role, and uses of ERG? (b) Define multifocal ERG and its importance
65. Pathogenesis, clinical features, diagnosis, and management of different grades of retinopathy in pregnancy-induced hypertension
66. (a) Intravitreal implants and indications for their use. (b) What are their possible side effects?
67. Describe the recent trend in the diagnostic modalities and their implications in the management of macular edema

NEURO-OPHTHALMOLOGY

1. Define scotoma. How do you differentiate between positive and negative scotoma? Discuss the approach to diagnosis in a patient presenting with left hemianopia
2. What is Horner's syndrome? Discuss clinical features, diagnosis, and management of syndrome
3. What are the common tumors of optic nerve in adults? Give clinical features to differentiate them clinically and give salient pathological features of these tumors
4. Describe anatomy and lesions of optic tracts, chiasma, and optic radiations*
5. (a) Signs of optic nerve dysfunction. (b) Various investigations available to assess the optic nerve function
6. (a) Various types of eye movements. (b) Various neuroanatomic pathways controlling eye movements
7. Blood supply of optic nerve head and intraorbital optic nerve with well-labeled diagrams and highlight their clinical importance
8. Describe the pupillary reflex pathways with a diagram.** Explain the causes, grading, and clinical importance of a relative afferent pupillary defect
9. (a) What is anisocoria and indications for its investigation? (b) Give the physiological basis and causes of light-near reflex dissociation. Discuss the approach to diagnosis of anisocoria*
10. (a) Visual pathway and the blood supply. (b) Anatomy of lateral geniculate body and visual cortex
11. (a) Describe the anatomy of optic nerve. (b) Draw a diagram to explain its blood supply and discuss its clinical significance
12. (a) Draw a labeled diagram of third cranial nerve nucleus. (b) Explain its clinical significance
13. Discuss the causes, features, investigations, and management of acute-onset third nerve palsy.** When will you decide surgical intervention in a case of third nerve palsy? What are the surgical techniques?

14. Describe etiology, clinical features, investigations, and management of sixth nerve palsy
15. Management options in a case of lateral rectus palsy with visually disabling diplopia
16. Discuss differential diagnosis of unilateral optic disk edema.* How will you differentiate each condition?
17. Describe pathogenesis and pathological features of papilledema
18. (a) Etiology, types, clinical features, diagnosis tests, and management of ocular myasthenia. (b) Important differential diagnosis and points to differentiate*
19. One and half syndrome—its cause and clinical features
20. (a) Neurofibromatosis-ocular manifestations.* (b) Differential diagnosis of optic nerve glioma
21. Differential diagnosis of painful ophthalmoplegia in a 40-year-old woman
22. (a) What is the clinical classification of mucormycosis? Describe the presentation of a case of rhino-orbital mucormycosis. (b) Indications, types, advantages, and disadvantages of various types of exenteration
23. Discuss the clinical features, investigations, differential diagnosis, and management of orbital apex syndrome
24. Optic neuritis—causes, types, symptoms, signs, and treatment*
25. Clinical features, investigations, and management of neuromyelitis optica (Devic's disease)
26. Classify ophthalmoplegia. Discuss causes and management of internuclear ophthalmoplegia
27. (a) Traumatic optic neuropathy. (b) Optic nerve sheath fenestration surgery
28. Discuss the risk factors, clinical features, evaluation, and management of ethambutol toxicity
29. Define gaze palsy. Discuss various forms of gaze palsy with their localization value
30. Ischemic optic neuropathy—diagnosis and management**
31. Give clinical presentation, causes, and diagnostic modality and treatment options in benign intracranial hypertension
32. What is visual evoked potential (VEP)? What are the types of VEP? What is the role of VEP in modern clinical practice? What are its limitations?
33. Describe sympathetic nerve supply to the eye with the help of a diagram. Describe various pharmacological tests to diagnose the abnormalities of the sympathetic system
34. (a) What are the main types of migraine? (b) Differential diagnoses of the visual phenomena that accompany an attack of migraine

35. Etiology, clinical features, diagnosis, and differential diagnosis of Horner's syndrome
36. (a) Draw a diagram showing the visual field defects in craniopharyngioma and occipital lobe lesion. (b) Discuss the management of a case of pulmonary tuberculosis who developed sudden decrease of vision
37. Discuss the anatomy of optic nerve and its blood supply

LIDS AND ADNEXA

1. Discuss the pharmacology, indications for use, and adverse effects of botulinum toxins in ophthalmology*
2. Describe clinical manifestations, pathology, differential diagnosis, and management of squamous cell carcinoma
3. Discuss clinical features, differential diagnosis, and management of lid tumor
4. (a) Enumerate malignant tumors of eyelid. (b) Clinical presentations and histopathology of sebaceous cell carcinoma. (c) Outline the management strategy for a 20 mm-sized sebaceous cell carcinoma of upper eyelid
5. Discuss the anatomy of eyelid and its blood supply, venous drainage, and lymphatic drainage. Discuss the clinical implications of blood supply.* Describe the anatomy of levator palpebrae superioris (LPS) and its clinical importance*
6. Anatomy of retractors of eyelids and its clinical significance
7. Discuss the preoperative assessment of entropion. Briefly discuss the surgical options for the correction of involutional entropion**
8. Discuss the surgical options for management of cicatricial entropion. Explain common techniques for correction of trachomatous upper lid entropion
9. Describe the types of orbital exenteration with their indications. Discuss the methods of rehabilitation
10. Describe the mechanism, causes, presentation, assessment, and management of senile ectropion*
11. Draw a labeled diagram of cut section of lid in relation to involutional ectropion. Describe the etiopathogenesis, clinical features, diagnosis, and surgical management of involutional ectropion
12. Classify chronic blepharitis. Describe its clinical features, etiology, and treatment*
13. A 65-year-old lady presents with progressively increasing upper lid mass (15 mm × 10 mm). Discuss differential diagnosis and management
14. A 75-year-old female presented with a painless ulcerated lesion on the medial side of left lower lid for 2 years, size 15 mm × 10 mm, involving 2/3rd of the lower lid. Discuss its differential diagnosis and management

15. Causes, evaluation, and management of lagophthalmos
16. A 6-year-old child is brought to the OPD by her parents with complaints of drooping of the left upper lid noticed 3 years ago. How would you evaluate this patient and decide on your course of management?
17. What are the principles of ptosis surgery? How will you manage a case of congenital ptosis with Marcus Gunn jaw-winking phenomenon?**
18. What is congenial ptosis? Describe the evaluation of ptosis and the management of congenital ptosis
19. Basic guidelines and management of ptosis in a 3-year-old child
20. Describe clinical features and management of blepharophimosis syndrome
21. Causes and management of a case of acquired ptosis
22. (a) What are the principles of lid reconstruction?* (b) Indications, technique, and complications of Cutler–Beard operation
23. (a) Meibomian gland dysfunction (MGD)—pathogenesis, clinical features, evaluation, and treatment. (b) Dry eye workshop 2 (DEWS2) definition of dry eyes. (c) What is intense pulsed light therapy? (d) Lipiflow

LACRIMAL APPARATUS

1. Causes, clinical features, special investigations, and management in a case of Sjogren's syndrome**
2. Discuss the components of tear film* and functions of each layer. Give Lemp's classification of dry eye syndrome. What are the methods to evaluate tear film disorders?* Describe the neural pathway for tear secretion by the lacrimal gland
3. (a) Classify various ocular lubricating agents used in the management of dry eye disease. (b) What is the role of preservatives used in them? (c) What are the various types of preservatives used in lubricating agents?
4. Describe the anatomy and development of the lacrimal drainage system*. Describe the developmental anomalies of lacrimal passages. Explain the mechanism of lacrimal pump
5. Describe relevant nasal anatomy in relation to endonasal dacryocystorhinostomy (DCR). Give the advantages and disadvantages of endonasal DCR versus external DCR
6. Discuss the indications, contraindications, and complications of conjunctivodacryocystorhinostomy. What are the various types of tubes available for the same?
7. (a) Discuss the contraindications of external DCR. What are the causes of failure of DCR surgery and steps taken to prevent it? (b) What is sump syndrome? How it can be prevented?

8. What is a physiological lacrimal pump? Describe clinical evaluation in a case of epiphora
9. Etiology, clinical features, and management of a case of pediatric epiphora
10. A 6-day-old neonate is brought with watering in both eyes. Discuss the differential diagnosis and management of the case
11. Discuss the causes of acquired nasolacrimal duct obstruction. Describe modalities of its treatment
12. Balloon-assisted lacrimal surgery. Implants used for orbital reconstruction—advantages and disadvantages
13. Describe the clinical features and management of lacrimal gland tumor
14. Describe the etiology, clinical features, differential diagnosis, and management of congenital nasolacrimal duct obstruction
15. (a) Describe techniques for repair of a canalicular injury. (b) Describe types of orbital implants and their advantages and disadvantages*

ORBIT AND OCULOPLASTY

1. Give differential diagnosis of painless progressive proptosis in a 35-year-old man. Describe clinical features, histopathology, and management of cavernous hemangioma
2. Discuss ophthalmic manifestation of thyrotoxicosis
3. Draw labeled diagrams depicting walls of the orbit. Describe in detail the medial wall of the orbit.** Describe the applied anatomy of the optic canal
4. Describe briefly origin, insertion, and actions of extraocular muscles with diagram
5. (a) Orbital spaces and their applied importance.** (b) Superior orbital fissure** and cavernous sinus: Anatomy and associated clinical features**
6. (a) Anatomy of the medial wall of orbit. (b) What is its importance in orbital decompression?* (c) What is the most common cause of severe bleed during external DCR?
7. (a) Genetics of retinoblastoma. (b) Histopathology of retinoblastoma
8. Give the international classification of retinoblastoma. Discuss the management of retinoblastoma with recent advances in detail*
9. Indications and complications of intra-arterial chemotherapy in retinoblastoma
10. A 2-month-old healthy infant was brought to the OPD by worried parents for evaluation as the elder sibling died of retinoblastoma at the age of 1 year. What are his chances of having the disease? How will you evaluate and manage?
11. Newer advances in the management of 2 DD unilateral retinoblastoma in the presenting eye and when presenting in the fellow eye in bilateral retinoblastoma

12. Describe clinical features and management of orbital cellulitis
13. Describe the origin, insertion, and actions of different extraocular muscles. What are the laws that govern the movements of extraocular muscles?
14. What is anophthalmic socket? What are the different types of orbital implants? What are the advantages and disadvantages of various implants?*
15. Discuss briefly various approaches in orbital surgery with specific indications in each approach. Enumerate four important complications of orbital surgery*
16. Describe in detail the diagnosis and management of idiopathic orbital inflammatory disease
17. Describe the causes, types, investigation, and management of a case of unilateral axial proptosis
18. A middle-aged female presents with unilateral proptosis of 1-year duration. Discuss differential diagnosis, evaluation, and management*
19. A 27-year-old driver developed left eye hypertropia following an accident. How will you diagnose and manage him?
20. A 27-year-old male presents with acute periorbital swelling, redness, and pain. How will you investigate, diagnose, and treat this case?
21. Give morphological classification of contracted socket. Discuss strategies for the management of contracted socket
22. A 3-year-old child presented with unilateral proptosis. Discuss differential diagnosis, evaluation, and management of this case
23. Define and classify the pseudotumor of the orbit. Enumerate the clinical features and differential diagnosis of the condition. Make a flowchart on the management of a 55-year-old man presenting with pseudotumor of the right eye
24. What is pure and impure blowout fracture? Describe mechanism, clinical features, investigations, and management of blowout fracture**
25. Describe clinical features, investigations, and management of a case of medial wall fracture of orbit
26. A 24-year-old male patient presented with mild proptosis and diplopia following blunt injury to the eye the previous day. The visual acuity was within normal limits. How will you evaluate and manage this case?
27. One month post-COVID, a 45-year-old diabetic male patient developed nasal congestion and painful ophthalmoplegia RE. Visual acuity RE was PL negative. Outline the evaluation and management
28. After giving 1 mL of a peribulbar anesthesia, there is sudden proptosis, pain, 5+5 subconjunctival hemorrhage, severe chemosis, and loss of vision with loss of all ocular movements and inability to close the eyelids
    (a) Describe what your further course of action would be
    (b) What are the signs of globe perforation during peribulbar block?

29. A 7-year-old presented with sudden painful proptosis with no history of trauma. Give differential diagnosis, evaluation, management
30. Carotid cavernous fistula—clinical features, evaluation, treatment; orbital hemangioma—clinical features, evaluation, treatment
31. Biologics in thyroid orbitopathy
32. Etiopathogenesis, clinical picture, differential diagnosis, and management of thyroid orbitopathy

OPTICS, REFRACTION, AND OPHTHALMIC EQUIPMENT

1. Describe in brief four clinical and therapeutic uses of prisms in ophthalmology.* What are Fresnel prisms, and mention one important application of these types of prisms?* Give principle of induction of prismatic effect through spectacle lens
2. Define range and amplitude of accommodation. Define manifest and latent hypermetropia. What are the different ways to uncover latent hypermetropia?
3. What are the different effects of keratorefractive surgery? Give a short description of each
4. What are spherical aberrations? How do spectacle lenses induce these aberrations? What modifications are done to minimize these spectacle-induced aberrations?
5. (a) What is the principle of indirect ophthalmology (IDO)? (b) What are the various lenses used for doing IDO, and what are their advantages and disadvantages? (c) Describe the lenses used for viewing the central retina on a slit lamp biomicroscope
6. Principles, composition, clinical applications, and advantages of an early treatment diabetic retinopathy study (ETDRS) visual acuity chart
7. (a) What is contrast sensitivity? (b) What are the various methods to measure it? (c) How do different types of IOLs influence contrast sensitivity?
8. (a) Theories of color vision.* (b) Methods of color vision defects evaluation.* (c) Differentiate between congenital and acquired color vision defects*
9. (a) Principles and optics of retinoscopy. (b) What are the problems of retinoscopy?
10. (a) Labeled diagram of Sturm's conoid. (b) Classify astigmatisms with example. (c) Methods to treat astigmatism
11. Classification and components of hypermetropia. Approach for subjective verification of refraction
12. Define abnormal retinal correspondence. Explain its development and methods of diagnosis
13. Optics of an operating microscope with a neat labeled diagram

14. (a) Mechanism of accommodation. (b) Anomalies of accommodation and their management*
15. (a) What are the principles of optical coherence biometry? (b) Which ophthalmic equipment uses this principle? (c) What are the advantages and disadvantages of this type of biometry?
16. (a) Enumerate various types of lasers used in ophthalmic practice.* (b) Uses of lasers in ocular disorders. (c) Safety precautions in LASER delivery
17. (a) Supranuclear control of ocular movements. (b) Grades of binocular vision*—its prerequisites and advantages. (c) Discuss theories of binocular vision and tests for evaluation of binocular vision*
18. Clinical manifestations and complications of myopia. Surgical correction for myopia*
19. Classify myopia. Write the indications, contraindications, and complications of phakic IOL* in the management of high myopia
20. What are the commonly used phakic IOLs in refractive surgery? What material are they made of? What are the indications of these lenses? How does one calculate their power and size?*
21. What are the various materials used for spectacle lenses and types of coatings given? Discuss briefly progressive and bifocal lens design and advantages and disadvantages of each design*
22. What is near point and range of accommodation of 4 D myope with an amplitude of 8? What are the tests to determine the AC/A ratio? Write a note on convergence insufficiency
23. (a) Explain Sturm's conoid with the help of a diagram. What is its clinical significance? (b) Discuss briefly the surgical management of astigmatism
24. Describe the principle and uses of ultrasonic biomicroscopy (UBM). Discuss its advantages and disadvantages over anterior segment OCT (AS-OCT)*
25. Describe the optics of specular microscope and discuss its uses
26. Write about the optical principle of pachymeter. Mention the types and uses in ophthalmic practice
27. Discuss the workup of a patient planned for refractive surgery.* Give relevance of each investigation. What are the absolute contradictions for laser refractive surgery?
28. What is a femtosecond laser? Discuss the use of the femtosecond laser system in ophthalmology. What are the current indications of femtosecond laser in corneal refractive surgery? What is opaque bubble laser?
29. What are the factors affecting the SIA (surgically induced astigmatism)? How do you manage these cases having preoperative astigmatism during cataract surgery?

30. What is the current management of postoperative astigmatism?
31. Recent advances in management of postoperative astigmatism
32. What is conductive keratoplasty? What is the mechanism, indications, advantages, and disadvantages of conductive keratoplasty?
33. Convergence—types, anomalies, and management
34. ATOM 1 and 2
35. Orthokeratology
36. Surgical and nonsurgical correction of presbyopia*
37. (a) What are the recent modalities available to treat presbyopia? (b) What are their advantages and limitations?
38. What is Badal's principle? Discuss its relevance to focimetry
39. How will you evaluate visual function in a patient with opaque media?
40. What is accommodation? Explain its clinical importance with the help of diagram(s)
41. What is Sturm conoid? Explain its clinical importance with the help of diagram(s)
42. Describe optics of jack-in-the-box phenomenon. How can you prevent it?
43. What is Scheimpflug's principle? How is it useful in ophthalmology? Name the appliance which uses this principle
44. What is a cross cylinder? Where all is it used during refractions? How can you create a cross cylinder by using lenses from the trial set? Please explain with an example
45. What is Donder's reduced eye? What are the cardinal points?
46. (a) Describe in brief various aberrations of the optical system of the eye. (b) What are the various corrective mechanisms built in the eye to overcome these?
47. Use of smartphone for ophthalmic imaging and teleophthalmology
48. Teleophthalmology
49. Discuss the indications, technique, intraoperative, and postoperative complications of small incision lenticule extraction (SMILE) surgery
50. What are the types of contact lenses? What is the principle of fitting contact lenses?
51. Laser interferometry

COMMUNITY OPHTHALMOLOGY, BIOSTATISTICS, AND MISCELLANEOUS

1. Discuss in detail the ocular manifestations of acquired immunodeficiency syndrome (AIDS). What is the impact of highly active antiretroviral therapy (HAART) on ocular features?**
2. Enumerate the various ocular manifestations of Hansen's disease*
3. Common systemic medications and ocular toxicity

4. Describe briefly the etiopathogenesis, classification, prophylaxis, and management of xerophthalmia.* Write measures to prevent the disease from occurring in the siblings of the patient
5. Write the definition of blindness as per World Health Organization (WHO) standards. Enumerate important causes of blindness as per four important surveys in India
6. What is incidence and prevalence of a disease? How will you calculate sample size and plan survey for cataract blindness?
7. (a) Discuss the microbiological profile in infective endophthalmitis with their antibiotic sensitivity profile. (b) Give doses and combinations of preferred intravitreal antibiotics. (c) What is the normal ocular flora?
8. Discuss disinfection of operation theater. What is the principle of laminar air-flow and its application in operation room? Discuss the methods of sterilization of linen, sharp instruments, and blunt instruments
9. Techniques, preparations, dosages, roles, indications, and advantages or disadvantages of periocular and intraocular steroids**
10. Classify antifungal drugs, their clinical uses, and side effects of each drug*
11. What are antiviral drugs? Describe the mechanism of action of acyclovir and dosages in different viral affections in eye
12. Role of antimetabolites and immunosuppressive drugs in ophthalmology
13. What are the objectives, strategies, approaches, and organization of Vision 2020 program?*
14. (a) Measures of central tendency in a series of observations. (b) Measures of variability of individual observations
15. Methods to increase the ocular bioavailability and efficacy of drugs used in the treatment of ocular disorders, along with examples
16. (a) Tests of significance. (b) Standard deviation. (c) Confidence interval
17. Enumerate causes of childhood blindness. How will you calculate sample size and plan survey of childhood blindness in India?
18. What are the types of prospective studies and their advantages?* What are the methods to avoid bias in a study?*
19. (a) What is a randomized controlled trial? (b) What is randomization and why is it required? (c) What are confounding factors in a study and how to avoid them?
20. (a) What are the various preservatives in eye drops?** (b) What are their advantages and side effects and how does one treat them?*
21. (a) Enumerate the microbiological techniques available to diagnose and identify the cause of intraocular infection. (b) Discuss the advantages and disadvantages of each technique
22. Discuss the mechanism of action of local anesthetic agents used in ophthalmology. What are the various routes of administration? What are the complications of peribulbar anesthesia?

23. Discuss clinical features, diagnosis, and management of intraocular and extraocular cysticercosis*
24. Describe clinical and laboratory diagnosis of trachoma. Discuss its management, complications, and prophylaxis. What is SAFE strategy?
25. (a) Etiopathogenesis of lid changes in trachoma. (b) Management outline of stage 2 trachoma
26. (a) Role of immunosuppressive drugs in ocular disorders. (b) Gene therapy
27. (a) Siderosis bulbi—clinical features.* (b) ERG changes on electrophysiology in siderosis
28. Discuss the role of genetics in ophthalmology
29. Principles of magnetic resonance imaging (MRI) and its role in practice of ophthalmology
30. To establish an ocular microbiology lab, which all medias are needed? Name the diseases in which each of these media is useful
31. Tabulate ophthalmic manifestations of COVID-19 infection. What are the protocols to be followed while conducting VR surgeries?
32. Role of oxidative stress in vision-threatening ophthalmic diseases
33. Answer the following:***
    - Define low vision as per WHO criteria
    - How do you evaluate a person with low vision?
    - What are the goals of visual rehabilitation?
    - Enumerate and discuss various management options (optical and nonoptical) of low vision.

CHAPTER 15

Instruments Used in Ophthalmology

SPECULUM

Barraquer Wire Speculum

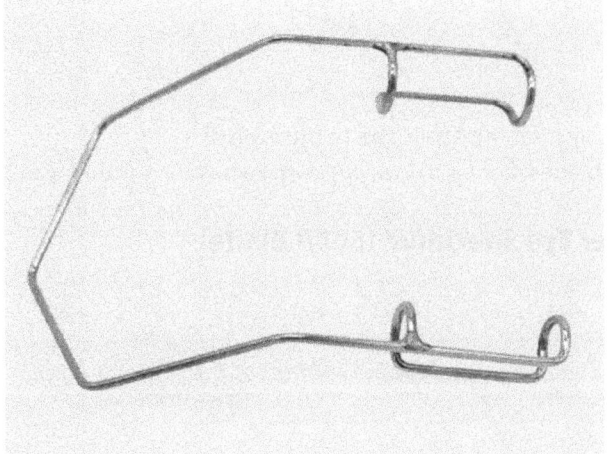

Characteristics:
- It is a universal speculum that can be used for both eyes
- It is used to separate eyelids for intraocular surgery
- Self-retaining
- Lightweight
- Adult size—16–18 mm, pediatric size—14 mm

Uses:
- Intraocular surgery—cataract and glaucoma surgery
- Extraocular surgery—squint and pterygium surgery
- Examination of the eye
- Removal of conjunctival and corneal foreign bodies
- Enucleation and evisceration surgery

Barraquer Eye Speculum (Fenestrated Blade)

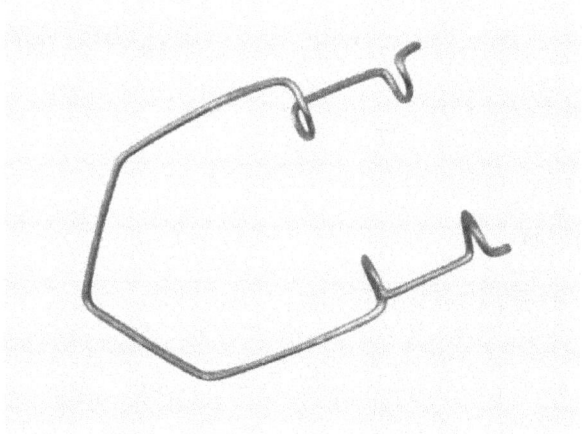

- It transmits minimal pressure to the eyeball
- It lacks blades; hence, it does not keep lashes away from the field of surgery

Barraquer Eye Speculum (Solid Blade)

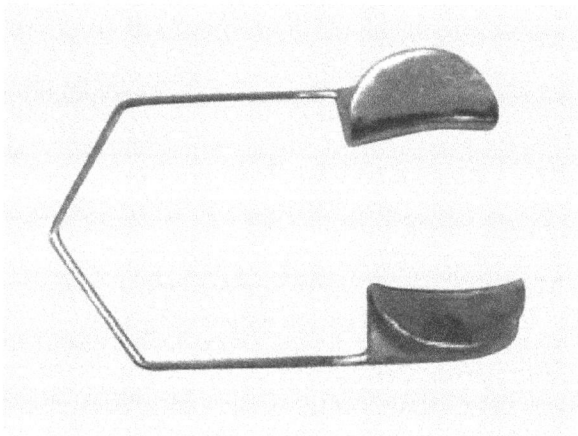

- The solid blades keep the eyelashes away from the field of surgery

Self-retaining Universal Eye Speculum

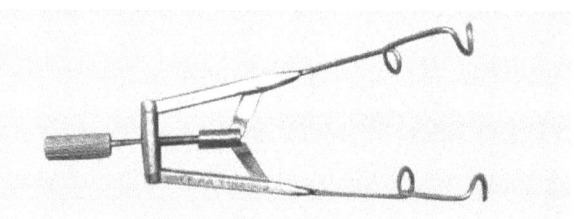

- The screw helps in giving desired exposure and can be adjusted as per the surgeon's preference according to each surgery
- It gives wide exposure and thus can be used in scleral buckling surgery
- The disadvantage is that the screw increases the pressure on the eyeball and can increase intraocular pressure; thus, it is not suitable for perforated cases

Murdoch Eye Speculum

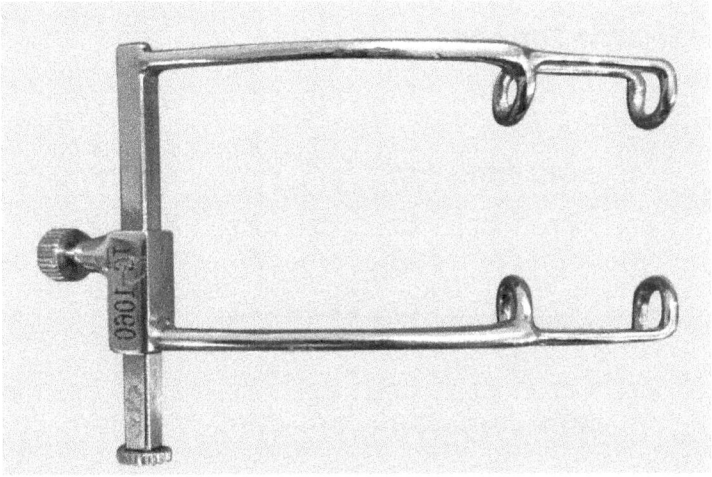

- It has cylindrical curved arms to follow the facial contour
- It has adjustable sliding bars to self-lock the blades
- It is useful in deep-set eyes

FORCEPS

Superior Rectus Holding Forceps

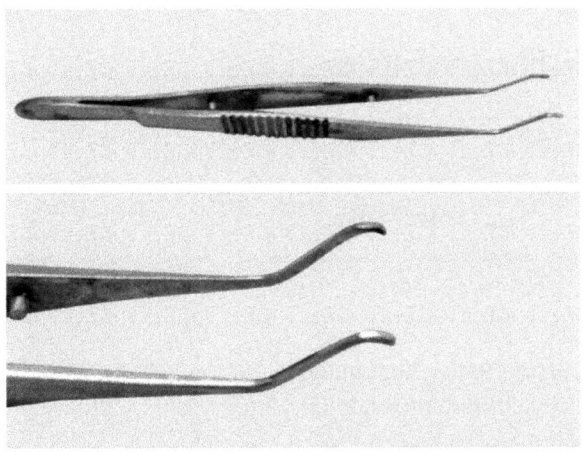

Characteristics:
- It is a forceps with a double curve at the end (S shaped)
- It has a single big tooth to hold the superior rectus muscle
- It has its first angle at 7.7 mm

Uses:
- It is used to hold the superior rectus muscle for passing bridle suture
- It helps to rotate the eyeball downward in cataract and glaucoma surgery
- It helps to fix the eyeball during surgery

Globe Fixation Forceps

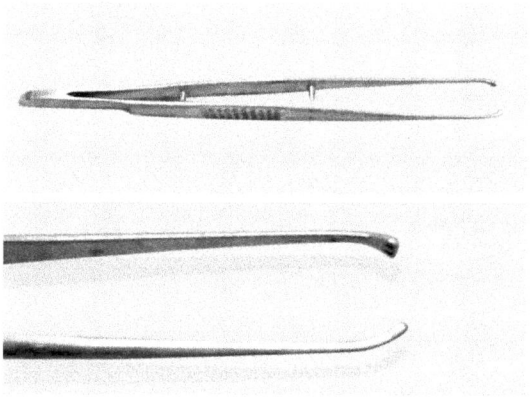

Characteristics:
- It has 2–3 or 3–4 teeth at its tip
- It holds the conjunctival tissue and episcleral tissue together

Uses:
- It is used to hold the conjunctiva for making a conjunctival flap with the use of a conjunctival scissor
- It is used to fix the globe while making a tunnel with a crescent

Kelman–McPherson Forceps

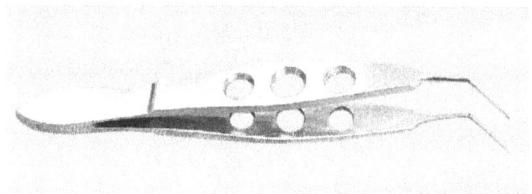

Characteristics:
- It is fine forceps with a bent blade
- It has an angled shaft of about 45°
- It is a nontoothed forceps

Uses:
- It is used to tear off the anterior capsule of the lens in cataract surgery
- It is used to hold the intraocular lens (IOL)
- It is used to hold the sutures

Lens-holding Forceps

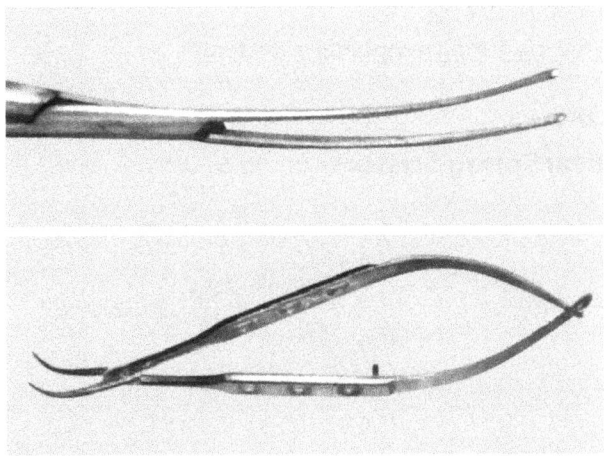

Characteristics:
- It is a spring action forceps
- It has blunt curved blades
- It does not have tooth

Use:
- It is used to hold the nonfoldable polymethyl methacrylate (PMMA) IOL during implantation

Utrata Forceps

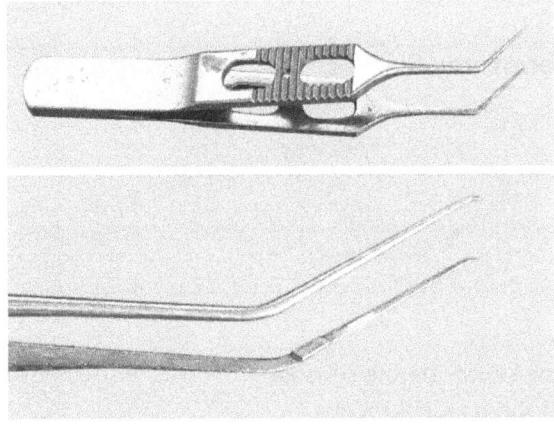

Characteristics:
- It is a fine long forceps with a curved sharp tip perpendicular to the body
- It is a nontoothed forceps

Uses:
It is used:
- In continuous curvilinear capsulorhexis
- To remove capsular tag
- To hold the iris during peripheral iridectomy

SCISSORS

Conjunctival Spring Scissors

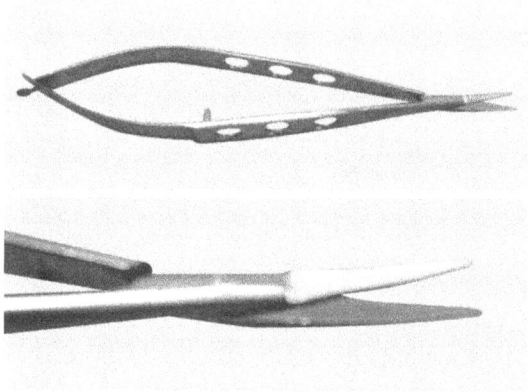

Characteristics:
- It may be straight or curved with a sharp or blunt tip
- It is a sleek longer scissor
- The blade is kept apart by spring action

Use:
- It is used to cut conjunctiva to make a conjunctival flap

Westcott Tenotomy Scissor

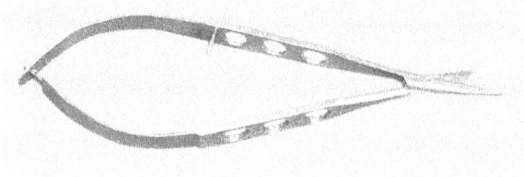

Characteristics:
- It is a spring handle thumb scissors
- It has both sharp and blunt tips

Uses:
- It is used in conjunctival dissection
- It is used in the opening of the orbital septum in levator advancement and upper eyelid blepharoplasty
- The blunt tips help in fine dissection during peritomy and protect the underlying structures

De Wecker Scissors

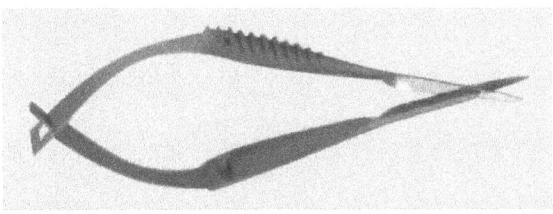

Characteristics:
- It has angled cutting blades
- It has a sharp and fine tip

Uses:
- It gives a greater field of view because of the angled blades
- It is used in iridectomy and iridotomy
- It is used for cutting vitreous strands

Vannas Scissors

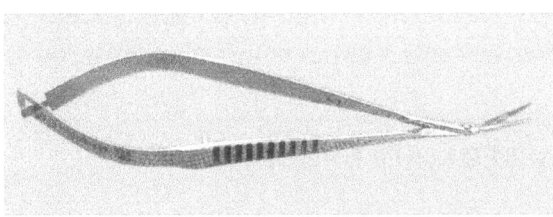

Characteristics:
- It is a fine, delicate scissors with small cutting blades kept apart by spring action
- It has a sharp tip with 7.5 mm blade
- Blades may be curved or straight
- It is angulated at about 45°

Uses:
It is used in:
- Surgical iridectomy
- Multiple sphincterotomies

- Anterior capsulotomy
- Manual vitrectomy
- Cutting sutures
- Cutting trabecular flap in trabeculectomy

Steven Tenotomy Scissors

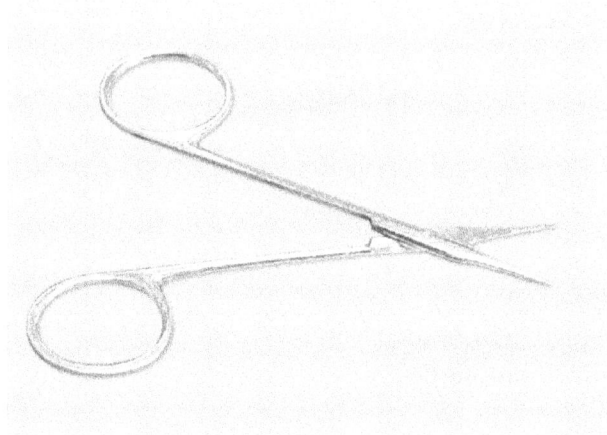

Characteristics:
- It is a fine blunt-tipped scissors
- It can be straight or curved

Uses:
- It is used to separate Tenon's from the underlying sclera
- It is used in buckling surgery, enucleation, evisceration, and squint surgery

BARD PARKER KNIFE HANDLE

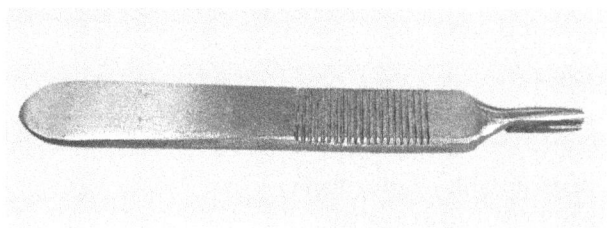

Characteristics:
- It is a flat handle in which 15 number disposable blade is loaded for cataract surgery
- It has a long handle with groove at its extreme end in which blade is loaded
- It gives pen-like grip

Uses:
- It is used to make corneoscleral gutter in cataract surgery
- It is used in dacryocystorhinostomy (DCR), ptosis, entropion, and ectropion surgeries for incision of the skin

CRESCENT KNIFE

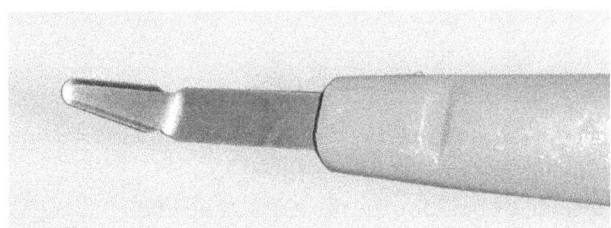

Characteristics:
- It is blunt-tipped which has a cutting action at the tip and both sides
- The blade is curved and mounted on a plastic handle

Use:
- It is used to make a self-sealing sclero-corneal tunnel after making the scleral gutter in cataract surgery

KERATOME

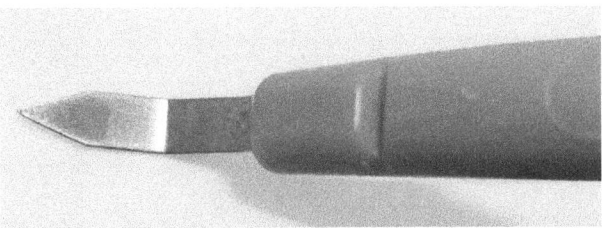

Characteristics:
- It has a thin diamond-shaped blade with a sharp apex
- It has two cutting edges
- It is mounted on a plastic handle at an angle of 45°
- Straight disposable keratomes are also available

Uses:
- It is used for making an entry in the anterior chamber after the tunnel is formed
- Bevel up keratome—phacoemulsification
- Bevel down keratome—small incision cataract surgery (SICS)

CYSTITOME

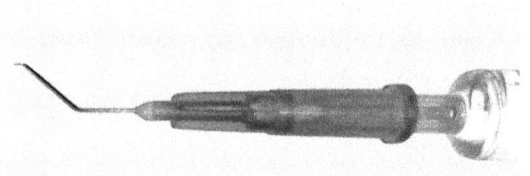

Characteristics:
- It has a tiny, sharp, and triangular flag-shaped tip
- It has two bends—the first bend is about 45°, and the second bend near tip is about 90°
- It can be made by bending the tip of a 26 G needle

Use:
- It is used for incising the anterior capsule of the lens by using the envelope method, can opener method or continuous curvilinear capsulorhexis

IRRIGATION WIRE VECTIS

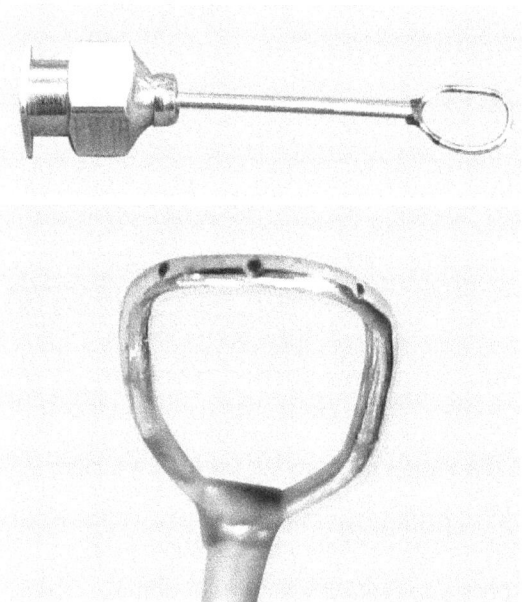

Characteristics:
- It is a modified Vectis in which the loop is made of hollow wire
- It has three openings of 0.3 mm in size for saline to pass through the anterior chamber (AC) and help in nucleus delivery. The three ports help in forming eddy currents and aid in nucleus delivery through tunnel

- The posterior end of the loop is continuous with a hollow handle to which an infusion set is attached

Uses:
- It is used to deliver the nucleus by introducing this Vectis from the tunnel and applying counterpressure at the 12 o'clock position

SIMCOE'S TWO-WAY IRRIGATION AND ASPIRATION CANNULA

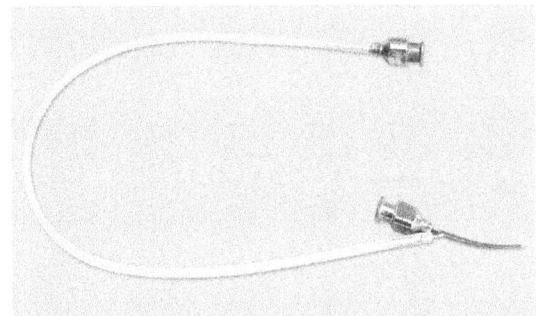

Characteristics:
- It has a curved thin-walled shaft with a double barrel
- The distal end has a straight or an angular blunt cannula. It has two ports—the one above is 0.3 mm for aspiration and the one below is for irrigation
- The proximal end has two inlets—one for fixing the 2 or 5 mL syringe and the other for infusion through tube

Uses:
- It is used for irrigation and suction of lens particles or cortical matter from the anterior chamber after nuclear delivery
- It can also be used for aspiration of hyphema

SINSKEY HOOK OR INTRAOCULAR LENS DIALER

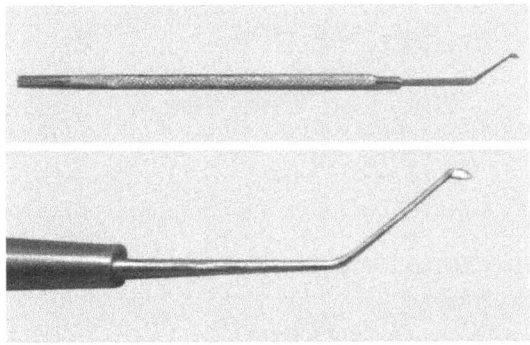

Characteristics:
- It is a pencil-like handle with a thin neck
- The neck is bent in between at 45°
- The tip is bent at 90°

Uses:
- It helps to wheel out the nucleus into AC
- The tip is engaged in the hole present in the optics of posterior chamber intraocular lens (PCIOL) and is used to rotate it into bag or sulcus

SPATULA

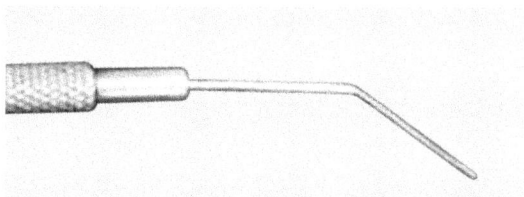

Characteristics:
- It is a flat malleable straight blade
- It is bent in between at 45°
- The edges are smooth
- The tip is attached to a handle

Uses:
- It is used to reposit the iris in the anterior chamber during surgery
- It is used to release synechiae at the pupillary border
- It is useful in the bimanual prolapse of the nucleus

NEEDLE HOLDER

Barraquer Needle Holder

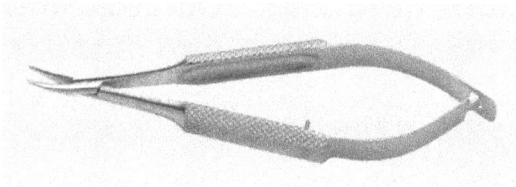

Characteristics:
- It is available:
  - In various sizes with straight or curved tips
  - In different shapes
  - With or without a locking system

- The jaws of the needle holder are finely serrated to hold the fine needles firmly

Use:
- Spring-type needle holders are used for passing sutures in the conjunctiva, cornea, sclera, and extraocular muscles

Castroviejo Needle Holder

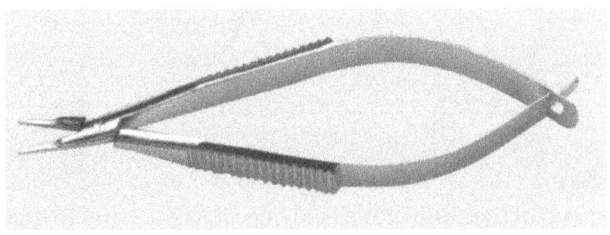

Characteristic:
- It is a medium-sized spring-action needle holder with an S-shaped locking system

Uses:
- It is generally used in extraocular surgery, e.g., conjunctival suturing and squint surgery
- It can also be used for intraocular surgery

Kalt Locking Needle Holder

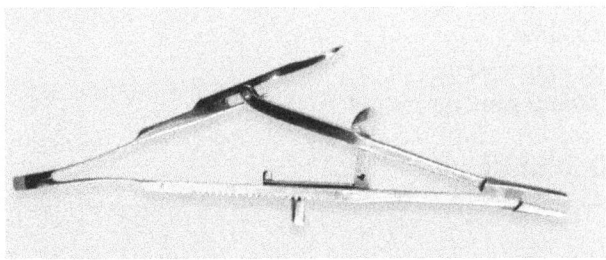

Characteristics:
- These are large needle holders
- The upper shank of these needle holders has a flat and broad plate to accommodate the surgeon's thumb
- These are available with and without a locking device

Use:
- These are very commonly used in lid surgery and also for passing superior rectus suture

PHACO TIP

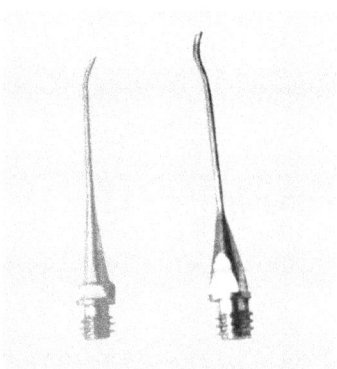

Characteristics:
- It is made up of titanium with distal opening of 0.9 mm in diameter
- The phaco needle fits onto the phaco handpiece directly
- The acoustic energy produced along the ultrasonic handpiece is then transmitted onto the phaco tip
- The angulation of the tip may vary from 0 to 60°
- The more the angulation, the cutting power is more, but the holding power is inversely proportional
- The most commonly used tips are angulated at 30 and 45°

Uses:
- It enhances emulsification and manipulation of the nucleus
- The important functions of the phaco tip are:
  - Holdability
  - Followability
  - Surge suppression
  - Maintaining energy output

PHACO SLEEVE

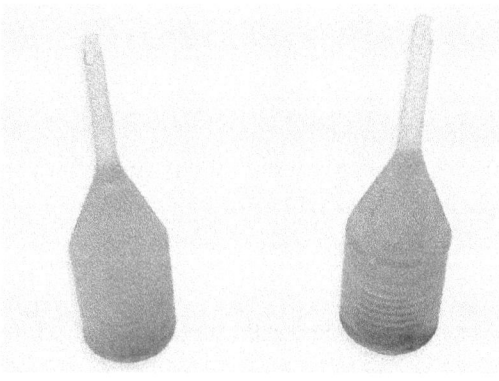

Characteristics:
- It is constructed of a thin stiff silicone material so that it remains rigid and does not twist and collapse at the incision
- It has two openings on the sides, 180° apart, through which irrigation fluid flows

Uses:
- It helps in irrigation around the phaco tip
- It lowers the resulting temperature and avoids wound burn
- It helps to fit snuggly at the tunnel to prevent leakage and maintain the anterior chamber

PHACO IRRIGATION AND ASPIRATION TIP

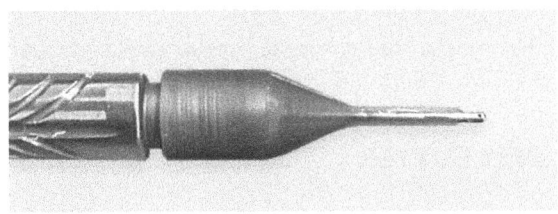

Characteristics:
- It has smooth edges with an opening port at one side, which is 0.3 mm in size
- It can be attached to the handpiece of the phaco probe
- There are three types of tips: (1) Straight tip, (2) angled tip, and (3) J-shaped tip
- The angled tip is about 45° to the shaft

CHOPPER

Characteristics:
- The angulation of the shaft to handle is 45°
- There are two types—horizontal and vertical
- Horizontal chopper—the cutting edge is perpendicular to the shaft
- Vertical chopper—short and sharp tip

Horizontal Chopper

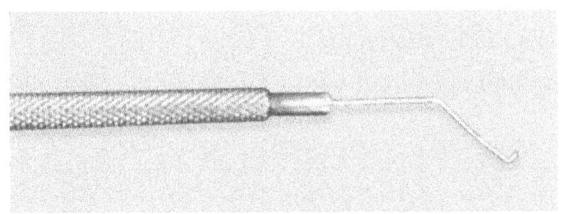

Vertical Chopper

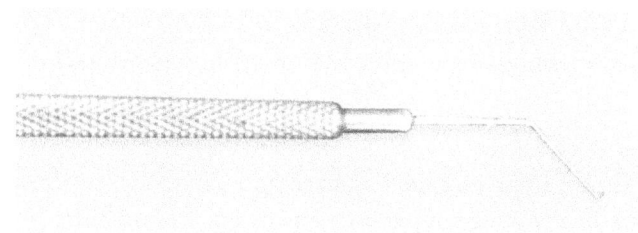

Uses:
- More efficient removal of hard nucleus, thus minimizing phacoemulsification energy
- During sculpting, chopping applies less force to zonules
- It is useful in complicated cases such as brunescent cataract and weak zonules

VITRECTOMY CUTTER

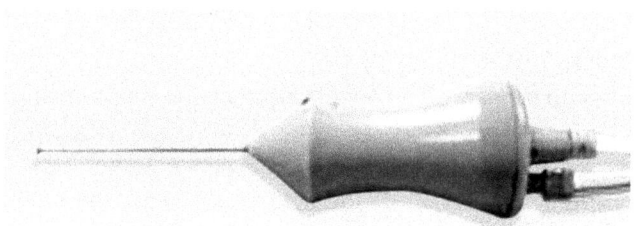

Characteristics:
- It has two channels on a pen-like handle:
  - For vitreous cutter
  - For vitreous aspiration
- Types:
  - Guillotine cutter
  - Rotatory cutter
  - Oscillatory cutter

Uses:
- It is used in anterior vitrectomy
- It helps in high-speed cutting of vitreous and controlled removal of vitreous

GLAUCOMA INSTRUMENTS
Kelly Descemet's Punch

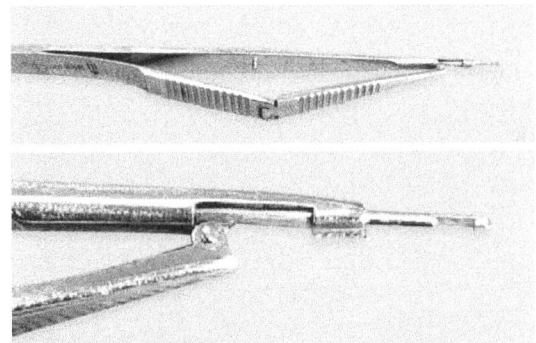

Characteristics:
- It has serrated squeeze action handles
- It has a mouth at the end
- It is found in two sizes: 0.75 mm and 1 mm punch

Uses:
- Creation of a dural window in optic nerve fenestration surgery
- Trabecular meshwork (TM) block excision in trabeculectomy
- Structures cut:
  - Descemet's membrane
  - TM and Schlemm's canal
  - Sclera
- Produces round punches without tissue tags

Iris Forceps

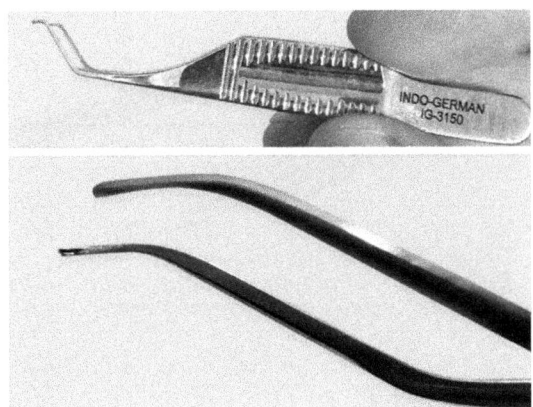

Characteristics:
- It is a toothed forceps
- It has an S-shaped curve

Use:
- It is used to grab and pull the iris during surgical iridectomy

Muscle Hook

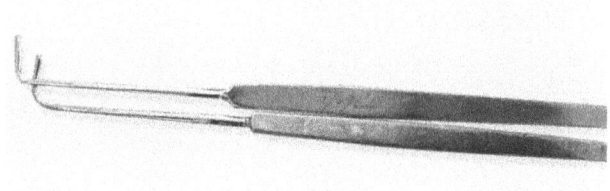

Characteristics:
- It has a thin, flat, blunt blade
- It is 10 mm long
- Blade is at right angle to the handle

Uses:
- During glaucoma drainage device (GDD) placement
- Identification and isolation of adjacent recti
- Blunt dissection
- To place the episcleral plate beneath the adjacent recti

Serrated Forceps

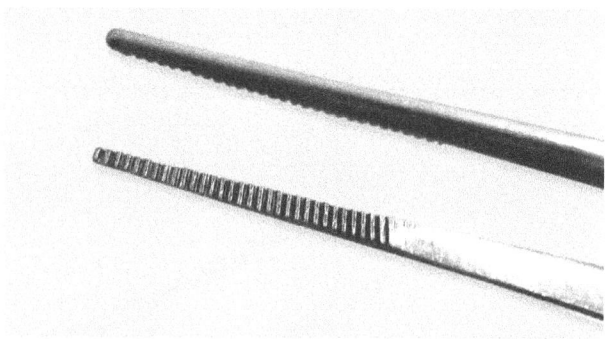

Characteristic:
- It has serrations at the tip

Uses:
- It is used to grip the tube of GDD and maneuver

Castroviejo Caliper

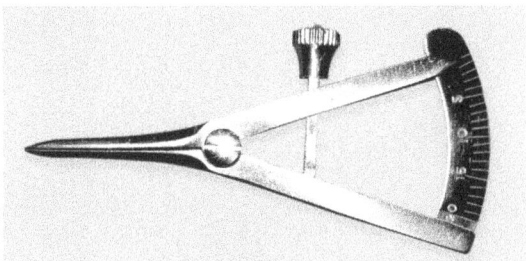

Characteristics:
- It is a divider-like instrument with a graduated scale at one end
- Its marking is in millimeters
- Other arm moves by a screw over the scale

Uses:
- Measuring the
  - Diameters of corneal button
  - Length of GDD tube to be resected
  - Mark site of muscle insertion on recession surgery
  - Mark site of pars plana entry

Harms Trabeculectomy Probe

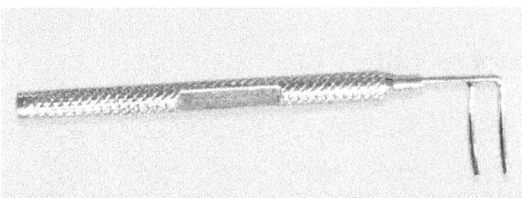

Characteristics:
- Radius—7 mm
- Double parallel prong design:
  - Probe
  - Guide
- Internal arm (probe) threaded into Schlemm's canal
- External arm is used as a guide
- Available in pair—left and right sided
- Pointed tips—0.3 mm diameter

Uses:
- Ab externo trabeculectomy—disruption of the internal wall of Schlemm's canal and TM—sweeping motion
- Done when the media is hazy

Straight Crescent Knife

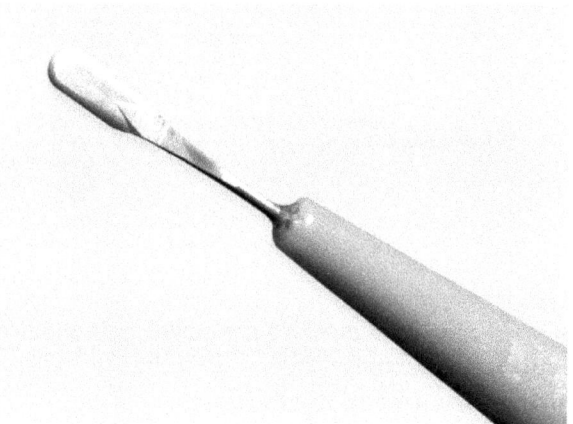

Characteristics:
- Bevel up
- 2.0 mm
- Straight blade

Use:
- It is used to create scleral flap in trabeculectomy and nonpenetrating deep sclerectomy

Fukasaku Hockey Knife

Characteristics:
- It has a long handle with hockey stick-shaped end
- One end is blunt and the other end is sharp

Uses:
- It is used to dissect Tenon's capsule prior to scleral incision in SICS and trabeculectomy
- If not done properly, it can lead to Tenon's cyst and uneven incision

Other—Tooke's knife

Diode Cyclophotocoagulation Probe

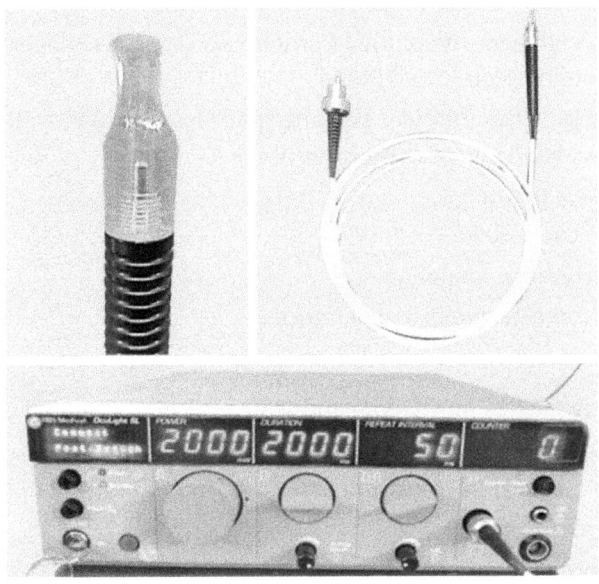

Characteristics:
- It uses a semiconductor solid-state laser
- Its wavelength is 810 μm
- G probe is used to deliver the laser
- It is indicated in intractable glaucoma
- Posterior edge is placed at the limbus
- Laser energy is delivered to the ciliary body 1.2 mm posterior to the limbus
- 16–24 spots circumferential, 3 and 9 o'clock hour spared—popping sound will be heard, which is the end point

Other—Ciliprobe

Ologen Implant

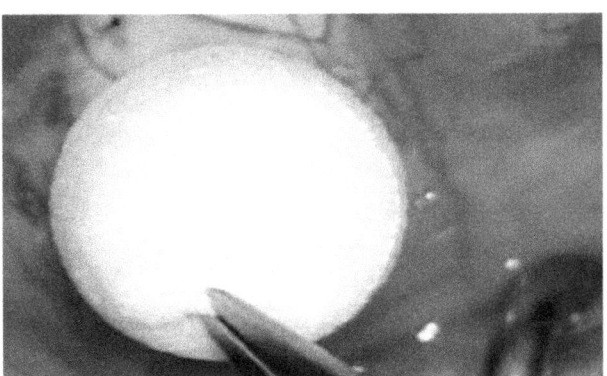

Characteristics:
- Biodegradable collagen matrix
- Porcine collagen—lyophilized crosslinked type 1 collagen (90%) and glycosaminoglycan (GAG) (10%)
- Scaffold provides irregular seeding space for fibroblasts—this prevents the formation of dense connective tissue
- Extensively porous
- Acts as a tissue sieve
- Helps in tissue remodeling
- Used in trabeculectomy when indicated

Indications:
- Risk of trabeculectomy failure and scarring is high
- Young patient
- Congenital/juvenile glaucoma
- High myopes
- Repeat procedure
- Uveitic glaucoma
- Poor mitomycin candidates—pregnancy, blebitis

ORBIT INSTRUMENTS
Kerrison Bone Rongeur Punch

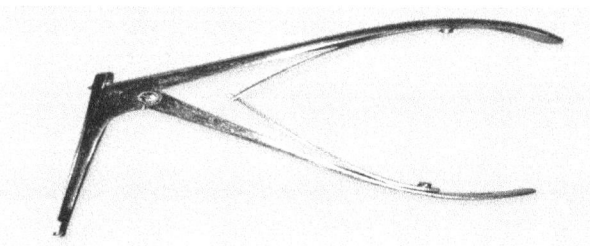

- It is used in DCR to enlarge the bony opening by punching bone from the margins of the opening
- The punch started at the junction of the lamina papyracea of the ethmoid and lacrimal bone
- Superiorly 2 mm above the medial canthus
- Inferiorly till nasolacrimal canal is partly deroofed
- Indicated in lacrimal duct obstruction
- Available in sizes from size 0 (1 mm) to size 4 (5 mm)
- Cutting end up or down design

Thudichum's Nasal Speculum

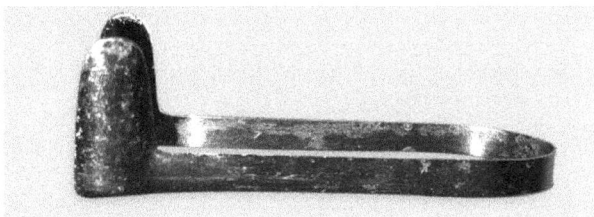

- During external DCR—for better visualization during nasal packing
- For examining the anterior nasal cavity
- For removal of foreign body

Tilley's Nasal Packing Forceps

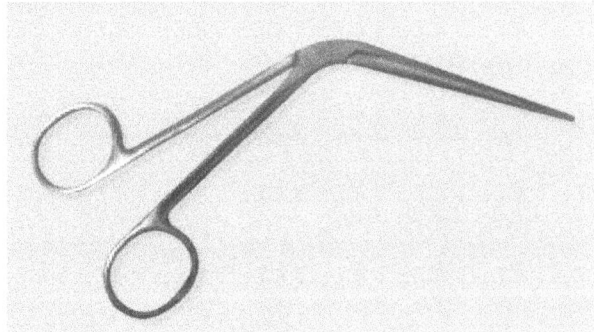

Characteristics:
- Bent nontoothed forceps used along with Thudichum's speculum
- To pack nose with a gauze strip during external DCR

Knapp's Lacrimal Sac Retractor

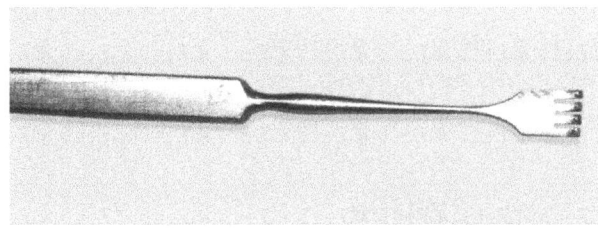

Characteristic:
- It has four wide blunt prongs

Use:
- It is used to retract tissues during dacryocystectomy (DCT) and DCR procedures

Lacrimal Sac Dissector and Curette

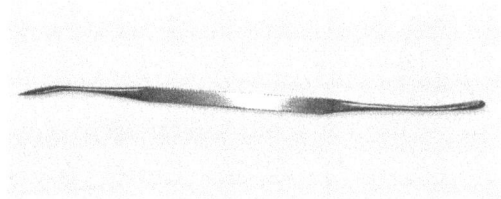

Characteristics:
- Cylindrical instrument
- One end—blunt tipped dissector
- Other end—curettage

Use:
- It is used to gently dissect lacrimal sac without damaging the sac

Bowman Lacrimal Probe

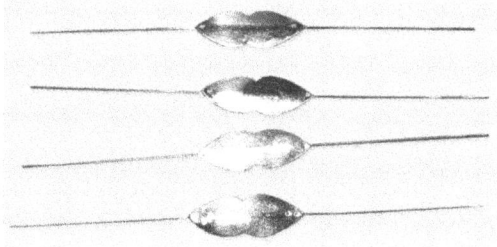

Characteristics:
- Metal wires of varying thicknesses with a blunt rounded end and a flattened central platform
- Size from 0000 to 4 (0 = 1 mm)

Uses:
- While checking patency—to determine
- Presence of hard stop or soft stop
- During DCT—to identify common canaliculus for cauterization after sac removal

Nettleship Lacrimal Dilator

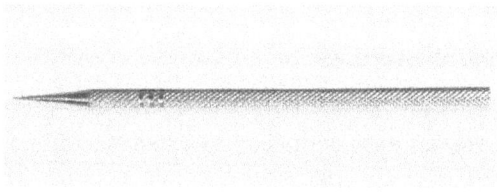

Characteristics:
- It has a conical pointed tip
- It is available in various sizes corresponding to probe size

Uses:
- To dilate punctum and canaliculus during:
  - Syringing
  - Probing
  - Dacryocystography
  - DCT and DCR

Desmarres Lid Retractor

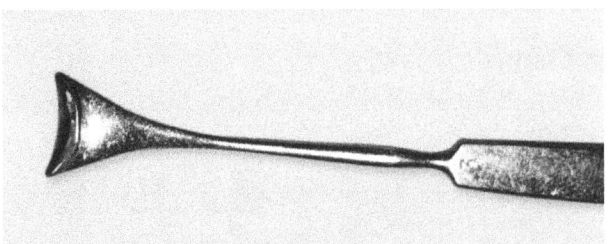

Characteristic:
- Curved configuration of tip with blunt ends

Uses:
- It is used in double eversion of eyelid
- It is used as a blunt retractor in minor surgical procedures

Hartman's Mosquito Forceps (Artery Forceps)

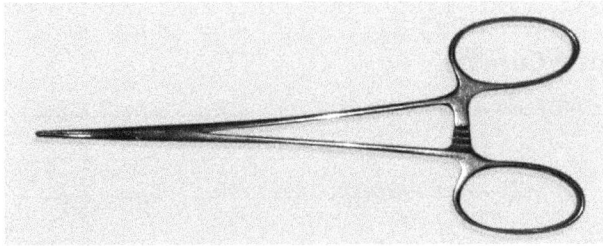

Characteristics:
- Scissor-like configuration with locking and multiple grooves

Uses:
- It is used to catch bleeding vessels—sac and lid surgery
- It is used to hold skin and muscle stay sutures
- It is used to hold gauze pieces while packing the socket

Chalazion Scoop

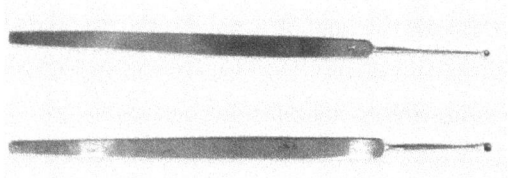

Characteristic:
- It is a small cup with sharp margins attached to a narrow handle

Use:
- It is used to scoop out chalazion contents during incision and curettage

Chalazion Clamp

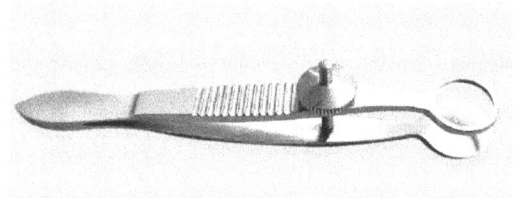

Characteristics:
- It consists of a circular disk
- It contains circular rim attached to each other with a handle that can be tightened with a screw

Use:
- It is used to fix chalazion and achieve hemostasis during incision and curettage

Evisceration Curette

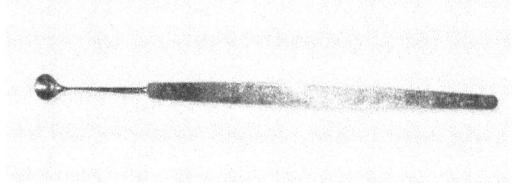

Characteristic:
- It contains a rounded shallow cup with blunt margins

Use:
- It is used to separate uvea from sclera prior to removing intraocular contents

Wells Enucleation Spoon

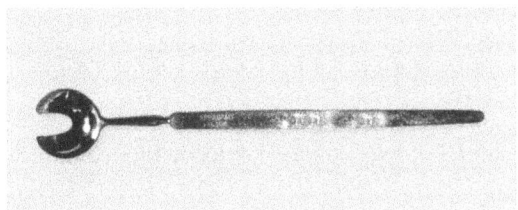

Characteristics:
- It is an optic nerve guide
- It is a spoon-shaped instrument with central cleavage

Use:
- It is used to engage optic nerve during enucleation

Enucleation Scissor

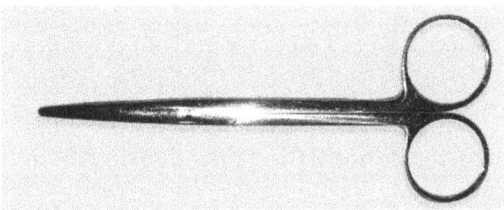

Characteristics:
- It is curved blunt scissors
- It is curved to facilitate reaching the optic nerve inside the orbital cavity

Use:
- It is used to cut the optic nerve that is engaged in enucleation spoon

Chisel

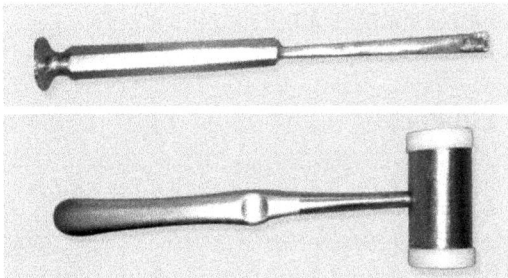

Characteristics:
- It is a blade with a sharp cutting straight edge with one surface beveled
- It has a long and stout handle

Use:
- It is used to cut bone during DCR and orbitotomy

Hammer

Characteristic:
- It is a small steel hammer attached to a corrugated handle

Use:
- It is used to hammer the chisel during DCR and orbitotomy

Freer Periosteal Elevator

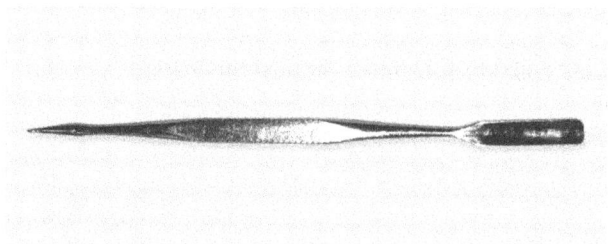

Characteristics:
- It is a long slender instrument that tapers into double end sharp and blunt blades
- The sharp end provides cutting capacity and the blunt end aids in lifting the periosteum from the bone

Uses:
- It is used to elevate the periosteum off the bone before performing osteotomy in sac surgeries, orbital fracture repair, orbitotomy, and orbital decompression
- It is used to initiate osteotomy in external DCR by breaking the innominate suture
- It is used to hold tissue away from the surgical site
- It is used for blunt dissection between the tumor and the orbital tissues

Khan Jaeger Lid Plate

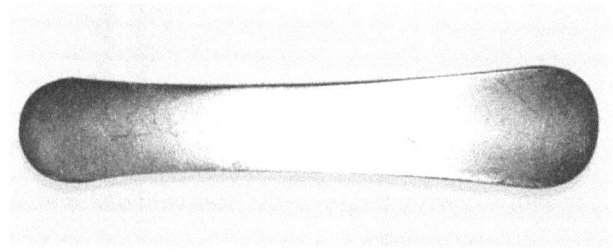

Characteristic:
- It is a stainless-steel concave plate

Use:
- It is used to protect the globe and support lid during:
  - Entropion
  - Ectropion
  - Ptosis and other lid surgeries

CORNEA INSTRUMENTS
Castroviejo Calipers

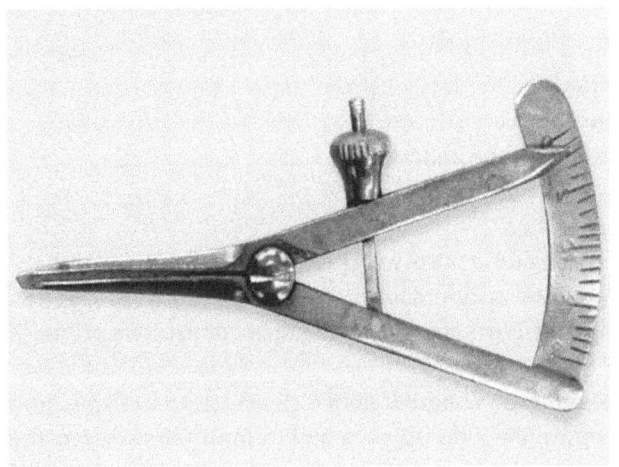

Characteristic:
- It is a dividers-like instrument with one fixed arm that is attached to a graduated curved scale in millimeters and another movable arm

Uses:
- Measurement during squint, ptosis, pterygium, scleral buckling, corneal surgeries
- To measure the size of the excised pterygium defect for calculating graft size
- Intraoperative measurement of the size of corneal opacity or lesion
- Determine the length of scleral incision in SICS
- Determine the distance from limbus for intravitreal injection and vitrectomy ports
- Measure corneal diameter

Advantages:
- It is portable and accurate when properly calibrated

BARRON'S ARTIFICIAL ANTERIOR CHAMBER

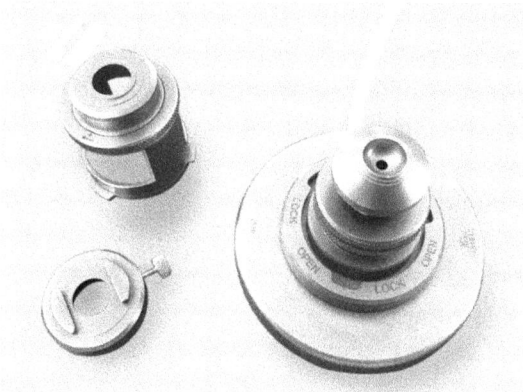

Characteristics:
- It has three parts:
  - Base with tissue pedestal
  - Tissue retainer
  - Locking ring
- It has two irrigation ports with pinch clamps
- It has a pedestal to mount the tissue epithelial side up, a tissue retainer, and a locking ring. Ports can be used to inject or aspirate saline, viscoelastics, or air
- The design of the chamber allows the surgeon to firmly hold the donor button epithelial side up on a bed of ophthalmic viscosurgical device (OVD), pressurize it, and perform lamellar dissection

Use:
- Manual lamellar dissection

LIEBERMAN TEFLON BLOCK

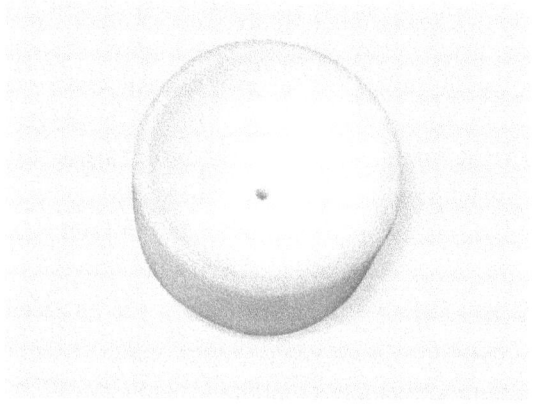

Characteristic:
- It is a white Teflon circular block with an internal concavity similar to the radius of curvature of the cornea and a drainage hole in the center

Uses:
- It is used for donor preparation and cutting. It is used as a base for trephination of donor tissue

Advantages:
- It approximates corneal shape and so reduces tissue distortion

Disadvantage:
- Slippage at the time of cutting

CORNEAL TREPHINE

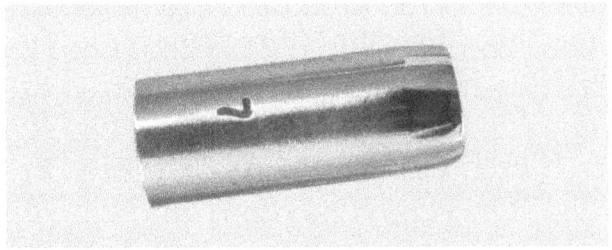

Disposable Trephine

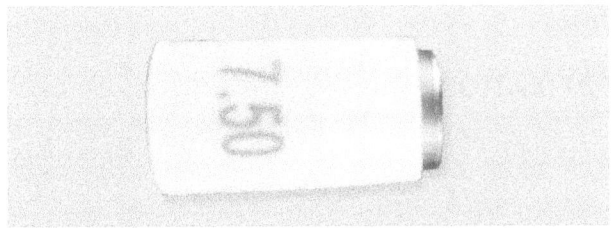

Characteristics:
- It is a cylindrical instrument that has three parts:
  - A circular blade
  - An adjustable inner core or "obturator"
  - A cover to protect the sharpness of the blade
- It is available in sizes from 3 to 17 mm in diameter
- Disposable trephine is also available

Use:
- Trephination of donor and recipient cornea

PIERSE HOSKIN FORCEPS

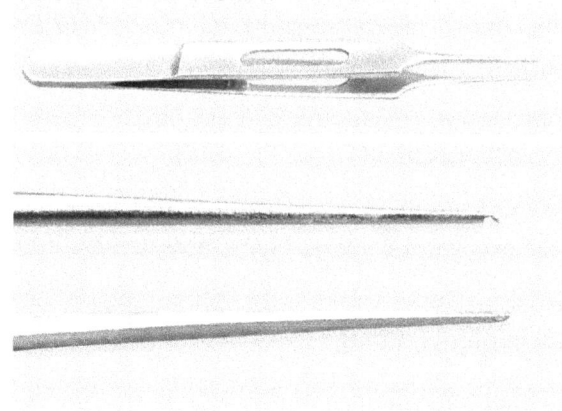

Characteristic:
- It is a small, fine forceps with a 6 mm platform and a 0.2 mm precision notched tip

Use:
- It is used to hold conjunctiva and muscles during extraocular and intraocular surgery

Advantage:
- Less traumatic than other forceps

Disadvantage:
- Less firm grip

GRAEFE FIXATION FORCEPS

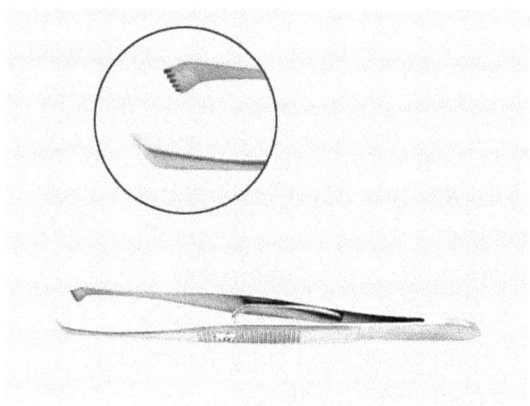

Characteristic:
- It is nontoothed forceps with a broad serrated end for good grasping

Uses:
- It is used to fix the eyeball during surgery
- It is used to hold the eyeball during forced duction test

OSHER NEUMAN CORNEAL RADIAL MARKER

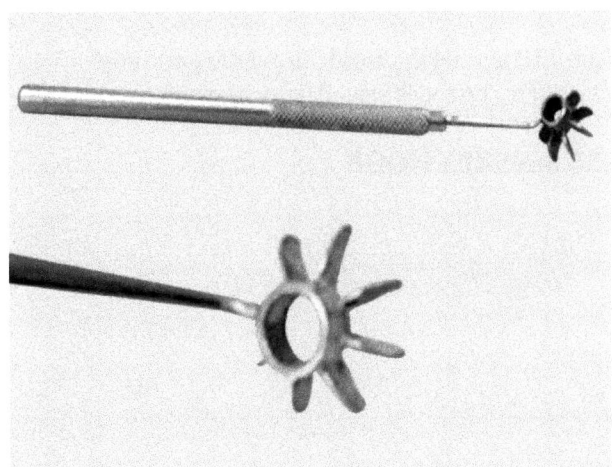

Characteristic:
- It has eight blades, on a central 4.5 mm ring, and a fixed round cross-serrated handle
- It marks radial lines 4 mm long
- To be used with skin marking pen

Uses:
- It helps in the orientation of sutures during keratoplasty
- It was previously used in radial keratectomy (RK), which is not done nowadays

Advantages:
- Its inner ring helps in centration and blunt blades allow minimal marking pressure

BORES U-SHAPED FIXATION FORCEPS

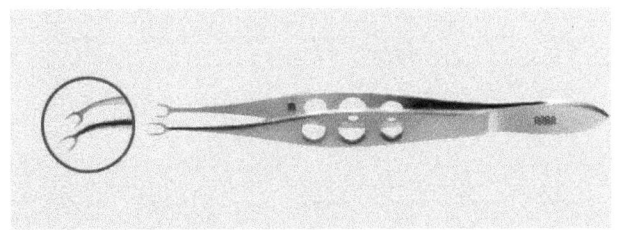

Characteristic:
- It can be either straight or curved. U-shaped spread, 1 × 2 teeth at each tip 0.12 mm

Use:
- It is used to firmly grasp the cornea while suturing

Advantages:
- Its delicate 0.12 mm teeth provide firm but gentle grip
- The U-shaped tip provides visualization during suturing

REVERSE SINSKEY HOOK

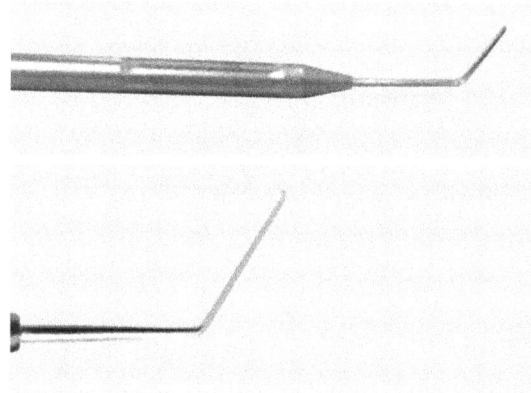

Characteristic:
- It is a long, slender instrument with 0.22 mm diameter blunt tip, 0.7 mm height pointing upward, 45° angled shaft with 10 mm length, and overall length 118 mm

Use:
- It is used for scoring of Descemet's membrane at the beginning of descemetorhexis

Advantage:
- It gently strips the membrane

GOROVOY DESCEMETORHEXIS FORCEPS

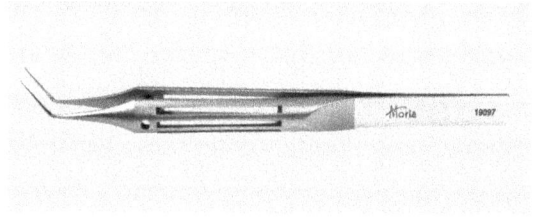

Characteristics:
- 90° bend at the tip pointing upward
- It has a blunt tip

Use:
- It is used to delaminate endothelium and Descemet's membrane

LAMELLAR DISSECTOR

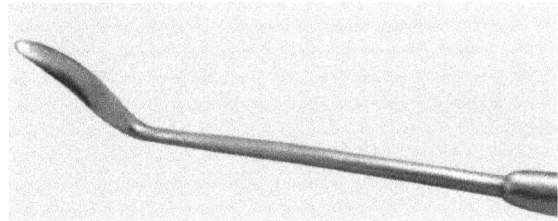

- It is used in dissecting the lamellar flap in deep anterior lamellar keratoplasty (DALK)
- It is used to initiate the dissection of the anterior stroma after partial trephination
- Blade contour matches the curvature of the cornea

TROUTMAN-KATZIN CORNEAL TRANSPLANT SCISSORS

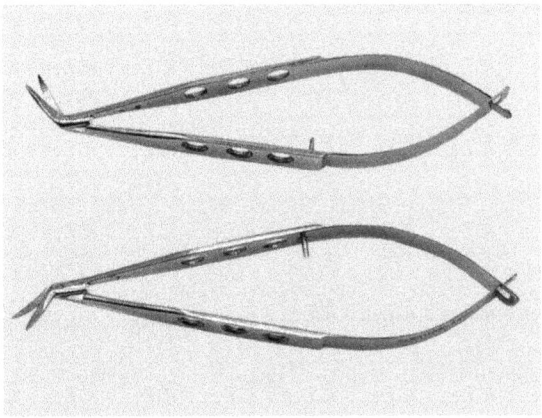

Characteristics:
- It is available as straight, right, and left scissors
- The lower blade in both right and left scissors is 0.5 mm longer than the upper blade—to match the curve of the limbus

Uses:
- Penetrating keratoplasty (PKP)
- DALK

Advantage:
- Its curved blade helps in the cutting of the cornea along its curvature

HOCKEY STICK MICROBLADE

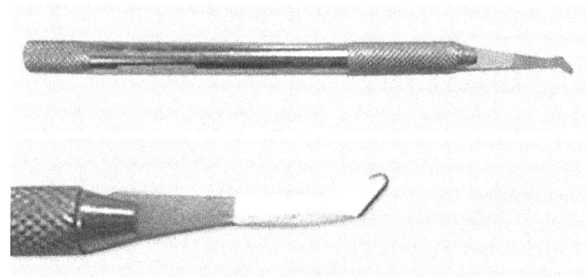

Characteristics:
- It is a hockey-shaped blade with width 1 mm and ultra-sharp cutting edges
- It is available in reusable as well as disposable variants
- It should be kept perpendicular to the corneal plane during dissection

Uses:
- It is used in epithelial debridement in procedures such as collagen cross-linking and photorefractive keratectomy (PRK)
- It is used for pterygium excision

Advantages:
- Nontraumatic, more control

FLIERINGA SCLERAL FIXATION RING

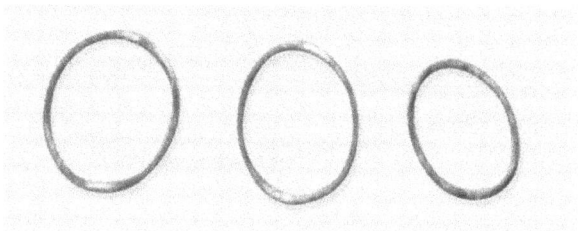

Characteristics:
- Scleral expansion rings made of stainless steel and polished finish
- Available as a set of eight rings from size 12 to 23 mm

Uses:
- They are sutured to the sclera with Vicryl sutures before keratoplasty
- They maintain the rigidity of the recipient's globe after trephination and prevent collapse of the eyeball

Advantage:
- Secure globe during open-sky procedures such as keratoplasty

DIAMOND BURR

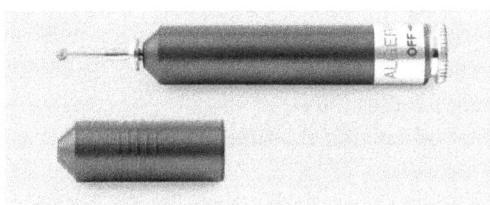

Characteristic:
- It consists of a handpiece with motor and batteries, a chuck, and a round, fine-grit diamond burr with a cap

Uses:
- It is used to smoothen the corneal surface in certain abnormalities involving the anterior layer of the cornea, such as:
  - Recurrent corneal erosions and epithelial basement membrane dystrophy
  - For rust ring removal
  - For polishing the cornea after pterygium excision

Advantage:
- It can be performed in the outpatient department using topical anesthesia

FIBRIN SEALANT KIT (RELISEAL)

Uses:
- Pterygium surgery
- Strabismus surgery—conjunctival closure
- Corneal surgery—sealing small perforation (2-3 mm), amniotic membrane transplant, limbal cell transplantation
- Glaucoma surgery—conjunctival closure, management of post trabeculectomy hypotony

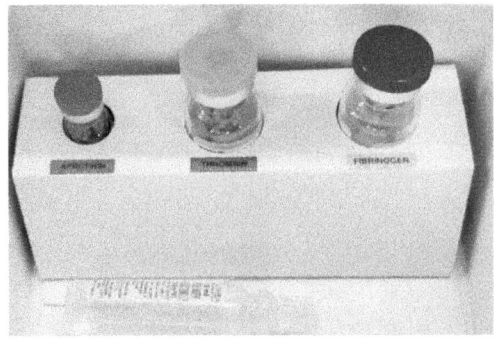

Reliseal—Kit:
- Contains three vials:
  - Red—Bovine aprotinin
  - Blue—thrombin
  - Yellow—fibrinogen
- Four sterile syringes (2 mL)
- Four sterile needles (21 G)
- Two application needles (20 G)
- One applicator with mixing chamber
- One 5 mL sterile water

Reliseal—Reconstitution:

Preparation of fibrinogen solution:
1. Remove the flip cap of two vials (red—aprotinin, yellow—fibrinogen)
2. Disinfect the rubber stopper
3. Aspirate aprotinin using the 21 G needle attached to the 2 mL syringe
4. Inject aprotinin into the yellow vial containing fibrinogen
5. Swirl in a circular fashion very gently until no more undissolved particles are seen

Preparation of thrombin solution:
1. Take 2 mL syringe (21 G needle attached), and aspirate 1 mL from the sterile water cartridge (5 mL)
2. Remove the flip cap of the thrombin vial (blue color)
3. Disinfect the rubber stopper
4. Inject the sterile water (1 mL) into the vial containing thrombin
5. Swirl in a circular fashion very gently until no more undissolved particles are seen

RETINA INSTRUMENTS

Trocar
- It is used in minimally invasive vitreoretinal surgery for making sclerotomy ports
- Different sizes are available: 20, 23, 25, and 27 G

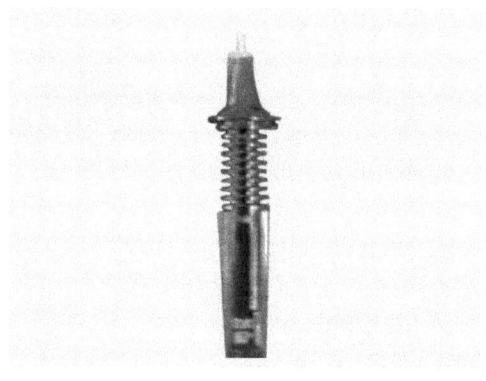

Light Source (Illuminator)

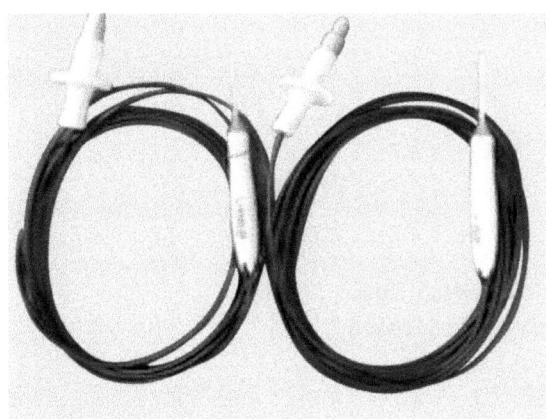

- Sizes available are 23 and 25 G
- It can be handheld or fixed
- Handheld—straight, bullet type, wedge type
- Fixed—chandelier system for surgeries with bimanual dissection

Endgripping Internal Limiting Membrane Peeling Forceps

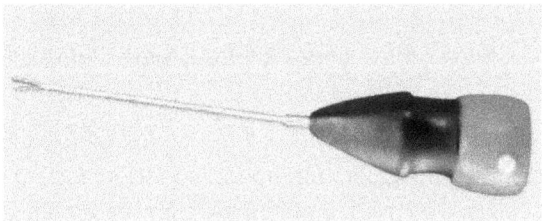

- It is used to grasp and peel internal limiting membrane (ILM)
- It is used to remove epiretinal membrane
- It is used to remove fine membranes

Membrane Peeling Forceps

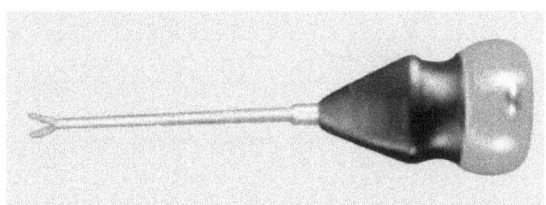

- It has a serrated grasping platform for tough membranes
- Its serrated tip allows for secure grasping of fibrous membranes
- Its wide opening allows for versatility

Charles Flute Handle

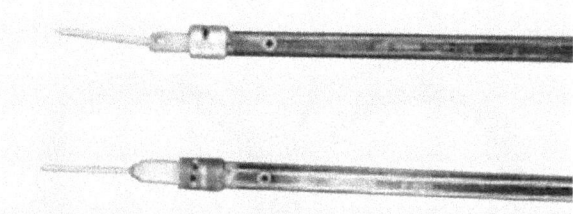

- Drainage of subretinal fluid
- Removal of preretinal blood
- Fluid-air/gas exchange
- 23 G—green
- 25 G—orange

Globe Indenter

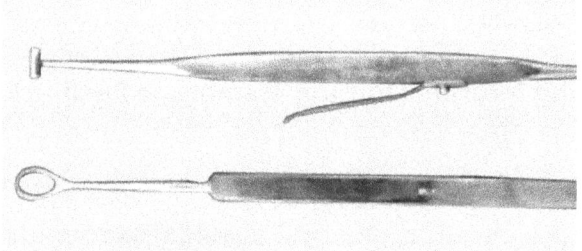

- It is used to indent the globe intraoperatively to locate tear/hole
- The Vectis can also be used to indent the globe in infants

Silicone Band

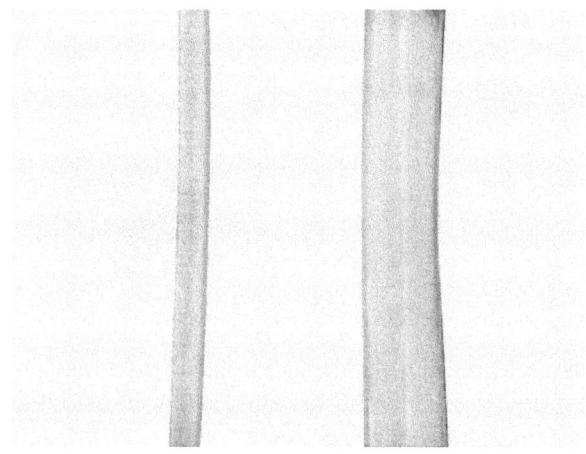

- This is a silicon band with scleral buckle
- Commonly used sizes of buckles are 276, 277, and 287
- Band—240, 42
- The band will fit inside the groove

Used in:
- Uncomplicated retinal detachment (RD)
- RD with indentable breaks
- Inferior and anterior breaks
- Young phakic patient without any posterior vitreous detachment (PVD)

Index

4:2:1 rule 437

A
Abducens nerve palsy 643, 645
Aberrant regeneration 633
Aberrations, peripheral 812
Abetalipoproteinemia 521, 960
Absorption 408
Acanthamoeba 102, 103
   keratitis 1008
      causes of 102
      differential diagnosis of 104
      pathogenesis of 102
      signs of 103
   life cycle of 102
Accelerated hypertension, hallmark of 459
Accommodation 820
   amplitude of 381, 820
   range of 820
   transient paralysis of 429
Acetaminophen 26
Acetazolamide 29, 263, 318, 319
Acetylcholinesterase inhibitors 654
Achromatopsia, congenital 864
Acquired immunodeficiency syndrome 41, 303
   ocular manifestations of 41
Actinomyces 505
Acyclovir 25
   ointment 1007
Adenine arabinoside 25
Adenoid squamous cell carcinoma 129
Adenovirus 39
   laboratory diagnosis of 39
   morphology of 39
Adherent leukoma 125, 126
   causes of 125
   development of 125
   signs of 125
   symptoms of 125
Adie's tonic pupil, characteristics of 564
Adjuvant antimetabolite therapy, indications of 357
Adnexa 182, 428, 1036, 1038, 1075, 1094
Adrenaline 723

Adrenergic agonists 262
Adrenergic receptors, types of 315
Advanced glaucoma intervention study 926
   results of 379
Advanced phaco systems 951
Aflibercept 535, 536, 905, 957
Age-related eye disease 922
   study classification 531
Age-related macular degeneration 530, 533, 557, 916, 917, 919, 920
   classification of 531
   clinical features of 530
   complications of 922
   treatment of 910
Ahmed glaucoma valve, mechanism of action of 366
Ahmed valve 305
Ahmed-Baerveldt study 929
Aicardi syndrome, features of 617
Alexander's law 660
Almond-shaped palpebral fissures 865
Alport's syndrome 960
Alström syndrome 960
Amaurosis fugax 464, 474, 587, 623, 682-684
   causes of 683
Amblyopia 789, 790, 822
   causes of 789
   treatment study 937
   types of 789
Amikacin 22-25, 510
   sulfate 512
Aminocaproic acid 879
   contraindications of 880
   side effects of 880
Amiodarone 965
Amphotericin
   B 23-25, 99, 512
   dose of 99
   mechanism of action of 99
Ampicillin 22, 513
Amyloid, components of 146
Anatomical limbus 343
Anderson's criteria 254
Anemia 880
Angiogenesis 285, 550

1146 Index

Angiogenic molecules 550
Angiogram 412
Angiography, anterior segment 420
Angioid streaks 406
Angioscotomas 246
Angiotensin-converting enzyme 212
   inhibitor 331
Angle kappa 793
Angle width, Van Herick estimate of 226
Angle-closure disease 259
Angle-closure glaucoma 256, 259, 260, 262,
     263, 266-268, 1017
   causes of 257, 286
   chronic 265
   differential diagnosis of acute 265
   management of 1017
   stage 264, 285
Angular artery 771
Aniridia 863, 865-867, 952
   ring 952
Aniseikonia 821
   etiology of 821
   symptoms of 821
   treatment for 822
Anisometropia 821
   types of 821
Anisometropic amblyopia 789
Anophthalmic socket 779, 780
Antazoline 331
Antegrade optic atrophy 602
Anterior chamber
   angle 274, 298
   biometry of 257
   depth, measurement of 224
   paracentesis 214, 477
Anterior ischemic optic neuropathy 620
Anterior lamellar
   defects 728
   keratoplasty 165
   repair 729
Anterior retinal cryotherapy 469
   indications of 455
Anti-acetylcholine receptor 654
Antiangiogenic factors 550
Antiapoptotic properties 961
Antiarrhythmic agents 965
Antibiotics 22
   sulfa-based 262
   systemic 512
Antibody, source of 649
Anticholinesterase 262
Antifibrinolytic agents, mechanism of
     action of 880
Antifungals 25, 98

Antiglaucoma medication 28, 315
Anti-infective dosage 22
Antimetabolites
   complications of 352
   indications of 363
   toxicity 363
Antinuclear antibodies 210
Anti-Parkinson drugs 961
Antireflection coating 835
Antitorque sutures 164
Anti-vascular endothelial growth
     factor 894, 898, 899
   agents 554
   complications of 555
   contraindications of 553
   indications of 553
   role of 88
Aphakia 393, 814
Aplasia 46
Apoptosis inhibitors 29
Applanation tonometer
   end point of 233
   principle of 232
   types of 232
Applanation tonometry 1024
   errors of 234
Apraclonidine 318
   over clonidine, advantages of 318
Aqueous drainage implants 1016
Aqueous humor 16, 270
   outflow, mechanism of 270
   role of 353
Aqueous shunt
   devices 364
   surgery, complications of 371
Arcuate scotoma
   differential diagnosis for 246
   double 247
Arcuate's area 246
Arcus senilis 94
Argon laser
   advantages of 453
   disadvantages of 453
   suture lysis, advantages of 353
   trabeculoplasty 338
     complications of 338
     indications of 337
   wavelength of 453
Argyll Robertson pupil,
     characteristics of 564
Arteriolar light reflex, causes of 457
Arteritic anterior ischemic optic
     neuropathy
   causes of 622
   clinical features of 623

Index **1147**

Artery
   attenuation of 967
   forceps 1127
A-scan 422
Aseptic cavernous sinus thrombosis 678
Aspergillus 43
   fumigatus 42
      habitat of 42
      morphology of 42
   infection, ocular manifestations of 43
   keratitis 886
Aspiration cannula 1113
Aspirin 26, 304
Asteroid hyalosis 423
Asthma 316
Astigmatic dial refraction 830
Astigmatic keratotomy 845, 846
   mechanism of 846
   technique of 846
Astigmatism 84, 234, 391, 789, 816, 817, 844, 846
   against-the-rule 817
   irregular 817
   oblique 817
   regular 817
   surgical techniques of correcting 845
   unilateral 949
Ataxia telangiectasia 867
Atherosclerosis 473
   features of 473
Atrial natriuretic peptide 30
Atrophic papilledema, clinical features of 588
Atrophy 46
Atropine 1002
   role of 288, 349, 652
   uses of 194
Auscultation 1024
Autofluorescence 416
Autoimmune 176
   diseases 654
   disorders 115
   vasculitis 463
Automated perimetry 252, 253
Autoregulation, significance of 572
Autosomal dominant disease 862
Autosomal recessive disease 863
Auxiliaries, uses of 62
Avastin 555, 916
Avellino corneal dystrophy 145, 146
Axenfeld-Rieger syndrome 863, 866
Axoplasmic flow, types of 271
Azathioprine 27, 654

B

Bacitracin 22
Bacteria
   gram-negative 97, 869
   gram-positive 97, 869
Bacterial corneal ulcer 95, 1002
   general principles 1003
   positive signs 1002
Bacterial keratitis
   characteristic features of 95
   typical features of 95
Baerveldt implant 366
Band keratopathy 122, 123
   causes of 122
   differential diagnosis of 123
   pathogenesis of 122
   signs of 123
   symptoms of 123
Bard Parker knife handle 1110
Bardet-Biedl syndrome 864, 960
Bare orbits, causes of 72
Barraquer eye speculum 1104
Barraquer needle holder 1114
Barraquer wire speculum 1103
Barron's artificial anterior chamber 1132
Basal cell carcinoma 48
   clinical types of 49
   histopathology of 49
   treatment of 49
Basal cell nevus syndrome 49
Basal tumors 645
Basement membrane, functions of 430
Basic fibroblast growth factor 961
Basopenia 205
Basophilia 205
Basophils 205
Bassen-Kornzweig syndrome 521
Batten-Spielmeyer-Vogt syndrome 521
Bean pot sign 277
Beaver dam eye study 947
Behçet's disease 201, 623
   Research Committee Criteria 201
Behçet's skin test 210
Bell's phenomenon 717, 718
   types of 718
Benedict's syndrome 634
Benign intracranial hypertension
   medical treatment for 597
   surgical treatment for 597
Berman's locator 856
Best disease 863
Best eye 1010
Beta 2 adrenergic agonists 29
Beta-blockers 28

Betamethasone 27
  sodium phosphate
    ointment 26
    solution 26
Betaxolol 28
  advantages of 317
Bevacizumab 291, 535, 536, 895, 898, 900, 905, 906, 916, 953, 957, 963
  intravitreal 905
Bevasiranib 536
Bevordex 898
Bielschowsky's head tilt test 638
Bietti's crystalline dystrophy 149
Bifocal glasses
  prentice rule in 835
  types of 835
Biguanides, mechanism of action of 104
Bimatoprost 28
Binocular single vision 790
  grades of 790
Bioblique astigmatism 817
Biointegrated implants
  advantages of 782
  disadvantages of 782
Biometry 390
Biopsy, indications of 755
Bitemporal hemianopia 668
  causes of 668
  clinical features of 669
Bitot's spot 848, 849
Bjerrum's area 246
Bjerrum's perimetry 248
Bjerrum's screen 250
Blanket therapy 874
Bleb failure 351
Bleb infection
  earliest evidence of 355
  treatment of 356
Bleb revision 401
Blepharitis 110
  types of 110
Blepharokeratoconjunctivitis 110
Blepharophimosis ptosis epicanthus inversus syndrome 720, 736, 867, 989
Blepharoptosis 714
  amount of 715
Blepharospasm 181
  treatment for 939
Blind spot 245, 248, 589
  enlargement of 589
  location of 248
  size of 249

Blindness 868, 874
  causes of 869
  day 515
  magnitude of 868
Blood
  coagulation disorders 471
  dyscrasias 319
  retinal barriers
    breakdown of 430
    inner 427
    outer 427
  tests 652
  vessel 240
Blowout fracture 73, 759-761
  management of 761
  surgery, complications of 764
  surgical management of 762
  symptoms in 760
Bluefield entopic phenomena 4
Blue-yellow defects, causes of acquired 14
Blunt injury 991
Boeck candy test 8
Bone
  destruction, causes of 74
  free method 856, 858
  spicule pigment deposits, causes of 516
Bonnet's sign 457, 471
Bony orbit 76
Bores U-shaped fixation forceps 1135
Botox 769
  mechanism of action of 769
  structure of 769
  use of 769
Botulinum toxin 262, 769, 770
  concentration 769
  injection 938, 939, 973
Bowen's disease 128, 129
  clinical forms of 128
Bowman's lacrimal probe 1126
Bowman's membrane 854
Brachytherapy 131
  complications of 131
Bradycardia 316
Brain-derived natriuretic peptide 30
Brainstem syndrome 645
Braley's test 745
Branch retinal vein occlusion 469, 905
Bridge procedure 732
Bridle sutures, purpose of 497
Brimonidine 317, 1009
Brinzolamide 29, 318
Brolene ointment 1008
Brolucizumab 536
Bronchospasm 316

Bronson's electromagnet 861
Brow suspension 722, 990
   ptosis repair 721, 724, 983, 985
   surgery, techniques of 726
Brown's syndrome 802, 825
   types of 802
Bruch's membrane, layers of 479
Bruckner test 794
Brunescent cataract 396
Bruns nystagmus, features of 662
B-scan 422
Buckling theory 759
Bull's eye maculopathy 406
Bullous keratopathy 157
Bumetanide 263
Buphthalmos 374
Burn
   duration 446
   intensity 446
Burnt-out stage 285

C

Cadaver enucleation 784
Cake decoration test 8
Calcific emboli 474
Calcification, causes of 71
Calcium channel blocker 29
Caldwell's view 69
Caloric nystagmus 663
Campbell's theory 293
Campimetry 247
Candida 505
   albicans 42
      morphology of 42
   infection
      diagnosis of 42
      treatment of 42
   ocular manifestations of 42
Candy-Stripe sign 882
Cannabinoids 30, 326
Canthal tendon
   integrity 702
   lateral 701
Cantholysis 731
Canthoplasty, medial 988
Capsular bag distension syndrome 397
Capsular delamination, differential
      diagnosis of 297
Capsular tear, intraoperative posterior 392
Capsular tension
   ring 396, 1059
   segment 994

Capsulopalpebral fascia 700
   assessment of 710
Carbachol 262
Carbenicillin 22
Carbon monoxide 965
Carbonic anhydrase inhibitors 29, 1009, 1011
Carcinoma in situ 129
Cardiovascular system 316
Carnay's locator 856
Caroticocavernous fistula 679, 681, 690
   clinical features of 691
   ocular manifestations of 680
Carotid artery 690
   compression 738
   occlusion 682
Carotid duplex scanning 685
Carteolol 28
Castroviejo caliper 1121, 1131
Castroviejo needle holder 1115
Cataract 381, 384, 386, 960, 1041, 1085
   bilateral 382, 949
   causes of 382
   characteristic types of 384
   complicated 189, 385, 386, 995, 996
   extraction 992
   formation, causes of 518
   incision, types of 391
   pediatric 383
   significant 1040
   surgery 302, 356, 382, 389, 391, 393, 395, 398, 399, 518, 844, 845, 869, 947, 950, 1013
      indications of 382, 384
      microincision 951
   traumatic 386, 991, 992
   types of 384
   unilateral 382
   white 396, 950
CATT trial 538
Cavernous hemangioma 863
Cavernous optic atrophy 605, 966
Cavernous sinus
   anatomy of 671
   lesion 630, 647
   meningiomas, features of 692
   syndrome 634, 640, 647, 688
   thrombosis 671, 675-677
      causes of 671
      clinical features of 672
      differential diagnosis of 674
Cefamandole 22
Cefazolin 22-25
   hydrochloride 512

Ceftazidime 24, 25, 510
  hydrochloride 511
Ceftriaxone 22, 23, 677
Celecoxib 263
Cells
  grading of 185
  types of 185
Central 30-2 test 253
Central crystalline dystrophy 148
  clinical features of 148
Central foveal thickness 894
Central nervous system 316
Central retinal artery occlusion 473, 623, 966
  causes of 473
  clinical features of 474
  incidence of 474
Central retinal artery supply 473
Central retinal vein occlusion 462, 905, 963, 1019
  causes of 462
  differential diagnosis of 470
  management of 469
  types of 462
Central scotoma 249
Central serous chorioretinopathy 546
  complications of 549
  differential diagnosis of 549
  risk factors of 546
Central vein occlusion study 902
  group, findings of 468
Central vision loss, causes of 515
Cephalosporium 505
Cerebellopontine angle lesions 643
Cerebral angiography 629
Cerebrospinal fluid
  cytologic examination of 629
  pathway of 583
Chalazion clamp 1128
Chalazion scoop 1128
Chalcosis, treatment of 861
CHARGE syndrome 863
Charles flute handle 1142
Chédiak-Higashi syndrome 867
Chemotherapeutic agents 527
Chemotherapy, role of 527
Cherry-red spot 405, 475
  causes of 475
Childhood blindness, causes of 873
Childhood malignancies 523
Chlamydia
  diagnostic tests for 39
  trachomatis 38, 869, 874
Chlamydial infection 39
Chlorambucil 27
Chloramphenicol 22, 965
Chlorhexidine digluconate 23
Chloroquine 965
Chlorothiazide 263
Chlorpropamide 262
Chlorthalidone 263
Cholesterol 474
Cholinergic crisis 262, 655
Chopper 1117
Chorioretinal biopsy
  complications of 215
  contraindications of 215
  indications of 215
  technique of 215
Chorioretinitis, causes of 193
Choroid
  blood supply of 480
  circulation 460
  detachment 494
  folds 406
  hemangioma 426
  layers of 479
  mass 492
  melanoma 49, 50, 425
Choroidal neovascular membrane 531, 533, 557
  differential diagnosis for 534
Choroidal neovascularization 909, 910, 919-921
  age-related 917
  trial 916
Choroiditis 180, 191
  active 191
  healed 191
  pigmentation 453
Chromatic aberration 811
Chromophilic adenoma 71
Chromosomal aberrations 865
Chromosomal disorders 865, 873
Chromosomes 862
Cicatricial component 703, 710
Cicatricial entropion 978
  causes of 709
  management of 713
Cicatrizing conjunctival disease, presence of 711
Ciliary artery, posterior 481
Ciliary block
  band 239
  changes 298
  glaucoma, treatment of 351
  melanoma 50

Ciliary ganglion 561, 627
  roots of 627
Ciliary neurotrophic factor 961
Cilioretinal artery 573
Ciliprobe 1123
Cionni ring 994
Ciprofloxacin 22, 23
Circumlinear vessels, baring of 275
Claude's syndrome 634
Cleaning, types of 883
Clivus lesions 643
Cloquet's canal 481
Clotrimazole 1008
Coats' disease 283, 434
Coats' white ring 854, 1059
Coca-cola sign 755
Cogan's syndrome 112
Coin test 9
Collagen cross-linkage 138
  mechanism of action of 138
Collagen vascular disorders 115
Collagenase activity 1005
Coloboma 952
Color blindness 12
  acquired 13
  congenital 12, 13
Color defects, acquired 12
Color tests 697
Color vision 11, 14
  defects 13
  loss 608
    specific 608
  neurophysiology of 13
  theories of 13
Colored haloes 264
Comberg's method 859
Combined cataract surgery,
    advantages of 356
Combined granular-lattice dystrophy,
    clinical features of 147
Combined surgery
  advantages of 1041
  disadvantages of 1041
Community ophthalmology 868,
    1065, 1100
Compressive optic neuropathy,
    diagnosis of 752
Computed tomography 75, 525
  indications of 75
  scan
    advantages of 860
    role of 596
Conbercept 536
Cones, types of 135

Congenital corneal opacity, differential
    diagnosis of 151
Congenital crescents 573
Congenital entropion, surgical procedure
    for 713
Congenital hereditary
    endothelial dystrophy 157
    stromal dystrophy 149
Congenital lacrimal drainage
    obstruction 771
Congenital nystagmus 662
  features of 660
Congenital ptosis 720, 982
  surgery for 725
Congenital rubella 873
  syndrome, clinical manifestations of 40
Congenital syphilis 111
  systemic features of 111
Congenital third nerve palsies,
    causes of 627
Congenital tilted disk syndrome,
    features of 617
Congestive attack, acute 264
Conjunctiva 182, 222, 360, 362, 386, 428,
    680, 1036, 1038, 1067, 1078
Conjunctival buttonhole 355
Conjunctival congestion 181
Conjunctival flaps 997
Conjunctival spring scissors 1108
Conjunctival xerosis 848, 849
Conjunctivitis
  chronic 128
  membranous 37
  neonatal 869
Consciousness, loss of 590
Consecutive optic atrophy 966, 1045
  causes of 604
Conserving tears 772
Contact delivery systems 377
Contact lens 95
  advantage of 837
  fitting, three-point touch technique
      of 137
  haptic 981
  method 859
  role of 135, 376
Continuous sutures, disadvantages of 164
Contracted socket 778
  types of 778
Contrast sensitivity 519
Conus 568
Convergence, test for 796
Copper wiring 458
Copper, reaction of 854

Cornea 15, 83, 86, 89, 93, 118, 132, 182,
    190, 222, 292, 360, 362, 429, 873,
    885, 1038, 1067, 1078
  dioptric power of 84
  histopathology of 136
  instruments 1131
  nerve supply of 89
  normal age-related changes of 122
  parts of 855
  periphery of 114
  proforma 1049
  spherical 84
  swirl staining of 134
Corneal allogenic intrastromal ring
    segments 142
Corneal anesthesia 89, 91
Corneal blindness
  causes of 873
  prevalence of 873
Corneal changes 298
Corneal compensation 243, 244
Corneal conditions 192
Corneal curvature, range of 84
Corneal degenerations 143
Corneal deposits 92
  causes of superficial 92
Corneal disease 866
Corneal donor study 889
Corneal dystrophies 143, 144, 150
  dominant 866
  inheritance of 145
Corneal edema 266
Corneal endothelial damage 371
Corneal erosions, recurrent 152
Corneal exposure 702
Corneal fistula, treatment of 127
Corneal graft rejection, acute 1046
Corneal guttae 158
Corneal hysteresis, concept of 279
Corneal incision 348, 846
  purpose of 347
Corneal lesions 110
Corneal neovascularization 88
Corneal opacities, types of 125
Corneal preservation, types of 170
Corneal refractive surgery 391
Corneal rust ring 1059
Corneal scars 849
Corneal sensation 90, 703
Corneal sensitivity 90
Corneal status 711
Corneal thickness, role of 279
Corneal transplant epidemiological
    study 888

Corneal trephine 1133
Corneal ulcer 96, 126, 848
  complications of 99
  trial 887
Corneal vascularization 86, 87
Corneal xerosis 848, 849
Corneoscleral graft 1004
Corpora amylacea 573
Cortical blindness 667
Corticosteroid 26, 512, 677
  intravitreal 936
  role of 359
Corynebacterium 505
  diphtheria 36
    characteristics of 36
    morphology of 36
Cotton wool spot 433, 458
  causes of 433
Cover test 792, 794
  alternate 794, 795
  monocular 795
  prerequisites for 794
  prism 794
  types of 794
Cover-uncover test 794
Cranial nerve
  examination of 1033
  palsy 680
Create chorioretinal adhesion 958
Crescent knife 1111
Crossed cylinder technique 696
Cryoablation 528
Cryoprobes, types of 376
Cryotherapy 105, 291
  indications of 498
  mechanism of 131
  principle of 498
  side effects of 131
  technique of 498
Curvature hypermetropia 814
Curved mirror, uses of 825
Cyclic guanosine monophosphate 30
Cyclitis 180
Cyclocryotherapy 374, 375
  additional effect of 374
  mechanism of action of 373
  role of 469
  technique of 374
Cyclodestruction 1016
Cyclodestructive procedure 290, 340, 373
  indications of 291
Cyclodestructive surgery 305
Cyclodiathermy 373
Cyclopentolate 789, 1002

Cyclophosphamide 27
Cyclophotocoagulation 289, 375
Cycloplegic refraction 792
    indications for 833
Cycloscopy 237
Cyclosporine 27, 654
Cyclotherapy 374
Cylindrical lenses, transposition of 825
Cylindrical refraction 830
Cylindrical streak reflex 829
Cystitome 1112
Cystoid edema outside macula,
    honeycomb appearance of 421
Cystoid macular edema 557, 961
    development of 960
    causes of 192
Cysts 739
Cytomegalovirus 40, 558
    infection, congenital 40
Cytoskeleton modulators 30

D

Dacryocystitis, chronic 95
Dacryocystorhinostomy 772, 774
    surgery, complications of 776
    surgical steps of external 773
    types of 773
Dapsone 262
Darkroom prone test 267
De Wecker scissors 1109
Decompression, indications of 598
Deep anterior lamellar keratoplasty 1000
    technique of 166
Deep lamellar endothelial
    keratoplasty 166
Deep vessels 87
Defective vision 1032
    causes of 190, 264, 431, 788
Degenerations 143
Demeclocycline 331
Demyelinating diseases 668
Dendritic keratitis 107
Dental infections 672
Depression 246, 316
Descemet's membrane 854, 1049
    endothelial keratoplasty,
        advantages of 167
Descemet's stripping
    automated endothelial
        keratoplasty 167
    endothelial keratoplasty 166, 167
Desmarres lid retractor 1127

Deviation
    quantify amount of 796
    vertical 793
Devic's disease 579
Dexamethasone 27, 510, 898, 957
    efficacy of 898
    implants 956
    intravitreal implant 897, 957
    phosphate
        ointment 26
        solution 26
Diabetes 894
    control and complications trial 891
    interventions, epidemiology of 891
    mellitus 427, 566
        insulin-dependent 427, 891
        noninsulin-dependent 427
        ocular manifestations of 428
Diabetic macular edema 559, 894-897,
        900, 956
    differential diagnosis for 440
    early stages of 469
    steroids for 897, 898
Diabetic maculopathy 435, 898
Diabetic microangiopathy,
    pathogenesis of 429
Diabetic ophthalmoplegia 688
Diabetic retinopathy 427, 443, 448, 891,
    892, 899
    clinical research
        network 449
        studies 436
    differential diagnosis of 801
    preproliferative stage of 434, 437
    study 801
        grid, treatment 954
        technique, early treatment 449
    vitrectomy study 893
Diagnostic ophthalmic ultrasonography,
    frequency of 422
Diamidines, mechanism of action of 105
Diamond burr 1139
Diathermy 373
    demerits of 373
Dibrompropamidine 1008
Dichlorphenamide 29
Dichromatic color vision 12
Diclofenac sodium 26
Diffuse macular edema 553
Digital pressure 354
    role of postoperative 353
    technique of 341
Digital tonometry, principle of 231
Digitalis 668, 965

1154 Index

Diluents, amounts of 769
Diminished vision 698
Diode cyclophotocoagulation
 complications of 342
 probe 1123
Diode laser transscleral
 cyclophotocoagulation 341
Dipivefrine 317
 side effects of 317
Diplopia 804, 1032
 charting 804
  disadvantages of 805
  indications for 804
  principle of 804
 horizontal 644
 tests 695, 792
Dipyridamole 304
Direct ophthalmoscope 60-62, 1057, 1058
 advantages of 62
 drawbacks of 62
 magnification of 62
 parts of 61
 therapeutic use of 61
Disciform keratitis, features of 108
Disinfection 883
Disk
 damage, types of 279
 edema, diagnosis of 597
 hemorrhage, significance of 276
 neovascularization of 455, 956
Diskiform
 keratitis 1006
 scar 533
Dispersive viscoelastics 387
Disposable trephine 1133
Distance acuity 6
Distant direct ophthalmoscopy 60, 1018, 1042, 1043
 applications of 60
Distraction test 702
Diuretics, sulfa-based 263
Diurnal variation
 causes of 271
 curves, types of 228
 measurement, use of 272
Donor cornea, use of 875
Donor tissue 168
Dorsal-nasal arteries 765
Dorzolamide 29, 318, 324
Double ring sign 1059
Double-flanged-haptic tension 950
Down's syndrome 135, 865
Downbeat nystagmus, features of 661
Doxycycline 1005

Drainage tube 369
Drugs
 antiglaucoma 316
 anti-inflammatory 26, 308
 antitubercular 965
 cholinergic 28
 immunosuppressive 654
 intravitreal 511
 neuroprotective 325
 rheumatological 263
 sensitivity 36
 sulfa-based 262
Drusen 532
Dry eye 110
 disease, severity of 888
 workshop study 888
Duane's syndrome 633, 798
Duochrome test 831
Dye laser 444
Dynamic contact tonometer 235
Dyschromatopsia 12, 576
Dysplasia 46
Dysthyroid optic neuropathy 976
Dystrophy 144
 types of 144

E

Eales' disease 283
Eccentric proptosis 742, 744
Echography, indications of 422
Eclipse technique 224
Ectopia lentis 311
 causes of 312, 383
 et papillae 864
 medical management of 312
 surgical treatment of 312
Ectropion 700-702, 979, 1027
 acquired 979
 cicatricial 706, 979
 clinical features of 702
 congenital 708, 979
 involutional 703, 979
 stage severity of 701
 uveae 283
Edelstein-Dryden procedure 706
Edinger-Westphal nucleus 561
 anatomy of 626
Edrophonium test 652, 653
Edrophonium, dose of 652
Eight-ball hyphema 877
Eikonometer 822
 types of 822
Electrical stimulation, controlled 961

Electrolyte imbalance 319
Electromagnet, Haab's type of 861
Electroretinography 685
Elevated episcleral venous pressure,
	causes of 227
Elschnig's pearls 397
Elschnig's spots 460
Elschnig's scleral ring 1059
Empty delta sign 78
Empty sella syndrome 72
Endogenous endophthalmitis 507,
	511, 512
	treatment of 511
Endonasal dacryocystorhinostomy
	contraindications of 775
	indications of 775
	surgical steps of 775
Endophthalmitis 424, 505, 507, 510,
	513, 1004
	bleb-related 356
	differential diagnosis of 506
	infectious 509
	postoperative 507, 511
	post-traumatic 511
	signs of 506
	sterile postoperative 510
	symptoms of 506
	traumatic 507
	treatment 507
	vitrectomy study 509, 922
Endoscopic surgery
	advantages of 776
	disadvantages of 776
Endothelial cell damage
	causes of 431
	sequelae of 160
Endothelial diseases 157
Endothelial disorders 157
Endothelial keratoplasty,
	indications for 888
Endothelial melanosis, causes of 94
Endothelial rejection 169
Endothelitis 1006
Endothelium cells, ratio of 430
Enlarged extraocular muscles 747
Enophthalmos 711, 737
	causes of 741
Entropion 709-711, 978, 1028
	acquired 978
	congenital 709, 710, 978
	involutional 709, 978
	nonsurgical management of 711
	surgery for 713

Enucleation 784, 1016
	indications of 784
	scissor 1129
	techniques 784
Enzyme-linked immunosorbent assay 211
	uses of 211
Eosinopenia 204
Eosinophilia 204
Eosinophils 204
Ephedrine 262
Epiblepharon 978
Epicanthus fold 987
Epikeratoplasty 138
Epinephrine
	eye drops 93
	side effects of 317
Epiretinal membrane, causes of 544
Episclera 1067, 1078
	venous pressure 227
Episcleritis 1007
Epithelial debridement 105
Epithelial keratitis 1006
Epithelial melanosis, causes of 94
Epithelium 1048
Eplerenone 548
Epstein-Barr virus infection 660
Erythrocyte sedimentation rate 206
	principle of 206
Escherichia coli 505
Esodeviation, types of 798
Esotropia
	concomitant 798
	essential infantile 799
	incomitant 799
	infantile 800
Ethacrynic acid 30
Ethambutol 965
Ethmoid vessels 765
Etodolac 26
Evisceration 785
	contraindications of 786
	curette 1128
	disadvantages of 786
	indications of 785
	over enucleation, advantages of 786
Excimer laser phototherapeutic
		keratectomy 138
Exenteration 786
	indications of 786
	surgery, types of 787
Exfoliation syndrome 287, 302
Exfoliative cytology 130
	advantages of 130
	disadvantages of 130

Exophthalmometry, types of 740, 744
Exophthalmos 737
Exotropia
  concomitant 798
  incomitant 798
  types of 798
Expulsive suprachoroidal hemorrhage, signs of 397
External beam radiotherapy, limitations of 529
External dacryocystorhinostomy
  advantages of 774
  contraindications of 772
  indications of 772
Extracellular matrix hydrolysis, activators of 30
Extraocular movement 429, 1036
Extraocular muscle 650, 750
  congenital fibrosis of 863
  enlargement 749
    causes of 76
  surgery, indications of 754
Extraocular vascular disorders 284
Eye 448, 795, 865
  anterior segment of 858
  bank 873, 876
    functions of 170, 875
  care 851
  disease 871, 874, 931
    acute 1007
    treatment of 177
  disorders of 863
  dissociation of 806
  emmetropic 65
  fundus 1053, 1054
  hypermetropic 65
  left 1010
  movement 229
    supranuclear control systems for 791
  muscles of 17, 650
  optical defects of 811
  pain 264
  postoperative evaluation of 349
  reduced 820
  right 995, 1010, 1023, 1027, 1037, 1042, 1055
  schematic 820
  surgeries 994
Eyeball 386
Eyelid 18, 222, 360, 362, 386, 701
  Defects
    causes of 727
    repair 730
  malignant tumor of 48
  margin 730
  reconstruction 727
    full-thickness 732
    principles of 727
  retraction 754
  skin, deficiency of 708
  splitting made, vertical 766
  surgical anatomy of 700

F

Face, infection of 671
Facial
  bone growth completes 780
  nerve 1034
  sling 707
  symmetry 1051
Faden's procedure 803
False fluorescence 414
Familial radial drusen 863
Far point 820
Faricimab 536
Fasanella-Servat operation 721, 722, 983
Fasanella-Servat surgery, modified 723, 983
Fascia lata sling 724, 985
Fascicular cavernous sinus portion 628
Fascicular midbrain portion 628
Fascicular orbital portion 628
Fascicular subarachnoid portion 628
Fascicular third nerve palsy 631
Fat suppression techniques 80
  types of 80
Femtosecond Descemet's stripping endothelial keratoplasty 167
Femtosecond laser
  assisted cataract surgery 401
  energy 402
Fetal alcohol syndrome 873
Fever 179
Fibers, topographic arrangement of 626
Fibrin sealant kit 1139
Fibrinogen solution, preparation of 1140
Fibrinolysis 476
Fibrinolytic agents 477
Fibrinous reactions 506
Fibrin-platelet emboli 474
Fibrovascular proliferation
  constituents of 438
  severe progressive 957
Filamentous fungal infection 99
Filtering surgery 290
  types of 343

Filtration, failure of 351
Fincham test 264
Fixation tests 696
Fixed combination
    advantages of 324
    disadvantages of 324
Flame-shaped hemorrhages, differential
        diagnosis of 458
Flashes 486
Fleck dystrophy, features of 149
Fleischer's ring 133, 1059
    clinical significance of 133
Flexner-Wintersteiner rosette 524
Flieringa ring 1059
Flieringa scleral fixation ring 1138
Floaters, significance of 486
Flow rate 388
Fluconazole 25, 1005
Flucytosine 25
Fluocinolone acetonide 27, 896
    uveitis study 935
Fluorescein
    angiogram 437, 685
    angiography 409, 410, 412, 533,
        953, 963
    biophysical properties of 408
    chemical properties of 408
    emission peaks of 408
    fundus angiography, contraindications
        of 411
    leak 287
    pattern 137
        abnormal 414
    solution, bacterial contaminant of 409
    true 414
Fluorometholone
    ointment 26
    suspension 26
Fluorouracil filtering surgery study 928
Flurbiprofen 26
Focal edema 435
Focal laser photocoagulation 548
Focal photocoagulation, side effects of 450
Focal therapy, indications of 528
Fogging tests 696
Forced duction test perimetry,
        advantages of 251
Forceps, serrated 1120
Foreign body
    sensitivity for 856
    types of 852
Forgetfulness 316
Forme fruste keratoconus 134
Fornix-based flap, advantages of 347

Fornix-based flap, disadvantages of 347
Fossa aneurysm, posterior 688
Foster-Kennedy syndrome 595
    treatment of 595
Four-dot test 797
Fourth nerve palsy 638, 640
    symptoms of 638
Fovea 479
    characteristic features of 432
Foveal avascular zone, pathologic
        enlargement of 953
Foveal thickness 435
Foveola 479
    characteristic features of 432
Foville's syndrome 645
Fractures
    medial 762
    posterior 762
Francois central cloudy dystrophy 149
Free tarsoconjunctival graft 730
Freer periosteal elevator 1130
Fresnel's prism 641
Frontalis sling 990
Fuchs' dystrophy 153, 155, 156
    clinical stages of 154
    diagnosis of 154
    differential diagnosis of 154
    epidemiology of 153
    features of 154
    medical management of 155
    pathogenesis of 153
    surgical management of 155
    symptoms of 153
Fuchs' endothelial dystrophy 153, 866, 873
Fuchs' heterochromic iridocyclitis 197, 287
    signs of 197
    symptoms of 197
Fuchs' heterochromic uveitis 178
Fukasaku hockey knife 1122
Fundus autofluorescence imaging 416
Fundus evaluation 792
Fundus examination 1019, 1037,
        1043-1045, 1057
    relevance of 1033
Fundus fluorescein angiography 408,
        547, 572
    adverse reactions of 413
    history of 409
    principle of 409
    side effects of 413
Fungal corneal ulcer 95, 99
    management of 1003
Fungal culture 98
Fungal keratitis, typical features of 98

Fungal ulcer 1004
Fungi 98
Furosemide 263
Fusarium 886, 887
   infection 43

G

Gadolinium 80
Gallium scan 216
Ganglion cell 272
   complex 1039
   die 272
   loss 278
   types of 273
Gas lasers 444
Gastrointestinal disturbances 319
Gatifloxacin 22
Gaze-evoked nystagmus, features of 661
Gel-forming solution, advantages of 316
Gene 862
   therapy, intravitreal 962
Genetic
   counseling 867, 1001
   testing, techniques for 867
Geniculate body, lateral 13
Genitourinary disturbances 319
Gentamicin 22-24, 513
   sulfate 512
Geometric construction 857
Ghost cell 881, 882
   arteritis 622
   glaucoma 881
      differential diagnosis of 882
Giant magnet 861
Giant tear 483
Giemsa's stain, use of 96
Ginkgo biloba extract 331
Glabellar flap 733
Glass prisms 795
Glaucoma 93, 158, 224, 230, 246, 255, 256,
      270-272, 275-282, 300, 307, 313,
      326, 333, 356, 361, 379, 463, 464,
      680, 866, 877, 880, 881, 924, 1035,
      1038, 1069, 1081
   absolute 265
   after cataract surgery, causes of 393
   angle recession 279
   basic examination of 224
   capsulare 297
   cases of neovascular 1015
   congenital 158, 866
   control of 304
   corticosteroid-induced 306
   damage, pathogenesis of 272
   development of 303
   diagnosis of 280
   diagnostic with variable corneal
      compensation, advantages
      of 244
   drainage devices 364
      indications of 365
      principle of 364
   evaluation of 280
   failed primary 365
   filtering surgeries 359, 361-363
      role of 5-fu in 361
   hemifield test 253
   incidence of 297
   instruments 1119
   inverse 265
   laser trial 927, 928
   lens induced 287, 309
   malignant 256, 340
   mechanism 269
   medical management of 313
   medical therapy for 313
   occurs, traumatic 881
   pigmentary 292, 299
   postpenetrating injury 882
   preperimetric 278
   secondary 311
   studies 379
   surgical procedures 290
   testing 252
   theories of 278
   types of 286, 382
   visual field defects 245, 251, 255
Glaucomatous cupping, differential
      diagnosis of 276
Glaucomatous damage 273
Glaucomatous optic nerve damage 277
Gliclazide 262
Glimepiride 262
Globe fixation forceps 1106
Glossopharyngeal nerve 1034
Glutamate, role of 278
Glycerol 29
Golden ring 1059
Goldmann applanation tonometer 235
Goldmann perimetry, features of 254
Goldmann-Favre syndrome 864
Goniophotocoagulation 288, 341
Gonioscopy 182, 237, 239, 241, 266,
      273, 1037
   clinical uses of 239
   compression 239
   diagnosis 1037
   direct 237, 238

indirect 237, 238
intraocular pressures 1037
principle of 237
Goodpasture syndrome 471
Gorlin syndrome 49, 863
Gorovoy descemetorhexis forceps 1136
Gradenigo's syndrome 646
Graefe fixation forceps 1134
Graft
   complications 713
   failure 170
      types of 169
   rejection, incidence of 887
      signs of 169
      symptoms of 169
Gram stain 96
Granular dystrophy 145
   differential diagnosis of 145
   features of 145
Granulomatous uveitis
   causes of
      bilateral 178
      unilateral 178
Graves' disease 597, 752
Graves' ophthalmopathy 78
Graves' orbitopathy 755
Green laser, disadvantages of 449
Guillain-Barré syndrome 653
Gunn's sign 457

H

Haemophilus influenza 34, 505
   cultural characteristics of 34
   morphology of 34
Hallervorden-Spatz syndrome 521
Haltia-Santavuori syndrome 521
Hand movements 3
Handwash disinfectants,
      components of 883
Haploscopic principle 806
Hard exudates 433, 458
   differential diagnosis of 458
Hartman's mosquito forceps 1127
Hassall-Henle bodies 158
Hayreh's theory 584
Head injury, ocular signs of 574
Headache 590, 600
   causes of 590
Heavy metals 965
Heidelberg retinal tomography
   advantages of 281
   disadvantages of 281
Helmholtz's instrument, modified 83

Hemiakinesia meter 563
Hemianopic pupillary reaction 562
Hemorrhage 406, 433, 765
   expulsive 398
   intraretinal 403
   flame-shaped 458
Hemostasis 774
Hepatic dysfunction 976
Hereditary optic atrophy 967
Hering's law 791, 806
Herpes simplex
   dendrite, characteristics of 107
   dendritic keratitis of 107
   keratitis, types of 107
   virus 39
      keratitis 1006
      laboratory diagnosis of 40
Herpes zoster
   dendrite, features of 108
   ophthalmicus 1006
      features of 108
   virus infection 623
Herpetic eye disease study 1006
   findings of 108
Hertel's exophthalmometry 1024
Hess chart 639, 644, 806, 807
   indications of 807
   interpretation of 808
   principles of 806
   uses of 809
Heterophoria method 800
Hippocampal gyrus herniation 631
Hirschberg test 793
Hockey stick microblade 1138
Hollenhorst plaques 474
Holmgren's wool test 14
Homatropine 1002
Homer-Wright rosette 524
Homocystinuria 384, 864
Homonymous hemianopia 667
   causes of 668
Horner's pupil, characteristics of 565
Horner's syndrome
   causes of 565
   characteristics of 565
Horopter 790
Horseshoe tear 483
Hounsfield units 76
Hudson-Stahli line 93
Hughes tarsoconjunctival flap 730
Human immunodeficiency virus 41
   retinopathy, features of 41
Human leukocyte antigen 887, 1059
Human plasma 270

Humphrey field analyzer 1010
Hunter's syndrome 864
Hutchinson's pupil 632
   characteristics of 564
Hutchinson's triad 112
Hyaloid face, taut posterior 955
Hydraulic theory 759
Hydrochloride 511
Hydrocortisone acetate
   ointment 26
   sodium succinate 27
   solution 26
   suspension 26
Hydrops, acute 133, 134
Hyperacuity 10
Hyperfluorescence, causes of 415
Hypermetropia 789, 814, 839
   axial 814
   causes of 814
   clinical features of 815
   components of 815
   optical changes of 814
   treatment for 819
Hyperosmotic agents 29
   contraindications for 321
   dosages of 322
   indications of 321
   mechanism of action of 321
   peak action of 323
   side effects of 322
Hyperplasia 46
Hypersensitivity 176
   reaction, type of 750
Hypertension
   malignant 461
   pregnancy-induced 599
Hypertensive arteriolosclerosis 460
Hypertensive choroidopathy 460
Hypertensive eye disease 459
Hypertensive optic neuropathy 461
   differential diagnosis of 461
Hypertensive retinopathy 457, 593
   classification of 457
   complications of 460
   management of 461
Hyperthyroidism, signs of 639
Hypertrophy 46
Hyphema 186, 371, 877
Hypofluorescence, causes of 415
Hypoglossal nerve 1034
Hypoplasia 46
Hypopyon 99, 186
Hypotony 371, 882
   causes of 368

I

Ibuprofen 26
Ice pack test 651
Ice syndrome 159
   pathogenesis of 159
   treatment of 160
Idiopathic hypertension trial,
      longitudinal 944
Idiopathic intracranial hypertension
   943, 969
Idiopathic pseudotumor 755
Illiterate E-cutout test 9
Imidazole 304
   mechanism of action of 99
Imipenem 24
Immune modulation 329
Immunohistochemistry, role of 51
Immunological tests 676
Immunosuppressants 221
   indications of 220
Immunosuppressive 121
   agents 304
   classes of 220
   use, indications for 995
Incision, types of 767
Indapamide 263
Indirect ophthalmoscope 62, 63, 65
   delivery 454, 455
Indirect ophthalmoscopy 1042, 1043
   advantages of 64
   disadvantages of 64
Indocyanine green angiography 420
Indomethacin 26, 304
Indoxyl 304
Infection
   acute phase of 1004
   mode of transmission of 44
   ocular manifestations of 38
Infectious diseases 848
Inferior meatus, level of 772
Inflammation
   control of 304
   level of 177
Inflammatory conditions 385, 526
Inflammatory vasculitis 463
Infraorbital foramen 765
Infusion cannula, normal length of 539
Injection, recommended sites for 556
Interferometers 4
Intermittent proptosis, causes of 737
Intermittent visual claudication, causes
   of 607
Internal capsule lesion,
      characteristics of 666

Internal jugular venous 738
International Uveitis Study Group 220
  classification 174
Interpupillary distance 832
Interrupted sutures
  advantages of 164
  disadvantages of 164
  indications of 163
Interstitial keratitis 110
  causes of 110
  complications of 111
Intracameral antibiotics 947
Intracameral hyaluronic acid, role of 370
Intracapsular lens extraction 993
Intracavernous carotid artery
      aneurysm 690
Intracorneal rings 141
Intracranial lesion 279
Intracranial mass lesions 653
Intracranial portion 567
Intracranial pressure 590
Intracranial tension, signs of raised 68
Intracranial tumor 585
Intraocular calcification 526
Intraocular foreign body 424, 852
  localization of 852
  management of 860
Intraocular gases, characteristics of 502
Intraocular invasion 130
Intraocular lens 194, 949
  dialer 1113
  implantation 993, 996
  place toric 846
  power calculation 390, 391
    formulae 391
  square-edge polymethylmethacrylate 948
  tackiness of 395
  types of 390, 399, 952
Intraocular malignancy 49, 523
Intraocular photocoagulation, types of 377
Intraocular pressure 183, 227, 374, 584, 877, 1037, 1058
  target 1010
Intraocular ranibizumab 914
Intraocular structure 1004
Intraocular surgery 305
Intraocular tumor 784
Intraorbital calcification, causes of 74
Intraorbital portion 567
Intraretinal microvascular
      abnormality 434
Intrastromal corneal ring segments 1059
  types of 141

Intravenous steroids
  dose of 220
  indications of 220
Intravitreal aflibercept 899
Intravitreal anti-vascular endothelial growth
      factor agents 954, 956, 963
Intravitreal injection 25, 439, 508, 552, 558, 469, 552, 954, 957
  material for 508
Intravitreal lucentis 915
Intravitreal stem cell transplantation 968
Intravitreal steroids
  complications of 553
  indications of 552
Intravitreous ranibizumab 900
Invasive procedures, indications of 215
Involutional ectropion,
      management of 704
Involutional entropion, treatment in 712
Ipratropium bromide 262
Ipsilateral Horner's syndrome 647
Ipsilateral synergists 791
Iridectomy 348
  types of peripheral 334
Iridociliary tumor 257
Iridocorneal endothelial syndromes 287
Iridocyclitis 1006
  complications of 192
Iridotomy
  penetration, signs of 336
  peripheral 334
Iridotrabecular contact 260
Iris 172, 429, 1036
  angiography 216
  atrophic patch of 187
  changes 186, 298
  coloboma 398, 399
    treatment of 398
  fluorescein angiography 299
  forceps 1119
  neovascularization of 1015
  nodules, differential diagnosis for 188
  retroillumination of 55
  transillumination defects 292
Iron staining, reasons for 93
Irrigation wire vectis 1112
Irritation 222, 360
Ischemic index 466
Ischemic neuropathy 594
Ischemic optic atrophy
  causes of 605
  mechanism of 605
Ischemic optic neuropathy, anterior 620

Ishihara chart 11, 14
Ishihara color testing 697
Isoniazid 965
Isopter 246
Isosorbide 29
  over glycerol, advantages of 322
Itraconazole 1005

J

Jackson's cross cylinder 830
Jaeger's chart 3
Jansky-Bielschowsky syndrome 521
Javal-Schiotz keratometer 84
Jaw movement 720
Jerk nystagmus 660
Jones procedure 712, 978
  modified 712
Junctional scotoma 666

K

Kalt locking needle holder 1115
Kayser-Fleischer ring 93, 1059
Kearns-Sayre syndrome 521, 865, 960
Keith-Wagener-Barker classification 457
Kelly Descemet's punch 1119
Kelman-McPherson forceps 1106
Kemeralopia 515
Kemp and Collin classification 710
Keratic precipitates, distribution of 184
Keratitis 95, 107
  infective 100
  marginal 110
  pathogenesis of 43
  ring 1059
  severe deep 1004
Keratoconus 84, 132, 135-137, 999, 1049
  clinical features of 140
  diagnosis of 136
  management of 137
  ocular associations of 135
  posterior 136
  signs of 132
  treatment 141
Keratoepithelioplasty 120
  rationale of 121
Keratoglobus 140
Keratome 1111
Keratometer 83, 84
  optical principle of 83
  types of 85
Keratometry 83-85, 136
  limitations of 85
Keratomileusis 819

Keratopathy, causes of exposure 748
Keratophakia 819
Keratoplasty 106, 161, 162, 876
  complications of 167
  indications of 100, 161, 1008
  technique of 1004
  types of 162
Kerrison bone rongeur punch 1124
Kestenbaum capillary number 602
Ketoconazole 25, 1008
Ketoprofen 26
Ketorolac tromethamine 26
Khan Jaeger lid plate 1130
Khodadoust line 169
Kinetic perimetry 245, 699
Knapp's classification 641
Knapp's lacrimal sac retractor 1125
Knudson's two-hit hypothesis 865
Krabbe's leukodystrophy 668
Krimsky test 794
Krypton laser
  advantages of 453
  disadvantages of 454
Kuhnt meniscus 570
Kuhnt-Szymanowski procedure 705
Kveim test 210

L

Lacrimal apparatus 18, 703, 1076, 1095
Lacrimal crest, anterior 773
Lacrimal gland 771
  biopsy 215
  function 711
Lacrimal sac 777
  curette 1126
  distension 771, 773
Lacrimal secretory 771
Lagophthalmos 703, 713, 718, 980
  causes of 718
  treatment 980
Lambert-Eaton syndrome 653
Lamellar keratectomy, superficial 121
Lamellar keratoplasty 165, 166
  disadvantages of 165
  indications of 165
  types of 162
Lamina cribrosa 277
Laminar dot sign 278
Laminar flow 412
Landcaster's red-green test 639
Landolt's testing chart 3
Lantern test 14
Larger graft, disadvantages of 163

Laser 333
  applications of 333
  cycloablation 376
  demarcation 958
  iridoplasty 339
  iridotomy 337
    indications of 334
  light, properties of 447
  modes of delivery of 454
  monotherapy 895
  parameters 339
  peripheral iridotomy
    complications of 337
    contraindications of 334
  photoablation 528
  photocoagulation 446, 448, 450, 455, 909, 953, 954
    advantages of 455
    indications of 448, 454
  ranibizumab-triamcinolone study 899
  retinopexy 498
  role of 340
  suturolysis 340
    complications of 341
    technique of 340
  tissue interaction, types of 443
  trabeculoplasty 305, 339
Latanoprost 28
Latent nystagmus 662
Lateral tarsal strip procedure 705
Latrunculin B 30
Lattice degeneration 483
Lattice dystrophy 146
  features of 146
  systemic features of 146
Laurence-Moon-Bardet-Biedl syndrome 521
Lead 965
  reaction of 855
Leber's congenital amaurosis 135
Leber's hereditary optic neuropathy 865
Leber's miliary aneurysm 283
Lens 16, 190, 285, 381, 429, 831, 1070, 1085
  achromatic 827
  aplanatic 827
  aspheric 63, 827
  aspiration 994
  biconvex 63
  capsule
    anterior 299, 854
    true exfoliation of 297
  coloboma, types of 382
  damage 371
  dislocated 506

effects of 818
holding forceps 1107
particle glaucoma 310
  clinical features of 310
  treatment of 310
parts of progressive addition 836
photochromatic 835
planoconvex 63
status 384
subluxation of 991, 993
types of 63
Lenticonus
  anterior 381
  posterior 381
Lenticular changes 298
Leprosy, ocular manifestations of 38
Lesions, level of 634
Leukocoria, differential diagnosis of 492, 524
Levator
  function 716
  resection 721, 722, 723, 725, 983, 984
Levobunolol 28, 317
Lid 182, 428, 1036, 1038, 1075, 1094
  crutches 981
  drooping of 1032
  elasticity 710
  elevation of 981
  fatigue test 651
  gaze dyskinesis 633
  infection 713
  instability 710
  laxity 702, 710
  margin 710
    defects, full-thickness 734
  necrosis 713
  retraction of 720, 747
Lieberman teflon block 1132
Light
  diffraction of 811
  perception of 3
  reflex pathway 561
Limbal relaxing incisions
  advantages of 845
  disadvantages of 845
Limbal ring test, limitations of 858
Limbal transition zone 128
Limbitis 105
Limbus-based flap
  advantages of 347
  disadvantages of 347
Lincoff's rule 488
Linear light 804
Linezolid 965

Index

Liquid lasers 444
Local anesthesia 1007
Loteprednol etabonate 26
Low vision aids 961
Lower canaliculi, causes of 771
Lower lid
   reconstruction 733
      techniques for 735
   retraction, causes of 747
   retractor 700
      disinsertion 703
      reinsertion 978
Lucentis 555
Lumbar puncture 629
   complications of 596
   indications of 217
Luminescence 408
Lymphocytopenia 205
Lymphocytosis 205
Lysergic acid diethylamide 668

M

Macrodisk 570
Macropsia 822
Macula 190, 405, 479, 518
   characteristic features of 431
   edema of 894
Macular atrophy 405
Macular chorioretinitis, causes of 193
Macular corneal dystrophy 1000, 1046
Macular degeneration
   age-related 533
   dry age-related 533
   neovascular age-related 915
Macular dystrophy 147, 148
   characteristics of 147
Macular edema 405, 435, 450, 468, 905, 953, 963
   clinically significant 435, 557, 559, 1018, 1019
   treatment of 449, 903, 905, 953
Macular fan 587
Macular hole surgery, steps of 544
Macular ischemia 436
Macular laser therapy 895
Macular photocoagulation study 909, 910
Macular polypoidal choroidal vasculopathy 920
Macular sparing, reasons for 667
Macular star 405, 459
   differential diagnosis of 459
Maddox rod test 797
   double 639, 797
Maddox wing 797

Magnets, types of 861
Mannitol 29
Manual perimeter, types of 248
Marcus Gunn jaw-winking syndrome 719
Marcus Gunn phenomenon
   degree of 720
   graded 720
Marcus Gunn pupil, characteristics of 564
Marfan's syndrome 384, 863, 867, 993, 994
   features of 383
Marina trial 537
Mass lesions 969
Mean deviation 253
Mechanical ectropion 708, 979
Mechanical theory 293
Medial canthal tendon 701, 773, 989
   laxity 710
   plication 705
Medical therapy, maximal 325
Medical treatment history, significance of 1033
Medrysone 26
Meesmann's corneal dystrophy 866
Mefenamic acid 263
Megalopapilla, features of 616
Meibomian gland function 711
Melanoma
   malignant 49, 491
   ring 50
Melatonin 331
Membrane peeling forceps 1141
Menace reflex 694
Mendelian inheritance 708
Meningioma 77
Mercury 965
Mescaline 668
Metabolic disorders 606
Metaplasia 46
Metastasis 50, 653
   sites of 130
Methazolamide 29, 318
Methicillin 22
Methotrexate 27
Methyl alcohol poisoning 609
   features of 609
   treatment of 610
Methylprednisolone 27
   acetate 27
Metipranolol 28
Metolazone 263
Metronidazole 677
Miconazole 25
Microaneurysm 432, 433
   size of 432

Microdisk 570
Microphthalmos 867
Micropsia 822
Microspherophakia 382
    causes of 382
Microsporidia 45
    habitat of 45
    keratitis 45
    morphology of 45
Microvascular leakage 430
Migraine 668
Millard-Gubler syndrome 645
Miniature toy test 9
Mirrors in retinoscope, types of 828
Misdirection syndrome 633
Mitochondrial deoxyribonucleic acid 864
Mitochondrial inheritance
            disorders 864, 865
Mitochondrial myopathy 521
Mitomycin C, administration of 359
Mittendorf dot 382
M-mode 422
Mobile scotoma 249
Mobius syndrome 802
Molteno implant 366
Monocular blindness 695
Monocular hemianopias 699
Monocular nystagmus, causes of 660
Monocytopenia 206
Monocytosis 205
Mooren's ulcer 113-116, 118, 121, 873
    clinical presentation of 113
    management of 119
    pathology of 117
    pathophysiology of 117
    symptoms of 113
    types of 114
Morning glory
    disk anomaly, features of 615
    syndrome 616
Motor signs 574
Movement disorders 659
Moxalactam 22
Moxifloxacin 22
Mucoepidermoid carcinoma 129
Mucopolysaccharidosis 521, 607, 960
Mucous membrane grafts 997
Multicenter uveitis steroid treatment
            trial 931
Multifocal intraocular lens
    disadvantages of 395
    implantation 949
    types of 394
Multiple pinhole 832

Munson's sign 133
Murdoch eye speculum 1105
Muscle
    enlargement, causes of 745
    entrapment, differential diagnosis
            of 760
    hook 1120
    sequelae, development of 807
Myasthenia 649, 650, 656
    gravis 639, 649, 974
    symptoms of 655
    transient neonatal 653
Myasthenic crisis 656
Myasthenic symptoms 653
Mycobacterium leprae 38
Mycobacterium tuberculosis 37
    morphology of 37
Mycophenolate mofetil 27, 654
Mycotic ulcer treatment trial 886
    results of 101
Mydriasis, reverse 833
Mydriatic cycloplegics 304
Mydriatic test 266
Mydricaine 194
Myelinated nerve fibers, features of 619
Myokymia 660
Myopathy 656
Myopia 280, 789, 815, 816
    causes of 815
    clinical features of 816
    complications of high 816
    evaluation trial, correction of 941
    optical changes of 815
    pathological 484
    simple 837
    spectacles in 837
    treatment for 819, 940
    types of 815
Myopic astigmatism, compound 840
Myopic crescents 573
Myopic eyes 65
Myositis 751
Myotonic dystrophy 863

N

Nagel's anomaloscope test 14
Nail-patella syndrome 866
Nanophthalmos 425
Naphazoline 262
Naproxen 26
Nasal mucosa, exposure of 773
Nasalization 276
Nasociliary nerve, branches of 89

Nasolacrimal duct 771
Nasopharyngeal tumors, features of 692
Natamycin 25, 886
　treatment 886
Natriuretic peptides 30
Near point 820
Near vision 3, 4, 1036
　Donder's rule for 844
Necrotizing keratitis, features of 108
Neisseria infection 34
　laboratory diagnosis of 34
Neoplasia 46
Neoplasms 176, 284
Neostigmine test 652
Neovascular glaucoma 283, 462, 543, 557, 956, 1011, 1015
　differential diagnosis of 287
　etiology of 283
　management 1015
Neovascularization 434, 437, 956, 963
　angle, absence of 1015
　anterior segment 468
　causes of 437
Neovasculogenesis, theories of 285
Nerve fibers 570
Nerve palsy
　benign transient isolated sixth 647
　causes of painful third 630
　chronic isolated sixth 647
　isolated fourth 640
　isolated sixth 647, 973
　isolated third 629
Nettleship lacrimal dilator 1126
Neuralgia, postherpetic 109, 1007
Neuro retinitis, causes of 188
Neurogenic defects 808
Neurological diseases 670
Neuro-ophthalmology 560, 665, 942, 1074, 1092
Neuroprosthetic devices 961
Neuroprotection 329
　methods for 329
Neuroprotective effects 317
Neuroprotector 329
Neuroretinal rim 568
　shape of 277
Neurotrophic keratitis, features of 108
Neutral density filters 566
Neutropenia 204
Neutrophils, raised 204
Night blindness 514, 848, 849, 1037
　progressive 514
Nitric oxide synthase inhibitors 29
Nocardia keratitis, laboratory diagnosis of 36

Nonarteritic anterior ischemic optic neuropathy, clinical features of 621
Nonaxial proptosis, causes of 742
Noncatecholamine adrenergic agonists 262
Noncontact tonometers, disadvantages of 235
Noncontact transscleral cyclophotocoagulation 376
Nongranulomatous uveitis, causes of unilateral 178
Nonhealing corneal ulcers 101
　causes of 100
　signs of 100
Nonintegrated implants 782
　disadvantages of 782
Nonpenetrating glaucoma surgeries, role of 268
Nonperfusion area 466
Nonproliferative diabetic retinopathy 953
　differential diagnosis for 440
　features of 431
　severe 1019
Nonsteroidal anti-inflammatory drugs 26, 304, 996
　role of 259
Nontrauma dialysis 483
Nuclear fascicular syndrome 640
Nuclear portion 628
Nuclear sclerosis, grade 2 1037
Nuclear third nerve palsy
　Daroff's rules for 636
　features of 631
Nucleus, location of 643
Nutritional amblyopia 606
Nyctalopia, causes of 514
Nystagmoid movements 659
Nystagmus 658, 659, 663
　anatomic basis of 659
　classification of 658
　degrees of 663
　types of 658
　upbeat 661

O

Occipital lesions 668
Occipital lobe 670
　lesions 667
Occludable angle 242
Occlusio pupillae 188
Occlusive vascular diseases 286
Ocular alignment, test for 793
Ocular angiography 408

Ocular anomalies 381
Ocular association 801
Ocular bobbing 659
Ocular causes 793
Ocular disease 45, 462, 476
Ocular dysmetria 660
Ocular examination 1022, 1026, 1030,
　　　　　1036, 1047, 1051, 1056
Ocular flutter 660
Ocular genetic disorders, congenital 867
Ocular hypertension treatment study 924
　　findings of 379
Ocular hypotensive agents 300, 326
Ocular infections 33, 37
　　types of 33
Ocular inflammation 283
Ocular ischemic syndrome 683, 685
　　clinical presentation of 683
　　features of 685
　　treatment of 686
Ocular lesions 44
Ocular massage 476
Ocular melanoma 935
Ocular motility 796
Ocular myasthenia 651
Ocular neovascularization 466
Ocular pythiosis 45
Ocular structures, embryologic
　　　　derivation of 21
Ocular surface 710
Ocular surgery 784, 837
Ocular tissue, reaction of 853
Ocular trauma 257
Ocular vascular diseases 283
Ocular vessels, chronic dilatation of 285
Oculocutaneous albinism 867
Oculomotor nerve 625
　　synkinesis, primary 634
Oculomotor sympathetic central
　　　　neuron 645
Oculomotor synkinesis 633
Oculoplethysmography 685
Oculosensory reflex 562
Ofloxacin 22, 23
Oguchi disease 864
Oil droplet sign 134
Ologen implant 1123
Onchocerca volvulus 874
Onchocerciasis 874
Open-angle glaucoma 257, 273, 300
　　diagnosis of 280
　　juvenile 866
　　stage 285
　　　　histopathological feature of 286
　　treatment of 280

Operative disk decompressions 599
Ophthalmia neonatorum 869
　　management of 869
Ophthalmia nodosa 855
Ophthalmic artery, branches of 19
Ophthalmic equipment 1098
Ophthalmic infections 39
Ophthalmic management 788
Ophthalmic pathology 46, 47
Ophthalmic plastic surgery 770
Ophthalmodynamometry 685
Ophthalmometalloscope 856
Ophthalmoplegia 687, 689, 1032
　　acute painful 689
　　delayed painful 689
　　external 521
　　features of 690, 691
　　types of 687
Opsoclonus 660
Optic 811, 837, 1098
Optic atrophy 222, 517, 601-603, 605-609,
　　　　　612, 965, 967
　　causes of 588
　　　　ascending 602
　　　　secondary 604
　　clinical features of 601
　　differential diagnosis of 607
　　earliest sign of 603
　　features of 601
　　histopathological hallmarks of 603
　　partial 608
　　pathology of 601
　　primary 603, 965
　　process 607
　　secondary 604, 966
　　tobacco-induced 606
　　types of 611
Optic canal 76
　　causes of small 71
　　erosion, causes of 71
　　expansion, causes of 71
Optic chiasma, lesions of 665
Optic disk 190, 429
　　anomalies 613, 614
　　　　congenital 613
　　coloboma 616
　　　　features of 615
　　composition of 601
　　drusen 593
　　　　features of 618
　　edema, causes of 594
　　findings 578
　　pit 617
　　saucerization of 276
　　size of 570

1168 Index

Optic foramen 77
   diameter of 77
   significance of 70
Optic nerve 77, 608-610, 747, 1033
   compressive lesions of 965
   disorders 608
   glioma 77, 758
   inflammation, classification of 575
   meningioma 82
   pathology 608
   sheath meningioma 758
   vessels 572
Optic nerve head 183, 267, 567
   lesions 670
   dimensions of 567
   features of 614
   parts of 567
   size of 275
   vascular supply of 571
Optic neuritis 82, 575-580, 592, 594
   causes of 575
   clinical signs of 577
   differential diagnosis of 579
   study, longitudinal 943
   symptoms of 576
   treatment trial 942
Optic pit, features of 617
Optic tract
   hemianopia, characteristics of 667
   lesions 666
Optical coherence tomography 258, 402, 963
   advantages of 258
   anterior segment 256, 397
   disadvantages of 258
   typical 547
Optical defects, causes of pathological 812
Optical instruments, prisms in 825
Optical keratoplasty, donor corneas for 876
Optokinetic nystagmus 662, 695
   features of 662
Oral acyclovir 886
Oral antifungals, indications of 99
Oral antiglaucoma medications 1011
Oral steroids 219
Orbicularis
   muscle tone 703
   reflex 562
Orbit 18, 428, 680, 700
   and oculoplasty 1076, 1096
   blowout fractures of 759
   causes of small 72
   contents of floor of 765

   diffuse osteolysis of 73
   enlargement of 74
   hyperostosis of 73
   instruments 1124
   lateral wall of 765
   surgical spaces of 757
   vascular supply of 19
   volume of 737
   walls of 765
Orbital apex syndrome 653
Orbital blowout fractures 759
Orbital bruit 755
Orbital color Doppler imaging 685
Orbital decompression 753
   complications of 753
   surgery, indications of 753
Orbital disease 72, 688
Orbital fracture 760
Orbital implants 763, 764, 781
Orbital mass 78
Orbital prosthesis 781
Orbital pseudotumor 755
Orbital surgery 756
Orbital syndrome 634, 640, 647
Orbital trauma 78
   primary malignant 51
Orbital wall decompression 753
Orbitomeatal line 70
Orbitotarsal disparity 703
Orbitotomy 765
   anterior 756
   inferior 756
   lateral 757
   medial 756
   superior 756
Orbitotonometry 739
Organic materials produce 854
Organic nitrates 331
Osher neuman corneal radial marker 1135
Osteogenesis imperfecta 863
Osteoporosis 976
Otis lee procedure 704
Otitis media 672
Oxacillin 677
Oxyphenbutazone 26

P

Paecilomyces 505
Pain
   causes of 453, 576
   mechanism of 180
   relief of 156
Painful ophthalmoplegia 688
   causes of 688

Pallor
    atrophy 967
    causes of 602
Palpable mass, differential diagnosis
        of 742
Palpation 1023, 1024
Palpebral fissure
    height 717
    width, alteration of 803
Palsy, truly isolated 635
Pannus 86
Panophthalmitis 127, 513
Panretinal photocoagulation 559, 893, 899
    complications of 452
Papilledema 574, 583-594, 596, 597, 599,
        967, 969, 1053
    causes of 584, 585
    chronic 587
    differential diagnosis of 592
    occurrence of 584
    pathogenesis of 584
    pathological features of 586
    regression of 598
    stages of 585
    staging system of 588
    theories of 584
    treatment of 591, 597, 598
Papillitis 592
Para pontine reticular fiber 645
Paracentral field defect 699
Paracentral scotoma 247, 249
Paralytic ectropion 707, 979
    management of 707
Parapapillary chorioretinal atrophy 569
Parasellar syndrome, causes of 688
Parietal lobe lesions 667, 670
Parinaud syndrome 564
Parks-Bielschowsky three-step test 796
Pars plana 183
Pars plana lensectomy 994
Pars plana vitrectomy 439, 953, 956, 994
    over open sky vitrectomy,
        advantages of 541
Partial thickness flap over full thickness,
        advantages of 344
Partial thickness operation 343
PAX6 gene 866
Pegaptanib 535, 957
    sodium 953
Pelli-Robson chart 577
Pellucid marginal degeneration 116, 140
Pen torch shadow 224
Pendular nystagmus, features of 661
Penetrating cyclodiathermy,
        technique of 373

Penetrating injury 992
Penetrating keratoplasty
    complications of 121
    indications of 221
Penicillin 22, 23
Penicillium 505
Pentagonal wedge resection 705
Perforation, advantages of 126
Peribulbar anesthesia
    advantages of 387
    complications of 387
    disadvantages of 387
Pericytes 430
Peri-injection management 555
Periocular chemotherapy 528
    side effects of 528
Periocular corticosteroids 936
Periocular steroids
    complications of 219
    indications of 219
    over drops, advantages of 219
Peripheral anterior synechiae 182, 240
    types of 187
Peripheral ulcerative keratitis
    clinical features of 114
    medical management of 119
    pathophysiology of 116
    surgical management of 120
Peritomy 497
Persistent epithelial defect 105
Peter's anomaly 866, 867
Petrous apex syndromes 646
Petrous bone fracture 646
Phaco aspiration tip 1117
Phaco irrigation tip 1117
Phaco sleeve 1116
Phaco tip 1116
Phacodynamics 388
Phacoemulsification 389
    machines 388
Phakoanaphylactic glaucoma 310
    clinical feature of 310
Phakolytic glaucoma 309, 310
    clinical features of 309
    mechanism of 309
Phakomorphic glaucoma 310, 311
    differential diagnosis for 311
    pathogenesis of 311
Phakonit 401
Pharmacotherapy, refractory to 955
Phenylbutazone 26
Phenylephrine 262
    pilocarpine test 267
Phlebitis 646

Phorias 792
Phosphorescence 408
Photoablation 443, 447
Photoactivation 443
Photocoagulation 333, 439, 443, 447, 455
  burns, intensity of 449
  indications of 448
  procedures 455
  refractory to 955
Photodisruption 333, 443
Photodynamic therapy 548, 910
Photophobia 181
Photopic stress test 685
Photoreceptor transplantation 961
Phototherapy 444
Phthisis 192
  bulbi, reasons of 126
Physiological cup 567
Phytanic acid storage disease 521
Pierre-Marie's hereditary cerebellar ataxia 521
Pierse Hoskin forceps 1134
Piezometry 739
Pigment dispersion
  glaucoma 292
  syndrome 292
Pigment epithelium detachment 533
Pigmentation, differential diagnosis of 293
Pigmented trabecular meshwork 240
Pigments, absorption spectrum of 447
Pilocarpine 262, 324
  acts 314
  adverse effects of 314
  mechanism of action of 314
  use of 314
Pinch test 702
Ping pong gaze 660
Pinhole
  principle of 831
  size of 5
  test 4, 5
  types of 5
Pituitary apoplexy 691
  classical triad of 692
Pituitary macroadenoma 82
Plastic prisms 795
Plateau iris 256
  configuration 261
  syndrome 261, 262
Pneumatic retinopexy 500, 958
  advantages of 501
  disadvantages of 501
Pneumococcal infection 33

Pneumoretinopexy
  complications of 501
  principle of 501
Poisons 668
Polar cataract, posterior 385
Polaroid glasses 697
Polycarbonate 834
Polyhexamethylene biguanide 24
Polymerase chain reaction 213
  uses of 213
Polymorphic light eruption 668
Polymyxin B 22
Pontine syndromes 643
Poor near acuity, causes of 6
Posner-Schlossman syndrome 304
  characteristic features of 192
Posterior capsular rent, signs of 392
Posterior capsule opacification 960
  types of 396
Posterior chamber intraocular lens implantation 994
Posterior hyaloid
  detachment of 436
  traction 957
Posterior lamellar graft 713, 729
  principle of 730
Posterior lamellar keratoplasty, disadvantages of 166
Posterior lamellar reconstruction 729
Posterior lamellar support, assessment of 711
Posterior polymorphous dystrophy 158
  associations of 159
  clinical manifestations 159
  management of 159
Postinjection procedure 557
Postmydriatic test 833
Post-trabeculectomy 1011, 1037
Prednisolone 27
  acetate suspension 26
  sodium phosphate solution 26
Prednisone 654
Preglaucoma stage 285
Prematurity, retinopathy of 558, 906
Prentice rule 825
Preproliferative retinopathy 956
Prerubeosis stage 285
Presbyopia 382, 839, 818
  treatment 819
Presbyopic correction 818
Presbyopic glasses 818
Preseptal orbicularis muscle override, assessment of 711

Primary closure-angle glaucoma 314
    acute congestive stage of 287
    classification of 260
Primary open-angle glaucoma 264, 270, 271,
        300, 314, 344, 1009, 1037, 1040
    causes of 603
    differential diagnosis of 279
Prism 823, 831
    dissociation tests 695
    notation 823
    uses of 824
Probenecid 263
Progressive addition lenses 836
    spectacles, types of 836
Progressive pannus 87
Proliferative diabetic retinopathy 427, 557,
        559, 899, 900, 956
    complications of 439
    differential diagnosis for 440
    high-risk 1018
    ocular management of 956
Promethazine 262
Prominent corneal nerves, causes of 142
Prone test 267
Prophylactic treatment 851
Prophylaxis 870
Propionibacterium acnes 505
Proptometry 744
Proptosis 737, 738, 741, 744, 750, 755, 1020
    axial 742
    causes of 743
        acute 737
        bilateral 740
        unilateral 738, 740
    etiology of 755
    evaluation of 1022
    physiological 737
Prostaglandins 320, 324
    benefits of 321
    contraindications for 320
    effects of 321
    indications of 320
    mechanism of action of 320
    side effects of 320
    synthetase inhibitors 304
Prostamides 325
Protein kinase inhibitors 30, 327
Proteus mirabilis 505
Protocol-T aflibercept 900
Pseudo-Argyll Robertson pupil 633
Pseudoexfoliation 297, 401
    differential diagnosis of 301
    glaucoma 297, 294, 1013
        right eye 1013

origin of 297
    syndrome, intraocular complications
        of 299
Pseudo-Fleischer's ring 1059
Pseudofluorescence 416
Pseudo-Foster-Kennedy syndrome 595
Pseudo-Gradenigo's syndrome 646
Pseudohypopyon, causes of 186
Pseudomonas aeruginosa 35, 505
    cultural characteristics of 35
    morphology of 35
Pseudo-orbital apex syndrome 632
Pseudopapilledema 592
Pseudophakic bullous keratopathy 160
Pseudoproptosis 741
    causes of 741
Pseudoptosis 719
Pseudosquint, causes of 792
Pseudotumor 426
Pseudo-von Graefe's sign 633, 750
Psychophysical tests 255
Pterygium 997
    excision 997
Ptosis 651, 714, 715, 725, 726, 747, 981,
        987, 1025
    acquired 720
    bilateral 721, 790, 983
    cases of bilateral 983
    causes of unilateral 714
    correction
        practiced surgery for 984
        techniques for 723
    cosmetic point 981
    evaluation of 1027
    functional point 981
    management of 981
    mild 983
    mild-to-moderate 981
    severe 981
    surgery for 982
        local anesthesia for 720
    unilateral 790
Ptosis repair 721
    options for 721
    procedures
        contraindications of 722
        indications of 722
Pulfrich effect 577
Pulmonary function test 653
Pulsating proptosis, causes of 738
Pulse-steroid therapy 976
Punctal ectropion 704
Punctal eversion 702
Punctal plugs, types of 772
Punctoplasty 704

Pupil 190, 298, 429, 560, 715, 1036
　abnormal 564
　changes 188
　size of 560, 563
Pupil-gaze dyskinesis 633
Pupillary abnormalities 666
Pupillary block 256
　reverse 294
Pupillary defect 564
Pupillary involvement 629
Pupillary light reaction 560
Pupillary reactions 562
Pupillary response 694
Pupillary signs 574
Pupillary sphincter 561
Pupillometer 563
　projection 563
Pupillometry, methods of 563
Pupil-sparing third nerve palsy,
　　causes of 632
Pure blowout fractures 759
Purkinje-Sanson images 823
Pyramidal tract 645
Pythiosis 45
Pythium insidiosum 45
　habitat of 45
　morphology of 45

Q

Q-switching 447
Quickert procedure 712, 978
Quinine 965

R

Rabinowitz's criteria 136
Raccoon eyes 748
Radial buckling, indications of 496
Radiation therapy, types of 528
Radiographic method, limitations of
　　direct 857
Radiotherapy 976
Ranibizumab 535, 536, 557, 559, 894, 896,
　　900, 903, 905, 908, 913-915, 953,
　　963
　monotherapy 895, 920
Raymond's syndrome 645
Rays, projection of 3
Rebleeding, risk factors for 878
Recession, principle of 802, 803
Recti muscles, weakening of 802
Rectus holding forceps, superior 1105
Rectus tendon, superior 348
Red Amsler grid test 698

Red blood cells 880
Red-green defects, causes of acquired 14
Reese-Ellsworth classification 526
Reflex distance, margin 715, 716
Reflex imply, movement of 829
Reflex pathway
　trace light 561
　trace near 562
Reflex tearing 694
Refraction 789, 811, 812, 832, 837,
　　1065, 1098
　relation to 813
　steps in 827
　subjective 838, 839, 841
Refractive accommodative esotropia 800
Refractive amblyopia 789
Refractive errors 744, 789, 822
　types of 837
Refsum disease 864, 960
Refsum's syndrome 521
Regression, signs of 438, 525
Regressive pannus 87
Rehabilitation 967
Reid's baseline 76
Relapsing polychondritis 623
Renal failure, chronic 411
Repetitive nerve stimulation test 652
Resolution charts, minimum angle of 2
Respiratory system 316
Restricted ocular movements 745
Retina 16, 403, 516, 889, 1072, 1088
　blood supply of 480
　degenerations, peripheral 483
　instruments 1140
　layers of 479
　peripheral 190
　pigmentary degeneration of 521
　thickest parts of 432
　total area of 466
　vascular changes of 407
Retinal artery
　anatomical layers of 427
　characteristic features of 427
　pulsation, significance of 569
Retinal break 482, 491, 498
　prophylactic management of 497
Retinal capillary, characteristics of 427
Retinal circulation 460
Retinal collaterals 434
Retinal deposits 404
Retinal detachment 479, 485
　incidence of 488
　studies 889
　surgery, principle of 495
　types of 486

Retinal dialysis 482
Retinal edema 435, 956
Retinal embryogenesis, abnormal 493
Retinal fibers, arrangement of 570
Retinal findings, differential
    diagnosis of 403
Retinal hypoxia 285
Retinal motility 491
Retinal neovascularization 403
Retinal pigment
    epithelial detachment 531
    epithelium 531, 533, 855
Retinal prosthesis 962
Retinal telangiectasia 404
Retinal thickening, moderate-to-severe 954
Retinal vascular tortuosity 404
Retinal vein occlusion
    corticosteroid for 902
    studies 901
    treatments for 905
Retinal vessel
    attenuation, causes of 516
    emergence of 569
    narrowing, differential diagnosis of 516
Retinaldehyde 847
    role of 847
Retinitis 191
Retinitis pigmentosa 514, 518, 863, 867,
    960, 961, 966
    bilateral 1045
    earliest presentation of 514
    medical treatment 960
    syndrome 865
    theories of 518
    treatment 522
        modalities 960
Retinoblasmic eye 527
Retinoblastoma 426, 523, 865
    incidence of 523
    management of 527
Retinochoroiditis, causes of 193
Retinoic acid 847
    role of 847
Retinopathy of prematurity 906, 908
Retinoschisis 484, 494
    X-linked 867
    types of 828
Retinoscopy 134, 750, 828, 842
    objective 828
    performing 829
    principal of 828
    reflex, characteristics of 829
    stages of 828

Retraction test 702
Retrobulbar alcohol injection 269, 1016
Retrobulbar anesthesia 387, 455
    complications of 387
Retrobulbar block 648, 648
Retrobulbar external compression 471
Retrobulbar optic neuritis 965
Reynolds–Braude phenomenon 42
Rhabdomyosarcoma 51
    treatment of 51
Rhegmatogenous retinal detachment 958,
    1042, 1043
    symptoms of 486
Rhese's view 70
Rhomboid flap 729
Rimexolone 26
Ring scotomas, causes of 515
Rizzuti's sign 133
Roenne's central nasal step 247
Roman test types 4
Romberg's test 1034
Roper Hall's locator 856
Roth spots 406
Rubella 40
Rubeosis 956
Rubeosis iridis 291

S

Salbutamol 262
Sallmann's folds 748
Salus's sign 457
Sampaolesi's line 240, 298
Sanders–Retzlaff–Kraff formula 389
Sanfilippo's syndrome 521
Sarcoidosis, diagnosis of 216
Scanning laser polarimetry 244
Scatter panretinal photocoagulation focal
    grid laser 956
Scheie's gonioscopic classification
    242, 457
Schie's syndrome 521
Schilder's disease 668
Schiotz tonometry 231, 232
    advantages of 231
    disadvantages of 231
Schlemm's canal 241
Schnyder's crystalline dystrophy 148
Schnyder's dystrophy sine crystals 148
Schocket device, modified 371
Schwalbe's line 239, 292
Schwartz syndrome 487
Scissoring reflex 134
Scissors 1108

1174 Index

Sclera 15, 360, 853, 1067, 1078
   identify perforation of 368
   indentation 1043
   weak areas of 481
Scleral buckling 499, 501, 504, 890, 959
   complications of 500
   surgery 496
Scleral indentation, role of 66
Scleral patch graft
   advantages of 370
   complications of 370
Scleral ring 568
Scleral spur 239
Sclerectomy 370
Scleritis 105, 1007
Sclerosis
   amyotrophic lateral 653
   multiple 653
Sclerostomy 347
   full-thickness 377
Sclerotic scatter 54
Scopolamine 349
Scotoma 246
   absolute 249
   annular 249
   classification of 249
   negative 249
   peripheral 249
   positive 249
   relative 249
Scotometry 247
Seclusio pupillae 188
Seesaw nystagmus, features of 661
Segmental circumferential buckling,
   indications of 496
Segmental optic atrophy 967
   causes of 604
Seidel's scotoma 247
Selective laser trabeculoplasty 279, 296
   contraindications for 339
   indications of 338
   mechanism of action of 339
Self-retaining universal eye
   speculum 1104
Sella turcica, normal dimensions of 71
Sella, enlargement of 71
Semiconductor diode lasers, advantages
   of 375
Semiconductor lasers 444
Septic cavernous sinus thrombosis 678
Serum
   calcium 212
   lactate dehydrogenase 213
   lysozyme 213

Setons 364
Shaffer's grading system 241
Sheridan's ball test 8
Sheridan's letter test 9
Sherrington's law 791
Short arm 11 deletion syndrome 865
Short-wavelength automated
   perimetry 251
Shunts 364, 434
   dural 679
Sickle cell
   anemia 880, 881
   retinopathy 283
   trait 880
Siderosis 854
   treatment of 861
Siegrist's streaks 460
Silicone band 1142
Silicone oil
   complications of 503
   mechanism of action of 503
   over intraocular gases, advantages
     of 503
   study 889
   use of 503
Silver wiring 458
Simcoe's two-way irrigation 1113
Single-gene defects 873
Sinskey hook 1113
   reverse 1136
Sinus thrombosis, lateral 646
Sinusitis 672
Sirna-027 therapy 537
Sirolimus 27, 932
Sixth nerve palsy 644, 647, 973
   causes of 643, 647
   clinical features of 644
Sjögren's syndrome 873
Skew deviation 639
Skin
   flaps, types of 729
   muscle flaps 732
   repair, direct 729
   tests 210
   role of 210
Skin graft 707
   full-thickness 729
   procedure 730
   types of 729
Skull, plain X-ray of 67
Sleep disorders 316
Sleep test 651
Sling surgery 724
   materials used 724

Slit-lamp 52, 146
    biomicroscope 52
    biomicroscopy 1054
    evaluation 1052
    examination 52, 850, 1042, 1043, 1052, 1057
    illumination, basic principles of 52
    optics of 57
Small-incision cataract surgery 950
Smith's lazy-T procedure 705
Smith's method 224, 226, 227
Smith's modification 705
Snail track degeneration 483
Snellen's chart 2
Snellen's near vision test 4
Socket disorders 778
Sodium
    hyposulfate 861
    thiosulfate 861
Soemmerring's ring 397, 1059
Soft shell technique 396
SoftPerm lens 137
Soper lens system 138
Sotalol 262
Spaeth classification 242
Spasmus nutans 662
Spastic entropion 978
Spatula 1114
Spectacle frames
    parts of 836
    types of 836
Spectral domain-optical coherence tomography
    advantages of 281
    disadvantages of 281
Specular microscopy 154, 299
Specular reflection 56
Speculum 1103
Sphenocavernous syndrome 632
Spherical aberration 811
Spherical refraction 830
Spheroidal degeneration 93
Spinal accessory nerve 1034
Spindle cell variant 129
Spindle procedure, medial 704
Spinocerebellar degenerations 521
Spironolactone 331
Split limbal technique 224
Spot size 446
Spurious night blindness 514
Squamous cell carcinoma 47, 129
    histopathology of 48
    types of 48

Squamous dysplasia 129
Squint 793
    alternation of 795
    paralytic 636
    surgery, indications for 802
Staphylococcus
    aureus 31, 505
        morphology of 31
    epidermidis 505
    infection 32
Staphyloma
    peripapillary 616
    treatment of anterior 127
Static perimetry 245
Static refraction 829
Stationary night blindness, congenital 514
Stem beads 968
Stem cell theory 128
Stereoacuity 10
Stereopsis 698
Stereoscope methods 857
Stereoscopic tests 698
Sterile pentamidine isethionate powder 1008
Sterilization 883
    monitor effectiveness of 884
    steps in 883
    techniques 883
Steroid 887
    drops, use of 306
    ocular complications of 221
    responsiveness 306
    role of 469, 655
    systemic complications of 222
    treatment 220
Steroid-induced glaucoma 306-308
    diagnosis of 307
    management of 308
Steven tenotomy scissors 1110
Stickler syndrome 863, 867
Stiles–Crawford effect 10
Strabismic amblyopia 789
Strabismus 725, 788, 791, 793
    horizontal 725
    surgery 754, 938
Straight crescent knife 1122
Streptococcus
    pneumoniae 32, 505
        habitat of 32
        morphology of 32
    viridans 505
Streptomycin 965
Stroma 1048
    anterior half of 1000

Stromal deposits, causes of 92
Stromal dystrophy 143, 150, 151, 873
  recommended sites for 145
Stromal keratitis 1006
  necrotizing 1006
Sturge-Weber syndrome 74, 1011
Sturm's conoid 817
Subarachnoid space syndrome 640, 645
Subconjunctival antibiotics 1002
Submacular surgery trial 911, 912
Subretinal choroidal
    neovascularization 403
Subretinal fluid drainage, advantages of
    spread of 499
Subretinal gene therapy 962
Sub-tenon triamcinolone acetonide,
    posterior 995
Sub-Tenon's anesthesia 387
Subthreshold micropulse laser 548
Sudden visual loss, causes of 478
Sulfadiazine 262
Sulfamethoxazole 262
Sulfasalazine 263
Sulfonamides 965
Sulfonylureas 262
Sumatriptan 262
Sump syndrome 777
Superior oblique paresis
  causes of 639
  management of 641
Superior orbital fissure 73, 687, 688
  anatomy of 687
  enlargement of 76
Superonasal placement, complications
    of 369
Superonasal quadrant 742
Superotemporal quadrant 743
Supplemental scleral buckle 959
Supranuclear control systems 791
Suprasellar calcification, causes of 72
Suprofen 26
Surgery
  contraindications of 982
  goals of 971
  indications for 986, 993
Surgical correction, srinciples of 982
Surgical iridectomy 337
Surgical limbus 343
Suture tarsorrhaphy, temporary 707
Suture technique 704
Suturing nonmarginal lid defects 733
Sweet's method 857
Sympathetic ophthalmia 195
  clinical features of 196
  pathology of 195

Sympathomimetics, mechanism of action
    of 317
Synchysis 482
Synechiae
  causes of 188
  posterior 1002
  types of 187
Syneresis 482
Synoptophore, uses of 798
Syphilis 211, 1059
Syringing test interpreted 772
Systemic antifungal indications 1004
Systemic bevacizumab therapy 915
Systemic immunosuppressive therapy 931
Systemic inflammatory disorders 471
Systemic steroid therapy, chronic 120
Systemic vascular disease 462

T

Tacrolimus 27
Tafluprost 28
Takayasu's arteritis 623
Takayasu's disease 434
Tangent screen 248
  examination 250
  material of 248
Target pressure 273, 313
Tarsal kink syndrome 978
Tarsal platform show, amount of 981
T-cell lymphocytes, inhibitors of 27
Tear drainage, normal 771
Tear-film
  loss of homeostasis of 889
  ocular surface 889
Telecanthus 987
  severe 989
Temporal flare, causes of 749
Temporal lobe lesions 666, 670
Temporalis sling repair 985
Temporalis transfer 708
Temporary ligature sutures, types of 368
Temporary sling 724
Tenon's cyst, treatment of 356
Tenon's steroids 953
Terrien's marginal
  degeneration 116
  keratitis 115
Tessler's classification 175
Tetracycline 331, 1005
  derivatives 331
Tetrahydrocortisol 331
Therapeutic keratoplasty 101
  indications for 1004

Therapeutic prism 824
  forms of 825
Therapeutic ultrasound, technique of 377
Thermokeratoplasty 138
Third nerve lesions, localization of 631
Third nerve nucleus
  anatomy of 625
  components of 625
Third nerve palsy 630, 633-636, 639, 971, 1029
  causes of 628
  differential diagnosis of 636
  investigations for 629
  types of 627
Three-port pars plana vitrectomy, technique of 541
Thrombin solution, preparation of 1140
Thudichum's nasal speculum 1125
Thymus gland, role of 649
Thyroid
  eye disease 745
  myopathy 426
  ophthalmopathy 639
  orbitopathy 737, 750, 754
Thyroid-related ophthalmopathy 737, 753
  hyperthyroid 746
  mild 975
  moderate 975
  severe 975
  signs 757
Thyroid-related orbitopathy 737, 975
  surgery for 976
Thyroid-related proptosis 737
Ticarcillin 22
Tilley's nasal packing forceps 1125
Timolol 28, 316, 324, 1009
  advantages of 324
  application 316
Tobacco amblyopia, treatment of 606
Tobramycin 22-24
Tolbutamide 262
Tolosa–Hunt syndrome, features of 692
Tonometers
  disinfection of 234
  types of 231
Tonometry 750
  basic examination of 224
Tonopen, advantages of 235
Tooke's knife 1122
Topiramate 262
Torchlight
  examination 849, 1051, 1056
  signs 574

Toric intraocular lens 389
  advantages of 845
  disadvantages of 845
  implantation 949
  rotation of 846
Toric lens, spherical equivalent of 827
Torque sutures 164
Torsion, tests for 792
Torsional deviation 793
Torsional imbalance 796
Towne's projection 70
Toxic
  amblyopia 222
    causes of 605
  maculopathies 406
  optic neuropathy 965
Toxocara canis 43, 44
Toxoplasma gondii 44
  ocular lesions of 44
Toxoplasmic retinochoroiditis 193
Toxoplasmosis 41, 44, 74
  laboratory diagnosis of 44
  serological tests for 211
Trabecular aspiration 302
Trabecular meshwork 239
  pigmentation, causes of 240
Trabeculectomy 338, 343-346, 348, 349, 352, 356, 359, 371, 927, 1014, 1016
  bleb 368
  complications of 354
  indications of 268, 344
  modified 290
  steps of 345
  surgery 348, 355
Trachoma 874
Traction optic atrophy, causes of 608
Tractional retinal detachment 490
Tranexamic acid 879
Transcaruncular incision 767
Transconjunctival incision 766, 767
Transcutaneous incision 766
Transient ischemic attack 682
Transillumination 492
Transmission defect 417
Transpupillary cyclophotocoagulation 377
  technique of 289, 377
Transpupillary thermotherapy 536
Transscleral cyclophotocoagulation 375, 376
  complications of 376
  indications of 341
  mechanism of action of 375
  techniques 289

Transscleral photocoagulation 375
Transsynaptic antegrade atrophy 603
Transverse sutures 711
Trapdoor fracture 761
Traquair's periosteal elevator 773
Traumatic hyphema 877-880
  complications of 878
Traumatic optic atrophy 607, 965
  mechanism of 607
Traumatic optic neuropathy 607
Travoprost 28
Treacher–Collins syndrome 863, 867
Triamcinolone 27
  acetate 957
  acetonide 27, 953, 956, 963
  diacetate 27
Trichromatic theory 13
Trifluorothymidine 25
Trigeminal nerve 1034
Trimethoprim 262
Triple test 267
Trivex 834
Trocar 1140
Tropias 792
Tropical amblyopia
  features of 606
  pathogenesis of 606
Tropicamide 262
Troutman-katzin corneal transplant
    scissors 1137
Trypan blue, use of 396
Tuberculin skin test 207
  reaction 209
Tuberculosis 1033, 1059
  laboratory diagnosis of 38
Tuberous sclerosis 74, 863
Tubular vision 515
Tumbling E test 9
Tumor 668, 739
  surgical resection of 727
Tzanck smear 40

U

Uhthoff's phenomenon 576
Ultrasonic biomicroscopy, advantages
    of 257
Ultrasonography 422
  disadvantages of 860
  role of 507
  uses of 217
Ultrasound 422
  biomicroscope 256
    disadvantages of 257

Ultraviolet light, chronic exposure to 997
Uncal herniation syndrome 634
Uncover test, monocular 795
Uniocular diplopia, causes of 805
Unoprostone 28
Upper canaliculi, causes of 771
Upper eyelid reconstruction 733
  techniques for 734
Upper lid
  ectropion 708
  elevation of 720
  level 715
  normal position of 715
  reconstruction 733
  retraction, causes of 747
  retractors 700
Urea 29
  advantages of 323
  disadvantages of 323
Urine culture, significance of 213
Usher's syndrome 521, 864, 960
  types of 522
Utrata forceps 1107
Uvea 15, 172, 361, 1055, 1071, 1083
Uveal melanoma 50
Uveitic conditions 191
Uveitic eye 194
Uveitic glaucoma 287, 303, 325, 1011
  management of 304
  mechanism of 303
Uveitic macular oedema trial 936
Uveitis 172-174, 177, 179, 180, 186-194,
    203, 210-218, 221, 325, 931, 995,
    996, 1059
  active 995
  acute generalized 178
  acute posterior 178
  causes of 178
    acute suppurative 178
  chronic posterior 178
  nomenclature, standardization of 177
  occurrence of 176
  signs of 182
  terminology, activity of 177
  therapeutic approach 932
  treatment of 218, 995

V

Vacuum 388
Valves 364
Van Herick's method 224, 225
Vancomycin 22-25, 510, 511, 513
Vannas scissors 1109

Vascular accidents 668
Vascular endothelial growth factor 531, 552, 559
　pathological roles of 551
　properties of 551
Vascular filling defects 415
Vasculitis, infectious 463
Vasodilation 476
Vasoinhibitory factors 285
Vein occlusion 300
Venous pulsation, significance of 569
Vernier acuity 4, 10
Vertebrobasilar insufficiency 668
Verteporfin 910
　photodynamic therapy 920
　plus ranibizumab 919, 920
Vertical chopper 1118
Vertical diplopia
　diagnoses of 639
　differential diagnosis of 639
Vessel wall, onion skin appearance of 460
Vessels, superficial 87
Vestibular nystagmus, features of 661
Vestibule cochlear 1034
Viral keratitis 107
Viscoelastics 387
Vision 7-9, 587
　2020, objectives of 871
　defective field of 1032
　loss, causes of 428, 464, 747, 761
　measurement of 1
　painful loss of 478
　painless loss of 478
　sudden loss of 465, 1038
　transient obscuration of 587
　unaided 1036
Visual acuity 1, 607, 698, 868, 788, 905
　best corrected 886, 892, 899
　during infancy 788
　minimal level of 450
　simulation of 698
Visual angle 1, 698
Visual field 217, 245, 247, 248, 515, 519, 665, 868
　normal 245
　sensitivity of 245
　significance of 487
　testing, types of 665
Visual field defects 278, 279, 515, 577, 582, 590, 748
　sequential progression of 246
　treatment of 670
Visual function 595
　tests of 519

Visual impairment 868
Visual loss
　preventing severe 892
　risk of severe 893
Visual prognosis 470
Visual symptoms 600
Visualization, direct 855
Visualize enlarged muscle 752
Vital 1030, 1051
Vital signs 1056
Vitamin A 847
　requirements of 847
　role of 847
　sources of 847
Vitamin A deficiency 847, 850, 851, 870
　etiology of 848
　prevention of 851
　primary 848
　risk factors of 848
　secondary 848
　subclinical signs of 850
Vitrectomy 504, 509, 539, 540, 959
　advantages of 508
　anterior 993
　contraindications of 544
　cutter 1118
　efficacy of 439
　indications of 221, 502, 509, 539
　intraoperative complications of 542
　primary 890
　types of 540
Vitreomacular traction syndrome 955
Vitreoretinal traction 489
Vitreoretinopathy
　familial exudative 863
　proliferative 889
Vitreous 190, 853
　aspiration 214
　base 480
　cells 189
　changes 189, 491
　characteristic features of 539
　detachment, posterior 425
　disturbance, traumatic cataract with 991
　hemorrhage 423, 957
　　acute 487
　humor 16
　liquefaction of 486
　particles 518
　transparent 481
Vitritis 178
Vogt's method 858
　indicators for 858

Vogt's striae 133
Vogt's triad 268
Vogt–Koyanagi–Harada syndrome 199, 490
von Graefe's sign 750
von Hippel–Lindau disease 74, 863
Voriconazole 23, 24, 512, 886, 887, 1005
   treated cases 886
Vortex vein, landmarks of 481
Vossius' ring 384, 1059
V-Y plasty 706, 729

W

Waardenburg syndrome 863, 960
Wagner disease 863
Wallerian degeneration 602
Wand's classification 286
Warwick's classification 625
Water's view 69, 73
Watson classification 114
Watson criteria 114
Wave, continuous 444
Waxy disk pallor 517
   causes of 517
Weber's syndrome 634
Wegener's granulomatosis 118
   ophthalmic manifestations of 116
Weill–Marchesani syndrome 864
Weiss classification 148
Weiss ring 485, 1059
Wells enucleation spoon 1129
Wernicke's syndrome, Hemianopic
      pupillary reaction of 562
Wessely immune ring 1059
Westcott tenotomy scissor 1108
White-eyed blowout fracture 761
Whitnall's ligament 715
Wies procedure 712, 978
Wilson's disease 239, 864, 1059
With-the-rule astigmatism 817
Wolfram syndrome 429, 864
Working distance 828

Worst Lovac contact lens 859
Worth four-dot test 797
Worth's Ivory ball test 8
Wound
   closure of 733
   dehiscence 713
   edges 728
   healing, modulation of 359
   modulation 353
Wound leak
   characteristics of 350
   treatment of 350

X

Xanthelasma 428
Xenon laser 893
Xerophthalmia 849
   classification of 848
   fundus 849, 850
X-linked congenital idiopathic
      nystagmus 867
X-linked recessive disease 864
X-ray skull 67
   advantages of 67
Xylocaine 723

Y

Yoke muscles 791
Y-V plasty 988

Z

Ziv-Aflibercept 536
Zonular dehiscence, traumatic cataract
      with 991
Zonular dialysis, grading of 991
Zonular weakness 298, 395
Zonules 298
Z-plasty 706, 729
   double 988

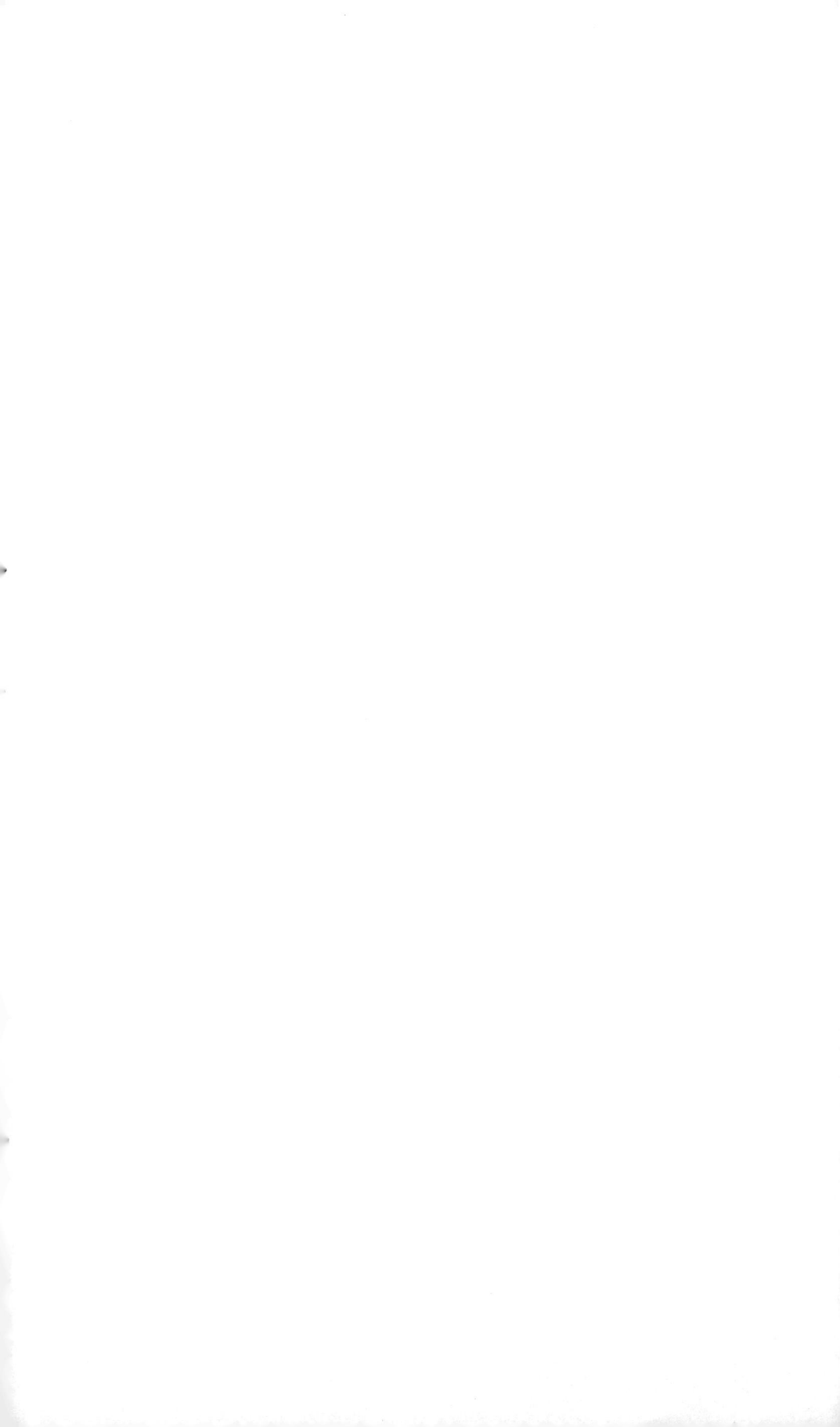

EU GSPR Authorised Reprsentative
Logos Europe, 9 rue Nicolas Poussin
1700, La Rochelle, France
Phone: +33 (0) 6 67 93 73 78
E-mail: contact@logoseurope.eu

www.ingramcontent.com/pod-product-compliance
Ingram Content Group UK Ltd.
Pitfield, Milton Keynes, MK11 3LW, UK
UKHW050056090825

461530UK00017B/160